The Intervertebral Disc

Irving M. Shapiro • Makarand V. Risbud
Editors

The Intervertebral Disc

Molecular and Structural Studies of the Disc in Health and Disease

Springer

Editors
Irving M. Shapiro
Department of Orthopaedic Surgery
and Graduate Program in Cell
and Developmental Biology
Jefferson Medical College
Thomas Jefferson University
Philadelphia
PA
USA

Makarand V. Risbud
Department of Orthopaedic Surgery
and Graduate Program in Cell
and Developmental Biology
Jefferson Medical College
Thomas Jefferson University
Philadelphia
PA
USA

ISBN 978-3-7091-1534-3 ISBN 978-3-7091-1535-0 (eBook)
DOI 10.1007/978-3-7091-1535-0
Springer Wien Heidelberg New York Dordrecht London

Library of Congress Control Number: 2013943012

Printed on acid-free paper

Springer is part of Springer Science+Business Media (www.springer.com)

Foreword

Current understandings of the biology of the intervertebral disc is predicated on comprehension of the processes of aging in the human body. Its generalized nature has often led to flawed surgical strategies with focal attention on what is now understood to be a widespread and universal process throughout the spine. The global nature of aging and degenerative changes of the spine has led to an epidemic of disease and disability affecting primarily the aged. As our population achieves greater longevity, these changes become increasingly manifest and the demands for improved understanding become more vital. Age changes in the disc are not dissimilar from those found throughout the connective tissues of the body including the skin, aorta, ligaments, and peripheral joints. Biomechanical weakness of the annulus can lead to local breakdowns in the integrity of the disc with nuclear herniation and nerve root compression. For those discs that are unresponsive to medical therapy, surgical intervention can be extraordinarily successful providing dramatic and usually lasting relief. When the annular changes are more generalized and the facet joints become incompetent, instability can occur provoking a condition known as degenerative spondylolisthesis. Rather than nerve root compression, this provokes instability and back pain and again is reasonably amenable to surgical stabilization. Generalized mechanical insufficiency can provoke arthritic changes, narrowing of the spine, and neurologic symptoms associated with the entity known as spinal stenosis. Again, if localized, this is amenable to surgical decompression and possible stabilization. Diffuse age-related disc degeneration is provocative of axial spine pain and substantial disability and yet is the least responsive to surgical and, indeed, nonsurgical intervention. This wide spectrum of degenerative changes are predicated on aging and matrix degeneration that only later provoke mechanical disorders.

Thus, a true understanding of spinal disease requires the study of the molecular and cell biology of the normal, aging, and pathologic spine and the pathogenesis of neurologic and non-neurologic pain syndromes and careful controlled studies of both surgical and nonsurgical interventions.

In this authoritative book, the reader is privileged to benefit from an elegant and careful educational process moving from basic biology to common disease entities and the intended hope for ultimate biologic regeneration. This should be a mandatory reading for all of those who hope to understand and effectively treat what is today's leading cause of skeletal disability, i.e., diseases of the intervertebral disc.

Richard H. Rothman, MD, PhD
James Edwards Professor and Founder,
The Rothman Institute at Thomas Jefferson University,
Philadelphia, PA, USA

Introduction

The major reason for embarking on the daunting task of editing a book on the intervertebral disc is that the available literature is either too clinical for most newcomers to the field or too fragmented for the expert. Accordingly, there is a critical need for a book that will provide a holistic overview of advanced topics in molecular, mechanical, developmental, and cellular aspects of intervertebral disc research, while serving as a useful text for graduate students, postdocs, and fellows. It should be noted that the target audience is not confined to basic scientists as the import of much of the information contained in the book impacts the need of many neurosurgeons and neurologists, orthopedic surgeons, pain and rehabilitation specialists, physicians, chiropractors, and kinesiologists. These individuals work tirelessly to understand and expand the repertoire of treatment modalities available to relieve the pain and loss of function associated with the degeneration of the intervertebral disc, a widespread condition that afflicts a huge percentage of the global population.

Indeed, in comparison with the plethora of books on the clinical management of spinal disease, only one book has been published within the past 50 years that is entirely focused on the disc. To provide continuity with the past, the preface of the current book is written by one of the authors, the eminent surgeon-clinician scientist, Dr. Richard Rothman. A comparison of his earlier book with the current volume shows just how far knowledge of the disc and the pathogenesis of disease has advanced in the past half century. However, even now, despite the explosion of interest in degenerative disc disease, from an investigative point of view and in comparison with cartilage and bone research, discal biology in health and disease can be regarded as the last frontier of connective tissue research. Obviously, there is still much to be accomplished and hopefully this book will energize investigators and clinicians to define the limits of current knowledge and to develop novel insights into the many outstanding questions concerning the function of the intervertebral disc and the cause of disease.

To assemble this book, the editors have brought together an international galaxy of experts, many of whom have influenced their own discipline in a very significant way. The contributors were asked to summarize the current state of their field while at the same time to critique current research strategies, approaches, and the interpretation of accepted and projected therapies. So as to preserve their "voice," the editors have tried to maintain, almost intact, each of the contributions. While this has allowed the reader to view the topic through the mind of the contributor, it has resulted in some duplication of the written word that hopefully will be forgiven.

The book is divided into three parts. The first section deals with the basic biology, developmental biology, and biomechanics of the normal healthy disc, topics that have received considerable study although some glaring gaps in knowledge still exist. For example, there is debate concerning cell type in the aging disc: does it contain viable and functional notochordal cells or are the embryonic cells replaced by other cell populations? The second part is devoted to intervertebral disc disease and disc herniation, raising questions concerning epidemiology and pathogenesis. The authors question whether discogenic pain is directly linked to the degenerative state. Following on from the discussion of discogenic pain are chapters dealing with surgical and nonsurgical modes of treatment. Authors of these chapters ask the following question: are the advances in knee and hip surgery transferable to the disc? Since all clinical treatments are dependent on the availability of model systems, the last section of the book discusses the value of in vitro systems and small and large animal models to mimic the environment of the human disc. Closely aligned with these concerns are discussions of the use of transgenic mouse models, stem cell biology, and gene therapy to promote disc repair. In the chapter on the future use of tissue engineering systems to effect biological repair, it is stated that the technology will likely be "personalized to the individual and influenced by the extent of disease." Concomitant with the development of tissue engineering approaches for biological repair, the important concept is reiterated that it is necessary to delineate the mechanism(s) leading to back pain so that the twin goals of all new therapies are to ameliorate pain and maintain function.

The editors have a number of people to thank for their help in preparing this book. First and foremost, they must acknowledge the responsiveness of the individual contributors who have risen to the challenge of preparing each of their chapter with such flare and imagination. The editors also thank F. Michael Angelo, MA, University Archivist for the reproduced images of rare books, courtesy of the Archives and Special Collections at Thomas Jefferson University, Philadelphia. Second, the authors thank Katrina Lenhart, Wilma McHugh, and the team at Springer for all of their help. Lastly the editors must thank their own families for giving up time for completion of this endeavor.

IMS dedicates this book to two unique individuals: Dr. Michael Bush OBE, *punnist extraordinaire* and a great friend and cousin, who devoted much of his life to preventing and treating AIDS in Africa. His untimely death brought great sadness to his family and to the patients who depended on him. And to Dr. Susan H. Shapiro who traded her spinal pain for resolution, hope, and courage. The fortitude with which she endured the pain now empowers her to follow her heart and intuition. MVR dedicates this book to his parents Swati V. and Vinayak Y. Risbud for their unconditional love. In addition, MVR thanks Rashmi, the love of his life, for her constant encouragement and support and Aditya and Akshay for the fun and happiness they generate each day.

Finally, appealing to our inner futurist, it is fun to contemplate the focus of a similar book on the disc published 50 years hence. Indeed, will there be a book or will new knowledge transmit directly from the bench into ganglia and neurons of the central nervous system? Will surgery be regarded as an inhuman and savage approach to treating a chronic health problem? Will the new molecular therapies be based on those described in this book or will there be approaches that are as yet unimaginable at this time? Or will nutrient excess and lack of exercise promote devolution of the human spine to the notochord of a sessile wormlike creature discussed in Chap. 1? If we can avoid the last scenario, there is reason to hope that the pain of disc disease will be like quinsy and polio, remnants of a bygone era eliminated by the groundbreaking work of many of the clinicians and scientists who contributed to this book.

March 2013 Irving M. Shapiro
Philadelphia, PA, USA Makarand V. Risbud

Contents

Part I

Biomechanical and Molecular Studies of the Intervertebral Disc

Introduction to the Structure, Function, and Comparative Anatomy of the Vertebrae and the Intervertebral Disc

1

Irving M. Shapiro and Makarand V. Risbud

The spine is composed of vertebrae, and it extends from the head down to the loins. The vertebrae are all perforated, and, above, the bony portion of the head is connected with the topmost vertebrae, and is designated the 'skull'.

Aristotle

Contents

I.M. Shapiro (✉) • M.V. Risbud
Department of Orthopaedic Surgery and Graduate Program in Cell and Developmental Biology,
Jefferson Medical College, Thomas Jefferson University,
1025 Walnut Street, Suite 511 College Bldg,
Philadelphia, PA 19107, USA
e-mail: makarand.risbud@jefferson.edu;
irving.shapiro@jefferson.edu

1.1 Introduction

1.1.1 Evolutionary Considerations

The goal of this introductory chapter is to provide an overview of the design, evolution, and basic characteristics of the disc and the vertebrae that comprise the human spine. As with any survey, the state of current knowledge reflects the work of earlier cohorts of individuals whose insightful observations relied almost entirely on observation, argument, and inductive reasoning. Over the centuries, sequential observations by men like Aristotle, Vesalius, Hunter, and Winslow have all contributed to understanding how the oversized human head can restrictively swivel on the multiple bones of the vertebrate spine and in doing so provide our species with its huge biological advantage.

It needs to be acknowledged that the spine as we know it with the intervening intervertebral discs is a relatively late phylogenetic development in the animal kingdom. It was preceded by the appearance of a stiff rodlike structure, the notochord. In animals that lack backbones, the notochord provides rigidity and some resilience to the organism, promotes formation of an extended shape, and protects the overlying spinal cord. The defining characteristic of vertebrates, the backbone, first appeared in the fossil record about 500 million years ago, during the Ordovician period. While details of the transition (notochord to spine) are missing, the 500-million-year-old tiny Middle Cambrian fossil chordate, *Pikaia*, possessed a notochord that separated the distinct head and tail regions; *Haikouichthys*—a small early Cambrian fish-like fossil—exhibited well-developed eyes as well as muscle blocks typical of early vertebrates (Shu et al. 2003). Box 1.1 shows the metameric structure of *Pikaia*.

I.M. Shapiro, M.V. Risbud (eds.), *The Intervertebral Disc*,
DOI 10.1007/978-3-7091-1535-0_1, © Springer-Verlag Wien 2014

Box 1.1

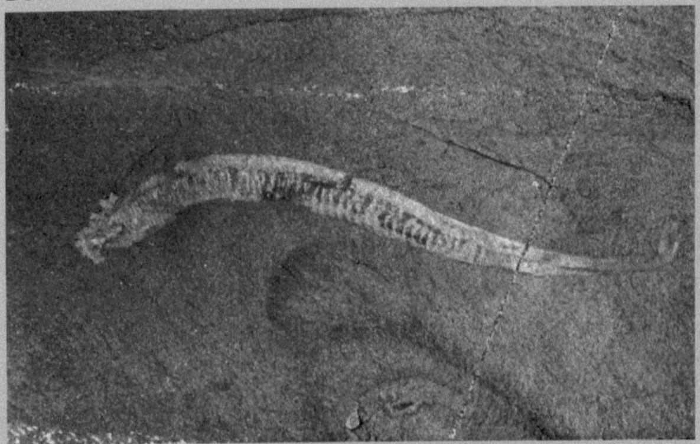

Fossil of *Pikaia gracilens*, a 505-million-year-old creature, found in the Burgess Shale fossil beds in Canada. There is evidence of a notochord, a dorsal nerve, and myotome-like structure. Pikaia was originally thought to be a chordate which would thus make it an early vertebrate ancestor (Courtesy of Smithsonian Institution)

The appearance of the spine probably signaled the most critical event in evolution of higher organisms. The stimulus for invertebrate chordates to develop the complex mineralized metameric structure that characterizes the vertebrate subphylum is still unknown; even less understood is how evolutionary pressures prompted the development of the intervertebral disc, an event that permitted rapid locomotion and flexion. Remarkably, evidence is mounting that this evolutionary jump might be the result of the development and expression of microRNAs (Iwama et al. 2013). Rather than viewing this type of transformation as a slow evolutionary process, Garstang (1928) has proposed that both cephalochordates and vertebrates evolved along separate pathways in prehistory. This worker proposed that as a result of neotenic[1] evolution, our ancestor may have been a sessile, ascidian wormlike organism.

As organisms evolved a mineralized vertebrate axial skeleton, the biological advantages offered by the spine motion segment provided functions that profoundly influenced the activities of other organ systems. Not surprisingly, aside from allowing extension of the body with some flexibility, the vertebral bone protects the spinal cord. Other advantages of the vertebral bones are that they provide sites for attachment of the axial skeleton to the appendicular bones via the pectoral and pelvic girdles; additionally, the attachment of muscles and ribs to vertebrae facilitates functional changes required for locomotion and respiration. With respect to the discs that separate each of the vertebrae, specific functions are to allow movement of the individual vertebrae, transmit forces between vertebrae, and serve as hydrodynamic shock absorbers.

In humans and other primates, the spine permitted adoption of a vertical posture facilitating the transition from arboreal to terrestrial locomotion. The upright bipedal stance afforded evolutionary advantages including extended three-dimensional vision: enhanced depth perception would be expected to enhance manual dexterity, which in turn would promote skills linked to tool creation. That these same influences also promoted weaponization added to the uniqueness of the human race and its determination to limit its own growth and development. Away from the appendicular skeleton, the stable, strong, flexible, and vertical spine permitted evolutionary changes in the bones of the skull, allowing marked cranial growth and development. Thus, over time, the head, albeit balanced precariously at the tip of the vertical spine, together with the bones of the arms, ribs, and legs, would undergo phenotypic alterations that characterize primates and humans. Moreover, the change in the biomechanical status of the appendicular skeleton would impact the size, shape, and depth of the pelvis. These evolutionary changes provided animals with an enormous biological advantage, moving the organism away from the wormlike characteristics of our distant ancestors to the frenetic and often random activities of modern day bipedal hominids.

Other chapters of this book will ask the following questions: Why did these transitions take place, and what or how are the biomechanical forces accommodated by the skeleton and the musculature? What gene clusters are altered to support this critical evolutionary change, and what is the fate of the notochord itself—can notochordal remnants influence the functional and developmental biology of the spine? Hopefully, insights generated by these developmental, molecular, mechanical, physiological, and biochemical studies of the spine will provide answers to questions concerning the health and function of the intervertebral disc—answers that could not be derived through extant anatomical and pathological analysis.

1.1.2 Development of the Vertebrae and Intervertebral Disc

The vertebrae develop from individual ossification centers which are well documented historically (Kerkring 1717; Albinus 1737; Rambaud and Renault 1864). Probably the most detailed report in the twentieth century was by Peacock (1951). The reader is urged to review the latter report for more details; the developmental biology of the intervertebral disc and the vertebrae is discussed in great detail in Chap. 3.

The vertebral bodies are formed by fusion of sclerotome from two adjacent somites: thus, tissue from the caudal

[1]Term used to describe the retention in the adult of traits or phenotype expressed in the immature state.

portion of one sclerotome fuses with cranial sclerotome of the succeeding somite. The dense connective tissue of the two halves of each sclerotome becomes two centers of chondrogenesis. At each putative vertebrae, two more chondrogenic centers appear laterally and grow backwards to form the cartilage precursor to the neural arch. During this phase of development, the notochord becomes compressed by the pressure exerted by the cartilage and may persist for a while as a "mucoid streak." However, between the developing vertebrae, notochordal tissue is retained and subsequently forms the intervertebral disc. At these sites, notochordal cells become enclosed in a dense ring of connective tissue, the putative annulus fibrosus. Noteworthy, some notochordal cells may remain in the cartilage; at a later time, cells buried in the bone of the centrum may serve as a site for tumor formation (see Chaps. 3 and 17). The nucleus pulposus is thus formed early in fetal life from notochordal elements and grows rapidly in late fetal life and early infancy. By birth, it occupies half of the intervertebral space in the lumbar region, and by 1 year it occupies almost three quarters of the space. It is thought that there is some remodeling of the intervertebral space early in life (Taylor 1975).

By the seventh week of life, the cartilage undergoes endochondral ossification. Dorsal and ventral blood vessels invade the two cartilage anlagen and trigger their replacement with bone. Subsequently, the anterior and posterior portions of the calcified centrum fuse. Along the anterior and lateral periphery of the vertebrae, cartilage plates appear to form the apophysis. This is the site for insertion of the fibers of the annulus fibrosus. As the centrum ossifies, the cartilage anlage of the neural arch is replaced by bone. The two sides of the arch fuse and then join together with the centrum. The process begins in the upper cervical region and extends caudally. The laminae are also formed in cartilage—they join together after birth and then fuse with the rest of the vertebrae between the third and seventh years of life. Vertebrae growth is mediated by chondrogenic activity at the growth plate. Actually, as the centrum has two centers of growth, it should be labeled as a synchondrosis. Histologically, prior to closure in the 17th–25th year, a well-defined zone of hypertrophic chondrocytes is visible. Once growth has ceased, the only remaining cartilage is the endplate.

1.2 Anatomical and Molecular Structure of the Intervertebral Discs

Medieval anatomists were the first to recognize that the vertebrae were separated by soft "gristle"-like structures, the intervertebral discs. In his intricate drawings of the spine, Winslow (1776) provided a detailed description of the disc, which considering the limitations posed by the distortions of hand lenses was remarkably accurate. Another analysis of spinal anatomy and the intervertebral disc in health and disease was performed by one of the most prolific anatomists of the nineteenth century, Hubert von Luschka. In his monograph *Die Halbgelenke des menschlichen Körpers* (1868), von Luschka described the gross and microscopic structure of the intervertebral discs from birth to death. Almost at the same time, Humphrey (1858) in his book *A Treatise on the Human Skeleton* provided a detailed description of each of the discs. He reported the looping fibrils of the annulus fibrosus and noted the absence of blood vessels in the nucleus and inner annulus fibrosus. Studies of age changes in the disc were subsequently noted by Henle (1872), Poirier and Charpy (1899), Fick (1904) and Petersen (1930), and Bohmig (1930). As far as we can tell, the earliest comment on the relationship of the disc to the notochord was reported by the Austrian anatomist Schaffer early in the twentieth century (1910).

1.2.1 Form and Function of the Intervertebral Discs

Depending on age, time of day, occupation, and disease state, the discs make up approximately 15–20 % of the length of the spinal column. Aside from absorbing biomechanical forces, each disc permits movement of the spinal column. Undoubtedly, flexibility decreases with age, while spinal movements at all stages of life can be severely limited by disease. Since vertebrae themselves are relatively inelastic, movement in the spine is mediated notably by the tissues of the intervertebral disc. Although the mobility of contiguous vertebrae (motion segments) can be viewed as limited, the integrated motion of the 33 intervertebral discs together with movement at the zygapophyseal joints permits all of the critical movements of the spine without compromising nerve or muscle function.

The famous English anatomist Henry Gray (1827–1861) classified articulations between vertebrae as "amphiarthroses in which the contiguous bony surfaces are either connected by broad flattened discs of fibrocartilage, of a more or less complex structure." By definition, these joints permit very little motion. Shapiro et al. (2012) compared the structure-function relationships of both the intervertebral disc and synovial joints. On first consideration, the intervertebral disc could be seen as being very different from the generic synovial joint. However, on reflection, the separate tissues of the intervertebral disc are very similar to that of the diarthrodial joint: both types of joints are lined by cartilage, they are limited by an external ligament, and the joint space contains molecules that promote lubrication (lubricin and hyaluronan) and elevate the osmotic pressure (aggrecan). Indeed, even the presence of a band of nucleus pulposus tissue across the joint is not out of line with what is known of complex diarthrodial joints that contain cartilage and fibrocartilage discs and menisci. Related to the function of the nucleus pulposus and the inner annulus, it is not yet clear whether a distinct synovial-like membrane exists in the intervertebral disc. Whether inner annulus is derived from the notochordal sheath has not been determined. Nevertheless, like the cells of the synovium, the resident disc cells do have the ability to mount a robust defense against bacterial attack (Nerlich et al. 2002; Jones et al. 2008).

In terms of movement, the current classification of the disc as an amphiarthrosis would indicate very limited mobility. However, biomechanical studies of the motion segment with or without contributions from the zygapophyseal joints indicate that there is wide range of motion between vertebrae. Moreover, the actual movement of the cervical, thoracic, and lumbar vertebrae includes flexion-extension, axial rotation, and lateral bending, as well as translatory motions. These three-dimensional movements are more in line with those of a diarthrodial joint rather than an amphiarthrosis where movements are slow and motion is limited. Probably the major difference between appendicular diarthrodial joints and the axial intervertebral joints lies in their development. Although the joints originate from different mesenchymal elements, the nucleus pulposus is derived from a unique embryonic tissue, the notochord; deletion studies indicate here too there are considerable similarities in the expression of genes that govern organ development and maturation. Recent investigations indicate that joint formation and even function are dependent on the expression of a number of genes including those of the Hox family, BMPs, and GDF5 (Brunet et al. 1998; Archer et al. 2003; Pacifici et al. 2005). Indeed, deletion of Ext1 influences not just the development of limb joints but also the formation of the intervertebral disc (Mundy et al. 2011). This topic is considered further in Chap. 3.

Based on the overt structural and functional similarities between the intervertebral disc and the synovial joint and recognizing that while some differences exist between these articulations, it would seem logical to place the disc in the same grouping as the diarthrodial joint. Further, since the intervertebral motion segment displays movement in three dimensions and the spine itself provides further rotatory movements, Shapiro et al. (2012) were of the opinion that it should be classified not as an amphiarthrosis, "a slightly moveable joint," but as a complex polyaxial joint.

1.2.2 Spinal Curvature

While the intervertebral discs and the zygapophyseal joints provide sites for vertebral motion, the overall shape of the spine as well as curvatures in specific regions of the spine is dependent on intrinsic genetic factors as well as

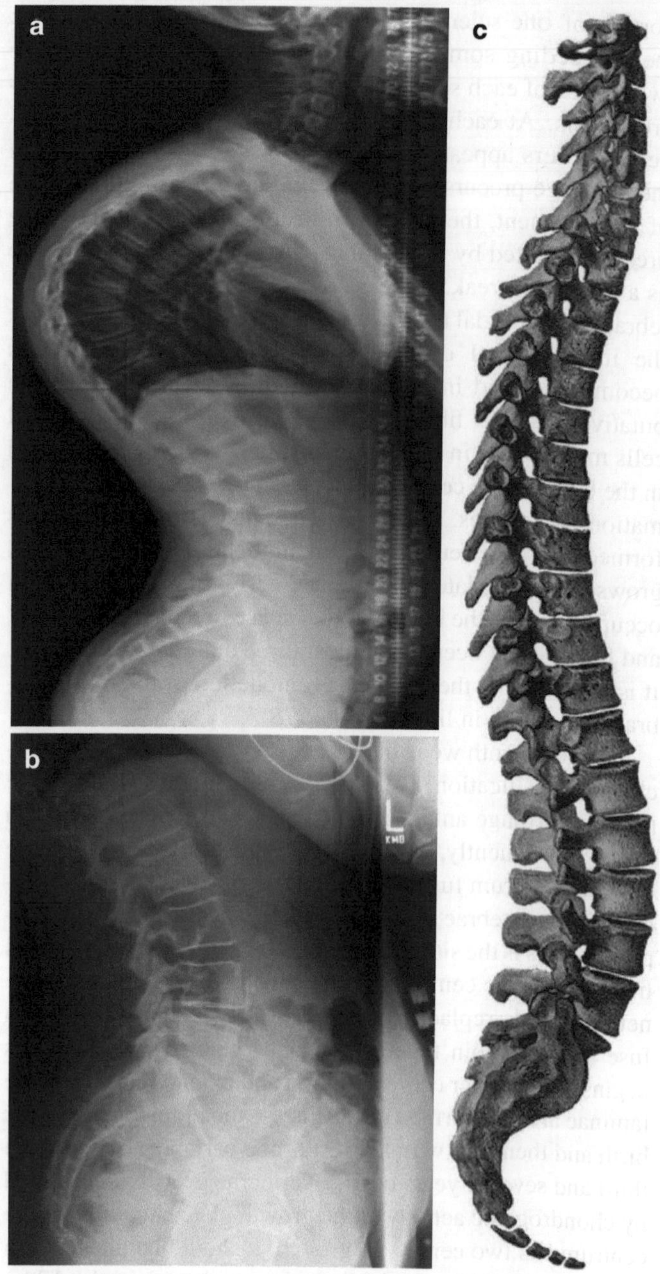

Fig. 1.1 Spinal curvature: kyphosis and lordosis. Anterior-posterior radiographs of the spine showing (**a**) kyphosis (excessive posterior bending of the thoracic motion segments) and (**b**) lordosis (extreme anterior bending of the lumbar and often the cervical spine). (**c**) The complete spine showing the natural curvature in the cervical, lumbar, and sacral regions (From Bougery and Jacob (1833). Plate 6)

biomechanical forces mediated through the pull of muscles, ligaments, and gravity. Encoded curvatures are seen in the cervical, lumbar, and sacral regions of the spine. On adoption of a vertical stance, and with maturation, these curvatures become more distinct (Fig. 1.1c). However, about 2–3 % of the population exhibit deficits in axial curvature, which vary from simple bending with little functional implications to excessive bending which impacts not just

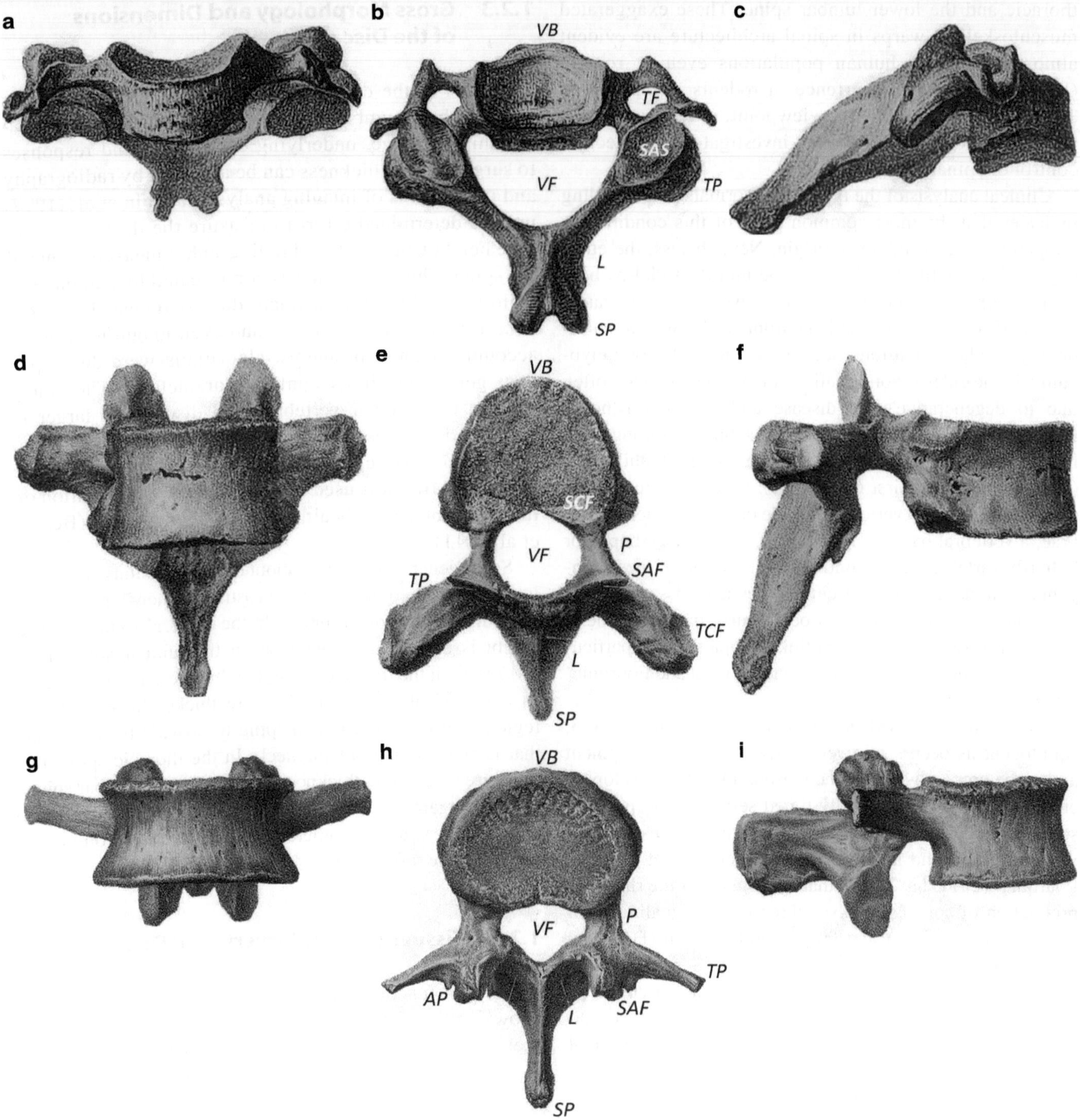

Fig. 1.2 Human vertebrae. (**a–c**) show vertebrae from the cervical spine (below C2); (**d–f**) show vertebrae from the thoracic region of the spine; (**g–i**) show lumbar vertebrae. **a**, **d**, and **g** anterior-posterior aspects of the vertebrae; **b**, **e**, and **h** are superior views; **c**, **f**, and **i** are lateral views of the spine. *VB* vertebral body or centrum, *P* pedicle, *L* lamina, *TP* transverse process, *VF* vertebral foramen, *SP* spinous process, *TF* transverse foramen, *SAS* superior articular surface, *SCF* superior costal facet, *TCF* transverse costal facet, *AP* accessory process, *SAF* superior articular facet (From Bougery and Jacob (1833). Plates 8 and 9)

locomotor activities, but other critical functions associated with the spinal nerves. The "hunchback" spine, kyphosis, is due to excessive posterior bending of the thoracic motion segments (Fig. 1.2a); when the cervical and lumbar anterior spinal curvatures become excessive, this condition is termed lordosis (Fig. 1.2b). While these latter conditions are deviation in the anterior-posterior (cephalic-caudal) axis of the spine, abnormal bending is also seen in the lateral (side-to-side) dimensions. Scoliosis can affect any part of the spine; the most common regions are in the thoracic and the lower lumbar spine. These exaggerated musculoskeletal warps in spinal architecture are evident almost entirely in human populations even in royalty (Richard III); their occurrence in rodents is infrequent. Thus, from an experimental viewpoint, rodents and lagomorphs make useful models to investigate the molecular control of spinal curvature.

Clinical analysis of the types of abnormal spinal bending indicates that the most common form of this condition is idiopathic, i.e., of unknown origin. Nevertheless, the etiology of this condition is likely to be multifactorial as both environmental and genetic factors have been implicated. A second form of scoliosis is neuromuscular which is secondary to other conditions, such as cerebral palsy or a myopathy. In the elderly, abnormalities in axial bending are often due to degenerative disc disease and spondylolisthesis. Possibly, the most intriguing form of scoliosis is congenital in origin, a rare condition that is evident early in childhood (usually within the first 6–8 weeks). Radiographically, the spine exhibits fused vertebrae, single or multiple hemivertebrae, a vertebral bar, block vertebrae, and wedge-shaped or butterfly vertebrae. If left untreated, almost all of these congenital anomalies result in deformities and loss of normal function. Since the anomalies occur early in development, this form of scoliosis has been linked to patterning, particularly during the period of somitogenesis (Chal and Pourquie' 2009).

As will be discussed in considerable detail in Chap. 3, somitogenesis occurs at a very early stage in development and is the process whereby the mesoderm of the developing embryo undergoes a carefully timed segmentation process; somites are generated that specify skeletal muscles, dermis, vertebrae, ribs, and annulus fibrosus. Very recent work by Pourquie' (2011) has shown that the trigger for the rhythmic production of somites involves three major signaling pathways: Notch (Jiang et al. 2000), Wnt/β-catenin (Dequeant et al. 2006), and fibroblast growth factor (Benazeraf et al. 2010) which are integrated into a molecular circuit. The oscillatory activities of this circuit generate a highly coordinated developmental event that serves as a traveling wave of gene expression along the anterior-posterior axis of the developing embryo. Pourquie' (2011) refers to this synchronized change in gene expression in the pre-mesodermal cells as the "segmentation clock." Clearly any activity that interferes with coordinated gene expression and the development of the waves of gene oscillations will impact somitogenesis which in turn will influence the subsequent formation of the vertebrae and the intrinsic curvature of the axial skeleton. Although this system was developed from studies in mice, it is most likely that these new understandings will impact our understanding and ultimately the treatment of congenital scoliosis.

1.2.3 Gross Morphology and Dimensions of the Disc

The sizes of the discs in the human skeleton have been assessed by a number of investigators, especially in relationship with age, underlying conditions, and responses to surgery. Disc thickness can be assessed by radiography and other forms of imaging analysis. Frobin et al. (1997) made a determined effort to measure the disc and vertebrae height using archived radiographic measurements of the spine. This approach was complicated by a number of factors that included artifacts due to image distortion, axial rotation and lateral tilt, and even magnification. To account for these problems, algorithms were developed that generated dimensionless parameters. The study showed that lumbar vertebrae and discs were larger in males and females and in males there appeared to be no or little impact of age. More recently, magnetic resonance imaging (MRI) was used to provide direct information on the discs of seven healthy males aged 22–30 (Belavý et al. 2011).

Some general comments about disc dimensions are as follows. Disc height (cephalic-rostral dimensions) varies according to the spinal region. In the cervical spine, the disc height is about 3 mm, whereas in the lumbar spine, it is 9–17 mm; in the thoracic spine, the thickness is about 5 mm. In the cervical spine, the discs are thicker in the anterior region than posterior, thus helping to provide the curvature that is characteristic of the neck. In the thoracic spine, the discs are of constant thickness, whereas in the lumbar spine, they are again thickest anteriorly. Radiographs have been used to assess disc parameters in animals most commonly used in spine research (O'Connell et al. 2007).

1.2.4 Tissues of the Intervertebral Disc

The major functional role of the disc is mechanical: it allows movements between the axial and appendicular skeleton and the head; it accommodates applied loads; and to some extent the disc protects the spinal cord and nerve roots. The discs themselves are complex tissues comprising an outer circumferential ring of fibrocartilage, the annulus fibrosus which encloses a central proteoglycan-rich core, the nucleus pulposus. The nucleus is sandwiched caudally and cephalically by the cartilage endplates of the contiguous vertebrae. Since details of the biochemical, developmental, and biomechanical aspects of each of the disc tissues are provided in considerable detail in other chapters of this book, the sections below merely highlight the major characteristics of the endplate cartilage, nucleus pulposus, and the annulus fibrosus.

1.2.4.1 Annulus Fibrosus

As an introduction to these topics, it is worth noting that the annulus can be divided into an inner fibrocartilagenous region and an outer or peripheral fibrous zone (Souter and Taylor 1970). It was reported that the outer annulus fibrosus is composed of very well-defined collagen I fibers that bundle to form long parallel concentric lamellae. Marchand and Ahmad (1990) showed that the number of fiber bundles varies from 20 to 62. The thickness of lamellae varies both circumferentially and radially and increases markedly with age, location, and vertebral type. The central annulus fibers are inserted into the endplate cartilage, while those at the periphery are anchored to the vertebral bone. In terms of collagen organization and cell content, this region is not unlike tendon or ligament.

The inner annulus fibrosus represents roughly 50 % of the total radial thickness. Designated by some workers as the transitional zone, it differs substantially from the outer region. Compared with the outer annulus where the cells are elongated and fusiform and extend in the long axis of the fibrils, the cells of the inner annulus are spherical in shape and many resemble chondrocytes. These cells are few in number with short processes. A further difference between the inner and outer annulus is their chemical composition. The inner annulus contains collagens I and II. While aggrecan is present in both regions of the annulus, decorin and biglycan are found mainly in the outer annulus. The other protein of significance is elastin which accounts for 2 % of the dry tissue weight.

1.2.4.2 Nucleus Pulposus

The nucleus pulposus is derived from the notochord and notochordal cells remain in the tissue after birth and into adult life. During development, the nucleus is highly cellular: after birth, the number of cells is reduced; in the adult, the cell density is very low. The histology of the nucleus pulposus cells is unique and complex: large cells arranged mainly in clusters and separated by an abundant extracellular matrix. Among the large notochordal cells, much smaller cells possibly derived from the notochordal sheath can also be seen. The large cells appear to have numerous vacuoles, which has prompted some authorities to describe them as "physaliphorous." Probably the most complete TEM analysis of the nucleus of the adult rabbits was described by Gan et al. (2003). These workers showed that the nucleus pulposus contained cell clusters embedded in a proteoglycan-collagen matrix. The cells exhibited a well-defined Golgi system, an extensive endoplasmic reticulum, and a complex vesicular system filled with beaded structures (proteoglycans). Neither necrotic nor apoptotic cells were evident. A remarkable finding was that the cells contain few if any mitochondria. A defining characteristic of the cells was the presence of numerous cytoplasmic processes.

With respect to the extracellular matrix, nucleus pulposus cells secrete aggrecan, as well as collagens I and II. The matrix also contains collagens IX and XI, and collagen X has also been reported to be present during degeneration. Because of the presence of aggrecan, the disc exhibits a high osmotic pressure; moreover, since it has no blood supply, the oxygen tension within the disc is very low. These limitations have prompted the Risbud group to note that nucleus pulposus cells "tune" their metabolism to the available oxygen supply (see Chap. 6 for details). In this case, nucleus pulposus cells evidence almost complete reliance on the glycolytic pathway to generate metabolic energy (Agrawal et al. 2007).

1.2.4.3 Endplate Cartilage

The caudal and cephalic ends of the disc are covered by a layer of cartilage, the endplate. This thin layer of hyaline cartilage is maximally thick in the newborn and thins with age; in the adult, the actual width is about 0.5–1 mm. It serves not just as an interface between the soft nucleus pulposus and the dense bone of the vertebrae, but as a biomechanical barrier that prevents the disc from applying pressure directly to the bone. It is the presence of the cartilage layer that provides the motion segment with its joint-like characteristics. Some authorities believe that the cartilage also plays a role in maintaining the viability of cells of the nucleus pulposus (Dahia et al. 2009). Structurally, the endplate resembles articular cartilage. Thus, it contains chondrocytes embedded in an aggrecan-rich and collagen II extracellular matrix. Although the cells do not undergo terminal differentiation, collagen X may be present in the central region of the endplate perhaps in relationship to focal areas of endochondral bone formation. The endplate transitions into bone through a region of calcified cartilage.

In his review of the cartilage, Moore noted that vascular channels penetrate the cartilage, but at maturity the vessels become narrow, constricted, or even obliterated. It is likely that this change impacts the nutrient supply to both the cartilage and the disc (Moore 2000). Crock and Yoshizawa (1976) reported that the central region of the endplate where there is a high concentration of channels is freely permeable to small molecules. On the other hand, Nachemson et al. (1970) noted that at the tissue periphery, the cartilage is much less permeable to low molecular weight dyes. Clinically, it is not uncommon to note that the central region undergoes sclerosis or mineralization with alterations in the mechanical properties of the cartilage. When this occurs, nucleus pulposus tissue can be forced through the endplate into the underlying bone of the vertebrae. This phenomenon is known as Schmorl's nodes which Schmorl himself considered to be linked to degenerative changes at the cartilage bone interface (see Box 1.2).

1.3 Vertebral Structure

Since the book is devoted to the intervertebral disc, there is little need to review the detailed anatomy of each of the vertebrae. Instead, we herein provide broad brush strokes that delineate the general features of human vertebrae; this is followed by a few comments about individual vertebrae and the sacrum. Detailed images of each of the vertebrae are shown in Figs. 1.2 and 1.3.

At first sight, the architecture of the vertebrae appears to be very complex, each bone being riddled with numerous nooks, crannies, protrusions, and extrusions. However, the basic organization of the 24 articulating bones of the spine is quite simple: the vertebral structure reflects its two primary functions, articulation with contiguous vertebrae and protection of the spinal cord. From an anatomical viewpoint, a canal is formed as bone is deposited around the cord. This canal, the vertebral foramen, houses and protects the spinal cord. The remaining structure of the vertebrae forms in the caudal-cephalic direction a boat-like shape (albeit designed by a drunken engineer), while the anterior-posterior axis exhibits a very inexact pyramidal-like structure (albeit designed by a heat-affected Pharaonic architect). The base of the pyramid is comprised of a robust bone, the centrum or body, while the sides of the pyramid form a bone arch or lamella (the hull) that surrounds the spinal cord. The apex of the arch extends backwards to form the spinous process (the keel). This process is very well developed in the thoracic spine where it serves as a site for attachment of the powerful muscles of the back. Projecting upwards and forwards from the base of the lamellae are transverse processes (retractable stabilizers) which are sites of origin of the pedicles that form a base for the articulating zygapophyseal (facet) joints: the superior (cephalic) articulating process articulates with the zygapophyseal joints of the contiguous cephalic vertebrae; projecting downwards and backwards from the laminae is the inferior articulating process from which a facet joint is formed with the contiguous caudal vertebrae. "Portholes" at the junction of the "fin" and the "lateral stabilizers" provide openings, "intervertebral foramina," for the nerves that flow from and into the spinal cord. In terms of general anatomy, other than C1 and C2, the largest portion of a typical vertebra is the bony centrum, the weight-bearing region of the vertebrae. With increasing distance from C3, there is a significant increase in the robustness of the centrum and the vertebrae, thus the lumbar vertebrae and its centrum are larger than vertebrae of either the thoracic or cervical spine. In cervical and even upper thoracic vertebrae, on the cephalic bone surface, a ring-like protuberance, the uncus, may be present. This ossified structure, the uncinate process, serves to limit movement at the intervertebral disc and forms the so-called uncovertebral joints (joints of von Luschka, see Box 1.2).

Box 1.2

Christian Georg Schmorl (1861–1932): To spine surgeons, the name Schmorl is synonymous with Schmorl's nodes, small protrusions of nucleus pulposus tissue which herniate through the endplate cartilage. They are often associated with degenerative disc disease, and while they can be painless, they can cause inflammatory changes in the underlying bone marrow. Details of the work that Schmorl performed come through the writings of Ormond A. Beagle, an American surgeon who spent time with Schmorl at the Friedrichstadt Krankenhaus in Dresden, Germany. He reported that Schmorl removed every spine for examination at postmortem. In a 5-year period, he had collected about 7,000 spines and many were preserved in the museum. Schmorl reported on many problems of the anatomy and pathology of the spine and the intervertebral disc.

Hubert von Luschka aka Hubert Luschka (1820–1875): Born in Konstanz, Germany, he is the eighth of 12 sons. He was a student of both pharmacology and medicine at the University of Freiburg and the University of Heidelberg. Luschka is considered among the major anatomists of the nineteenth century and was the author of a multivolume textbook on surgical anatomy and numerous research publications. Testaments to the extent of his work are the multitude of structures named after him, especially the recurrent nerves of Luschka (meningeal branches of spinal nerves that pass through the intervertebral foramen and innervate the zygapophyseal facet joints and the annulus). He described what are now considered to be tears of the annulus. Also with regard to the spine, he found that individuals lose height when they stand and that the height of an individual decreases with age. He discovered the uncovertebral joints (Luschka joints) which he called "half joints" present in the cervical spine usually between C3 and C6. These pseudo joints are formed between the vertebrate bodies of contiguous vertebrae.

From Tubbs et al. (2011)

1.3.1 Cervical Vertebrae (Figs. 1.2 and 1.3)

In line with the generalized numbering system of the individual regions of the spine, the cervical vertebrae are sequentially numbered from rostral to caudal (C1 to C7); C1 and C2, the atlas and axis vertebrae, respectively, form the joint complex that permits the spinal column to articulate with the head via the occipital condyles. Neither of these vertebrae have a well-defined body; indeed, the atlas can be viewed as a ring of dense membrane bone. Bound to the skull by very

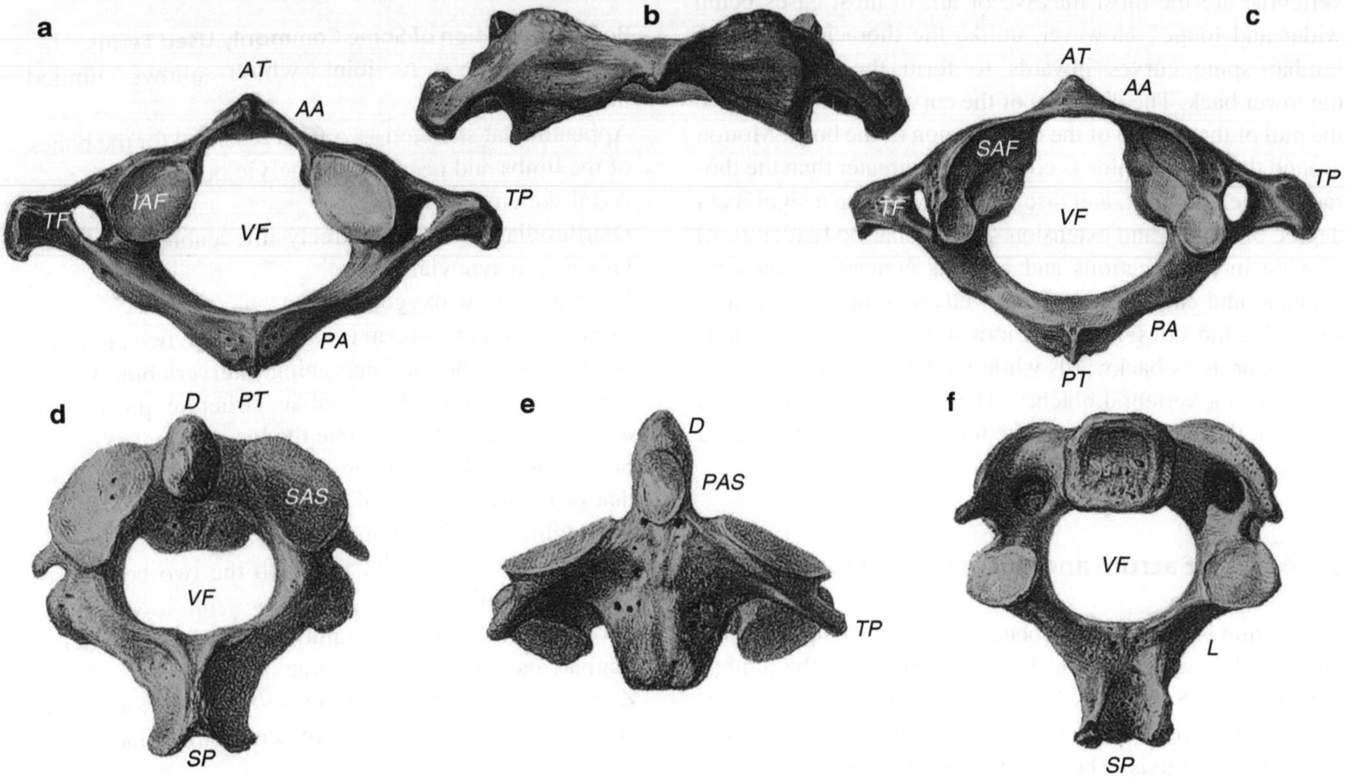

Fig. 1.3 Human cervical vertebrae: atlas and axis. (**a–c**) show the atlas (C1) and (**d–f**) indicate the axis (C2) vertebrae. (**a, d**) are superior views; (**c, f**) show inferior views; (**b, e**) are lateral aspects of the vertebrae. *VF* vertebral foramen, *AT* anterior tubercle, *PT* posterior tubercle, *AA* anterior arch, *PA* posterior arch, *TF* transverse foramen, *TP* posterior tubercle, *SAF* superior articulating facet, *SAS* superior articulating surface, *PAS* posterior articulating surface, *L* lamina, *SP* spinous process, *D* dens or odontoid process (From Bougery and Jacob (1833). Plate 7)

strong ligaments, these vertebrae allow a range of motion that permits up and down as well as rotational movements of the skull. Thus, the joint between the atlas (named after the God who balanced the world on his shoulders) and the occiput ("hole in the head"), the atlanto-occipital joint, permits flexion and extension (basically nodding), while the atlanto-axial joint (C1 and C2) allows nodding, gliding, and rotation. Rotation of the head and with it the atlas is mediated by the odontoid process or dens, a bony peg-like extension of C2 into C1. The actual interaction between C1 and C2 is complex with a number of centers of movement: the pivoting odontoid process of the axis and the gliding facet joints between the axis and atlas vertebrae. Noteworthy there is no disc between the occiput and the atlas or between the axis and the atlas; the first intervertebral disc is between the axis C2 and C3. The detailed anatomy of the axis and atlas are shown in Fig. 1.3; the anatomy of C4–C7 is shown in Fig. 1.2.

1.3.2 Thoracic Vertebrae

In general, the twelve thoracic vertebrae have the same functional role as the other axial vertebrae. They are larger in size than in the cervical spine, but smaller than those of the lumbar region. Common architectural features of the thoracic vertebrae are that the body (centrum) and the spinous processes are large and unlike vertebrae of the lumbar region, the spinous processes point downwards (see Fig. 1.2f, i). A major function of the thoracic spine is stability and through articulations with the ribs provides protection for the lungs and the heart. Of the bones that comprise the rib cage, the seven cephalic thoracic vertebrae are attached to the sternum via 12 pairs of ribs. As such, each sternal rib articulates with two vertebrae: sites of attachment are through joints on the inferior and superior aspects of the centrum and a third facet located at the end of the transverse process (costal facets). The remaining thoracic vertebrae are attached to the unanchored ribs (also known as floating ribs) by similar types of articulations.

1.3.3 Lumbar Spine (Fig. 1.2)

Like the thoracic spine, the robustness of the lumbar vertebrae increases from L1 to L5. When compared with the vertebrae of the other regions of the spine, the individual lumbar vertebrae are the most massive of all: in most cases being wider and longer. However, unlike the thoracic spine, the lumbar spine curves inwards to form the concavity in the lower back. The direction of the curve is probably due to the pull of the viscera of the lower region of the body. Motion around the lumbar spine is considerably greater than the thoracic spine, the facet, and disc joints, permitting a significant degree of flexion and extension. The lumbar body (centrum) is wide in all directions and exhibits concavities on both cephalic and caudal surfaces as well as being slightly constricted at the sides. Like the thoracic vertebrae, the spinous process projects backwards while the large pedicles display deep inferior vertebral notches. The L2 segment is the level at which the spinal nerves come together to form the cauda equina.

1.3.4 The Sacrum and Coccygeal Bones (Fig. 1.4)

The sacrum is a very strong robust multibone triangular complex (S1–S5) which is joined at its upper end to the lumbar vertebrae at L5 while its lower portion associates with the coccyx. The five fused bones of the sacrum integrate the two halves of the pelvis. The sacrum is united to the ileum by fibrocartilage which accommodates and transmits the weight of the upper body mass. The inferior end of the sacrum articulates with the five fused bones of the coccyx. Intervertebral discs are not present in the bones of the sacrum or the coccyx (Box 1.3).

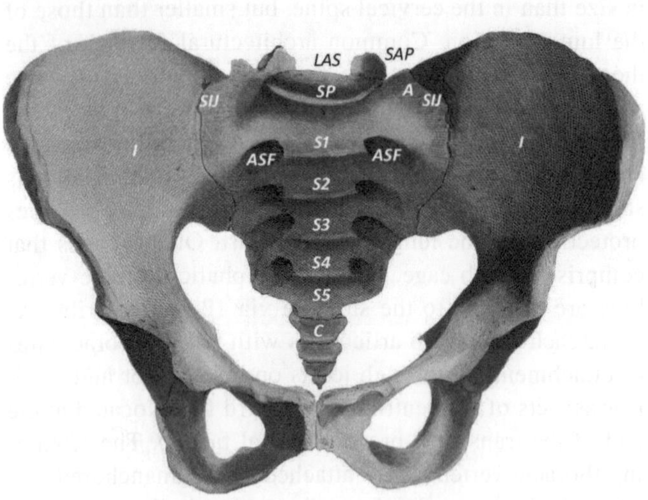

Fig. 1.4 Human sacrum and coccygeal bones. The ala (*A*) of the sacrum articulates with the ileum (*I*) of the pelvis at the sacroiliac joints (*SIJ*). The sacrum consists of five fused vertebrae (*S1–S5*). The superior portion of the sacrum articulates with L5 (lumbar sacrum articulation, *LSA*) while the inferior aspect fuses with the bones of the coccyx (C1–C5). Running through the sacrum is a continuation of the vertebral canal from which the sacral nerves emerge through both anterior (*ASF*) and posterior foramina. *SAP* superior articulating process, *SP* sacral promontory, *AS* apex of sacrum (From Lizars (1857). Plate III, Bones of the pelvis)

Box 1.3 Definition of Some Commonly Used Terms

Amphiarthroses—A joint which allows limited motion
Appendicular skeleton—A term reserved for the bones of the limbs and pectoral and pelvic bones
Axial skeleton—Spine
Diarthrodial joints—A freely moveable joint also known as a synovial joint
Hypoxia—Low oxygen tension
Motion segment—Term used to describe two contiguous vertebrae and the intervening intervertebral disc
Notochord—A flexible rodlike structure present in chordates that helps to define the longitudinal axis
Sclerotome—The portion of the embryonic somite that gives rise to the axial skeleton
Spondylitis—Inflammation of the vertebrae
Synchondrosis—A joint in which the two bones are joined by cartilage
Vertebral formula—The number of cervical, thoracic, lumbar, and coccygeal vertebrae
Zygapophyseal or facet joints—Synovial joints on each vertebra that permit movement of the spine

1.4 Vertebrae and Intervertebral Discs of Animals

1.4.1 Anatomical Considerations

While considerable space is devoted to the sand rat (see Chap. 20) as well as other quadrupeds (see Chap. 18), it is worthwhile summarizing some key features of small animals that are used extensively in studies of the intervertebral disc. In contrast to the vertically orientated human vertebral column, the almost horizontal spine of quadrupeds is subjected to a different series of biomechanical forces. Discussing the cat spine, Macpherson and Ye note, “Not surprisingly, the force vectors on all of the vertebrae differ substantially from the human. The axial skeleton may be considered as a segmented beam with the legs as pillar supports and two overhanging regions, the head-neck segments and the tail” (Macpherson and Ye 1998). At the rostral end of the spine, the animal’s head is supported through the muscles and ligaments of the cervical spine. The first two vertebrae are ring shaped and are organized to allow for controlled movements of the head. Like the human, these vertebrae do not have the robust body, but exhibit all of the articulations for spinal movement. Macpherson and Ye (1998) propose that the support for the head is provided by muscles that join the spine with the scapula. These muscles include the levator scapulae and serratus ventralis, which are inserted into the transverse

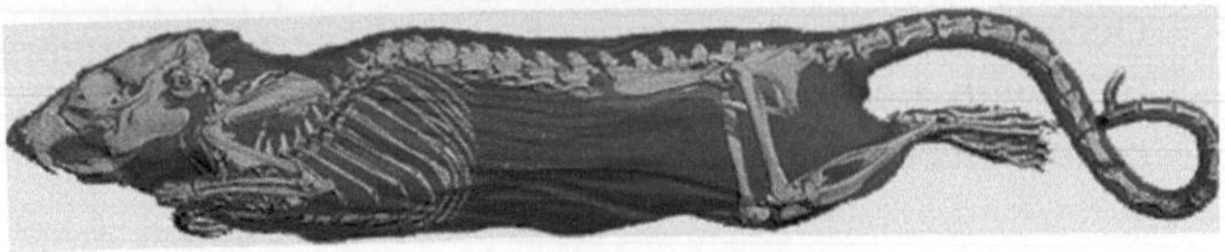

Fig. 1.5 Axial skeleton of the rat. Micro-CT analysis of the rat. Note the 12 thoracic vertebrae form an S-shaped curve with facets for articulation with the ribs. The last lumbar vertebra articulates with the sacrum which articulates with the pelvis through the ilium, thereby transferring the weight of the posterior region of the body to the femurs and the almost vertical legs. The tail is composed of 28–30 vertebrae which, with increasing distance from the sacrum, exhibits a progressive loss of centrum mass and decrease in the identity of articulating surfaces, processes, and foramina. Eventually, the neural arch becomes fused with the centrum (Figure provided with kind permission by Dr. Rasesh Kapadia, Scanco Medical, Switzerland)

Table 1.1 Vertebral formula for animals and man

Species	Cervical	Thoracic	Lumbar	Sacral	Coccygeal
Man	7	12	5	5	5
Rat	7	13	6	4	28–36
Mouse	7	13	6	4	24–28
Dog	7	13	7	3	Var
Horse	7	18	6	5	18
Swan	22–25	?	?	8	?
Giraffe	7	12	5	5	4
Frog	1	8		1	Urostyle
Snake	350	4–7	2–10		1
Plesiosaur	40	?	?	?	?

The number of coccygeal vertebrae in the dog is variable (*var*), frogs are tailless (anurans) and the final vertebrae form a long bone-like structure, the urostyle. ? unknown

processes of C3 to T9/10, and the rhomboids which join the scapula to the spinous process of C4 to T4. Together these muscles "suspend the trunk from the scapulae much like the wires on a suspension bridge."

In the rat, the 12 thoracic vertebrae form an S-shaped curve (see Fig. 1.5). These vertebrae display well-developed long spinous processes that are intermediate in size between cervical and lumbar, and they exhibit facets for articulation with the ribs. Like the human spine, the lumbar vertebrae are the most massive in the rat with very well-defined intervertebral discs. The last lumbar vertebra articulates with the sacrum. The body of these composite vertebrae forms a slab of bone in which there is loss of intervertebral discs and the zygapophyses and lateral processes are fused (Fig. 1.5). The sacrum articulates with the pelvis through the ilium, thereby transferring the weight of the posterior region of the body to the femurs. Thus, forces applied to the animal's body are transmitted across the almost horizontal sacrum (usually at S1 and often S2) to the vertical legs.

Composed of a variable number of vertebrae (about 28–30), the tail represents the final region of the spine. While the first few vertebrae are anatomically complete, with increasing distance from the sacrum, there is a change in vertebra size and complexity. There is a progressive loss of centrum mass and decrease in the identity of articulating surfaces and processes and foramina. Eventually, the neural arch becomes fused with the centrum, while the diameter of the intervertebral foramen becomes narrowed and indistinct. Since some studies of the intervertebral disc are performed in the caudal region of the spine, these anatomical limitations need to be taken into account when devising studies of the caudal intervertebral discs.

1.4.2 Conservation of Vertebral Number

The vertebral formula for humans is surprisingly constant: 7 cervical, 12 thoracic, 5 lumbar, 5 fused vertebrae that make up the sacrum, and 4 or 5 coccygeal bones. Details of the vertebral formula for a number of common mammals are shown in Box 1.2. In nonmammalian species, considerable differences exist in the vertebral formula. Snakes have a large number of thoracic (between 100 and 200) and caudal (between 15 and 140) vertebrae; the extinct marine *Plesiosaurus* had more than 70 cervical vertebrae (Narita and Kuratani 2005).

For both humans and many mammals, the number of vertebrae in the cervical region of mammals appears to be constant. Galis (1999) analyzed the vertebral formula data for mammals from the *Descriptive Catalogue of the Osteological Series Contained in the Museum of the Royal College of Surgeons of England* compiled by Richard Owen in 1853. This catalogue contains data of 133 species from 15 orders of mammals and showed that a very high percentage of animals, possibly with the exception of carnivores, expressed seven cervical vertebrae (Table 1.1).

Galis (1999) reported that occasionally, there is a loss of a single cervical vertebra (C7) with a concomitant increase in the number of thoracic vertebrae and the appearance of a cervical rib. Associated with this change, in the space between the clavicle and the rib (the thoracic outlet), there is often nerve and blood vessel compression, a condition described as thoracic outlet syndrome (TOS) (Makhoul and Machleder 1992). Correlated with cervical rib formation, Schumacher et al. (1992) reported that there was an increase in childhood cancer including neuroblastoma, Wilms tumor, Ewing sarcoma, and lymphoblastic and myeloid leukemia. It is likely that this developmental anomaly is a result of aberrant Hox gene expression. Thus, a higher incidence of cervical rib is seen in the phenotype of Hoxa-4, Hoxd-4, Hoxa-5, and Hoxa-6 knockouts or overexpression of Hoxb-7 or Hoxb-8 D (Aubin et al. 1998). The relationship between Hox expression and development of the axial skeleton in mammals is developed in more detail in Chap. 3.

As an aside, while a vertebrae-dependent increase in rib number is correlated with disease, loss of a rib has biblical implications.

> But for Adam, no suitable helper was found. So the LORD God caused the man to fall into a deep sleep; and while he was sleeping, he took one of the man's ribs and closed up the place with flesh. Then the LORD God made a woman from the rib he had taken out of the man, and brought her to the man.

Whether Adam had TOS or suffered from headaches due to cervical tension or loss of a rib is not known. For a discussion of this and other biblical possibilities including the emergence of the baculum (ossified penis bone), please read Gilbert and Zevit (2001).

1.5 Summary of Critical Concepts Discussed in the Chapter

- The intervertebral disc/vertebrae were preceded phylogenetically by the notochord which provided rigidity and some resilience to the organism, promoted formation of an extended shape, and protected the overlying spinal cord.
- The vertebral bodies are formed by fusion of sclerotome from two adjacent somites: following formation of the neural arch, remnants of the notochord subsequently form the nucleus pulposus of the intervertebral disc.
- Synchronized change in gene expression in the pre-mesodermal cells activates the "segmentation clock." The coordinated expression of a limited number of genes provides waves of gene oscillations which control somitogenesis. Disturbances in this system influence the subsequent formation of the vertebrae and the intrinsic curvatures of the axial skeleton.
- The discs comprise an outer circumferential ring of fibrocartilage, the annulus fibrosus. The annulus encloses a central proteoglycan-rich core known as the nucleus pulposus and bounded by the cartilage endplates of the contiguous vertebrae.
- As a joint, the disc is classified as an amphiarthrosis with very limited mobility. Biomechanical studies indicate that there is wide range of motion between vertebrae that are more in line with those of a diarthrodial joint rather than an amphiarthrosis.
- The vertebrae protect the spinal cord and serve as sites for connection of the pectoral and pelvic girdles and as bone for attachment of muscle and rib for functional changes that enhanced locomotion and respiration. Specific functions of the discs include acting as hydrodynamic shock absorbers as well as providing flexibility to the whole spine.
- The vertebral formula for primates is well conserved: in humans 7 cervical, 12 thoracic, 5 lumbar, 5 fused vertebrae that make up the sacrum, and 4 or 5 coccygeal bones. Occasionally, there is a loss of a single cervical vertebra (C7) with a concomitant increase in the number of thoracic vertebrae and the appearance of a cervical rib.

Acknowledgments The authors would like to thank Dr. Chris Keppler for the radiographs shown in Fig. 1.2, the Smithsonian Institution for the permission to reproduce the image of Pikaia (Box 1.1), Scanco Medical for the use of the microCT image shown in Fig. 1.5, and F. Michael Angelo, MA, for use of the plates shown in Figs. 1.1, 1.2, 1.3, and 1.4. Lastly, the authors wish to thank the NIH and NIAMS for the ongoing support through grants AR050087 and AR055655.

References

Agrawal A, Guttapalli A, Narayan S, Albert TJ, Shapiro IM, Risbud MV (2007) Normoxic stabilization of HIF-1alpha drives glycolytic metabolism and regulates aggrecan gene expression in nucleus pulposus cells of the rat intervertebral disk. Am J Physiol Cell Physiol 293:C621–C631

Archer CW, Dowthwaite GP, Francis-West P (2003) Development of synovial joints. Birth Defects Res C Embryo Today 69:144–155

Aubin J, Lemieux M, Tremblay M, Behringer RR, Jeannotte L (1998) Transcriptional interferences at the Hoxa4/Hoxa5 locus: importance of correct Hoxa5 expression for the proper specification of the axial skeleton. Dev Dyn 212:141–156

Belavý DL, Bansmann PM, Böhme G, Frings-Meuthen P, Heer M, Rittweger J, Zange J, Felsenberg D (2011) Changes in intervertebral disc morphology persist 5 mo after 21-day bed rest. J Appl Physiol 111:1304–1314

Benazeraf B, Francois P, Baker RE, Denans N, Little CD, Pourquie' O (2010) A random cell motility gradient downstream of FGF controls elongation of an amniote embryo. Nature 466:248–252

Bougery JM, Jacob NH (1833) Atlas of complete treatise on human anatomy comprising operative medicine. C.A. Delaunay, Paris

Brunet LJ, McMahon JA, McMahon AP, Harland RM (1998) Noggin, cartilage morphogenesis, and joint formation in the mammalian skeleton. Science 280:1455–1457

Chal J, Pourquie' O (2009) Patterning and differentiation of the vertebrate spine. In: Pourquie O (ed) The skeletal system. Cold Spring Harbor Laboratory Press, Cold Spring Harbor, pp 41–116

Crock HV, Yoshizawa H (1976) The blood supply of the lumbar vertebral column. Clin Orthop Relat Res 115:6–21

Dahia CL, Mahoney EJ, Durrani AA, Wylie C (2009) Intercellular signaling pathways active during intervertebral disc growth, differentiation, and aging. Spine (Phila Pa 1976) 34:456–462

Dequeant ML, Glynn E, Gaudenz K, Wahl M, Chen J, Mushegian A, Pourquie' O (2006) A complex oscillating network of signaling genes underlies the mouse segmentation clock. Science 314:1595–1598

Frobin W, Brinckmann P, Biggemann M, Tillotson M, Burton K (1997) Precision measurement of disc height, vertebral height and sagittal plane displacement from lateral radiographic views of the lumbar spine. Clin Biomech (Bristol, Avon) 12(Suppl 1):S1–S63

Galis F (1999) Why do almost all mammals have seven cervical vertebrae? Developmental constraints, Hox genes, and cancer. J Exp Zool 285:19–26

Gan JC, Ducheyne P, Vresilovic EJ, Swaim W, Shapiro IM (2003) Intervertebral disc tissue engineering I: characterization of the nucleus pulposus. Clin Orthop Relat Res 411:305–314

Garstang W (1928) The morphology of the tunicata, and its bearings on the phylogeny of the chordata. Q J Microsc Sci 72:51–187

Gilbert SF, Zevit Z (2001) Congenital human baculum deficiency: the generative bone of Genesis 2:21–23. Am J Med Genet 101:284–285

Iwama H, Kato K, Imachi H, Murao K, Masaki T (2013) Human microRNAs originated from two periods at accelerated rates in mammalian evolution. Mol Biol Evol 30(3):613–626

Jiang YJ, Aerne BL, Smithers L, Haddon C, Ish-Horowicz D, Lewis J (2000) Notch signalling and the synchronization of the somite segmentation clock. Nature 408(6811):475–9

Jones P, Gardner L, Menage J, Williams GT, Roberts S (2008) Intervertebral disc cells as competent phagocytes in vitro: implications for cell death in disc degeneration. Arthritis Res Ther 10:R86

Lizars J (1857) A system of anatomical plates of the human body; accompanied with descriptions, and physiological, pathological, and surgical observations. Lizars, Edinburgh

Macpherson JM, Ye Y (1998) The cat vertebral column: stance configuration and range of motion. Exp Brain Res 119:324–332, RESEARCH ARTICLE

Makhoul RG, Machleder HI (1992) Developmental anomalies at the thoracic outlet: an analysis of 200 consecutive cases. J Vasc Surg 16:534–542

Marchand F, Ahmed AM (1990) Investigation of the laminate structure of lumbar disc anulus fibrosus. Spine (Phila Pa 1976) 15:402–410

Moore RJ (2000) The vertebral end-plate: what do we know? Eur Spine J 9:92–96

Mundy C, Yasuda T, Kinumatsu T, Yamaguchi Y, Iwamoto M, Enomoto-Iwamoto M et al (2011) Synovial joint formation requires local Ext1 expression and heparan sulfate production in developing mouse embryo limbs and spine. Dev Biol 351:70–81

Nachemson A, Lewin T, Maroudas A, Freeman MA (1970) In vitro diffusion of dye through the end-plates and the annulus fibrosus of human lumbar inter-vertebral discs. Acta Orthop Scand 41: 589–607

Narita Y, Kuratani S (2005) Evolution of the vertebral formulae in mammals: a perspective on developmental constraints. J Exp Zool B Mol Dev Evol 304:91–106

Nerlich AG, Weiler C, Zipperer J, Narozny M, Boos N (2002) Immunolocalization of phagocytic cells in normal and degenerated intervertebral discs. Spine 27:2484–2490

O'Connell GD, Vresilovic EJ, Elliott DM (2007) Comparison of animals used in disc research to human lumbar disc geometry. Spine (Phila Pa 1976) 32:328–333

Pacifici M, Koyama E, Iwamoto M (2005) Mechanisms of synovial joint and articular cartilage formation: recent advances, but many lingering mysteries. Birth Defects Res C Embryo Today 75: 237–248

Peacock A (1951) Observations on the pre-natal development of the intervertebral disc in man. J Anat 85(Pt 3):260–274

Pourquie' O (2011) Vertebrate segmentation from cyclic gene networks to scoliosis. Cell 145:651–663

Schumacher R, Mai A, Gutjahr P (1992) Association of rib anomalies and malignancy in childhood. Eur J Pediatr 151:432–434

Shapiro IM, Vresilovic EJ, Risbud MV (2012) Is the spinal motion segment a diarthrodial polyaxial joint: what a nice nucleus like you doing in a joint like this? Bone 50:771–776

Shu DG, Morris SC, Han J, Zhang ZF, Yasui K, Janvier P, Chen L, Zhang XL, Liu JN, Li Y, Liu HQ (2003) Head and backbone of the Early Cambrian vertebrate Haikouichthys. Nature 421(6922): 526–529

Souter WA, Taylor TK (1970) Sulphated acid mucopolysaccharide metabolism in the rabbit intervertebral disc. J Bone Joint Surg Br 52:371–384

Taylor JR (1975) Growth of human intervertebral discs and vertebral bodies. J Anat 120(Pt 1):49–68

Tubbs RS, Vahedi P, Loukas M, Shoja MM, Cohen-Gadol AA (2011) Hubert von Luschka (1820–1875): his life, discoveries, and contributions to our understanding of the nervous system: Historical vignette. J Neurosurg 114:268–272

The Intervertebral Disc: Overview of Disc Mechanics

2

Daniel H. Cortes and Dawn M. Elliott

Contents

D.H. Cortes • D.M. Elliott, PhD (✉)
Department of Biomedical Engineering,
University of Delaware,
125 E Delaware Avenue, Newark, DE 19716, USA
e-mail: delliott@udel.edu

I.M. Shapiro, M.V. Risbud (eds.), *The Intervertebral Disc*,
DOI 10.1007/978-3-7091-1535-0_2, © Springer-Verlag Wien 2014

2.1 Introduction

The vertebral column is the main structural element of the spine and is composed of the vertebrae and the intervertebral discs. The function of the vertebral column is to provide rigidity to the axial skeleton while allowing limited rotation and bending. The vertebrae are the osseous elements of the vertebral column and the spine. Each vertebra is composed of a vertebral body and posterior elements. The vertebral bodies resemble boxes of cortical bone filled with trabecular bone. They are separated by the intervertebral discs, which are attached to the relatively flat surfaces at the top and bottom of the vertebral body. On the posterior side of the vertebral bodies, a bony structure composed of pedicles and processes, known as the posterior elements, serves as anchor points for tendons and ligaments. Anatomical details of each of the vertebrae that comprise the spine are presented in Chap. 1. Definition of technical terms can be found in Box 2.1.

The zygapophysial joint is an articular joint between the inferior and posterior articular processes of adjacent vertebrae. Like most articular joints, the zygapophysial joint comprises a capsule filled with synovial fluid. Inside this capsule, the bones are covered by a thin layer of articular cartilage separated by the fibroadipose meniscoids. The zygapophysial joints play an important role in the mechanics of the spine. These joints prevent excessive axial rotation between the vertebral bodies, resist forward sliding of the superior vertebra, limit the amount of extension by the contact of the inferior articular process and the lamina of the vertebra below, and contribute to the transmission of a fraction of the load. The ligaments and the joints connecting the vertebral bodies provide some passive stability; the muscles surrounding the vertebral column, through an active mechanism, provide most of the stability of the spine during physical activity. A detailed description of spine muscle anatomy, forces, and lines of action is outside of the scope of this chapter, but can be found in Adams et al. (2006).

The intervertebral disc is the soft tissue in between the vertebral bodies. It is composed of three distinct tissues: nucleus pulposus, annulus fibrosus, and the cartilaginous

Box 2.1 Glossary of Mechanical Terms

Stress Stress is the force intensity and is calculated as applied load divided by area over which it is applied. Stress is classified into normal (perpendicular to the surface) and shear (along the surface) stresses.

Strain Strain is a measurement of deformation. Similar to stress, there are normal and shear strains. Normal strain is defined as change in length divided by original length. Shear strains are related to the change in angle.

Poisson's ratio When a sample is stretched it contracts in the lateral direction. The Poisson's ratio is the lateral contraction divided by the longitudinal stretch. This mechanical property is related to the compressibility of the material. A material with a Poisson's ratio of 0.0 does not exhibit any lateral contraction, while a material with a Poisson's ratio of 0.5 is incompressible.

Stiffness The stiffness is a measure of the resistance to deformation. It is defined as force divided elongation. The stiffness depends not only on the material itself, but also on the size of the object.

Modulus The modulus is related to the stiffness, except that the effects of object size are eliminated, therefore, the modulus is a material property. Modulus is calculated as stress divided by strain.

Anisotropy A material is anisotropic if its mechanical properties are different depending on direction of load. For instance, in the annulus fibrosus or other fibrous tissues, collagen fibers create direction-dependent anisotropy.

Viscoelasticity A material is viscoelastic when its mechanical behavior changes over time or as a function of the speed at which the loads are applied. The viscoelastic properties of a material are usually measured using *creep* or *stress relaxation tests*. In a creep test, a load is applied to the material and the deformation increases over time. In a stress relaxation test, a deformation is applied and the stress decreases over time.

endplates. Each of these tissues has a characteristic composition and structure which provide them with special mechanical properties to perform their function. Their interaction enables the intervertebral disc to transmit loads while allowing a constrained flexibility between vertebral bodies. In a healthy disc, the nucleus pulposus is a highly hydrated gel-like material which is surrounded by the annulus fibrosus and the cartilaginous endplates (Fig. 2.1). The main function of the nucleus pulposus is to support mechanical loads through hydraulic and osmotic pressure. The cartilaginous endplates are thin layers of cartilage that cover the central area of the vertebral body (Fig. 2.1a). At the periphery of the vertebral body, not covered by the cartilaginous endplate, is the ring apophysis. The cartilaginous endplates have an important role on the exchange of nutrients, waste products, and other metabolites between the nucleus and the blood vessels in the vertebral bodies. The annulus fibrosus is composed of series of concentric layers with collagen fibers in alternating orientations (Fig. 2.1b). The outer lamellae of the collagen fibers attach directly to the vertebral bodies while the inner lamellae attach to the cartilaginous endplates. The annulus fibrosus provides a lateral confinement of the nucleus pulposus, supports vertical loads, and limits the amount of motion between the vertebral bodies.

The intervertebral disc undergoes biochemical and structural changes due to aging and degeneration. Biochemical changes include a decrease of proteoglycan content, an increase in protein cross-linking, and changes in the collagen type and distribution. The biochemical changes during degeneration are similar to those of aging; they are characterized by occurring in a faster rate and accompanied by structural changes that impair disc function. Structural changes observed during degeneration include a decrease in disc height, inward and outward bulging of the annulus fibrosus, and loss of its lamellar organization. The objective of this chapter is to describe the mechanical behavior of the individual tissues of the intervertebral disc and then analyze how they work together in different loading scenarios. In addition, the effects of degeneration on the mechanics at the tissue and disc levels are described.

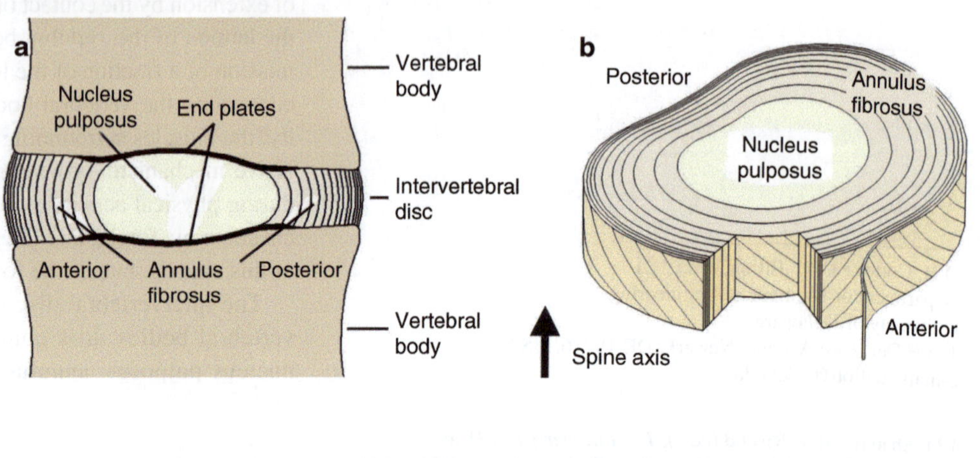

Fig. 2.1 Schematic representations of the adult intervertebral disc. (**a**) Midsagittal cross section showing anatomical regions. (**b**) Three-dimensional view illustrating AF lamellar structure (Adapted from Smith et al. 2011)

2.2 Structure–Function of Intervertebral Disc Tissues

Although many studies have shed light on the structure–function relationships for the tissues that form the intervertebral disc, this is still an ongoing research topic, the aim of which is to describe the mechanical behavior of healthy tissues, the effects of degeneration, and the implications of disc mechanics on the cell biology. Recent findings on the structure–function relationships of the tissues of the intervertebral disc are presented in the following sections.

2.2.1 Osmotic Effects

The tissues of the intervertebral disc are mainly composed of water, proteoglycans, and collagen (Eyre 1979). The relative content of each of these components differs from tissue to tissue. For instance, the nucleus pulposus has the highest proteoglycan content, while the annulus fibrosus has the highest collagen content (see Chaps. 3 and 4) (Eyre and Muir 1976). The differences in relative content of these individual components and their organization provide these disc tissues with their special mechanical properties. For example, it is well known that due to its higher collagen content and fiber organization, the annulus fibrosus has a superior tensile loading capacity. In a similar way, the high proteoglycan content of the nucleus pulposus provides the tissue with high compressive properties. However, since the tissues in the disc have similar components, they also share some mechanical behaviors, specifically, the osmotic effects which reflect the proteoglycan high negative charge density (Urban and Maroudas 1981). The osmotic effects have important implications on the mechanics of the disc. For instance, the osmotic pressure causes a deformation of the tissue usually known as osmotic swelling. This swelling pressure induces tensile stresses and increases the stiffness of the tissue. This osmotic swelling also draws water into these tissues keeping the disc hydrated. Since the osmotic effects play an important role in the mechanics of all disc tissues, this section provides a brief description of the relationship between composition and osmotic effects.

The osmotic effects are mediated by the proteoglycan content of the tissue (Maroudas and Bannon 1981; Urban et al. 1979). Proteoglycans are large molecules composed of many glycosaminoglycan units attached to a long core protein. Glycosaminoglycans are chains of polysaccharides that at a physiological pH present an excess of negatively charged ions (Comper and Laurent 1978). The molecular structure of proteoglycans and glycosaminoglycans is discussed in great detail in Chap. 4. Due to their large size, proteoglycans are trapped in the network of collagen fibers. Therefore, collagen and proteoglycans form a charged, porous, deformable solid material which is embedded in a solution of water and ions (Urban and Maroudas 1981). The amount of negative charges attached to the solid is quantified by the fixed charge density. At equilibrium, the balance of chemical potentials results in an increase of osmotic pressure (p), which is a function of the fixed charge density and the ionic strength of the surrounding fluid (Overbeek 1956). Assuming an ideal solution for the interstitial fluid and external solution, the osmotic pressure can be expressed as

$$p = RT\left(\sqrt{c_{\mathrm{fc}}^2 + 4c_{\mathrm{b}}^2} - 2c_{\mathrm{b}}\right) \qquad (1)$$

where R is the universal gas constant, T is the absolute temperature, c_{fc} is the fixed charge density, and c_{b} is osmolarity of the surrounding fluid bath.

The osmotic pressure and the external applied forces result in deformation of the solid component of the tissue, which in turn alter the fixed charge density (c_{fc}). That change can be quantified by

$$C_{\mathrm{fc}} = \frac{c_{\mathrm{fc0}}\phi_{\mathrm{f}}^{0}}{\left(J - 1 + \phi_{\mathrm{f}}^{0}\right)} \qquad (2)$$

where c_{fc0} and ϕ_{f}^{0} are the fixed charge density and the water content at the reference configuration, respectively, and J is the ratio between the volume at the deformed and reference configurations. The reference configuration, usually defined as the configuration where stresses are zero, plays an important role in the calculation of the osmotic pressure.

2.2.2 Nucleus Pulposus

The nucleus pulposus is the gelatinous core of the intervertebral disc and it is composed of water (70–85 % of total weight), proteoglycans (30–50 % of dry weight), collagen (20 % of dry weight), and other minor proteins (Adams and Muir 1976; Eyre 1979). Aggrecan is the most abundant proteoglycan in the nucleus pulposus, followed by other proteoglycans such as decorin (Melrose et al. 2001). Aggrecan contains keratan and chondroitin sulfate chains which interact with hyaluronic acid filaments forming large molecules that are trapped in the collagen network (Kiani et al. 2002). These side chains are negatively charged; consequently, positively charged Na^+ ions bind to these chains creating an accumulation of cations inside the nucleus pulposus. Since the glycosaminoglycans are not able to diffuse out of the nucleus pulposus, there is a permanent difference of the concentration of cations compared to the surrounding environment. This unbalance of cations is the cause of the osmotic pressure in the disc.

Collagen II is the most abundant type of collagen in the nucleus pulposus and other compression-bearing tissues such as articular cartilage (Eyre and Muir 1976). Unlike articular cartilage, collagen II forms an unorganized fiber network in the nucleus pulposus. A recent study showed that long fibers in the nucleus pulposus continuously connect both endplates (Wade et al. 2011). In an intact disc, these fibers are much longer than the disc height; they fold in a rather arbitrary configuration and can withstand substantial tension when unfolded. Experimentally, however, since it was necessary to cut the annulus fibrosus to separate the endplates, it is unlikely that the nucleus pulposus fibers experience high levels of tension under physiological conditions. This is different from articular cartilage, where fibers are highly organized and experience substantial tension due to the osmotic swelling (Ateshian et al. 2009; Cavalcante et al. 2005). In the case of the nucleus pulposus, the osmotic and hydrostatic pressure is supported axially by the endplates and radially by tensile (hoop) stresses in the annulus fibrosus. Consequently, fibers are not required to hold the nucleus pulposus in place as is the case in articular cartilage.

Due to its high levels of hydration and gelatinous consistency, the mechanical behavior of the nucleus pulposus has characteristics of both a fluid and a solid (Iatridis et al. 1996). Consequently, the nucleus pulposus is usually treated as a viscoelastic material. The mechanical properties of the nucleus pulposus have been investigated mainly through torsion and compression tests (Heneghan and Riches 2008a, b; Iatridis et al. 1997a, b; Johannessen and Elliott 2005; Perie et al. 2005). Confined compression has been typically used to measure several mechanical properties of the nucleus pulposus such as aggregate modulus and permeability coefficients (Johannessen and Elliott 2005). It is measured by axially compressing a cylindrical sample in a chamber that prevents lateral expansion. Although physiologically the nucleus pulposus is not fully confined or fully unconfined, confined compression tests have been generally accepted to characterize its compressive behavior. For small deformations (around 5 %), the nucleus pulposus can be considered to have a constant permeability and exhibits a linear relationship between stresses and strains (Johannessen and Elliott 2005). However, the properties are strain dependent (i.e., nonlinear) for moderate and large strains (Heneghan and Riches 2008a). Table 2.1 presents a summary of nucleus pulposus values obtained using confined compression.

The elastic behavior of the nucleus pulposus can be apportioned in terms of the contribution of osmotic (ionic) and solid tissue (nonionic) effects. The contribution of the osmotic effects to the compressive properties has been measured by eliminating the osmotic effects using a surrounding medium with high osmolarity or by reducing the proteoglycan content via enzymatic digestion (Heneghan and Riches 2008a; Perie et al. 2006b). When a high ionic concentration medium was used, the compressive properties of the bovine nucleus pulposus were reduced to 20–30 % of the value measured in isotonic (physiological) medium concentrations. Therefore, the contribution of the osmotic effects to the stiffness and load support of the nucleus pulposus is approximately 70–80 %. The contribution of the osmotic effects was almost constant through a wide range of applied deformations (0–70 % compressive strains). If the proteoglycans are removed by enzymatic digestion, a reduction of 20- to 30-fold was observed in the compressive properties of the nucleus pulposus (Perie et al. 2006b). This suggests that the proteoglycans also have a nonionic contribution to the mechanics of the nucleus pulposus. Evidence of the nonionic contribution of the proteoglycans has been reported for other tissues such as articular cartilage (Canal Guterl et al. 2010).

Viscoelastic or frequency-dependent properties of the nucleus pulposus have been analyzed using torsion tests (Iatridis et al. 1997a, b). Stress relaxation tests measured an instantaneous shear modulus around 11 kPa. However, the shear stress rapidly relaxed to near-zero values suggesting a fluid-like behavior. In dynamic torsion tests, a shear modulus of ~20 kPa and a phase shift (the delay between strain and stress measured in terms of degrees) of ~30° were measured. For comparison, the dynamic modulus of articular cartilage is 600–1,000 kPa, the modulus for the meniscus is 540 kPa, while proteoglycan solutions are 0.01 kPa (Hardingham et al. 1987; Zhu et al. 1993, 1994). Values of phase shift of 13° for cartilage, 22° for meniscus, and 65° for proteoglycan solutions have been reported. Since the phase shift for the nucleus is lower than 45°, it suggests a more solid-like dynamic behavior.

The studies discussed above illustrate the complexity of the mechanical behavior and structure–function relationships of the nucleus pulposus. The contribution of osmotic pressure

Table 2.1 Aggregate modulus (H_A) as a function of the stretch ratio (λ) and glycosaminoglycan content for the nucleus pulposus

Study	H_A (kPa)	λ	NP tissue	s-GAG (% dry wt.)
Heneghan and Riches (2008a)	69–1,650	1.0–0.3	Bovine tail	24
Perie et al. (2005)	350–520	1.0–0.8	Bovine tail	
Perie et al. (2006a)	~600	1.0–0.6	Bovine tail	~35
Perie et al. (2006b)	~400–510	1.0–0.8	Bovine tail	~42
Johannessen and Elliott (2005)	1,010	0.95	Human	44

and the blend between exhibiting characteristics of fluid and solid mechanics pose a difficult challenge to model and also complicate the prediction of deformations during physiological loading. Nonetheless, it is important to understand and characterize the mechanics of the nucleus pulposus as it influences cell function and impacts predictions related to mechanically induced injuries and regeneration.

2.2.3 Annulus Fibrosus

Similar to the nucleus pulposus, the annulus fibrosus is composed mainly of proteoglycans and collagen, although the relative content and organization of its components are substantially different. In the healthy human annulus fibrosus, the water content is 50 %, collagen is approximately 70 % of the dry weight, and proteoglycans make up to 10 % of the dry weight (Eyre and Muir 1976; Eyre 1979). The annulus fibrosus is subjected to both tensile and compressive stresses during physiological loading. Consequently, it has high collagen content similar to other tension-bearing tissues such as tendon and ligaments. Proceeding from the outer to the inner annulus, there is an decrease in the ratio of collagens I to II, and the amount of proteoglycan rises. This profile reflects a change in the loading environment from more tension in the outer annulus fibrosus to more compression towards the nucleus pulposus (Eyre and Muir 1976). In a similar way, in the outer annulus fibrosus, collagen fibers insert directly to the cortical bone of the vertebrae and not to the endplate as in the case of inner annulus fibrosus, again probably reflecting the higher tensile loads present in the outer annulus fibrosus (Nachemson 1963; Wu and Yao 1976).

Noteworthy, in the annulus, collagen fibers are arranged in concentric lamellae with alternating orientations (Fig. 2.1b). The angle between fiber directions of adjacent lamellae changes from ~60° to the spinal axis in the outer annulus fibrosus to ~90° in the inner annulus fibrosus (Cassidy et al. 1989; Guerin and Elliott 2006a; Hickey and Hukins 1980). This arrangement provides the annulus with a series of important mechanical properties, including anisotropy (direction dependence). Since the fibers play such an important role in the mechanics of the annulus fibrosus, this tissue can be analyzed as a combination of fibers and an isotropic material known as extrafibrillar matrix (Spencer 1984). As its name indicates, the extrafibrillar matrix represents all the solid components of the annulus fibrosus, except fibers.

One of the more important characteristics of the mechanics of collagenous tissues is nonlinearity. The nonlinearity of the fibers is characterized by a low stiffness region for small deformations, known as toe region, followed by a transition (heel) region and a much stiffer linear region (Guerin and Elliott 2007; Wu and Yao 1976). Collagen fibers, in most tension-bearing tissues, have a hierarchical organization from fibrils to large collagen bundles or fascicles (Kastelic et al. 1978). Collagen fibers in these tissues have a wavy or zigzag shape commonly known as crimp (Diamant et al. 1972; Kastelic and Baer 1980). When the fibers are stretched, the fibers progressively straighten with minimal resistance; i.e., a negligible force is required to uncrimp the fibers. The amount of stretch required to straighten the fiber is known as uncrimping stretch. Once a fiber is straight, it starts taking load (Fig. 2.2). The uncrimping stretch is not same for all fibers in a tissue. For small deformations, few fibers with a small uncrimping stretch are straightened as they accommodate the load. Consequently, the stiffness of the tissue is low. Progressively, all the fibers stretch and contribute to load support resulting in high tissue stiffness (Fig. 2.2). If the tissue is further stretched, fibers will fail by several possible mechanisms including breakage and fiber pullout.

All the other components of the annulus fibrosus (except the fibers) are usually treated as a single material known as extrafibrillar matrix. Since the fibers contribute to the mechanics of the annulus fibrosus when they are in tension, the matrix characterizes the compressive properties of the annulus fibrosus. Other properties, including permeability and diffusivity of solutes, are also attributed to matrix. For simplicity, the elasticity of the matrix has been considered isotropic, which means that the elastic properties (i.e., Young modulus and Poisson's ratio) are same in all directions. Although the matrix includes some fibrillar components such as elastin and protein cross bridges, their content

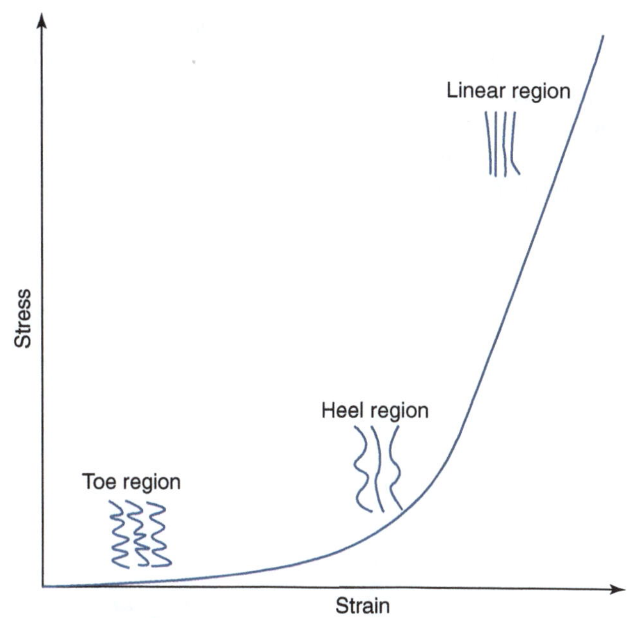

Fig. 2.2 The tensile stress–strain response of collagenous tissues, such as annulus fibrosus, can be divided into several regions, corresponding to different mechanisms. In the toe region, the contribution of fibers is small due to fiber crimping. In the heel region, the increase in stiffness is due to fiber straightening. In the linear region, most of the fibers are straight and contributing to the high tensile stiffness

is small and unlikely to significantly alter the assumption of isotropy. However, transport properties such as permeability and diffusivities have been shown to be anisotropic (Gu et al. 1999; Travascio and Gu 2011), which means that there are directions where the fluid and solutes can flow or move with less resistance.

The tensile properties of the annulus fibrosus have been characterized using uniaxial and biaxial tension tests (Jacobs et al. 2013; Nerurkar et al. 2010). In uniaxial tests, a strip of tissue is cut from the annulus fibrosus in a given orientation (circumferential, axial, radial, or along the fibers), and the force required to stretch the sample is recorded as a function of the applied strain. The Poisson's ratio can be measured by recording the lateral contraction of the sample during the test. The Young modulus is calculated from the slope of the stress–strain response. A summary of these properties is presented in Table 2.2. The Young modulus is higher in the disc's circumferential direction than the axial. This is expected since the fibers are oriented closer in the circumferential direction; therefore, fibers are not stretched during axial loading so that modulus is primarily due to the matrix.

Biaxial loading is another tensile test used to quantify annulus fibrosus mechanics. It is thought that biaxial loading more closely resembles multiaxial physiological loading of the annulus fibrosus (Bass et al. 2004; Gregory and Callaghan 2011; Huyghe 2010; Jacobs et al. 2013; O'Connell et al. 2012). For this test, a rectangular thin sample is gripped on all four sides and loads are applied in two directions (Fig. 2.3). Two-dimensional deformations are optically recorded during the test. Unlike a uniaxial test, there is not a direct relationship between the slope of these curves and the elastic properties of the annulus fibrosus; the forces (or stress) in one direction are affected by the deformation applied to the other direction (O'Connell et al. 2012). Consequently, the data from biaxial tests are analyzed through the use of a model. The advantage of using biaxial experiments to characterize the mechanics of the fibers is that the values obtained through these types of tests can be used to predict the response of the annulus fibrosus in uniaxial tests and with other biaxial strain ratios (O'Connell et al. 2012).

Since the collagen fibers only contribute to the mechanics of the annulus fibrosus in tension, the elastic properties of the extrafibrillar matrix can be measured through confined compression tests (Cortes and Elliott 2012; Drost et al. 1995; Klisch and Lotz 2000; Perie et al. 2005). This test provides the aggregate modulus, measured as a function of strain. Similar to the nucleus pulposus, the mechanical behavior of the matrix depends on contributions from the osmotic pressure and the nonionic extrafibrillar matrix (Cortes and Elliott 2012). In this manner, the mechanical properties of this extrafibrillar matrix can be measured in tension and compression by applying osmotic swelling and confined compression simultaneously. The nonionic extrafibrillar matrix is nonlinear with a higher stiffness in compression (~50 kPa) than in tension (~10 kPa), and the contribution of the osmotic pressure in the support of the applied loads is high (~70 % of total) when the EFM is in compression and low (~25 %) when in tension.

Table 2.2 Linear region moduli of nongenerated (ND) and degenerated (D) annulus fibrosus tissue (Elliott and Setton 2001; Guerin and Elliott 2006b)

	Circumferential		Axial		Radial	
	ND	D	ND	D	ND	D
Inner anterior	5.6–10.0	5.0	1.0	–	–	–
Outer anterior	17.0–29.0	22.0–29.0	0.8	–	0.4–0.5	0.4
Inner posterior	2.0–6.0	4.0	–	–	0.5	–
Outer posterior	13.0–19.0	8.0	–	–	–	–

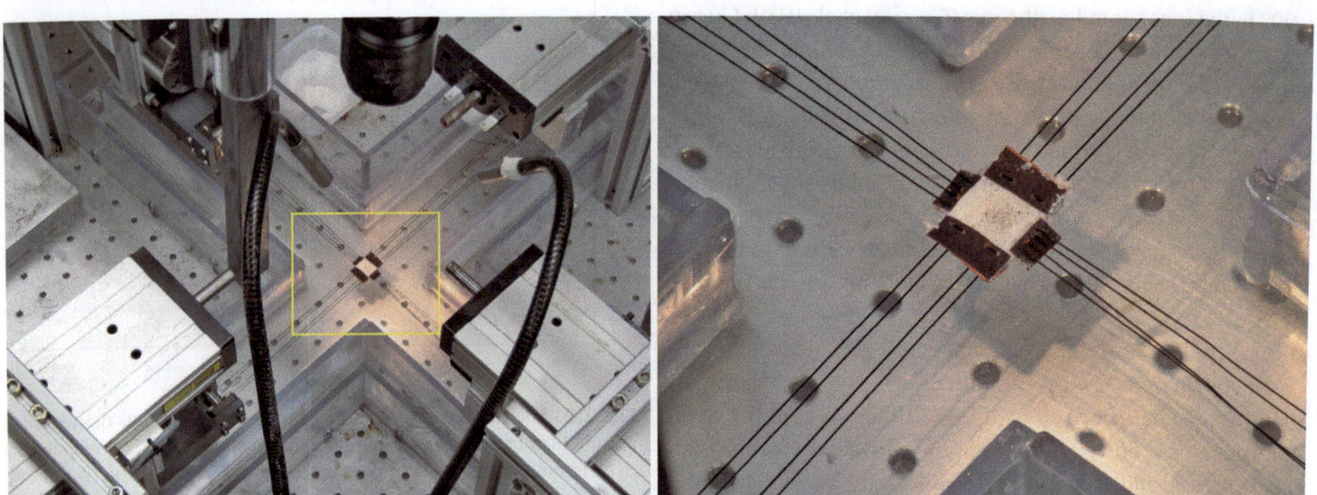

Fig. 2.3 In a biaxial test of annulus fibrosus, a sample is loaded simultaneously in the axial and circumferential direction

Table 2.3 Shear modulus (kPa) of human annulus fibrosus: effects of sample orientations and location and type of test

		Orientation		
Type of test	Location	Circ-radial	Circ-axial	Radial-axial
Simple shear – compressive preload	Anterior	28.92	58.56	40.16
Simple shear – compressive preload	Posterolateral	22.2	53.6	25.1
Simple shear – tensile preload	Anterior	–	193.6	–
Torsion shear – equilibrium	Anterior	20–100	–	–
Torsion shear – dynamic	Anterior	100–280	–	–

Shear tests have been used to determine elastic and viscoelastic properties of the annulus fibrosus. Elastic shear properties have been measured by applying simple shear tests (Fujita et al. 2000; Hollingsworth and Wagner 2011; Iatridis et al. 1999; Jacobs et al. 2011). Since the fibers have a contribution during this test, the shear modulus is anisotropic with a higher modulus in the circumferential–axial plane where the fibers experience stretches (Table 2.3). On the other hand, torsion tests have been used to measure viscoelastic properties of the annulus fibrosus (Iatridis et al. 1999). The dynamic modulus increases with frequency. Both equilibrium and dynamic modulus decrease with shear strain amplitude. The highly viscoelastic nature of the annulus fibrosus is evidenced by the threefold increase of the dynamic modulus over the equilibrium modulus.

Although separating the mechanics of the annulus fibrosus into fibers and matrix is very convenient and describes much of the mechanical behavior of annulus fibrosus, there are interactions between these components. Specifically, the stiffness of the matrix increases with the stretch of the fibers (Guo et al. 2012). To account for these effects, several fiber–matrix and fiber–fiber interactions have been formulated in terms of the strain perpendicular and along the fibers (Guerin and Elliott 2007; O'Connell et al. 2009, 2012; Wagner and Lotz 2004). These interactions have more accurately described the mechanical behavior of the annulus fibrosus. It has also been suggested that shear interactions are essential to obtain a good simultaneous prediction of uniaxial, biaxial, and shear experimental data (Hollingsworth and Wagner 2011; O'Connell et al. 2012).

While many aspects of the mechanical behavior of the annulus fibrosus have been well described, this is still an active area of research. Special attention needs be given to relations between interactions and composition of the annulus fibrosus and the contribution of these interactions to mechanics of the disc. Additionally, these interactions between components should be replicated in engineered tissues that are currently being investigated as therapeutic alternatives (Mauck et al. 2009; Nerurkar et al. 2010).

2.2.4 Cartilaginous Endplate

The biomechanics of the cartilaginous endplate has been far less studied than other disc tissues. The endplate is the interface between the nucleus pulposus and inner annulus fibrosus with the vertebral bodies (Fig. 2.1a). It covers most of the vertebral endplate except for a small ring in the periphery called the ring apophysis. The thickness of the cartilaginous endplate varies: it is thinnest in the center (~0.2 mm) and thickest in the periphery (~0.9 mm) (Moon et al. 2013). The composition of the cartilaginous endplate is similar to that of hyaline cartilage, which is characterized by a high proteoglycan and collagen II content. The water content of human endplate is 58 % of the wet weight, the s-GAG content is 17 % of the dry weight, and the total collagen content is 60–80 % of dry weight (Setton et al. 1993). The cartilaginous endplate plays an important role in the transport of nutrients and other metabolites into the nucleus pulposus and the inner portion of the annulus fibrosus.

The mechanics of the cartilaginous endplate has been measured using confined compression tests (Setton et al. 1993). The aggregate modulus of the baboon endplate is 0.44 MPa. The hydraulic permeability (14.3×10^{-14} m^4/Ns) is considerably higher than values of 0.09×10^{-14} m^4/Ns and 0.153×10^{-14} m^4/Ns for the human annulus fibrosus and nucleus pulposus, respectively. The high permeability value suggests that its main function is to allow the transport of fluids, nutrients, and waste products to the cells in the nucleus pulposus and part of the annulus fibrosus.

2.3 Intervertebral Disc Mechanics

In the previous sections, the mechanics of individual disc tissues were described separately. However, these tissues interact with each other providing the disc with a special mechanical behavior. In a similar way, a disruption or a change in mechanical properties of one of these tissues causes an impairment of the mechanical function of the overall disc. In this section, disc mechanics are presented as the contribution of individual tissues during a given loading scenario. First, the residual stresses in the unloaded disc are briefly described. Then, the mechanics of the intervertebral disc are analyzed for three of the most important loads: axial compression, bending, and torsion.

2.3.1 Stress and Strain in the Unloaded Disc

Before analyzing the mechanics of the disc under different types of loading scenarios, it is important to understand the impact of internal stresses and strains on the unloaded disc. As described above, at the tissue level, the osmotic pressure is balanced by tensile or "residual" stresses. In a similar way, at the disc level, there are residual stresses and strains due to osmotic effects caused by tissue proteoglycans, are present even in the absence of applied loads. When external loads are applied to the disc, additional stress builds up above that of the residual stress. There are several mechanisms, at different scales, contributing to residual stress (Lanir 2009). At the micro-level, the interaction between proteoglycans, ions, water, and the collagen network produces an osmotic pressure that contributes to the total stress of the tissue. At the meso-level, residual stress arises from inhomogeneities within the tissues, e.g., the gradient of proteoglycan and collagen content from inner and outer annulus. Residual stress at meso-level has been recently measured in terms of the opening angle after a radial cut in bovine annulus fibrosus rings (Michalek et al. 2012). This effect is similar to that observed in aortic arteries, where differences in proteoglycan content between the media and the adventitia contribute to this component of the residual stress (Azeloglu et al. 2008; Chuong and Fung 1986). At the disc level, residual stress is also generated by the interaction between different tissues (nucleus pulposus, annulus fibrosus, endplates, and vertebral bodies). The high proteoglycan content of the nucleus pulposus results in a significant osmotic pressure. This pressure has been measured in vitro and in vivo using a needle pressure gauge (Nachemson 1981; Panjabi et al. 1988; Wilke et al. 1996, 1999). The radial expansion of the nucleus is constrained by the annulus fibrosus through tensile stresses in the circumferential direction (hoop stress) and compression stress in the radial direction. Similarly, the osmotic pressure in the nucleus tends to vertically separate the vertebral bodies, which are held in place by tensile stresses in the annulus fibrosus in the axial direction. All these contributions to the residual stress of the disc create a multidirectional and inhomogeneous initial state of stresses and strains that must be considered for the analysis of disc mechanics.

2.3.2 Compression Mechanics

Axial compression loading of the spine is of major physiological importance and arises from the weight of the upper body and by forces exerted by the muscles in the trunk during common daily activities. Compression loads are transmitted from vertebra to vertebra through the intervertebral disc and the zygapophysial joints in proportion to body posture. For instance, 84 % of the compressive load is transmitted through the intervertebral disc in the erect standing posture, whereas 100 % of the load is transmitted through the disc in the erect sitting posture (Adams and Hutton 1980). Although the compressive load to the intervertebral disc changes with posture and activity, the mechanism by which the different tissues of the intervertebral disc interact to support this load is the same. In this section, the interaction between disc tissues is described for compressive loads over short and long periods of time.

After a compression load is applied to the disc, the immediate mechanics are different from that measured at longer time intervals. Immediately after the load has been applied, the tissues in the disc can be considered to be incompressible materials; due to the low permeability of the disc tissues, there is insufficient time for interstitial fluid flow (Ateshian et al. 2007). In this loading state, the interstitial fluid in the nucleus pulposus pressurizes, supporting a fraction of the load. Since the nucleus pulposus behaves as an incompressible material, it tends to expand radially. However, since it is contained by the annulus fibrosus, there is a large tensile strain in the circumferential direction and outward bulging of the annulus (Tsantrizos et al. 2005). The applied load is supported by the lamellae through compressive stress in the axial direction. As a result, the compressive load causes the lamellae in the inner annulus fibrosus to buckle towards the nucleus pulposus; of course, this is opposed by the outward pressure exerted by the nucleus pulposus. Inward buckling of the inner annulus fibrosus is evident in the degenerate disc due to a decrease in the internal pressure of the nucleus pulposus associated with altered osmotic pressure and permeability changes (Sasaki et al. 2001; Sato et al. 1999; Wang et al. 2010). From this perspective, pressurization of the nucleus pulposus is of critical importance not only to carry part of the compressive load but also to provide stability to the lamellae in the radial direction.

During the diurnal loading cycle, the disc is subjected to a prolonged period of compression followed by a period of low-load recovery. If the load on the disc is maintained for some hours, the pressurized interstitial fluid will flow to regions of lower pressure through the annulus fibrosus and the endplate (van der Veen et al. 2007). During this process, the disc height decreases while the outward bulging of the annulus fibrosus increases (O'Connell et al. 2007). In addition, the nucleus pulposus depressurizes, reducing its contribution to load and increasing the axial compression of the annulus fibrosus (O'Connell et al. 2007). In this "relaxed" state, the tissues in the disc interact, as described above for instantaneous loading; however, the relative contribution of each of the tissues changes. After relaxation, the osmotic pressure in the healthy nucleus pulposus does not vanish completely. In fact, due to osmotic effects the remaining intradiscal pressure is largely responsible for hydration recovery and mechanics during the resting period of the diurnal cycle (O'Connell et al. 2011; van der Veen et al. 2007).

Nutrient and metabolite exchange during loading and unloading is essential for disc cell viability. In this process, nutrients and metabolites are brought to, and waste byproducts expelled from, the disc by diffusion and convection (Das et al. 2009; Ferguson et al. 2004; Holm et al. 1981; Shirazi-Adl et al. 2010; Soukane et al. 2007; Urban et al. 1978, 1982, 2004). The rate at which fluid leaves the disc depends on the hydraulic permeability and diffusivity of its component tissues. Since the hydraulic permeability of the endplate is higher than the annulus fibrosus, it should enhance aqueous flow through the endplate (Setton et al. 1993). Moreover, from the periphery (endplates and outer annulus) to the center of the disc, there is a change in metabolite concentration. Numerical simulations have also shown that the concentrations of glucose and oxygen are low close to the center of the disc, whereas lactic acid, which is the major metabolite, has a reverse distribution (Jackson et al. 2011; Soukane et al. 2007). Recent studies are aimed at improving the accuracy of the numerical models by considering anisotropy and nonlinearity of elastic, flow, and diffusion properties (Chuang et al. 2010; Jackson et al. 2008).

2.3.3 Flexion/Extension and Lateral Bending

Flexion/extension and lateral bending are spine movements required for many daily activities. Flexion and extension are terms used when the trunk bends forward and backward, respectively. In a well-aligned spine, a neutral position is observed when standing upright. However, the natural curvature of the spine changes during daily activities such as sitting or lifting a weight. This curvature change is the sum of the relative rotations between each of the vertebral bodies, each of which produce internal strains and stresses in the disc. To quantify the mechanics of the disc under this type of motion, the forces and moments can be estimated by monitoring muscle activity. However, this approach has been shown to be inconsistent (Potvin et al. 1991). A better approach to estimating forces and bending moments consists of determining the correlation between in vivo and in vitro measurements (Adams and Dolan 1991).

A common kinematic characteristic of flexion/extension and lateral bending is that the axis of rotation is perpendicular to the axis of spine. Therefore, flexion, extension, and lateral bending produce a similar pattern of internal deformations to the disc. During flexion, the axial compression in the anterior portion of the annulus fibrosus is increased. Consequently, there is an increase in the bulging of the outer region of the annulus and buckling of the lamellae in the inner portion of the anterior annulus fibrosus. On the other hand, the posterior region experiences tension in the axial direction. Additionally, the nucleus pulposus is shifted to the opposite side of bending, and there is an increase in intradiscal pressure (Nachemson 1981; Wilke et al. 1999). When the spine is in extension, the reverse effects are observed: tension in the anterior annulus fibrosus, compression of the posterior annulus, and shifting of the nucleus in the anterior direction. Lateral bending produces a similar pattern of strains in the disc; however, the compression and tension regions are located in the lateral annulus fibrosus (Costi et al. 2007; Tsantrizos et al. 2005).

The stiffness and range of motion of disc segments can be obtained by applying a known force and/or bending moment. The range of motion is defined as the relative rotation of the vertebral bodies when a pure moment is applied in the sagittal or coronal plane. On the other hand, the stiffness can be calculated as the slope of the moment–rotation curve at the end of the range of motion. Due to the asymmetric shape of the disc and the effect of the posterior elements, measurements of the range of motion and stiffness are different in flexion and extension. For instance, an increase of the compression strain from 2.7 to 6.7 % for an applied force of 500 N was reported for human L2/L3 spine segments when the posterior elements were removed (Heuer et al. 2008). In a similar way, the range of motion increased from 5.2° to 6.9° in flexion and from 3.4° to 8.2° in extension for a pure applied moment of 7.5 Nm (Heuer et al. 2008). The stiffness of disc segments has been measured on the principal axes of the disc and on multidirectional axes (Spenciner et al. 2006). It was concluded that the experimentally measured stiffness along the multidirectional axes do not match with the analytical predictions from the stiffness along principal axes (Spenciner et al. 2006).

2.3.4 Torsion

During a twisting motion of the trunk, torsion becomes another important component of the loading of intervertebral discs. Similar to flexion/extension, torsion is defined as the relative rotation of consecutive vertebral bodies; however, the axis of rotation is parallel to the axis of the spine. Consequently, the strains in the disc are substantially different. During physical activity, the rotation between vertebral bodies is about 1°–3° which is very small compared to the rotations observed during flexion or extension (Pearcy et al. 1984). The torsion range of motion is constrained by contact of the zygapophysial joints, which also increases the stiffness of intact spine segments (Adams and Hutton 1981). In vitro and numerical studies have reported a range of motion of 4°–8° for intact spinal segments. The removal of the posterior elements of the spine increases the range of motion twofold (Shirazi-Adl et al. 1986).

Shear strains are the main component of deformation during torsion. Deformation results in tensile stretch of one of the fiber populations, and while not contributing to torsion support due to fiber buckling, the other experiences compression. The tensile stretch on the fibers increases radially; consequently, the maximum fiber stretch is found in the outermost lamella. Removing the posterior elements of the spine resulted in an increase in the maximum fiber stretch from 3.1 to 11.4 % for an applied torque of 7.5 Nm (Heuer et al. 2008). From in vitro experiments, there is a reduction of the outward bulging of the annulus fibrosus and an increase of disc height and intradiscal pressure (Heuer et al. 2008; van Deursen et al. 2001a, b). The decrease of outward bulging can be directly linked to the high tensile fiber stresses in the outer lamellae. The decrease of lateral bulging also explains the increase of disc height and intradiscal pressure. Although the strains observed in torsion may be too small to cause significant damage to the disc, a decrease in the failure loads have been observed when torsion is combined with compression and flexion/extension.

2.4 Effect of Degeneration on Disc Mechanics

Intervertebral disc degeneration can be defined as a post-traumatic cell-mediated cascade of biochemical, mechanical, and structural changes that affect the function of the disc (Adams and Roughley 2006) (Fig. 2.4). Compositional changes during disc degeneration are mainly loss of proteoglycans, increased cross-linking, and an increase in the amount of collagen I over collagen II. These changes are first noticeable in the nucleus pulposus and later spread outwards to the annulus fibrosus. Although the causes remain largely unclear, factors that include structural injury, genetic heritance, age, inadequate metabolite transport, and loading history have been associated with the onset and progression of disc degeneration (Adams and Roughley 2006; Battié et al. 2008; Buckwalter 1995; Hsu et al. 1990; Pye et al. 2007; Rannou et al. 2004). In this section we limit our discussion to the effect of degeneration on the mechanics at the tissue and disc levels. A brief review of total disc replacements, which is of the treatments for disc degeneration, is presented in Box 2.2.

Numerous studies have measured the changes in the mechanical behavior of the disc tissues at several stages of degeneration. The compositional changes in the nucleus pulposus include a decrease in proteoglycan content and an increase in collagen I cross-links. These changes exert contradictory effects on the mechanics of the nucleus pulposus. On one hand, the loss of proteoglycans causes a decrease in the osmotic pressure and consequently a reduction in tissue stiffness. On the other hand, the increase in cross-linking and collagen content causes tissue stiffening. Experimentally, it has been noted that there is an overall decrease in the compression properties of nucleus pulposus (Johannessen and Elliott 2005). This observation is in accord with other studies that show that proteoglycans contribute approximately 80 % to the compressive properties of the nucleus pulposus with degeneration (Heneghan and Riches 2008a; Perie et al. 2006b). However, there is also a significant increase in the shear modulus (Iatridis et al. 1997b). Transport properties of the nucleus pulposus are also affected by degeneration as there

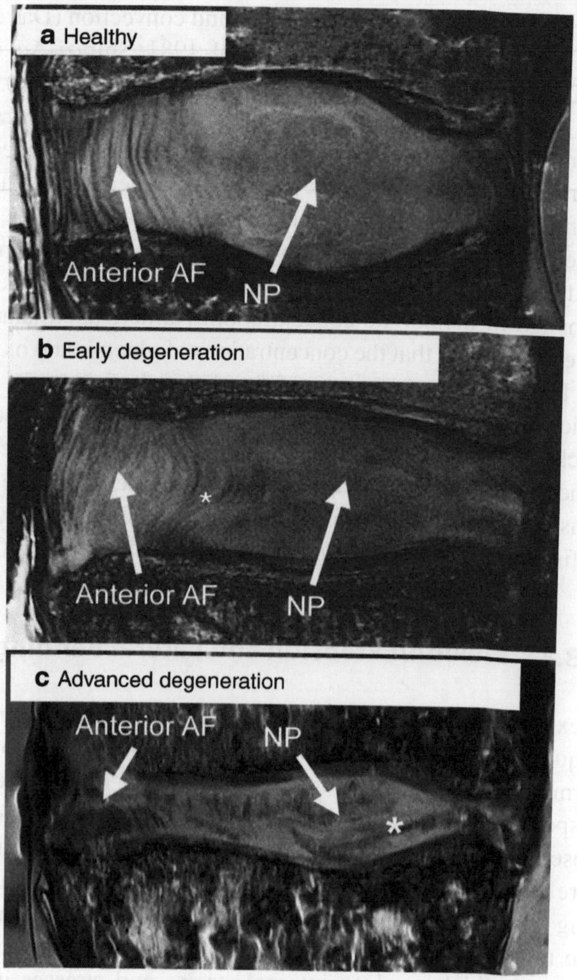

Fig. 2.4 Magnetic resonance images illustrating different stages of human lumbar disc degeneration. (**a**) Healthy disc exhibiting distinct AF lamellae (*AF*) and central NP region (*NP*). (**b**) Disc exhibiting early stages of degeneration, including moderate height reduction, decreased NP signal intensity, and inward bulging of AF lamellae (*). (**c**) Disc exhibiting advanced stages of degeneration, including severely reduced height, large fissure (*), and generalized structural deterioration. Images obtained using 7T Siemens scanner and a turbo spin echo sequence at 200 μm isotropic voxel resolution (Adapted from Smith et al. 2011)

is an increase in the hydraulic permeability (Johannessen and Elliott 2005).

The annulus fibrosus undergoes mechanical changes with degeneration. The modulus at the toe region increases with degeneration, probably due to changes in the water content and the increase in collagen I levels (Guerin and Elliott 2006a).The Poisson's ratio decreases about 50 % with degeneration (Acaroglu et al. 1995; Elliott and Setton 2001; Guerin and Elliott 2006a), as does the shear modulus (Iatridis et al. 1999). Additionally, fiber reorientation decreases, while interaction between fibers and extrafibrillar matrix increases with degeneration (Guerin and Elliott 2006a; O'Connell et al. 2009). That fiber–matrix interactions increase with

Box 2.2 Total Disc Replacements

Total disc replacement (TDR) is a relatively new treatment for discogenic pain that may be used instead of fusion in some patients. In a TDR, a mechanical device replaces the disc and aims to permit motion between the vertebrae, as opposed to fusion where there is no motion. Rational for TDR are related to perceived advantages over fusion for reduced surgical time, improved patient recovery, and long-term improved mechanics to prevent degeneration at other sites in the disc. An ideal artificial disc should have the same range of motion and mechanical properties as a healthy disc. However, this is generally not the case. Metallic spheres were the first intervertebral disc replacements and were implanted in patients in the early 1960s. The most common complication was subsidence, or penetration of the ball into the endplate and vertebral body, and this device was abandoned. The Acroflex, from the 1970s, consists of two porous plates separated by a hyperelastic polymer. The design was revolutionary in the sense that the porous plate allowed integration with the bone and the polymer provided controlled flexibility. Unfortunately short-term failure of the polymeric material stopped wide clinical use. The Charite, introduced in the 1980s, has two metallic endplates articulating against a polymeric core similar to a ball-and-socket articulation. Although this device has been very popular in Europe, long-term studies have reported several complications including migration, subsidence, ejection, and wear of the core. Recent designs similar to the Charite include the ProDisc and FlexiCore. These devices all permit motion, but generally do not mimic normal disc mechanics in terms of have axial compression motion, energy absorption, and resistance to torsion. While the FDA has approved some models for use, they are not widely used in patients. Total disc replacement in the cervical spine, which requires more motion and less axial load, appears to be more widely applied and successful. A more detailed review of total disc replacements and other devices can be found in "*Intervertebral disc properties: challenges for biodevices*" by Costi et al. (2011).

degeneration is evident from biaxial tests (O'Connell et al. 2012).

All the degenerative changes observed at the tissue level have an effect on the mechanics at the disc level. Of all of the tissues in the intervertebral disc, the most mechanically affected with degeneration is the nucleus pulposus. The loss of osmotic pressure and hydration in the center of disc leads to a reduction of the disc height and an increase in instability of the disc measured by an increase in the range of motion and neutral zone (Mimura et al. 1994; O'Connell et al. 2007). The decrease of disc height causes an increase in the compression load in the axial direction which in turn results in buckling of the lamellae, increase of outward and inner bulging of the annulus fibrosus, and loss of organization of the lamellae structure (O'Connell et al. 2007, 2010). The decrease in osmotic pressure also causes a reduction in fluid exchange during the diurnal cycle (Massey et al. 2011). The fluid exchange reduction affects the transport of metabolites such as glucose and lactic acid, thereby influencing cellular function.

2.5 Mechanically Induced Injury of the Intervertebral Disc

In a healthy person, the loads applied to the intervertebral disc are not likely to exceed its strength limits. However, in some cases such as trauma, a single high-magnitude load causes a mechanical disruption of the structure of the spine. Usually, in such events, the posterior elements of the spine such as the zygapophysial joints are damaged before the disc is affected. However, under certain conditions, damage to the intervertebral disc in the form of disc prolapse, fracture of the vertebral endplate, or tears in the annulus fibrosus or nucleus pulposus can be observed. Such catastrophic changes can cause a permanent change on the internal distribution of stresses and strains, thereby affecting the normal functioning of disc. In addition, such changes in the mechanical environment trigger a cell mediate cascade of biochemical, structural, and morphological changes known as degenerative disc disease that further impairs disc function. Another case of abnormal loading occurs when a low-magnitude load is applied a great number of times. This repeating loading event, known as fatigue, is believed to be linked to the onset and propagation of tears in the disc and is a cause of herniation. In this section, recent studies analyzing the relationship between abnormal loading and injury of the intervertebral disc are discussed.

2.5.1 Herniation

Herniation is characterized by the prolapse of the nucleus pulposus through the annulus fibrosus. In vitro, herniation can be produced by a single high-intensity load or the repetitive application of forces with lower intensity (Callaghan and McGill 2001; Iencean 2000). Herniation has been induced mechanically by applying a compressive force in the order of 5.4 kN to the disc in an anterolateral flexion position. This results in extrusion of the nucleus pulposus in a posterolateral radial direction (Aultman et al. 2005). The internal strains developed during flexion/extension and lateral bending show tensile strains in the axial direction and thinning of the annulus fibrosus at the opposite direction of bending (Costi et al. 2008; Tsantrizos et al. 2005). Therefore, a radial protrusion in posterolateral direction occurs when there is anterolateral flexion. Non-degenerated, highly hydrated discs have higher risk of herniation than severely degenerated discs (Gallagher 2002; Simunic et al. 2001). This is probably due to the reduction of intradiscal pressure in the nucleus pulposus with degeneration. However, when mechanical disruption is caused by artificially increasing the nucleus pressure (instead of applying a compressive load), degenerated discs fails at a lower rupture pressure (Iencean 2000).

Herniation has also been induced in vitro when cyclic flexion/extension motion is applied to the disc (Callaghan and McGill 2001). In this case, the herniation pathway is in a posterolateral radial direction. Increasing the compression load decreases the number of cycles required to cause disc damage. Similarly, the application of a static torque moment shortens the disc cycle life (Drake et al. 2005). The increase in intradiscal pressure due to the applied torque may accelerate the susceptibility of intervertebral discs to injury. The shape of the disc has also been found to influence the herniation pathway in repetitive flexion/extension bending (Yates et al. 2010). Specifically, limacon-shaped discs had a defined posterolateral herniation pathway, whereas oval-shaped discs had a more diffuse herniation pathway.

2.5.2 Endplate Fracture

Another mechanically driven injury is the fracture of the vertebral endplate. The endplate is the cortical bone on the superior and inferior (cranial and caudal sides, respectively) aspects of the vertebral body. On one side, the vertebral endplate is in contact with the intervertebral disc through the cartilaginous endplate; on the other side, it is supported by the trabecular bone inside the vertebral body. The main component of the load applied to the vertebral endplate comes from the intradiscal pressure. However, tension and shear forces are also applied by traction of the annulus fibrosus (Baranto et al. 2005). Fracture of the vertebral endplate occurs when the strains exceed the strength of the vertebral endplate (Fields et al. 2010). Endplate strength has been correlated with the density of the supporting trabecular bone (Adams and Dolan 2011; Ordway et al. 2007; Zhao et al. 2009). In fact, due to lower density of the cranial trabecular bone, there is a greater incidence of fractures in this endplate. The degree of degeneration of the intervertebral disc also affects the loads at which endplate fracture occurs: a higher force is required to cause endplate fracture in degenerated discs (Baranto et al. 2005). The rationale behind this observation is that healthy, hydrated discs have a higher intradiscal pressure; in degenerated discs there is a lower compression stress in the center of the disc, while the posterior elements transmit a larger portion of the compressive load (Adams and Dolan 2011).

2.6 Summary of Critical Concepts Discussed in the Chapter

- The mechanics of the intervertebral disc is determined by the interaction between the annulus fibrosus, nucleus pulposus, and endplates in different loading scenarios.
- The osmotic pressure plays an important role in the transmission of forces through the spine as well as in the stability of the intervertebral disc structure.
- Nonlinearity is an important mechanical characteristic of disc tissues. Nonlinearity is evident in the spine's relatively lax neutral zone mechanics and stiffer linear region response in motion segment tests. Nonlinearity is important to permit both disc motion and stability.
- Anisotropy (see Box 2.1) is an important mechanical characteristic of the annulus fibrosus and comes from the structural organization of collagen fibers.
- The viscoelastic behavior of the disc can be explained in part by the interstitial fluid flow during loading and unloading and the intrinsic viscoelasticity of disc tissues.
- Degeneration affects the mechanics of disc tissues, which is then reflected on the mechanics of the entire disc. One major effect of degeneration is an increase of the range of motion.
- Several modes of injury, such as herniation and endplate fracture, are closely related to the pressure in the nucleus pulposus and are more frequent in healthy discs.

Acknowledgments This chapter is funded by research grants from the National Institutes of Health R01 AR 050052, R21 AR061751, and R01 EB 002425.

References

Acaroglu ER, Iatridis JC, Setton LA, Foster RJ, Mow VC, Weidenbaum M (1995) Degeneration and aging affect the tensile behavior of human lumbar anulus fibrosus. Spine (Phila Pa 1976) 20(24):2690–2701

Adams MA, Dolan P (1991) A technique for quantifying the bending moment acting on the lumbar spine in vivo. J Biomech 24(2):117–126

Adams MA, Dolan P (2011) Biomechanics of vertebral compression fractures and clinical application. Arch Orthop Trauma Surg 131(12):1703–1710

Adams MA, Hutton WC (1980) The effect of posture on the role of the apophysial joints in resisting intervertebral compressive forces. J Bone Joint Surg Br 62(3):358–362

Adams MA, Hutton WC (1981) The relevance of torsion to the mechanical derangement of the lumbar spine. Spine (Phila Pa 1976) 6(3):241–248

Adams P, Muir H (1976) Qualitative changes with age of proteoglycans of human lumbar discs. Ann Rheum Dis 35(4):289–296

Adams MA, Roughley PJ (2006) What is intervertebral disc degeneration, and what causes it? Spine (Phila Pa 1976) 31(18):2151–2161

Adams MA, Bogduk N, Burton K, Dolan P (2006) The biomechanics of back pain, 2nd edn. Churchill Livingstone Elsevier, London, pp 29–48

Ateshian GA, Ellis BJ, Weiss JA (2007) Equivalence between short-time biphasic and incompressible elastic material responses. J Biomech Eng 129(3):405–412

Ateshian GA, Rajan V, Chahine NO, Canal CE, Hung CT (2009) Modeling the matrix of articular cartilage using a continuous fiber angular distribution predicts many observed phenomena. J Biomech Eng 131(6):061003

Aultman CD, Scannell J, McGill SM (2005) The direction of progressive herniation in porcine spine motion segments is influenced by the orientation of the bending axis. Clin Biomech (Bristol, Avon) 20(2):126–129

Azeloglu EU, Albro MB, Thimmappa VA, Ateshian GA, Costa KD (2008) Heterogeneous transmural proteoglycan distribution provides a mechanism for regulating residual stresses in the aorta. Am J Physiol Heart Circ Physiol 294(3):H1197–H1205

Baranto A, Ekstrom L, Hellstrom M, Lundin O, Holm S, Sward L (2005) Fracture patterns of the adolescent porcine spine: an experimental loading study in bending-compression. Spine (Phila Pa 1976) 30(1):75–82

Bass EC, Ashford FA, Segal MR, Lotz JC (2004) Biaxial testing of human annulus fibrosus and its implications for a constitutive formulation. Ann Biomed Eng 32(9):1231–1242

Battié MC, Videman T, Levälahti E, Gill K, Kaprio J (2008) Genetic and environmental effects on disc degeneration by phenotype and spinal level: a multivariate twin study. Spine (Phila Pa 1976) 33(25):2801–8. doi: 10.1097/BRS.0b013e31818043b7

Buckwalter JA (1995) Aging and degeneration of the human intervertebral disc. Spine (Phila Pa 1976) 20(11):1307–1314

Callaghan JP, McGill SM (2001) Intervertebral disc herniation: studies on a porcine model exposed to highly repetitive flexion/extension motion with compressive force. Clin Biomech (Bristol, Avon) 16(1):28–37

Canal Guterl C, Hung CT, Ateshian GA (2010) Electrostatic and non-electrostatic contributions of proteoglycans to the compressive equilibrium modulus of bovine articular cartilage. J Biomech 43(7):1343–1350

Cassidy JJ, Hiltner A, Baer E (1989) Hierarchical structure of the intervertebral disc. Connect Tissue Res 23(1):75–88

Cavalcante FS, Ito S, Brewer K, Sakai H, Alencar AM, Almeida MP et al (2005) Mechanical interactions between collagen and proteoglycans: implications for the stability of lung tissue. J Appl Physiol 98(2):672–679

Chuang SY, Popovich JM Jr, Lin LC, Hedman TP (2010) The effects of exogenous crosslinking on hydration and fluid flow in the intervertebral disc subjected to compressive creep loading and unloading. Spine (Phila Pa 1976) 35(24):E1362–E1366

Chuong CJ, Fung YC (1986) On residual stresses in arteries. J Biomech Eng 108(2):189–192

Comper WD, Laurent TC (1978) Physiological function of connective tissue polysaccharides. Physiol Rev 58(1):255–315

Cortes DH, Elliott DM (2012) Extra-fibrillar matrix mechanics of annulus fibrosus in tension and compression. Biomech Model Mechanobiol 11(6):781–790

Costi JJ, Stokes IA, Gardner-Morse M, Laible JP, Scoffone HM, Iatridis JC (2007) Direct measurement of intervertebral disc maximum shear strain in six degrees of freedom: motions that place disc tissue at risk of injury. J Biomech 40(11):2457–66

Costi JJ, Stokes IA, Gardner-Morse M, Laible JP, Scoffone HM, Iatridis JC (2008) Direct measurement of intervertebral disc maximum shear strain in six degrees of freedom: motions that place disc tissue at risk of injury. J Biomech 40(11):2457–66

Costi JJ et al (2011) Intervertebral disc properties: challenges for biodevices. Expert Rev Med Devices 8(3):357–376

Das DB, Welling A, Urban JP, Boubriak OA (2009) Solute transport in intervertebral disc: experiments and finite element modeling. Ann N Y Acad Sci 1161:44–61

Diamant J, Keller A, Baer E, Litt M, Arridge RG (1972) Collagen; ultrastructure and its relation to mechanical properties as a function of ageing. Proc R Soc Lond B Biol Sci 180(60):293–315

Drake JD, Aultman CD, McGill SM, Callaghan JP (2005) The influence of static axial torque in combined loading on intervertebral joint failure mechanics using a porcine model. Clin Biomech (Bristol, Avon) 20(10):1038–1045

Drost MR, Willems P, Snijders H, Huyghe JM, Janssen JD, Huson A (1995) Confined compression of canine annulus fibrosus under chemical and mechanical loading. J Biomech Eng 117(4):390–396

Elliott DM, Setton LA (2001) Anisotropic and inhomogeneous tensile behavior of the human anulus fibrosus: experimental measurement and material model predictions. J Biomech Eng 123(3):256–263

Eyre DR (1979) Biochemistry of the intervertebral disc. Int Rev Connect Tissue Res 8:227–291

Eyre DR, Muir H (1976) Types I and II collagens in intervertebral disc. Interchanging radial distributions in annulus fibrosus. Biochem J 157(1):267–270

Ferguson SJ, Ito K, Nolte LP (2004) Fluid flow and convective transport of solutes within the intervertebral disc. J Biomech 37(2):213–221

Fields AJ, Lee GL, Keaveny TM (2010) Mechanisms of initial endplate failure in the human vertebral body. J Biomech 43(16): 3126–3131

Fujita Y, Wagner DR, Biviji AA, Duncan NA, Lotz JC (2000) Anisotropic shear behavior of the annulus fibrosus: effect of harvest site and tissue prestrain. Med Eng Phys 22(5):349–357

Gallagher S (2002) Letters. Spine (Phila Pa 1976) 27(12):1378

Gregory DE, Callaghan JP (2011) A comparison of uniaxial and biaxial mechanical properties of the annulus fibrosus: a porcine model. J Biomech Eng 133(2):024503

Gu WY, Mao XG, Foster RJ, Weidenbaum M, Mow VC, Rawlins BA (1999) The anisotropic hydraulic permeability of human lumbar anulus fibrosus. Influence of age, degeneration, direction, and water content. Spine (Phila Pa 1976) 24(23):2449–2455

Guerin HA, Elliott DM (2006a) Degeneration affects the fiber reorientation of human annulus fibrosus under tensile load. J Biomech 39(8):1410–1418

Guerin HA, Elliott DM (2006b) Structure and properties of soft tissues in the spine. In: Kurtz SM, Edidin AA (eds) SPINE: technology handbook. Elsevier Academic Press, Amsterdam/Boston

Guerin HL, Elliott DM (2007) Quantifying the contributions of structure to annulus fibrosus mechanical function using a nonlinear, anisotropic, hyperelastic model. J Orthop Res 25(4): 508–516

Guo Z, Shi X, Peng X, Caner F (2012) Fibre-matrix interaction in the human annulus fibrosus. J Mech Behav Biomed Mater 5(1): 193–205

Hardingham TE, Muir H, Kwan MK, Lai WM, Mow VC (1987) Viscoelastic properties of proteoglycan solutions with varying proportions present as aggregates. J Orthop Res 5(1):36–46

Heneghan P, Riches PE (2008a) The strain-dependent osmotic pressure and stiffness of the bovine nucleus pulposus apportioned into ionic and non-ionic contributors. J Biomech 41(11):2411–2416

Heneghan P, Riches PE (2008b) Determination of the strain-dependent hydraulic permeability of the compressed bovine nucleus pulposus. J Biomech 41(4):903–906

Heuer F, Schmidt H, Wilke HJ (2008) The relation between intervertebral disc bulging and annular fiber associated strains for simple and complex loading. J Biomech 41(5):1086–1094

Hickey DS, Hukins DW (1980) Relation between the structure of the annulus fibrosus and the function and failure of the intervertebral disc. Spine (Phila Pa 1976) 5(2):106–116

Hollingsworth NT, Wagner DR (2011) Modeling shear behavior of the annulus fibrosus. J Mech Behav Biomed Mater 4(7): 1103–1114

Holm S, Maroudas A, Urban JP, Selstam G, Nachemson A (1981) Nutrition of the intervertebral disc: solute transport and metabolism. Connect Tissue Res 8(2):101–119

Hsu K, Zucherman J, Shea W, Kaiser J, White A, Schofferman J et al (1990) High lumbar disc degeneration. Incidence and etiology. Spine (Phila Pa 1976) 15(7):679–682

Huyghe JM (2010) Biaxial testing of canine annulus fibrosus tissue under changing salt concentrations. An Acad Bras Cienc 82(1):145–151

Iatridis JC, Weidenbaum M, Setton LA, Mow VC (1996) Is the nucleus pulposus a solid or a fluid? Mechanical behaviors of the nucleus pulposus of the human intervertebral disc. Spine (Phila Pa 1976) 21(10):1174–1184

Iatridis JC, Setton LA, Weidenbaum M, Mow VC (1997a) The viscoelastic behavior of the non-degenerate human lumbar nucleus pulposus in shear. J Biomech 30(10):1005–1013

Iatridis JC, Setton LA, Weidenbaum M, Mow VC (1997b) Alterations in the mechanical behavior of the human lumbar nucleus pulposus with degeneration and aging. J Orthop Res 15(2):318–322

Iatridis JC, Kumar S, Foster RJ, Weidenbaum M, Mow VC (1999) Shear mechanical properties of human lumbar annulus fibrosus. J Orthop Res 17(5):732–737

Iencean SM (2000) Lumbar intervertebral disc herniation following experimental intradiscal pressure increase. Acta Neurochir (Wien) 142(6):669–676

Jackson AR, Yuan TY, Huang CY, Travascio F, Yong Gu W (2008) Effect of compression and anisotropy on the diffusion of glucose in annulus fibrosus. Spine (Phila Pa 1976) 33(1):1–7

Jackson AR, Huang CY, Gu WY (2011) Effect of endplate calcification and mechanical deformation on the distribution of glucose in intervertebral disc: a 3D finite element study. Comput Methods Biomech Biomed Engin 14(2):195–204

Jacobs NT, Smith LJ, Han WM, Morelli J, Yoder JH, Elliott DM (2011) Effect of orientation and targeted extracellular matrix degradation on the shear mechanical properties of the annulus fibrosus. J Mech Behav Biomed Mater 4(8):1611–1619

Jacobs NT, Cortes DH, Vresilovic EJ, Elliott DM (2013) Biaxial tension of fibrous tissue: using finite element methods to address experimental challenges arising from boundary conditions and anisotropy. J Biomech Eng 135(2):021004. doi:10.1115/1.4023503

Johannessen W, Elliott DM (2005) Effects of degeneration on the biphasic material properties of human nucleus pulposus in confined compression. Spine (Phila Pa 1976) 30(24):E724–E729

Kastelic J, Baer E (1980) Deformation in tendon collagen. Symp Soc Exp Biol 34:397–435

Kastelic J, Galeski A, Baer E (1978) The multicomposite structure of tendon. Connect Tissue Res 6(1):11–23

Kiani C, Chen L, Wu YJ, Yee AJ, Yang BB (2002) Structure and function of aggrecan. Cell Res 12(1):19–32

Klisch SM, Lotz JC (2000) A special theory of biphasic mixtures and experimental results for human annulus fibrosus tested in confined compression. J Biomech Eng 122(2):180–188

Lanir Y (2009) Mechanisms of residual stress in soft tissues. J Biomech Eng 131(4):044506

Maroudas A, Bannon C (1981) Measurement of swelling pressure in cartilage and comparison with the osmotic pressure of constituent proteoglycans. Biorheology 18(3–6):619–632

Massey CJ, van Donkelaar CC, Vresilovic E, Zavaliangos A, Marcolongo M (2011) Effects of aging and degeneration on the human intervertebral disc during the diurnal cycle: a finite element study. J Orthop Res 30(1):122–128

Mauck RL, Baker BM, Nerurkar NL, Burdick JA, Li WJ, Tuan RS et al (2009) Engineering on the straight and narrow: the mechanics of nanofibrous assemblies for fiber-reinforced tissue regeneration. Tissue Eng Part B Rev 15(2):171–193

Melrose J, Ghosh P, Taylor TK (2001) A comparative analysis of the differential spatial and temporal distributions of the large (aggrecan, versican) and small (decorin, biglycan, fibromodulin) proteoglycans of the intervertebral disc. J Anat 198(Pt 1):3–15

Moon SM, Yoder JH, Wright AC, Smith LJ, Vresilovic EJ, Elliott DM (2013) Evaluation of intervertebral disc cartilaginous endplate structure using magnetic resonance imaging. Eur Spine J doi:10.1007/s00586-013-2798-1

Michalek AJ, Gardner-Mose MG, Iatridis JC (2012). Large residual strains are present in the intervertebral disc annulus fibrosus in the unloaded state. J Biomech 45(7):1227–1231

Mimura M, Panjabi MM, Oxland TR, Crisco JJ, Yamamoto I, Vasavada A (1994) Disc degeneration affects the multidirectional flexibility of the lumbar spine. Spine (Phila Pa 1976) 19(12):1371–1380

Nachemson A (1963) The influence of spinal movements on the lumbar intradiscal pressure and on the tensil stresses in the annulus fibrosus. Acta Orthop Scand 33:183–207

Nachemson AL (1981) Disc pressure measurements. Spine (Phila Pa 1976) 6(1):93–97

Nerurkar NL, Elliott DM, Mauck RL (2010) Mechanical design criteria for intervertebral disc tissue engineering. J Biomech 43(6):1017–1030

O'Connell GD, Johannessen W, Vresilovic EJ, Elliott DM (2007) Human internal disc strains in axial compression measured noninvasively using magnetic resonance imaging. Spine (Phila Pa 1976) 32(25):2860–2868

O'Connell GD, Guerin HL, Elliott DM (2009) Theoretical and uniaxial experimental evaluation of human annulus fibrosus degeneration. J Biomech Eng 131(11)

O'Connell GD, Vresilovic EJ, Elliott DM (2010) Human intervertebral disc internal strain in compression: the effect of disc region, loading position, and degeneration. J Orthop Res 29(4):547–555

O'Connell GD, Jacobs NT, Sen S, Vresilovic EJ, Elliott DM (2011) Axial creep loading and unloaded recovery of the human intervertebral disc and the effect of degeneration. J Mech Behav Biomed Mater 4(7):933–942

O'Connell GD, Sen S, Elliott DM (2012) Human annulus fibrosus material properties from biaxial testing and constitutive modeling are altered with degeneration. Biomech Model Mechanobiol 11(3–4):493–503

Ordway NR, Lu YM, Zhang X, Cheng CC, Fang H, Fayyazi AH (2007) Correlation of cervical endplate strength with CT measured subchondral bone density. Eur Spine J 16(12):2104–2109

Overbeek JT (1956) The Donnan equilibrium. Prog Biophys Biophys Chem 6:57–84

Panjabi M, Brown M, Lindahl S, Irstam L, Hermens M (1988) Intrinsic disc pressure as a measure of integrity of the lumbar spine. Spine (Phila Pa 1976) 13(8):913–917

Pearcy M, Portek I, Shepherd J (1984) Three-dimensional x-ray analysis of normal movement in the lumbar spine. Spine (Phila Pa 1976) 9(3):294–297

Perie D, Korda D, Iatridis JC (2005) Confined compression experiments on bovine nucleus pulposus and annulus fibrosus: sensitivity of the experiment in the determination of compressive modulus and hydraulic permeability. J Biomech 38(11):2164–2171

Perie D, Iatridis JC, Demers CN, Goswami T, Beaudoin G, Mwale F et al (2006a) Assessment of compressive modulus, hydraulic permeability and matrix content of trypsin-treated nucleus pulposus using quantitative MRI. J Biomech 39(8):1392–1400

Perie DS, Maclean JJ, Owen JP, Iatridis JC (2006b) Correlating material properties with tissue composition in enzymatically digested bovine annulus fibrosus and nucleus pulposus tissue. Ann Biomed Eng 34(5):769–777

Potvin JR, McGill SM, Norman RW (1991) Trunk muscle and lumbar ligament contributions to dynamic lifts with varying degrees of trunk flexion. Spine (Phila Pa 1976) 16(9):1099–1107

Pye SR, Reid DM, Lunt M, Adams JE, Silman AJ, O'Neill TW (2007) Lumbar disc degeneration: association between osteophytes, end-plate sclerosis and disc space narrowing. Ann Rheum Dis 66(3):330–333

Rannou F, Lee TS, Zhou RH, Chin J, Lotz JC, Mayoux-Benhamou MA et al (2004) Intervertebral disc degeneration: the role of the mitochondrial pathway in annulus fibrosus cell apoptosis induced by overload. Am J Pathol 164(3):915–924

Sasaki M, Takahashi T, Miyahara K, Hirosea T (2001) Effects of chondroitinase ABC on intradiscal pressure in sheep: an in vivo study. Spine (Phila Pa 1976) 26(5):463–468

Sato K, Kikuchi S, Yonezawa T (1999) In vivo intradiscal pressure measurement in healthy individuals and in patients with ongoing back problems. Spine (Phila Pa 1976) 24(23):2468–2474

Setton LA, Zhu W, Weidenbaum M, Ratcliffe A, Mow VC (1993) Compressive properties of the cartilaginous end-plate of the baboon lumbar spine. J Orthop Res 11(2):228–239

Shirazi-Adl A, Ahmed AM, Shrivastava SC (1986) Mechanical response of a lumbar motion segment in axial torque alone and combined with compression. Spine (Phila Pa 1976) 11(9):914–927

Shirazi-Adl A, Taheri M, Urban JP (2010) Analysis of cell viability in intervertebral disc: effect of endplate permeability on cell population. J Biomech 43(7):1330–1336

Simunic DI, Broom ND, Robertson PA (2001) Biomechanical factors influencing nuclear disruption of the intervertebral disc. Spine 26(11):1223–1230

Smith LJ, Nerurkar NL, Choi KS, Harfe BD, Elliott DM (2011) Degeneration and regeneration of the intervertebral disc: lessons from development. Dis Model Mech 4(1):31–41

Soukane DM, Shirazi-Adl A, Urban JP (2007) Computation of coupled diffusion of oxygen, glucose and lactic acid in an intervertebral disc. J Biomech 40(12):2645–2654

Spencer AJM (1984) Continuum theory of the mechanics of fibre-reinforced composites. Springer, Wien/New York

Spenciner D, Greene D, Paiva J, Palumbo M, Crisco J (2006) The multidirectional bending properties of the human lumbar intervertebral disc. Spine J 6(3):248–257

Travascio F, Gu WY (2011) Simultaneous measurement of anisotropic solute diffusivity and binding reaction rates in biological tissues by FRAP. Ann Biomed Eng 39(1):53–65

Tsantrizos A, Ito K, Aebi M, Steffen T (2005) Internal strains in healthy and degenerated lumbar intervertebral discs. Spine 30(19):2129–2137

Urban JP, Maroudas A (1981) Swelling of the intervertebral disc in vitro. Connect Tissue Res 9(1):1–10

Urban JP, Holm S, Maroudas A (1978) Diffusion of small solutes into the intervertebral disc: as in vivo study. Biorheology 15(3–4):203–221

Urban JP, Maroudas A, Bayliss MT, Dillon J (1979) Swelling pressures of proteoglycans at the concentrations found in cartilaginous tissues. Biorheology 16(6):447–464

Urban JP, Holm S, Maroudas A, Nachemson A (1982) Nutrition of the intervertebral disc: effect of fluid flow on solute transport. Clin Orthop Relat Res 170:296–302

Urban JP, Smith S, Fairbank JC (2004) Nutrition of the intervertebral disc. Spine (Phila Pa 1976) 29(23):2700–2709

van der Veen AJ, van Dieen JH, Nadort A, Stam B, Smit TH (2007) Intervertebral disc recovery after dynamic or static loading in vitro: is there a role for the endplate? J Biomech 40(10): 2230–2235

van Deursen DL, Snijders CJ, Kingma I, van Dieen JH (2001a) In vitro torsion-induced stress distribution changes in porcine intervertebral discs. Spine (Phila Pa 1976) 26(23):2582–2586

van Deursen DL, Snijders CJ, van Dieen JH, Kingma I, van Deursen LL (2001b) The effect of passive vertebral rotation on pressure in the nucleus pulposus. J Biomech 34(3):405–408

Wade KR, Robertson PA, Broom ND (2011) A fresh look at the nucleus-endplate region: new evidence for significant structural integration. Eur Spine J 20(8):1225–1232

Wagner DR, Lotz JC (2004) Theoretical model and experimental results for the nonlinear elastic behavior of human annulus fibrosus. J Orthop Res 22(4):901–909

Wang C, Witschey W, Elliott MA, Borthakur A, Reddy R (2010) Measurement of intervertebral disc pressure with T 1rho MRI. Magn Reson Med 64(6):1721–1727

Wilke HJ, Wolf S, Claes LE, Arand M, Wiesend A (1996) Influence of varying muscle forces on lumbar intradiscal pressure: an in vitro study. J Biomech 29(4):549–555

Wilke HJ, Neef P, Caimi M, Hoogland T, Claes LE (1999) New in vivo measurements of pressures in the intervertebral disc in daily life. Spine (Phila Pa 1976) 24(8):755–762

Wu HC, Yao RF (1976) Mechanical behavior of the human annulus fibrosus. J Biomech 9(1):1–7

Yates JP, Giangregorio L, McGill SM (2010) The influence of intervertebral disc shape on the pathway of posterior/posterolateral partial herniation. Spine (Phila Pa 1976) 35(7):734–739

Zhao FD, Pollintine P, Hole BD, Adams MA, Dolan P (2009) Vertebral fractures usually affect the cranial endplate because it is thinner and supported by less-dense trabecular bone. Bone 44(2): 372–379

Zhu W, Mow VC, Koob TJ, Eyre DR (1993) Viscoelastic shear properties of articular cartilage and the effects of glycosidase treatments. J Orthop Res 11(6):771–781

Zhu W, Chern KY, Mow VC (1994) Anisotropic viscoelastic shear properties of bovine meniscus. Clin Orthop Relat Res 306:34–45

Development of the Intervertebral Disc

3

Megan K. Cox and Rosa Serra

Contents

M.K. Cox • R. Serra (✉)
Department of Cell, Developmental, and Integrative Biology, University of Alabama at Birmingham,
1918 University Blvd. 660 MCLM, Birmingham, AL 35294, USA
e-mail: mkcox@uab.edu, rserra@uab.edu

3.1 Overview

Intervertebral discs are derived from embryonic structures called the sclerotome and notochord (Paavola et al. 1980; Theiler 1988; Rufai et al. 1995). The nucleus pulposus, the cushioning core of the mature intervertebral disc, is derived from the notochord, while the annulus fibrosus, which provides the structural properties of the disc, is derived from sclerotome (Christ et al. 2004, 2007; Christ and Scaal 2008). The sclerotome is derived from the somites, transient structures that determine the segmented nature of the embryo. In response to signals from the notochord and floor plate of the neural tube, the maturing somites undergo dorsal-ventral compartmentalization establishing the dermomyotome and sclerotome, the latter forming most of the connective tissues of the future axial skeleton. The development of the sclerotome is characterized by proliferation and expansion of cells as well as the formation of three subcompartments: ventral, lateral, and dorsal. The ventral sclerotome gives rise to the vertebral bodies and annulus fibrosus and is made up of Pax-1-expressing cells that have invaded the perinotochordal space (Monsoro-Burq et al. 1994; Peters et al. 1999).

In addition to dorsal-ventral compartmentalization, each sclerotome segment demonstrates rostral to caudal polarity (Christ et al. 2007; Christ and Scaal 2008). This polarity is morphologically apparent in the ventral sclerotome as a condensed caudal portion and loose rostral portion within each segment. Due to resegmentation of sclerotome during development, the caudal domain of the sclerotome will form the anterior structures of each vertebra and the rostral domain forms the posterior structures (Huang et al. 2000). The annulus fibrosus will form from the cells in the sclerotome adjacent to the border, sometimes called von Ebner's fissure, between the sclerotome halves. These cells can be traced back to somitocoele cells at the center of the somite before the formation of the sclerotome. This subcompartment of the sclerotome has been termed the arthrotome (Mittapalli et al. 2005).

I.M. Shapiro, M.V. Risbud (eds.), *The Intervertebral Disc*,
DOI 10.1007/978-3-7091-1535-0_3, © Springer-Verlag Wien 2014

Endochondral bonc formation follows the expansion, migration, and patterning of the sclerotome to form the vertebral body. As the vertebral bodies undergo chondrogenesis, notochord cells are removed from the vertebral region and expand into the intervertebral disc region to form the nucleus pulposus. The annulus fibrosus develops into a fibrocartilage structure and does not normally undergo endochondral ossification. The annulus fibrosus can be further divided into an inner portion and a more fibrous outer portion. TGF-ß3 is one of the earliest markers of the developing intervertebral disc within the sclerotome (Pelton et al. 1990). Later, it is preferentially expressed in the outer annulus. In the adult, the annulus fibrosus is bound by the spinal ligaments, which insert into the bone to form the entheses. It is likely that the ligament is also derived from the sclerotome although this has not been addressed directly. Tendons in the axial skeleton are derived from a subcompartment of the sclerotome call the syndetome (Brent et al. 2003; Schweitzer et al. 2001). The adult disc is juxtaposed to the cartilage end plate of the adjacent vertebra, which consists of hyaline cartilage similar to that found in the peripheral joints. The fibrocartilage of the adult annulus fibrosus, the cartilage-like matrix of the nucleus pulposus, and the hyaline cartilage of the vertebrae have distinct and overlapping properties. All contain collagen II and aggrecan. The annulus fibrosus also contains collagen I with higher levels in the outer annulus. Versican and fibromodulin (Fmod) are preferentially expressed in the annulus fibrosus relative to cartilage (Smits and Lefebvre 2003; Shi et al. 2003; Sohn et al. 2010). Versican is also present in ligaments and entheses (Shi et al. 2003) (see Chap. 4). Keratin 8, Keratin 18, Keratin 19, and NCAM1 have recently been identified as markers to distinguish the nucleus pulposus from the annulus fibrosus and hyaline cartilage (Sakai et al. 2009; Lee et al. 2007; Minogue et al. 2010). Brachyury/T is also considered a marker for the notochord as well as the nucleus pulposus (Kispert et al. 1994).

Insight into the mechanisms of pathology in the spine can be provided through an understanding of the development of the axial skeleton. Since the intervertebral disc is derived from the notochord, somites, and sclerotome, alterations in the development of any of these tissues can result in human developmental disorders that affect the intervertebral disc. Alterations in the segmentation of the somites can lead to congenital defects in the formation of the vertebrae and the disc resulting in fusion of vertebrae (Turnpenny 2008; Shifley and Cole 2007). Genetic variations involved in increased susceptibility to intervertebral disc degeneration can be associated with subtle developmental abnormalities (Jin et al. 2011; Dahia et al. 2009). In addition to providing insight into the etiology of disorders of the spine, an understanding of developmental biology can provide a basis for treatment, repair, or regeneration strategies. Information about how the axial skeleton develops in the first place would also be the basis for tissue engineering protocols (Lenas et al. 2009a, 2011; Gadjanski et al. 2012). Recently, the concept of "developmental engineering" has been used to generate chondrocytes from embryonic stem cells (Oldershaw et al. 2010). This concept could also be used in the future to engineer the intervertebral disc (Box 3.1). This chapter will cover the molecular mechanisms governing the major steps of intervertebral disc development with an emphasis on processes important for understanding human disease and potential for tissue engineering.

Box 3.1: Developmental Engineering and the Intervertebral Disc

Developmental biology can provide insights into novel strategies for repair, regeneration, or engineering of tissues. The effort to develop in vitro processes that mimic normal development was recently termed "developmental engineering" (Lenas et al. 2011, 2009a, b; Gadjanski et al. 2012). The term is used to emphasize the concept that it is not the tissue, but rather the process of development that needs to be engineered. Noteworthy, conventional tissue engineering has been an empirical discipline, the goal of which is to generate functional tissues using scaffold, cells, and signaling molecules. By incorporating information on development, a rational methodology can be developed to generate tissues in vitro.

Developmental engineering aims to build on the most significant aspects of embryonic development: the highly regulated spatiotemporal organization of cells into complex tissues. This approach would thus allow the separate sequential steps that correspond to varying stages of development to generate tissue intermediates that can act as modular functional units of the engineered tissue (Lenas et al. 2011, 2009a). This gradual and stepwise process is inherently stable and can be controlled for quality at each step. The early stages of development would be given the highest scrutiny since subsequent development could progress naturally and in many cases would be semiautonomous. In addition, care would need to be taken not to interfere with normal cell-cell interactions or morphogen gradients since this would disrupt the architecture of the final product. Functional modules can then be used to generate more complex organs (Lenas et al. 2011).

Early forms of developmental engineering have been used to direct human embryonic stem cells to chondrocytes and to recapitulate endochondral bone formation using mesenchymal stem cells (Oldershaw et al. 2010; Scotti et al. 2010). In both cases, the stepwise approach mimicking normal development was used. Although the intervertebral disc is more complex than cartilage or bone, the use of a stepwise processes based on information about embryonic development would facilitate the disc tissue engineering process. Special consideration would have to be given to gradients within the tissue and integration of the annulus fibrosus and the nucleus pulposus with each other and with the surrounding end plate and ligaments. The pathways controlling these aspects of intervertebral disc development are starting to be elucidated.

3.2 Development of the Notochord and the Formation of the Nucleus Pulposus

The notochord is a transient rodlike mesodermal structure that is located under the neural tube and spans most of the length of the embryo (Stemple 2005). It serves as a primitive support structure for the embryo and as a signaling center, directing development of surrounding structures including the sclerotome. In mice and humans, the notochord will eventually develop into the nucleus pulposus of the intervertebral disc (Fig. 3.1). The notochord forms during embryonic gastrulation. Cells that migrate through the primitive streak will form the endoderm and mesoderm. Some of the migrating cells will form the notochordal process, which integrates transiently with the endoderm to form the notochordal plate. The notochordal plate buds off of the endoderm to finally form the notochord, which lies between the roof of the primitive gut and the floor of the developing neural tube (Moore and Oersaud 2003).

3.2.1 Development and Maintenance of the Notochord

Mutations in 19 genes resulting in absence of the notochord have been catalogued by the Mouse Genome Informatics (MGI) database (www.informatics.jax.org). The most well characterized is the *T* gene, encoding the brachyury protein (Kispert et al. 1994). Brachyury is the prototype T-box transcription factor. It is also considered a marker of primitive mesoderm and notochord. It starts out being expressed in all mesodermal cells. Later, it becomes restricted to the notochord where expression is maintained. Mice with homozygous mutations in T have defects in the formation of mesoderm, and the trunk notochord is not established (Dobrovolskaia-Zavadskaia 1927). Subsequent malformations in the spine and allantois lead to the early demise of the embryo. Mice with a dominant-negative mutation in T (*Tc*) survive but demonstrate abnormal nucleus pulposus morphology (Stott et al. 1993). Brachyury is also a marker for chordomas, rare malignant tumors along the spine thought to arise from persistent remnants of the notochord (Vujovic et al. 2006). Duplications in the *T* gene in humans have been associated with susceptibility to

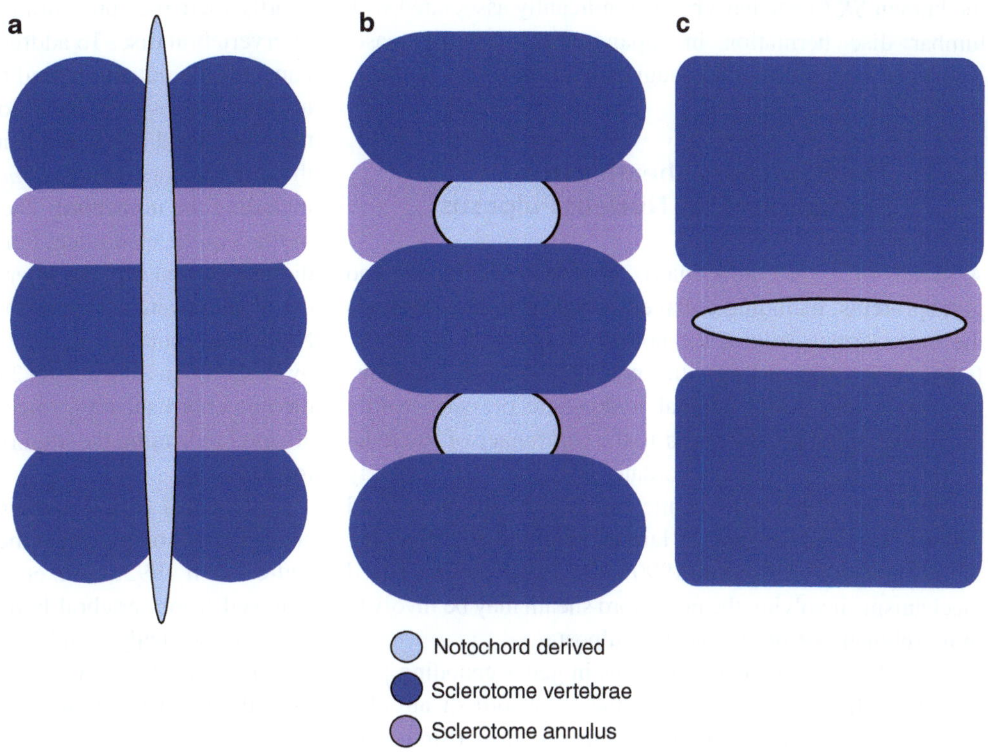

Fig. 3.1 Development of the notochord and nucleus pulposus. (**a**) The nucleus is derived from the notochord, a rod-shaped embryonic structure that lies under the neural tube. Sclerotome condenses around the notochord to form the vertebrae and annulus fibrosus of the intervertebral disc. Brachyury/T, Sd, Shh, and Sox5/6/9 are required for the formation of notochord and notochord sheath. (**b**) Once the vertebrae and disc start to form, the notochord contracts from the vertebral body and expands into the area of the future disc. The notochord sheath and collagen II, which helps to maintain osmotic pressure in the vertebral cartilage, are required for the expansion of the notochord and formation of the nucleus pulposus. (**c**) Growth and maintenance of the nucleus pulposus is in part controlled by the *Skt* gene

chordoma (Yang et al. 2009). For a complete discussion of chordomas, see Chap. 18.

While mice with mutations in *T* fail to establish the notochord, Danforth's short-tail (*Sd*) mutation results in failure to maintain the notochord (Paavola et al. 1980). Sd mice arose from a spontaneous mutation in a yet unknown gene. Sd mice have abnormal nucleus pulposus morphology likely due to defects in the formation and maintenance of the notochord early in development. In Sd mice the notochord is discontinuous and becomes increasingly fragmented, eventually disappearing in mice homozygous for the mutant allele. In heterozygous mice, the intervertebral disc forms but the nucleus pulposus is absent and the disc is occupied with fibrous tissue similar to the annulus fibrosus (Semba et al. 2006).

Mutations in the Sickle tail gene (*Skt*), on the same chromosome as *Sd*, have nucleus pulposi; however, the nuclei are shifted to the periphery of the disc (Semba et al. 2006). The boundary between the nucleus pulposus and the annulus fibrosus is altered, and the annulus exhibits thin fibrous layers relative to control mice. The sequence of the *Skt* gene was identified using the gene-trapped ES clone from which it was derived. The protein product is predicted to have a proline-rich region in the N-terminus and a coiled-coil domain in the middle. The coiled-coil domain was similar to those found in a large number of scaffold proteins including keratins. It was suggested that while *Sd* is required at early stages of notochord development, *Skt* is required later in development for proper growth, differentiation, and maintenance of the nucleus pulposus. Furthermore, specific polymorphisms in the human *SKT* gene have been significantly associated with lumbar disc herniation in Japanese and Finnish case-controlled populations (Karasugi et al. 2009).

3.2.2 The Notochord Sheath and Formation of the Nucleus Pulposus

A sheath of extracellular matrix containing collagens and glycoproteins, including collagen II and laminin, surrounds the mesodermal cells of the notochord (Gotz et al. 1995). It has been proposed that the notochord sheath functions to contain and direct internal hydrostatic pressure within the notochord. The notochord is the forerunner of the axial skeleton in non-vertebrate chordates (Box 3.2). During early Xenopus development, osmotic inflation of the notochord against the sheath results in lengthening and straightening of the embryo (Adams et al. 1990). Similar mechanics-based mechanisms involving the notochord sheath may be involved in morphogenesis of the nucleus pulposus.

It has been shown that mutations in genes encoding proteins that affect the formation of the notochord sheath also affect the development of the nucleus pulposus (Smits and Lefebvre 2003; Choi and Harfe 2011). Sox5 and Sox6 are Sry-related HMG box transcription factors that cooperate with Sox9 to mediate chondrogenesis (Lefebvre 2002). Inactivation of Sox5 and Sox6 result in dramatic chondrodysplasia with impaired chondrocyte differentiation (Smits et al. 2001). Sox5/6 is also required for the formation of the notochord sheath and subsequent survival of the notochord and development of the nucleus pulposus (Smits and Lefebvre 2003). The sheath contains many matrix proteins that are also found in cartilage including collagen II and proteoglycans containing sulfated glycosaminoglycans like aggrecan and perlecan. The aggrecan and perlecan content in the notochord sheath from *Sox5/6* mutant mice was dramatically reduced, whereas collagen II was not affected. It was suggested that Sox5/6 promotes the formation of the notochord sheath by regulating matrix gene expression in the notochord cells. Failure to maintain the sheath matrix resulted in premature death of notochord cells and an aberrant nucleus pulposus.

Shh, a secreted signaling molecule important for several aspects of development, is also required for the formation and maintenance of the notochordal sheath (Choi and Harfe 2011). Shh is secreted by the notochord as well as the nucleus pulposus in embryonic and postnatal life (Dahia et al. 2009; DiPaola et al. 2005). Shh binds to its receptor, Ptc, on nearby cells, thus relieving repression of Smoothened, Smo, a transmembrane protein that is required to transmit the Shh signal (Ingham and McMahon 2001). In mice containing a germ line null allele of *Shh*, the notochord was formed, but was not maintained (Chiang et al. 1996). The embryos died shortly thereafter preventing analysis of development of the intervertebral disc. To address the role of Shh in the maintenance of the notochord and the subsequent formation of the nucleus pulposus, a conditionally deleted allele of *Smo* in mice was used (Choi and Harfe 2011). In these experiments the investigators removed *Smo* from all Shh-expressing cells, including the notochord. The notochord sheath was missing in the *Smo*-deleted mice. Furthermore, the nucleus pulposus did not expand into the intervertebral disc region, and notochord cells were scattered throughout the vertebral column. Notochord remnants in the vertebral body could be marked by ROSA26 in ShhCreERT2 mice. If *Smo* was removed after the notochord sheath formed, the nucleus pulposus was not affected indicating the importance of the sheath in this tissue formation.

Collagen II (Col2) is the major collagen in cartilage and an important component of the notochordal sheath (Swiderski and Solursh 1992; Gotz et al. 1995). The notochord is not removed from vertebral bodies, and intervertebral discs do not form normally in mice with a null mutation in *Col2a1* (Aszódi et al. 1998). Cartilage proteins including collagens IX and XI, aggrecan, and COMP appear to be expressed in these mice, but collagens I and II are inappropriately expressed in the cartilage of the presumptive vertebrae. As a result, the collagen fibers in cartilage are disorganized. It was proposed that this disorganization would lead to a weakened structure unable to contain the cartilage osmotic pressure. The reduction in internal pressure within the vertebral body could be responsible for the failure of the notochord to be removed from the vertebrae and expand into the intervertebral disc (Adams et al. 1990), as a result, the nucleus pulposus would not form. Mutations in other genes that are expressed in the sclerotome and affect the development of the vertebral body including Nkx3.2 and Pax1/9 also affect the removal of the notochord from the vertebral body and development of the nucleus pulposus, further supporting the requirement of mechanical pressure for removal/expansion of the nucleus pulposus (Peters et al. 1999; Lettice et al. 1999; Tribioli and Lufkin 1999).

Box 3.2: Evolution of the Intervertebral Disc

The notochord is the forerunner of the axial skeleton in early non-vertebrate chordates. In basal vertebrates including lamprey and fish (teleosts), most of the axial skeleton is derived from the notochord (Koob and Long 2000; Ytteborg et al. 2012; Haga et al. 2009; Dale and Topczewski 2011; Inohaya et al. 2007). Sclerotome is not detected in non-vertebrate chordates. A primitive sclerotome, however, is observed in the most basal vertebrates and teleosts (Scaal and Wiegreffe 2006; Keller 2000; Koob and Long 2000; Inohaya et al. 2007). Development of the axial skeleton in teleosts, including salmon, medaka, and zebra fish, begins with patterned mineralization of the notochord sheath where the vertebrae will form (Ytteborg et al. 2012; Haga et al. 2009; Dale and Topczewski 2011; Inohaya et al. 2007). In adult fish, the disc consists of a central core, similar to the nucleus pulposus, containing cells with large fluid-filled vacuoles derived from the notochord, a fibrous layer derived from the notochord sheath, and an elastic membrane or ligament that is likely derived from the primitive sclerotome (Ytteborg et al. 2012; Haga et al. 2009; Dale and Topczewski 2011; Inohaya et al. 2007).

Comparative anatomy suggests the sclerotome evolved further in amphibians. In some, the sclerotome composes a large portion of the differentiating somite, and segmentation is independent of the notochord (Scaal and Wiegreffe 2006; Keller 2000). By the time amniotes evolved, they already had a well-developed intervertebral disc with a nucleus-like tissue derived from the notochord and an annulus-like fibrous tissue derived from an evolving sclerotome. It was recently shown that some adult reptiles and birds, including chicken and quail, lack a nucleus pulposus and there is limited, if any, contribution of the notochord to the adult axial skeleton (Bruggeman et al. 2012). Since the contribution of the notochord to the axial skeleton and development of a nucleus pulposus-like structure occurred very early in vertebrate evolution, before significant contribution of sclerotome derived tissues, it seems likely that the nucleus pulposus was lost during the evolution of reptiles and birds. This loss could have been due to either selective pressure to lose the nucleus pulposus or lack of pressure to keep it. Perhaps as the sclerotome evolved, it was able to take over all of the functions of the adult axial skeleton that were previously served by the notochord.

The line that would lead to mammals (synapsids) and that of reptiles and birds (saurapsids) diverged from the basal amniotes some 320 million years ago. Whatever the reason (pressures related to gait or mechanical loading), mammals retained the notochord-derived structure. Of course, proof of this model will require additional fossil evidence, which is scarce for unmineralized tissue; more complete comparative anatomy of existing species; and further experimentation, including lineage tracing and molecular biology, on the development of the intervertebral disc in multiple species.

3.2.3 Evidence for Lineage of the Nucleus Pulposus

The lineage of the cells in the adult nucleus pulposus has been the source of much debate (Risbud et al. 2010; Erwin 2010; Shapiro and Risbud 2010). It has been proposed that the notochord forms the initial central part of the intervertebral disc, but as this compartment matures, these large notochord cells are replaced with smaller cells that more closely resemble chondrocytes, perhaps recruited from the end plate or the inner annulus (Wamsley 1953; Kim et al. 2003). However, more recently, evidence has accumulated to suggest that all of the cells within the nucleus pulposus are indeed derived from the notochord.

Shh is highly expressed in the notochord and later in the nucleus pulposus (Dahia et al. 2009; DiPaola et al. 2005; Choi et al. 2008). Mice that express an inducible Cre under the control of the Shh promoter were used in fate mapping studies of the notochord (Choi et al. 2008). To exclude the possibility that Shh-Cre would mark cells in the notochord and then again in a new nucleus pulposus cell population, a tamoxifen-inducible Cre was employed. Notochord cells were "pulse labeled" by administration of tamoxifen at an early stage of development and then followed over time with ß-galactosidase staining through Cre-mediated activation of the ROSA26-LacZ locus. When mouse embryos were pulse labeled at E8.0 days of gestation and examined at E13.5, it was clear that all of the cells of the nucleus pulposus were labeled. Furthermore, when old mice (19 months) were examined, all of the cells of the nucleus pulposus were labeled with no labeling observed in the annulus fibrosus. More recently, notochord cells were traced using a Noto-Cre mouse (McCann et al. 2012). Noto is a highly conserved transcription factor with expression limited to the node and early notochord. Again, when cells were marked by activation of the ROSA26-LacZ locus by Noto-Cre, all of the nucleus pulposus cells in the adult, after dramatic changes in cellular morphology, were still labeled although only a subset of adult nucleus cells stained for K8, a putative marker for nucleus pulposus cells. The fate mapping studies strongly suggest the nucleus pulposus is derived completely from the notochord.

Evidence that the nucleus pulposus is derived from the notochord also comes from gene profiling studies. Recent studies used microarray technology to compare the gene expression patterns in human, bovine, canine, and rodent nucleus pulposus, annulus fibrosus, and articular cartilage (Minogue et al. 2010; Lee et al. 2007; Sakai et al. 2009). Brachyury/T, K8, K18, and K19 were highly expressed in the nucleus pulposus. Brachyury/T is known as a marker of the notochord and also a marker of chordoma, notochord tumors, suggesting that the nucleus pulposus could be derived from these embryonic cells. More importantly, gene expression patterns significantly overlapped, and expression of the above nucleus pulposus markers was similar in the large notochord-like cells and the smaller chondrocytic cells within the nucleus pulposus. In contrast to this result, another group showed heterogeneity in the nucleus pulposus with regard to K8 expression (Gilson et al. 2010). Heterogeneity in K8 expression was also observed in the Noto-Cre cell fate mapping studies described above, even though all of the nucleus pulposus cells were clearly derived from Noto-expressing cells (McCann et al. 2012). A likely explanation is that the notochord can differentiate into all of the cell types including K8-expressing and K8-non-expressing cells, within the nucleus pulposus. This idea is supported by studies showing that notochord cells from rabbit can differentiate into cells with varying morphological characteristics similar to those observed in the adult nucleus pulposus (Kim et al. 2009). Taken together, there is now considerable evidence indicating that all of the cell types in the adult nucleus pulposus are derived from the notochord.

3.3 Somitogenesis

Somites are transient structures formed from the presomitic mesoderm (PSM) that define the anterior-posterior segmented pattern of the embryo. They are essentially balls of cells composed of an outer epithelial layer surrounding a mesenchymal core, the somitocoele (Ferrer-Vaquer et al. 2010). The formation of somites is tightly controlled during development both spatially and temporally. Somite pairs bud off from the anterior end of the PSM at time intervals specific to the species (Pourquie 2011; Brand-Saberi et al. 2008). Somite nomenclature is based on the relationship of the somite to the anterior end of the PSM with the closest somite labeled number SI followed by SII, SIII, etc., counting toward the anterior end of the embryo (Christ and Ordahl 1995). Future somites in the presomitic mesoderm are labeled S0 and SI. These somites have not budded off the PSM, but can be seen histologically or with molecular markers and are frequently referred to as somitomeres. It is important to note that the first five somites to bud off are destined to fuse and form the occipital bone (Couly et al. 1993). The remaining somites will progress into the components of the axial skeleton and skeletal muscle. Disruptions to somitogenesis and segmentation of the somites result in birth defects that can severely affect the function of the spine by disrupting the formation and shape of both vertebral bodies and intervertebral disc (Box 3.3; Turnpenny 2008).

Box 3.3: Human Pathologies Associated with Segmentation Defects: Klippel-Feil Syndrome

Many congenital defects of the spine are caused by problems in segmentation of the somites (Turnpenny 2008; Shifley and Cole 2007). Some of these are linked to teratogens such as retinoic acid (RA) which can cause axial skeleton abnormalities by interfering with the normal retinoid signaling and thus affecting the normal timing and location of segment formation (Alexander and Tuan 2010). Various types of spondylocostal dysostosis have been linked to the clock genes Dll3, Lnfg, Hes7, and Mesp2 (Pourquie 2011). Alagille syndrome, which is characterized by misshapen "butterfly" vertebrae caused by dorsal fusion failure, has been linked to mutations in Jagged1, a Notch ligand (Oda et al. 1997; Li et al. 1997). Segmentation defects can also affect the intervertebral disc as well as the vertebra. Most prominently, the disc is completely absent with fused block vertebrae and pushed to one side when only partial vertebral fusion occurs (Turnpenny 2008; Shifley and Cole 2007). Unfortunately, many clinical observations fail to include discal analysis, most likely due to inability to visualize it by earlier imaging methods.

Klippel-Feil syndrome (KFS) is one of the clearest examples of a disc development defect in humans. KFS is primarily characterized by congenital cervical synostosis due to an absence of the disc and resulting in fusion of adjacent vertebrae. First identified in 1912 by Klippel and Feil, it was described as limited head range of motion, low posterior hairline, and absence of neck (Klippel and Feil 1975; Willard and Nicholson 1934). KFS is currently categorized into three types as follows (Tracy et al. 2004; Kaplan et al. 2005):

- Type I – multiple cervical fusions
- Type II – 1–2 cervical fusions
- Type III – cervical fusion combined with lumbar fusions

After a screen of 63 affected individuals showed 6 with potential deleterious mutations in *PAX1*, it was proposed that defects in PAX1 function resulting in somite segmentation defects were the major cause of KFS (McGaughran et al. 2003). More recently, genetic analysis of both inherited and sporadic cases of KFS identified two missense mutations (L298P and A249E) in the *GDF6* gene and an inversion (q22.2q23.3) 623 kb 3′ of *GDF6* (Clarke et al. 1995; Tassabehji et al. 2008). GDF6 (also known as BMP13) is a member of the TGF-ß protein family that clusters with GDF5 and GDF7 (BMP14, BMP12) and is structurally related to BMP2 and BMP4 (Rider and Mulloy 2010). Knockdown of GDF6 in zebra fish and Xenopus results in KFS-like phenotypes (Asai-Coakwell et al. 2009; Tassabehji et al. 2008). Deletion of GDF6 in mice does not result in any obvious spinal phenotypes; however, the additional deletion of GDF5 results in a KFS-like scoliosis phenotype suggesting some redundancy in the function of GDF5 and GDF6 (Asai-Coakwell et al. 2009; Settle et al. 2003). It is also important to note that even with the double deletion, these mice do not exhibit vertebral fusions. It has been shown that GDF6 can inhibit endochondral ossification of mesenchymal stem cells in culture suggesting that GDF6 may normally help to specify or maintain the disc space in the sclerotome (Shen et al. 2009). Furthermore, it has been shown that GDF6 prevents the effects of annular injury in an ovine model and may act as a protective agent for the annulus fibrosus (Wei et al. 2009). These only cover a few of the many abnormalities associated with segmentation, but future genetic screening promises to link more cases with the genes involved in somitogenesis.

3.3.1 Clock and Wavefront

The first step in the formation of the somite from the PSM is the determination and timing of the segmentation site. This anterior-posterior segmentation and patterning of the PSM was originally hypothesized by Cooke and Zeeman (1976) to occur via a "clock and wavefront" mechanism (Fig. 3.2). This model proposed that the tightly controlled size and number of somites is due to the cycling of expression for specific genes within the PSM cells. Cycling of gene expression within individual cells provides the "clock," and the presence of a morphogen gradient across the anterior-posterior axis of the embryo provides the "wavefront." This gradient in combination with the timing of genes expressed through the clock leads to the formation of a boundary where the somite will separate from the PSM. Commitment and differentiation of cells is also modulated as they pass through this boundary. Additional experimental evidence over the years has supported and expanded upon the "clock and wavefront" model so that now many of the molecular details have been elucidated (Pourquie 2011; Brand-Saberi et al. 2008).

3.3.1.1 Clock Regulation

Two major signaling pathways are involved in regulating the "clock" that helps determine where and when each somite will separate from the PSM. The first is the Notch pathway. Notch1 has a critical role in the segmentation and epithelialization of somites (Conlon et al. 1995; Swiatek et al. 1994). Although Notch1 is expressed throughout the PSM, activated Notch signals where segmentation will occur (Reaume et al. 1992) and other pathway members that regulate Notch activity, such as delta1(Dll1) (Bettenhausen et al. 1995), Hes1 (Palmeirim et al. 1997; Dequeant et al. 2006), Hes7 (Bessho et al. 2003), and lunatic fringe (Lfng) (Evrard et al. 1998; Johnston et al. 1997; Forsberg et al. 1998; Zhang and Gridley 1998), exhibit cyclic expression patterns in the PSM. The pattern of expression has been compared to waves washing up on shore. Expression starts at the posterior end of the PSM and moves in a wave to the point where the next somite will form, then expression starts back at the posterior domain. The timing of the cycle is species dependent. Mesp2, an inhibitor of Notch signaling, also has a cyclic expression pattern in the PSM, and its expression becomes restricted to, and maintained in, the anterior portion of the SI somite at each cycle (Morimoto et al. 2005). This sets up a sharp boundary of Notch activity that is high in the posterior end of the S0 somite and low in the anterior end of the future SI somite, thus defining the segmentation site for the S0 somite (Morimoto et al. 2005; Saga 2007; Sasaki et al. 2011; Saga et al. 1997).

The second signaling pathway shown to be involved in the clock system and in regulating its cyclic pattern of gene expression is that of Wnt. Axin2, a negative regulator of the Wnt pathway, has an oscillating pattern of expression that is not in synchrony with genes of the Notch family (Aulehla et al. 2003; Dequeant et al. 2006). Disruption of the Notch pathway does not disrupt Axin2 expression, although disruption of Wnt3a disrupts Lnfg, an inhibitor of Notch signaling (Aulehla et al. 2003, 2008). This suggests that cyclic Wnt

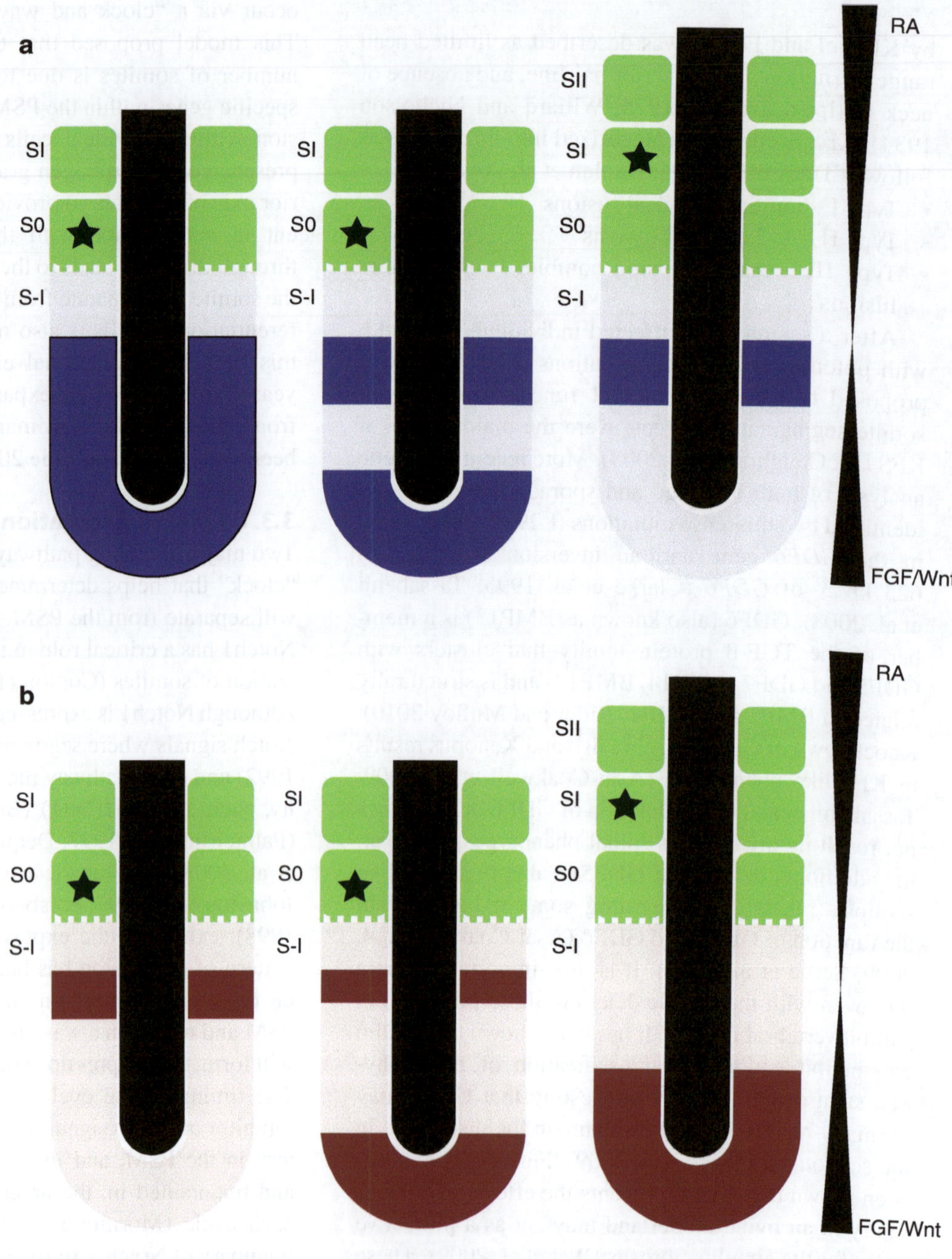

Fig. 3.2 Somitogenesis (segmentation). Somites (*green*) bud off at evenly spaced time intervals, the period of which is determined by species, from the anterior PSM. Counter gradients of RA and FGF/Wnt signaling determine the location of the determination front near the posterior boundary of somite SI. The two main "clock" signaling pathways cycle on and off synchronously with somite formation yet slightly out of phase with each other. (**a**) *Blue stripes* are representative of Wnt pathway gene cycling within the PSM during the period of one somite generation. (**b**) *Red* stripes are representative of Notch pathway gene cycling within the PSM during the period of one somite generation. *The star* indicates the position of a single cell during the period of formation for one somite

signaling is occurring upstream of the cyclic Notch signaling. This cycling of gene expression seems to allow the cells of the PSM to respond to the "wavefront" signals at the appropriate time initiating the cellular shape and adhesion changes that permit the somite to "bud off" from the PSM.

3.3.1.2 Wavefront

The concept of the "wavefront," a point of abrupt transition leading to somite formation, has evolved to include two counteracting morphogen gradients (Brand-Saberi et al. 2008; Pourquie 2011). The first identified was that of fibroblast growth factor (FGF) signaling. FGF8 was found to be present at high levels in the posterior PSM and gradually decreases toward the anterior PSM (Dubrulle et al. 2001). More recently, FGF4 was seen expressed in a similar pattern (Naiche et al. 2011). Experiments implanting beads soaked in Fgf8 have demonstrated the ability of Fgf8 concentration to regulate the size of the developing somites (Sawada et al. 2001). Deletion of Fgfr1, the only FGF receptor expressed in the PSM, results in loss of cyclic gene expression and failure of somite segmentation (Wahl et al. 2007). The FGF8 gradient has been determined to be due to the instability of the RNA transcripts that leads to a gradual decrease in Fgf8 protein (Dubrulle and Pourquie 2004), thus allowing for the tight temporal and spatial control of the segmentation boundary. In addition to FGF, Wnt signaling shows a similar gradient, as evidenced by localization of β-catenin protein, that acts both through and parallel to FGF signaling (Aulehla et al. 2008). This Wnt signaling gradient also suggests a mechanism of cross talk between the "clock" and "wavefront" as Wnt signaling can control the Notch pathway. It has been suggested that the gradient and cyclic expression of Wnt acts as a bridge between the wavefront and clock (Brand-Saberi et al. 2008; Pourquie 2011).

The counter gradient to FGF is a retinoic acid (RA) gradient that extends in an anterior to posterior direction along the developing embryo and is inhibited by Fgf8 through repression of Raldh2, a gene required for RA synthesis (Diez del Corral et al. 2003). In turn, RA is then able to repress FGF signaling (Diez del Corral et al. 2003). Cyp26, an enzyme that degrades RA, is expressed in the tail bud (Sakai et al. 2001) providing a mechanism to keep the diffusion of RA localized. This method of gradient formation is known as a source-sink mechanism (Aulehla and Pourquié 2010) in contrast to the mRNA decay used to control the FGF gradient. It is currently thought that the boundary of the "wavefront" is determined by the transition from high FGF/Wnt and low RA signaling to low FGF/Wnt and high RA signaling.

The bilateral symmetry of the somite pairs produced during somitogenesis is also controlled by RA signaling (Kawakami et al. 2005; Vermot et al. 2005; Vilhais-Neto et al. 2010; Vermot and Pourquie 2005; Sirbu and Duester 2006). During normal embryonic development, the asymmetric expression of various genes, such as *Nodal* and *Pitx2*, occurs directing the organization of the internal organs. It has been proposed that RA acts to insulate somitogenesis from surrounding signals driving the left-right asymmetry seen throughout the body cavity (Brent 2005; Brend and Holley 2009). This work links the genes involved in somitogenesis directly to the control of body symmetry.

3.3.2 Epithelialization

As somites bud off of the anterior end of the PSM, the outer cell layer undergoes a mesenchymal to epithelial transition (MET). The two primary transcription factors involved in MET are Pax3 and Paraxis. In vitro overexpression of Pax3 results in epithelialization of mesenchymal cell lines (Wiggan et al. 2002), while deletion of *Pax3* in the PSM results in somites that are unable to maintain epithelial integrity (Mansouri et al. 2001). Loss of *Paraxis* also disrupts epithelialization of the somite (Burgess et al. 1996) although it does not affect segmentation and future differentiation. The first evidence for MET during somitogenesis came from a finding in 1978 that cells from the segmented mesoderm showed a greater adhesiveness than those of the unsegmented PSM (Bellairs et al. 1978). Various adhesion molecules are expressed in the developing somite such as N-cadherin, fibronectin, cytoactin, and neural cell adhesion molecule (Duband et al. 1987; Crossin et al. 1986). These molecules are known to be involved in the formation of epithelia. N-cadherin is necessary for the production of stable somites with its loss resulting in irregular and loosely attached somites (Radice et al. 1997) as well as lack of adhesion in culture (Duband et al. 1987). EphA4/Ephrin signaling is also required for proper epithelialization of the somite. Ablation of EphA4/Ephrin signaling in the form of a dominant-negative, truncated EphA4 results in somite boundaries, but no epithelial layer formation (Barrios et al. 2003). This process results in epithelia forming only on the outer boundary of each somite sphere. It is not clear how high Notch signaling from the segmentation clock translates into MET, but Notch regulates the expression of a transcription factor called Hes1 that regulates Ephrin expression (Glazier et al. 2008).

3.3.3 Segment Identity

Hox genes control the patterning of the PSM, which will ultimately lead to the differences in cranial to sacral vertebrae identity (Iimura et al. 2009; Wellik 2009). Originally discovered in drosophila segmentation, Hox genes are located in clusters that are arranged from 3′ to 5′ in the order of their expression from anterior to posterior domains. In mammals, there are four clusters Hox A, B, C, and D each containing up to 13 Hox genes (Wellik 2009). Hox genes with the same number across clusters are called paralogous groups (e.g., *Hoxa1*, *Hoxb1*, and *Hoxd1*). The expression domains of individual Hox genes have been shown to line up with specific vertebral segments (Burke et al. 1995). Although the colinearity of the Hox genes is easily demonstrated in drosophila with deletions resulting in anterior homeotic transformations, in the mouse, *Hox* deletions result in both the expected anterior homeotic transformations and posterior homeotic transformations (Wellik 2007). The reason for this variation seen in mice is thought to be due to the activity of paralogous Hox genes. Deletion of multiple paralogous Hox genes consistently results in anterior homeotic transformations (Wellik 2007). The term "Hox code" is used to describe the phenomenon in which a very specific complement of Hox expression determines the identity of a specific vertebral segment (Kessel and Gruss 1991; Iimura et al. 2009). In the mouse, the anterior boundaries of Hox gene expression are set by embryonic day 12.5 (Wellik 2007). There has been some indication that Hox gene expression is linked to the somite clock (Zakany et al. 2001; Kmita and Duboule 2003) allowing additional layers of specification in the patterning of the spine. RA has also been linked to the control of Hox gene expression during specific stages of development with ectopic RA causing homeotic transformations in the vertebrae (Kessel and Gruss 1991). Thus, there is cross talk between the signaling pathways in the "wavefront" and those required for location specification. This activity emphasizes how all of the signaling pathways that regulate development of the axial skeleton overlap and intertwine.

3.4 Formation of Sclerotome

Differentiation begins starting with the anterior-most somite. The dorsal epithelium of the somite will form the dermomyotome, which will later differentiate into the dermis of the back and skeletal muscle. The somitocoele and the ventral epithelium of the somite will undergo an epithelial to mesenchymal transition (EMT) to generate sclerotome, which will form all of the connective tissues of the axial skeleton. The division of sclerotome and dermomyotome begins when the somite reaches SIII (Christ and Ordahl 1995) although the sclerotome segment is still plastic until a much later stage (Dockter and Ordahl 2000). Shh secreted from the notochord and ventral floor plate is the primary inductive signal controlling the delamination of the epithelial somite to form the sclerotome (Borycki et al. 1998; Fan and Tessier-Lavigne 1994; Murtaugh et al. 1999; Dockter 2000; Chiang et al. 1996; Marcelle et al. 1999). Pax3 and Pax7 are expressed in the unsegmented PSM but are downregulated in the ventral somite and somitocoele as the sclerotome differentiates. The expression of Pax1 and Pax9, markers of sclerotome, increases (Brand-Saberi and Christ 2000). Shh has been shown to induce Pax1, a marker of sclerotome, when present ectopically (Fan and Tessier-Lavigne 1994; Johnson et al. 1994). A second permissive signal is also required for the formation of sclerotome (Stafford et al. 2011). BMP from the lateral plate mesoderm normally interrupts differentiation of sclerotome and interferes with Shh signaling, allowing the sclerotome to differentiate only from the ventral medial side of the somite. Several extracellular BMP antagonists are expressed regionally that carefully restrict BMP activity (Stafford et al. 2011; Rider and Mulloy 2010). Noggin (Nog) and Gremlin1 (Grem1) cooperate to antagonize BMP signaling, permitting sclerotome differentiation in the presence of Shh (Stafford et al. 2011). Deletion of *Nog* and *Grem1* in mice results in the complete failure of sclerotome differentiation. Dermomyotome was not affected in these mice. Inhibition of BMP alone is not sufficient to specify sclerotome or expand sclerotome differentiation in vivo suggesting antagonism of BMP is a permissive factor for sclerotome differentiation (Rider and Mulloy 2010). Very recently, using notochord deficient *Sd* mice, it was shown that the floor plate alone is sufficient for the development of the sclerotome (Ando et al. 2011). Shh from the floor plate could replace Shh from the notochord to allow differentiation of sclerotome in the absence of notochord.

3.5 Resegmentation

Resegmentation of the sclerotome was first proposed by Remak in 1855 (Bagnall et al. 1988) after observing that in relationship to the original somites, there was half-segment realignment of the vertebrae. The initial studies followed somite development in chick embryos through lineage tracing using quail/chick chimeras (Bagnall et al. 1988; Goldstein and Kalcheim 1992), vital dye (Bagnall 1992), or viral transduction (Ewan and Everett 1992). The consensus from these studies was that the sclerotome derived from one somite divides into rostral and caudal halves with the rostral half of one segment joining with the caudal half of the segment immediately rostral to it forming the vertebral body. Accordingly, the intervertebral disc would be derived from the sclerotome at the junction of the two half segments (Fig. 3.3). Since those early reports, it has been determined that resegmentation occurs after the sclerotome differentiates from the ventral portion of the somite. Resegmentation results in a one half-segment stagger between the sclerotome and myotome allowing for the alternating pattern between the musculature and the vertebral body in the axial skeleton. Phenotypes indicative of alterations in resegmentation include fusion of vertebrae where joints should be, split vertebrae and ribs, alterations in migration of neural crest through the sclerotome and disorganization of the dorsal root ganglia. Several mouse models demonstrate these types of resegmentation defects including deficiencies in RAB23 (*opb* mutant) (Sporle and Schughart 1998), *Paraxis* (Johnson et al. 2001), and *Tgfbr2* (Baffi et al. 2006). Ablation of the neural tube after sclerotome formation also results in resegmentation failure suggesting a role for signals from the neural tube in directing resegmentation (Colbjorn Larsen et al. 2006). Much of the molecular mechanisms defining the process of resegmentation remain to be elucidated.

3.6 Sclerotome Derivatives

Sclerotome contains multipotent progenitor cells that differentiate into all of the connective tissue cell types of the axial skeleton (Monsoro-Burq 2005). Sclerotome can differentiate into cartilage that will subsequently undergo endochondral ossification to form the bony vertebrae of the spine. It will also differentiate into the annulus fibrosus of the intervertebral disc and the tendons that link the vertebrae to the muscle. Which cell type is specified is determined by the location of cells within the sclerotome and complex interactions of growth factors (Fig. 3.4). How these factors interact with each other to specify cell lineage in the axial skeleton is just beginning to be determined.

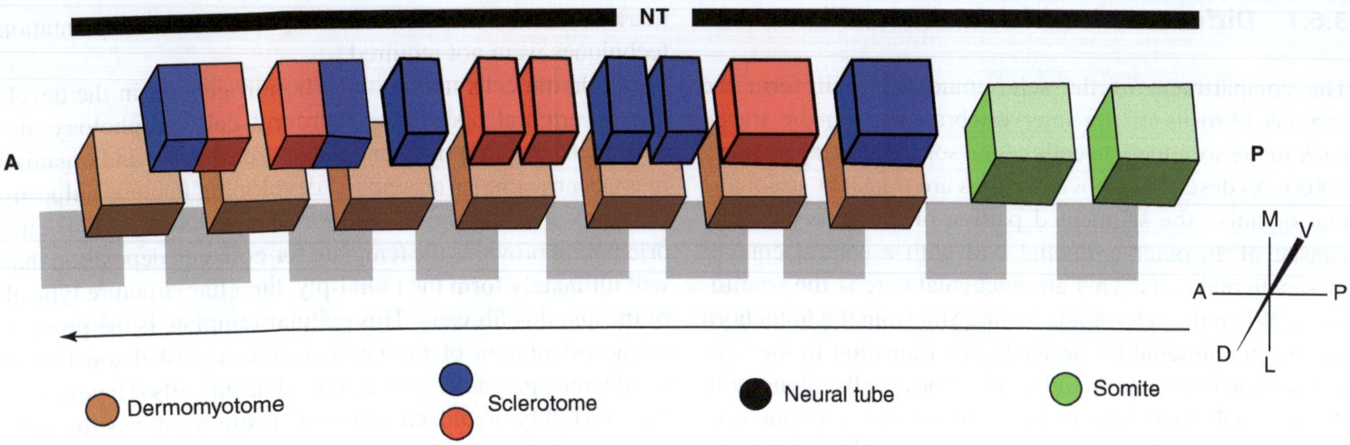

Fig. 3.3 Sclerotome resegmentation. Resegmentation begins with the dorsal-ventral division of the somite into the dermomyotome (*brown*) and sclerotome (*red and blue*), respectively. The sclerotome then proceeds to divide into anterior and posterior regions that can be seen as alternating loose and condensed mesenchyme. The anterior region of one sclerotome then associates with the posterior region of the sclerotome directly anterior to form what will later become an individual vertebral body. In this way the vertebral body and muscle segment will be staggered by one half segment. *Arrow* indicates direction of cell fate determination. *NT* Neural Tube

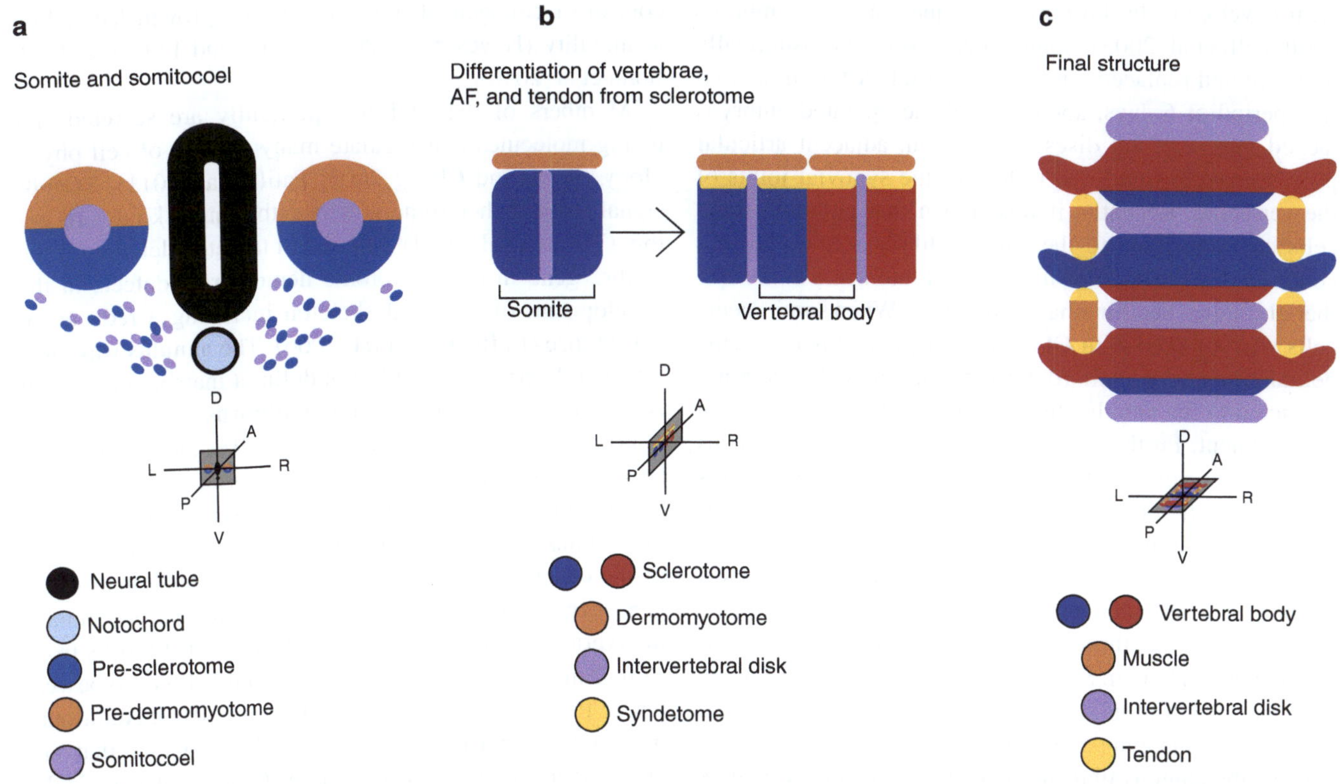

Fig. 3.4 Derivatives of the sclerotome. (**a**) Sclerotome is derived from the ventral medial portion of the somite. In response to Shh, cells from the somite and somitocoele migrate toward the notochord and differentiate into sclerotome. (**b**) Cells from the somitocoele end up at the border between the rostral and caudal halves of each segment. After resegmentation, these cells lie in between the developing vertebral bodies and will become the annulus fibrosus (*AF*) of the intervertebral disc. Cells at the dorsal border of the sclerotome differentiate into tendon in response to factors from the myotome. (**c**) In the final structure, the disc is situated between the vertebral bodies, which are staggered by one half segment from the muscle and connected to the muscle though the tendons

3.6.1 Differentiation of the Annulus Fibrosus

The compartment of the sclerotome that will form the annulus fibrosus of the intervertebral disc can be traced back to the somitocoele cells of the somite (Mittapalli et al. 2005). As described above, somites are transient structures that organize the segmented pattern of the embryo. They consist of an outer epithelial ball with a central core of mesenchymal cells. This mesenchymal core is the somitocoele. When the sclerotome forms, Shh from the notochord causes an epithelial to mesenchymal transition in the ventral portion of the epithelial somite, these cells, along with the mesenchymal cells of the somitocoele, migrate ventrally to surround the notochord and form the sclerotome (Monsoro-Burq 2005). The cells from the somitocoele end up in the caudal half of the sclerotome adjacent to von Ebner's fissure, the domain that marks the border between the two sclerotome halves (Williams 1910; Christ et al. 2000). After resegmentation, this is the area that will end up in between the vertebrae as the annulus fibrosus. The importance of this compartment for the formation of the intervertebral disc as well as the zygapophysial joints (synovial joints of the vertebrae) was determined using classical developmental biology techniques in chick embryos (Mittapalli et al. 2005). Somitocoeles were microsurgically removed and replaced with an inert bead. After an incubation period of 6 days, about half of the operated embryos lacked intervertebral discs. In addition, adjacent articular processes were fused due to loss of the synovial joints of the vertebrae. Recently, it was shown that although these cells can contribute to the annulus fibrosus, they are not committed to the annulus fibrosus cell fate while in the epithelial somite (Senthinathan et al. 2012). When somitocoele cells were marked with GFP and transplanted between the neural tube and notochord, GFP-expressing cells were not restricted to the annulus fibrosus or vertebral body later in development. Furthermore, expression of annulus fibrosus markers was not found in the vertebral bodies. The results suggest that the annulus cells are likely specified by their location within the sclerotome.

It is clear that the annulus fibrosus is derived from cells at the border of sclerotome halves; however, there is some dispute about whether the annulus arises from the rostral or caudal side of this border. Somitocoele cells normally end up on the caudal side of this boundary (Mittapalli et al. 2005), and previous fate mapping and peanut agglutinin binding studies suggest the annulus fibrosus arises from the caudal domain (Bagnall and Sanders 1989; Huang et al. 1994). In contrast, experiments using chick-quail grafting experiments and, more recently, dye-labeling studies suggest the annulus arises from the rostral sclerotome (Goldstein and Kalcheim 1992; Bruggeman et al. 2012). The advantage of the dye-labeling studies was that two discrete cell populations could be marked within the same somite and precise cell transplantation techniques were not required.

While the cells undergoing chondrogenesis in the developing vertebral body adopt a round cell morphology, the cells in the presumptive annulus are fibroblastic and organize in concentric circles around the developing nucleus pulposus (Peacock 1951; Rufai et al. 1995; Hayes et al. 2011). This orientation provides the template for collagen deposition that will ultimately form the radial-ply, lamellar structure typical of the annulus fibrosus. This cellular template is the product of the orientation of the cellular actin cytoskeleton linked to adherens junctions connecting adjacent cells (Hayes et al. 1999). Highly organized matrix deposition follows this cellular orientation phase. The organized deposition of the collagen matrix may be similar to that seen in other connective tissues like the tendon: collagen fibrils self-assemble in the cell, then larger fibers are formed in membrane-bound compartments between cells (Birk and Trelstad 1986); small leucine-rich proteoglycans (SLRPs) control collagen fiber formation as well as regulate the availability of growth factors, including TGF-ß. Fibromodulin is strongly expressed in the annulus fibrosus relative to the vertebral cartilage and may play an important role in its development through its control of collagen fiber formation and growth factor bioavailability (Hayes et al. 2011; Smits and Lefebvre 2003; Sohn et al. 2010).

Members of the TGF-ß superfamily are secreted signaling molecules that regulate many aspects of cell physiology (Serra and Chang 2003; Patil et al. 2011). TGF-ßs signal through heteromeric serine/threonine kinase receptors (Wrana et al. 1994). Mice with targeted deletion of the Tgfbr2 gene in the sclerotome demonstrate defects in the development of the axial skeleton including a reduced or absent disc (Baffi et al. 2004, 2006). The annulus was most affected. Expression of fibromodulin, a matrix protein that is highly enriched in the annulus fibrosus, was reduced or missing. The mature form of collagen IIB, indicating vertebral development, was ectopically expressed in the presumptive annulus fibrosus and peanut agglutinin, which normally only stains the presumptive vertebrae, stained the length of the developing spine. Furthermore, a global analysis of gene expression comparing wild-type and Tgfbr2 mutant intervertebral discs indicated that the annulus fibrosus from Tgfbr2 mutant mice more closely resembled wild-type vertebrae than annulus fibrosus (Sohn et al. 2010). Additional microarray experiments also showed that genes that are enriched in the annulus fibrosus were stimulated in TGF-ß-treated sclerotome (Sohn et al. 2010). A separate study using rat annulus cells in culture showed that TGF-ß could upregulate proteins associated with fibrocartilage including collagen I and II (Hayes and Ralphs 2011). Together the results suggest that TGF-ß could (a) allow formation of the intervertebral disc by preventing differentiation of vertebral cartilage in the disc space and/or (b) directly stimulate annulus differentiation.

Klippel-Feil syndrome (KFS; OMIM#118100) is a congenital malformation characterized by cervical synostosis due to lack of intervertebral disc resulting in fusion of adjacent vertebrae. It was recently shown that KFS is associated with mutations in the *GDF6* gene (Tassabehji et al. 2008). GDF6/BMP13 is a member of the BMP subgroup within the TGF-ß/BMP family of secreted signaling molecules. The mechanism of GDF6 action in development of the intervertebral disc is not known, but it has been speculated to regulate specification of where the disc will form within the sclerotome (Box 3.3).

3.6.2 Differentiation of Vertebral Cartilage

Vertebral chondrocyte cell fate is specified early when the sclerotome first forms (Murtaugh et al. 1999). Shh secreted from the notochord, which induces delamination of cells from the somite and initial differentiation of the sclerotome, can also prime the cells to respond to the chondrogenic actions of BMP. Shh induces expression of the transcription factors Pax1 and Pax9, which can also be considered markers of the early sclerotome (Muller et al. 1996). Shh and Pax1/9 regulate the expression of a transcriptional repressor called Nkx3.2 (Zeng et al. 2002; Rodrigo et al. 2003). Nkx3.2 is one of the earliest markers of prechondrogenic cells in the axial skeleton, and it induces the expression of Sox9, a master regulator of chondrogenesis, in a BMP-dependent manner (Zeng et al. 2002; Tribioli and Lufkin 1999). Since Nkx3.2 is a transcriptional repressor, induction of Sox9 is likely mediated by derepression, with Nkx3.2 inhibiting an as yet unidentified repressor of Sox9. Nkx3.2 and Smad1/Smad4 interact directly to recruit histone deacetylase/Sin3a to DNA, thus acting to inhibit gene expression (Kim and Lassar 2003). These results demonstrated that Smads act as transcriptional repressors in the context of specific binding partners like Nkx3.2. In this way, BMP and Nkx3.2 cooperate to regulate chondrogenesis. Once Sox9 expression and chondrogenesis are initiated in the axial skeleton, chondrocyte differentiation and endochondral bone formation occur in the vertebral bodies in a manner similar to that seen in the limbs. When the bony vertebra is formed, hyaline cartilage is maintained at the end plate, adjacent to the intervertebral disc.

3.6.3 Boundary Between Vertebral Body and Annulus Fibrosus

After resegmentation, the sclerotome is organized into a patterned structure of alternating loose and dense mesenchyme. The dense mesenchyme represents the future annulus fibrosus of the intervertebral disc, and the loose mesenchyme is where the vertebral cartilage will form. A sharp boundary exists between the two compartments. High concentrations of BMP activity are required to generate the vertebral cartilage. Deletion of BMP receptors results in an overall disruption to chondrogenesis and endochondral bone formation (Yoon et al. 2005). Nevertheless, BMP mRNA is synthesized in the cells that will become the disc (Zakin et al. 2008, 2010). To generate the morphogenetic field that defines disc and vertebrae within the sclerotome, BMP activity must be relocalized and concentrated. Two BMP interacting proteins, Crossveinless-2 (Cv-2) and Chordin (Chd), are required (Zakin et al. 2008, 2010). Loss of Cv-2 or Chd results in small vertebral bodies and slightly increased intervertebral space. Cv-2 mRNA is made in cells in the presumptive vertebrae. The protein is attached to cells via heparin sulfate proteoglycans and resides in the vertebral compartment. Chd mRNA is made in the presumptive intervertebral disc; however, most of the protein is localized to the vertebral compartment. Chordin binds to and inactivates BMP in the developing disc, but it also moves BMP to the developing vertebral body. Once in the vertebral compartment, Chd binds to Cv-2, the Chd is cleaved by a tolloid-like protease, releasing BMP. Strong BMP activity in the vertebral body is indicated by the presence of phospho-Smad1, which is low to absent in the intervertebral disc compartment. The movement and concentration of BMP activity within the sclerotome help to set up the compartments and boundaries that define where the vertebrae and disc will form.

In addition, examination of mouse embryos with a conditional deletion of *Tgfbr2* in the sclerotome indicated that Tgfbr2 was required to maintain the sharp boundary between the developing vertebrae and annulus fibrosus (Baffi et al. 2006). Pax1/9 is important for specifying and maintaining boundaries in developing tissues, and the expression domain of Pax1/9 was expanded in Tgfbr2 mutant mice. As TGF-ß can antagonize BMP activity, it is possible that loss of TGF-ß results in inappropriate BMP signaling in the presumptive intervertebral disc where BMP mRNA is synthesized (Candia et al. 1997; Li et al. 2006). TGF-ß may also interfere with the relocalization of BMP activity through Chd and Cv-2.

3.6.4 Syndetome (Tendon)

The tendons of the axial skeleton are formed from a compartment of the sclerotome called the syndetome (Brent et al. 2003). Since tendons link the vertebrae to the muscle, localization during development is critical. When the sclerotome separates from the somite, the epithelial dermomyotome is formed from the most dorsal part of the somite. The future muscle cells then separate to form the myotome, which expresses master regulators of muscle development,

MyoD and Myf5. The myotome is immediately dorsal and adjacent to the sclerotome and secretes fibroblast growth factors (FGF) 4 and 6. Receptors for FGF are located on the sclerotome and FGF signaling stimulates expression of Scleraxis (Scx), marking developing tendon. High levels of Shh on the ventral side of the sclerotome from the notochord prevent tendon formation and promote the formation of the vertebral bodies; thus, the tendon forms in between and adjacent to the vertebrae and muscle (Brent et al. 2003, 2005).

3.7 Developmental Pathways Involved in Maintenance of Postnatal Disc

Several signaling pathways that regulate development are also involved in maintaining the intervertebral disc structure in the adult. For example, Tgfb is expressed in the intervertebral disc and end plate cartilage into maturity (Dahia et al. 2009). Mice expressing a dominant-negative Tgfbr2 (DNIIR) show kyphoscoliosis by 3 months of age (Serra et al. 1997), while postnatal deletion of the Tgfbr2 in the annulus fibrosus of the intervertebral disc and the end plate cartilage results in signaling changes that suggest accelerated degeneration (Jin et al. 2011). Together, these studies indicate that functional TGF-ß signaling is necessary for the maintenance of a healthy intervertebral disc well after the original development has ended. Another example is Wnt signaling: inappropriate activation of Wnt/ß-catenin signaling via disruption of the inhibitors Axin1 and Axin2 results in scoliosis and fusions in lumbar vertebrae (Dao et al. 2010). Likewise, transient activation of Wnt signaling by expression of a constitutively active ß-catenin resulted in postnatal deterioration of the annulus fibrosus (Kondo et al. 2011). Many other pathways important to intervertebral disc development continue to be active in the postnatal state including Shh, Wnt, FGF, and BMP (Dahia et al. 2009). Future studies will elucidate molecular mechanism through which these developmentally important pathways maintain the postnatal disc.

3.8 Closing

Understanding of signals involved in the embryonic development of the axial skeleton provides insight into mechanisms of spinal pathology. For this purpose, it is necessary to understand how cells with specialized functions are derived from undifferentiated cells and how cells interact with each other and their environment to form tissues and organs. In addition, a clear understanding of how the skeletal system develops directly impacts regeneration and tissue engineering strategies as well as understanding the pathogenesis of diseases of the spine.

3.9 Summary of Critical Concepts Discussed in the Chapter

- The intervertebral disc is derived from two embryonic structures, somites and notochord.
- Notochordal cells form the nucleus pulposus.
- Somites are transient structures that determine the segmented pattern of the embryo.
- Somites differentiate into sclerotome and dermomyotome. The sclerotome will form all of the connective tissues of the spine.
- The sclerotome resegments after it differentiates from the somite so that the muscle and vertebral segments are staggered by one half segment.
- The annulus fibrosus is derived from a subcompartment of the sclerotome known as the arthrotome, which can be traced to the somitocoele of the somite.
- Tendons are derived from a subcompartment of the sclerotome known as the syndetome.
- Defects in formation or maintenance of the notochord, segmentation of somites, formation of sclerotome, resegmentation, and differentiation of annulus fibrosus result in disorders of the spine that affect intervertebral disc.
- Understanding how the intervertebral disc develops will lead to novel strategies for developmental engineering of this complex organ.

Acknowledgments Spine research in Dr. Serra's laboratory is supported by a grant from the National Institutes of Health, R01AR053860. MC is supported by NIDCR Training Grant (DART) T32-DE0176707. The authors would like to thank Zak Kosan for the help with the figures.

References

Adams DS, Keller R, Koehl MA (1990) The mechanics of notochord elongation, straightening and stiffening in the embryo of Xenopus laevis. Development 110(1):115–130

Alexander PG, Tuan RS (2010) Role of environmental factors in axial skeletal dysmorphogenesis. Birth Defects Res C Embryo Today 90(2):118–132

Ando T, Semba K, Suda H, Sei A, Mizuta H, Araki M, Abe K, Imai K, Nakagata N, Araki K, Yamamura K (2011) The floor plate is sufficient for development of the sclerotome and spine without the notochord. Mech Dev 128(1–2):129–140

Asai-Coakwell M, French CR, Ye M, Garcha K, Bigot K, Perera AG, Staehling-Hampton K, Mema SC, Chanda B, Mushegian A, Bamforth S, Doschak MR, Li G, Dobbs MB, Giampietro PF, Brooks BP, Vijayalakshmi P, Sauve Y, Abitbol M, Sundaresan P, van Heyningen V, Pourquie O, Underhill TM, Waskiewicz AJ, Lehmann OJ (2009) Incomplete penetrance and phenotypic variability characterize Gdf6-attributable oculo-skeletal phenotypes. Hum Mol Genet 18(6):1110–1121

Aszódi A, Chan D, Hunziker E, Bateman JF, Fässler R (1998) Collagen II is essential for the removal of the notochord and the formation of intervertebral discs. J Cell Biol 143(5):1399–1412

Aulehla A, Pourquié O (2010) Signaling gradients during paraxial mesoderm development. Cold Spring Harb Perspect Biol 2(2)
Aulehla A, Wehrle C, Brand-Saberi B, Kemler R, Gossler A, Kanzler B, Herrmann BG (2003) Wnt3a plays a major role in the segmentation clock controlling somitogenesis. Dev Cell 4(3):395–406
Aulehla A, Wiegraebe W, Baubet V, Wahl MB, Deng C, Taketo M, Lewandoski M, Pourquie O (2008) A [beta]-catenin gradient links the clock and wavefront systems in mouse embryo segmentation. Nat Cell Biol 10(2):186–193
Baffi MO, Slattery E, Sohn P, Moses HL, Chytil A, Serra R (2004) Conditional deletion of the TGF-beta type II receptor in Col2a expressing cells results in defects in the axial skeleton without alterations in chondrocyte differentiation or embryonic development of long bones. Dev Biol 276(1):124–142
Baffi MO, Moran MA, Serra R (2006) Tgfbr2 regulates the maintenance of boundaries in the axial skeleton. Dev Biol 296(2):363–374
Bagnall KM (1992) The migration and distribution of somite cells after labelling with the carbocyanine dye, Dil: the relationship of this distribution to segmentation in the vertebrate body. Anat Embryol (Berl) 185(4):317–324
Bagnall KM, Sanders EJ (1989) The binding pattern of peanut lectin associated with sclerotome migration and the formation of the vertebral axis in the chick embryo. Anat Embryol (Berl) 180(5): 505–513
Bagnall KM, Higgins SJ, Sanders EJ (1988) The contribution made by a single somite to the vertebral column: experimental evidence in support of resegmentation using the chick-quail chimaera model. Development 103(1):69–85
Barrios A, Poole RJ, Durbin L, Brennan C, Holder N, Wilson SW (2003) Eph/Ephrin signaling regulates the mesenchymal-to-epithelial transition of the paraxial mesoderm during somite morphogenesis. Curr Biol 13(18):1571–1582
Bellairs R, Curtis AS, Sanders EJ (1978) Cell adhesiveness and embryonic differentiation. J Embryol Exp Morphol 46:207–213
Bessho Y, Hirata H, Masamizu Y, Kageyama R (2003) Periodic repression by the bHLH factor Hes7 is an essential mechanism for the somite segmentation clock. Genes Dev 17(12):1451–1456
Bettenhausen B, Hrabe de Angelis M, Simon D, Guenet JL, Gossler A (1995) Transient and restricted expression during mouse embryogenesis of Dll1, a murine gene closely related to Drosophila Delta. Development 121(8):2407–2418
Birk DE, Trelstad RL (1986) Extracellular compartments in tendon morphogenesis: collagen fibril, bundle, and macroaggregate formation. J Cell Biol 103(1):231–240
Borycki AG, Mendham L, Emerson CP (1998) Control of somite patterning by Sonic hedgehog and its downstream signal response genes. Development 125(4):777–790
Brand-Saberi B, Christ B (2000) Evolution and development of distinct cell lineages derived from somites. Curr Top Dev Biol 48:1–42
Brand-Saberi B, Rudloff S, Gamel AJ (2008) Avian somitogenesis: translating time and space into pattern. Adv Exp Med Biol 638:42–57
Brend T, Holley SA (2009) Balancing segmentation and laterality during vertebrate development. Semin Cell Dev Biol 20(4):472–478
Brent AE (2005) Somite formation: where left meets right. Curr Biol 15(12):R468–R470
Brent AE, Schweitzer R, Tabin CJ (2003) A somitic compartment of tendon progenitors. Cell 113(2):235–248
Brent AE, Braun T, Tabin CJ (2005) Genetic analysis of interactions between the somitic muscle, cartilage and tendon cell lineages during mouse development. Development 132(3):515–528
Bruggeman BJ, Maier JA, Mohiuddin YS, Powers R, Lo Y, Guimaraes-Camboa N, Evans SM, Harfe BD (2012) Avian intervertebral disc arises from rostral sclerotome and lacks a nucleus pulposus: implications for evolution of the vertebrate disc. Dev Dyn 241(4): 675–683
Burgess R, Rawls A, Brown D, Bradley A, Olson EN (1996) Requirement of the paraxis gene for somite formation and musculoskeletal patterning. Nature 384(6609):570–573
Burke AC, Nelson CE, Morgan BA, Tabin C (1995) Hox genes and the evolution of vertebrate axial morphology. Development 121(2):333–346
Candia AF, Watabe T, Hawley SH, Onichtchouk D, Zhang Y, Derynck R, Niehrs C, Cho KW (1997) Cellular interpretation of multiple TGF-beta signals: intracellular antagonism between activin/BVg1 and BMP-2/4 signaling mediated by Smads. Development 124(22): 4467–4480
Chiang C, Litingtung Y, Lee E, Young KE, Corden JL, Westphal H, Beachy PA (1996) Cyclopia and defective axial patterning in mice lacking Sonic hedgehog gene function. Nature 383(6599):407–413
Choi K-S, Harfe BD (2011) Hedgehog signaling is required for formation of the notochord sheath and patterning of nuclei pulposi within the intervertebral discs. Proc Natl Acad Sci 108(23):9484–9489
Choi KS, Cohn MJ, Harfe BD (2008) Identification of nucleus pulposus precursor cells and notochordal remnants in the mouse: implications for disk degeneration and chordoma formation. Dev Dyn 237(12):3953–3958
Christ B, Ordahl CP (1995) Early stages of chick somite development. Anat Embryol (Berl) 191(5):381–396
Christ B, Scaal M (2008) Formation and differentiation of avian somite derivatives. Adv Exp Med Biol 638:1–41
Christ B, Huang R, Wilting J (2000) The development of the avian vertebral column. Anat Embryol (Berl) 202(3):179–194
Christ B, Huang R, Scaal M (2004) Formation and differentiation of the avian sclerotome. Anat Embryol (Berl) 208(5):333–350
Christ B, Huang R, Scaal M (2007) Amniote somite derivatives. Dev Dyn 236(9):2382–2396
Clarke RA, Singh S, Mckenzie H, Kearsley JH, Yip MY (1995) Familial Klippel-Feil syndrome and paracentric inversion Inv(8)(Q22.2q23.3). Am J Hum Genet 57(6):1364–1370
Colbjorn Larsen K, Fuchtbauer EM, Brand-Saberi B (2006) The neural tube is required to maintain primary segmentation in the sclerotome. Cells Tissues Organs 182(1):12–21
Conlon RA, Reaume AG, Rossant J (1995) Notch1 is required for the coordinate segmentation of somites. Development 121(5): 1533–1545
Cooke J, Zeeman EC (1976) A clock and wavefront model for control of the number of repeated structures during animal morphogenesis. J Theor Biol 58(2):455–476
Couly GF, Coltey PM, Le Douarin NM (1993) The triple origin of skull in higher vertebrates: a study in quail-chick chimeras. Development 117(2):409–429
Crossin KL, Hoffman S, Grumet M, Thiery JP, Edelman GM (1986) Site-restricted expression of cytotactin during development of the chicken embryo. J Cell Biol 102(5):1917–1930
Dahia CL, Mahoney EJ, Durrani AA, Wylie C (2009) Intercellular signaling pathways active during intervertebral disc growth, differentiation, and aging. Spine (Phila Pa 1976) 34(5):456–462
Dale RM, Topczewski J (2011) Identification of an evolutionarily conserved regulatory element of the zebrafish col2a1a gene. Dev Biol 357(2):518–531
Dao DY, Yang X, Flick LM, Chen D, Hilton MJ, O'Keefe RJ (2010) Axin2 regulates chondrocyte maturation and axial skeletal development. J Orthop Res 28(1):89–95
Dequeant ML, Glynn E, Gaudenz K, Wahl M, Chen J, Mushegian A, Pourquie O (2006) A complex oscillating network of signaling genes underlies the mouse segmentation clock. Science 314(5805):1595–1598
Diez del Corral R, Olivera-Martinez I, Goriely A, Gale E, Maden M, Storey K (2003) Opposing FGF and retinoid pathways control ventral neural pattern, neuronal differentiation, and segmentation during body axis extension. Neuron 40(1):65–79

DiPaola CP, Farmer JC, Manova K, Niswander LA (2005) Molecular signaling in intervertebral disk development. J Orthop Res 23(5):1112–1119. doi:10.1016/j.orthres.2005.03.008

Dobrovolskaia-Zavadskaia N (1927) Sur la mortification spotanee de la chez la souris nouvau-nee et sur l'existence d'un caractere (facteur) herededitaire, non-viable. CR Soc Biol 97:114–116

Dockter JL (2000) Sclerotome induction and differentiation. Curr Top Dev Biol 48:77–127

Dockter J, Ordahl CP (2000) Dorsoventral axis determination in the somite: a re-examination. Development 127(10):2201–2206

Duband JL, Dufour S, Hatta K, Takeichi M, Edelman GM, Thiery JP (1987) Adhesion molecules during somitogenesis in the avian embryo. J Cell Biol 104(5):1361–1374

Dubrulle J, Pourquie O (2004) fgf8 mRNA decay establishes a gradient that couples axial elongation to patterning in the vertebrate embryo. Nature 427(6973):419–422

Dubrulle J, McGrew MJ, Pourquie O (2001) FGF signaling controls somite boundary position and regulates segmentation clock control of spatiotemporal Hox gene activation. Cell 106(2):219–232

Erwin WM (2010) The enigma that is the nucleus pulposus cell: the search goes on. Arthritis Res Ther 12(3):118

Evrard YA, Lun Y, Aulehla A, Gan L, Johnson RL (1998) Lunatic fringe is an essential mediator of somite segmentation and patterning. Nature 394(6691):377–381

Ewan KB, Everett AW (1992) Evidence for resegmentation in the formation of the vertebral column using the novel approach of retroviral-mediated gene transfer. Exp Cell Res 198(2):315–320

Fan C-M, Tessier-Lavigne M (1994) Patterning of mammalian somites by surface ectoderm and notochord: evidence for sclerotome induction by a hedgehog homolog. Cell 79(7):1175–1186

Ferrer-Vaquer A, Viotti M, Hadjantonakis A-K (2010) Transitions between epithelial and mesenchymal states and the morphogenesis of the early mouse embryo. Cell Adh Migr 4(3):447–457

Forsberg H, Crozet F, Brown NA (1998) Waves of mouse Lunatic fringe expression, in four-hour cycles at two-hour intervals, precede somite boundary formation. Curr Biol 8(18):1027–1030

Gadjanski I, Spiller K, Vunjak-Novakovic G (2012) Time-dependent processes in stem cell-based tissue engineering of articular cartilage. Stem Cell Rev 8(3):863–881

Gilson A, Dreger M, Urban JP (2010) Differential expression level of cytokeratin 8 in cells of the bovine nucleus pulposus complicates the search for specific intervertebral disc cell markers. Arthritis Res Ther 12(1):R24

Glazier JA, Zhang Y, Swat M, Zaitlen B, Schnell S (2008) Coordinated action of N-CAM, N-cadherin, EphA4, and ephrinB2 translates genetic prepatterns into structure during somitogenesis in chick. Curr Top Dev Biol 81:205–247

Goldstein RS, Kalcheim C (1992) Determination of epithelial half-somites in skeletal morphogenesis. Development 116(2):441–445

Gotz W, Osmers R, Herken R (1995) Localisation of extracellular matrix components in the embryonic human notochord and axial mesenchyme. J Anat 186(Pt 1):111–121

Haga Y, Dominique VJ, Du SJ (2009) Analyzing notochord segmentation and intervertebral disc formation using the twhh:gfp transgenic zebrafish model. Transgenic Res 18(5):669–683

Hayes AJ, Ralphs JR (2011) The response of foetal annulus fibrosus cells to growth factors: modulation of matrix synthesis by TGF-beta1 and IGF-1. Histochem Cell Biol 136(2):163–175

Hayes AJ, Benjamin M, Ralphs JR (1999) Role of actin stress fibres in the development of the intervertebral disc: cytoskeletal control of extracellular matrix assembly. Dev Dyn 215(3):179–189

Hayes AJ, Isaacs MD, Hughes C, Caterson B, Ralphs JR (2011) Collagen fibrillogenesis in the development of the annulus fibrosus of the intervertebral disc. Eur Cell Mater 22:226–241

Huang R, Zhi Q, Wilting J, Christ B (1994) The fate of somitocoele cells in avian embryos. Anat Embryol (Berl) 190(3):243–250

Huang R, Zhi Q, Brand-Saberi B, Christ B (2000) New experimental evidence for somite resegmentation. Anat Embryol (Berl) 202(3):195–200

Iimura T, Denans N, Pourquié O (2009) Chapter 7, Establishment of Hox vertebral identities in the embryonic spine precursors. In: Olivier P (ed) Current topics in developmental biology, vol 88. Academic, New York, pp 201–234

Ingham PW, McMahon AP (2001) Hedgehog signaling in animal development: paradigms and principles. Genes Dev 15(23):3059–3087

Inohaya K, Takano Y, Kudo A (2007) The teleost intervertebral region acts as a growth center of the centrum: in vivo visualization of osteoblasts and their progenitors in transgenic fish. Dev Dyn 236(11):3031–3046

Jin H, Shen J, Wang B, Wang M, Shu B, Chen D (2011) TGF-beta signaling plays an essential role in the growth and maintenance of intervertebral disc tissue. FEBS Lett 585(8):1209–1215

Johnson RL, Laufer E, Riddle RD, Tabin C (1994) Ectopic expression of Sonic hedgehog alters dorsal-ventral patterning of somites. Cell 79(7):1165–1173

Johnson J, Rhee J, Parsons SM, Brown D, Olson EN, Rawls A (2001) The anterior/posterior polarity of somites is disrupted in paraxis-deficient mice. Dev Biol 229(1):176–187, S0012-1606(00)99969-X [pii]

Johnston SH, Rauskolb C, Wilson R, Prabhakaran B, Irvine KD, Vogt TF (1997) A family of mammalian Fringe genes implicated in boundary determination and the Notch pathway. Development 124(11):2245–2254

Kaplan KM, Spivak JM, Bendo JA (2005) Embryology of the spine and associated congenital abnormalities. Spine J 5(5):564–576

Karasugi T, Semba K, Hirose Y, Kelempisioti A, Nakajima M, Miyake A, Furuichi T, Kawaguchi Y, Mikami Y, Chiba K, Kamata M, Ozaki K, Takahashi A, Makela P, Karppinen J, Kimura T, Kubo T, Toyama Y, Yamamura K, Mannikko M, Mizuta H, Ikegawa S (2009) Association of the tag SNPs in the human SKT gene (KIAA1217) with lumbar disc herniation. J Bone Miner Res 24(9):1537–1543

Kawakami Y, Raya A, Raya RM, Rodriguez-Esteban C, Belmonte JC (2005) Retinoic acid signalling links left-right asymmetric patterning and bilaterally symmetric somitogenesis in the zebrafish embryo. Nature 435(7039):165–171

Keller R (2000) The origin and morphogenesis of amphibian somites. Curr Top Dev Biol 47(47):183–244

Kessel M, Gruss P (1991) Homeotic transformations of murine vertebrae and concomitant alteration of Hox codes induced by retinoic acid. Cell 67(1):89–104

Kim DW, Lassar AB (2003) Smad-dependent recruitment of a histone deacetylase/Sin3A complex modulates the bone morphogenetic protein-dependent transcriptional repressor activity of Nkx3.2. Mol Cell Biol 23(23):8704–8717

Kim KW, Lim TH, Kim JG, Jeong ST, Masuda K, An HS (2003) The origin of chondrocytes in the nucleus pulposus and histologic findings associated with the transition of a notochordal nucleus pulposus to a fibrocartilaginous nucleus pulposus in intact rabbit intervertebral discs. Spine (Phila Pa 1976) 28(10):982–990

Kim JH, Deasy BM, Seo HY, Studer RK, Vo NV, Georgescu HI, Sowa GA, Kang JD (2009) Differentiation of intervertebral notochordal cells through live automated cell imaging system in vitro. Spine (Phila Pa 1976) 34(23):2486–2493

Kispert A, Herrmann BG, Leptin M, Reuter R (1994) Homologs of the mouse Brachyury gene are involved in the specification of posterior terminal structures in Drosophila, Tribolium, and Locusta. Genes Dev 8(18):2137–2150

Klippel M, Feil A (1975) The classic: a case of absence of cervical vertebrae with the thoracic cage rising to the base of the cranium (cervical thoracic cage). Clin Orthop Relat Res 109:3–8

Kmita M, Duboule D (2003) Organizing axes in time and space; 25 years of colinear tinkering. Science 301(5631):331–333

Kondo N, Yuasa T, Shimono K, Tung W, Okabe T, Yasuhara R, Pacifici M, Zhang Y, Iwamoto M, Enomoto-Iwamoto M (2011) Intervertebral disc development is regulated by Wnt/beta-catenin signaling. Spine (Phila Pa 1976) 36(8):E513–E518

Koob TJ, Long JH (2000) The vertebrate body axis: evolution and mechanical function. Am Zool 40(1):1–18

Lee CR, Sakai D, Nakai T, Toyama K, Mochida J, Alini M, Grad S (2007) A phenotypic comparison of intervertebral disc and articular cartilage cells in the rat. Eur Spine J 16(12):2174–2185

Lefebvre V (2002) Toward understanding the functions of the two highly related Sox5 and Sox6 genes. J Bone Miner Metab 20(3):121–130

Lenas P, Moos M, Luyten FP (2009a) Developmental engineering: a new paradigm for the design and manufacturing of cell-based products. Part I: from three-dimensional cell growth to biomimetics of in vivo development. Tissue Eng Part B Rev 15(4):381–394

Lenas P, Moos M, Luyten FP (2009b) Developmental engineering: a new paradigm for the design and manufacturing of cell-based products. Part II: from genes to networks: tissue engineering from the viewpoint of systems biology and network science. Tissue Eng Part B Rev 15(4):395–422

Lenas P, Luyten FP, Doblare M, Nicodemou-Lena E, Lanzara AE (2011) Modularity in developmental biology and artificial organs: a missing concept in tissue engineering. Artif Organs 35(6):656–662

Lettice LA, Purdie LA, Carlson GJ, Kilanowski F, Dorin J, Hill RE (1999) The mouse bagpipe gene controls development of axial skeleton, skull, and spleen. Proc Natl Acad Sci U S A 96(17):9695–9700

Li L, Krantz ID, Deng Y, Genin A, Banta AB, Collins CC, Qi M, Trask BJ, Kuo WL, Cochran J, Costa T, Pierpont ME, Rand EB, Piccoli DA, Hood L, Spinner NB (1997) Alagille syndrome is caused by mutations in human Jagged1, which encodes a ligand for Notch1. Nat Genet 16(3):243–251

Li TF, Darowish M, Zuscik MJ, Chen D, Schwarz EM, Rosier RN, Drissi H, O'Keefe RJ (2006) Smad3-deficient chondrocytes have enhanced BMP signaling and accelerated differentiation. J Bone Miner Res 21(1):4–16

Mansouri A, Pla P, Larue L, Gruss P (2001) Pax3 acts cell autonomously in the neural tube and somites by controlling cell surface properties. Development 128(11):1995–2005

Marcelle C, Ahlgren S, Bronner-Fraser M (1999) In vivo regulation of somite differentiation and proliferation by sonic hedgehog. Dev Biol 214(2):277–287

McCann MR, Tamplin OJ, Rossant J, Seguin CA (2012) Tracing notochord-derived cells using a Noto-cre mouse: implications for intervertebral disc development. Dis Model Mech 5

McGaughran JM, Oates A, Donnai D, Read AP, Tassabehji M (2003) Mutations in PAX1 may be associated with Klippel-Feil syndrome. Eur J Hum Genet 11(6):468–474

Minogue BM, Richardson SM, Zeef LA, Freemont AJ, Hoyland JA (2010) Characterization of the human nucleus pulposus cell phenotype and evaluation of novel marker gene expression to define adult stem cell differentiation. Arthritis Rheum 62(12):3695–3705

Mittapalli VR, Huang R, Patel K, Christ B, Scaal M (2005) Arthrotome: a specific joint forming compartment in the avian somite. Dev Dyn 234(1):48–53

Monsoro-Burq AH (2005) Sclerotome development and morphogenesis: when experimental embryology meets genetics. Int J Dev Biol 49(2–3):301–308

Monsoro-Burq AH, Bontoux M, Teillet MA, Le Douarin NM (1994) Heterogeneity in the development of the vertebra. Proc Natl Acad Sci U S A 91(22):10435–10439

Moore KL, Oersaud TVN (2003) Before we are born, 6th edn. Saunders, Philadelphia

Morimoto M, Takahashi Y, Endo M, Saga Y (2005) The Mesp2 transcription factor establishes segmental borders by suppressing Notch activity. Nature 435(7040):354–359. doi:10.1038/nature03591

Muller TS, Ebensperger C, Neubuser A, Koseki H, Balling R, Christ B, Wilting J (1996) Expression of avian Pax1 and Pax9 is intrinsically regulated in the pharyngeal endoderm, but depends on environmental influences in the paraxial mesoderm. Dev Biol 178(2):403–417

Murtaugh LC, Chyung JH, Lassar AB (1999) Sonic hedgehog promotes somitic chondrogenesis by altering the cellular response to BMP signaling. Genes Dev 13(2):225–237

Naiche LA, Holder N, Lewandoski M (2011) FGF4 and FGF8 comprise the wavefront activity that controls somitogenesis. Proc Natl Acad Sci 108(10):4018–4023

Oda T, Elkahloun AG, Pike BL, Okajima K, Krantz ID, Genin A, Piccoli DA, Meltzer PS, Spinner NB, Collins FS, Chandrasekharappa SC (1997) Mutations in the human Jagged1 gene are responsible for Alagille syndrome. Nat Genet 16(3):235–242

Oldershaw RA, Baxter MA, Lowe ET, Bates N, Grady LM, Soncin F, Brison DR, Hardingham TE, Kimber SJ (2010) Directed differentiation of human embryonic stem cells toward chondrocytes. Nat Biotechnol 28(11):1187–1194

Paavola LG, Wilson DB, Center EM (1980) Histochemistry of the developing notochord, perichordal sheath and vertebrae in Danforth's short-tail (sd) and normal C57BL/6 mice. J Embryol Exp Morphol 55:227–245

Palmeirim I, Henrique D, Ish-Horowicz D, Pourquié O (1997) Avian hairy gene expression identifies a molecular clock linked to vertebrate segmentation and somitogenesis. Cell 91(5):639–648

Patil AS, Sable RB, Kothari RM (2011) An update on transforming growth factor-beta (TGF-beta): sources, types, functions and clinical applicability for cartilage/bone healing. J Cell Physiol 226(12):3094–3103

Peacock A (1951) Observations on the prenatal development of the intervertebral disc in man. J Anat 85(3):260–274

Pelton RW, Dickinson ME, Moses HL, Hogan BL (1990) In situ hybridization analysis of TGF beta 3 RNA expression during mouse development: comparative studies with TGF beta 1 and beta 2. Development 110(2):609–620

Peters H, Wilm B, Sakai N, Imai K, Maas R, Balling R (1999) Pax1 and Pax9 synergistically regulate vertebral column development. Development 126(23):5399–5408

Pourquie O (2011) Vertebrate segmentation: from cyclic gene networks to scoliosis. Cell 145(5):650–663

Radice GL, Rayburn H, Matsunami H, Knudsen KA, Takeichi M, Hynes RO (1997) Developmental defects in mouse embryos lacking N-cadherin. Dev Biol 181(1):64–78

Reaume AG, Conlon RA, Zirngibl R, Yamaguchi TP, Rossant J (1992) Expression analysis of a Notch homologue in the mouse embryo. Dev Biol 154(2):377–387

Rider CC, Mulloy B (2010) Bone morphogenetic protein and growth differentiation factor cytokine families and their protein antagonists. Biochem J 429(1):1–12

Risbud MV, Schaer TP, Shapiro IM (2010) Toward an understanding of the role of notochordal cells in the adult intervertebral disc: from discord to accord. Dev Dyn 239(8):2141–2148

Rodrigo I, Hill RE, Balling R, Munsterberg A, Imai K (2003) Pax1 and Pax9 activate Bapx1 to induce chondrogenic differentiation in the sclerotome. Development 130(3):473–482

Rufai A, Benjamin M, Ralphs JR (1995) The development of fibrocartilage in the rat intervertebral disc. Anat Embryol (Berl) 192(1):53–62

Saga Y (2007) Segmental border is defined by the key transcription factor Mesp2, by means of the suppression of notch activity. Dev Dyn 236(6):1450–1455

Saga Y, Hata N, Koseki H, Taketo MM (1997) Mesp2: a novel mouse gene expressed in the presegmented mesoderm and essential for segmentation initiation. Genes Dev 11(14):1827–1839

Sakai Y, Meno C, Fujii H, Nishino J, Shiratori H, Saijoh Y, Rossant J, Hamada H (2001) The retinoic acid-inactivating enzyme CYP26 is essential for establishing an uneven distribution of retinoic acid along the anterio-posterior axis within the mouse embryo. Genes Dev 15(2):213–225

Sakai D, Nakai T, Mochida J, Alini M, Grad S (2009) Differential phenotype of intervertebral disc cells: microarray and immunohistochemical analysis of canine nucleus pulposus and anulus fibrosus. Spine (Phila Pa 1976) 34(14):1448–1456

Sasaki N, Kiso M, Kitagawa M, Saga Y (2011) The repression of Notch signaling occurs via the destabilization of mastermind-like 1 by Mesp2 and is essential for somitogenesis. Development 138(1):55–64

Sawada A, Shinya M, Jiang YJ, Kawakami A, Kuroiwa A, Takeda H (2001) Fgf/MAPK signalling is a crucial positional cue in somite boundary formation. Development 128(23):4873–4880

Scaal M, Wiegreffe C (2006) Somite compartments in anamniotes. Anat Embryol (Berl) 211(Suppl 1):9–19

Schweitzer R, Chyung JH, Murtaugh LC, Brent AE, Rosen V, Olson EN, Lassar A, Tabin CJ (2001) Analysis of the tendon cell fate using Scleraxis, a specific marker for tendons and ligaments. Development 128(19):3855–3866

Scotti C, Tonnarelli B, Papadimitropoulos A, Scherberich A, Schaeren S, Schauerte A, Lopez-Rios J, Zeller R, Barbero A, Martin I (2010) Recapitulation of endochondral bone formation using human adult mesenchymal stem cells as a paradigm for developmental engineering. Proc Natl Acad Sci U S A 107(16):7251–7256

Semba K, Araki K, Li Z, Matsumoto K, Suzuki M, Nakagata N, Takagi K, Takeya M, Yoshinobu K, Araki M, Imai K, Abe K, Yamamura K (2006) A novel murine gene, Sickle tail, linked to the Danforth's short tail locus, is required for normal development of the intervertebral disc. Genetics 172(1):445–456

Senthinathan B, Sousa C, Tannahill D, Keynes R (2012) The generation of vertebral segmental patterning in the chick embryo. J Anat 220(6):591–602

Serra R, Chang C (2003) TGF-beta signaling in human skeletal and patterning disorders. Birth Defects Res C Embryo Today 69(4):333–351

Serra R, Johnson M, Filvaroff EH, LaBorde J, Sheehan DM, Derynck R, Moses HL (1997) Expression of a truncated, kinase-defective TGF-b type II receptor in mouse skeletal tissue promotes terminal chondrocyte differentiation and osteoarthritis. J Cell Biol 139:541–552

Settle SH Jr, Rountree RB, Sinha A, Thacker A, Higgins K, Kingsley DM (2003) Multiple joint and skeletal patterning defects caused by single and double mutations in the mouse Gdf6 and Gdf5 genes. Dev Biol 254(1):116–130

Shapiro IM, Risbud MV (2010) Transcriptional profiling of the nucleus pulposus: say yes to notochord. Arthritis Res Ther 12(3):117

Shen B, Bhargav D, Wei A, Williams LA, Tao H, Ma DD, Diwan AD (2009) BMP-13 emerges as a potential inhibitor of bone formation. Int J Biol Sci 5(2):192–200

Shi S, Ciurli C, Cartman A, Pidoux I, Poole AR, Zhang Y (2003) Experimental immunity to the G1 domain of the proteoglycan versican induces spondylitis and sacroiliitis, of a kind seen in human spondylarthropathies. Arthritis Rheum 48(10):2903–2915

Shifley ET, Cole SE (2007) The vertebrate segmentation clock and its role in skeletal birth defects. Birth Defects Res C Embryo Today 81(2):121–133

Sirbu IO, Duester G (2006) Retinoic-acid signalling in node ectoderm and posterior neural plate directs left-right patterning of somitic mesoderm. Nat Cell Biol 8(3):271–277

Smits P, Lefebvre V (2003) Sox5 and Sox6 are required for notochord extracellular matrix sheath formation, notochord cell survival and development of the nucleus pulposus of intervertebral discs. Development 130(6):1135–1148

Smits P, Li P, Mandel J, Zhang Z, Deng JM, Behringer RR, de Crombrugghe B, Lefebvre V (2001) The transcription factors L-Sox5 and Sox6 are essential for cartilage formation. Dev Cell 1(2):277–290

Sohn P, Cox M, Chen D, Serra R (2010) Molecular profiling of the developing mouse axial skeleton: a role for Tgfbr2 in the development of the intervertebral disc. BMC Dev Biol 10(1):29

Sporle R, Schughart K (1998) Paradox segmentation along inter- and intrasomitic borderlines is followed by dysmorphology of the axial skeleton in the open brain (opb) mouse mutant. Dev Genet 22(4):359–373

Stafford DA, Brunet LJ, Khokha MK, Economides AN, Harland RM (2011) Cooperative activity of noggin and gremlin 1 in axial skeleton development. Development 138(5):1005–1014

Stemple DL (2005) Structure and function of the notochord: an essential organ for chordate development. Development 132(11):2503–2512

Stott D, Kispert A, Herrmann BG (1993) Rescue of the tail defect of Brachyury mice. Genes Dev 7(2):197–203

Swiatek PJ, Lindsell CE, del Amo FF, Weinmaster G, Gridley T (1994) Notch1 is essential for postimplantation development in mice. Genes Dev 8(6):707–719

Swiderski RE, Solursh M (1992) Localization of type II collagen, long form alpha 1(IX) collagen, and short form alpha 1(IX) collagen transcripts in the developing chick notochord and axial skeleton. Dev Dyn 194(2):118–127. doi:10.1002/aja.1001940205

Tassabehji M, Fang ZM, Hilton EN, McGaughran J, Zhao Z, de Bock CE, Howard E, Malass M, Donnai D, Diwan A, Manson FDC, Murrell D, Clarke RA (2008) Mutations in GDF6 are associated with vertebral segmentation defects in Klippel-Feil syndrome. Hum Mutat 29(8):1017–1027

Theiler K (1988) Vertebral malformations. Adv Anat Embryol Cell Biol 112:1–99

Tracy MR, Dormans JP, Kusumi K (2004) Klippel-Feil syndrome: clinical features and current understanding of etiology. Clin Orthop Relat Res 424:183–190

Tribioli C, Lufkin T (1999) The murine Bapx1 homeobox gene plays a critical role in embryonic development of the axial skeleton and spleen. Development 126(24):5699–5711

Turnpenny PD (2008) Defective somitogenesis and abnormal vertebral segmentation in man. Adv Exp Med Biol 638:164–189

Vermot J, Pourquie O (2005) Retinoic acid coordinates somitogenesis and left-right patterning in vertebrate embryos. Nature 435(7039):215–220

Vermot J, Gallego Llamas J, Fraulob V, Niederreither K, Chambon P, Dolle P (2005) Retinoic acid controls the bilateral symmetry of somite formation in the mouse embryo. Science 308(5721):563–566

Vilhais-Neto GC, Maruhashi M, Smith KT, Vasseur-Cognet M, Peterson AS, Workman JL, Pourquie O (2010) Rere controls retinoic acid signalling and somite bilateral symmetry. Nature 463(7283):953–957

Vujovic S, Henderson S, Presneau N, Odell E, Jacques TS, Tirabosco R, Boshoff C, Flanagan AM (2006) Brachyury, a crucial regulator of notochordal development, is a novel biomarker for chordomas. J Pathol 209(2):157–165

Wahl MB, Deng C, Lewandoski M, Pourquié O (2007) FGF signaling acts upstream of the NOTCH and WNT signaling pathways to control segmentation clock oscillations in mouse somitogenesis. Development 134(22):4033–4041

Wamsley R (1953) Development and growth of the intervertebral disc. Edinb Med J 60:341–363

Wei A, Williams LA, Bhargav D, Shen B, Kishen T, Duffy N, Diwan AD (2009) BMP13 prevents the effects of annular injury in an ovine model. Int J Biol Sci 5(5):388–396

Wellik DM (2007) Hox patterning of the vertebrate axial skeleton. Dev Dyn 236(9):2454–2463

Wellik DM (2009) Chapter 9, Hox genes and vertebrate axial pattern. In: Olivier P (ed) Current topics in developmental biology, vol 88. Academic, New York, pp 257–278

Wiggan O, Fadel MP, Hamel PA (2002) Pax3 induces cell aggregation and regulates phenotypic mesenchymal-epithelial interconversion. J Cell Sci 115(Pt 3):517–529

Willard DP, Nicholson JT (1934) The Klippel-Feil syndrome. Ann Surg 99(4):561–567

Williams LW (1910) The somites of the chick. Am J Anat 11:55–100

Wrana JL, Attisano L, Wieser R, Ventura F, Massague J (1994) Mechanism of activation of the TGF-beta receptor. Nature 370(6488):341–347

Yang XR, Ng D, Alcorta DA, Liebsch NJ, Sheridan E, Li S, Goldstein AM, Parry DM, Kelley MJ (2009) T (brachyury) gene duplication confers major susceptibility to familial chordoma. Nat Genet 41(11):1176–1178

Yoon BS, Ovchinnikov DA, Yoshii I, Mishina Y, Behringer RR, Lyons KM (2005) Bmpr1a and Bmpr1b have overlapping functions and are essential for chondrogenesis in vivo. Proc Natl Acad Sci U S A 102(14):5062–5067

Ytteborg E, Torgerson J, Baeverfjord G, Takle H (2012) Chapter 14, The Atlantic salmon (Salmo salar) vertebra and cellular pathways to vertebral deformities. In: Carvalho ED, David GS, Silva RJ (eds) Health and environment in aquaculture. Intech, Rijeka

Zakany J, Kmita M, Alarcon P, de la Pompa JL, Duboule D (2001) Localized and transient transcription of Hox genes suggests a link between patterning and the segmentation clock. Cell 106(2):207–217

Zakin L, Metzinger CA, Chang EY, Coffinier C, De Robertis EM (2008) Development of the vertebral morphogenetic field in the mouse: interactions between Crossveinless-2 and Twisted Gastrulation. Dev Biol 323(1):6–18

Zakin L, Chang EY, Plouhinec JL, De Robertis EM (2010) Crossveinless-2 is required for the relocalization of Chordin protein within the vertebral field in mouse embryos. Dev Biol 347(1):204–215

Zeng L, Kempf H, Murtaugh LC, Sato ME, Lassar AB (2002) Shh establishes an Nkx3.2/Sox9 autoregulatory loop that is maintained by BMP signals to induce somitic chondrogenesis. Genes Dev 16(15):1990–2005. doi:10.1101/gad.1008002

Zhang N, Gridley T (1998) Defects in somite formation in lunatic fringe-deficient mice. Nature 394(6691):374–377

Proteoglycans of the Intervertebral Disc

4

James Melrose and Peter Roughley

Contents

J. Melrose (✉)
Kolling Institute (B6), Level 10,
Royal NorthShore Hospital,
St. Leonards, New South Wales 2065, Australia
e-mail: james.melrose@sydney.edu.au

P. Roughley
Genetics Unit, Shriners Hospital for Children,
1529 Cedar Avenue, Montreal, QC, Canada H3G 1A6
e-mail: proughley@shriners.mcgill.ca

I.M. Shapiro, M.V. Risbud (eds.), *The Intervertebral Disc*,
DOI 10.1007/978-3-7091-1535-0_4, © Springer-Verlag Wien 2014

4.1 Introduction

Proteoglycans are present within the extracellular matrix (ECM) of the intervertebral disc and on the surface of its cells. The disc possesses many matrix proteoglycans, with most also being present in hyaline cartilages. The best studied of these are aggrecan and versican (members of the hyalectan/lectican family) and decorin, biglycan, fibromodulin, lumican, PRELP, and chondroadherin (members of the small leucine-rich repeat protein/SLRP family). More recently, the disc has also been shown to contain perlecan and lubricin, which were previously thought to be characteristic of basement membranes and the surface of articular cartilage, respectively. Much less is known about the disc cell-associated proteoglycans, though it is likely that several members of the syndecan (Tkachenko et al. 2005) and glypican (Fransson et al. 2004) families will be present, together with other unrelated proteoglycans such as NG2 (Akeda et al. 2007; Stallcup 2002). While little is known concerning the specific function of the cell-associated proteoglycans within the disc, it has been shown that syndecan-4 expression is increased when elevated levels of interleukin-1 (IL-1) or tumor necrosis factor-α (TNF-α) are present (Wang et al. 2011), and that it may play a role in promoting aggrecanase-mediated proteolysis within the disc. However, due to the scarcity of information on disc cell-associated proteoglycans, this chapter will focus on the matrix proteoglycans, in particular aggrecan.

4.2 Glycosaminoglycan Structure and Function

Proteoglycans can be considered as specialized glycoproteins and are a ubiquitous component of all tissues. They are distinguished from other glycoproteins by the substitution of their core protein with sulfated glycosaminoglycan (GAG) chains (Box 4.1), though they may also possess more typical *O*-linked and N-linked oligosaccharides (Nilsson et al. 1982). The sulfated GAGs can be divided into three families – chondroitin sulfate/dermatan sulfate (CS/DS), keratan sulfate (KS), and heparan sulfate/heparin (HS/Hep) (Jackson et al. 1991). While many proteoglycans possess GAGs from only one family, some proteoglycans possess GAGs from different families.

CS is a copolymer of glucuronic acid and *N*-acetylgalactosamine, with the latter commonly being sulfated at the 4 or 6 position. DS is initially synthesized as CS, but during processing in the Golgi, some of the glucuronic acid is epimerized to iduronic acid, which may be sulfated at the 2 position. KS is a copolymer of galactose and *N*-acetylglucosamine and may be sulfated at the 6 position on either residue. HS is a copolymer of glucuronic acid or iduronic acid and *N*-acetylglucosamine, in which the iduronic acid may be sulfated at its 2 position and the *N*-acetylglucosamine may be sulfated at the 3 and 6 positions. On some glucosamine residues, N-sulfation may replace the N-acetyl group. In heparin, the presence of iduronic acid and O- and N-sulfation is high. As there is no template for GAG synthesis, GAG chain length, degree and position of sulfation, and degree of epimerization can vary enormously, both between different proteoglycans and on the same proteoglycan at different sites.

GAG chains have traditionally been considered structural electrorepulsive entities of connective tissues. This is due to their repeating charged disaccharide and sulfated sugar motifs or as agents which provide a high fixed charge density in the tissues. As such due to GAG-associated counterions and the Donnan equilibrium effect, they are responsible for the water-regain properties of tissues. With the emerging concept of the sugar code, with the realization that dynamic structural changes in HS produce a characteristic (nonrandom) heparanome, these charged sugars may also be involved in information storage and transfer (Cummings 2009). The biological importance of chondroitin sulfation during mammalian development and growth factor signaling is poorly understood (Caterson 2012; Caterson et al. 1990), although chondroitin 4-*O*-sulfation is required for proper CS localization and modulation of distinct signaling pathways during growth plate morphogenesis (Kluppel et al. 2005). On this basis, chondroitin sulfation has emerging biological roles in mammalian development. The elucidation of the intimate interplay of GAG chains with a variety of specific bioactive binding partners triggering cell signaling, cell proliferation, matrix production, and differentiation underscores the range of functionalities which may all be affected (Turnbull 2010). Accordingly, GAG chains are versatile tools for information storage and transfer and represent a new paradigm in developmental biology.

Due to differences in either synthesis or degradation, each proteoglycan does not possess a unique structure: both the core protein and the GAG chains may vary with site, age, and pathology. Synthetic changes occurring within the cell are most commonly associated with the GAG chains, but splicing variations (Fulop et al. 1993) or the use of alternative transcription start sites (Muragaki et al. 1990) may also influence the structure of the core protein of some proteoglycans. In contrast, degradative changes occurring within the matrix are most commonly associated with processing of the core proteins by proteinases, although modification of GAGs by extracellular sulfatases or glycosidases has been reported (Vlodavsky et al. 1999). Irrespective of their origin, all types of structural change have the potential to influence proteoglycan function.

Proteoglycans have been classified by the type of GAG chain that they possess or by their location within the tissue. In terms of location, the division is commonly between proteoglycans that reside in the ECM and those associated with the cell. Matrix proteoglycans are often substituted with CS, DS, or KS, whereas cell-associated proteoglycans are often linked with HS. Heparin is usually only defined in relationship to the serglycin proteoglycan present within mast cells (Humphries and Stevens 1992) but can be structurally similar to regions of highly sulfated and epimerized HS present on other proteoglycans (Girardin et al. 2005). CS and HS may replace one another at the same site on some proteoglycans, as they share the same amino acid substitution motif (Ser-Gly) and linkage oligosaccharide (Xyl-Gal-Gal-GlcA). In contrast, KS has two different substitution motifs and linkage oligosaccharides, which it shares with *O*-linked and N-linked oligosaccharides.

Box 4.1: A Historical Perspective of Glycosaminoglycans and Proteoglycans

The existence of glycosaminoglycans has been known since the 1860s when chondroitin sulfate was first described in cartilage. Discovery of the other glycosaminoglycans did not occur until the twentieth century, with many owing their discovery to the work of Karl Meyer. Meyer described the existence of hyaluronic acid in the vitreous humor of the eye in 1934, dermatan sulfate in skin in 1941, and keratan sulfate in the cornea in 1953. Heparin was first described in 1916 because of its anticoagulant activity, and the structurally related heparan sulfate in 1948. However, modern terminology was not in use by the 1950s when the glycosaminoglycans were referred to as mucopolysaccharides which formed the ground substance of connective tissues. This name persists today with "the mucopolysaccharidoses," a group of heritable disorders due to gene defects in specific lysosomal glycosyltransferases, glycosidases, and sulfatases responsible for glycosaminoglycan assembly and catabolism. Similarly, the original terminology for some of the mucopolysaccharides was also different, with dermatan sulfate being referred to as chondroitin sulfate B and heparan sulfate as heparitin sulfate or heparin monosulfate. Once the structure of all the mucopolysaccharides was established, and it was appreciated that they were all copolymers of a sugar and an amino sugar, the term glycosaminoglycan came into use. In addition, until the 1950s it was not appreciated that the sulfated glycosaminoglycans were attached to protein, and considerable effort was made to purify them from this "contamination." It was in 1958 that Helen Muir proved that chondroitin sulfate in cartilage was covalently attached to protein via a serine residue, and the proteoglycan era was born. However, initially the term protein polysaccharide was used. In 1966, Lennart Roden described the structure of the trisaccharide which links the chondroitin sulfate with its serine core protein attachment point. This attachment region is now known to be common to all the sulfated glycosaminoglycans, with the exception of keratan sulfate, irrespective of the proteoglycan core to which the glycosaminoglycan is attached.

4.3 Aggrecan

Aggrecan is a KS/CS proteoglycan that was originally isolated from hyaline cartilage and the gene was cloned from chondrosarcoma cells (Doege et al. 1987). It was later shown to be present in the intervertebral disc and to be synthesized by disc cells. On a weight basis, aggrecan is the most abundant proteoglycan in both the disc and cartilage and has probably been more extensively studied than any other proteoglycan. Aggrecan belongs to the family of hyaluronan (HA)-binding proteoglycans, together with versican, neurocan, and brevican (Margolis and Margolis 1994). All family members possess an amino terminal globular domain responsible for interaction with HA and a carboxy terminal globular domain containing a lectin homology domain. These common features give rise to the alternative family names of hyalectins and lecticans. The interaction with HA permits the formation of proteoglycan aggregates (Morgelin et al. 1988), and it was this ability to form proteoglycan aggregates that led to the name aggrecan.

Aggrecan provides the disc with its ability to resist compressive loading on the spine, causing the disc to swell and keep the vertebrae apart. The acquisition of a biped vertical posture resulted in loading of the spine due to gravity. Partial removal of this load at night and the imbibition of tissue fluid result in swelling of the disc, which accounts for the diurnal variation in disc height (Botsford et al. 1994). The swelling properties of aggrecan are related to its abundance, degree of sulfation, and ability to form proteoglycan aggregates. The swelling is driven principally by the sulfate groups on the GAGs, which attract water into the disc by osmosis. As more water enters the disc, the osmotic properties of the aggrecan decrease, and an equilibrium is attained in which the swelling of the disc is counterbalanced by the tension induced in the collagenous framework of the tissue. On subjecting the disc to compressive load, water is displaced, effectively increasing the aggrecan concentration and its swelling potential. On removal of the load, the increased swelling potential is dissipated by re-imbibition of water into the disc and restoration of the equilibrium state. In addition to the symmetric loading due to gravity, the disc experiences asymmetric compressive loading upon bending. Under asymmetric loading it is essential that the aggrecan cannot diffuse from the site of compression if optimal restoration of disc height is to occur following straightening. The diffusion of aggrecan is related to its size and is minimized by the formation of large proteoglycan aggregates. This topic is discussed further in Chap. 5.

Aggrecan is located throughout the disc, though its abundance at different sites varies greatly with age. In the fetal human spine, aggrecan is prominently immunolocalized in the cartilaginous vertebral rudiment cartilages and in the developing intervertebral disc space (Fig. 4.1) (Smith et al. 2009). The fetal vertebral rudiment cartilages are transient developmental scaffolds which are transformed into ossified structures in the adult spine, while the discs remain as permanent cartilaginous entities. In the human, aggrecan predominates in the nucleus pulposus in the young juvenile. The aggrecan content of the nucleus pulposus increases during juvenile growth and reaches a maximum in the late adolescent/early adult period. During adult life the aggrecan content of the nucleus pulposus declines (Fig. 4.2a). Aging is also associated with an increase in aggrecan abundance in the annulus fibrosus, particularly the inner annulus, and in the mature adult the aggrecan content of the annulus fibrosus may surpass that of the nucleus pulposus. Thus, in the mature adult, the annulus fibrosus is as important as the nucleus pulposus for resisting compression.

4.3.1 Aggrecan Protein Structure and Function

The aggrecan core protein possesses about 2,300 amino acids, which form three disulfide-bonded globular regions with two intervening extended regions (Fig. 4.3a) (Sandy et al. 1990; Watanabe et al. 1998). The amino terminal globular region (G1) responsible for interaction with HA possesses three disulfide-bonded loops. The first loop allows interaction with a link protein (LP) that stabilizes the proteoglycan aggregate (Neame and Barry 1993), and this is

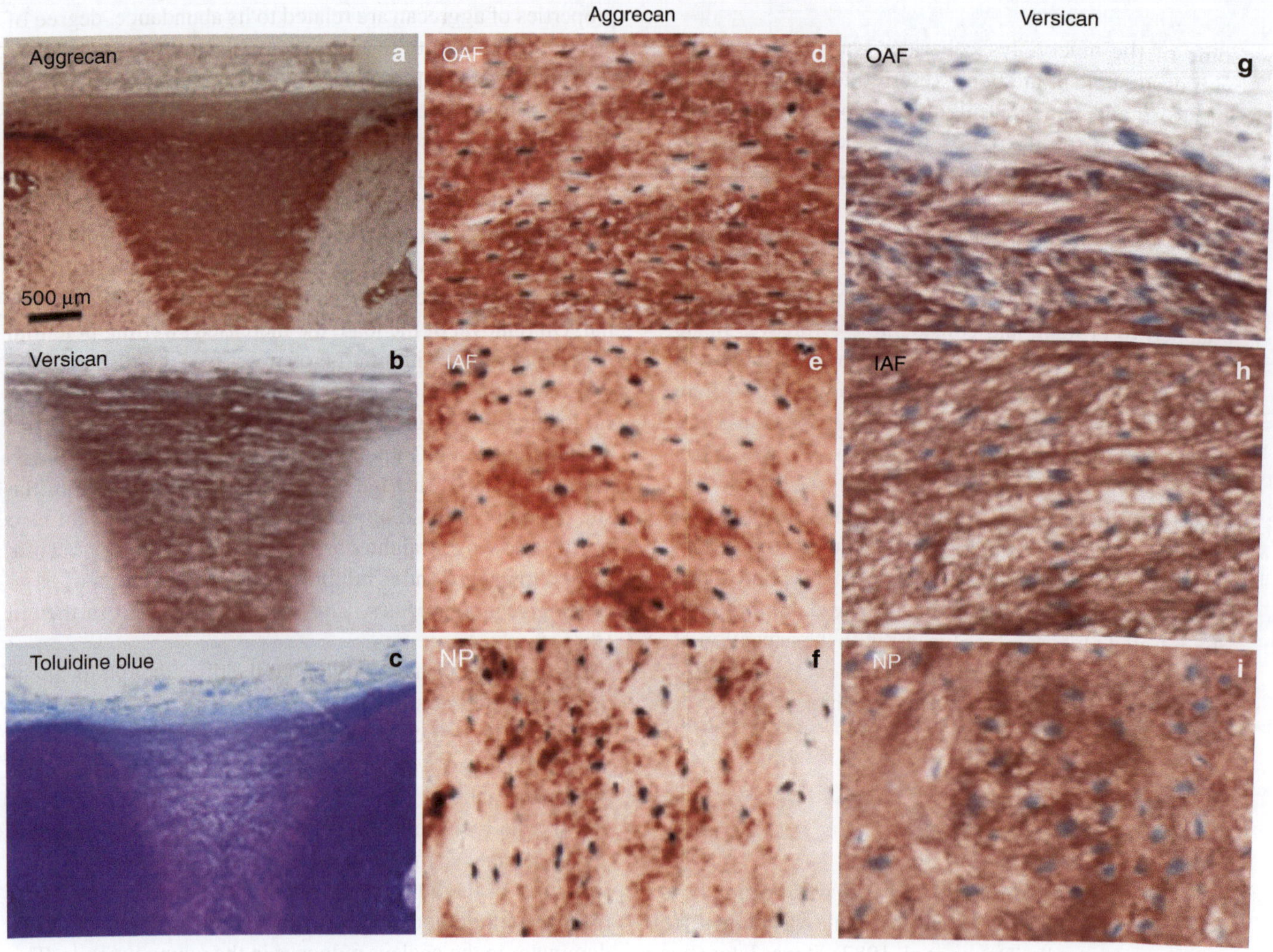

Fig. 4.1 Immunolocalization of aggrecan (**a**), versican (**b**), and toluidine blue-stained proteoglycan (**c**) in a 14-week gestational age fetal human intervertebral disc and adjacent cartilaginous vertebral body rudiment cartilages. Higher-power images of the outer annulus fibrosus (*OAF*), inner annulus fibrosus (*IAF*), and nucleus pulposus (*NP*) are also presented in selected areas of the aggrecan (**d–f**) and versican (**g–i**) immunolocalizations

followed by a pair of loops responsible for the interaction with HA (Watanabe et al. 1997). The second globular region (G2) possesses two disulfide-bonded loops that share structural homology with the HA-binding loops of the G1 region. However, they do not facilitate interaction with HA (Fosang and Hardingham 1989), and their function is presently unclear. The G1 and G2 regions are separated by a short interglobular domain (IGD). After the G2 region, there is a long extended region to which the majority of GAG chains are attached. There may be over 100 GAG chains attached to each core protein, accounting for about 90 % of the molecular weight of aggrecan.

The GAG-attachment region may be divided into three domains. The domain closest to the G2 region is responsible for the attachment of KS (KS domain), and this is followed by two domains responsible for the attachment of CS (CS1 and CS2 domains). The KS and CS chains provide the aggrecan with osmotic properties essential for its function in resisting disc compression. While the CS chains are confined to the CS1 and CS2 domains, KS chains may also be present on the G1, IGD, and G2 regions (Barry et al. 1995). The CS2 domain is followed by the carboxy terminal globular domain (G3), which possesses disulfide-bonded loops having homology to epidermal growth factor (EGF), C-type lectin, and complement regulatory protein (CRP) sequences. The G3 region facilitates transit of the aggrecan through the cell during synthesis (Zheng et al. 1998) and via its lectin domain also facilitates the interaction with other components of the extracellular matrix, such as fibulins and tenascins (Day et al. 2004). It is not clear if these G3 region interactions are of functional significance in vivo, but they could potentially link proteoglycan aggregates to one another.

Both the abundance and structure of aggrecan change with age, due to variations in intracellular synthesis and extracellular degradation. Apart from possible variations in gene expression, the synthesis changes are confined to

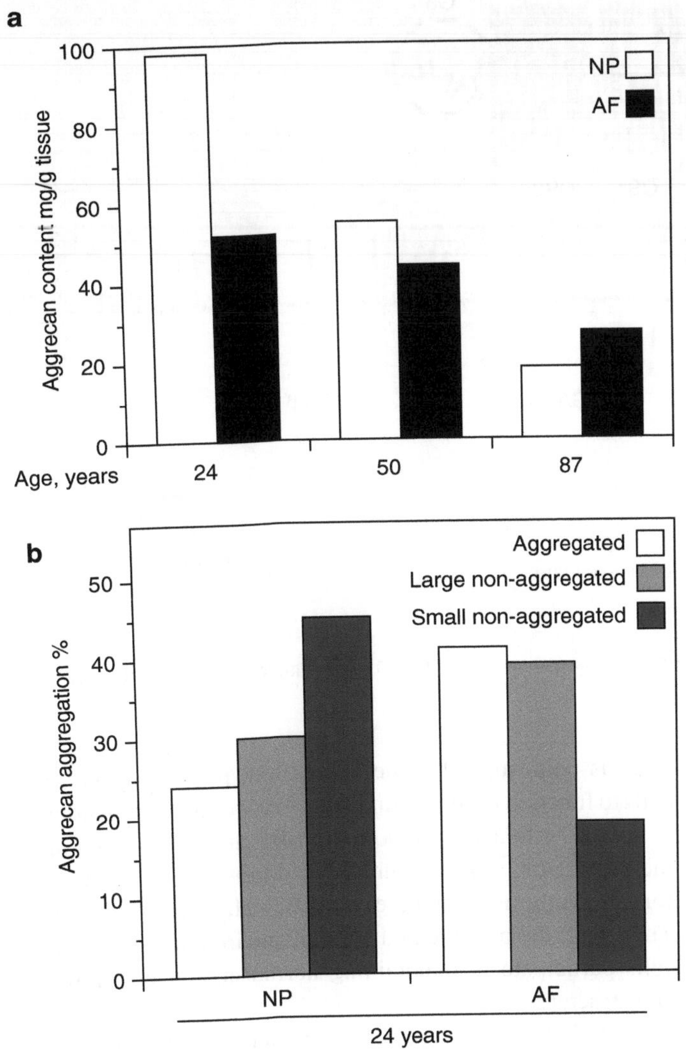

Fig. 4.2 Variation in aggrecan content (**a**) and aggregation (**b**) in the human intervertebral disc. Aggrecan content declines with age throughout the disc but at a faster rate in the nucleus pulposus than the annulus fibrosus. Aggrecan aggregation is lower and the proportion of small aggrecan fragments is greater in the nucleus pulposus (*NP*) than the annulus fibrosus (*AF*)

posttranslational modification of the core protein, particularly the synthesis of KS and CS (Brown et al. 1998; Roughley and White 1980). With age, the chain length of KS increases, while that of CS decreases. This could be viewed as a compensation mechanism for maintaining the sulfation of aggrecan and its swelling properties. The sulfation position of CS also changes with age, with the level of 4-sulfation decreasing and 6-sulfation increasing. It is not clear whether this variation in sulfation position has any functional significance. Currently, there is no evidence for the extracellular degradation of CS or KS, and degradative changes in aggrecan are confined to the proteolytic cleavage of its core protein (Roughley et al. 2006). Each proteolytic cleavage generates one fragment possessing a G1 region that remains bound to HA (aggregated) and one fragment that is no longer bound to HA (non-aggregated) and is free to diffuse within the disc. In articular cartilage the latter fragments are rapidly lost into the synovial fluid, but in the disc they accumulate as their diffusion is impeded by the vertebral end plates and the outer fibrous layers of the AF. With increasing age, the abundance of the non-aggregated fragments may exceed that of the aggregated fragments (Fig. 4.2b), and ongoing proteolysis further decreases the size of both the aggregated and non-aggregated fragments. Ultimately, the aggregated fragments are cleaved to their G1 region, which appears to be relatively resistant to proteolysis. As the size of the non-aggregated fragments declines, they are eventually lost from the tissue, and the total aggrecan content declines. The G1 fragments may also be eventually lost from the tissue as the size of the aggregates decreases due to depolymerization of the HA by extracellular hyaluronidases (Durigova et al. 2011b) or free radicals (Roberts et al. 1987). The average half-life of both the aggregated and non-aggregated aggrecan fragments within the disc is about 20 years (Sivan et al. 2006).

Aggrecans from different species do not possess identical structures, and there are differences in the structure of both their core proteins and GAG chains. The major core protein differences relate to the number of repeats in both the KS and CS1 domains (Barry et al. 1994; Doege et al. 1997). Of particular note is the absence of an extended KS domain in the mouse and rat, though it is unclear whether this is of functional importance. The largest species differences are in the GAG chains, which can differ enormously in chain length and degree and position of sulfation. In addition, there is variation in the abundance of aggrecan within the discs of different species. While changes in aggrecan structure and abundance are likely to have functional consequences, it is unclear whether such changes render some species more susceptible to disc or cartilage degeneration.

4.3.2 Aggrecan Gene Organization, Expression, and Mutations

The human aggrecan gene (ACAN, AGC1, CSPG1) resides on chromosome 15 (Korenberg et al. 1993) and is composed of 19 exons (Valhmu et al. 1995). Exon 1 encodes the 5′-untranslated region (UTR), exon 2 encodes the signal peptide, exons 3–6 encode the G1 region, exon 7 encodes the IGD, exons 8–10 encode the G2 region, exons 11 and 12 encode the GAG-attachment region, exons 13–18 encode the G3 region, and exon 19 encodes the 3′-UTR. The G3 region does not possess a unique structure, as the exons encoding its two EGF-like sequences and its one CRP-like sequence may undergo alternative splicing (Doege et al. 1991; Fulop et al.

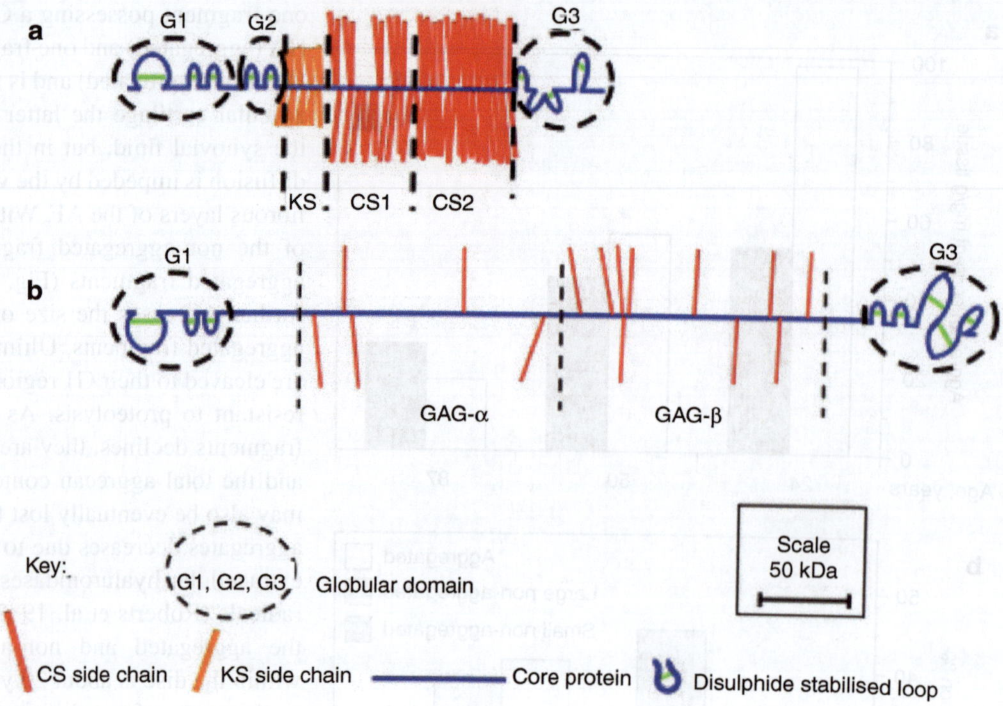

Fig. 4.3 Schematic depiction of the structural organization of aggrecan (**a**) and versican (**b**) drawn to scale

1993). All alternatively spliced forms of aggrecan do, however, possess a G3 region with a lectin-like sequence, and hence may participate in ECM interactions. It is not clear whether absence of the EGF and CRP domains influences the function of the G3 domain in vivo, but this has been suggested (Day et al. 2004). Exon 12, which encodes the CS1 and CS2 domains, exhibits a unique length polymorphism within the sequence encoding the CS1 domain in the human (Doege et al. 1997). The human CS1 domain is composed of repeats of 19 amino acids, each of which bears consensus sequences for the attachment of two CS chains. The number of repeats has been reported to vary between 13 and 33, with most individuals possessing 26–28 repeats. This type of polymorphism can influence the number of CS chains present on each aggrecan molecule, and it has therefore been suggested that this may influence aggrecan function; it is predicted that those aggrecan molecules bearing less repeats are functionally inferior (Roughley 2006). This led to the prediction that individuals possessing aggrecan with a low number of CS1 repeats would be more susceptible to degeneration of both the intervertebral disc and articular cartilage. While some evidence does support this conclusion (Kawaguchi et al. 1999), it is likely that other predisposing factors must also be present.

Aggrecan gene expression is regulated by a number of factors that relate to the unique environment within the disc. TonEBP, an osmoregulatory protein present in nucleus pulposus cells, interacts with two conserved TonE motifs within the aggrecan gene promoter and promotes aggrecan synthesis, thereby allowing the nucleus pulposus cells to adapt to their hyperosmotic environment (Tsai et al. 2006). HIF-1α also enhances aggrecan promoter activity and increases nucleus pulposus cell gene expression, permitting the disc cells to function normally under low oxygen tension (Agrawal et al. 2007). In addition, both TonEBP and HIF-1α regulate the expression of the glucuronic acid transferase responsible for CS synthesis (Gogate et al. 2011; Hiyama et al. 2009). Thus, both the osmotic and hypoxic environment of the disc cells participate in maintaining normal aggrecan synthesis and structure.

Mutations in the aggrecan gene and genes involved in GAG sulfation give rise to a variety of chondrodysplasias, which affect not only the hyaline cartilages but also the intervertebral disc. In humans some forms of spondyloepiphyseal dysplasia (SED) and spondyloepimetaphyseal dysplasia (SEMD) are associated with mutations in the aggrecan gene (Gleghorn et al. 2005; Tompson et al. 2009). A nonsense mutation is responsible for nanomelia in chickens (Li et al. 1993), and a 7bp deletion in exon 5 causing a frameshift and a premature stop in exon 6 is responsible for cartilage matrix deficiency (cmd) in mice (Watanabe et al. 1994). Aggrecan is deficient in the extracellular matrix of the mutant tissues, probably due to a combination of nonsense-mediated decay of the message and impaired secretion and intracellular degradation of any truncated product. Mutations in the DSDST sulfate transporter gene are responsible for diastrophic dysplasia, atelosteogenesis type II, and achondrogenesis type 1B in humans (Karniski 2001; Superti-Furga et al. 1996), and a mutation in the APS kinase, responsible for sulfate donor (PAPS) synthesis in cartilage, gives rise to brachymorphism in mice (Kurima et al. 1998). Chondrocytes and disc cells require large amounts of sulfate for aggrecan synthesis, and when absent, an undersulfated product is formed. These disorders add credence to the view that disc function requires both a high tissue content of aggrecan and a high degree of sulfation.

4.3.3 Aggrecan Degradation in the Degenerate Disc

The interglobular domain of aggrecan is particularly susceptible to proteolysis and is cleaved by most proteinases in vitro (Fosang et al. 1992). Analysis of in vivo degradation products indicates two predominant naturally occurring cleavage sites, which could be cleaved by aggrecanases (ADAMTS4 and ADAMTS5) and matrix metalloproteinases (MMPs) (Sztrolovics et al. 1997). Both aggrecanases and several MMPs have been detected in the disc (Roberts et al. 2000), and it is currently unclear as to which family members are predominantly responsible for causing aggrecan damage in vivo. However, in vitro studies indicate that ADAMTS5 is more efficient than ADAMTS4 at cleaving within the aggrecan IGD (Gendron et al. 2007) and that MMP-3, MMP-7, and MMP-12 are the most efficient MMPs (Durigova et al. 2011a). Aggrecanases are also able to cleave within the CS2 region of aggrecan, and five cleavage sites within this region have been identified (Tortorella et al. 2002). MMPs may also cleave at sites outside the IGD, but at present the extent of their cleavage is not fully understood. One of the initial events in aggrecan degradation, following its secretion into the extracellular matrix, is removal of the G3 region (Flannery et al. 1992), and it is unclear whether aggrecanases or MMPs are responsible.

Proteolytic cleavage of aggrecan and its loss are detrimental to disc function and are thought to be directly involved with intervertebral disc degeneration (Roughley 2004). Not only does degradation and loss of aggrecan lessen the ability of the disc to swell, it may also predispose it to mechanical damage. Indeed, there may be a vicious circle in which overloading of the disc stimulates aggrecan degradation via the production of proteinases by the disc cells, which in turn renders the disc susceptible to material damage. Such material damage may be irreversible and distinguish disc degeneration from normal aging (Adams and Roughley 2006). Loss of aggrecan can also promote angiogenesis (Johnson et al. 2005) and may be a prelude to blood vessel and nerve invasion of the disc with the onset of discogenic pain (Johnson et al. 2002). Structural changes in aggrecan are also associated with the discs present in the scoliotic spine. This may also be a consequence of abnormal loading, but this time in an asymmetric manner. Indeed, aggrecan changes do vary between the concave and convex sides of the scoliotic disc. It has been suggested that dietary supplementation with CS and glucosamine may help prevent aggrecan loss in articular cartilage (Box 4.2), and if true this may also be relevant to the disc.

Box 4.2: The Therapeutic Use of Chondroitin Sulfate and Glucosamine

For the past two decades, nutraceutical companies have been promoting oral supplements of glucosamine and chondroitin sulfate (CS) for the treatment of osteoarthritis. The original theory behind this treatment was that CS was a building block for aggrecan and that glucosamine was a building block for CS and that their supplementation would therefore promote aggrecan production or their presence in the bloodstream would somehow tolerize the body to these components, thus preventing autoantibody production which is prevalent in some forms of immune-driven inflammatory arthritis. As loss of aggrecan is associated with a deterioration in the functional properties of articular cartilage in osteoarthritis, it seemed reasonable that an increase in aggrecan production would be beneficial. Indeed it may be, but the question is whether CS and glucosamine aid in this process. Aggrecan synthesis does not involve the addition of intact CS chains to its protein core, and CS synthesis does not utilize glucosamine to produce its *N*-acetyl galactosamine component. Commercial sources of glucosamine are derived from the chitin component (poly-*N*-acetyl glucosamine) of crustacean shells, and while it may make more sense to administer galactosamine as a therapeutic agent, there is no readily available commercial source of this material. Furthermore, it is likely that much of the CS entering the circulation would be degraded to its constituent monosaccharides by the liver. It is therefore not surprising that there is much skepticism concerning the ability of CS and glucosamine to promote cartilage repair, particularly given the high doses of these components required to elicit a positive response. There is however some evidence that CS and glucosamine therapy can aid in the relief of joint pain in arthritic patients, although the mechanism for this effect is not clear. If this is true, then CS and glucosamine therapy may be an attractive alternative to more conventional nonsteroidal anti-inflammatory drug (NSAID) therapy, as the former have few side effects. It does however remain to be shown whether all formulations of CS plus glucosamine are equally effective and whether CS plus glucosamine formulations are more effective than glucosamine alone.

4.4 Versican

Versican was originally identified in fibroblasts and recognized to encode a CS proteoglycan (Zimmermann and Ruoslahti 1989). Versican has a much wider tissue distribution than aggrecan and together with HA has been suggested to provide tissue hydration and viscoelasticity (Hasegawa et al. 2007). In the fetal intervertebral disc, versican is prominently expressed throughout the tissue, but not in the adjacent cartilaginous vertebral body rudiments, and it prominently demarcates the margins of the developing disc from adjacent structures (Fig. 4.1) (Smith et al. 2009). In the mature intervertebral disc, versican is present throughout the tissues, being diffusely distributed within the nucleus pulposus, and most prominent between the lamellae of the annulus fibrosus (Melrose et al. 2001). Although versican is less abundant than aggrecan in the disc, its abundance is greater than in articular cartilage (Sztrolovics et al. 2002). It is unclear whether versican serves a unique function throughout the disc, but it could provide viscoelastic properties to the outer annulus fibrosus where aggrecan is depleted. However, the function of versican may not be restricted to a structural role within the extracellular matrix, as it is also known to influence cell function, particularly in cancer (Ricciardelli et al. 2009). The versican G3 region has also been shown to influence disc cell function (Yang et al. 2003).

4.4.1 Versican Protein Structure and Function

Versican is structurally related to aggrecan, possessing terminal domains analogous to the G1 and G3 regions of aggrecan (Fig. 4.3b), although there is no evidence for alternative splicing in the versican G3 region (Grover and Roughley 1993). There is also no analogous IGD or G2 region, and the central GAG-attachment region is completely different in its amino acid sequence and GAG organization. Likewise, a domain for the attachment of KS does not exist, although KS may be present on the G1 region, and there are many fewer CS chains. The G1 region of versican has functional HA-binding and LP-binding domains, and is able to form proteoglycan aggregates, but it is uncertain whether versican and aggrecan can reside on the same aggregate. Interestingly, the four hyalectan genes reside in tandem with an LP gene (Spicer et al. 2003), suggesting that coordinated gene expression may occur. Somewhat surprisingly, versican interacts best with the LP adjacent to the aggrecan gene, whereas aggrecan interacts best with the LP adjacent to the versican gene (Shi et al. 2004). As with aggrecan, the lectin domain within the G3 region of versican has the ability to interact with fibulins and tenascins (Olin et al. 2001). The presence of multiple protein-binding motifs and the resulting possibility of versatility in function led to the name versican.

The versican core protein possesses different splice variants, which alter the size of its GAG-attachment region. The core protein of the common V1 form of versican is of a similar length to that of aggrecan, whereas that of the V0 form of versican is much larger than aggrecan, having a core protein with about 3,400 amino acids. Versican undergoes extensive proteolytic modification (Sztrolovics et al. 2002), which has hampered its purification from aggrecan. As a result, there is little information on the structure of its CS chains and whether they may change in structure with age in the disc. Although versican is commonly referred to as a CS proteoglycan, the presence of DS cannot be discounted at all ages. The spectrum of versican core protein sizes within the disc is of a similar range to those of aggrecan, varying from free G1 regions to intact molecules (Sztrolovics et al. 2002).

4.4.2 Versican Gene Organization and Mutation

The human versican gene (VCAN, CSPG2) resides on chromosome 5 (Iozzo et al. 1992) and is composed of 15 exons (Naso et al. 1994). Exon 1 encodes the 5′-UTR, exon 2 encodes the signal peptide, exons 3–6 encode the G1 region, exons 7 and 8 encode the GAG-attachment region, exons 9–14 encode the G3 region, and exon 15 encodes the 3′-UTR. The region encoded by exon 7 is referred to as GAGα and that encoded by exon 8 is referred to as GAGβ. The exons encoding the GAG-attachment region may undergo alternative splicing (Dours-Zimmermann and Zimmermann 1994), giving rise to four versican mRNAs. The presence of both the GAGα and GAGβ regions gives rise to the V0 form of versican, the presence of only the GAGβ region gives rise to the V1 form, the presence of only the GAGα region gives rise to the V2 form, and the absence of both the GAGα and GAGβ regions gives rise to the V3 form. The V1 form of versican appears to be the most common form in most tissues, including the disc (Sztrolovics et al. 2002). Whether the different forms of versican serve unique functions is unknown, but it is likely that the V3 form, being devoid of CS, may differ in function from the other forms. The V0 form of versican is analogous to PG-M, which was identified in chick limb bud mesenchyme (Ito et al. 1995).

Mutations in the human versican gene give rise to the dominantly inherited Wagner syndrome, and in the original index case, this was due to a base substitution at the exon 8/intron 8 splice junction affecting the splicing of exon 8 (Kloeckener-Gruissem et al. 2006). Additional mutations affecting the intron7/exon 8 splice junction have also been reported in other families with Wagner syndrome (Mukhopadhyay et al. 2006). Defective splicing of exon 8 results in a decrease in the V1 form of versican and an increase in the V2 and V3 forms. Wagner syndrome is classified as a vitreoretinopathy, and its ocular features are probably associated with perturbation in the role played by versican in gelling of the human vitreous. However, in accord with the widespread tissue distribution of versican, Wagner syndrome patients also exhibit extraocular features, including skeletal defects similar to those reported in Stickler syndrome. Accordingly, it is likely that perturbation in intervertebral disc formation and function will also occur.

4.4.3 Versican Degradation in the Degenerate Disc

The V1 form of versican can be cleaved by ADAMTS1 and ADAMTS4 to yield a product of 441 amino acids that includes the G1 region (Sandy et al. 2001). Thus, aggrecanases could potentially play a role in versican degradation within the disc in vivo. However, the size of this product appears to be larger than that of the free G1 region present in vivo, suggesting that other proteinases are also active. The MMPs would be the most likely candidates to fulfill this role. As with aggrecan, it is likely that premature or excessive proteolytic degradation of versican is associated with intervertebral disc degeneration. Peptide sequences within both the versican and aggrecan G1 regions have also been associated with the development of autoimmune spondyloarthropathies (Shi et al. 2003).

4.5 Perlecan

Perlecan was named for its appearance when first visualized by rotary shadowing electron microscopy, where it appeared as multiple globular domains considered to resemble a string of pearls on a chain. Perlecan has a widespread distribution throughout the developing human fetal intervertebral disc and vertebral cartilaginous rudiment cartilages, where it displays a pericellular localization pattern. However, it is also prominent in the territorial and interterritorial matrix of the developing disc (Fig. 4.4) (Smith et al. 2009). Perlecan expression is elevated in hypertrophic chondrocytes surrounding the ossification center of the developing vertebral body and in terminally differentiated growth plate chondrocytes (Smith et al. 2009). In the neonatal and adult disc, perlecan is cell associated in the pericellular matrix of the nucleus pulposus, inner and outer annulus fibrosus, cartilaginous end plates, and vertebral growth plates (Fig. 4.5). However, its relative abundance diminishes with the decline in cell number evident in the aging intervertebral disc.

Perlecan interacts with a number of growth factors and morphogens, including FGF-1, FGF-2, FGF-7, FGF-9, and FGF-18; platelet-derived growth factor (PDGF); vascular endothelial cell growth factor (VEGF); hepatocyte growth factor; BMP-1, BMP-2, BMP-4, and BMP-7; hedgehog (Hh); and Wnt, and through these molecules influences cell proliferation and differentiation and matrix production (Whitelock et al. 2008). Perlecan also interacts with a number of cell attachment proteins, including laminin, fibronectin, thrombospondin, and $\alpha5\beta1$ and $\alpha2\beta1$ integrin, and thereby plays an important role in cell attachment and recruitment during tissue development and remodeling. Through its ability to interact with a number of matrix components, including PRELP; WARP; types IV, VI, XIII, and XVIII collagen; fibrillin-1 and fibrillin-2; nidogen-1 and nidogen-2; latent transforming growth factor-beta binding protein-2 (LTBP-2); and tropoelastin, perlecan modulates extracellular matrix assembly and stabilization (Hayes et al. 2011c; Iozzo 1994, 1998; Melrose et al. 2008b). Via these interactions, perlecan participates in disc development and in conversion of the cartilaginous vertebral rudiment cartilages into bone during spine development (Smith et al. 2009). This is consistent

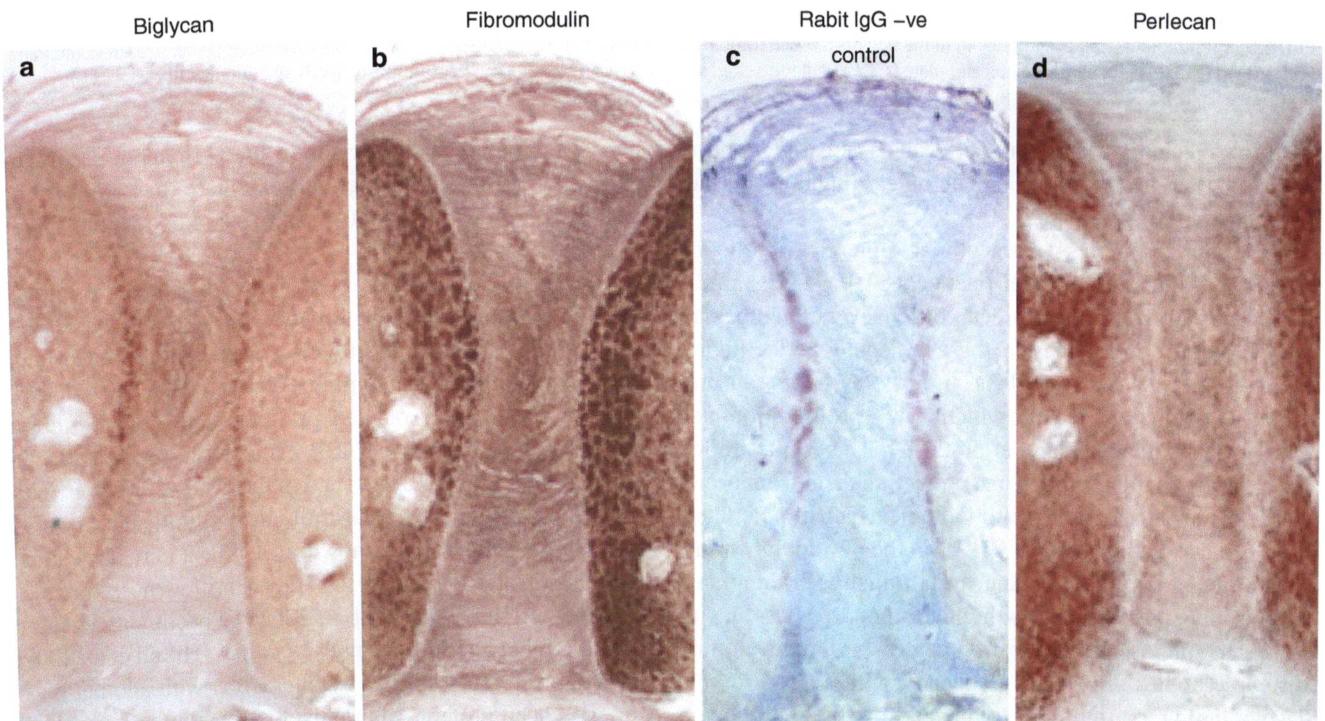

Fig. 4.4 Immunolocalization of biglycan (**a**), fibromodulin (**b**), nonimmune rabbit IgG negative control (**c**), and perlecan (**d**) in a 14-week gestational age fetal human intervertebral disc and adjacent cartilaginous vertebral body rudiment cartilages

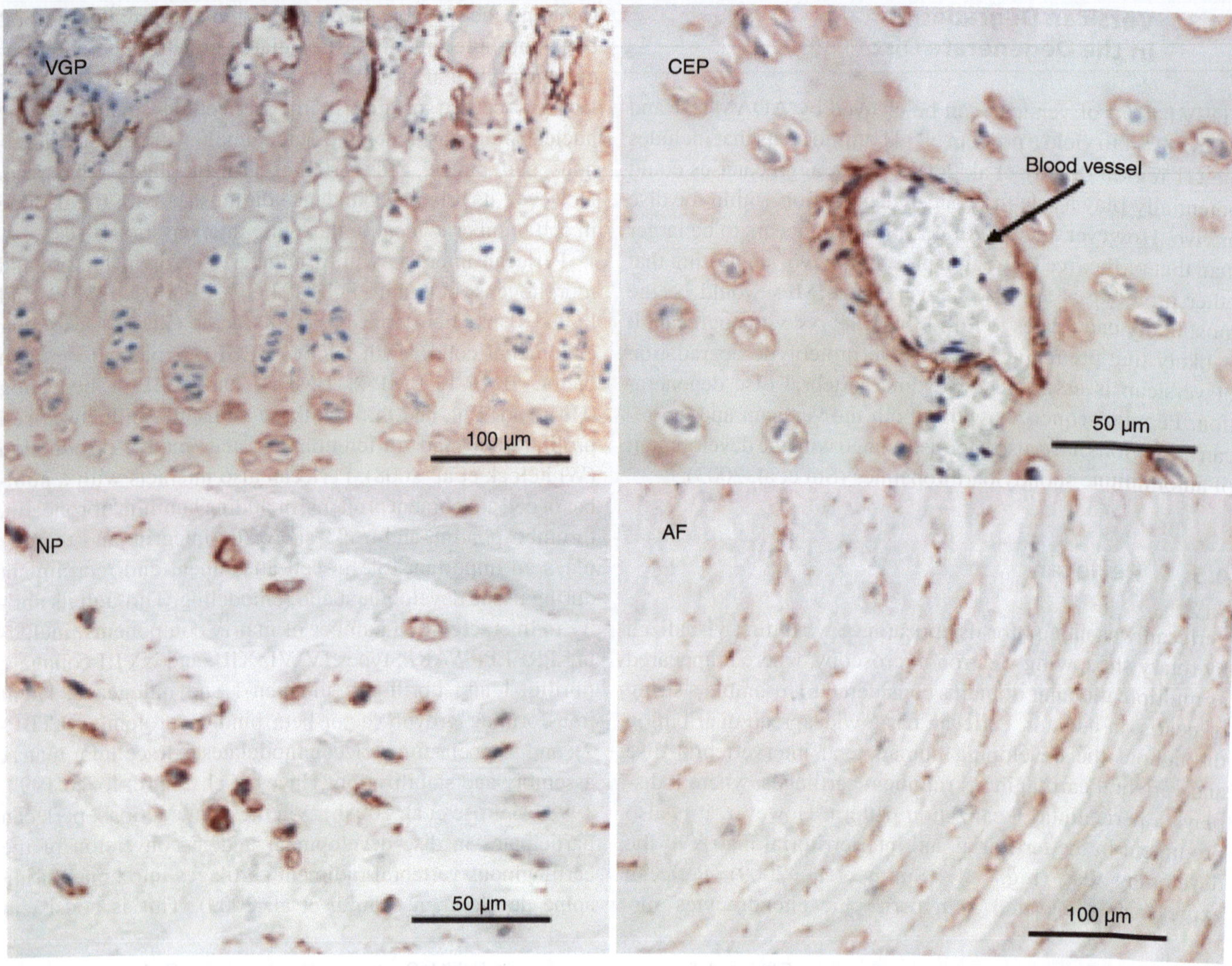

Fig. 4.5 Immunolocalization of perlecan in the newborn ovine lumbar intervertebral disc. Perlecan is present as a pericellular proteoglycan in the vertebral growth plate (*VGP*), cartilaginous end plate (*CEP*), a blood vessel within the CEP, and the nucleus pulposus (*NP*) and annulus fibrosus (*AF*)

with roles recently ascribed to perlecan as an early chondrogenic marker in the development of cartilaginous tissues (Smith et al. 2010).

Perlecan promotes extracellular matrix production through its interactions with members of the FGF family. Perlecan is a low-affinity co-receptor for several members of the FGF family and sequesters these molecules pericellularly for later presentation to FGFRs. In this way, FGF can promote cell signaling events which drive proliferation and matrix production (Chuang et al. 2010). This sequestration process also stabilizes the FGFs, protecting them from proteolysis in situ and extending their biological half-life. Perlecan has been co-localized with FGF-18 in the developing spine, with an overexpression evident in terminally differentiated hypertrophic vertebral growth plate chondrocytes and in cells surrounding the ossification centers in the developing vertebral bodies. Perlecan associates with FGF-2 in the developing intervertebral disc interspace in the fetal human spine. Thus, FGF-18 promotes terminal differentiation of chondrocytes, leading eventually to bone formation, whereas FGF-2 maintains chondrocytes in the permanent cartilages in a delayed state of differentiation, where they are responsible for the replenishment of matrix components to effect tissue homeostasis.

Recent studies have also shown that the HS chains of perlecan are important in fibrillin and elastin assembly (Hayes et al. 2011a, c) and support earlier observations concerning basement membrane assembly. Perlecan is localized to a number of elastin-associated proteins in the intervertebral disc (Hayes et al. 2011c). LTBP-2 interacts with the perlecan HS chains (Parsi et al. 2010) and in the disc co-localizes with perlecan pericellularly. The biological significance of this localization is not known; however, LTBP-2 may have some regulatory role to play in the microfibrillogenesis process (Hirai et al. 2007; Hirani et al. 2007) by occupying sites on fibrillin-1 that LTBP-1 normally occupies (Hirani et al. 2007; Vehvilainen et al. 2009) or by interaction with another elastin-associated protein. Alternatively, by acting as a competitive substrate for the HS chains in perlecan domain I, it may regulate growth factor binding to perlecan.

4.5.1 Perlecan Protein Structure

Perlecan is a large modular HS-proteoglycan composed of five distinct domains with homology to growth factors and to protein modules involved in lipid metabolism, cell adhesion, and homotypic and heterotypic interactions involved in matrix assembly and stabilization (Melrose et al. 2008b; Murdoch and Iozzo 1993) (Box 4.3). The N-terminal domain I contains three HS attachment sites, through which HS-mediated growth factor and morphogen interactions occur. Consensus regions for GAG attachment have also been identified in the C-terminal domain V (Fig. 4.6a). The N-terminal domain is unique to perlecan, whereas domain II exhibits homology to the low-density lipoprotein receptor and domain III bears homology to the L4 laminin-type IV domain and LE laminin EGF domain. Domain IV, the largest domain in perlecan, contains multiple immunoglobulin repeats, although this domain is truncated by about 20 kDa in mouse perlecan (Melrose et al. 2008b; Murdoch and Iozzo 1993). The C-terminal domain V bears homology to the LG laminin-type G domain and contains three LG domains separated by EGF-like domains. The perlecan core protein is large (467 kDa) and highly aggregative under associative conditions, leading to the formation of higher molecular weight forms of about 800 kDa in free solution.

The perlecan core protein can contain three HS chains in the N-terminal domain, and additional GAG consensus attachment points have been identified in domain V; however, it has yet to be definitively shown that these are occupied in the intervertebral disc. Disc cells synthesize a hybrid HS/CS proteoglycan form of perlecan, with at least one of the HS chains replaced by a chondroitin-4-sulfate (C4S) chain. In the fetal and newborn disc, this C4S chain is capped by a unique developmental CS motif identified by MAb 7D4 (Hayes et al. 2011b). However, the abundance of this 7D4 epitope on perlecan diminishes with aging, and it is not clear if this has any functional consequence.

Box 4.3: Perlecan and Its Interactive Components

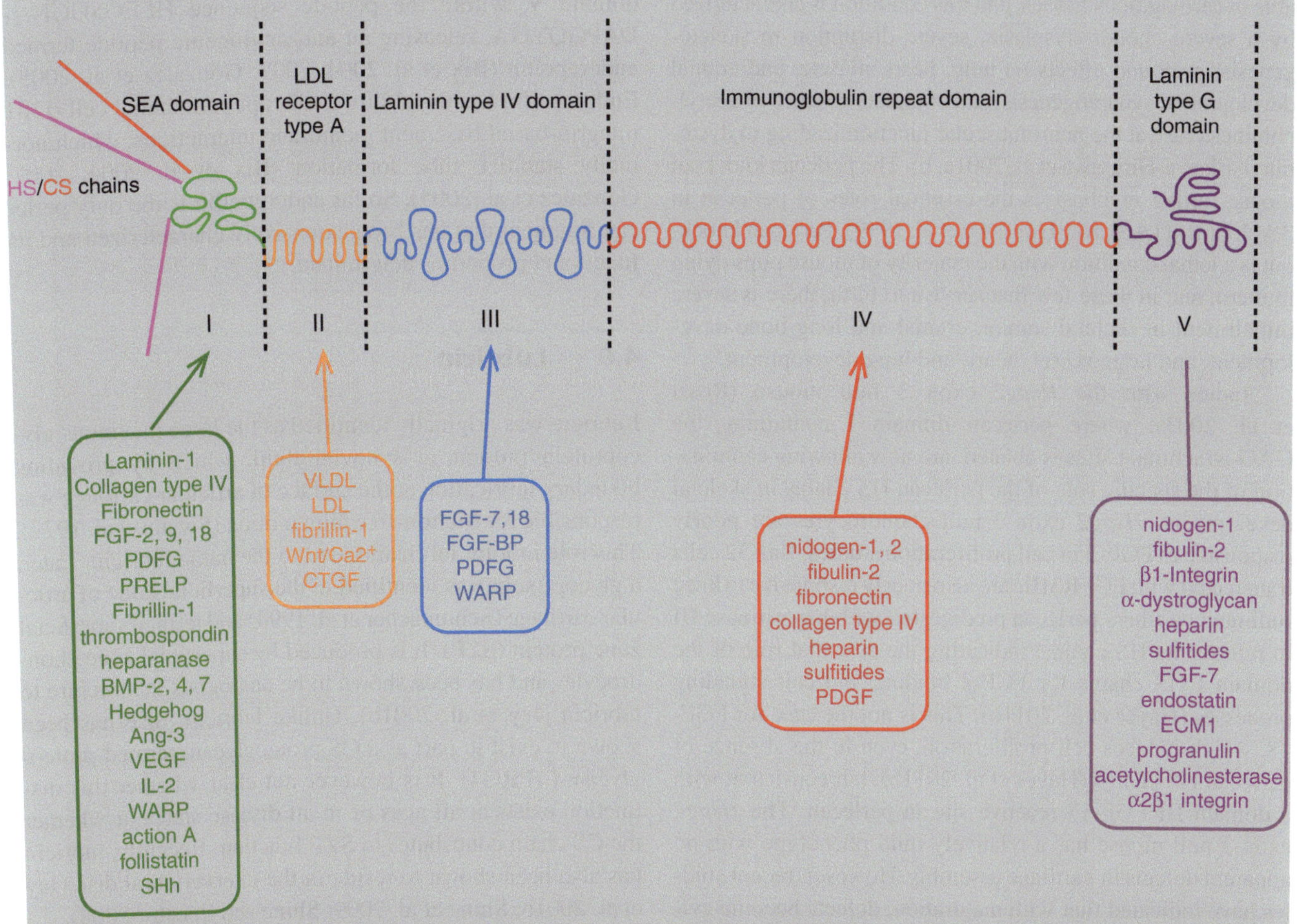

Abbreviations: *FGF* fibroblast growth factor, *PDGF* platelet derived growth factor, *PRELP* proline/arginine-rich and leucine-rich repeat protein/prolargin, *BMP* bone morphogenetic protein, *Ang* angiopoietin, *SHh* sonic hedgehog, *VLDL* very low density lipoprotein, *LDL* low density lipoprotein, *Wnt* a morphogenic ligand, hybrid abbreviation of Int (integration-1) and Wg (wingless), *CTGF* connective tissue growth factor, *FGF-BP* FGF binding protein, *WARP* von Willebrand factor A domain-related protein.

4.5.2 Perlecan Gene Organization and Mutation

The perlecan gene (*HSPG2*) is encoded by 94 exons located on chromosome 1p36–34 (Cohen et al. 1993; Kallunki and Tryggvason 1992; Murdoch et al. 1992; Noonan et al. 1991), with each of the structural domains being encoded by multiple exons.

The importance of perlecan in skeletogenesis (Arikawa-Hirasawa et al. 1999), vasculogenesis, and muscle and nerve development is evident from analyses of two naturally occurring mutations in the human *HSPG2* gene. Schwartz-Jampel syndrome is a relatively mild skeletal condition, which arises from missense, splicing, exon skipping, and deletion mutations. These events result in partial loss of domain IV and total loss of domain V, complete loss of domain V only, or defective disulfide bonding in domain III of perlecan (Arikawa-Hirasawa et al. 2002). As a result, there are reduced functional levels of perlecan in cartilaginous tissues, chondrodysplasia, myotonia, impairment in the endochondral ossification process, and short stature. In the more severe condition of dyssegmental dysplasia, Silverman-Handmaker type, perlecan is almost undetectable in cartilaginous tissues, and this condition is characterized by a severe chondrodysplasia; severe disruption in skeletogenesis; profound effects on lung, heart, muscle, and cranial development; synaptogenesis; and complete absence of acetylcholinesterase at the neuromuscular junction leading to dystonia (Arikawa-Hirasawa et al. 2001a, b). The perlecan knockout mouse further emphasizes the essential roles of perlecan in development (Arikawa-Hirasawa et al. 1999). Perlecan knockout is a lethal condition with the majority of mouse pups dying in utero, and in those few that survive to birth, there is severe impairment in skeletal stature, cranial and long bone development, and large vessel, heart, and lung development.

Studies with the *Hspg2* exon 3 null mouse (Rossi et al. 2003), where perlecan domain I containing the GAG-attachment sites is ablated, are now allowing examination of the specific role of the perlecan HS chains in skeletal development. *Hspg2* exon 3 null chondrocytes are poorly responsive to FGF-2 in cell proliferation studies. Baf-32 cells transfected with FGFR3IIIc are also poorly responsive to knee rudiment cartilage perlecan predigested with heparitinase III to remove its HS chains, indicating the essential role of the domain I HS chains for FGF-2 binding and cell signaling processes (Hayes et al. 2011b). This is not the case for FGF-18, which induces cell proliferation, even in the absence of perlecan HS chains (Hayes et al. 2011b), but consistent with a domain III FGF-18 reactive site in perlecan. The *Hspg2* exon 3 null mouse has a relatively mild phenotype with no apparent defects in cartilage assembly. However, recent studies have indicated that with maturation, defects become evident in cartilaginous tissues, and its reparative ability after a traumatic challenge also appears to be impaired. Fibrillin-1 assembly and deposition is also impaired in the *Hspg2* exon 3 null mutant mouse intervertebral disc (Hayes et al. 2013).

4.5.3 Perlecan Degradation

Little is known about the mechanism by which perlecan is processed in the intervertebral disc. Gel electrophoresis separates full-length perlecan from three other perlecan species in newborn and young adult ovine discs. The latter three species are smaller than full-length perlecan, devoid of GAG, and detectable using a MAb to perlecan domain I. Thus, they represent fragments cleaved from the domain I carboxy terminal to the HS chains. However, the cleavage sites themselves still await detailed characterization. Perlecan fragmentation has also been observed by Western blotting of newborn and 2-year-old intervertebral disc extracts using a domain I-specific MAb, with one major and four minor species evident (Fig 4.6b). A similar range of perlecan fragments has been observed in extracts of human knee joint articular cartilage (Melrose et al. 2006).

In vitro digestion of endothelial cell perlecan with MMP-1, MMP-3, and plasmin has demonstrated the susceptibility of perlecan to cleavage in domains IV and V (Whitelock et al. 1996). Tolloid-like metalloprotease (BMP-1) also cleaves perlecan between the LG2 and LG3 domains of domain V, within the peptide sequence HLEGSGGN-↓-DAPGQYGA, releasing an anti-angiogenic peptide termed endorepellin (Bix et al. 2004, 2007; Gonzalez et al. 2005). Endorepellin has the ability to disrupt endothelial cell $\alpha 2\beta 1$ integrin-based basement membrane interactions, which normally stabilize tube formation (Bix et al. 2004, 2007; Gonzalez et al. 2005). So far endorepellin is the only perlecan fragment that has been extensively characterized and its functional properties determined.

4.6 Lubricin

Lubricin was originally identified as the large mucinous glycoprotein present in synovial fluid, which by providing boundary lubrication at the surface of articular cartilage was responsible for friction-free joint motion (Swann et al. 1977). This role in joint lubrication led to the name lubricin. Later, a glycoprotein was identified in the superficial zone of articular cartilage (Schumacher et al. 1994) and termed superficial zone protein (SZP). It is produced by superficial zone chondrocytes and has been shown to be analogous in structure to lubricin (Jay et al. 2001b). Unlike lubricin, SZP has been shown to exist in part as a CS proteoglycan, termed proteoglycan 4 (PRG4). It is however not clear whether this distinction exists at all ages or in all disease states or whether the CS chain contributes to SZP function. Recently, lubricin has also been shown to reside in the intervertebral disc (Jay et al. 2001b; Shine et al. 2009; Shine and Spector 2008).

Lubricin is present in all regions of the disc but appears to be most abundant in the nucleus pulposus (Shine et al. 2009). Its core protein undergoes extensive proteolytic degradation, with accumulation of the degradation products in the tissue;

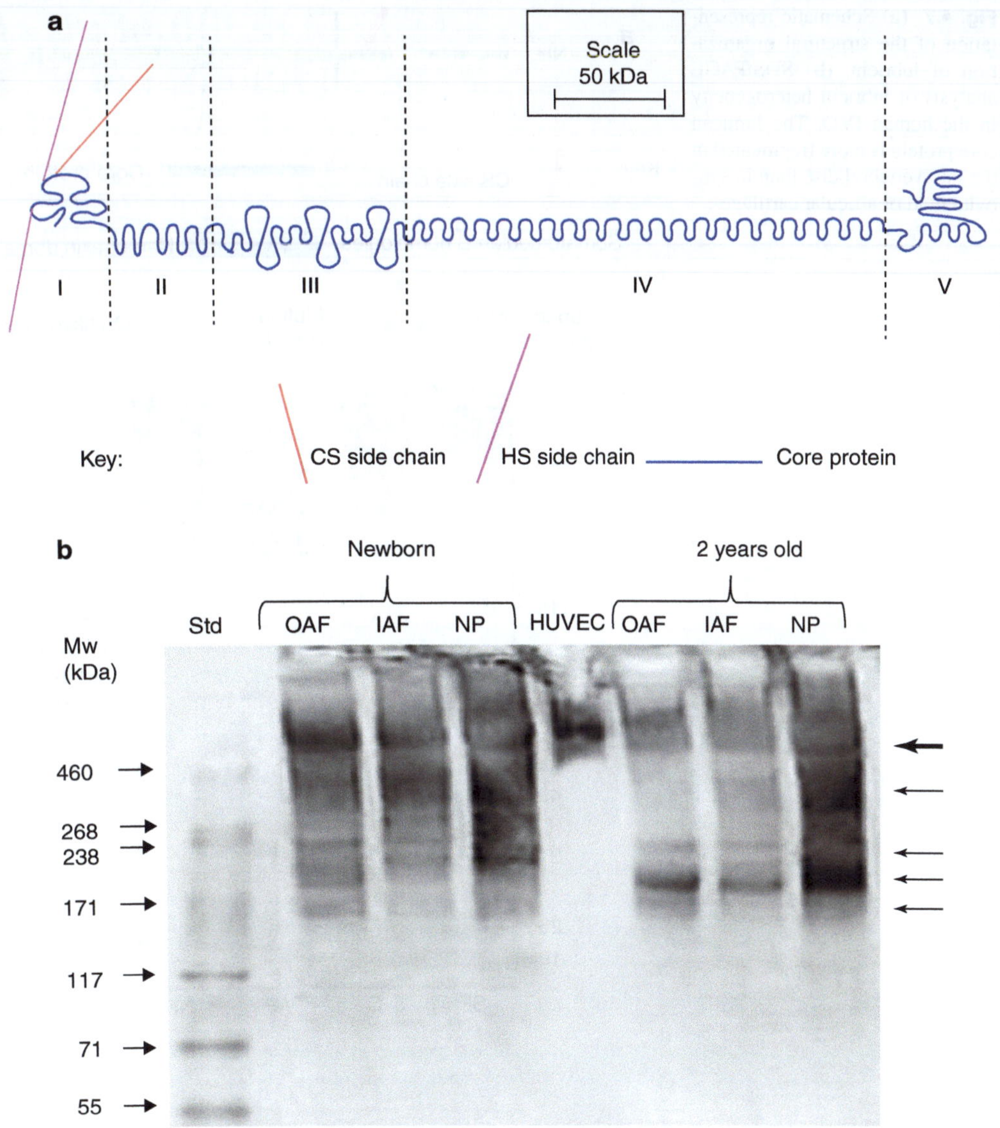

Fig. 4.6 (**a**) Schematic representation of the structural organization of perlecan. (**b**) SDS/PAGE analysis of perlecan heterogeneity in newborn and 2-year-old ovine intervertebral disc samples. Note the extensive fragmentation of disc perlecan compared to that from human vascular endothelial cells (*HUVEC*). The multiple perlecan species that are discernible in the disc are identified by arrows in the right hand margin. *OAF* outer annulus fibrosus, *IAF* inner annulus fibrosus, *NP* nucleus pulposus

it has a polydisperse size distribution comparable to other tissue sources, such as synovial fluid or articular cartilage (Fig. 4.7b). It is not known which proteinases are responsible for cleavage in vivo, but they are likely to be the same as those involved in aggrecan and versican degradation. In this respect, MMPs have been demonstrated to degrade lubricin in vitro (Elsaid et al. 2005). Also unknown is the precise function of lubricin in the disc and how proteolysis may affect lubricin function. One possibility is a role in lubricating motion between adjacent annulus fibrosus lamellae.

4.6.1 Lubricin Protein Structure

Intact lubricin has a molecular weight of about 240 kDa, of which about 50 % is contributed by O-linked mucin-like oligosaccharides (Swann et al. 1981b), which reside in a long central domain. This mucin-like domain is flanked by N- and C-terminal cysteine-rich domains that resemble domains of vitronectin. Domains possessing somatomedin B homology and a heparin-binding domain may reside at its N-terminus, and a hemopexin domain resides at its C-terminus (Fig. 4.7a). There is a single consensus sequence for the attachment of CS near the N-terminus of the mucin-like domain. In its SZP form, lubricin has also been reported to contain KS, but it is unclear where this resides. The lubricating properties of lubricin are conferred by its mucin-like domain (Jay et al. 2001a), but the other domains provide the potential for extracellular interactions and cell associations. The terminal domains appear to be important, as their reduction and alkylation impairs lubricin function (Swann et al. 1981a).

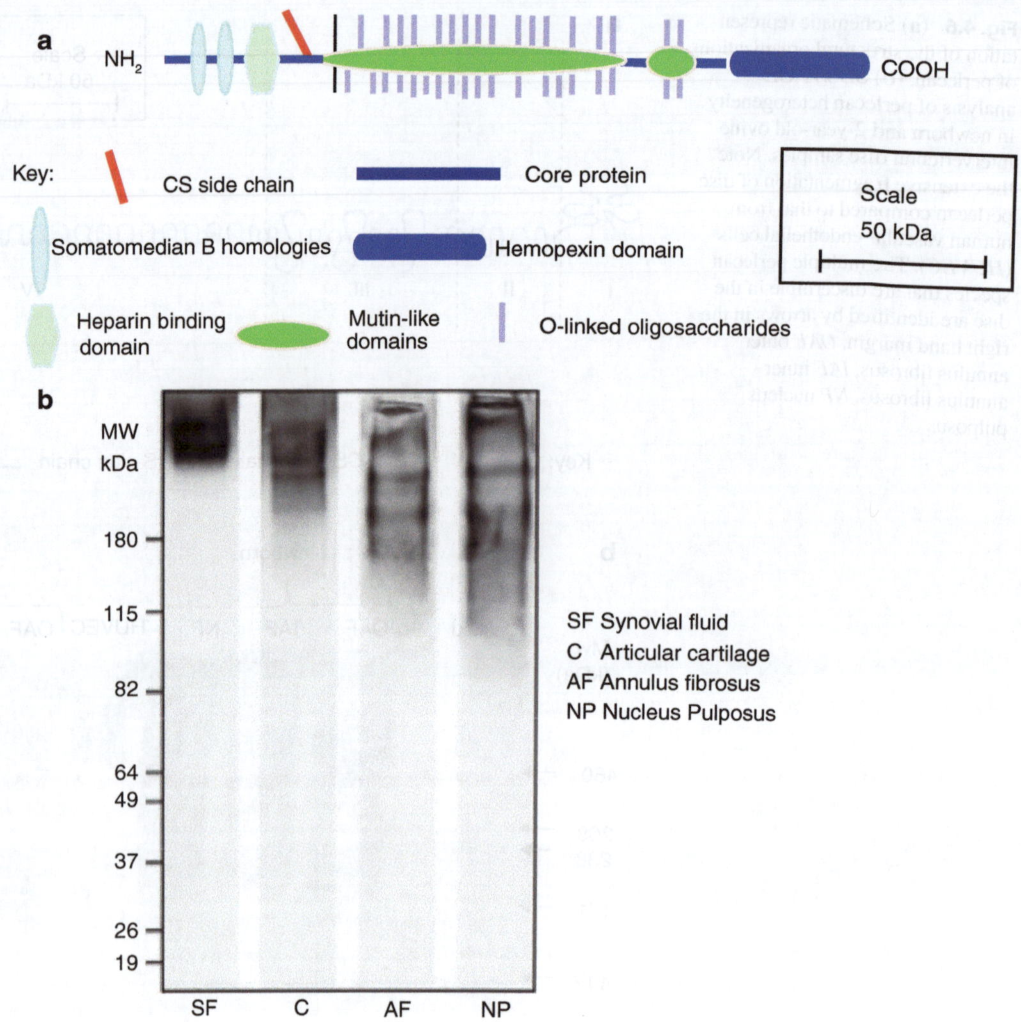

Fig. 4.7 (a) Schematic representation of the structural organization of lubricin. (b) SDS/PAGE analysis of lubricin heterogeneity in the human IVD. The lumican core protein is more fragmented in the intervertebral disc than in synovial fluid or articular cartilage

4.6.2 Lubricin Gene Organization and Mutation

The mRNA encoding lubricin/SZP has been shown to originate by alternative splicing of the megakaryocyte stimulating factor (MSF) precursor gene (PRG4) (Flannery et al. 1999). The human PRG4 gene resides on chromosome 1 and possesses 12 exons (Merberg et al. 1993). Exon 1 encodes the signal peptide, exons 2 and 3 encode domains with somatomedin B homology, and exons 4 and 5 encode a region containing a heparin-binding domain. Exon 6 encodes the mucin-like domain, possessing about 80 potential attachment sites for O-linked oligosaccharides and a single potential attachment site for CS. Exons 7–12 encode the carboxy terminus of the molecule, which contains a domain with hemopexin-like homology. Both synovial lubricin and cartilage SZP are derived by alternative splicing of a combination of PRG4 exons 2, 4, and 5 to yield several messages. Thus, there is no unique structure for the lubricin core protein, but all forms possess at least one somatomedin B-like domain and a hemopexin-like domain flanking the central mucin-like domain. This heterogeneity accounts for the variable size of intact lubricin.

Mutations in the human PRG4 gene give rise to the autosomal recessive camptodactyly-arthropathy-coxa vara-pericarditis syndrome (CACP) (Marcelino et al. 1999). Most of the originally identified mutations causing frameshifts or nonsense substitution near the end of exon 6 or in subsequent exons result in truncation of the hemopexin domain. These mutations result in a lack of lubricin in synovial fluid and a lack of lubricin production by cultured synoviocytes (Rhee et al. 2005b). Many of the features of CACP are recapitulated in the lubricin knockout mouse (Rhee et al. 2005a), supporting the concept that deficient production of lubricin is responsible for the CACP phenotype. The wide range of symptoms associated with CACP show that lubricin function is not restricted to joint motion but also influences tendons and the heart. While patients with CACP have spine abnormalities (Faivre et al. 2000), it is not clear whether disc function is also affected in these individuals.

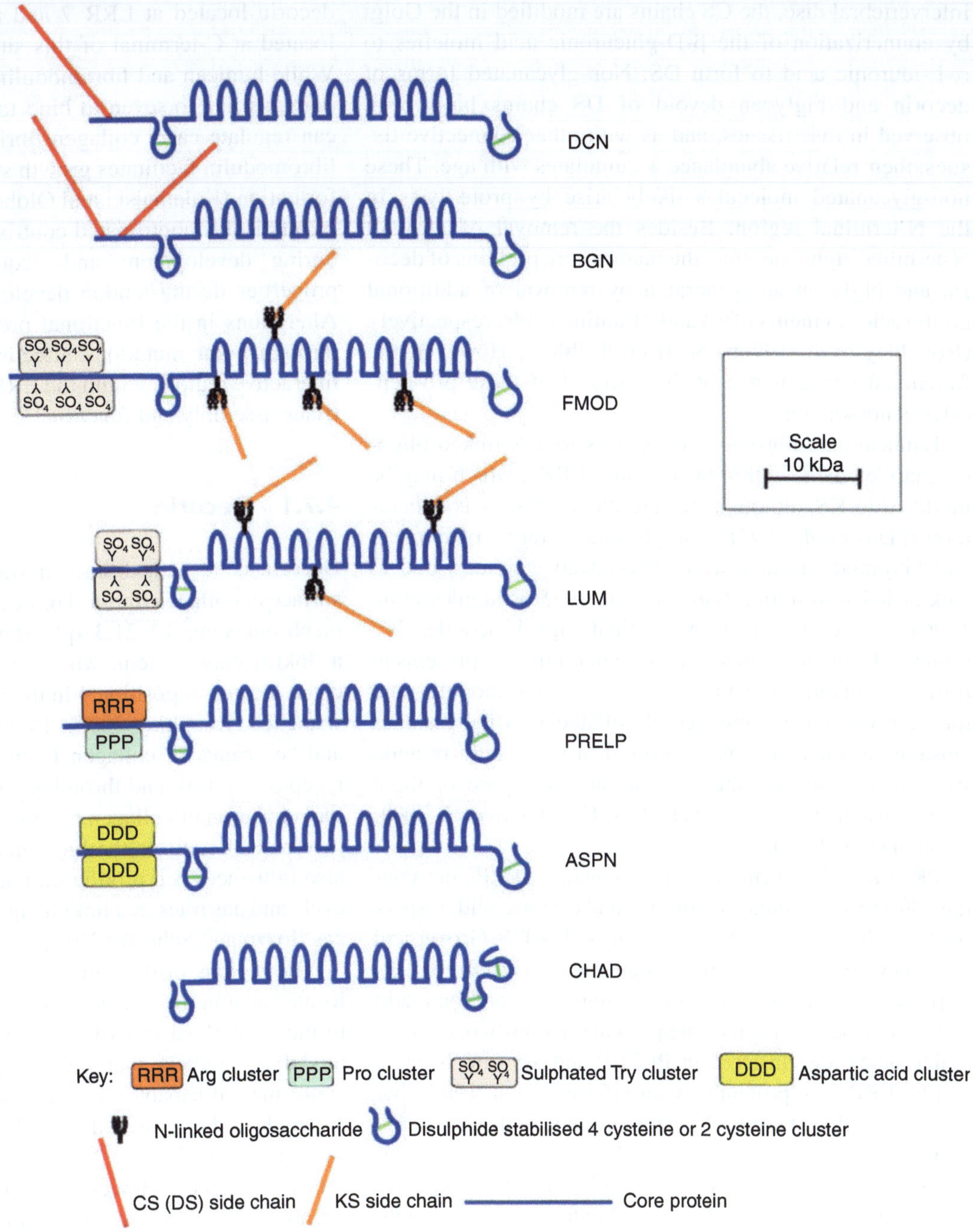

Fig. 4.8 Schematic representation of the structural organization of SLRPs found in the intervertebral disc

4.7 The Small Leucine-Rich Repeat Proteoglycans (SLRPS)

The SLRPs are members of a large family of leucine-rich repeat (LRR) proteins, which contain multiple adjacent 24 amino acid domains bearing a common leucine-rich motif (Hocking et al. 1998). The SLRPs have been categorized into a number of subfamilies on the basis of their gene organization, number of LRRs, type of GAG substitutions, and general structural organization (Kalamajski and Oldberg 2010). Eight SLRPs have been identified in the intervertebral disc, including the CS-/DS-substituted decorin and biglycan; KS-substituted lumican, fibromodulin, and keratocan; and non-glycanated proline/arginine-rich protein (PRELP, prolargin), chondroadherin, and asporin (Fig. 4.8). These SLRPs contain ten LRRs, which are flanked by amino and carboxy terminal disulfide-bonded regions.

Decorin and biglycan possess attachment sites for their CS/DS side chains within the extreme amino terminus of their core proteins. In decorin, there is one such site, whereas biglycan contains two GAG substitution sites (Roughley and White 1989). In most connective tissues, including the intervertebral disc, the CS chains are modified in the Golgi by epimerization of the β-D-glucuronic acid moieties to α-L-iduronic acid to form DS. Non-glycanated forms of decorin and biglycan devoid of DS chains have been observed in disc tissues, and as with other connective tissues, their relative abundance accumulates with age. These non-glycanated molecules likely arise by proteolysis in the N-terminal region. Besides the removal of a small N-terminal signal peptide, the mature core proteins of decorin and biglycan are generated by removal of additional amino acid segments of 14 and 21 amino acids, respectively (Roughley et al. 1996b; Scott et al. 2000). However, the functional consequence of the removal of these pro-peptides is not known.

Lumican and fibromodulin possess four N-linked oligosaccharide chains within their central LRRs, which may be modified to KS, although substitution at all sites is uncommon (Plaas et al. 1990). Non-glycanated forms of lumican and fibromodulin also occur in connective tissues, due to lack of KS substitution (Grover et al. 1995; Roughley et al. 1996a). Only the small N-terminal signal peptides are removed from the lumican and fibromodulin core proteins to form the mature core proteins in situ. Fibromodulin and lumican also have a number of sulfated tyrosine residues clustered at their extreme N-termini in the mature protein, which may also contribute to the anionic nature of these SLRPs in situ (Antonsson et al. 1991; Onnerfjord et al. 2004; Tillgren et al. 2009).

PRELP and asporin are non-glycanated SLRPs but contain clusters of arginine and proline and aspartic acid, respectively, at their N-termini (Bengtsson et al. 1995; Grover and Roughley 1998, 2001). PRELP is unique amongst the SLRPs in possessing a cationic N-terminal region. Chondroadherin is devoid of an N-terminal core protein region where charged amino acids are clustered in PRELP and asporin. It has a similar LRR core protein structure (Grover et al. 1997), but differs from the other SLRPs in the structure of its C-terminal region.

SLRPs have important roles to play as tissue organizers based on how they affect the orientation and assembly of collagenous matrices and how they interact with growth factors and cell surface receptors during tissue development and matrix remodeling (Iozzo et al. 2011). They display diversified and overlapping functional properties with a level of redundancy between SLRP members. Asporin binds to collagen with an affinity in the low nanomolar ranges, as does decorin (Kalamajski et al. 2009). Asporin and decorin bind to the same region in fibrillar collagen and can effectively compete with one another for this site when applied at equimolar concentrations, whereas biglycan cannot (Kalamajski and Oldberg 2010). The collagen-binding sites on asporin and decorin differ, with the binding site for decorin located at LRR 7 and the binding site on asporin located at C-terminal of this site (Kalamajski et al. 2009). While lumican and fibromodulin both utilize leucine repeat domains five to seven to bind to fibrillar collagen and both can regulate early collagen fibril assembly processes, only fibromodulin facilitates growth steps leading to mature fibril formation (Kalamajski and Oldberg 2009). Decorin and biglycan display coordinated control of collagen fibrillogenesis during development and acquisition of biomechanical properties during tendon development (Iozzo et al. 2011). Alterations in the functional properties of SLRP members through point mutations affecting the structure of critical interactive regions within the LRRs can give rise to impaired tissue assembly and function.

4.7.1 Decorin

Decorin is so named since it was found to "decorate" the surface of collagen fibrils. The decorin gene (DCN) is located on chromosome 12q21.3–q23. It possesses 8 exons encoding a 36kDa core protein, which contains a single CS or DS chain located at position 4 in the mature human core protein sequence (Roughley 2006). Decorin interacts with the "d" and "e" bands of collagen I fibrils, fibronectin, C1q, EGF receptor, TGF-β, and thrombospondin. Thus, it has roles in the regulation of collagen fibrillogenesis in vitro and fibrosis in vivo and controls the bioavailability of TGF-β. Decorin also influences cell proliferation at certain stages of the cell cycle and has roles as a linking module in collagenous matrices (Iozzo and Schaefer 2010).

The regions of decorin which interact with collagen are located within the leucine-rich repeats at dissimilar regions to those involved in its interaction with TGF-β. Molecular modeling predicts that decorin possesses a "horseshoe" conformation capable of accommodating a single collagen molecule at the surface of the collagen fibrils within its concave face (Orgel et al. 2009; Scott 1996, 2003; Scott and Stockwell 2006). However, X-ray diffraction analysis of decorin crystals indicates that it exists as a dimer with interlocking concave faces (Scott et al. 2004), although it is not clear whether decorin dimers represent the functional form in solution and how this impacts its interactions with other molecules. Decorin, together with biglycan, fibromodulin, and lumican, also interacts with collagen VI, XII, and XIV (Nareyeck et al. 2004; Wiberg et al. 2002), fibronectin and elastin, and growth factors and cytokines such as EGF, IGF, TGF-β, and TNF-α. SLRP GAG chain interactions with growth factors sequester them in the matrix surrounding cells in cartilaginous matrices, with the possibility that SLRPs play a role in the regulation of the bioavailability of these growth factors.

The decorin core protein is susceptible to cleavage by MMPs in vitro (Imai et al. 1997; Monfort et al. 2006) and is fragmented in an ovine annular lesion model of intervertebral disc degeneration (Melrose et al. 2007) and in an ovine meniscectomy model of osteoarthritis in areas undergoing remodeling processes (Young et al. 2005). Fragmentation of decorin is also evident in meniscal and articular cartilages from osteoarthritic knees and hips (Melrose et al. 2008a). Decorin is processed by three isoforms of BMP-1 (von Marschall and Fisher 2010) and MT1-MMP (Mimura et al. 2009). However, by acting as a sacrificial substrate on the surface of collagen fibers or through steric exclusion effects which prevent the collagenase from accessing the collagen substrate, its presence may protect the protein from cleavage by collagenases (Geng et al. 2006).

4.7.2 Biglycan

The biglycan gene (BGN) is located on chromosome Xq28 (McBride et al. 1990). It possesses eight exons encoding the 38 kDa biglycan core protein, which has two CS/DS chains located at amino acids five and ten of the mature human core protein sequence. Non-glycanated forms of biglycan have been detected and appear to be the result of proteolysis within the amino terminal region of the core protein. Mature biglycan is cleaved by MMPs (Monfort et al. 2006), and probiglycan by BMP-1 (Scott et al. 2000). Extensive biglycan fragmentation is also evident in models of osteoarthritis induced by meniscectomy (Young et al. 2005), in an annular lesion model of experimental disc degeneration (Melrose et al. 2007), and in pathological meniscal and articular cartilage from osteoarthritic knees and hips (Melrose et al. 2008a).

Unlike the interaction of decorin, fibromodulin, and lumican with collagen fibrils, the association of biglycan with collagen fibrils is sensitive to environmental conditions. This may explain the differences observed in the distribution of biglycan, which is more of a cell-associated SLRP than the other SLRP members. Biglycan interacts with the lattice-forming collagen VI to form chondron basketlike structures around cells in cartilaginous matrices and the intervertebral disc. Biglycan has a widespread distribution in the developing human fetal disc and prominently demarcates its margins with the cartilaginous vertebral body rudiment cartilages, where it is also prominently localized. As such, its position delineates the margins of the developing intervertebral disc interspace from the presumptive cartilage end plate (Fig. 4.4). Biglycan also interacts with BMPs and TGF-β. Biglycan plays a role in the initiation of the inflammatory response during tissue stress, by binding to BMP/TGF-β, and may modulate their activities, influencing fibrosis and skeletal cell differentiation. Biglycan also has emerging roles as a signaling molecule, with an extensive repertoire of molecular interactions with growth factors and receptors, which regulate cell growth, morphogenesis, and immunity (Iozzo and Schaefer 2010).

4.7.3 Asporin

The naming of asporin reflects its unique N-terminal aspartic acid cluster (Henry et al. 2001; Lorenzo et al. 2001). Asporin is also known as periodontal-associated protein-1 (PLAP-1). The asporin gene (ASPN) is located at chromosome 9q21–23 and possesses eight exons that encode a 43 kDa non-glycanated core protein. The asporin core protein exhibits polymorphism within its N-terminal region, which contains 9–20 aspartic acid repeats. An association of the ASPN D14 allele has been observed with disc degeneration (Gruber et al. 2009; Song et al. 2008). Asporin is a cell-associated SLRP and is found predominantly in the outer annulus fibrosus (Gruber et al. 2009).

4.7.4 Fibromodulin

The fibromodulin gene (FMOD) is located on chromosome 1q32 (Antonsson et al. 1993; Sztrolovics et al. 1994) and possesses three exons encoding the 42 kDa fibromodulin core protein. Fibromodulin is a KS-substituted SLRP which shares significant amino acid sequence homology with decorin and biglycan (Antonsson et al. 1993; Oldberg et al. 1989) but contains four N-linked oligosaccharide sites within the LRR domains, which can potentially be substituted with KS. Fibromodulin also possesses a cluster of amino terminal sulfated tyrosine residues which impart an anionic character to the molecule and allow this region to interact with clusters of basic residues in a variety of heparin-binding proteins, including a number of bioactive factors (Onnerfjord et al. 2004; Tillgren et al. 2009). Non-glycanated forms of fibromodulin can accumulate in tissues (Grover et al. 1995; Roughley et al. 1996a), due to an age-dependent decline in KS synthesis.

Fibromodulin interacts with collagen I and II fibrils and inhibits fibrillogenesis in vitro (Chen et al. 2010; Ezura et al. 2000). Fibromodulin also interacts with TGF-β and C1q and may have roles in TGF-β sequestration, in inflammation, in the regulation of the assembly of collagen I and II fibrils in vivo, and in the bio-regulation of TGF-β activity. The use of fibromodulin knockout mice has demarcated the significant functional roles of fibromodulin in cartilaginous tissues with regard to collagen assembly and in the regulation of the fibrillogenesis (Chakravarti 2002; Goldberg et al. 2006; Svensson et al. 1999).

Fibromodulin is prominently immunolocalized in the cartilaginous vertebral rudiment cartilages of the human fetal spine and also the developing disc, and its distribution in the fetal spine prominently demarcates the margins of the developmental intervertebral disc with the vertebral rudiment cartilages (Fig. 4.4). In the mature disc, fibromodulin is localized with collagenous structures pericellularly and in the interstitial matrix. It occurs throughout the intervertebral disc, but predominantly in the annulus fibrosus.

When bound to collagen, fibromodulin is susceptible to cleavage by MMP-13 which removes the N-terminal sulfated tyrosine cluster (Heathfield et al. 2004). Soluble fibromodulin is not, however, susceptible to cleavage by MMP-13, neither is it degraded by MMP-2, MMP-8, and MMP-9. The MMP-13 cleavage site is contained within a 10 kDa N-terminal peptide, Gln19-Lys 98, which is located adjacent to the sulfated tyrosine cluster (Heathfield et al. 2004). Fibromodulin is extensively fragmented in pathological meniscal and articular cartilage from osteoarthritic knees and hip (Melrose et al. 2008a), in an ovine annular lesion model of intervertebral disc degeneration in areas undergoing remodeling (Melrose et al. 2007), and in an ovine meniscectomy model of osteoarthritis (Young et al. 2005).

4.7.5 Lumican

The lumican gene (LUM) is located at chromosome 12q21.3–q22 (Danielson et al. 1999; Grover et al. 1995) and possesses three exons encoding the 38 kDa lumican core protein, which has four N-linked sites within the LRR domain that potentially can be substituted with KS. Lumican interacts with similar partners to those outlined for fibromodulin and displays similar roles to those of fibromodulin in tissues. Lumican and fibromodulin have homologous sequences in the 5–7 LRRs which compete for collagen binding (Kalamajski and Oldberg 2009), and they bind to the same regions of collagen I fibrils (Svensson et al. 2000). However, despite the significant similarities between lumican and decorin, they have dissimilar binding sites on collagen I (Hedbom and Heinegard 1993) and modulate collagen fibrillogenesis independently (Neame et al. 2000).

As with fibromodulin and decorin, lumican is also susceptible to degradation by MMPs, but apparently to a lesser extent, and it is also cleaved by MT1-MMP (Li et al. 2004). Fragmentation of lumican is a prominent feature in pathological meniscal and articular cartilages from osteoarthritic knees and hips (Melrose et al. 2008a) and has also been observed in an ovine annular lesion model of disc degeneration in areas undergoing remodeling (Melrose et al. 2007). Although it does not contain KS, lumican expression is, however, upregulated in an ovine meniscectomy model of osteoarthritis, with increased levels of lumican core protein evident (Young et al. 2005).

4.7.6 PRELP

PRELP is a 55 kDa non-glycanated SLRP (Bengtsson et al. 1995) encoded by the PRELP gene which is located on chromosome 1q32 and possesses three exons (Grover et al. 1996). Its name PRELP is based on the presence of a unique cluster of N-terminal arginine and proline residues. PRELP binds to perlecan and collagens and may act as a basement membrane anchor or as a linking molecule bringing together collagenous tissue networks (Bengtsson et al. 2002). The N-terminus of PRELP binds to heparin and HS and thereby promotes interactions with the HS-proteoglycan perlecan (Bengtsson et al. 2000).

4.7.7 Chondroadherin

Chondroadherin is a developmentally regulated SLRP (Shen et al. 1998) closely related to decorin, biglycan, fibromodulin, lumican, and PRELP (Neame et al. 1994). The chondroadherin gene (CHAD) is located on chromosome 17q21.33 and possesses 4 exons encoding the 36 kDa non-glycanated chondroadherin core protein (Grover et al. 1997), which contains 10 LRRs (Neame et al. 1994). Chondroadherin interacts with collagen II (Mansson et al. 2001) and $\alpha 2\beta 1$ integrin (Camper et al. 1997; Haglund et al. 2011) and plays a role in the attachment of connective tissue cells to matrix components; in this way it could maintain the cellular phenotype and regulate tissue homeostasis. Depletion and proteolytic fragmentation of chondroadherin occurs in scoliotic intervertebral discs and appears to be associated with disc matrix remodeling (Haglund et al. 2009).

4.7.8 SLRP Knockout Mice and Gene Mutations

A number of human diseases are associated with SLRP mutations, and mouse knockout models have identified pathological consequences resulting from the ablation of SLRP genes. Examples of pathological features induced by SLRP gene ablation and human SLRP gene mutations are described in Tables 4.1 and 4.2. Thus far, asporin is the only SLRP specifically associated with human disc disease and the disc phenotype. The intervertebral disc nevertheless exhibits similarities in collagenous organization to tensional and weight-bearing connective tissues which display phenotypes in SLRP knockout mouse models. It is highly probable that SLRPs have specific roles to play in disc degeneration which await detailed elucidation.

Table 4.1 Pathological consequences of targeted ablation of SLRP genes in mouse models

Ablated gene	Pathology	Phenotype	References
Decorin	Collagen fibril structure in skin and tendon abnormal	Skin fragility Reduced tendon function	Danielson et al. (1997)
Biglycan	Decreased bone mass, structural collagen fibril abnormalities in medial aorta	Osteoporosis Spontaneous aortic dissection/rupture	Heegaard et al. (2007) and Xu et al. (1998)
Lumican	Abnormal collagen fibril organization in cornea and dermis	Skin fragility Corneal opacity	Chakravarti et al. (1998)
Fibromodulin	Abnormal collagen fibril organization in tendon	Lax tendons with reduced biomechanical function	Svensson et al. (1999)
Biglycan/decorin	Abnormal collagen fibril formation in bone, tendon, dermis	Similar to progeroid form of Ehlers-Danlos syndrome	Corsi et al. (2002)
Biglycan/fibromodulin	Maturational structural/biomechanical abnormalities in collagen fibrils in tendon	Gait impairment, ectopic calcification, premature OA	Ameye and Young (2002)
Lumican/fibromodulin	Abnormal collagen maturation and structure of tendons	Joint laxity and impaired tendon function	Jepsen et al. (2002)
Asporin	Reduced inhibition of periodontal ligament mineralization	Diminished negative regulation of periodontal ligament cell cytodifferentiation by point mutations disrupting asporin LRR5-mediated interactions with BMP-2	Tomoeda et al. (2008) and Yamada et al. (2007)

Table 4.2 Human diseases linked to mutations in SLRP genes

Gene	Type of mutation	Pathology/clinical phenotype	References
Decorin	Frameshift mutation generating a C-terminal truncated core protein	Corneal opacity, congenital stromal dystrophy of cornea	Bredrup et al. (2005)
Lumican, fibromodulin, PRELP	Intronic variations, single-nucleotide polymorphisms in promoter	Corneal detachment, choroidal neovascularization, high myopia	Chen et al. (2009), Majava et al. (2007), andWang et al. (2006)
Asporin	Asporin D4 allele polymorphisms affecting N-terminal of core protein	Early onset of OA and disc degeneration	Gruber et al. (2009) and Song et al. (2008)

4.8 Summary of Critical Concepts Discussed in the Chapter

Role of Proteoglycans in Disc Function

- Aggrecan provides the disc with its ability to swell and resist compressive loads. This property is dependent on two features of aggrecan: first, its ability to form large proteoglycan aggregates in association with HA, which limit its diffusion within the matrix, and second, the osmotic properties and water binding are due to its substitution with numerous CS and KS chains. Aggrecan swelling maintains disc height underload and is responsible for the diurnal variation in disc height associated with daily life.
- Versican and lubricin are present throughout the intervertebral disc, but their precise functions are unclear. The high abundance of versican in the immature disc may suggest a role in disc development during fetal life, and it has been suggested that lubricin plays a role in enhancing motion between adjacent lamellae within the annulus fibrosus.
- Perlecan promotes and stabilizes matrix assembly through its interaction with a diverse repertoire of matrix components. Roles are now also emerging for perlecan in fibrillin-1 and elastin assembly in the disc, with the HS chains of perlecan being important. The HS chains of perlecan also sequester a number of bioactive growth factors and morphogens of relevance to developmental and remodeling processes in the disc through their abilities to regulate cell proliferation and differentiation. Furthermore, the ability of perlecan to interact with a number of cell attachment proteins may regulate cellular recruitment during development and remodeling of the disc.
- The SLRPs have important regulatory roles to play in collagen fibrillogenesis and are important for disc extracellular matrix assembly and repair. Emerging interactive roles of SLRPs with cytokines and bioactive growth factors implicate them in cell signaling, affecting a diverse range of biological processes, including fibrosis, inflammation, and the immune response.

Role of Proteoglycans in Disc Disease

- Aggrecan degradation is associated with disc degeneration in the adult and probably in the juvenile with scoliosis. The proteolytic degradation of aggrecan results in fragments that are no longer able to interact with HA; these are slowly lost as their size is further decreased by continuing proteolysis. This decline in aggrecan content of the degenerate disc may facilitate blood vessel and nerve ingrowth and contribute to discogenic pain. Mutations in the aggrecan gene result in osteochondrodysplasia, the features of which include developmental abnormalities in the disc.

- Versican and lubricin undergo extensive proteolytic fragmentation throughout life, which is likely caused by the same proteinases responsible for aggrecan degradation. It is, however, unclear whether this contributes to disc pathology.
- Perlecan also undergoes extensive fragmentation within the disc, though little is known as to how this occurs or whether the released perlecan fragments provide new functional biological properties. An exception to this is the C-terminal peptide, endorepellin, which has anti-angiogenic properties due to its ability to destabilize tube formation by endothelial cells. In degenerate discs, if the fragments are not lost or further degraded, these properties might be expected to maintain the avascular nature of the disc.
- A number of the SLRPs are also fragmented in degenerate discs, and the loss of the CS/DS chains in decorin and biglycan may adversely affect their abilities to interact with cytokines and growth factors and thus their participation in cell regulatory processes. Fragmentation of lumican and fibromodulin is also evident in the degenerate disc, but it is not known how this impacts tissue function.

Acknowledgements We would like to thank the Shriners of North America and the Canadian Institutes of Health Research for support of the work described in this chapter. Support from the National Health and Medical Research Council of Australia is also gratefully acknowledged.

References

Adams MA, Roughley PJ (2006) What is intervertebral disc degeneration, and what causes it? Spine (Phila Pa 1976) 31:2151–2161

Agrawal A, Guttapalli A, Narayan S, Albert TJ, Shapiro IM, Risbud MV (2007) Normoxic stabilization of HIF-1alpha drives glycolytic metabolism and regulates aggrecan gene expression in nucleus pulposus cells of the rat intervertebral disk. Am J Physiol Cell Physiol 293:C621–C631

Akeda K, An HS, Pichika R, Patel K, Muehleman C, Nakagawa K, Uchida A, Masuda K (2007) The expression of NG2 proteoglycan in the human intervertebral disc. Spine (Phila Pa 1976) 32: 306–314

Ameye L, Young MF (2002) Mice deficient in small leucine-rich proteoglycans: novel in vivo models for osteoporosis, osteoarthritis, Ehlers-Danlos syndrome, muscular dystrophy, and corneal diseases. Glycobiology 12:107R–116R

Antonsson P, Heinegard D, Oldberg A (1991) Posttranslational modifications of fibromodulin. J Biol Chem 266:16859–16861

Antonsson P, Heinegard D, Oldberg A (1993) Structure and deduced amino acid sequence of the human fibromodulin gene. Biochim Biophys Acta 1174:204–206

Arikawa-Hirasawa E, Watanabe H, Takami H, Hassell JR, Yamada Y (1999) Perlecan is essential for cartilage and cephalic development. Nat Genet 23:354–358

Arikawa-Hirasawa E, Wilcox WR, Le AH, Silverman N, Govindraj P, Hassell JR, Yamada Y (2001a) Dyssegmental dysplasia, Silverman-Handmaker type, is caused by functional null mutations of the perlecan gene. Nat Genet 27:431–434

Arikawa-Hirasawa E, Wilcox WR, Yamada Y (2001b) Dyssegmental dysplasia, Silverman-Handmaker type: unexpected role of perlecan in cartilage development. Am J Med Genet 106:254–257

Arikawa-Hirasawa E, Le AH, Nishino I, Nonaka I, Ho NC, Francomano CA, Govindraj P, Hassell JR, Devaney JM, Spranger J, Stevenson RE, Iannaccone S, Dalakas MC, Yamada Y (2002) Structural and functional mutations of the perlecan gene cause Schwartz-Jampel syndrome, with myotonic myopathy and chondrodysplasia. Am J Hum Genet 70:1368–1375

Barry FP, Neame PJ, Sasse J, Pearson D (1994) Length variation in the keratan sulfate domain of mammalian aggrecan. Matrix Biol 14:323–328

Barry FP, Rosenberg LC, Gaw JU, Koob TJ, Neame PJ (1995) N- and O-linked keratan sulfate on the hyaluronan binding region of aggrecan from mature and immature bovine cartilage. J Biol Chem 270:20516–20524

Bengtsson E, Neame PJ, Heinegard D, Sommarin Y (1995) The primary structure of a basic leucine-rich repeat protein, PRELP, found in connective tissues. J Biol Chem 270:25639–25644

Bengtsson E, Aspberg A, Heinegard D, Sommarin Y, Spillmann D (2000) The amino-terminal part of PRELP binds to heparin and heparan sulfate. J Biol Chem 275:40695–40702

Bengtsson E, Morgelin M, Sasaki T, Timpl R, Heinegard D, Aspberg A (2002) The leucine-rich repeat protein PRELP binds perlecan and collagens and may function as a basement membrane anchor. J Biol Chem 277:15061–15068

Bix G, Fu J, Gonzalez EM, Macro L, Barker A, Campbell S, Zutter MM, Santoro SA, Kim JK, Hook M, Reed CC, Iozzo RV (2004) Endorepellin causes endothelial cell disassembly of actin cytoskeleton and focal adhesions through alpha2beta1 integrin. J Cell Biol 166:97–109

Bix G, Iozzo RA, Woodall B, Burrows M, McQuillan A, Campbell S, Fields GB, Iozzo RV (2007) Endorepellin, the C-terminal angiostatic module of perlecan, enhances collagen-platelet responses via the alpha2beta1-integrin receptor. Blood 109:3745–3748

Botsford DJ, Esses SI, Ogilvie-Harris DJ (1994) In vivo diurnal variation in intervertebral disc volume and morphology. Spine (Phila Pa 1976) 19:935–940

Bredrup C, Knappskog PM, Majewski J, Rodahl E, Boman H (2005) Congenital stromal dystrophy of the cornea caused by a mutation in the decorin gene. Invest Ophthalmol Vis Sci 46:420–426

Brown GM, Huckerby TN, Bayliss MT, Nieduszynski IA (1998) Human aggrecan keratan sulfate undergoes structural changes during adolescent development. J Biol Chem 273:26408–26414

Camper L, Heinegard D, Lundgren-Akerlund E (1997) Integrin alpha-2beta1 is a receptor for the cartilage matrix protein chondroadherin. J Cell Biol 138:1159–1167

Caterson B (2012) Fell-Muir lecture: chondroitin sulphate glycosaminoglycans: fun for some and confusion for others. Int J Exp Pathol 93:1–10

Caterson B, Mahmoodian F, Sorrell JM, Hardingham TE, Bayliss MT, Carney SL, Ratcliffe A, Muir H (1990) Modulation of native chondroitin sulphate structure in tissue development and in disease. J Cell Sci 97(Pt 3):411–417

Chakravarti S (2002) Functions of lumican and fibromodulin: lessons from knockout mice. Glycoconj J 19:287–293

Chakravarti S, Magnuson T, Lass JH, Jepsen KJ, LaMantia C, Carroll H (1998) Lumican regulates collagen fibril assembly: skin fragility and corneal opacity in the absence of lumican. J Cell Biol 141: 1277–1286

Chen ZT, Wang IJ, Shih YF, Lin LL (2009) The association of haplotype at the lumican gene with high myopia susceptibility in Taiwanese patients. Ophthalmology 116:1920–1927

Chen S, Oldberg A, Chakravarti S, Birk DE (2010) Fibromodulin regulates collagen fibrillogenesis during peripheral corneal development. Dev Dyn 239:844–854

Chuang CY, Lord MS, Melrose J, Rees MD, Knox SM, Freeman C, Iozzo RV, Whitelock JM (2010) Heparan sulfate-dependent signaling of fibroblast growth factor 18 by chondrocyte-derived perlecan. Biochemistry 49:5524–5532

Cohen IR, Grassel S, Murdoch AD, Iozzo RV (1993) Structural characterization of the complete human perlecan gene and its promoter. Proc Natl Acad Sci USA 90:10404–10408

Corsi A, Xu T, Chen XD, Boyde A, Liang J, Mankani M, Sommer B, Iozzo RV, Eichstetter I, Robey PG, Bianco P, Young MF (2002) Phenotypic effects of biglycan deficiency are linked to collagen fibril abnormalities, are synergized by decorin deficiency, and mimic Ehlers-Danlos-like changes in bone and other connective tissues. J Bone Miner Res 17:1180–1189

Cummings RD (2009) The repertoire of glycan determinants in the human glycome. Mol Biosyst 5:1087–1104

Danielson KG, Baribault H, Holmes DF, Graham H, Kadler KE, Iozzo RV (1997) Targeted disruption of decorin leads to abnormal collagen fibril morphology and skin fragility. J Cell Biol 136:729–743

Danielson KG, Siracusa LD, Donovan PJ, Iozzo RV (1999) Decorin, epiphycan, and lumican genes are closely linked on murine chromosome 10 and are deleted in lethal steel mutants. Mamm Genome 10:201–203

Day JM, Olin AI, Murdoch AD, Canfield A, Sasaki T, Timpl R, Hardingham TE, Aspberg A (2004) Alternative splicing in the aggrecan G3 domain influences binding interactions with tenascin-C and other extracellular matrix proteins. J Biol Chem 279: 12511–12518

Doege K, Sasaki M, Horigan E, Hassell JR, Yamada Y (1987) Complete primary structure of the rat cartilage proteoglycan core protein deduced from cDNA clones. J Biol Chem 262:17757–17767

Doege KJ, Sasaki M, Kimura T, Yamada Y (1991) Complete coding sequence and deduced primary structure of the human cartilage large aggregating proteoglycan, aggrecan. Human-specific repeats, and additional alternatively spliced forms. J Biol Chem 266:894–902

Doege KJ, Coulter SN, Meek LM, Maslen K, Wood JG (1997) A human-specific polymorphism in the coding region of the aggrecan gene. Variable number of tandem repeats produce a range of core protein sizes in the general population. J Biol Chem 272: 13974–13979

Dours-Zimmermann MT, Zimmermann DR (1994) A novel glycosaminoglycan attachment domain identified in two alternative splice variants of human versican. J Biol Chem 269:32992–32998

Durigova M, Nagase H, Mort JS, Roughley PJ (2011a) MMPs are less efficient than ADAMTS5 in cleaving aggrecan core protein. Matrix Biol 30:145–153

Durigova M, Troeberg L, Nagase H, Roughley PJ, Mort JS (2011b) Involvement of ADAMTS5 and hyaluronidase in aggrecan degradation and release from OSM-stimulated cartilage. Eur Cell Mater 21:31–45

Elsaid KA, Jay GD, Warman ML, Rhee DK, Chichester CO (2005) Association of articular cartilage degradation and loss of boundary-lubricating ability of synovial fluid following injury and inflammatory arthritis. Arthritis Rheum 52:1746–1755

Ezura Y, Chakravarti S, Oldberg A, Chervoneva I, Birk DE (2000) Differential expression of lumican and fibromodulin regulate collagen fibrillogenesis in developing mouse tendons. J Cell Biol 151:779–788

Faivre L, Prieur AM, Le Merrer M, Hayem F, Penet C, Woo P, Hofer M, Dagoneau N, Sermet I, Munnich A, Cormier-Daire V (2000) Clinical variability and genetic homogeneity of the camptodactyly-arthropathy-coxa vara-pericarditis syndrome. Am J Med Genet 95:233–236

Flannery C, Stanescu V, Morgelin M, Boynton R, Gordy J, Sandy J (1992) Variability in the G3 domain content of bovine aggrecan from cartilage extracts and chondrocyte cultures. Arch Biochem Biophys 297:52–60

Flannery CR, Hughes CE, Schumacher BL, Tudor D, Aydelotte MB, Kuettner KE, Caterson B (1999) Articular cartilage superficial zone protein (SZP) is homologous to megakaryocyte stimulating factor precursor and is a multifunctional proteoglycan with potential growth-promoting, cytoprotective, and lubricating properties in cartilage metabolism. Biochem Biophys Res Commun 254:535–541

Fosang AJ, Hardingham TE (1989) Isolation of the N-terminal globular protein domains from cartilage proteoglycans. Identification of G2 domain and its lack of interaction with hyaluronate and link protein. Biochem J 261:801–809

Fosang AJ, Neame PJ, Last K, Hardingham TE, Murphy G, Hamilton JA (1992) The interglobular domain of cartilage aggrecan is cleaved by PUMP, gelatinases, and cathepsin B. J Biol Chem 267: 19470–19474

Fransson LA, Belting M, Cheng F, Jonsson M, Mani K, Sandgren S (2004) Novel aspects of glypican glycobiology. Cell Mol Life Sci 61:1016–1024

Fulop C, Walcz E, Valyon M, Glant TT (1993) Expression of alternatively spliced epidermal growth factor-like domains in aggrecans of different species. Evidence for a novel module. J Biol Chem 268:17377–17383

Gendron C, Kashiwagi M, Lim NH, Enghild JJ, Thogersen IB, Hughes C, Caterson B, Nagase H (2007) Proteolytic activities of human ADAMTS-5: comparative studies with ADAMTS-4. J Biol Chem 282:18294–18306

Geng Y, McQuillan D, Roughley PJ (2006) SLRP interaction can protect collagen fibrils from cleavage by collagenases. Matrix Biol 25:484–491

Girardin EP, Hajmohammadi S, Birmele B, Helisch A, Shworak NW, de Agostini AI (2005) Synthesis of anticoagulantly active heparan sulfate proteoglycans by glomerular epithelial cells involves multiple 3-O-sulfotransferase isoforms and a limiting precursor pool. J Biol Chem 280:38059–38070

Gleghorn L, Ramesar R, Beighton P, Wallis G (2005) A mutation in the variable repeat region of the aggrecan gene (AGC1) causes a form of spondyloepiphyseal dysplasia associated with severe, premature osteoarthritis. Am J Hum Genet 77:484–490

Gogate SS, Nasser R, Shapiro IM, Risbud MV (2011) Hypoxic regulation of beta-1,3-glucuronyltransferase 1 expression in nucleus pulposus cells of the rat intervertebral disc: role of hypoxia-inducible factor proteins. Arthritis Rheum 63:1950–1960

Goldberg M, Septier D, Oldberg A, Young MF, Ameye LG (2006) Fibromodulin-deficient mice display impaired collagen fibrillogenesis in predentin as well as altered dentin mineralization and enamel formation. J Histochem Cytochem 54:525–537

Gonzalez EM, Reed CC, Bix G, Fu J, Zhang Y, Gopalakrishnan B, Greenspan DS, Iozzo RV (2005) BMP-1/Tolloid-like metalloproteases process endorepellin, the angiostatic C-terminal fragment of perlecan. J Biol Chem 280:7080–7087

Grover J, Roughley PJ (1993) Versican gene expression in human articular cartilage and comparison of mRNA splicing variation with aggrecan. Biochem J 291(Pt 2):361–367

Grover J, Roughley PJ (1998) Characterization of the human proline/arginine-rich end leucine-rich repeat protein (PRELP) gene promoter and identification of a repressor element. Biochem J 336(Pt 1):77–82

Grover J, Roughley PJ (2001) Characterization and expression of murine PRELP. Matrix Biol 20:555–564

Grover J, Chen XN, Korenberg JR, Roughley PJ (1995) The human lumican gene. Organization, chromosomal location, and expression in articular cartilage. J Biol Chem 270:21942–21949

Grover J, Chen XN, Korenberg JR, Recklies AD, Roughley PJ (1996) The gene organization, chromosome location, and expression of a 55-kDa matrix protein (PRELP) of human articular cartilage. Genomics 38:109–117

Grover J, Chen XN, Korenberg JR, Roughley PJ (1997) The structure and chromosome location of the human chondroadherin gene (CHAD). Genomics 45:379–385

Gruber HE, Ingram JA, Hoelscher GL, Zinchenko N, Hanley EN Jr, Sun Y (2009) Asporin, a susceptibility gene in osteoarthritis, is expressed at higher levels in the more degenerate human intervertebral disc. Arthritis Res Ther 11:R47

Haglund L, Ouellet J, Roughley P (2009) Variation in chondroadherin abundance and fragmentation in the human scoliotic disc. Spine (Phila Pa 1976) 34:1513–1518

Haglund L, Tillgren V, Addis L, Wenglen C, Recklies A, Heinegard D (2011) Identification and characterization of the integrin alpha-2beta1 binding motif in chondroadherin mediating cell attachment. J Biol Chem 286:3925–3934

Hasegawa K, Yoneda M, Kuwabara H, Miyaishi O, Itano N, Ohno A, Zako M, Isogai Z (2007) Versican, a major hyaluronan-binding component in the dermis, loses its hyaluronan-binding ability in solar elastosis. J Invest Dermatol 127:1657–1663

Hayes A, Lord MS, Smith SM, Smith MM, Whitelock JM, Weiss AS, Melrose J (2011a) Colocalization in vivo and association in vitro of perlecan and elastin. Histochem Cell Biol 136:437–475

Hayes AJ, Hughes CE, Ralphs JR, Caterson B (2011b) Chondroitin sulphate sulphation motif expression in the ontogeny of the intervertebral disc. Eur Cell Mater 21:1–14

Hayes AJ, Smith SM, Gibson MA, Melrose J (2011c) Comparative immunolocalisation of the elastin fibre associated proteins fibrillin-1, LTBP2 and MAGP-1 with components of the collagenous and proteoglycan matrix of the foetal human IVD. Spine (Phila Pa 1976) 36:E1365–E1372

Hayes AJ, Smith SM, Melrose J (2013) Comparative immunolocalisation of fibrillin-1 and perlecan in the human foetal and HS deficient Hspg2 exon 3 null mutant mouse intervertebral disc. Histochem Cell Biol 139:1–11

Heathfield TF, Onnerfjord P, Dahlberg L, Heinegard D (2004) Cleavage of fibromodulin in cartilage explants involves removal of the N-terminal tyrosine sulfate-rich region by proteolysis at a site that is sensitive to matrix metalloproteinase-13. J Biol Chem 279:6286–6295

Hedbom E, Heinegard D (1993) Binding of fibromodulin and decorin to separate sites on fibrillar collagens. J Biol Chem 268:27307–27312

Heegaard AM, Corsi A, Danielsen CC, Nielsen KL, Jorgensen HL, Riminucci M, Young MF, Bianco P (2007) Biglycan deficiency causes spontaneous aortic dissection and rupture in mice. Circulation 115:2731–2738

Henry SP, Takanosu M, Boyd TC, Mayne PM, Eberspaecher H, Zhou W, de Crombrugghe B, Hook M, Mayne R (2001) Expression pattern and gene characterization of asporin. A newly discovered member of the leucine-rich repeat protein family. J Biol Chem 276: 12212–12221

Hirai M, Horiguchi M, Ohbayashi T, Kita T, Chien KR, Nakamura T (2007) Latent TGF-beta-binding protein 2 binds to DANCE/fibulin-5 and regulates elastic fiber assembly. EMBO J 26:3283–3295

Hirani R, Hanssen E, Gibson MA (2007) LTBP-2 specifically interacts with the amino-terminal region of fibrillin-1 and competes with LTBP-1 for binding to this microfibrillar protein. Matrix Biol 26: 213–223

Hiyama A, Gajghate S, Sakai D, Mochida J, Shapiro IM, Risbud MV (2009) Activation of TonEBP by calcium controls {beta}1,3-glucuronosyltransferase-I expression, a key regulator of glycosaminoglycan synthesis in cells of the intervertebral disc. J Biol Chem 284:9824–9834

Hocking AM, Shinomura T, McQuillan DJ (1998) Leucine-rich repeat glycoproteins of the extracellular matrix. Matrix Biol 17:1–19

Humphries DE, Stevens RL (1992) Regulation of the gene that encodes the peptide core of heparin proteoglycan and other proteoglycans that are stored in the secretory granules of hematopoietic cells. Adv Exp Med Biol 313:59–67

Imai K, Hiramatsu A, Fukushima D, Pierschbacher MD, Okada Y (1997) Degradation of decorin by matrix metalloproteinases: identification of the cleavage sites, kinetic analyses and transforming growth factor-beta1 release. Biochem J 322(Pt 3):809–814

Iozzo RV (1994) Perlecan: a gem of a proteoglycan. Matrix Biol 14:203–208

Iozzo RV (1998) Matrix proteoglycans: from molecular design to cellular function. Annu Rev Biochem 67:609–652

Iozzo RV, Schaefer L (2010) Proteoglycans in health and disease: novel regulatory signaling mechanisms evoked by the small leucine-rich proteoglycans. FEBS J 277:3864–3875

Iozzo RV, Naso MF, Cannizzaro LA, Wasmuth JJ, McPherson JD (1992) Mapping of the versican proteoglycan gene (CSPG2) to the long arm of human chromosome 5 (5q12-5q14). Genomics 14:845–851

Iozzo R, Goldoni S, Berendsen AD, Young MF (2011) Small leucine rich proteoglycans. In: Mecham R (ed) The extracellular matrix: an overview, Biology of extracellular matrix. Springer, Berlin/Heidelberg, pp 197–231

Ito K, Shinomura T, Zako M, Ujita M, Kimata K (1995) Multiple forms of mouse PG-M, a large chondroitin sulfate proteoglycan generated by alternative splicing. J Biol Chem 270:958–965

Jackson RL, Busch SJ, Cardin AD (1991) Glycosaminoglycans: molecular properties, protein interactions, and role in physiological processes. Physiol Rev 71:481–539

Jay GD, Harris DA, Cha CJ (2001a) Boundary lubrication by lubricin is mediated by O-linked beta(1-3)Gal-GalNAc oligosaccharides. Glycoconj J 18:807–815

Jay GD, Tantravahi U, Britt DE, Barrach HJ, Cha CJ (2001b) Homology of lubricin and superficial zone protein (SZP): products of megakaryocyte stimulating factor (MSF) gene expression by human synovial fibroblasts and articular chondrocytes localized to chromosome 1q25. J Orthop Res 19:677–687

Jepsen KJ, Wu F, Peragallo JH, Paul J, Roberts L, Ezura Y, Oldberg A, Birk DE, Chakravarti S (2002) A syndrome of joint laxity and impaired tendon integrity in lumican- and fibromodulin-deficient mice. J Biol Chem 277:35532–35540

Johnson WE, Caterson B, Eisenstein SM, Hynds DL, Snow DM, Roberts S (2002) Human intervertebral disc aggrecan inhibits nerve growth in vitro. Arthritis Rheum 46:2658–2664

Johnson WE, Caterson B, Eisenstein SM, Roberts S (2005) Human intervertebral disc aggrecan inhibits endothelial cell adhesion and cell migration in vitro. Spine (Phila Pa 1976) 30:1139–1147

Kalamajski S, Oldberg A (2009) Homologous sequence in lumican and fibromodulin leucine-rich repeat 5–7 competes for collagen binding. J Biol Chem 284:534–539

Kalamajski S, Oldberg A (2010) The role of small leucine-rich proteoglycans in collagen fibrillogenesis. Matrix Biol 29:248–253

Kalamajski S, Aspberg A, Lindblom K, Heinegard D, Oldberg A (2009) Asporin competes with decorin for collagen binding, binds calcium and promotes osteoblast collagen mineralization. Biochem J 423:53–59

Kallunki P, Tryggvason K (1992) Human basement membrane heparan sulfate proteoglycan core protein: a 467-kD protein containing multiple domains resembling elements of the low density lipoprotein receptor, laminin, neural cell adhesion molecules, and epidermal growth factor. J Cell Biol 116:559–571

Karniski LP (2001) Mutations in the diastrophic dysplasia sulfate transporter (DTDST) gene: correlation between sulfate transport activity and chondrodysplasia phenotype. Hum Mol Genet 10:1485–1490

Kawaguchi Y, Osada R, Kanamori M, Ishihara H, Ohmori K, Matsui H, Kimura T (1999) Association between an aggrecan gene polymorphism and lumbar disc degeneration. Spine (Phila Pa 1976) 24: 2456–2460

Kloeckener-Gruissem B, Bartholdi D, Abdou MT, Zimmermann DR, Berger W (2006) Identification of the genetic defect in the original Wagner syndrome family. Mol Vis 12:350–355

Kluppel M, Wight TN, Chan C, Hinek A, Wrana JL (2005) Maintenance of chondroitin sulfation balance by chondroitin-4-sulfotransferase 1 is required for chondrocyte development and growth factor signaling during cartilage morphogenesis. Development 132:3989–4003

Korenberg JR, Chen XN, Doege K, Grover J, Roughley PJ (1993) Assignment of the human aggrecan gene (AGC1) to 15q26 using fluorescence in situ hybridization analysis. Genomics 16:546–548

Kurima K, Warman ML, Krishnan S, Domowicz M, Krueger RC Jr, Deyrup A, Schwartz NB (1998) A member of a family of sulfate-activating enzymes causes murine brachymorphism. Proc Natl Acad Sci USA 95:8681–8685

Li H, Schwartz NB, Vertel BM (1993) cDNA cloning of chick cartilage chondroitin sulfate (aggrecan) core protein and identification of a stop codon in the aggrecan gene associated with the chondrodystrophy, nanomelia. J Biol Chem 268:23504–23511

Li Y, Aoki T, Mori Y, Ahmad M, Miyamori H, Takino T, Sato H (2004) Cleavage of lumican by membrane-type matrix metalloproteinase-1 abrogates this proteoglycan-mediated suppression of tumor cell colony formation in soft agar. Cancer Res 64:7058–7064

Lorenzo P, Aspberg A, Onnerfjord P, Bayliss MT, Neame PJ, Heinegard D (2001) Identification and characterization of asporin. a novel member of the leucine-rich repeat protein family closely related to decorin and biglycan. J Biol Chem 276:12201–12211

Majava M, Bishop PN, Hagg P, Scott PG, Rice A, Inglehearn C, Hammond CJ, Spector TD, Ala-Kokko L, Mannikko M (2007) Novel mutations in the small leucine-rich repeat protein/proteoglycan (SLRP) genes in high myopia. Hum Mutat 28:336–344

Mansson B, Wenglen C, Morgelin M, Saxne T, Heinegard D (2001) Association of chondroadherin with collagen type II. J Biol Chem 276:32883–32888

Marcelino J, Carpten JD, Suwairi WM, Gutierrez OM, Schwartz S, Robbins C, Sood R, Makalowska I, Baxevanis A, Johnstone B, Laxer RM, Zemel L, Kim CA, Herd JK, Ihle J, Williams C, Johnson M, Raman V, Alonso LG, Brunoni D, Gerstein A, Papadopoulos N, Bahabri SA, Trent JM, Warman ML (1999) CACP, encoding a secreted proteoglycan, is mutated in camptodactyly-arthropathy-coxa vara-pericarditis syndrome. Nat Genet 23:319–322

Margolis RU, Margolis RK (1994) Aggrecan-versican-neurocan family proteoglycans. Methods Enzymol 245:105–126

McBride OW, Fisher LW, Young MF (1990) Localization of PGI (biglycan, BGN) and PGII (decorin, DCN, PG-40) genes on human chromosomes Xq13-qter and 12q, respectively. Genomics 6:219–225

Melrose J, Ghosh P, Taylor TK (2001) A comparative analysis of the differential spatial and temporal distributions of the large (aggrecan, versican) and small (decorin, biglycan, fibromodulin) proteoglycans of the intervertebral disc. J Anat 198:3–15

Melrose J, Roughley P, Knox S, Smith S, Lord M, Whitelock J (2006) The structure, location, and function of perlecan, a prominent pericellular proteoglycan of fetal, postnatal, and mature hyaline cartilages. J Biol Chem 281:36905–36914

Melrose J, Smith SM, Fuller ES, Young AA, Roughley PJ, Dart A, Little CB (2007) Biglycan and fibromodulin fragmentation correlates with temporal and spatial annular remodelling in experimentally injured ovine intervertebral discs. Eur Spine J 16:2193–2205

Melrose J, Fuller ES, Roughley PJ, Smith MM, Kerr B, Hughes CE, Caterson B, Little CB (2008a) Fragmentation of decorin, biglycan, lumican and keratocan is elevated in degenerate human meniscus, knee and hip articular cartilages compared with age-matched macroscopically normal and control tissues. Arthritis Res Ther 10:R79

Melrose J, Hayes AJ, Whitelock JM, Little CB (2008b) Perlecan, the "jack of all trades" proteoglycan of cartilaginous weight-bearing connective tissues. Bioessays 30:457–469

Merberg D, Fitz LJ, Temple P, Giannotti J, Murtha P, Fitzgerald M, Scaltreto H, Kelleher K, Preissner K, Kriz R, Jacobs K, Turner K (1993) A comparison of vitronectin and megakaryocyte stimulating factor. In: Rosenblatt S, Kost C, Wegerhoff J, Mosher DF, Preissner KT (eds) Biology of vitronectins and their Receptors. Elsevier, Amsterdam, pp 45–54

Mimura T, Han KY, Onguchi T, Chang JH, Kim TI, Kojima T, Zhou Z, Azar DT (2009) MT1-MMP-mediated cleavage of decorin in corneal angiogenesis. J Vasc Res 46:541–550

Monfort J, Tardif G, Reboul P, Mineau F, Roughley P, Pelletier JP, Martel-Pelletier J (2006) Degradation of small leucine-rich repeat proteoglycans by matrix metalloprotease-13: identification of a new biglycan cleavage site. Arthritis Res Ther 8:R26

Morgelin M, Paulsson M, Hardingham TE, Heinegard D, Engel J (1988) Cartilage proteoglycans. Assembly with hyaluronate and link protein as studied by electron microscopy. Biochem J 253:175–185

Mukhopadhyay A, Nikopoulos K, Maugeri A, de Brouwer AP, van Nouhuys CE, Boon CJ, Perveen R, Zegers HA, Wittebol-Post D, van den Biesen PR, van der Velde-Visser SD, Brunner HG, Black GC, Hoyng CB, Cremers FP (2006) Erosive vitreoretinopathy and wagner disease are caused by intronic mutations in CSPG2/Versican that result in an imbalance of splice variants. Invest Ophthalmol Vis Sci 47:3565–3572

Muragaki Y, Nishimura I, Henney A, Ninomiya Y, Olsen BR (1990) The alpha 1 (IX) collagen gene gives rise to two different transcripts in both mouse embryonic and human fetal RNA. Proc Natl Acad Sci USA 87:2400–2404

Murdoch AD, Iozzo RV (1993) Perlecan: the multidomain heparan sulphate proteoglycan of basement membrane and extracellular matrix. Virchows Arch A Pathol Anat Histopathol 423:237–242

Murdoch AD, Dodge GR, Cohen I, Tuan RS, Iozzo RV (1992) Primary structure of the human heparan sulfate proteoglycan from basement membrane (HSPG2/perlecan). A chimeric molecule with multiple domains homologous to the low density lipoprotein receptor, laminin, neural cell adhesion molecules, and epidermal growth factor. J Biol Chem 267:8544–8557

Nareyeck G, Seidler DG, Troyer D, Rauterberg J, Kresse H, Schonherr E (2004) Differential interactions of decorin and decorin mutants with type I and type VI collagens. Eur J Biochem 271:3389–3398

Naso MF, Zimmermann DR, Iozzo RV (1994) Characterization of the complete genomic structure of the human versican gene and functional analysis of its promoter. J Biol Chem 269:32999–33008

Neame PJ, Barry FP (1993) The link proteins. Experientia 49:393–402

Neame PJ, Sommarin Y, Boynton RE, Heinegard D (1994) The structure of a 38-kDa leucine-rich protein (chondroadherin) isolated from bovine cartilage. J Biol Chem 269:21547–21554

Neame PJ, Kay CJ, McQuillan DJ, Beales MP, Hassell JR (2000) Independent modulation of collagen fibrillogenesis by decorin and lumican. Cell Mol Life Sci 57:859–863

Nilsson B, De Luca S, Lohmander S, Hascall VC (1982) Structures of N-linked and O-linked oligosaccharides on proteoglycan monomer isolated from the Swarm rat chondrosarcoma. J Biol Chem 257:10920–10927

Noonan DM, Fulle A, Valente P, Cai S, Horigan E, Sasaki M, Yamada Y, Hassell JR (1991) The complete sequence of perlecan, a basement membrane heparan sulfate proteoglycan, reveals extensive similarity with laminin A chain, low density lipoprotein-receptor, and the neural cell adhesion molecule. J Biol Chem 266:22939–22947

Oldberg A, Antonsson P, Lindblom K, Heinegard D (1989) A collagen-binding 59-kd protein (fibromodulin) is structurally related to the small interstitial proteoglycans PG-S1 and PG-S2 (decorin). EMBO J 8:2601–2604

Olin AI, Morgelin M, Sasaki T, Timpl R, Heinegard D, Aspberg A (2001) The proteoglycans aggrecan and Versican form networks with fibulin-2 through their lectin domain binding. J Biol Chem 276:1253–1261

Onnerfjord P, Heathfield TF, Heinegard D (2004) Identification of tyrosine sulfation in extracellular leucine-rich repeat proteins using mass spectrometry. J Biol Chem 279:26–33
Orgel JP, Eid A, Antipova O, Bella J, Scott JE (2009) Decorin core protein (decoron) shape complements collagen fibril surface structure and mediates its binding. PLoS One 4:e7028
Parsi MK, Adams JR, Whitelock J, Gibson MA (2010) LTBP-2 has multiple heparin/heparan sulfate binding sites. Matrix Biol 29:393–401
Plaas AH, Neame PJ, Nivens CM, Reiss L (1990) Identification of the keratan sulfate attachment sites on bovine fibromodulin. J Biol Chem 265:20634–20640
Rhee DK, Marcelino J, Al-Mayouf S, Schelling DK, Bartels CF, Cui Y, Laxer R, Goldbach-Mansky R, Warman ML (2005a) Consequences of disease-causing mutations on lubricin protein synthesis, secretion, and post-translational processing. J Biol Chem 280: 31325–31332
Rhee DK, Marcelino J, Baker M, Gong Y, Smits P, Lefebvre V, Jay GD, Stewart M, Wang H, Warman ML, Carpten JD (2005b) The secreted glycoprotein lubricin protects cartilage surfaces and inhibits synovial cell overgrowth. J Clin Invest 115:622–631
Ricciardelli C, Sakko AJ, Ween MP, Russell DL, Horsfall DJ (2009) The biological role and regulation of versican levels in cancer. Cancer Metastasis Rev 28:233–245
Roberts CR, Mort JS, Roughley PJ (1987) Treatment of cartilage proteoglycan aggregate with hydrogen peroxide. Relationship between observed degradation products and those that occur naturally during aging. Biochem J 247:349–357
Roberts S, Caterson B, Menage J, Evans EH, Jaffray DC, Eisenstein SM (2000) Matrix metalloproteinases and aggrecanase: their role in disorders of the human intervertebral disc. Spine (Phila Pa 1976) 25:3005–3013
Rossi M, Morita H, Sormunen R, Airenne S, Kreivi M, Wang L, Fukai N, Olsen BR, Tryggvason K, Soininen R (2003) Heparan sulfate chains of perlecan are indispensable in the lens capsule but not in the kidney. EMBO J 22:236–245
Roughley PJ (2004) Biology of intervertebral disc aging and degeneration: involvement of the extracellular matrix. Spine (Phila Pa 1976) 29:2691–2699
Roughley PJ (2006) The structure and function of cartilage proteoglycans. Eur Cell Mater 12:92–101
Roughley PJ, White RJ (1980) Age-related changes in the structure of the proteoglycan subunits from human articular cartilage. J Biol Chem 255:217–224
Roughley PJ, White RJ (1989) Dermatan sulphate proteoglycans of human articular cartilage. The properties of dermatan sulphate proteoglycans I and II. Biochem J 262:823–827
Roughley PJ, White RJ, Cs-Szabo G, Mort JS (1996a) Changes with age in the structure of fibromodulin in human articular cartilage. Osteoarthritis Cartilage 4:153–161
Roughley PJ, White RJ, Mort JS (1996b) Presence of pro-forms of decorin and biglycan in human articular cartilage. Biochem J 318(Pt 3):779–784
Roughley PJ, Melching LI, Heathfield TF, Pearce RH, Mort JS (2006) The structure and degradation of aggrecan in human intervertebral disc. Eur Spine J 15(Suppl 3):S326–S332
Sandy JD, Flannery CR, Boynton RE, Neame PJ (1990) Isolation and characterization of disulfide-bonded peptides from the three globular domains of aggregating cartilage proteoglycan. J Biol Chem 265:21108–21113
Sandy JD, Westling J, Kenagy RD, Iruela-Arispe ML, Verscharen C, Rodriguez-Mazaneque JC, Zimmermann DR, Lemire JM, Fischer JW, Wight TN, Clowes AW (2001) Versican V1 proteolysis in human aorta in vivo occurs at the Glu441-Ala442 bond, a site that is cleaved by recombinant ADAMTS-1 and ADAMTS-4. J Biol Chem 276:13372–13378
Schumacher BL, Block JA, Schmid TM, Aydelotte MB, Kuettner KE (1994) A novel proteoglycan synthesized and secreted by chondrocytes of the superficial zone of articular cartilage. Arch Biochem Biophys 311:144–152
Scott JE (1996) Proteodermatan and proteokeratan sulfate (decorin, lumican/fibromodulin) proteins are horseshoe shaped. Implications for their interactions with collagen. Biochemistry 35:8795–8799
Scott JE (2003) Elasticity in extracellular matrix 'shape modules' of tendon, cartilage, etc. A sliding proteoglycan-filament model. J Physiol 553:335–343
Scott JE, Stockwell RA (2006) Cartilage elasticity resides in shape module decoran and aggrecan sumps of damping fluid: implications in osteoarthrosis. J Physiol 574:643–650
Scott IC, Imamura Y, Pappano WN, Troedel JM, Recklies AD, Roughley PJ, Greenspan DS (2000) Bone morphogenetic protein-1 processes probiglycan. J Biol Chem 275:30504–30511
Scott PG, McEwan PA, Dodd CM, Bergmann EM, Bishop PN, Bella J (2004) Crystal structure of the dimeric protein core of decorin, the archetypal small leucine-rich repeat proteoglycan. Proc Natl Acad Sci USA 101:15633–15638
Shen Z, Gantcheva S, Mansson B, Heinegard D, Sommarin Y (1998) Chondroadherin expression changes in skeletal development. Biochem J 330(Pt 1):549–557
Shi S, Ciurli C, Cartman A, Pidoux I, Poole AR, Zhang Y (2003) Experimental immunity to the G1 domain of the proteoglycan versican induces spondylitis and sacroiliitis, of a kind seen in human spondylarthropathies. Arthritis Rheum 48:2903–2915
Shi S, Grothe S, Zhang Y, O'Connor-McCourt MD, Poole AR, Roughley PJ, Mort JS (2004) Link protein has greater affinity for versican than aggrecan. J Biol Chem 279:12060–12066
Shine KM, Spector M (2008) The presence and distribution of lubricin in the caprine intervertebral disc. J Orthop Res 26:1398–1406
Shine KM, Simson JA, Spector M (2009) Lubricin distribution in the human intervertebral disc. J Bone Joint Surg Am 91:2205–2212
Sivan SS, Tsitron E, Wachtel E, Roughley PJ, Sakkee N, van der Ham F, DeGroot J, Roberts S, Maroudas A (2006) Aggrecan turnover in human intervertebral disc as determined by the racemization of aspartic acid. J Biol Chem 281:13009–13014
Smith SM, Whitelock JM, Iozzo RV, Little CB, Melrose J (2009) Topographical variation in the distributions of versican, aggrecan and perlecan in the foetal human spine reflects their diverse functional roles in spinal development. Histochem Cell Biol 132: 491–503
Smith SM, Shu C, Melrose J (2010) Comparative immunolocalisation of perlecan with collagen II and aggrecan in human foetal, newborn and adult ovine joint tissues demonstrates perlecan as an early developmental chondrogenic marker. Histochem Cell Biol 134:251–263
Song YQ, Cheung KM, Ho DW, Poon SC, Chiba K, Kawaguchi Y, Hirose Y, Alini M, Grad S, Yee AF, Leong JC, Luk KD, Yip SP, Karppinen J, Cheah KS, Sham P, Ikegawa S, Chan D (2008) Association of the asporin D14 allele with lumbar-disc degeneration in Asians. Am J Hum Genet 82:744–747
Spicer AP, Joo A, Bowling RA Jr (2003) A hyaluronan binding link protein gene family whose members are physically linked adjacent to chondroitin sulfate proteoglycan core protein genes: the missing links. J Biol Chem 278:21083–21091
Stallcup WB (2002) The NG2 proteoglycan: past insights and future prospects. J Neurocytol 31:423–435
Superti-Furga A, Hastbacka J, Rossi A, van der Harten JJ, Wilcox WR, Cohn DH, Rimoin DL, Steinmann B, Lander ES, Gitzelmann R (1996) A family of chondrodysplasias caused by mutations in the diastrophic dysplasia sulfate transporter gene and associated with impaired sulfation of proteoglycans. Ann N Y Acad Sci 785:195–201
Svensson L, Aszodi A, Reinholt FP, Fassler R, Heinegard D, Oldberg A (1999) Fibromodulin-null mice have abnormal collagen fibrils, tissue organization, and altered lumican deposition in tendon. J Biol Chem 274:9636–9647

Svensson L, Narlid I, Oldberg A (2000) Fibromodulin and lumican bind to the same region on collagen type I fibrils. FEBS Lett 470:178–182

Swann DA, Sotman S, Dixon M, Brooks C (1977) The isolation and partial characterization of the major glycoprotein (LGP-I) from the articular lubricating fraction from bovine synovial fluid. Biochem J 161:473–485

Swann DA, Hendren RB, Radin EL, Sotman SL, Duda EA (1981a) The lubricating activity of synovial fluid glycoproteins. Arthritis Rheum 24:22–30

Swann DA, Slayter HS, Silver FH (1981b) The molecular structure of lubricating glycoprotein-I, the boundary lubricant for articular cartilage. J Biol Chem 256:5921–5925

Sztrolovics R, Chen XN, Grover J, Roughley PJ, Korenberg JR (1994) Localization of the human fibromodulin gene (FMOD) to chromosome 1q32 and completion of the cDNA sequence. Genomics 23:715–717

Sztrolovics R, Alini M, Roughley PJ, Mort JS (1997) Aggrecan degradation in human intervertebral disc and articular cartilage. Biochem J 326(Pt 1):235–241

Sztrolovics R, Grover J, Cs-Szabo G, Shi SL, Zhang Y, Mort JS, Roughley PJ (2002) The characterization of versican and its message in human articular cartilage and intervertebral disc. J Orthop Res 20:257–266

Tillgren V, Onnerfjord P, Haglund L, Heinegard D (2009) The tyrosine sulfate-rich domains of the LRR proteins fibromodulin and osteoadherin bind motifs of basic clusters in a variety of heparin-binding proteins, including bioactive factors. J Biol Chem 284: 28543–28553

Tkachenko E, Rhodes JM, Simons M (2005) Syndecans: new kids on the signaling block. Circ Res 96:488–500

Tomoeda M, Yamada S, Shirai H, Ozawa Y, Yanagita M, Murakami S (2008) PLAP-1/asporin inhibits activation of BMP receptor via its leucine-rich repeat motif. Biochem Biophys Res Commun 371:191–196

Tompson SW, Merriman B, Funari VA, Fresquet M, Lachman RS, Rimoin DL, Nelson SF, Briggs MD, Cohn DH, Krakow D (2009) A recessive skeletal dysplasia, SEMD aggrecan type, results from a missense mutation affecting the C-type lectin domain of aggrecan. Am J Hum Genet 84:72–79

Tortorella MD, Liu RQ, Burn T, Newton RC, Arner E (2002) Characterization of human aggrecanase 2 (ADAM-TS5): substrate specificity studies and comparison with aggrecanase 1 (ADAM-TS4). Matrix Biol 21:499–511

Tsai TT, Danielson KG, Guttapalli A, Oguz E, Albert TJ, Shapiro IM, Risbud MV (2006) TonEBP/OREBP is a regulator of nucleus pulposus cell function and survival in the intervertebral disc. J Biol Chem 281:25416–25424

Turnbull JE (2010) Heparan sulfate glycomics: towards systems biology strategies. Biochem Soc Trans 38:1356–1360

Valhmu WB, Palmer GD, Rivers PA, Ebara S, Cheng JF, Fischer S, Ratcliffe A (1995) Structure of the human aggrecan gene: exon-intron organization and association with the protein domains. Biochem J 309(Pt 2):535–542

Vehvilainen P, Hyytiainen M, Keski-Oja J (2009) Matrix association of latent TGF-beta binding protein-2 (LTBP-2) is dependent on fibrillin-1. J Cell Physiol 221:586–593

Vlodavsky I, Friedmann Y, Elkin M, Aingorn H, Atzmon R, Ishai-Michaeli R, Bitan M, Pappo O, Peretz T, Michal I, Spector L, Pecker I (1999) Mammalian heparanase: gene cloning, expression and function in tumor progression and metastasis. Nat Med 5:793–802

von Marschall Z, Fisher LW (2010) Decorin is processed by three isoforms of bone morphogenetic protein-1 (BMP1). Biochem Biophys Res Commun 391:1374–1378

Wang IJ, Chiang TH, Shih YF, Hsiao CK, Lu SC, Hou YC, Lin LL (2006) The association of single nucleotide polymorphisms in the 5′-regulatory region of the lumican gene with susceptibility to high myopia in Taiwan. Mol Vis 12:852–857

Wang J, Markova D, Anderson DG, Zheng Z, Shapiro IM, Risbud MV (2011) TNF-alpha and IL-1beta promote a disintegrin-like and metalloprotease with thrombospondin type I motif-5-mediated aggrecan degradation through syndecan-4 in intervertebral disc. J Biol Chem 286:39738–39749

Watanabe H, Kimata K, Line S, Strong D, Gao LY, Kozak CA, Yamada Y (1994) Mouse cartilage matrix deficiency (cmd) caused by a 7 bp deletion in the aggrecan gene. Nat Genet 7:154–157

Watanabe H, Cheung SC, Itano N, Kimata K, Yamada Y (1997) Identification of hyaluronan-binding domains of aggrecan. J Biol Chem 272:28057–28065

Watanabe H, Yamada Y, Kimata K (1998) Roles of aggrecan, a large chondroitin sulfate proteoglycan, in cartilage structure and function. J Biochem 124:687–693

Whitelock JM, Murdoch AD, Iozzo RV, Underwood PA (1996) The degradation of human endothelial cell-derived perlecan and release of bound basic fibroblast growth factor by stromelysin, collagenase, plasmin, and heparanases. J Biol Chem 271:10079–10086

Whitelock JM, Melrose J, Iozzo RV (2008) Diverse cell signaling events modulated by perlecan. Biochemistry 47:11174–11183

Wiberg C, Heinegard D, Wenglen C, Timpl R, Morgelin M (2002) Biglycan organizes collagen VI into hexagonal-like networks resembling tissue structures. J Biol Chem 277:49120–49126

Xu T, Bianco P, Fisher LW, Longenecker G, Smith E, Goldstein S, Bonadio J, Boskey A, Heegaard AM, Sommer B, Satomura K, Dominguez P, Zhao C, Kulkarni AB, Robey PG, Young MF (1998) Targeted disruption of the biglycan gene leads to an osteoporosis-like phenotype in mice. Nat Genet 20:78–82

Yamada S, Tomoeda M, Ozawa Y, Yoneda S, Terashima Y, Ikezawa K, Ikegawa S, Saito M, Toyosawa S, Murakami S (2007) PLAP-1/asporin, a novel negative regulator of periodontal ligament mineralization. J Biol Chem 282:23070–23080

Yang BL, Yang BB, Erwin M, Ang LC, Finkelstein J, Yee AJ (2003) Versican G3 domain enhances cellular adhesion and proliferation of bovine intervertebral disc cells cultured in vitro. Life Sci 73:3399–3413

Young AA, Smith MM, Smith SM, Cake MA, Ghosh P, Read RA, Melrose J, Sonnabend DH, Roughley PJ, Little CB (2005) Regional assessment of articular cartilage gene expression and small proteoglycan metabolism in an animal model of osteoarthritis. Arthritis Res Ther 7:R852–R861

Zheng J, Luo W, Tanzer ML (1998) Aggrecan synthesis and secretion. A paradigm for molecular and cellular coordination of multiglobular protein folding and intracellular trafficking. J Biol Chem 273:12999–13006

Zimmermann DR, Ruoslahti E (1989) Multiple domains of the large fibroblast proteoglycan, versican. EMBO J 8:2975–2981

Svensson L, Näslund I, Oldberg A (2000) Fibromodulin and lumican bind to the same region on collagen type I fibrils. FEBS Lett 470:178–182

Swann DA, Sotman S, Dixon M, Brooks C (1977) The isolation and partial characterization of the major glycoprotein (LGP-I) from the articular lubricating fraction from bovine synovial fluid. Biochem J 161:473–485

Swann DA, Hendren RB, Radin EL, Sotman SL, Duda EA (1981) The lubricating activity of synovial fluid glycoproteins. Arthritis Rheum 24:22–30

Swann DA, Slayter HS, Silver FH (1981) The molecular structure of lubricating glycoprotein-I, the boundary lubricant for articular cartilage. J Biol Chem 256:5921–5925

Sztrolovics R, Chen XN, Grover J, Roughley PJ, Korenberg JR (1994) Localization of the human fibromodulin gene (FMOD) to chromosome 1q32 and completion of the cDNA sequence. Genomics 23:715–717

Sztrolovics R, Alini M, Roughley PJ, Mort JS (1997) Aggrecan degradation in human intervertebral disc and articular cartilage. Biochem J 326(Pt 1):235–241

Sztrolovics R, Grover J, Cs-Szabo G, Shi SL, Zhang Y, Mort JS, Roughley PJ (2002) The characterization of versican and its message in human articular cartilage and intervertebral disc. J Orthop Res 20:257–266

Tillgren V, Onnerfjord P, Haglund L, Heinegard D (2009) The tyrosine sulfate-rich domains of the LRR proteins fibromodulin and osteoadherin bind motifs of basic clusters in a variety of heparin-binding proteins, including bioactive factors. J Biol Chem 284:28543–28553

Tkachenko E, Rhodes JM, Simons M (2005) Syndecans: new kids on the signaling block. Circ Res 96:488–500

Tomoeda M, Yamada S, Shirai H, Ozawa Y, Yanagita M, Murakami S (2008) PLAP-1/asporin inhibits activation of BMP receptor via its leucine-rich repeat motif. Biochem Biophys Res Commun 371:191–196

Tompson SW, Merriman B, Funari VA, Fresquet M, Lachman RS, Rimoin DL, Nelson SF, Briggs MD, Cohn DH, Krakow D (2009) A recessive skeletal dysplasia, SEMD aggrecan type, results from a missense mutation affecting the C-type lectin domain of aggrecan. Am J Hum Genet 84:72–79

Tortorella MD, Liu R-Q, Burn T, Newton RC, Arner E (2002) Characterization of human aggrecanase 2 (ADAM-TS5): substrate specificity studies and comparison with aggrecanase 1 (ADAM-TS4). Matrix Biol 21:499–511

Tran CM, Fujita N, Huang BL, Ong JR, Lyons KM, Shapiro IM, Risbud MV (2013) Hypoxia-inducible factor (HIF)-1α and CCN2 form a regulatory circuit in hypoxic nucleus pulposus cells: CCN2 suppresses HIF-1α level and transcriptional activity. J Biol Chem 288:12654–12666

Turnbull JE (2010) Heparan sulfate glycomics: towards systems biology strategies. Biochem Soc Trans 38:1356–1360

Valhmu WB, Palmer GD, Rivers PA, Ebara S, Cheng JF, Fischer S, Ratcliffe A (1995) Structure of the human aggrecan gene: exon-intron organization and association with the protein domains. Biochem J 309(Pt 2):535–542

Van Damme EJ, Hattori M, Raaf OG, Hansen MR (?) [illegible] as receptor of [illegible] binding protein-2 [illegible] dependent [illegible]. J Cell Physiol [illegible]

Vlodavsky I, Friedmann Y, Elkin M, Aingorn H, Atzmon R, Ishai-Michaeli R, Bitan M, Pappo O, Peretz T, Michal I, Spector L, Pecker I (1999) Mammalian heparanase: gene cloning, expression and function in tumor progression and metastasis. Nat Med 5:793–802

von Marschall Z, Fisher LW (2010) Decorin is processed by three isoforms of bone morphogenetic protein-1 (BMP1). Biochem Biophys Res Commun 391:1374–1378

Wang IJ, Chiang TH, Shih YF, Hsiao CK, Lu SC, Hou YC, Lin LL (2006) The association of single nucleotide polymorphisms in the 5′-regulatory region of the lumican gene with susceptibility to high myopia in Taiwan. Mol Vis 12:852–857

Wang J, Markova D, Anderson DG, Zheng Z, Shapiro IM, Risbud MV (2011) TNF-alpha and IL-1beta promote a disintegrin-like and metalloprotease with thrombospondin type I motif-5-mediated aggrecan degradation through syndecan-4 in intervertebral disc. J Biol Chem 286:39738–39749

Watanabe H, Kimata K, Line S, Strong D, Gao LY, Kozak CA, Yamada Y (1994) Mouse cartilage matrix deficiency (cmd) caused by a 7 bp deletion in the aggrecan gene. Nat Genet 7:154–157

Watanabe H, Cheung SC, Itano N, Kimata K, Yamada Y (1997) Identification of hyaluronan-binding domains of aggrecan. J Biol Chem 272:28057–28065

Watanabe H, Yamada Y, Kimata K (1998) Roles of aggrecan, a large chondroitin sulfate proteoglycan, in cartilage structure and function. J Biochem 124:687–693

Whitelock JM, Murdoch AD, Iozzo RV, Underwood PA (1996) The degradation of human endothelial cell-derived perlecan and release of bound basic fibroblast growth factor by stromelysin, collagenase, plasmin, and heparanases. J Biol Chem 271:10079–10086

Whitelock JM, Melrose J, Iozzo RV (2008) Diverse cell signaling events modulated by perlecan. Biochemistry 47:11174–11183

Wiberg C, Heinegard D, Wenglen C, Timpl R, Morgelin M (2002) Biglycan organizes collagen VI into hexagonal-like networks resembling tissue structures. J Biol Chem 277:49120–49126

Xu T, Bianco P, Fisher LW, Longenecker G, Smith E, Goldstein S, Bonadio J, Boskey A, Heegaard AM, Sommer B, Satomura K, Dominguez P, Zhao C, Kulkarni AB, Robey PG, Young MF (1998) Targeted disruption of the biglycan gene leads to an osteoporosis-like phenotype in mice. Nat Genet 20:78–82

Yamada S, Tomoeda M, Ozawa Y, Yoneda S, Terashima Y, Ikezawa K, Ikegawa S, Saito M, Toyosawa S, Murakami S (2007) PLAP-1/asporin, a novel negative regulator of periodontal ligament mineralization. J Biol Chem 282:23070–23080

Yang BL, Yang BB, Erwin M, Ang LC, Finkelstein J, Yee AJ (2003) Versican G3 domain enhances cellular adhesion and proliferation of bovine intervertebral disc cells cultured in vitro. Life Sci 73:3399–3413

Young AA, Smith MM, Smith SM, Cake MA, Ghosh P, Read RA, Melrose J, Sonnabend DH, Roughley PJ, Little CB (2005) Regional assessment of articular cartilage gene expression and small proteoglycan metabolism in an animal model of osteoarthritis. Arthritis Res Ther 7:R852–R861

Zheng J, Luo W, Tanzer ML (1998) Aggrecan synthesis and secretion. A paradigm for molecular and cellular coordination of multiglobular protein folding and intracellular trafficking. J Biol Chem 273:12999–13006

Zimmermann DR, Ruoslahti E (1989) Multiple domains of the large fibroblast proteoglycan, versican. EMBO J 8:2975–2981

Collagen and Other Proteins of the Nucleus Pulposus, Annulus Fibrosus, and Cartilage End Plates

5

Fackson Mwale

Contents

F. Mwale
Division of Orthopaedic Surgery,
Lady Davis Institute for Medical Research, McGill University,
3755 Chemin de la Cote Ste-Catherine, Montreal,
QC H3T 1E2, Canada

I.M. Shapiro, M.V. Risbud (eds.), *The Intervertebral Disc*,
DOI 10.1007/978-3-7091-1535-0_5, © Springer-Verlag Wien 2014

5.1 Introduction

5.1.1 Evolutionary Considerations

Characterized by the presence of at least one triple-helical domain, members of the collagen family are the most abundant proteins in the animal kingdom. From a phylogenetic perspective, while the triple-helical domain is present in bacteria and fungi and even some viruses, collagen and collagen-like proteins have been identified in all metazoa. With the appearance of the phylum Chordata, the notochord provided a "first" skeleton which enabled the organism to assume a longitudinal shape and provided support for the digestive tube and the nerve cord. This notochordal structure is sheathed in collagen; postembryonic remnants of the notochord in vertebrates form the nucleus pulposus of the intervertebral discs. Zhang et al. (2009) have put forward the hypothesis that the vertebrate chondrocytes that all express the type II gene may have evolved from notochordal cells. In vertebrates, collagen fibrils formed the template for deposition of mineral and the development of bone and cartilage of the axial and appendicular skeleton.

5.1.2 Brief Overview of the Anatomical Characteristics of the Intervertebral Disc

The discs typically are composed of three morphologically distinct major structural regions – the peripheral collagen-rich annulus fibrosus, surrounding the proteoglycan-rich central nucleus pulposus, and the cartilage end plates interfacing the disc and the vertebral body. The junctional zone between vertebral bone and annulus fibrosus is a type of enthesis. The cartilage end plates in the juvenile are responsible for longitudinal vertebral growth. In the adult, the intervertebral discs are avascular and receive most of their nutrients from the vertebral bone vasculature by diffusion through the cartilage end plates. Collagens provide the structural framework of the intervertebral discs and are responsible for its biomechanical properties such as torsion and resistance to pressure or tension. Proteoglycans, such as decorin, fibromodulin, and biglycan together with other matrix constituents, have important influences on collagen fibril formation.

Box 5.1 Abbreviation List

C-NC domain	Carboxyl-terminal noncollagenous domain (same as C-propeptide)
COMP	Cartilage oligomeric matrix protein
DDR	Discoidin domain receptors
ECM	Extracellular matrix
ED-A	Extra domain A
EGF	Epidermal growth factor
ER	Endoplasmic reticulum
FACIT	Fibril-associated collagen with interrupted triple helices
GAG	Glycosaminoglycan
IVDD	Intervertebral disc degeneration
MACIT	Membrane-associated collagen with interrupted triple helices
MMP	Matrix metalloproteinases
Multiplexin	Multiple triple-helix domains and interruptions
NC	Noncollagenous
N-NC domain	Amino-terminal noncollagenous domain (same as N-propeptide)
RER	Rough endoplasmic reticulum
RUNX2	Runt-related transcription factor 2
TIMP	Tissue inhibitors of metalloproteinases

5.1.2.1 Annulus Fibrosus

The annulus fibrosus makes up the peripheral portion of the disc structure (Fig. 5.1). In the mature lumbar disc, there are up to 25 lamellae that comprise regular concentric bundles of parallel collagen fibers arranged around the central gelatinous nucleus pulposus (Roberts 2002). Collagen fibers in a particular lamella run in one direction, while fibers in an adjacent lamella run in the opposite direction. The thickness of the lamellae varies from 200 to 400 μm, increasing from inside to outside (Inoue 1973). This alternating pattern is designed to withstand torsional stresses. The key functions of the collagen fibrils in the annulus are retaining the nucleus and taking up and distributing the load exerted by the disc.

5.1.2.2 Nucleus Pulposus

The nucleus pulposus is a soft jellylike, highly hydrophilic tissue occupying the central region of the disc. The disc contains proteoglycans (predominantly aggrecan; see Chap. 4), randomly organized fibrillar collagens (Inoue 1981), radially arranged elastin fibers (Yu et al. 2002), and water. The proportion and organization of water, fibrillar collagens, and proteoglycans vary not only with the position across the disc, but with age and level (Antoniou et al. 1996; Scott et al. 1994; Demers et al. 2004; Mwale et al. 2004; Antoniou et al. 1996). The nucleus pulposus has a higher concentration of proteoglycans and water than other regions of the disc, whereas the highest levels of collagen are in the outer annulus and the lowest concentration in the nucleus (Mwale et al. 2004; Inkinen et al. 1998). The collagen content of the nucleus pulposus is greatest in cervical discs and lowest in lumbar discs. In contrast, the proteoglycan content of the nucleus pulposus peaks in lumbar discs and is lowest in cervical discs (Scott et al. 1994).

5.1.2.3 Cartilage End Plates

The end plates in the human disc consist of a thin horizontal layer of hyaline cartilage, usually less than 1 mm thick, which separate the nucleus pulposus and annulus fibrosus from the adjacent vertebral bone. In the adult, the cartilage end plate is narrow, and often calcified, leading to disturbances to the nutrient supply to the nucleus pulposus (Maroudas et al. 1975; Nachemson et al. 1970). The collagen fibers within the end plates run parallel to the vertebral bodies, with the fibers continuing into the disc (Roberts et al. 1989).

5.2 Protein Composition of the Intervertebral Discs

5.2.1 Collagenous Protein Structure

Collagen, the most abundant fibrous protein of the disc, is the name for a family of rope-like polypeptidic molecules (Fig. 5.1) that have a linear structure containing regions of repeating triplets of amino acids ($Gly_{aa}X_{aa}Y_{aa}$) with glycine (G_{aa}) at every third position and X and Y often being proline and hydroxyproline, respectively. These two amino acids constitute about 1/6 with glycine accounting for 1/3 of the sequence. Since glycine is the smallest amino acid with no side chain, it is positioned at every third position in the chain. The high glycine content stabilizes the collagen helix, facilitating hydrogen bonding and the formation of intermolecular cross-links (Eyre et al. 1984; Pokharna and Phillips 1998; Berg and Prockop 1973). The ring structures of proline and

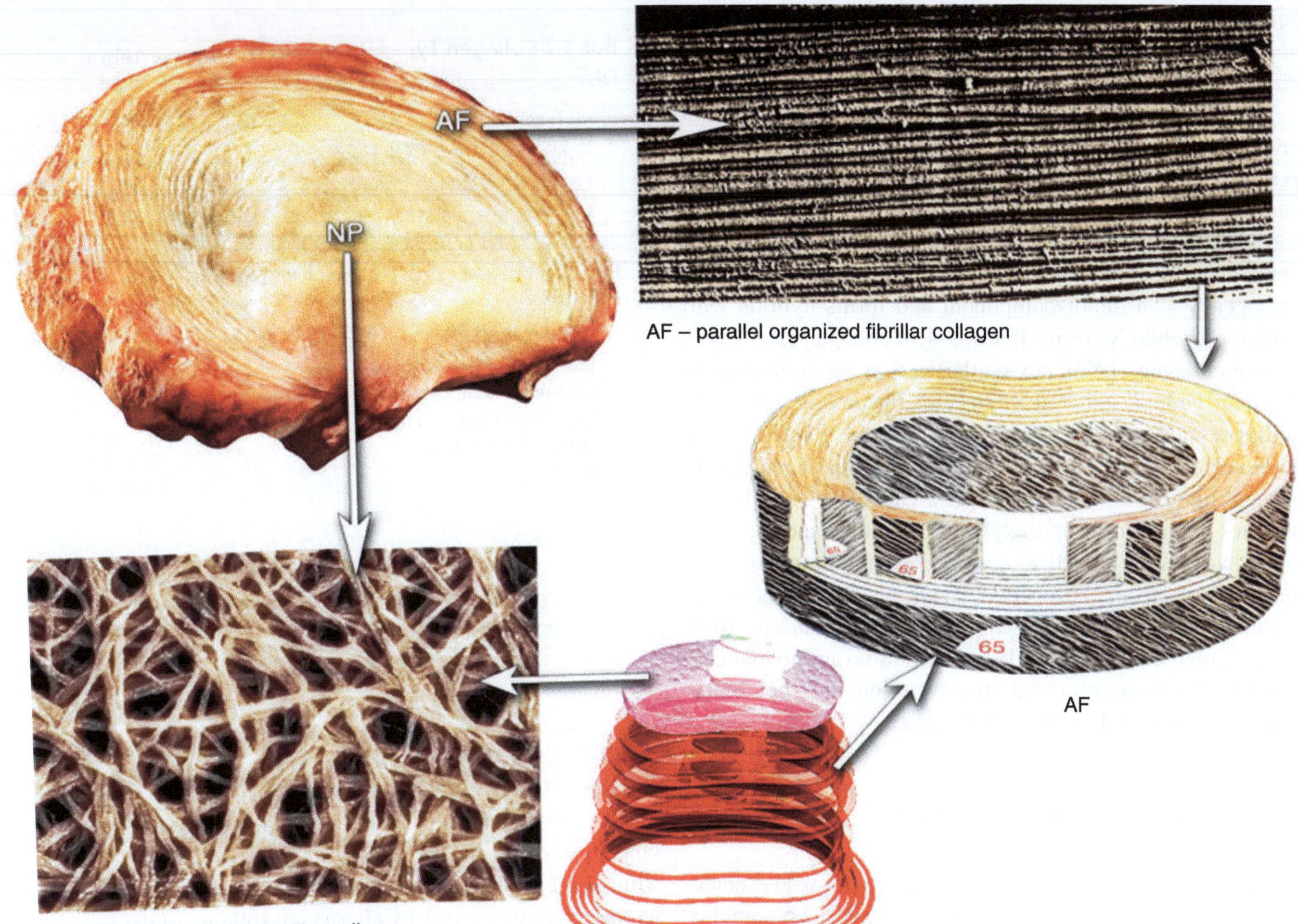

Fig. 5.1 Schematic illustration of the organization of fibrillar collagens in the annulus fibrosus (*AF*) and nucleus pulposus (*NP*) of a human intervertebral disc

hydroxyproline occupy the outer positions where they interact with neighboring collagen molecules. The hydroxyl groups of 4-hydroxyproline are essential for the formation of intramolecular hydrogen bonds and determine the thermal stability of each collagen chain (Berg and Prockop 1973).

The collagen molecule is formed from three α-chains wound together in a triple helix. These helices are twisted together into a right-handed coiled coil stabilized by hydrogen bonds and woven together to form a left-handed helix (Hulmes and Miller 1981). This uninterrupted triple-helix molecule is approximately 300 nm in length and 1.5 nm in diameter – a cable-like structure that provides significant tensile strength to skin, tendons, ligaments, and other cartilaginous structures, making them tough and flexible. The amino acid hydroxylysine is responsible for stabilizing the side-to-side packing of the chains into fibrils. The collagen molecule contains three structural domains, the amino- and carboxyl-terminal extra-helical regions and the major triple-helical rodlike domain. Collagens I–V are considered to be the major collagens, since they comprise 98 % of the total connective tissue protein. There is considerable complexity and diversity in the 28 different types of collagen.

In the lumbar disc, there are up to 25 lamellae that comprise regular concentric bundles of parallel collagen fibers arranged around the central gelatinous nucleus pulposus (Roberts 2002). Collagen fibers in a particular lamella run in one direction, while fibers in an adjacent lamella run in the opposite direction. The thickness of the lamellae varies from 200 to 400 μm, increasing from inside to outside (Inoue 1973). This alternating pattern is designed to withstand torsional stresses. The key functions of the collagen fibrils in the annulus are retaining the nucleus and taking up and distributing the load exerted by the disc. The fibril-forming collagens I and II form an important network in the disc. Collagen I forms hybrids with other fibrillar collagens, particularly collagen V. Co-fibril formation with collagen I is believed to regulate the diameter of fibrils because of the partial processing of the N-propeptide of collagen V. With disc aging and degeneration, there are profound alterations in collagen cross-links (Pokharna and Phillips 1998).

The proportion of collagen II and I varies gradually and inversely across the disc, with exclusively collagen I at the extreme outermost layers of the annulus fibrosus and the nucleus pulposus possessing mostly collagen type II (Eyre and Muir 1976). Under physiological conditions, collagen II fibrils contain more water than I fibrils (Grynpas et al. 1980). Collagen V is a minor component and forms hybrids with collagen I, while XI forms hybrids with collagen II.

The collagen chains are synthesized as procollagens. In the rough endoplasmic reticulum (ER), the procollagen chain undergoes a series of processing reactions. First, as with other secreted proteins, glycosylation of procollagen occurs in the rough ER and Golgi complex. Galactose and glucose residues are added to hydroxylysine residues, and long oligosaccharides are added to specific asparagine residues in the carboxyl-terminal propeptide, a segment at the carboxyl-terminus of a procollagen molecule that is absent from mature collagen. Generally, the propeptides (amino and carboxyl terminal) are removed after secretion, and then collagen fibrils form in the extracellular space.

Box 5.2 Collagen Types Present in the Intervertebral Disc

Fibril forming
- Type I (COL1 α1, COL1α2)
- Type II (COL2α1)
- Type III
- Type V (COL5α1, COL5α2, COL5α3)

FACIT (fibril-associated collagen with interrupted triple helices)
- Type IX (COL9α1, COL9α2, COL9α3)
- Type XII (COL12α1)

Basement membrane (basal membrane)
- Type IV (COL4α1, COL4α2, COL4α3, COL4α4, COL4α5, COL4α6)

Multiplexin
- None

Other
- Type VI (COL6α1,COL6α2, COL6α3, COL6α4)
- Type X (COL10α1, COL10α2, COL10α3)
- Type XI (COL11α1, COL11α2)

5.2.2 Classification of Collagens

The disc contains many different collagen types whose abundance changes with age (Roughley 2004). The annulus fibrosus is composed primarily of collagen I and to a lesser extent II, III, V, VI, IX, XI, XII, and XIV. The nucleus pulposus is rich in collagen II, but it also contains collagen I, VI, and IX (Eyre and Muir 1976, 1977; Wu et al. 1987; Eyre et al. 2002). Collagens I and II constitute about 80 % of the collagens in the disc (Eyre and Muir 1977) (for details of the collagen species, see Box 5.2).

5.2.2.1 Collagen I

The structure of procollagen I is similar to other fibrillar collagens, and it comprises three polypeptide α-chains, which form a unique triple-helical structure (Fig. 5.2). It is a heterotrimer of two α1 and one α2 chains. It contains an uninterrupted triple-helical domain flanked by short non-helical telopeptides. The telopeptides, which do not have a repeating Gly–X–Y structure and do not adopt a triple-helical conformation, account for 2 % of the molecule. Many macromolecules such as COMP, fibromodulin, matrilin, and decorin attach to collagen I (Fig. 5.3). Collagen I molecules form D-periodic ($D = 67$ nm, the characteristic axial periodicity of collagen) cross-striated fibrils in the extracellular space, giving the tissue its mechanical strength and providing the major biomechanical scaffold for cell attachment and anchorage of macromolecules (Fig. 5.4).

5.2.2.2 Collagen II

Collagen II fibrils in the nucleus pulposus appear to be organized randomly (Fig. 5.1). In the adult, these collagen molecules are joined by hydroxypyridium cross-links (Eyre and Muir 1976). There is evidence that procollagen II can be expressed in two forms by alternative splicing of the primary gene transcript. The two mRNAs either include (IIA) or exclude (IIB) exon 2, so that procollagen II can be synthesized with or without exon 2 encoding the major portion of the amino propeptide (Sandell et al. 1991; Ryan and Sandell 1990). This polymorphism is thought to influence cell morphology, with the cells expressing procollagen IIA being narrow, elongated, and "fibroblastic" in appearance, while the cells expressing procollagen IIB are large and round. The expression of procollagen IIB appears to be correlated with abundant synthesis and accumulation of aggrecan (Sandell et al. 1991). Procollagen IIA may function in the annulus fibrosus and nucleus pulposus, particularly during development.

5.2.2.3 Collagen VI

Collagen VI accounts for 10–20 % of the total collagen and is particularly prominent in the nucleus pulposus and the end plate cartilage (Roberts et al. 1991). It resembles collagens IX and X in that it is a shorter chain collagen than collagen II. It consists of α-chains that form a highly branched filamentous network based on the formation of tetramers but does not appear to form cross-links with other matrix molecules (Wu et al. 1987). The beaded filaments of collagen VI represent another important network in the disc matrix (Feng et al. 2006).

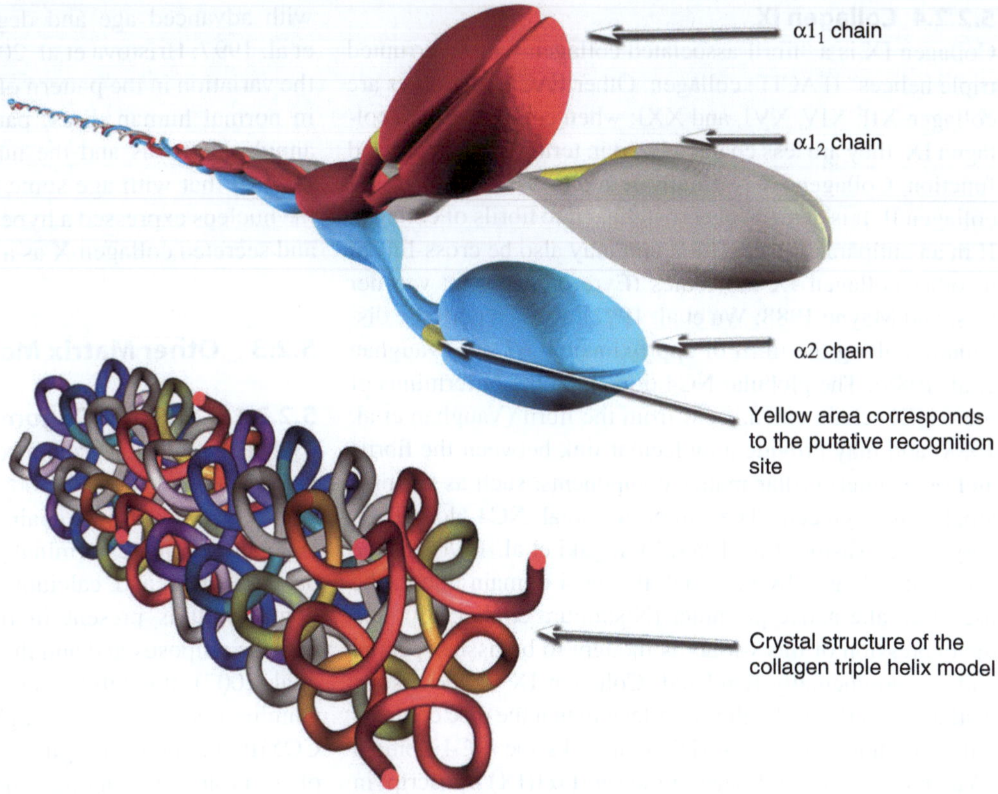

Fig. 5.2 Schematic illustration of type 1 collagen α-chains, recognition site in the C-NC domain, and the crystal structure of the collagen intertwined α-chains (the *upper image* was generated in 3D Studio Max, while the *lower image* was generated in CN3D ver. 4.3 using data for Crystal Structure of the Collagen Triple Helix Model [(Pro-Pro-Gly)10]3 from the Protein Data Bank rcsb.org DOI:10.2210/pdb1k6f/pdb)

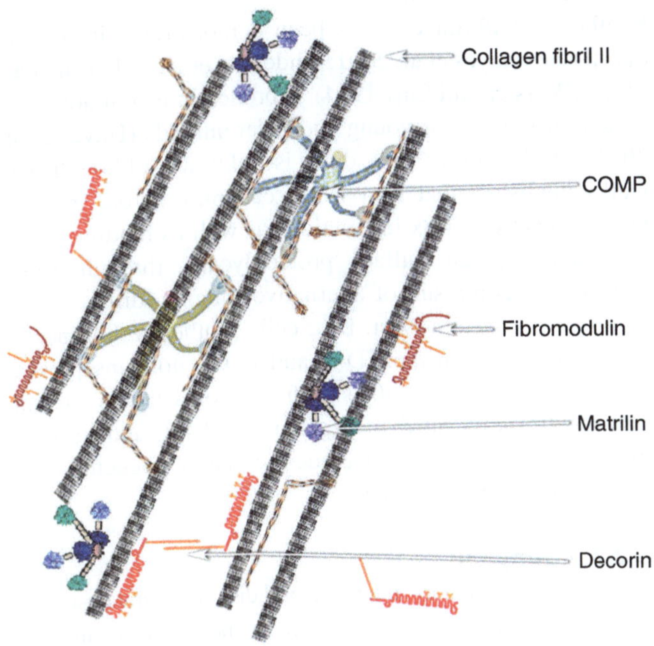

Fig. 5.3 Schematic illustration of assemblies of cross-striated collagen fibrils and cartilage oligomeric matrix protein (*COMP*), fibromodulin, matrilin, and decorin in the intervertebral disc (The figure was modified with permission from Feng et al. (2006))

It forms a tetramer of two pairs of antiparallel collagen VI molecules arranged such that two N-terminal ends are exposed at either end of the unit. Further assembly occurs both by

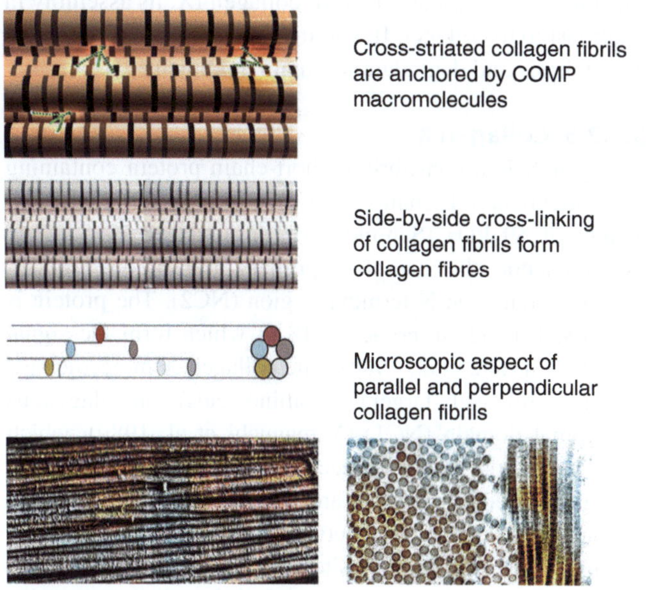

Fig. 5.4 Computer visualization model, schematics, and simulated microscopic images of normal collagen fibrils showing the association with COMP, side-by-side cross-linking of collagen fibrils, and microscopic aspects of collagen fibrils

end-to-end and side-to-side associations catalyzed by proteoglycans such as biglycan and decorin. These ligands (collagen VI tetramers) are also bound to molecules such as PRELP, fibronectin, and matrilin-1, -2, or -3, which in turn are bound to a collagen fiber, a procollagen molecule, or aggrecan.

5.2.2.4 Collagen IX

Collagen IX is a "fibril-associated collagen with interrupted triple helices" (FACIT) collagen. Other FACIT members are collagen XII, XIV, XVI, and XXI; when compared with collagen IX, they are less characterized in terms of structure and function. Collagen IX is usually found in tissues containing collagen II. It is extensively cross-linked to fibrils of collagen II in an antiparallel orientation and may also be cross-linked to other collagen IX molecules (Eyre et al. 1988; van der Rest and Mayne 1988; Wu et al. 1992). It has a periodic distribution along the fibril of approximately 67 nm (Vaughan et al. 1988). The globular NC4 domain at the N-terminus of the α1(IX) chain extends out from the fibril (Vaughan et al. 1988) and may provide a molecular link between the fibrils and other interfibrillar matrix components, such as the proteoglycan aggrecan. The amino-terminal NC4 domain is very basic (Vasios et al. 1988; Muragaki et al. 1990). Some forms of collagen IX may lack the NC4 domain due to the use of an alternative promoter (Nishimura et al. 1989), and the expression of this variant is thought to be tissue specific and developmentally regulated. Collagen IX of the disc is distinct from that of hyaline cartilage in that the disc contains only the short form of α1(IX) that lacks the NC4 domain (Wu and Eyre 2003). Usage of the short α1(IX) transcript in disc tissue has no apparent effect on cross-linking behavior. The precise biological role(s) of collagen IX, its assembly in relationship to collagen II, and the mechanisms that regulate its synthesis and degradation remain unknown.

5.2.2.5 Collagen X

Collagen X is a non-fibrillar short-chain protein containing three identical α1 chains [$\alpha1(X)_3$] with a low molecular weight of 59 kDa (Schmid and Linsenmayer 1985). Two exons encode the complete primary translation product, which contains the N-terminal region (NC2). The protein is comprised of 52 amino acids, 18 of which form the signal peptide (LuValle et al. 1988). The collagen X molecule also contains a relatively larger (162 amino acids) noncollagenous C-terminal domain (NC1) (Yamaguchi et al. 1989), which plays a key role in the intracellular assembly of the triple-helical collagen X molecules and may be necessary for aggregation to form extracellular networks. The presence of several functional RUNX2 binding sites within the promoter region of the COL10A1 genes suggests that it is a direct transcriptional target of RUNX2 during chondrogenesis (Zheng et al. 2003). It forms pericellular mats and is also closely associated with the fibrils of collagen II (Linsenmayer et al. 1998).

Collagen X is synthesized by hypertrophic chondrocytes during endochondral ossification in the growth plate (Mwale et al. 2000; Tchetina et al. 2003). It was shown to be present in human lumbar discs during aging and degeneration by Boos et al. (1997) and Xi et al. (2004). In addition, nucleus pulposus chondrocytes express collagen X in association with advanced age and degenerative disc lesions (Nerlich et al. 1997; Hristova et al. 2011). Aigner et al. (1998) studied the variation in the pattern of collagen X expression with age in normal human discs, particularly the cells of the inner annulus fibrosus and the nucleus pulposus. These workers showed that with age some cells from the inner annulus or the nucleus expressed a hypertrophic chondrocyte phenotype and secreted collagen X as a component of the disc matrix.

5.2.3 Other Matrix Molecules

5.2.3.1 Cartilage Oligomeric Matrix Protein (COMP)

COMP is a 524-kD protein composed of five identical glycoprotein subunits each of 100–120 kD held together by a five-stranded coiled-coil domain in the N-terminal portion and exposing unique C-terminal globular domains. Each subunit has EGF-like and calcium-binding (thrombospondin-like) domains. It is present in the extracellular matrix of the nucleus pulposus and annulus fibrosus (Ishii et al. 2006; Lee et al. 2007). It exhibits a lamellar distribution pattern in the annulus fibrosus region. Higher nucleus pulposus levels of COMP are found in aging discs (Lee et al. 2007). COMP plays a role in regulating collagen fibril assembly.

5.2.3.2 Fibronectin

Synthesis of fibronectin has been demonstrated in healthy disc tissue (Hayes et al. 2001; Anderson et al. 2010) and cartilage (Wurster and Lust 1984). Fibronectin is a minor component of the disc of young and older animals (Hayes et al. 2001). Its function in the discs is unknown, although it is well established that fibronectin can play a role in cell–matrix, matrix–matrix interactions as well as binding collagen and heparan sulfate proteoglycans through RGD sequences. As a result of alternative splicing, different isoforms of fibronectin exist. Disc cells synthesize fibronectin with either or both the ED-B and ED-A domains present (Anderson et al. 2010), the significance of which is unclear. Fibronectin is elevated in degenerated discs, and its fragments induce the cell to degrade the matrix (Oegema et al. 2000, Anderson et al. 2004).

5.2.3.3 Amyloid

Amyloid deposits in the intervertebral disc were first described by Bywaters and Dorling (1970). In the annulus, amyloid deposits are found lying between thick bundles of collagen fibers, while a diffuse nodular distribution is found in the nucleus pulposus, in proximity to cells (Ladefoged 1985). The incidence of amyloid deposition in discs increases with advancing age, although it is also found in the young disc (Ladefoged 1985; Yasuma et al. 1992). Amyloid deposits of different morphological types have been observed in the disc (Mihara et al. 1994). At the ultrastructu ral level, amyloid deposits are seen composed of 10-nm-wide nonbranching fibrils (Mihara et al. 1994). Changes in matrix glycosaminoglycans, particularly strongly sulfated glycosaminoglycans such as keratan sulfate, may play a role in the pathogenesis of localized and systemic amyloid deposition (Athanasou et al. 1995).

5.2.3.4 Tenascin

Tenascin has also been called hexabrachion (Erickson and Inglesias 1984) and myotendinous antigen (Chiquet and Fambrough 1984). The tenascins are a family of extracellular matrix glycoproteins with repeated structural domains homologous to epidermal growth factor (EGF), fibronectin type III, and the fibrinogens. It has been shown that aggrecan can interact with certain matrix proteins containing EGF-repeats, including tenascins, the fibrillins, as well as the fibulins, (Day et al. 2004) to form higher order networks. Tenascin is a large extended "octopus"-like molecule, in which six arms radiate out from a central point, with each arm having an Mr of 200 kDa and composed of a single polypeptide chain. The domain structure of the cloned molecule supports the finding that it can interact with multiple ligands (Nies et al. 1991). It is a hemagglutinin and can bind, directly or indirectly, with a variety of disc matrix molecules. In discs, it is present in young and adult annulus fibrosus and nucleus pulposus, where it is confined to the pericellular matrix (Gruber et al. 2002, 2006) and its expression can be modulated by mechanical strain (Benjamin and Ralphs 2004). It is thought to have a role in disc aging and degeneration, possibly by modulating fibronectin cell interactions and causing alterations in the shape of disc cells (Gruber et al. 2002).

5.2.3.5 Elastin

Earlier studies reported that the elastic fiber network of the disc was sparse and irregular. Thus, elastic fibers were generally considered to play no significant role in the mechanical functioning of the disc. However, recent studies have shown that the network is highly organized and that the distribution and orientation of elastic fibers varies from region to region (Yu et al. 2002, 2005). In the annulus fibrosus, elastin fibers appear densely distributed in the region between the lamellae and also in "bridges" across the lamellae. Elastin molecules are also present in the center of the nucleus, where long fibers are radially oriented and anchor perpendicularly or obliquely to the cartilaginous end plate (Yu et al. 2002, 2007). They form a network, as is fibrillin, and constitute the amorphous component of the nucleus pulposus that is responsible for its elastic properties. Individual elastin polypeptide chains (tropoelastin) are covalently cross-linked producing an insoluble protein and presumably forming random coil-like structures. With such coupling, elastic fibers could play a significant mechanical role even though overall elastin is less than 5 % of the total dry weight of the disc. Its content correlates with degenerative grade and age (Cloyd and Elliott 2007).

5.3 Biosynthesis of Collagen Proteins

5.3.1 Intracellular Processing and Posttranslational Modifications

The synthesis of collagen involves a cascade of unique posttranslational modifications of the original procollagen polypeptide. The many steps in collagen biosynthesis can be interrupted or changed by mutant enzymes or by disease processes. With procollagen synthesis on the RER, there is hydroxylation of proline and lysine, an initial glycosylation step and formation of triple helices. Hydroxylation begins after the peptide chain has reached a certain minimum length and is still bound to the ribosomes. The two enzymes involved are peptidyl prolyl hydroxylase and peptidyl lysyl hydroxylase. Glycosylation of lysine occurs after its hydroxylation. Each of the collagen isoforms has differing levels of carbohydrate in the form of galactose or glycosylgalactose linked to hydroxylysine. Terminal glycosylation takes place in the Golgi apparatus, and the molecule is packaged into secretory vesicles and secreted by exocytosis. Outside of the cell, procollagen peptidase removes the non-helical domains of procollagen.

5.3.2 Chaperone-Assisted Folding of Individual Chains into a Triple-Helical Structure

Assembly begins with α-chains' trimerization to form a triple-helical protomer. Protomers are usually heterotrimers, composed of up to three different α-chains. For example, collagen I is composed of α1 and α2 chains, forming an α1α1α2 heterotrimer. They have in common at least one triple-helical collagenous domain of varying length and two noncollagenous domains C-NC and C-NC that are positioned at the N and C ends. Thus, the N-propeptide from the N-NC domain and the C-propeptide from the C-NC domain act as molecular chaperones. The C-propeptide at the C-NC domain for both α1 and α2 chains contains five subdomains (Hulmes 2002). They are involved in the protection of nascent proteins on the ribosome; folding of newly synthesized or membrane-translocated proteins; protection and refolding of misfolded, partially unfolded, or aggregated proteins; and most importantly the maintenance of procollagen in a partially unfolded state for binding effectors or crossing membranes.

5.3.3 Mechanisms of Collagen Chain Selection, Intracellular Transport, and Secretion

Each chain is synthesized with an extra length of peptides called registration peptides on both the N-terminal and C-terminal end (Fig. 5.5). Registration peptides ensure that

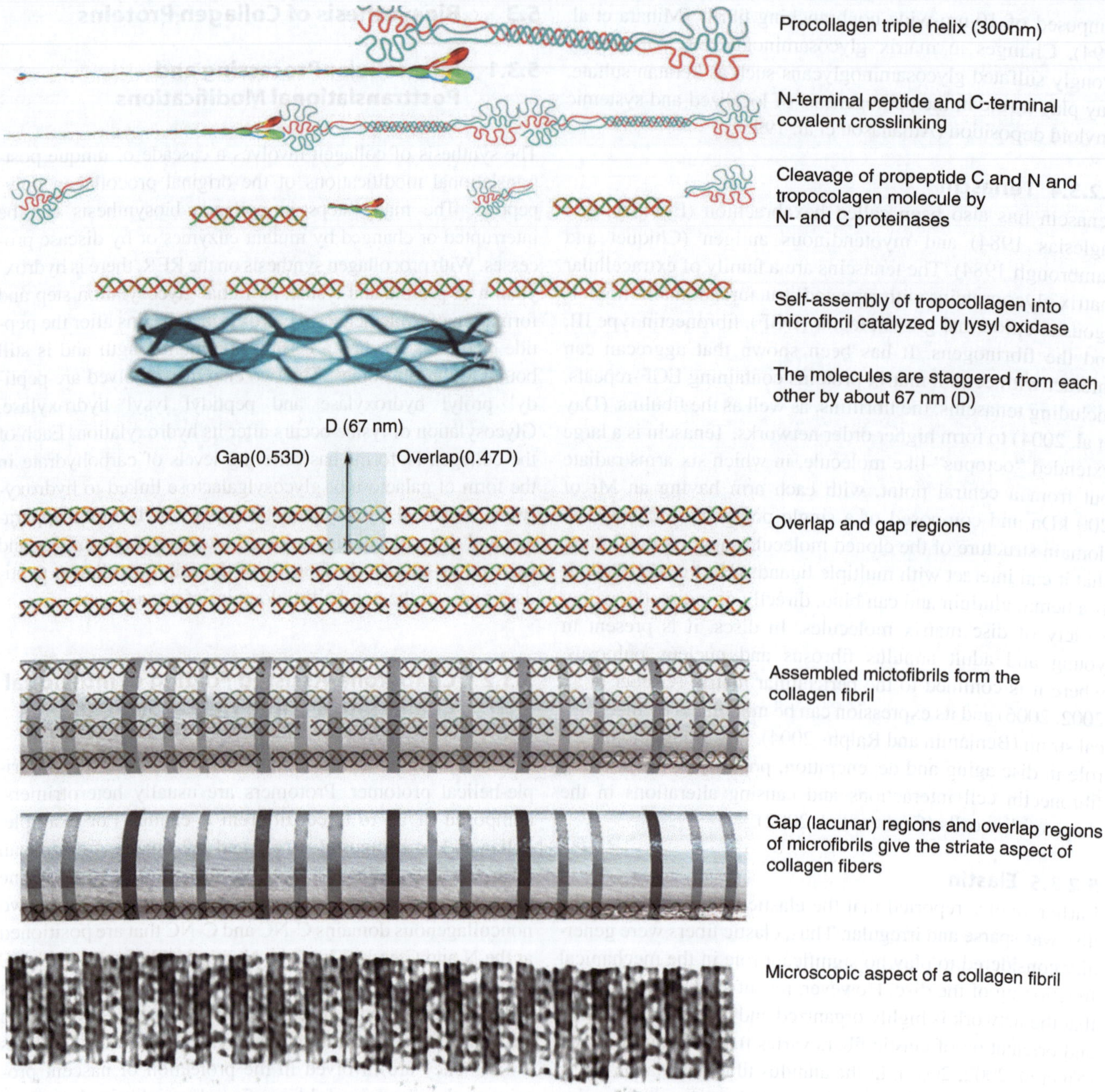

Fig. 5.5 Schematic illustration of the formation of tropocollagen, showing procollagen, cross-linking, propeptide cleavage, self-assembly, overlaps, and GAP regions of microfibrils

the chains assemble in the correct position as a triple helix. The terminal N and C domains are then excised, modified, or incorporated directly into the final structure, depending on protomer and function. Subsequently, specific protomers oligomerize into distinct suprastructures involving interactions that form end-to-end connections, lateral associations, and supercoiling of helices. An additional function of the extra peptides is to maintain the solubility of the procollagen molecule and prevent its premature intracellular assembly and precipitation as collagen fibrils. The C-NC domain is the key domain required for heterotrimer assembly. Disulfide bonding in the α2 C-NC domain is crucial for heterotrimer formation (Fig. 5.2). As discussed previously, the domain structure consists of a central collagenous triple-helical domain flanked by two noncollagenous domains, carboxy-terminus (NC1 domain) and amino-terminus (NC2 domain) (Fig. 5.4). The terminal NC domains function as recognition modules. This happens at the different subdomains (Telo, Ia, Ib, II, IV, III, and V) of the C-NC domain of the α1 and α2 chains. The selection, binding, and registration of the three α-chains for assembly of the triple-helical protomers at these subdomain sites are characterized by interactions based on complementarity of shape, electrostatic charge distribution, and hydrophobic selection of cognate α-chains (Khoshnoodi 2006). Domain I of the collagen molecule folds into subdomains Ia and Ib without α-helical or β-sheet conformations, inconsistent with suggestions that subdomain Ia participates in trimerization by forming α-helical coiled coils (McAlinden et al. 2003). Subdomain Ib contains the interchain disulfide bonds in the assembled C-NC trimer. Domains II and IV fold into globular regions G1 and G2, respectively. These are linked by an antiparallel sheet assembled from domains III and V.

Folding is initiated at the C-terminus by bimolecular association of the α2 and α12, peptide chains near the junction of domain III and domain IV-G2, and proceeds towards the N-terminus (Malone et al. 2005). The α2 C-NC domain, specifically domain V, provides the driving force for heterotrimer formation. Trimerization proceeds via a second interaction between the α2–α12 dimer and the α11 at domain II-G1 after which the interchain disulfide bonds become established in domain Ib. Folding of domain Ia is the last and slowest folding step, but eventually it drives the folding through the C–telo–Ia junction (Malone et al. 2004). Putative trimerization control sequences have been located within the C-NC domains.

5.4 Extracellular Processing of Collagens/Procollagens

5.4.1 Enzymes Involved in Processing of Procollagens

The formation and passage of correctly folded triple-helical collagen molecules through the secretory pathway involve chaperone proteins such as disulfide isomerase or binding proteins that are involved in the recognition of the C-propeptide which may be a mechanism for the retention of incorrectly folded collagen molecules in the cell (Bottomley et al. 2001). The major collagen-binding protein of the rough endoplasmic reticulum is HSP47, sometimes called gp46, or colligin (Tasab et al. 2002) and acts along with other chaperones during collagen passage from the rough endoplasmic reticulum to the Golgi apparatus. Outside of the cell registration peptides are cleaved and tropocollagen is formed by procollagen peptidase (Fig. 5.5). Multiple tropocollagen molecules form collagen fibrils, via covalent cross-linking (aldol reaction) by lysyl oxidase which links hydroxylysine and lysine residues. Multiple collagen fibrils form into collagen fibers.

5.4.2 Procollagen N and Procollagen C Proteinases

Fibrillar procollagens contain a C-propeptide that is completely removed by a C proteinase after secretion leading to polymerization of their triple-helical domains (Fig. 5.5) (Prockop et al. 1997/1998). In contrast, the extent to which their amino propeptide (N-propeptide) is removed by N procollagen proteinases is different. With certain types of collagens, such as collagens I and II, the N-propeptide is completely removed, whereas for collagens V and XI most of the N-propeptides are left attached on the triple-helical domains. As such, this may allow them to regulate fibril assembly by hindering the addition of molecules at fibril surfaces.

5.5 Self-Assembly of Collagen Fibrils

5.5.1 Homotypic Collagen–Collagen Interactions

The altered protein after cleavage, known as tropocollagen, is able to assemble into polymeric collagen fibrils (Fig. 5.5). Hydroxyproline residues contribute to the stability of the tropocollagen triple helix, forming hydrogen bonds between its polypeptide chains.

5.5.2 Heterotypic Collagen–Collagen and Collagen–Other Molecules

Collagen fibrils aggregate spontaneously to form fibers. Proteoglycans and structural glycoproteins play an important role in the aggregation of tropocollagen to form fibrils and in the formation of fibers from fibrils. Collagen may be attached to cell membranes via several types of proteins, including fibronectin and integrin.

5.5.3 Fibril Formation

Formation of collagen fibrils occurs by self-aggregation of tropocollagen molecules in a staggered array (Fig. 5.5). Collagen fibrils are stabilized by the formation of lysine-derived cross-links between tropocollagen molecules catalyzed by lysyl oxidase. The fibrillar structure is reinforced by the formation of covalent cross-links between tropocollagen molecules.

5.5.4 Cross-Link Formation

Side-by-side cross-linking of collagen fibrils to form a collagen fiber is mediated by proteoglycans and FACIT collagens. For correct assembly and/or turnover of collagen fibrils, other molecules, such as tenascin-X, are also required.

5.6 Collagen Fibril–Cell Interactions

5.6.1 Collagen–Integrin Binding

Heterodimers of four integrins, namely, $\alpha_1\beta_1$, $\alpha_2\beta_1$, $\alpha_{10}\beta_1$, and $\alpha_{11}\beta_1$, form a special subclass of cell adhesion receptors. They are all collagen receptors, and they recognize their ligands with an inserted domain (I domain) in their α-subunit. Integrin $\alpha_1\beta_1$ also known as VLA-1 or CD49a–CD29 is strongly expressed during development. Integrin $\alpha_2\beta_1$ was originally thought to be the only collagen receptor. Ligand binding to this receptor triggers intracellular signaling, which include the p38 MAP kinase activation.

5.6.2 Collagen–Discoidin Domain Receptor (DDR) Binding

Discoidin domain receptors (DDRs) DDR1 and DDR2 are receptor tyrosine kinases with the unique ability among receptor tyrosine kinases to respond to collagen. They are distinguished from other members of the receptor tyrosine kinase family by a discoidin homology repeat in their extracellular domains that is also found in a variety of other transmembrane and secreted proteins.

5.6.3 Integrin-Dependent and DDR-Dependent Signaling

Integrins are receptors that mediate the attachment between a cell and the tissues that surround it, such as other cells or the extracellular matrix. They are involved in cell signaling and the regulation of cell survival, differentiation, and response to environmental stimuli in the disc. However, little is known of the discoidin cell surface receptors that directly bind to and interact with these matrix proteins in the intervertebral disc.

5.7 Homeostasis of Collagenous Matrices

5.7.1 Degeneration of Collagenous Matrices

With age, the proportion of aggrecan to water in the nucleus pulposus falls steeply, while the proportion of collagen to aggrecan rises. A similar change is seen in degenerate discs. These changes appear to arise from loss of aggrecan rather than an increase in the amount of secreted collagen (Antoniou et al. 1996). The matrix metalloproteinase (MMP) family has been implicated in the breakdown of collagen and other matrix proteins.

5.7.2 Regulation of Collagen Expression

Besides the general protease inhibitors, mainly α2-macroglobulin and α1-antiprotease, the activities of matrix metalloproteinases (MMPs) are limited by specific inhibitors, the tissue inhibitors of metalloproteinases (TIMP-1–4) which binds to the substrate-binding site of the MMPs. In addition, TIMP-2 is a cofactor in the activation of MMP2 by membrane-type MMPs. TIMPs are produced by a broader range of cell types than the proteases, and TIMP-2 is often constitutively expressed. TIMP-3, in particular, appears to act as a pro-apoptotic factor. The expression of most TIMPs is additionally regulated at the transcriptional level. In general, the same factors that induce MMPs are involved, but additional cytokines such as TNFα as well as glucocorticoids and retinoids are active, at least in the regulation of TIMP-1.

5.8 Collagen-Related Diseases

5.8.1 Hereditary Disorders

While a considerable number of collagen diseases have been documented (a number of the more common diseases are shown in Table 5.1 and Box 5.3), in this chapter the focus is on those with a phenotype in the intervertebral disc.

Collagen IX: Recent reports have suggested the importance of genetic factors in disc disease. Mutations in collagen IX are associated with premature disc degeneration in mice (Kimura et al. 1996) and a predisposition to disc disorders in humans. Transgenic mice expressing mutant collagen alpha 1(IX) develop progressive joint degeneration with age as well as accelerated intervertebral disc degeneration (Kimura et al. 1996; Boyd et al. 2008). The changes include shrinkage or disappearance of the nucleus pulposus and fissures in the annulus fibrosus, which sometimes lead to herniation of disc material and osteophyte formation. Degeneration in the end plate is associated with cell proliferation, cartilage disorganization, and new bone formation (Boyd et al. 2008).

MMP-3: Matrix metalloproteinase-3 (MMP-3, stromelysin-1) is involved in the pathogenesis of disc disease (Takahashi et al. 2001). Polymorphisms in MMP3 as well as TIMP-1 were associated with the radiographic progression of disc degeneration (Valdes et al. 2005).

Table 5.1 Clinical phenotypes of collagen gene mutations

Gene or protein	Clinical phenotype
COL1A1, COLlA2 (collagen 1 αl, α2 chains)	Family: Osteogenesis imperfecta
COL2A1 (collagen 2 αl chain)	Family: achondrogenesis 2, hypochondrogenesis, congenital spondyloepiphyseal dysplasia (SEDC), Kniest, Stickler arthro-ophthalmopathy, familial osteoarthritis, other variants
COL9Al,COL9A2, C0L9A3 (collagen 9 α1, α2, α3 chains)	Multiple epiphyseal dysplasia (MED; two or more variants)
COLl0A1 (collagen 10)	Metaphyseal dysplasia (Schmid alchain)
COII IAI, Co111A2 (collagen 11 αl, α2 chains)	Oto-spondylo-megaepiphyseal dysplasia (OSMED); Stickler (variant), Marshall syndrome
COMP	Pseudoachondroplasia, multiple epiphyseal dysplasia (MED; one form)
MATN3 (matrilin-3)	Multiple epiphyseal dysplasia (MED; one variant)
Perlecan	Schwartz–Jampel type 1; dyssegmental dysplasia

Box 5.3 Clinical Disorders Resulting from Defects in Collagen Synthesis

Disorder	Defect	Symptoms
Ehlers–Danlos type III	Mutations in either one or two separate genes (also involved in Vascular EDS and tenascin-X deficiency)	Joint hypermobility
Ehlers–Danlos type IV (vascular EDS)	Faulty transcription or translation of type III	Aortic and/or intestinal rupture
Ehlers–Danlos type VI	Faulty lysine hydroxylation	Augmented skin elasticity, rupture of eyeball
Ehlers–Danlos type VII	Decrease in procollagen peptidase activity	Increased articular mobility, frequent luxation
Scurvy	Lack of vitamin C (cofactor for proline hydroxylase)	Ulceration of gums, hemorrhages
Osteogenesis imperfect	Change of one nucleotide in genes for collagen type I	Spontaneous fractures, cardiac insufficiency

5.8.2 Other Collagen-Related Diseases

See Table 5.1 and Box 5.3.

5.9 Summary of Critical Concepts Discussed in the Chapter

- Collagens provide the structural framework of the intervertebral discs and are responsible for biomechanical properties, including torsion and resistance to pressure or tension.
- Proteoglycans, such as decorin, fibromodulin, and biglycan together with other matrix constituents, influence collagen fibril formation.
- In the annulus, collagen lamellae are formed consisting of concentric bundles of parallel collagen fibers arranged around the central gelatinous nucleus pulposus.
- With age, the proportion of aggrecan to water in the nucleus pulposus falls steeply, while the proportion of collagen to aggrecan rises. A similar change is seen in degenerate discs. These changes appear to arise from loss of aggrecan rather than an increase in the amount of secreted collagen.
- Collagen II fibrils in the nucleus pulposus are organized randomly joined by hydroxypyridium cross-links. Procollagen II is expressed in two forms by alternative splicing with or without exon 2.
- The fibril-forming collagens I and II form an important network in the disc. Collagen I forms hybrids with other fibrillar collagens, particularly collagen V. Co-fibril formation with collagen I regulates the fibril diameter.
- The collagen chains are synthesized as procollagens. Glycosylation of procollagen occurs in the rough ER and Golgi complex. Galactose and glucose residues are added to hydroxylysine residues, and long oligosaccharides are added to specific asparagine residues in the C-propeptide.
- The formation and passage of correctly folded triple-helical collagen molecules through the secretory pathway involve disulfide isomerase that recognizes the C-propeptide. The major collagen-binding protein in the RER is HSP47.
- Outside of the cell, registration peptides are cleaved and tropocollagen is formed by procollagen peptidase. Multiple tropocollagen molecules form collagen fibrils, via covalent cross-linking by lysyl oxidase.
- Mutations in collagen IX are associated with premature disc degeneration in mice and a predisposition to disc disorders in humans.
- Noncollagenous fibrous proteins in the disc include COMP, fibronectin, amyloid, tenascin, and elastin.
- Collagen cell interactions are mediated via discoidin domain receptors and integrin $\alpha_2\beta_1$. Ligand binding to this receptor triggers p38 MAP kinase activation.

Acknowledgments Dr. Mwale is funded by AO Spine, Canadian Institute of Health Research (CIHR), and North American Spine Society (NASS). The author thanks Drs. Shapiro and Risbud for critically reading the manuscript and providing valuable suggestions and Dr. Ovidiu Ciobanu for generating the figures and helping with the manuscript.

References

Aigner T, Gresk-Otter KR, Fairbank JC, von der Mark K, Urban JP (1998) Variation with age in the pattern of type X collagen expression in normal and scoliotic human intervertebral discs. Calcif Tissue Int 63:263–268

Anderson ET, Fletcher L, Severin A, Murphy E, Baker SM, Matsuka YV (2004) Identification of factor XIIIA-reactive glutamine acceptor and lysine donor sites within fibronectin-binding protein (FnbA) from Staphylococcus aureus. Biochemistry 43(37):11842–11852, PubMed PMID: 15362870

Anderson DG, Markova D, Adams SL, Pacifici M, An HS, Zhang Y (2010) Fibronectin splicing variants in human intervertebral disc and association with disc degeneration. Spine 35:1581–1588

Antoniou J, Steffen T, Nelson F, Winterbottom N, Hollander AP, Poole RA, Aebi M, Alini M (1996) The human lumbar intervertebral disc: evidence for changes in the biosynthesis and denaturation of the extracellular matrix with growth, maturation, ageing, and degeneration. J Clin Invest 98:996–1003

Athanasou NA, Kokubun S, West L, Sallie B, Puddle B (1995) Glycosaminoglycans in intervertebral disc amyloid deposits. Eur Spine J 4:308–312

Benjamin M, Ralphs JR (2004) Biology of fibrocartilage cells. Int Rev Cytol 233:1–45

Berg RA, Prockop DJ (1973) The thermal transition of a non-hydroxylated form of collagen. Evidence for a role for hydroxyproline in stabilizing the triple-helix of collagen. Biochem Biophys Res Commun 52:115–120

Boos N, Nerlich AG, Wiest I, von der Mark K, Aebi M (1997) Immunolocalization of type X collagen in human lumbar intervertebral discs during ageing and degeneration. Histochem Cell Biol 108:471–480

Bottomley MJ, Batten MR, Lumb RA (2001) Quality control in the endoplasmic reticulum: PDI mediates the ER retention of unassembled procollagen C-propeptides. Curr Biol 11:1114–1118

Boyd LM, Richardson WJ, Allen KD, Flahiff C, Jing L, Li Y, Chen J, Setton LA (2008) Early-onset degeneration of the intervertebral disc and vertebral end plate in mice deficient in type IX collagen. Arthritis Rheum 58:164–171

Bywaters EGL, Dorling J (1970) Amyloid deposits in articular cartilage. Ann Rheum Dis 29:294–306

Chiquet M, Fambrough DM (1984) Chick myotendinous antigen. II. A novel extracellular glycoprotein complex consisting of large disulfide-linked subunits. J Cell Biol 98:1937–1946

Cloyd JM, Elliott DM (2007) Elastin content correlates with human disc degeneration in the annulus fibrosus and nucleus pulposus. Spine 32:1826–1831

Day JM, Olin AI, Murdoch AD, Canfield A, Sasaki T, Timpl R, Hardingham TE, Aspberg A (2004) Alternative splicing in the aggrecan G3 domain influences binding interactions with tenascin-C and other extracellular matrix proteins. J Biol Chem 279:12511–12518

Demers CN, Antoniou J, Mwale F (2004) Value and limitations of using the bovine tail as a model for the human lumbar spine. Spine 29(24):2793–2799

Doyle SA, Smith BD (1998) Role of the pro-alpha2(I) COOH-terminal region in assembly of type I collagen: disruption of two intramolecular disulfide bonds in pro-alpha2(I) blocks assembly of type I collagen. J Cell Biochem 71(2):233–242

Erickson HP, Inglesias JL (1984) A six-armed oligomer isolated from cell surface fibronectin preparations. Nature 311:267–269

Eyre DR (1979) Biochemistry of the intervertebral disc. Int Rev Connect Tissue Res 8:227–291

Eyre DR, Muir H (1976) Types I and II collagens in intervertebral disc. Interchanging radial distributions in annulus fibrosus. Biochem J 157:267–270

Eyre DR, Dickson IR, Van Ness K (1988) Collagen cross-linking in human bone and articular cartilage. Age-related changes in the content of mature hydroxypyridinium residues. Biochem J 252(2):495–500

Eyre DR, Koob TJ, Van Ness KP (1984) Quantitation of hydroxypyridinium crosslinks in collagen by high-performance liquid chromatography. Anal Biochem 137:380–388

Eyre DR, Matsui Y, Wu JJ (2002) Collagen polymorphisms of the intervertebral disc. Biochem Soc Trans 30(Pt 6):844–848

Feng H, Danfelter M, Stromqvist B, Heinegard D (2006) Extracellular matrix in disc degeneration. J Bone Joint Surg Am 88(Suppl 2):25–29

Gruber HE, Ingram JA, Hanley EN Jr (2002) Tenascin in the human intervertebral disc: alterations with aging and disc degeneration. Biotech Histochem 77:37–41

Gruber HE, Ingram JA, Hanley EN Jr (2006) Immunolocalization of thrombospondin in the human and sand rat intervertebral disc. Spine 31:2556–2561

Grynpas MD, Eyre DR, Kirschner DA (1980) Collagen type II differs from type I in native molecular packing. Biochim Biophys Acta 626:346–355

Hayes AJ, Benjamin M, Ralphs JR (2001) Extracellular matrix in development of the intervertebral disc. Matrix Biol 20:107–121

Hristova GI, Jarzem P, Ouellet JA, Roughley PJ, Epure LM, Antoniou J, Mwale F (2011) Calcification in human intervertebral disc degeneration and scoliosis. J Orthop Res 29:1888–1895

Hulmes DJS (2002) Building collagen molecules, fibrils, and suprafibrillar structures. J Struct Biol 137:10

Hulmes DJ, Miller A (1981) Molecular packing in collagen. Nature 293:239–240

Inkinen RI, Lammi MJ, Lehmonen S, Puustjarvi K, Kaapa E, Tammi MI (1998) Relative increase of biglycan and decorin and altered chondroitin sulfate epitopes in the degenerating human intervertebral disc. J Rheumatol 25:506–514

Inoue H (1973) Three-dimensional observation of collagen framework of intervertebral discs in rats, dogs and humans. Arch Histol Jpn 36:39–56

Inoue H (1981) Three-dimensional architecture of lumbar intervertebral discs. Spine 6:139–146

Khoshnoodi J, Cartailler J-P, Alvares K, Veis A, Hudson BG (2006) Molecular recognition in the assembly of collagens: terminal noncollagenous domains are key recognition modules in the formation of triplehelical protomers. J Biol Chem 281:38117–38121

Kimura T, Nakata K, Tsumaki N, Miyamoto S, Matsui Y, Ebara S, Ochi T (1996) Progressive degeneration of articular cartilage and intervertebral discs. An experimental study in transgenic mice bearing a type IX collagen mutation. Int Orthop 20:177–181

Ladefoged C (1985) Amyloid in intervertebral discs. A histopathological investigation of intervertebral discs from 30 randomly selected autopsies. Appl Pathol 3:96–104

Lee CR, Sakai D, Nakai T, Toyama K, Mochida J, Alini M, Grad S (2007) A phenotypic comparison of intervertebral disc and articular cartilage cells in the rat. Eur Spine J 16:2174–2185

Linsenmayer TF, Long F, Nurminskaya M et al (1998) Type X collagen and other up-regulated components of the avian hypertrophic cartilage program. Prog Nucleic Acid Res Mol Biol 60:79

LuValle P, Ninomiya Y, Rosenblum ND, Olsen BR (1988) The type X collagen gene. Intron sequences split the 5'-untranslated region and separate the coding regions for the non-collagenous amino-terminal and triple-helical domains. J Biol Chem 263:18378–18385

Malone JP, George A, Veis A (2004) Type I collagen N-Telopeptides adopt an ordered structure when docked to their helix receptor during fibrillogenesis. Proteins 54:206–215

Malone JP, Alvares K, Veis A (2005) Structure and assembly of the heterotrimeric and homotrimeric C-propeptides of type I collagen: significance of the α2(I) chain. Biochemistry 44:15269–15279

Maroudas A, Stockwell RA, Nachemson A, Urban J (1975) Factors involved in the nutrition of the human lumbar intervertebral disc: cellularity and diffusion of glucose in vitro. J Anat 120(Pt 1): 113–130

McAlinden A, Smith TA, Sandell LJ, Ficheux D, Parry DA, Hulmes DJ (2003) Alpha-helical coiled-coil oligomerization domains are almost ubiquitous in the collagen superfamily. J Biol Chem 278: 42200–42207

Mihara S, Kawai S, Gondo T, Ishihara T (1994) Intervertebral disc amyloidosis: histochemical, immunohistochemical and ultrastructural observations. Histopathology 25:415–420

Muragaki Y, Kimura T, Ninomiya Y, Olsen BR (1990) The complete primary structure of two distinct forms of human alpha 1 (IX) collagen chains. Eur J Biochem 192:703–708

Mwale F, Billinghurst C, Wu W, Alini M, Webber C, Reiner A, Ionescu M, Poole J, Poole AR (2000) Selective assembly and remodelling of collagens II and IX associated with expression of the chondrocyte hypertrophic phenotype. Dev Dyn 218:648–662

Mwale F, Roughley P, Antoniou J (2004) Distinction between the extracellular matrix of the nucleus pulposus and hyaline cartilage: a requisite for tissue engineering of intervertebral disc. Eur Cell Mater 8:58–63, discussion 63–54

Nachemson A, Lewin T, Maroudas A, Freeman MA (1970) In vitro diffusion of dye through the end-plates and the annulus fibrosus of human lumbar inter-vertebral discs. Acta Orthop Scand 41: 589–607

Nerlich AG, Schleicher ED, Boos N (1997) Volvo award winner in basic science studies. Immunohistologic markers for age-related changes of human lumbar intervertebral discs. Spine 22: 2781–2795

Nies DE, Hemesath TJ, Kim JH, Gulcher JR, Stefansson K (1991) The complete cDNA sequence of human hexabrachion (tenascin). A multidomain protein containing unique epidermal growth factor repeats. J Biol Chem 266:2818–2823

Nishimura I, Muragaki Y, Olsen BR (1989) Tissue-specific forms of type IX collagen-proteoglycan arise from the use of two widely separated promoters. J Biol Chem 264:20033–20041

Oegema TR Jr, Johnson SL, Aguiar DJ, Ogilvie JW (2000) Fibronectin and its fragments increase with degeneration in the human intervertebral disc. Spine 25:2742–2747

Pokharna HK, Phillips FM (1998) Collagen crosslinks in human lumbar intervertebral disc aging. Spine 23:1645–1648

Prockop DJ, Sieron AL, Li SW (1997/1998) Procollagen N-proteinase and procollagen C-proteinase Two unusual metalloproteinases that are essential for procollagen processing probably have important roles in development and cell signaling. Matrix Biol 16:399–408

Roberts S (2002) Disc morphology in health and disease. Biochem Soc Trans 30(Pt 6):864–869

Roberts S, Menage J, Urban JP (1989) Biochemical and structural properties of the cartilage end-plate and its relation to the intervertebral disc. Spine 14:166–174

Roberts S, Ayad S, Menage PJ (1991) Immunolocalisation of type VI collagen in the intervertebral disc. Ann Rheum Dis 50:787–791

Roughley PJ (2004) Biology of intervertebral disc aging and degeneration: involvement of the extracellular matrix. Spine 29(23):2691–2699

Ryan MC, Sandell LJ (1990) Differential expression of a cysteine-rich domain in the amino-terminal propeptide of type II (cartilage) procollagen by alternative splicing of mRNA. J Biol Chem 265:10334–10339

Sandell LJ, Morris N, Robbins JR, Goldring MB (1991) Alternatively spliced type II procollagen mRNAs define distinct populations of cells during vertebral development: differential expression of the amino-propeptide. J Cell Biol 114:1307–1319

Schmid TM, Linsenmayer TF (1985) Immunohistochemical localization of short chain cartilage collagen (type X) in avian tissues. J Cell Biol 100:598–605

Scott JE, Bosworth TR, Cribb AM, Taylor JR (1994) The chemical morphology of age-related changes in human intervertebral disc glycosaminoglycans from cervical, thoracic and lumbar nucleus pulposus and annulus fibrosus. J Anat 184(Pt 1):73–82

Takahashi M, Haro H, Wakabayashi Y, Kawa-uchi T, Komori H, Shinomiya K (2001) The association of degeneration of the intervertebral disc with 5a/6a polymorphism in the promoter of the human matrix metalloproteinase-3 gene. J Bone Joint Surg Br 83(4):491–495

Tasab M, Jenkinson L, Bulleid NJ (2002) Sequence-specific recognition of collagen triple helices by the collagen-specific molecular chaperone hsp47. J Biol Chem 277:35007–35012

Tchetina E, Mwale F, Poole AR (2003) Distinct phases of coordinated early and late gene expression in growth plate chondrocytes in relationship to cell proliferation, matrix assembly, remodeling, and cell differentiation. J Bone Miner Res 18:844–851

Valdes AM, Hassett G, Hart DJ, Spector TD (2005) Radiographic progression of lumbar spine disc degeneration is influenced by variation at inflammatory genes: a candidate SNP association study in the Chingford cohort. Spine 30:2445–2451

van der Rest M, Mayne R (1988) Type IX collagen proteoglycan from cartilage is covalently cross-linked to type II collagen. J Biol Chem 263(4):1615–1618

Vasios G, Nishimura I, Konomi H, van der Rest M, Ninomiya Y, Olsen BR (1988) Cartilage type IX collagen-proteoglycan contains a large amino-terminal globular domain encoded by multiple exons. J Biol Chem 263:2324–2329

Vaughan L, Mendler M, Huber S, Bruckner P, Winterhalter KH, Irwin MI, Mayne R (1988) D-periodic distribution of collagen type IX along cartilage fibrils. J Cell Biol 106:991–997

Wu JJ, Eyre DR (2003) Intervertebral disc collagen. Usage of the short form of the alpha1(IX) chain in bovine nucleus pulposus. J Biol Chem 278:24521–24525

Wu JJ, Eyre DR, Slayter HS (1987) Type VI collagen of the intervertebral disc. Biochemical and electron- microscopic characterization of the native protein. Biochem J 248:373–381

Wu JJ, Woods PE, Eyre DR (1992) Identification of cross-linking sites in bovine cartilage type IX collagen reveals an antiparallel type II-type IX molecular relationship and type IX to type IX bonding. J Biol Chem 267:23007–23014

Wurster NB, Lust G (1984) Synthesis of fibronectin in normal and osteoarthritic articular cartilage. Biochim Biophys Acta 800: 52–58

Yamaguchi N, Benya PD, van der Rest M, Ninomiya Y (1989) The cloning and sequencing of alpha 1 (VIII) collagen cDNAs demonstrate that type VIII collagen is a short chain collagen and contains triple-helical and carboxyl-terminal non-triple-helical domains similar to those of type X collagen. J Biol Chem 264:16022–16029

Yasuma T, Arai K, Suzuki F (1992) Age-related phenomena in the lumbar intervertebral discs. Lipofuscin and amyloid deposition. Spine 17:1194–1198

Yu J, Winlove PC, Roberts S, Urban JP (2002) Elastic fibre organization in the intervertebral discs of the bovine tail. J Anat 201: 465–475

Yu J, Fairbank JC, Roberts S, Urban JP (2005) The elastic fiber network of the annulus fibrosus of the normal and scoliotic human intervertebral disc. Spine 30:1815–1820

Yu J, Tirlapur U, Fairbank J, Handford P, Roberts S, Winlove CP, Cui Z, Urban J (2007) Microfibrils, elastin fibres and collagen fibres in the human intervertebral disc and bovine tail disc. J Anat 210:460–471

Zhang G, Eames BF, Cohn MJ (2009) Chapter 2. Evolution of vertebrate cartilage development. Curr Top Dev Biol 86:15–42

Zheng Q, Zhou G, Chen Y, Garcia-Rojas X, Lee B (2003) Type X collagen gene regulation by Runx2 contributes directly to its hypertrophic chondrocyte-specific expression in vivo. J Cell Biol 162: 833–842

Microenvironmental Control of Disc Cell Function: Influence of Hypoxia and Osmotic Pressure

6

Makarand V. Risbud and Irving M. Shapiro

The action of this principle is exactly like that of the centrifugal governor of the steam engine, which checks and corrects any irregularities almost before they become evident; and in like manner no unbalanced deficiency in the animal kingdom can ever reach any conspicuous magnitude, because it would make itself felt at the very first step, by rendering existence difficult and extinction almost sure soon to follow

Alfred Russell Wallace

Contributions to the Theory of Natural Selection 1858

Contents

M.V. Risbud (✉) • I.M. Shapiro
Department of Orthopaedic Surgery and Graduate Program in Cell and Developmental Biology,
Jefferson Medical College, Thomas Jefferson University,
1025 Walnut Street, Suite 511 College Bldg,
Philadelphia, PA 19107, USA
e-mail: makarand.risbud@jefferson.edu; irving.shapiro@jefferson.edu

6.1 Defining the Intervertebral Disc Niche

The intervertebral disc is a complex structure that displays many of the characteristics of a diarthrodial polyaxial joint in that it separates opposing cartilage-covered bones (vertebrae), permits a range of motions, and accommodates high biomechanical forces. The nature of this joint has been described in detail in Chap. 1 and in a recent review by Shapiro et al. (2012). While discs from the different anatomical regions of the spine vary in shape and volume, their architecture is generally similar. At the disc periphery, the outer annulus fibrosus layer forms a ligamentous structure, composed of tightly packed parallel collagen I fibrils that are inserted into contiguous superior and inferior vertebral bodies. The inner surface of the annulus fibrosus comprises a poorly organized fibrocartilage containing collagen II fibrils. The annulus and the cartilaginous endplates enclose the nucleus pulposus, an aggrecan-rich gel-like tissue that is sparsely populated with cells. Although embryologically distinct, cells of the nucleus pulposus are often mistakenly compared with chondrocytes. The nucleus pulposus is derived from the notochord, whereas annulus fibrosus and endplate cartilage are sclerotomal in origin (see Chap. 3 for further details concerning the ontology of disc cells). Throughout this chapter, cells of this notochordal-derived tissue are described as cells of the nucleus pulposus.

The interaction between the semifluid nucleus pulposus and the tight molecular lattice of the annulus fibrosus provides the biomechanical properties necessary for spinal stability. Disturbing this relationship by compromising the stability of the nucleus pulposus, the annulus fibrosus, or the endplate cartilage results in disc degeneration, a condition that can lead to excruciating pain and loss of function and which often results in costly surgical interventions. Because the degenerative process is chronic, the nucleus pulposus cells are required to function for long time periods in what

I.M. Shapiro, M.V. Risbud (eds.), *The Intervertebral Disc*,
DOI 10.1007/978-3-7091-1535-0_6, © Springer-Verlag Wien 2014

can be described as a suboptimal microenvironmental niche; the goal of this chapter is to consider those conditions that enhance nucleus pulposus cell survival as well as factors that disregulate the disc microenvironment and promote degenerative disc disease.

Herein, we use the term niche to describe the confines of the nucleus, bounded laterally and medially by the annulus and superiorly and inferiorly by the endplate cartilage. Although the concept of a niche was originally directed at anatomical structures, more recently the term has been used to describe interactions between communities of cells that are in close proximity to each other. For example, within the bone marrow niche, stem cell commitment to a particular lineage is dependent on local microenvironmental conditions that regulate the interactions between resident hematopoietic as well as stromal cells.

Although the clinical outcomes of degenerative disc disease are well documented, biological events that regulate nucleus pulposus cell survival are not understood. One overriding aspect of disc cell biology is that cells of the nucleus pulposus and cells residing in the inner annulus are removed from the blood supply. For example, blood vessels originating in the vertebral body traverse the superficial region of the endplates; none of these vessels infiltrate the nucleus pulposus. Urban, Maroudas, and colleagues pioneered the studies of solute transport and biophysical properties of the disc (Urban et al. 1977). Several modeling studies and biochemical measurements of glycolytic pathway metabolites by these workers predict that the oxygen tension (pO_2) within the disc is low and that metabolism is primarily anaerobic (Bartels et al. 1998), even if the oxygen tension is raised (Holm et al. 1981). With respect to the annulus, Gruber et al. (2005) pointed out that this tissue is avascular except for small discrete capillary beds in the dorsal and ventral surfaces; in no case, does the annulus vasculature enter the nucleus pulposus. Microangiographical and immunohistochemical studies of the human disc lend strong support to the notion that the nucleus pulposus is avascular in nature (Hassler 1969; Rudert and Tillmann 1993). Moreover, even during disc degeneration vascular invasion of the nucleus pulposus is not seen, suggesting that vascular in-growth is not a defining feature of disc disease (Nerlich et al. 2007). Lee and colleagues examined hypoxic nature of the rat disc using 2-nitroimidazole, EF5, a drug that at low pO_2 forms covalent product with cellular proteins (Lee et al. 2007). These studies revealed that the transition zone and not the nucleus pulposus exhibited the highest level of EF5 binding. The authors concluded that the disc cells adapt to the local environment by limiting the consumption of oxygen. To further investigate this concept, Schipani and colleagues generated and characterized hypoxia-inducible reporter mice (5XHRE-LacZ reporter) (Fig. 6.1). Labeling with hypoxia marker EF5 clearly showed a robust signal in the presumptive intervertebral disc indicating a hypoxic environment. Based on these and other studies, it is now widely accepted that the nucleus pulposus cells reside in a hypoxic tissue niche.

Another important environmental factor that characterizes the disc niche is the elevated osmolarity. Although sparse, cells in the nucleus pulposus secrete a complex extracellular matrix that contains collagens and the proteoglycan aggrecan as well as versican. Glycosaminoglycan (GAG) chains of the aggrecan molecule provide a robust hydrodynamic system that serves to accommodate applied biomechanical forces (Feng et al. 2006; Setton and Chen 2006). In the nucleus pulposus, the principle GAG is chondroitin sulfate. Bound to the aggrecan core protein and associated with hyaluronic acid, the chondroitin sulfate chains form a giant polydispersed supramolecular structure with a net negative charge; this serves as a driving force for binding cations especially Na^+, thereby elevating tissue osmolarity (this topic is discussed further in Chaps. 2 and 4). The high osmotic pressure of the aggregate contains the forces applied to the spine (Ng et al. 2003). We have shown that nucleus pulposus cells responded to changes in osmotic pressure by upregulating the transcription factor, TonEBP (tonicity enhancer-binding protein) (Tsai et al. 2006), the only known mammalian transcription factor that responds to changes in osmolarity. In the following sections, we will describe in detail the activities of this interesting protein and its importance in maintenance of disc cell function. In addition to osmolarity and hypoxia, several other morphogenic proteins including those of the TGF-β superfamily play an important role in niche maintenance. Towards the end of the chapter, the activities of TGF-β in the postnatal nucleus pulposus are briefly discussed.

6.2 Role of HIF Proteins in the Intervertebral Disc Niche

If the concept of a regulatory niche, composed of a number of cell types responsive to local microenvironmental conditions, is valid, then this begs the question: is cell survival in the hypoxic niche hypoxia-inducible factor (HIF) dependent? Thanks to the brilliant studies of Semenza and colleagues, it is now recognized that the critical molecule regulating energy metabolism and survival activity under hypoxia is HIF-1 (Semenza et al. 1994). HIF is a member of the basic helix–loop–helix (bHLH)–PER–ARNT–SIM (PAS) family of proteins and composed of a constitutively expressed β-subunit and an α-subunit. In most cells, the latter subunit is stable under hypoxic conditions but is rapidly degraded in normoxia (Wang et al. 1995). Transactivation of HIF-1 target genes involves dimerization of the two subunits and binding to an enhancer, the hypoxia-response element in target genes. HIF-1 serves as a key transcription factor that

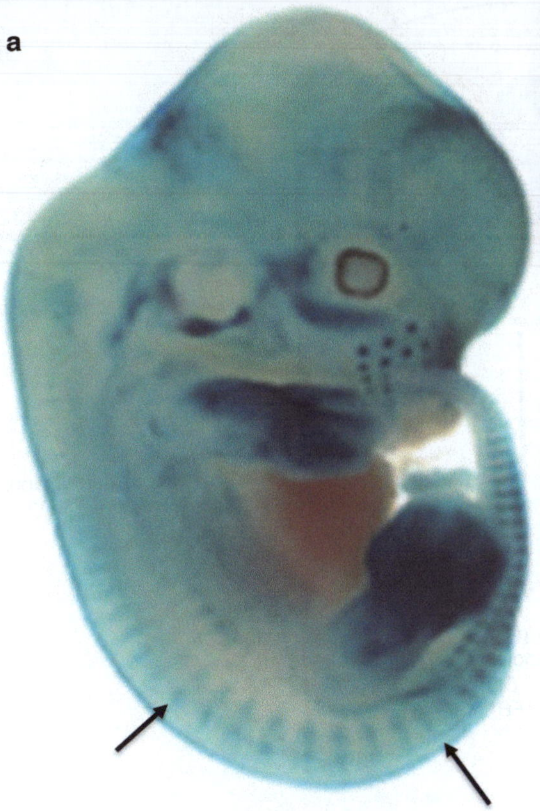

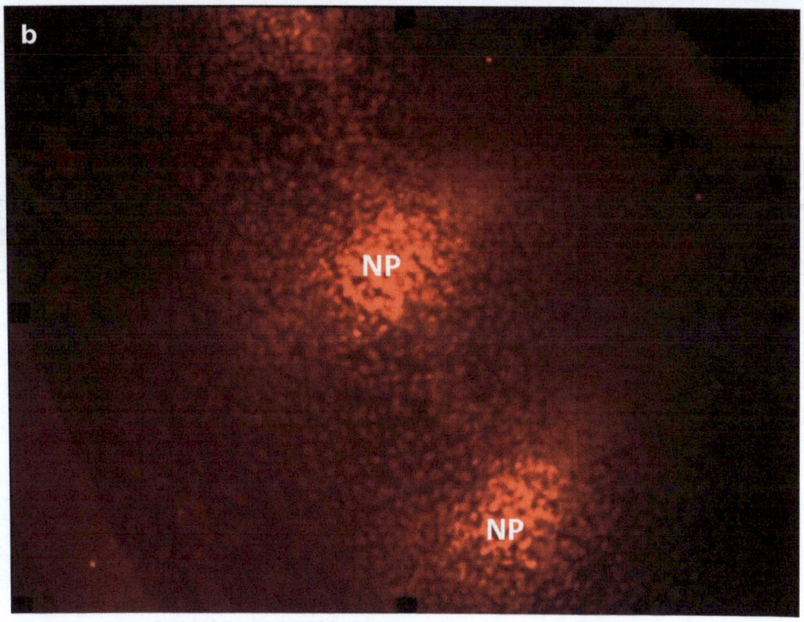

Fig. 6.1 The axial skeleton is hypoxic and expresses HIF-1α. (**a**) Characterization of hypoxia- inducible reporter mice (5XHRE-LacZ reporter). Note activation of the reporter construct in mesenchymal condensations by β-gal staining (*black arrows*). (**b**) Staining with hypoxia marker EF5 confirms that the nucleus pulposus (NP) of the presumptive intervertebral disc is hypoxic (Images kindly provided by Dr. Ernestina Schipani, Indiana University)

regulates the expression of enzymes concerned with glycolysis, the activity of the TCA cycle, and oxidative phosphorylation (Semenza et al. 1994; Papandreou et al. 2006; Fukuda et al. 2007). Additional target genes include those required for survival, apoptosis, autophagy, and matrix synthesis (Schipani et al. 2001; Zhang et al. 2008; Hofbauer et al. 2003). Details of these relationships are shown schematically in Fig. 6.2. It should be added that other isoforms exist, the most important being HIF-2α. Recent evidence suggests that HIF-1α and HIF-2α are not redundant and that the relative importance of each of the homologues, in response to hypoxia, varies among different cell types (Sowter et al. 2003). For example, unlike HIF-1, HIF-2 regulates expression of a number of unique genes including superoxide dismutase 2 (SOD2), catalase, frataxin, and cited2 (Scortegagna et al. 2003; Oktay et al. 2007; Aprelikova et al. 2006).

In addition to the genes mentioned above, the Sox family of transcription factors that are essential for the development and function of the nucleus pulposus are hypoxia and HIF sensitive (Smits and Lefebvre 2003; Lafont et al. 2007; Khan et al. 2007; Kanichai et al. 2008). Lafont et al. (2007) showed that HIF-2, but not HIF-1, regulated the expression of Sox9 and the phenotype of primary human chondrocytes. Similarly, expression of Sox9, Sox5, and Sox6 is hypoxia- (5 % O_2) and HIF-2-sensitive during chondrogenic differentiation of stem cells derived from the infrapatellar fat pads of osteoarthritic patients (Khan et al. 2007). In contrast, using marrow mesenchymal stem cells, Kanichai et al. (2008) showed involvement of HIF-1α in regulating Sox9 expression during chondrogenesis under hypoxia. However, the relationship between Sox proteins and HIF in the hypoxic niche of the disc is not as yet known (Box 6.1).

Box 6.1: Oxygen, Hypoxia and HIF

Over a billion years ago, the primitive atmosphere of the earth held very small amounts of dioxygen. Through the extraordinary activities of photosynthetic plants and organisms, over an enormous time period, the level of oxygen increased rapidly: a mere 200 million years ago, the oxygen content increased to about 16 %. Today, despite a huge elevation in manmade and natural oxidative activities, the gas level has held constant around 21 %.

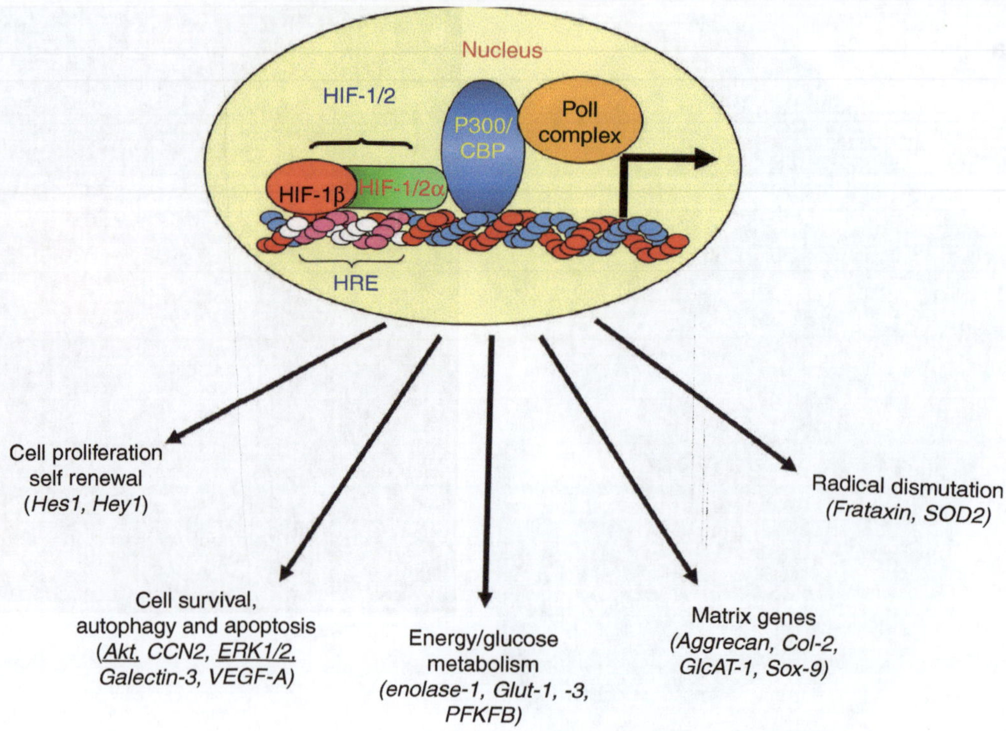

Fig. 6.2 Functional activity of HIF target genes. Critical functions include energy metabolism, angiogenesis, cell survival, autophagy and apoptosis, matrix synthesis, proliferation, self-renewal and differentiation, radical dismutation, and pH regulation. Many of these functions are critical for survival and functioning of the nucleus pulposus cells in the avascular niche of the intervertebral disc. Hypoxia-/HIF-sensitive proteins that are identified in the nucleus pulposus cells are shown in *parentheses* (Reproduced from Risbud et al. (2010). With permission from Elsevier)

The life-supporting activities of the gas was recognized by the Greeks who postulated that there were only four natural elements, air – along with earth, water, and fire. At the time of the American Revolution, there was a convergence of intellectual thought on the notion that air was a mixture of gases, especially the vital gas, oxygen. Among those charged with the discovery of oxygen were Joseph Priestley, Carl Wilhelm Scheele, and Antoine Lavoisier. Priestley, an Englishman, who for religious and political reasons settled in Pennsylvania, and was a good friend of Benjamin Franklin, found that a gas generated from metal oxides could keep a mouse alive longer than a similar volume of air. Priestley called his discovery "dephlogisticated air." Almost at the same time, Scheele isolated the same gas which he termed "fire air." A Frenchman, Antoine Lavoisier, labeled the gas "acid-maker" or "oxygen," viewing it as part of the air that was free to combine with other elements. Of note, Priestly found that the "dephlogisticated air" had the property of changing dark venous blood to bright red arterial blood.

We now know that red blood cells carry dioxygen to all of the tissues of the body so as to power metabolic reactions, particularly those concerned with maintenance of redox and high-energy intermediates such as ATP. Oxygen sensor systems exist within tissues: for example, in the carotid body and in mitochondria. A family of enzymes, prolyl hydroxylases, monitors the oxemic state of the cell and enhances adaptation to hyperoxic and hypoxic conditions.

The term hypoxia is a generalized term used to describe the fall in oxygen to levels that are necessary to sustain most animal life. In some tissues, the blood oxygen concentration can be normoxic, but the cells experience hypoxia due to a high cell density, elevated metabolic activity, or poor vascularization. If hypoxia develops, a family of transcription factors is activated. Hypoxia-inducible factors or HIFs serve to change the metabolic activities of the cell so as to accommodate the available oxygen concentration.

6.2.1 Control of HIF-α Stability in the Disc

To return to the question raised above concerning the importance of the HIF system, a considerable number of reports now clearly show that there is a robust HIF response by cells of the nucleus pulposus. The response is evident across species; it is seen in vivo and in vitro, and more importantly, HIF-1α activity is unresponsive to the oxemic state of the tissue (Rajpurohit et al. 2002; Risbud et al. 2006a, b; Agrawal et al. 2007). Accordingly, when compared with most other tissues, there are substantive underlying differences in the HIF status and reactivity of disc cells: HIF-1α expression and activity is always "on." This unusual response suggests that stabilization of HIF-1α in cells of the nucleus pulposus ensures that transcriptional activity is a major determinant of cell function. The second HIF homologue, HIF-2α, is robustly expressed by nucleus pulposus cells. Like HIF-1α, steady-state protein levels are similar in both hypoxia and normoxia, suggesting that it too is constitutively expressed (Agrawal et al. 2008).

Before leaving this topic, it is important to comment on mechanisms of stabilization and turnover of HIF-1α and HIF-2α in nucleus pulposus cells. HIF-1a can be stabilized in a number of different ways. For example, von Hippel-Lindau protein activity can be suppressed, or O_2 sensing by one or more of the prolyl hydroxylase (PHD) enzymes, members of the 2-oxoglutarate/Fe^{2+}-dependent dioxygenase superfamily, could be low (Appelhoff et al. 2004). Importantly, since the activity of PHDs depends on the tissue oxygen tension, these molecules serve as sensors that control the cellular abundance of HIF-α proteins. It is known that PHD proteins hydroxylate specific prolyl residues in the oxygen-dependent degradation domain of HIF-α subunits. The hydroxylated proteins are bound by the ubiquitin ligase von Hippel–Lindau tumor suppressor protein (pVHL), which targets them for rapid ubiquitination and 26S proteasomal degradation (Maxwell et al. 1999). We reported recently that expression of PHD1-3 is higher in cells of the nucleus pulposus than in cells of the annulus fibrosus (Fujita et al. 2012a). Noteworthy, unlike other cells, our studies clearly showed that in nucleus pulposus cells, stability of HIF-α-oxygen-dependent degradation domain (ODD) is independent of oxemic tension. In addition, mutagenesis studies suggest that hydroxylation reaction may not control HIF-2α degradation in these cells (Köditz et al. 2007; Fujita et al. 2012a). Again these findings are different from articular chondrocytes that exhibit responsiveness of HIF-2α degradation to PHD function in vitro suggesting a cell type-specific response (Thoms and Murphy 2010).

Further investigations found that both HIF-1α and HIF-2α were degraded through the 26S proteasome pathway. Since all PHDs mediate proteasomal HIF-α degradation, but differ in their ability to hydroxylate HIF-1α in vivo, we investigated their individual role in HIF-α turnover in nucleus pulposus cells (Minamishima et al. 2008; Takeda et al. 2006). The high relative expression of PHD2 in nucleus pulposus tissue suggests that this isoform may play an important role in HIF-α turnover. These studies indicate that PHD2 controls to a limited extent HIF-1α degradation even under hypoxic conditions, indicating preservation of PHD2 enzymatic activity at low O_2 tension. This finding is in marked contrast to previous reports demonstrating HIF-1α stabilization at low oxygen tensions because of inhibition of PHD enzymatic activity (Epstein et al. 2001). Moreover, this observation highlights the unique physiology of the nucleus pulposus cells and suggests that

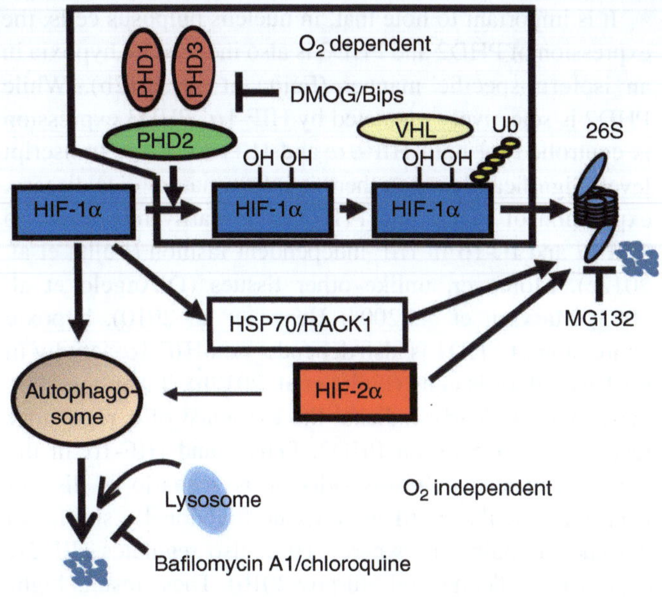

Fig. 6.3 A schematic model of the unique regulation of HIF-1α and HIF-2α degradation in nucleus pulposus cells. PHD2 controls a limited oxygen-dependent degradation of HIF-1α through 26S proteasome pathway. Oxygen-independent mechanisms through 26S proteasome as well as lysosomal pathway are active in HIF-1α turnover. In contrast, HIF-2α is unresponsive to oxidative degradation and is also turned over though 26S and lysosomal pathway (Reproduced from Fujita et al. (2012a). With permission of the American Society for Bone and Mineral Research)

there is very low cellular utilization of O_2, an adaptive response to the hypoxic niche (Bibby et al. 2005; Lee et al. 2007). The limited involvement of PHD2 in HIF-1α degradation implies that it is not a major regulator of HIF-1α turnover. Furthermore, it lends support to the hypothesis that HIF-1α levels are regulated primarily by oxygen-independent pathways.

In contrast to HIF-1α, the turnover of HIF-2α through 26S proteasome is largely independent of PHD function; there is also a limited involvement of the lysosomal pathway. Relevant to this discussion, recent studies by Gogate et al. (2012) indicate that Hsp70 modulates HIF-1α protein stability and transcriptional activity. In nucleus pulposus, Hsp70 was shown to interact with HIF-1α under hypoxic conditions and promoted degradation through the proteasomal pathway (Gogate et al. 2012). These findings strongly suggest that nucleus pulposus cells are functionally adapted to their avascular, hypoxic microenvironment and rely mostly on oxygen-independent pathways for controlling HIF-1α and HIF-2α levels. With respect to regulation, in hypoxia, PHD3 promotes HIF-1α transcriptional activity (Fujita et al. 2012b); this observation is in line with a recent report that describes a crucial role of the PHD3–PKM2 complex in enhancing HIF-1α interaction with p300, an important transcriptional coactivator (Luo et al. 2011). The possible pathways involved in HIF-α turnover in nucleus pulposus cells are demarcated in Fig. 6.3.

It is important to note that, in nucleus pulposus cells, the expression of PHD2 and PHD3 is also induced by hypoxia in an isoform-specific manner (Fujita et al. 2012b). While PHD2 is selectively regulated by HIF-1α, PHD3 expression is controlled by both HIF-1α and HIF-2α at the transcript level. Significantly when there is inflammatory disc disease, expression of PHD2 and PHD3 is primarily responsive to TNF-α and IL-1β in HIF independent fashion (Fujita et al. 2012c). Moreover, unlike other tissues (D'Angelo et al. 2003; Marxsen et al. 2004; Henze et al. 2010), hypoxic expression of PHD1 is also dependent on HIF-1α activity in nucleus pulposus cells (Fujita et al. 2012b). Taken together, these studies clearly indicate the existence of a regulatory feedback loop between PHD2, PHD3, and HIF-1α in the hypoxic nucleus pulposus cells. This scenario is distinct from the articular cartilage, a tissue functionally similar to the nucleus pulposus, where PHD2 also regulates HIF-2α degradation (Thoms and Murphy 2010). These results highlight the unique nature and control of the HIF-PHD system in nucleus pulposus cells and for the first time provide a biochemical rationale for normoxic stabilization and maintenance of steady-state levels of these proteins in the nucleus pulposus. Whether stabilization of HIF-α proteins is related to the unique embryonic origins of the tissue is currently unknown. However, it is important to note that because discs are hypoxic in vivo, stabilization of HIF-α expression would serve to maintain cell metabolism and functional activities when disc integrity is breached during disc herniation (Ha et al. 2006) or at an early stage of degeneration (Roberts et al. 2006).

6.2.2 Role of HIF-1 in Energy Conservation by Cells of the Nucleus Pulposus

Earlier classical biochemical studies have shown that when the pO_2 is low, there is almost complete reliance on glycolysis to generate ATP and reducing equivalents. As indicated in the previous section, one of the consequences of low oxygen tension in the nucleus pulposus is the reliance on glycolysis for energy generation (Agrawal et al. 2007; Holm et al. 1981). Glycolysis may be viewed as a relatively inefficient process: it generates 2 mol of ATP/mol glucose; in contrast, mitochondrial metabolism is slow, but it creates about 30 mol of ATP/mol glucose. In the trade-off between rate and yield, the glycolytic pathway generates a small number of ATP molecules at a very fast rate and maintains the reducing status of the cell. In this way, glycolysis provides sufficient energy for both housekeeping functions and for protein synthesis.

One of the logical outcomes of stabilization of HIF-1α is the robust expression of glucose transporters and enzymes required for anaerobic glycolysis. When the expression of three target genes (glucose transporter [GLUT]-1 and –3 and GAPDH) at 2–21 % O_2 were evaluated, it was found that the activities are comparable and remain constant over time (Agrawal et al. 2007). Although these genes were not responsive to the oxemic state of the culture, we have observed a small induction in enolase-1 and phosphofructokinase 2 (PFKFB) promoter activities. This result is surprising as the later protein is regarded as the glycolytic "pacemaker"; however, because this intermediary step is sensitive to a number of hormones, and metabolic intermediates, it is more than likely that induction is in response to other regulatory factors. Nevertheless, the muted response does not detract from the conclusion that the glycolytic flux in disc cells, even in normoxia, is high.

In normoxia, the basal concentration of ATP in nucleus pulposus cells is between 20 and 25 nmol/L/mg protein (Agrawal et al. 2007). These values are comparable with levels reported for articular chondrocytes, another cell type that uses glycolysis to generate energy (Pfander et al. 2003). In the presence of 2-deoxyglucose, a potent inhibitor of glycolysis, ATP generation is suppressed by almost 80 % (Agrawal et al. 2007). The sensitivity of the cells to this inhibitor emphasizes the reliance on glycolysis for energy generation. Based on this observation, it is likely that the oxemic stability of HIF-1α in nucleus pulposus cells is optimal for survival in an environment where there are frequent shifts in vascular supply and O_2 delivery; in the intervertebral disc, these shifts may reflect minute to minute or day/night variations in biomechanical forces applied to the spinal units.

Although glycolysis is clearly the major ATP-generating pathway, the possibility exists that some high-energy intermediates may be produced through mitochondrial oxidative phosphorylation. However, current studies indicate that inhibitors of mitochondrial function do not influence ATP production nor nucleus pulposus cell viability (Agrawal et al. 2007). As for a role, if any, for mitochondria, little is known. Gan et al. (2003) have reported that although nucleus pulposus cells contain mitochondria with normal architecture, the total number of organelles per cell is low. Nevertheless, nucleus pulposus cells can perform mitochondrial oxidative metabolism: thus, they oxidize fatty acid and generate ATP (Agrawal et al. 2007). Based on all of these studies, there is strong support for the notion that although glucose and anaerobic glycolysis represent the major fuel and pathway for energy generation, respectively, mitochondria in the nucleus pulposus are functional; they retain the capacity to metabolize fatty acids through mitochondrial oxidative metabolism.

The conclusion that disc cell energy metabolism is dependent on glycolysis fits well with current observations concerning the regulatory functions of HIF-1. It is known that HIF-1 plays a major role in directing the interplay between glycolysis and oxidative phosphorylation. HIF-1 inhibits mitochondrial function by *trans*-activating the gene encoding pyruvate dehydrogenase kinase 1. Because this protein suppresses pyruvate dehydrogenase, pyruvate cannot be converted into acetyl-CoA, and as a result the TCA cycle is blocked (Papandreou et al. 2006). Moreover Fukuda et al. (2007) showed that HIF-1 reciprocally regulates mitochondrial cytochrome c oxidase (COX)-4 subunit expression by activating transcription of the genes encoding COX4-2 and a protease that is required for COX4-1 degradation. Thus, HIF regulates not just the entry of reducing equivalents into the mitochondria but also oxidative phosphorylation. Based on these observations, it is concluded that although mitochondrial function is retained by cells of the intervertebral disc, it is reasonable to assume that normoxic expression of HIF-1α by nucleus pulposus cells serves to suppress oxidative phosphorylation and promotes glycolytic ATP generation. More than likely, nucleus pulposus mitochondria are required for non-energy-related metabolic functions, while oxidative phosphorylation is used to a very minor degree.

6.2.3 Role of Hypoxia and HIF in Promoting Cell Survival and Function in the Disc

If the premise is correct that the HIF signaling network serves to promote nucleus pulposus function, then the cells should be adapted to survive and grow in a hypoxic environment. Studies from our lab (Risbud et al. 2005a, b; Agrawal et al. 2007; Zeng et al. 2007) and other groups (Mwale et al. 2011; Feng et al. 2013) show that hypoxia, possibly through HIF-1, enhances the expression of important matrix genes and the phenotype of nucleus pulposus cells. Experiments have also been performed in which nucleus pulposus cells were treated with low levels of common apoptogens and survival measured (Risbud et al. 2005a, b). Notably, when the pO_2 was below 5 %, there was maximum disc cell survival. Studies of nucleus pulposus and chondrocytes showed that when HIF-1α is partially silenced, viability is maintained in the face of an O_2 challenge (Fujita et al. 2012b; Bohensky et al. 2007). On the other hand, complete deletion of HIF-1 in growth plate chondrocytes results in massive cell death highlighting the requirement of HIF-1 for cell survival in the hypoxic niche (Schipani et al. 2001). However, it is possible that some effects of hypoxia on nucleus pulposus survival are probably mediated by other signaling molecules in an HIF-1-independent fashion. The latter observation raises the question: which signaling pathways are upregulated in hypoxia? Work from a number of labs suggests that a variety of hypoxia-responsive proteins exist, including vascular endothelial growth factor (VEGF) (Fujita et al. 2008; Agrawal et al. 2008), galectin-3 (Zeng et al. 2007), and Akt/PI3K (Risbud et al. 2005a, b). Our work has shown that expression levels of phospho-Akt in nucleus pulposus cells are high in hypoxia and when serum-starved confers resistance to apoptosis (Risbud et al. 2005a, b). Activation of this protein is of considerable interest as it has been shown to modulate apoptosis by inactivating Bad and caspase-9 and modulating the transcription of proapoptotic transcription factors (Duronio 2008). Relevant to nucleus pulposus cells, activation of PI3K/Akt signaling has been shown to regulate HIF-1α protein levels in other cell types (Kanichai et al. 2008). Like Akt, extracellular signal-regulated kinase (ERK)1/2 is induced in hypoxic nucleus pulposus cells. Because activation of ERK has been linked to survival, possibly by regulating nitric oxide synthase and caspase activities, the it is probable that activation of ERK in concert with Akt serves to maintain the viability of the disc cells at a low pO_2 (Risbud et al. 2005a, b).

Like HIF-1, one of the critical functions of Akt is regulation of glucose metabolism. It is thought that Akt may promote cell survival by maintaining GLUT-1 transcription under conditions of growth factor withdrawal (serum starvation) (Rathmell et al. 2003). Indeed, the high level of expression of GLUT-1 protein by nucleus pulposus cells in vivo (Rajpurohit et al. 2002; Richardson et al. 2008) indicates that this tissue may adapt to its hypoxic environment by increasing glucose uptake. This activity would serve to promote and enhance glycolysis, thereby preventing ischemia-induced injury. Taken together, these studies suggest that the PI3K-Akt and ERK signaling pathways in conjunction with HIF-1 provide a mechanism by which nucleus pulposus cells remain viable and maintain their specialized physiological function, despite environmental limitations in O_2 and possibly changes in nutrient availability.

Two proteins that have been linked to nucleus pulposus survival in hypoxia are VEGF-A and galectin-3. In disc cells, it has been reported that HIF-1 regulates galectin-3 expression (Zeng et al. 2007). From a functional perspective, by forming complexes with integrins, externalized galectin-3 influences cell adhesion and spreading (Sasaki et al. 1998). Accordingly, galectin-3 is most likely involved with matrix stability and in concert with HIF-1 provides the discal cells with both a mechano-transduction and a survival function. Other studies have shown that galectin-3 regulates survival by suppressing signaling through the TNF family of proteins (Oka et al. 2005). This finding is particularly pertinent to disc disease, as TNF-α together with other cytokines is known to play a major role in the etiology, as well as progression, of the degenerative state. Based on these findings, it is possible that in the hypoxic intervertebral disc, the robust expression of HIF-1α serves to maintain galectin-3 levels, which then serve to promote cell survival and disc function (Zeng et al. 2007).

With respect to VEGF-A, not surprisingly, levels of this protein are high in herniated discs or in degenerative discs where there is evidence of neovascularization

(Kokubo et al. 2008). In the normative state, because the disc environment is avascular, it would be reasonable to assume that VEGF expression is low. However, this is not the case as there is robust expression of this protein and its receptor in the nucleus pulposus (Fujita et al. 2008; Agrawal et al. 2008). Most likely, the level of expression is related to both HIF-1 and HIF-2, as both isoforms upregulate VEGF-A expression and promoter activity (Agrawal et al. 2008). This observation begs the question: in the disc, what is the function of VEGF? Clearly, it cannot serve to promote angiogenesis as this activity would promote vascularization and compromise disc function. There is some information to indicate that VEGF supports cell survival (Zelzer et al. 2004). Indeed, Fujita et al. (2008) confirmed that VEGF and its receptors are expressed by nucleus cells in hypoxia and showed that this protein promoted nucleus pulposus survival. Thus, from a functional viewpoint, VEGF could serve as to maintain nucleus pulposus viability in the face of shifts in environmental pO_2.

As indicated above, there is growing interest in the second HIF homologue, HIF-2α. This protein is robustly expressed by nucleus pulposus cells. With respect to functional activities, unlike most other tissues, hypoxia failed to increase the transcriptional activities of SOD2 and frataxin, two common HIF-2 target genes concerned with radical dismutation (Scortegagna et al. 2003; Oktay et al. 2007). This finding could explain why this tissue is susceptible to radical attack associated with annular lesions or nucleus herniation. Notably, there is evidence to indicate that kyphosis, scoliosis, and radiculopathies are linked to defective radical dismutation (Murakami and Kameyama 1963; Sparrow et al. 2012), whereas Friedreich's ataxia is now known to be attributable to low frataxin levels and loss of antioxidant defenses (Gakh et al. 2006). It would be important to know whether these conditions are also linked to the inability of vertebral tissues to mount a robust HIF-2-dependent scavenging response.

Notably, both HIF-1 and HIF-2 are involved in survival of endplate chondrocytes by activation of the autophagic pathway (Bohensky et al. 2009; Srinivas et al. 2009). Recent studies suggest that autophagy is active in the nucleus pulposus (Ye et al. 2011; Jiang et al. 2012). The importance of this system for removal of misfolded proteins and damaged organelles has been emphasized by a number of workers, and its role in directing the maturation of connective tissue cells has been discussed by Srinivas and his colleagues (Srinivas et al. 2009). Noteworthy, although autophagy is viewed as a survival pathway, there is little doubt that continued macromolecular breakdown, while serving as a source of nutrients and energy for the stressed cell, inevitably leads to increased susceptibility to apoptosis (type II apoptosis). Hence, HIF activity and ultimately HIF targets serve as key proteins that straddle both the apoptotic and survival pathways.

Bohensky et al. (2009) pointed out that HIF-2 was involved in regulating survival by modulating autophagy. HIF-2 was expressed abundantly by cells in human and murine articular cartilage, hypertrophic cartilage, and in the endplate cartilage. When HIF-2α was suppressed, ROS generation was elevated, and there was a decrease in the activity of the ROS dismutating enzymes catalase and superoxide dismutase. Suppression of HIF-2α was associated with decreased Akt-1, reduced Bcl-x(L) expression, and a robust autophagic response, even under nutrient-replete conditions (Bohensky et al. 2009). In addition, Semenza and colleagues have demonstrated important contributions of HIF-1α to autophagy (Zhang et al. 2008). Relevant to disc disease, it is generally agreed that the degenerative state is exacerbated by a decrease in the permeability of the endplate cartilage and the concomitant reduction in nutrient availability. It is possible that under these nutritionally challenging conditions, increased HIF-1/-2 expression may serve to maintain nucleus pulposus survival by promoting the induction of autophagy (Box 6.2).

Box 6.2: HIF, Hypoxia, and Human Populations

Oxidative metabolism and the availability of oxygen have powered evolutionary processes that have permitted animals to populate almost every region of the planet. At high altitudes and in the depth of the ocean, the partial pressure of oxygen is low; nevertheless, organisms have evolved mechanisms to adapt to these nonphysiologic conditions. The question that has intrigued scientists is: what type of adaptation mechanism exists to enable humans and animals to reside in harsh environments characterized by the high Andean, Tibetan, and Ethiopian plateaus? For humans living at high altitudes, there may be genetic selection pressures for phenotypes characterized by raised oxygen hemoglobin saturation; one problem here is that a change in blood viscosity can elicit profound medical problems. However, studies of Tibetans living at very high altitudes show that they exhibit an SNP close to the region encoding HIF-2. Beall et al. (2010) have proposed that this mutation causes a "blunted erythropoietic response." In this case, the change in viscosity would be minimal. There is evidence that HIF-1 isoform may also be involved. Studying the Naqu Yak, an animal that has lived on the Tibetan plateau for more than million years at an altitude of 9,000–15,000 ft above sea level, Wang et al. (2006) reported that HIF-1 is expressed at high levels in the brain, lung, and kidney. Since HIF-1 targets EPO (erythropoietin) as well as many other genes concerned with erythropoiesis, these animals would have an enhanced ability to transport oxygen in the blood stream. In summary, both animal and humans have adapted to hypoxia by expressing genes that modify oxygen transport and erythropoiesis.

References

Beall CM, Cavalleri GL, Deng L, Elston RC, Gao Y, Knight J, Li C, Li JC, Liang Y, McCormack M, Montgomery HE, Pan H, Robbins PA, Shianna KV, Tam SC, Tsering N, Veeramah KR, Wang W, Wangdui P, Weale ME, Xu Y, Xu Z, Yang L, Zaman MJ, Zeng C, Zhang L, Zhang X, Zhaxi P, Zheng YT (2010) Natural selection on EPAS1 (HIF2alpha) associated with low hemoglobin concentration in Tibetan highlanders. Proc Natl Acad Sci U S A 107(25):11459–11464

Wang DP, Li HG, Li YJ, Guo SC, Yang J, Qi DL, Jin C, Zhao XQ (2006) Hypoxia-inducible factor 1alpha cDNA cloning and its mRNA and protein tissue specific expression in domestic yak (Bos grunniens) from Qinghai-Tibetan plateau. Biochem Biophys Res Commun 15:348(1):310–349

6.3 Contribution of TonEBP to the Maintenance of the Osmotic Niche

For disc cells, the second major environmental challenge is the high osmotic pressure of the niche (this topic is also discussed in Chap. 2). As pointed out earlier, the biomechanical function of the nucleus pulposus is primarily attributed to the water binding and unique osmotic properties of the tissue. Osmotic pressurization of the nucleus pulposus balances the loads experienced by the spine. Studies by Urban and colleagues indicate that the tissue osmolarity is substantially higher than that of plasma and is in the range of 400–500 mosmol/kg (Urban and Maroudas 1981; Ishihara et al. 1997).

Until recently, the mechanism by which cells of the nucleus pulposus and annulus fibrosus control their intracellular osmotic properties was not known. Drawing on information relevant to other tissues, it was noted that cellular adaptation to hyperosmotic stress is mediated by the tonicity enhancer-binding protein (TonEBP), also called OREBP (Miyakawa et al. 1999) or NFAT5 (Lopez-Rodríguez et al. 1999). TonEBP/NFAT5 belongs to the 5-member NFAT protein subfamily (NFAT1-5) which is part of the larger Rel superfamily of proteins. Similar to other members of the Rel family, it contains the Rel homology domain, a conserved DNA-binding domain. However, no similarities are seen between TonEBP and NF-κB or NFAT1-4 outside of the Rel homology domain. It lacks the binding site for calcineurin necessary for NFAT1-4 dephosphorylation and subsequent nuclear translocation (Lopez-Rodríguez et al. 1999). It is the largest Rel family member and unlike monomeric members of the NFAT family exists as a homodimer and forms stable dimers with DNA. Upon activation, TonEBP binds to the tonicity-responsive enhancer element (TonE) of genes required for osmotolerance and cell survival. These genes include the betaine/γ-aminobutyric acid transporter, sodium myo-inositol co-transporter (Ko et al. 1997; Miyakawa et al. 1998; Rim et al. 1998), taurine transporter (Zhang et al. 2003; Ito et al. 2004), and aldose reductase (Lopez-Rodríguez et al. 1999). By regulating levels of betaine, myo-inositol, taurine, and sorbitol, these genes control the osmotic properties of the cytosol. Hsp70, a molecular chaperone that maintains cellular function under hypertonic stress is also induced by TonEBP (Woo et al. 2002; Shim et al. 2002). Most homozygous TonEBP knockout mice evidence midgestational lethality. Of the few that survive, all exhibit severe growth retardation and kidney dysfunction (Lopez-Rodriguez et al. 2004). A transgenic mouse expressing a dominant-negative form of TonEBP (DN-TonEBP) in collecting duct epithelial cells demonstrated an absolute requirement of TonEBP for expression of the urea transporter gene and aquaporin-2 (Lam et al. 2004).

Aside from osmoregulation, TonEBP is required for T cell proliferation and function (Trama et al. 2000; Go et al. 2004), and it is implicated in cancer cell migration and metastasis (Jauliac et al. 2002). A study by Wang et al. (2005) showed that expression of DN-TonEBP in lens fiber cells promoted cataract formation by causing defects in their elongation. Since TonEBP is expressed by a number of cell types, it is reasonable to assume that it serves a variety of physiologic functions, especially those that impact on tissue hydration and the osmotic environment (Maouyo et al. 2002).

TonEBP and its downstream target genes are robustly expressed in the nucleus pulposus and the annulus fibrosus (see Fig. 6.4). Importantly, TonEBP is critical for maintenance of nucleus pulposus survival under hyperosmotic conditions (Tsai et al. 2006). The observed increase in apoptosis is in agreement with studies of TonEBP null mice and transgenic animals expressing DN-TonEBP in the thymus and in the lens (Trama et al. 2000; Go et al. 2004; Wang et al. 2005). In both these conditions, there was an acceleration of cell death through apoptosis. Very importantly, recent studies in C. elegans demonstrating selective and pronounced expression of TonEBP in the notochord suggest that its osmoregulatory function first evolved in the primitive axial skeleton prior to diversification to other tissues (José-Edwards et al. 2011). The relationship between TonEBP and cell death and its expression in the notochord lends strength to the notion that this transcription factor is of critical importance in the life history of cells of the nucleus pulposus.

One of the primary responses of cells to variations in local osmolarity is a change in regulatory cell volume. Disc cells and chondrocytes alike adapt to these osmotic shifts by remodeling their cytoskeleton and by catalyzing the

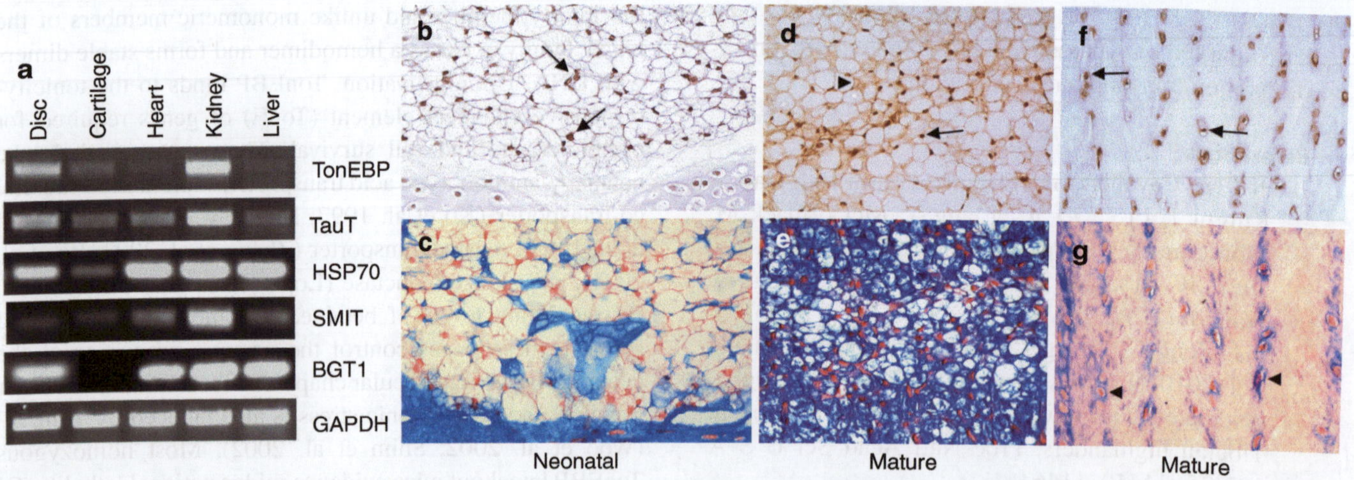

Fig. 6.4 (**a**) Expression level of TonEBP and other osmotically active genes in the intervertebral disc and other rat tissues. mRNA was extracted from disc tissue, costochondral cartilage, heart, kidney, and liver of adult rats and subjected to RT-PCR analysis. Note there is robust expression of TonEBP and its target genes: HSP-70, BGT-1, and SMIT mRNA. Cartilage another aggrecan-rich skeletal tissue contains lower levels of TonEBP mRNA than the disc. Kidney maximally expresses TonEBP as well as the target genes. (**b–g**) Sagittal and longitudinal sections of disc tissue from neonatal (**b**) and mature rat (**d–f**) spines that were treated with anti-TonEBP antibody or counterstained with alcian blue, eosin, and propidium iodide (**c–g**). Note that nucleus pulposus cells in the neonatal (**b**) as well as skeletally mature disc cells (**d**) express TonEBP protein; much of the staining is localized to the nucleus (**b**, *arrows*). Some staining is also evident in the cytosol of the nucleus pulposus cells of mature discs (**d**, *arrowhead*). Furthermore, annulus fibrosus cells localized in a narrow zone of alcian blue-positive matrix (**g**, *arrowhead*) express TonEBP protein (**f**, *arrow*). Magnification: ×20 (This research was originally published in Tsai et al. (2006). © the American Society for Biochemistry and Molecular Biology)

transport of osmotically active molecules and water across the plasma membrane (Pritchard et al. 2002; Tsai et al. 2006, 2007; Hall and Bush 2001). Water transport is regulated by a large family of channel-forming proteins, aquaporins (AQP) (Fu and Lu 2007). AQP2, an arginine vasopressin regulated channel, plays an important role in water reabsorption by connecting tubules and collecting ducts of the kidney (Verkman 2006). When activated, phosphorylation of critical serine residues in AQP2 results in its translocation from cytoplasmic vesicles to the apical membrane. Intercalated with membrane proteins, AQP2 enhances water influx into the cell (Verkman 2006). It has been suggested that in the kidney, expression of AQP2 is regulated by TonEBP (Hasler et al. 2006; Li et al. 2007; Jeon et al. 2006). Studies by Li et al. (2007) suggest that calcium ions with calcineurin-NFAT participate in regulation of AQP2 expression. Related to the functional importance of this system, Pritchard et al. (2002) have documented the presence of calcium transients in disc cells exposed to osmotic stress. In recent studies, we clearly showed that in both the rat and the human, nucleus pulposus cells express AQP2 protein (Gajghate et al. 2009). Importantly, unlike kidney, osmotic pressure and calcium modulate AQP2 expression through TonEBP in calcineurin–NFAT-independent fashion. This finding lends credence to the view that by regulating the hydration status of the disc, TonEBP maintains cell function in a hyperosmotic mechanically stressed environment.

6.3.1 Control of TonEBP Expression and Activity in the Nucleus Pulposus

Before leaving this topic, it is important to comment on several mechanisms unique to the disc niche that control TonEBP expression and activity. The mechanism of activation of TonEBP is complex and not completely understood, especially whether it is mediated by protein phosphorylation (Woo et al. 2002). In T cells and kidney cells, there is some evidence to indicate that regulation may be mediated by a phosphatase, calcineurin, which is activated by calcium ions (Trama et al. 2000). Studies from our lab suggest that although Ca^{2+} is involved in TonEBP activation, the downstream mechanisms and contribution of calcineurin may be cell type specific (Hiyama et al. 2009). Treatment of nucleus pulposus cells with cyclosporine A and FK506, inhibitors of calcineurin signaling, failed to block induction of TonEBP or change the promoter activity of the TonEBP target gene, taurine transporter. Other niche factors like hypoxia, TGF-β, and BMP-2 have been shown to modulate TonEBP expression (Hiyama et al. 2010). Gogate et al. (2012) showed that hypoxia causes a small increase in TonEBP protein levels. Importantly, in hypoxia, there was increased phosphorylation and activation of TonEBP-TAD. Likewise, BMP-2 or TGF-β increased protein levels of TonEBP and there was a significant activation of TAD. Since calcium regulates TonEBP activity and as one effect of TGF-β is the initiation of calcium transients, this raises the question: are these transients required for TGF-β-mediated TonEBP activation? Nevertheless, it is clear that irrespective of changes in Ca^{2+} flux, TGF-β and BMP-2 serve to upregulate TonEBP expression as well as its transcriptional activity possibly in a cell-/tissue-specific manner. The notion that TonEBP expression and activity is controlled by tissue- and cell-specific niche factors in addition to osmolarity was supported by a recent study of smooth muscle cells by Halterman and colleagues (Halterman et al. 2011). In these cells, angiotensin II promoted TonEBP nuclear translocation and activity, while PDGF-BB elevated TonEBP protein levels.

6.4 Niche Factors Control Matrix Synthesis by Nucleus Pulposus Cells

6.4.1 Control of Proteoglycan Synthesis

Although a considerable number of water-binding molecules contribute to the regulation of the osmotic pressure, aggrecan is the major polyelectrolyte. The charged COO− and SO_4^{2-} groups of N-acetylgalactosamine, glucuronic acid, and other substituted sugars bind hydrated Na^+ ions, thereby regulating the osmotic properties of the disc. While it is known that aggrecan transcription and oxemic tension as well as osmotic pressure are linked (Ishihara et al. 1997; Risbud et al. 2006a, b; Wuertz et al. 2007), details of the relationship are obscure. Promoter analysis of aggrecan provided a new insight into this relationship. We showed the presence of two TonE sites at −390 and −912 bp in the mouse aggrecan promoter (Tsai et al. 2006). A similar motif was noted in the human aggrecan promoter. The observation that the human TonE was at −890 bp probably reflects differences in species specific organization of the aggrecan promoter sequence. The presence of these conserved motifs provides a direct link between aggrecan expression and tissue osmolarity. Subsequent loss-of-function studies clearly showed that aggrecan promoter is responsive to TonEBP (Tsai et al. 2006). Important to this discussion of aggrecan regulation, studies from our lab (Risbud et al. 2005a, b; Agrawal et al. 2007) and Feng et al. (2013) showed that hypoxia and HIF-1α positively controls aggrecan gene expression in nucleus pulposus cells. These findings strongly indicate that aside from Sox9 and other transcriptionally active proteins, TonEBP and HIF-1 serve as regulators of aggrecan expression, a critically functional component of the disc matrix.

6.4.2 Control of GAG Synthesis by Niche Factors

As the water binding capacity of the proteoglycan matrix is dependent on the GAG side chains, it raises the question whether disc niche factors also regulate GAG and in particular chondroitin sulfate synthesis. Other workers have shown that galactose-β1,3-glucuronysltransferase-1 (GlcAT-I) activity is required for GAG chain synthesis (Kitagawa et al. 1996); hence, there is the possibility that this enzyme serves as the rate-limiting step in GAG synthesis for nucleus pulposus cells as well as chondrocytes (Venkatesan et al. 2004; Bai et al. 1999). Related to this point, it is now known that IL-1β suppresses GAG biosynthesis by downregulating GlcAT-I expression and activity (Gouze et al. 2001). A second factor regulating aggrecan as well as GAG synthesis is the intracellular Ca^{2+} concentration (Alford et al. 2003; Parvizi et al. 2002; Vijayagopal and Subramaniam 2001; Fagnen et al. 1999); it is speculated that Ca^{2+} ions controlled a common early step in the GAG biosynthetic pathway. Building on these observations, we performed studies to investigate the role of Ca^{2+} and TonEBP in GlcAT-I expression. Our studies clearly demonstrated that TonEBP regulates GlcAT-I expression and that regulation is dependent on intracellular Ca^{2+} ions (Hiyama et al. 2009). We also showed that Ca^{2+}-dependent calcineurin (Cn)-NFAT signaling serves as a negative regulator of GlcAT-I expression in these cells. From this perspective, by controlling GAG as well as aggrecan synthesis, TonEBP permits nucleus pulposus cells to autoregulate the osmotic environment of the disc. However, in contrast to TonEBP, HIF-1 serves as a negative regulator of GlcAT-I expression (Gogate et al. 2011). This observation was surprising as hypoxia serves to increase GAG synthesis by the nucleus pulposus cells (Gogate et al. 2011; Feng et al. 2013). Thus, TonEBP and HIF-1 may in some instances counter each other's activities.

6.4.3 Hypoxia, HIF-1, and CCN2 Expression

Previous work has shown that CCN2/CTGF, a matricellular protein is expressed by nucleus pulposus cells and is critical for matrix homeostasis. In nucleus pulposus cells, CCN2 promotes expression of aggrecan and collagen II (Tran et al. 2010; Erwin et al. 2006). Relevant to the niche of the intervertebral disc, low oxygen tension is known to regulate CCN2 in several cell types (Higgins et al. 2004; Hong et al. 2006; Kondo et al. 2006). Interestingly, CCN2 regulation by hypoxia is cell type specific and complex, with hypoxia promoting production of CCN2 in most cells; in some, CCN2 expression is downregulated.

Higgins et al. (2004) were the first to demonstrate that hypoxic induction of CCN2 in tubular epithelial cells required two HREs in the murine CCN2 promoter located at −1558/−1554 and −3745/−3741 bp. It was concluded that HIF-1α induces CCN2 transcription in response to hypoxia and that both of the HRE binding sites were necessary for promoter activation. Although the latter HRE lies within an evolutionary conserved region (ECR) of the promoter, these HREs are not conserved in location in the human CCN2 promoter, begging the question: are HREs in the human promoter functional and required for controlling expression in the nucleus pulposus?

To address this question and study the regulation of CCN2 in nucleus pulposus cells, we analyzed the proximal 5 kb of the human CCN2 promoter with an experimentally validated HRE matrix using the JASPAR database and found three putative HREs located at −640/−634,−2010/−2006, and −2264/−2258 bp, of which, the −2010/−2006 bp site lies within an ECR. In nucleus pulposus cells, we observed that hypoxia decreased CCN2 transcription. Interestingly, mutagenesis of the putative HREs in both human and mouse promoter showed that the suppressive effect of hypoxia may not involve direct binding of HIF-1α to these sites and suggests a complex regulation of CCN2 by hypoxia and HIF-1α in nucleus pulposus cells (Tran et al. 2013). This is not surprising given the unique stabilization of HIF-1α and a similar mode of regulation of other HIF-1α target genes in the nucleus pulposus (Fujita et al. 2012a; Gogate et al. 2012). Moreover, TGF-β, another important morphogenic factor, robustly induced CCN2 and is active in the disc from development to maturation. We have shown that TGF-β can still induce CCN2 expression under hypoxia. Although the magnitude of induction is decreased it supports the idea that hypoxic suppression of CCN2 in nucleus pulposus cells may serve to prevent excessive CCN2 production (Tran et al. 2013). The fact that the locations of HREs in the CCN2 promoter are not conserved in vertebrates suggests that regulation by hypoxia is not only cell type specific, but may also be species specific.

6.5 Role of Niche Factors in Promoting Disc Cell Renewal

In this chapter, attention has been drawn to the critical role of the tissue oxygen tension on the function and survival of cells of the intervertebral disc. We have focused on the mechanisms by which the hypoxia-sensitive transcription factors HIF-1 and HIF-2 influence energy metabolism and expression of survival proteins. In addition, we have discussed how cells of the nucleus respond to hypoxia-sensitive proteins, galectin-3, Akt, and VEGF-A. Where applicable, we have extended these discussions to include the impact of these molecules and hypoxia on degenerating resident cells in the intervertebral niche. It should be stated that in concert with most connective tissues, cell turnover within the disc niche is slow. Moreover, like most of these tissues, progenitor cells are present in the disc that can differentiate along the mesengenic pathway to replace resident cells (Risbud et al. 2007; Sakai et al. 2012) (also see Chap. 23). Thus, tissue renewal in the intervertebral disc is dependent on the ability of progenitor cells to commit to the nucleus pulposus lineage and undergo terminal differentiation.

The notch signaling pathway is central to these progenitor activities, and pertinent to the ideas discussed earlier, the notch signaling pathway is responsive to hypoxia. In skeletal tissues, disruption of notch signaling markedly increases trabecular bone mass: with aging, the mice become osteopenic due to a sharp reduction in mesenchymal progenitor populations (Engin et al. 2008; Hilton et al. 2008). Hypoxia also increases the expression of known notch target genes such as Hes1 and Hey1 (Gustafsson et al. 2005). Recent studies by Hiyama and colleagues showed that the cells of the nucleus pulposus and annulus fibrosus expressed genes of the notch signaling pathway (Hiyama et al. 2011). Moreover, in both tissues, hypoxia increased notch1 and notch4 expression. Interestingly, some tissue specificity was also noticed in that Jagged1 was induced by hypoxia only in the annulus fibrosus, while Jagged2 expression was highly sensitive to hypoxia in both tissues. Importantly, inhibition of notch signaling blocked disc cell proliferation. Relevant to disc disease, this study clearly showed increased expression of notch signaling genes in degenerated human discs (Hiyama et al. 2011).

Central to this discussion, HIF-1α has been shown to interact with the intracellular domain of the notch protein and results in inhibition of differentiation of myogenic and neural precursor cells (Gustafsson et al. 2005). Accordingly, in the nucleus, HIF-1α may directly interact with the notch intracellular domain and direct cell fate. Based on what is known of cell replacement in other tissues, this HIF-1-regulated pathway is a critical component of cell renewal and replacement.

From a disease viewpoint, an oxemic shift possibly mediated by alterations in the vascular supply to the endplate cartilage or even the annulus fibrosus would be expected to lead to a failure in progenitor cell activation and a decrease in the number of differentiated cells. In turn, this would lead to decrements in function and enhancement of the effect of agents that are known to promote disc degeneration. From a therapeutic viewpoint, it should be possible to modulate the niche environment to enhance renewal and promote differentiation of precursors into functional cells of the nucleus or the annulus. Accordingly, rather than relying on surgical and other interventional strategies, which may themselves damage the disc or cause infection, it should be possible to promote tissue repair by manipulating oxemic conditions within the niche or use proteins of the notch signaling pathway to reactivate the endogenous progenitor cells in the annulus fibrosus or nucleus pulposus. Restoration of disc cell function and prevention of degeneration remains the ultimate goal of current intervertebral disc research.

6.6 Summary of Critical Concepts Discussed in the Chapter

- The tissues of the intervertebral disc form a specialized niche which is avascular and hypoxic; the osmotic pressure within the niches is raised due to the high concentration of aggrecan and other proteoglycans.

- In the disc niche, nucleus pulposus activities are controlled by HIF and TonEBP, two major transcription factors.
- HIF-α stability in the nucleus pulposus is primarily controlled by oxygen-independent pathways. PHD2 plays a limited role in HIF-1α turnover, while HIF-2α turnover is refractory to prolyl hydroxylation.
- Nucleus pulposus cells are obligate glycolytic and require HIF-1 for energy generation.
- Hypoxia, HIF, and other hypoxia-sensitive protein play an important role in maintenance of cell survival activities in the disc.
- In the hyperosmolar and mechanically stressed environment of the disc, both nucleus pulpous and annulus fibrosus cells robustly express TonEBP protein which is critical for the maintenance of cell survival.
- Osmolarity and other niche factors such as hypoxia, TGF-β family proteins, and Ca^{2+} control TonEBP expression and activity in the nucleus pulposus.
- Homeostatic maintenance of proteoglycan-rich matrix in the intervertebral disc is TonEBP and HIF dependent.
- Niche factors acting through the notch pathway may promote disc cell proliferation and differentiation.

Acknowledgements This work is supported by grants AR050087 and AR055655 from the National Institutes of Health (NIAMS). The authors wish to thank Dr. Ernestina Schipani for the use of the images of the 5XHRE reporter mouse (Fig. 6.1).

References

Agrawal A, Guttapalli A, Narayan S, Albert TJ, Shapiro IM, Risbud MV (2007) Normoxic stabilization of HIF-1alpha drives glycolytic metabolism and regulates aggrecan gene expression in nucleus pulposus cells of the rat intervertebral disk. Am J Physiol Cell Physiol 293:C621–C631

Agrawal A, Gajghate S, Smith H, Anderson DG, Albert TJ, Shapiro IM et al (2008) Cited2 modulates hypoxia-inducible factor-dependent expression of vascular endothelial growth factor in nucleus pulposus cells of the rat intervertebral disc. Arthritis Rheum 58:3798–808

Alford AI, Yellowley CE, Jacobs CR, Donahue HJ (2003) Increases in cytosolic calcium, but not fluid flow, affect aggrecan mRNA levels in articular chondrocytes. J Cell Biochem 90:938–944

Appelhoff RJ, Tian YM, Raval RR, Turley H, Harris AL, Pugh CW et al (2004) Differential function of the prolyl hydroxylases PHD1, PHD2, and PHD3 in the regulation of hypoxia-inducible factor. J Biol Chem 279:38458–38465

Aprelikova O, Wood M, Tackett S, Chandramouli GV, Barrett JC (2006) Role of ETS transcription factors in the hypoxia-inducible factor-2 target gene selection. Cancer Res 66:5641–5647

Bai X, Wei G, Sinha A, Esko JD (1999) Chinese hamster ovary cell mutants defective in glycosaminoglycan assembly and glucuronosyltransferase I. J Biol Chem 274:13017–13024

Bartels EM, Fairbank JC, Winlove CP, Urban JP (1998) Oxygen and lactate concentrations measured in vivo in the intervertebral discs of patients with scoliosis and back pain. Spine 23:1–7

Bibby SR, Jones DA, Ripley RM, Urban JP (2005) Metabolism of the intervertebral disc: effects of low levels of oxygen, glucose, and pH on rates of energy metabolism of bovine nucleus pulposus cells. Spine 30:487–496

Bohensky J, Shapiro IM, Leshinsky S, Terkhorn SP, Adams CS, Srinivas V (2007) HIF-1 regulation of chondrocyte apoptosis: induction of the autophagic pathway. Autophagy 3:207–214

Bohensky J, Terkhorn SP, Freeman TA, Adams CS, Garcia JA, Shapiro IM, Srinivas V (2009) Regulation of autophagy in human and murine cartilage: hypoxia-inducible factor 2 suppresses chondrocyte autophagy. Arthritis Rheum 60:1406–1415

D'Angelo G, Duplan E, Boyer N, Vigne P, Frelin C (2003) Hypoxia up-regulates prolyl hydroxylase activity: a feedback mechanism that limits HIF-1 responses during reoxygenation. J Biol Chem 278: 38183–38187

Duronio V (2008) The life of a cell: apoptosis regulation by the PI3K/PKB pathway. Biochem J 415:333–344

Engin F, Yao Z, Yang T, Zhou G, Bertin T, Jiang MM et al (2008) Dimorphic effects of notch signaling in bone homeostasis. Nat Med 14:299–305

Epstein AC, Gleadle JM, McNeill LA, Hewitson KS, O'Rourke J, Mole DR et al (2001) C. Elegans EGL-9 and mammalian homologs define a family of dioxygenases that regulate HIF by prolyl hydroxylation. Cell 107:43–54

Erwin WM, Ashman K, O'Donnel P, Inman RD (2006) Nucleus pulposus notochord cells secrete connective tissue growth factor and upregulate proteoglycan expression by intervertebral disc chondrocytes. Arthritis Rheum 54:3859–3867

Fagnen G, Phamantu NT, Bocquet J, Bonnamy PJ (1999) Inhibition of transmembrane calcium influx induces decrease in proteoglycan synthesis in immature rat sertoli cells. J Cell Biochem 76:322–331

Feng H, Danfelter M, Strömqvist B, Heinegård D (2006) Extracellular matrix in disc degeneration. J Bone Joint Surg Am 88:25–29

Feng G, Li L, Liu H, Song Y, Huang F, Tu C et al (2013) Hypoxia differentially regulates human nucleus pulposus and annulus fibrosus cell extracellular matrix production in 3D scaffolds. Osteoarthritis Cartilage 21:582–588.

Fu D, Lu M (2007) The structural basis of water permeation and proton exclusion in aquaporins. Mol Membr Biol 24:366–374

Fujita N, Imai J, Suzuki T, Yamada M, Ninomiya K, Miyamoto K et al (2008) Vascular endothelial growth factor-a is a survival factor for nucleus pulposus cells in the intervertebral disc. Biochem Biophys Res Commun 372:367–372

Fujita N, Chiba K, Shapiro IM, Risbud MV (2012a) HIF-1α and HIF-2α degradation is differentially regulated in nucleus pulposus cells of the intervertebral disc. J Bone Miner Res 27:401–412

Fujita N, Markova D, Anderson DG, Chiba K, Toyama Y, Shapiro IM et al (2012b) Expression of prolyl hydroxylases (PHDs) is selectively controlled by HIF-1 and HIF-2 proteins in nucleus pulposus cells of the intervertebral disc: distinct roles of PHD2 and PHD3 proteins in controlling HIF-1α activity in hypoxia. J Biol Chem 287:16975–16986

Fujita N, Gogate SS, Chiba K, Toyama Y, Shapiro IM, Risbud MV (2012c) Prolyl hydroxylase 3 (PHD3) modulates catabolic effects of tumor necrosis factor-α (TNF-α) on cells of the nucleus pulposus through co-activation of nuclear factor κB (NF-κB)/p65 signaling. J Biol Chem 287:39942–39953

Fukuda R, Zhang H, Kim JW, Shimoda L, Dang CV, Semenza GL (2007) HIF-1 regulates cytochrome oxidase subunits to optimize efficiency of respiration in hypoxic cells. Cell 129:111–122

Gajghate S, Hiyama A, Shah M, Sakai D, Anderson DG, Shapiro IM et al (2009) Osmolarity and intracellular calcium regulate aquaporin2 expression through TonEBP in nucleus pulposus cells of the intervertebral disc. J Bone Miner Res 24:992–1001

Gakh O, Park S, Liu G, Macomber L, Imlay JA, Ferreira GC et al (2006) Mitochondrial iron detoxification is a primary function of frataxin that limits oxidative damage and preserves cell longevity. Hum Mol Genet 15:467–479

Gan JC, Ducheyne P, Vresilovic EJ, Swaim W, Shapiro IM (2003) Intervertebral disc tissue engineering I: characterization of the nucleus pulposus. Clin Orthop Relat Res 411:305–314

Go WY, Liu X, Roti MA, Liu F, Ho SN (2004) NFAT5/TonEBP mutant mice define osmotic stress as a critical feature of the lymphoid microenvironment. Proc Natl Acad Sci U S A 101:10673–10678

Gogate SS, Nasser R, Shapiro IM, Risbud MV (2011) Hypoxic regulation of β-1,3-glucuronyltransferase I expression in nucleus pulposus cells of the rat intervertebral disc: role of hypoxia-inducible factor proteins. Arthritis Rheum 63:1950–1960

Gogate SS, Fujita N, Skubutyte R, Shapiro IM, Risbud MV (2012) Tonicity enhancer binding protein (TonEBP) and hypoxia-inducible factor (HIF) coordinate heat shock protein 70 (Hsp70) expression in hypoxic nucleus pulposus cells: role of Hsp70 in HIF-1α degradation. J Bone Miner Res 27:1106–1117

Gouze JN, Bordji K, Gulberti S, Terlain B, Netter P, Magdalou J et al (2001) Interleukin-1 beta down-regulates the expression of glucuronosyltransferase I, a key enzyme priming glycosaminoglycan biosynthesis: influence of glucosamine on interleukin-1beta-mediated effects in rat chondrocytes. Arthritis Rheum 44:351–360

Gruber HE, Ashraf N, Kilburn J, Williams C, Norton HJ, Gordon BE et al (2005) Vertebral endplate architecture and vascularization: application of micro-computerized tomography, a vascular tracer, and immunocytochemistry in analyses of disc degeneration in the aging sand rat. Spine 30:2593–2600

Gustafsson MV, Zheng X, Pereira T, Gradin K, Jin S, Lundkvist J et al (2005) Hypoxia requires notch signaling to maintain the undifferentiated cell state. Dev Cell 9:617–628

Ha KY, Koh IJ, Kirpalani PA, Kim YY, Cho YK, Khang GS et al (2006) The expression of hypoxia inducible factor-1alpha and apoptosis in herniated discs. Spine 31:1309–1313

Hall AC, Bush PG (2001) The role of a swelling-activated taurine transport pathway in the regulation of articular chondrocyte volume. Pflugers Arch 442:771–781

Halterman JA, Kwon HM, Zargham R, Bortz PD, Wamhoff BR (2011) Nuclear factor of activated T cells 5 regulates vascular smooth muscle cell phenotypic modulation. Arterioscler Thromb Vasc Biol 31:2287–2296

Hasler U, Jeon US, Kim JA, Mordasini D, Kwon HM, Féraille E et al (2006) Tonicity-responsive enhancer binding protein is an essential regulator of aquaporin-2 expression in renal collecting duct principal cells. J Am Soc Nephrol 17:1521–1531

Hassler O (1969) The human intervertebral disc. A micro-angiographical study on its vascular supply at various ages. Acta Orthop Scand 40:765–772

Henze AT, Riedel J, Diem T, Wenner J, Flamme I, Pouyseggur J et al (2010) Prolyl hydroxylases 2 and 3 act in gliomas as protective negative feedback regulators of hypoxia-inducible factors. Cancer Res 70:357–366

Higgins DF, Biju MP, Akai Y, Wutz A, Johnson RS, Haase VH (2004) Hypoxic induction of ctgf is directly mediated by Hif-1. Am J Physiol Renal Physiol 287:F1223–F1232

Hilton MJ, Tu X, Wu X, Bai S, Zhao H, Kobayashi T et al (2008) Notch signaling maintains bone marrow mesenchymal progenitors by suppressing osteoblast differentiation. Nat Med 14:306–314

Hiyama A, Gajghate S, Sakai D, Mochida J, Shapiro IM, Risbud MV (2009) Activation of TonEBP by calcium controls β1,3-glucuronosyltransferase-I expression, a key regulator of glycosaminoglycan synthesis in cells of the intervertebral disc. J Biol Chem 284: 9824–9834

Hiyama A, Gogate SS, Gajghate S, Mochida J, Shapiro IM, Risbud MV (2010) BMP-2 and TGF-beta stimulate expression of beta1,3-glucuronosyl transferase 1 (GlcAT-1) in nucleus pulposus cells through AP1, TonEBP, and Sp1: role of MAPKs. J Bone Miner Res 25:1179–1190

Hiyama A, Skubutyte R, Markova D, Anderson DG, Yadla S, Sakai D et al (2011) Hypoxia activates the notch signaling pathway in cells of the intervertebral disc: implications in degenerative disc disease. Arthritis Rheum 63:1355–1364

Hofbauer KH, Gess B, Lohaus C, Meyer HE, Katschinski D, Kurtz A (2003) Oxygen tension regulates the expression of a group of procollagen hydroxylases. Eur J Biochem 270:4515–4522

Holm S, Maroudas A, Urban JP, Selstam G, Nachemson A (1981) Nutrition of the intervertebral disc: solute transport and metabolism. Connect Tissue Res 8:101–119

Hong K, Yoo S, Kang S, Choi J, Kim W, Cho C (2006) Hypoxia induces expression of connective tissue growth factor in scleroderma skin fibroblasts. Clin Exp Immunol 146:362–370

Ishihara H, Warensjo K, Roberts S, Urban JP (1997) Proteoglycan synthesis in the intervertebral disk nucleus: the role of extracellular osmolality. Am J Physiol 272:C1499–C1506

Ito T, Fujio Y, Hirata M, Takatani T, Matsuda T, Muraoka S et al (2004) Expression of taurine transporter is regulated through the TonE (tonicity-responsive element)/TonEBP (TonE-binding protein) pathway and contributes to cytoprotection in HepG2 cells. Biochem J 382:177–182

Jauliac S, Lopez-Rodriguez C, Shaw LM, Brown LF, Rao A, Toker A (2002) The role of NFAT transcription factors in integrin-mediated carcinoma invasion. Nat Cell Biol 4:540–544

Jeon US, Kim JA, Sheen MR, Kwon HM (2006) How tonicity regulates genes: story of TonEBP transcriptional activator. Acta Physiol (Oxf) 187:241–247

Jiang L, Zhang X, Zheng X, Ru A, Ni X, Wu Y et al (2012) Apoptosis, senescence, and autophagy in rat nucleus pulposus cells: implications for diabetic intervertebral disc degeneration. J Orthop Res. doi:10.1002/jor.22289

José-Edwards DS, Kerner P, Kugler JE, Deng W, Jiang D, Di Gregorio A (2011) The identification of transcription factors expressed in the notochord of Ciona intestinalis adds new potential players to the brachyury gene regulatory network. Dev Dyn 240:1793–1805

Kanichai M, Ferguson D, Prendergast PJ, Campbell VA (2008) Hypoxia promotes chondrogenesis in rat mesenchymal stem cells: a role for AKT and hypoxia-inducible factor (HIF)-1alpha. J Cell Physiol 216:708–715

Khan WS, Adesida AB, Hardingham TE (2007) Hypoxic conditions increase hypoxia-inducible transcription factor 2alpha and enhance chondrogenesis in stem cells from the infrapatellar fat pad of osteoarthritis patients. Arthritis Res Ther 9:R55

Kitagawa H, Ujikawa M, Sugahara K (1996) Developmental changes in serum UDP-GlcA:chondroitin glucuronyltransferase activity. J Biol Chem 271:6583–6585

Ko BC, Ruepp B, Bohren KM, Gabbay KH, Chung SS (1997) Identification and characterization of multiple osmotic response sequences in the human aldose reductase gene. J Biol Chem 272:16431–16437

Köditz J, Nesper J, Wottawa M, Stiehl DP, Camenisch G, Franke C et al (2007) Oxygen-dependent ATF-4 stability is mediated by the PHD3 oxygen sensor. Blood 110:3610–3617

Kokubo Y, Uchida K, Kobayashi S, Yayama T, Sato R, Nakajima H et al (2008) Herniated and spondylotic intervertebral discs of the human cervical spine: histological and immunohistological findings in 500 en bloc surgical samples. Laboratory investigation. J Neurosurg Spine 9:285–295

Kondo S, Kubota S, Mukudai Y, Moritani N, Nishida T, Matsushita H et al (2006) Hypoxic regulation of stability of connective tissue growth factor/CCN2 mRNA by 3′-untranslated region interacting with a cellular protein in human chondrosarcoma cells. Oncogene 25:1099–1110

Lafont JE, Talma S, Murphy CL (2007) Hypoxia-inducible factor 2alpha is essential for hypoxic induction of the human articular chondrocyte phenotype. Arthritis Rheum 56:3297–3306

Lam AK, Ko BC, Tam S, Morris R, Yang JY, Chung SK et al (2004) Osmotic response element-binding protein (OREBP) is an essential regulator of the urine concentrating mechanism. J Biol Chem 279:48048–48054

Lee DC, Adams CS, Albert TJ, Shapiro IM, Evans SM, Koch CJ (2007) In situ oxygen utilization in the rat intervertebral disc. J Anat 210:294–303

Li SZ, McDill BW, Kovach PA, Ding L, Go WY, Ho SN et al (2007) Calcineurin-NFATc signaling pathway regulates AQP2 expression in response to calcium signals and osmotic stress. Am J Physiol Cell Physiol 292:C1606–C1616

Lopez-Rodríguez C, Aramburu J, Rakeman AS, Rao A (1999) NFAT5, A constitutively nuclear NFAT protein that does not cooperate with Fos and Jun. Proc Natl Acad Sci U S A 96:7214–7219

Lopez-Rodriguez C, Antos CL, Shelton JM, Richardson JA, Lin F, Novobrantseva TI et al (2004) Loss of NFAT5 results in renal atrophy and lack of tonicity-responsive gene expression. Proc Natl Acad Sci U S A 101:2392–2397

Luo W, Hu H, Chang R, Zhong J, Knabel M, O'Meally R et al (2011) Pyruvate kinase M2 is a PHD3-stimulated coactivator for hypoxia-inducible factor 1. Cell 145:732–744

Maouyo D, Kim JY, Lee SD, Wu Y, Woo SK, Kwon HM (2002) Mouse TonEBP-NFAT5: expression in early development and alternative splicing. Am J Physiol 282:F802–F809

Marxsen JH, Stengel P, Doege K, Heikkinen P, Jokilehto T, Wagner T et al (2004) Hypoxia-inducible factor-1 (HIF-1) promotes its degradation by induction of HIF-alpha-prolyl-4-hydroxylases. Biochem J 381:761–767

Maxwell PH, Wiesener MS, Chang GW, Clifford SC, Vaux EC, Cockman ME et al (1999) The tumour suppressor protein VHL targets hypoxia-inducible factors for oxygen-dependent proteolysis. Nature 399:271–275

Minamishima YA, Moslehi J, Bardeesy N, Cullen D, Bronson RT, Kaelin WG (2008) Somatic inactivation of the PHD2 prolyl hydroxylase causes polycythemia and congestive heart failure. Blood 111:3236–3244

Miyakawa H, Woo SK, Chen CP, Dahl SC, Handler JS, Kwon HM (1998) Cis- and trans-acting factors regulating transcription of the BGT1 gene in response to hypertonicity. Am J Physiol 274:F753–F761

Miyakawa H, Woo SK, Dahl SC, Handler JS, Kwon HM (1999) Tonicity-responsive enhancer binding protein, a rel-like protein that stimulates transcription in response to hypertonicity. Proc Natl Acad Sci U S A 96:2538–2542

Murakami U, Kameyama Y (1963) Vertebral malformation in the mouse foetus caused by maternal hypoxia during early stage of pregnancy. J Embryol Exp Morphol 11:107–118

Mwale F, Ciobanu I, Giannitsios D, Roughley P, Steffen T, Antoniou J (2011) Effect of oxygen levels on proteoglycan synthesis by intervertebral disc cells. Spine (Phila Pa 1976) 36:E131–E138

Nerlich AG, Schaaf R, Wälchli B, Boos N (2007) Temporo-spatial distribution of blood vessels in human lumbar intervertebral discs. Eur Spine J 16:547–555

Ng L, Grodzinsky AJ, Patwari P, Sandy J, Plaas A, Ortiz C (2003) Individual cartilage aggrecan macromolecules and their constituent glycosaminoglycans visualized via atomic force microscopy. J Struct Biol 143:242–257

Oka N, Nakahara S, Takenaka Y, Fukumori T, Hogan V, Kanayama HO et al (2005) Galectin-3 inhibits tumor necrosis factor-related apoptosis-inducing ligand-induced apoptosis by activating Akt in human bladder carcinoma cells. Cancer Res 65:7546–7553

Oktay Y, Dioum E, Matsuzaki S, Ding K, Yan LJ, Haller RG et al (2007) Hypoxia-inducible factor 2 alpha regulates expression of the mitochondrial aconitase chaperone protein frataxin. J Biol Chem 282:11750–11756

Papandreou I, Cairns RA, Fontana L, Lim AL, Denko NC (2006) HIF-1 mediates adaptation to hypoxia by actively downregulating mitochondrial oxygen consumption. Cell Metab 3:187–197

Parvizi J, Parpura V, Greenleaf JF, Bolander ME (2002) Calcium signaling is required for ultrasound-stimulated aggrecan synthesis by rat chondrocytes. J Orthop Res 20:51–57

Pfander D, Cramer T, Schipani E, Johnson RS (2003) HIF-1alpha controls extracellular matrix synthesis by epiphyseal chondrocytes. J Cell Sci 116:1819–1826

Pritchard S, Erickson GR, Guilak F (2002) Hyperosmotically induced volume change and calcium signaling in intervertebral disk cells: the role of the actin cytoskeleton. Biophys J 83:2502–2510

Rajpurohit R, Risbud MV, Ducheyne P, Vresilovic EJ, Shapiro IM (2002) Phenotypic characteristics of the nucleus pulposus: expression of hypoxia inducing factor-1, glucose transporter-1 and MMP-2. Cell Tissue Res 308:401–407

Rathmell JC, Fox CJ, Plas DR, Hammerman PS, Cinalli RM, Thompson CB (2003) Akt-directed glucose metabolism can prevent Bax conformation change and promote growth factor-independent survival. Mol Cell Biol 23:7315–7328

Richardson SM, Knowles R, Tyler J, Mobasheri A, Hoyland JA (2008) Expression of glucose transporters GLUT-1, GLUT-3, GLUT-9 and HIF-1alpha in normal and degenerate human intervertebral disc. Histochem Cell Biol 129:503–511

Rim JS, Atta MG, Dahl SC, Berry GT, Handler JS (1998) Kwon HM (1998) transcription of the sodium/myo-inositol cotransporter gene is regulated by multiple tonicity-responsive enhancers spread over 50 kilobase pairs in the 5′-flanking region. J Biol Chem 273: 20615–20621

Risbud MV, Fertala J, Vresilovic EJ, Albert TJ, Shapiro IM (2005a) Nucleus pulposus cells upregulate PI3K/Akt and MEK/ERK signaling pathways under hypoxic conditions and resist apoptosis induced by serum withdrawal. Spine 30:882–889

Risbud MV, Guttapalli A, Albert TJ, Shapiro IM (2005b) Hypoxia activates MAPK activity in rat nucleus pulposus cells: regulation of integrin expression and cell survival. Spine 30:2503–2509

Risbud MV, Guttapalli A, Stokes DG, Hawkins D, Danielson KG, Schaer TP et al (2006a) Nucleus pulposus cells express HIF-1alpha under normoxic culture conditions: a metabolic adaptation to the intervertebral disc microenvironment. J Cell Biochem 98:152–159

Risbud MV, Di Martino A, Guttapalli A, Seghatoleslami R, Denaro V, Vaccaro AR et al (2006b) Toward an optimum system for intervertebral disc organ culture: TGF-beta 3 enhances nucleus pulposus and annulus fibrosus survival and function through modulation of TGF-beta-R expression and ERK signaling. Spine 31:884–890

Risbud MV, Guttapalli A, Tsai TT, Lee JY, Danielson KG, Vaccaro AR et al (2007) Evidence for skeletal progenitor cells in the degenerate human intervertebral disc. Spine 32:2537–2544

Risbud MV, Schipani E, Shapiro IM (2010) Hypoxic regulation of nucleus pulposus cell survival: from niche to notch. Am J Pathol 176:1577–1583

Roberts S, Evans H, Trivedi J, Menage J (2006) Histology and pathology of the human intervertebral disc. J Bone Joint Surg Am 88: 10–14

Rudert M, Tillmann B (1993) Lymph and blood supply of the human intervertebral disc. Cadaver study of correlations to discitis. Acta Orthop Scand 64:37–40

Sakai D, Nakamura Y, Nakai T, Mishima T, Kato S, Grad S et al (2012) Exhaustion of nucleus pulposus progenitor cells with ageing and degeneration of the intervertebral disc. Nat Commun 3:1264. doi:10.1038/ncomms2226

Sasaki T, Brakebusch C, Engel J, Timpl R (1998) Mac-2 binding protein is a cell-adhesive protein of the extracellular matrix which self-assembles into ring-like structures and binds beta1 integrins, collagens and fibronectin. EMBO J 17:1606–1613

Schipani E, Ryan HE, Didrickson S, Kobayashi T, Knight M, Johnson RS (2001) Hypoxia in cartilage: HIF-1 alpha is essential for chondrocyte growth arrest and survival. Genes Dev 15:2865–2876

Scortegagna M, Ding K, Oktay Y, Gaur A, Thurmond F, Yan LJ et al (2003) Multiple organ pathology, metabolic abnormalities and impaired homeostasis of reactive oxygen species in Epas1–/– mice. Nat Genet 35:331–340

Semenza GL, Roth PH, Fang HM, Wang GL (1994) Transcriptional regulation of genes encoding glycolytic enzymes by hypoxia-inducible factor 1. J Biol Chem 269:23757–23763

Setton LA, Chen J (2006) Mechanobiology of the intervertebral disc and relevance to disc degeneration. J Bone Joint Surg Am 88:52–57

Shapiro IM, Vresilovic EJ, Risbud MV (2012) Is the spinal motion segment a diarthrodial polyaxial joint: what a nice nucleus like you doing in a joint like this? Bone 50:771–776

Shim EH, Kim JI, Bang ES, Heo JS, Lee JS, Kim EY et al (2002) Targeted disruption of hsp70.1 Sensitizes to osmotic stress. EMBO Rep 3:857–861

Smits P, Lefebvre V (2003) Sox5 and Sox6 are required for notochord extracellular matrix sheath formation, notochord cell survival and development of the nucleus pulposus of intervertebral discs. Development 130:1135–1148

Sowter HM, Raval RR, Moore JW, Ratcliffe PJ, Harris AL (2003) Predominant role of hypoxia-inducible transcription factor (Hif)-1 alpha versus Hif-2 alpha in regulation of the transcriptional response to hypoxia. Cancer Res 63:6130–6134

Sparrow DB, Chapman G, Smith AJ, Mattar MZ, Major JA, O'Reilly VC et al (2012) A mechanism for gene-environment interaction in the etiology of congenital scoliosis. Cell 149:295–306

Srinivas V, Bohensky J, Zahm AM, Shapiro IM (2009) Autophagy in mineralizing tissues: microenvironmental perspectives. Cell Cycle 8:391–393

Takeda K, Ho VC, Takeda H, Duan LJ, Nagy A, Fong GH (2006) Placental but not heart defects are associated with elevated hypoxia-inducible factor alpha levels in mice lacking prolyl hydroxylase domain protein 2. Mol Cell Biol 26:8336–8346

Thoms BL, Murphy CL (2010) Inhibition of hypoxia-inducible factor-targeting prolyl hydroxylase domain-containing protein 2 (PHD2) enhances matrix synthesis by human chondrocytes. J Biol Chem 285:20472–20480

Trama J, Lu Q, Hawley RG, Ho SN (2000) The NFAT-related protein NFATL1 (TonEBP/NFAT5) is induced upon T cell activation in a calcineurin-dependent manner. J Immunol 165:4884–4894

Tran CM, Markova D, Smith HE, Susarla B, Ponnappan RK, Anderson DG et al (2010) Regulation of CCN2/CTGF expression in the nucleus pulposus of the intervertebral disc: role of smad and AP1 signaling. Arthritis Rheum 62:1983–1992

Tran CM, Fujita N, Huang BL, Ong J, Lyons KM, Shapiro IM et al (2013) HIF-1α and CCN2 form a regulatory circuit in hypoxic nucleus pulposus cells: CCN2 suppresses HIF-1α level and transcriptional activity. J Biol Chem 288:12654–12666

Tsai TT, Danielson KG, Guttapalli A, Oguz E, Albert TJ, Shapiro IM et al (2006) TonEBP/OREBP is a regulator of nucleus pulposus cell function and survival in the intervertebral disc. J Biol Chem 281:25416–25424

Tsai TT, Guttapalli A, Agrawal A, Albert TJ, Shapiro IM, Risbud MV (2007) MEK/ERK signaling controls osmoregulation of nucleus pulposus cells of the intervertebral disc by transactivation of TonEBP/OREBP. J Bone Miner Res 22:965–974

Urban JP, Maroudas A (1981) Swelling of the intervertebral disc in vitro. Connect Tissue Res 9:1–10

Urban JP, Holm S, Maroudas A, Nachemson A (1977) Nutrition of the intervertebral disk. An in vivo study of solute transport. Clin Orthop Relat Res 129:101–114

Venkatesan N, Barré L, Benani A, Netter P, Magdalou J, Fournel-Gigleux S et al (2004) Stimulation of proteoglycan synthesis by glucuronosyltransferase-I gene delivery: a strategy to promote cartilage repair. Proc Natl Acad Sci U S A 101:18087–18092

Verkman AS (2006) Roles of aquaporins in kidney revealed by transgenic mice. Semin Nephrol 26:200–208

Vijayagopal P, Subramaniam P (2001) Effect of calcium channel blockers on proteoglycan synthesis by vascular smooth muscle cells and low density lipoprotein–proteoglycan interaction. Atherosclerosis 157:353–360

Wang GL, Jiang BH, Rue EA, Semenza GL (1995) Hypoxia-inducible factor 1 is a basic-helix-loop-helix-PAS heterodimer regulated by cellular O2 tension. Proc Natl Acad Sci U S A 92:5510–5514

Wang Y, Ko BC, Yang JY, Lam TT, Jiang Z, Zhang J et al (2005) Transgenic mice expressing dominant-negative osmotic-response element-binding protein (OREBP) in lens exhibit fiber cell elongation defect associated with increased DNA breaks. J Biol Chem 280:19986–19991

Woo SK, Lee SD, Na KY, Park WK, Kwon HM (2002) TonEBP/NFAT5 stimulates transcription of HSP70 in response to hypertonicity. Mol Cell Biol 22:5753–5760

Wuertz K, Urban JP, Klasen J, Ignatius A, Wilke HJ, Claes L et al (2007) Influence of extracellular osmolarity and mechanical stimulation on gene expression of intervertebral disc cells. J Orthop Res 25:1513–1522

Ye W, Xu K, Huang D, Liang A, Peng Y, Zhu W et al (2011) Age-related increases of macroautophagy and chaperone-mediated autophagy in rat nucleus pulposus. Connect Tissue Res 52:472–478

Zelzer E, Mamluk R, Ferrara N, Johnson RS, Schipani E, Olsen BR (2004) VEGFA is necessary for chondrocyte survival during bone development. Development 131:2161–2171

Zeng Y, Danielson KG, Albert TJ, Shapiro IM, Risbud MV (2007) HIF-1 alpha is a regulator of galectin-3 expression in the intervertebral disc. J Bone Miner Res 22:1851–1861

Zhang Z, Ferraris JD, Brooks HL, Brisc I, Burg MB (2003) Expression of osmotic stress-related genes in tissues of normal and hyposmotic rats. Am J Physiol 285:F688–F693

Zhang H, Bosch-Marce M, Shimoda LA, Tan YS, Baek JH, Wesley JB et al (2008) Mitochondrial autophagy is an HIF-1-dependent adaptive metabolic response to hypoxia. J Biol Chem 283:10892–10903

The Effects of Mechanical Forces on Nucleus Pulposus and Annulus Fibrosus Cells

7

Jeffrey C. Lotz and Adam H. Hsieh

Contents

J.C. Lotz (✉)
Orthopaedic Bioengineering Laboratory, Department of Orthopaedic Surgery, University of California, San Francisco, 513 Parnassus Ave, 11th Floor, S1157, San Francisco, CA 94143-0514, USA
e-mail: jeffrey.lotz@ucsf.edu

A.H. Hsieh
Orthopaedic Mechanobiology Laboratory, Fischell Department of Bioengineering, University of Maryland, College Park, Jeong H. Kim Engineering Building, Rm 3242, College Park, MD 20742, USA
e-mail: hsieh@umd.edu

I.M. Shapiro, M.V. Risbud (eds.), *The Intervertebral Disc*,
DOI 10.1007/978-3-7091-1535-0_7, © Springer-Verlag Wien 2014

7.1 Introduction

The relationship between mechanical loading and intervertebral disc health and disease has long been recognized (Panel on Musculoskeletal Disorders and the Workplace 2001). While it is well established that mechanical factors can significantly influence cell function (Nelson et al. 2005; Hoffman and Crocker 2009), how this process influences nucleus pulposus and annulus fibrosus activity in the intervertebral disc is complex and confounded by multiple, hierarchical mechanisms by which load affects the human body. At the whole-body level, spinal forces depend on body mass, external loads, posture, muscle function, and body resonant frequencies. At the organ level, disc loads vary with duration, spinal level, and posture. At the tissue level, stress and strains are heterogeneously distributed within the disc in a time-dependent manner. Ultimately, disc cells convert local physical cues into biochemical signals and integrate these into cellular responses. Adding further complexity is the fact that local cellular responses influence the entire spinal system by modifying disc material properties (thereby altering organ-level behaviors) or triggering pain (thereby altering muscle function and whole-body mechanics). This chapter dissects this highly complex process and identifies patterns in disc mechanobiology at various levels of scale, disc regions, and cell types. Clarification of these relationships is relevant to understanding disease mechanisms and for developing treatments for patients with spinal pathology.

7.2 Organ and Tissue Levels

Discussion of mechanotransduction by nucleus pulposus and annulus fibrosus cells must begin at the level of the functional spinal unit, since the transmission of loads through the spinal column dictates the magnitude and types of intervertebral disc stress. At each spinal level, loads are shared between the intervertebral disc anteriorly and the

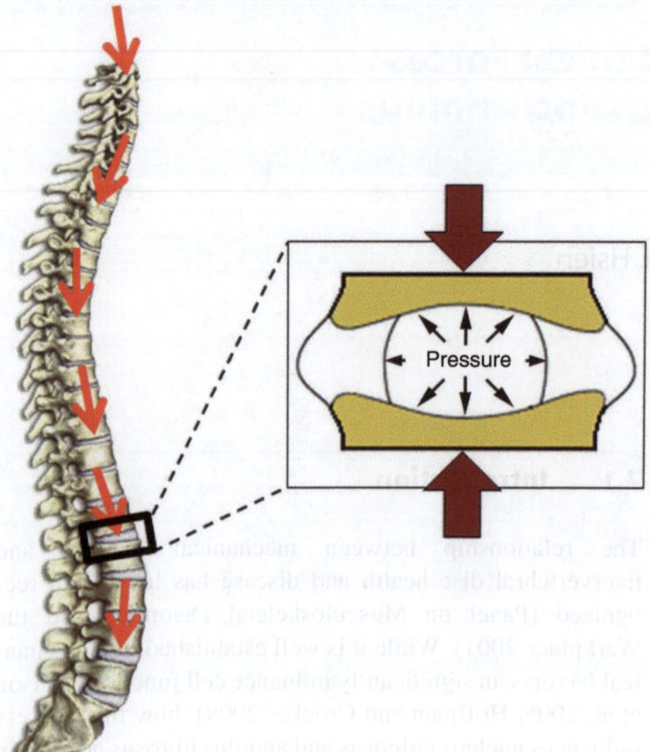

Fig. 7.1 Static loading of the spine under a follower load configuration, resulting in a primarily axial compression of the intervertebral disc

two facet joints posteriorly. Generally speaking, the disc's principal mechanical role is to support compressive forces, while the facets resist shear and guide segmental rotations during spinal movements (Shirazi-Adl and Drouin 1987). Disc/facet interactions vary between the multiple spinal levels as the biomechanical behaviors change from the cervical (high rotation/low compression) to lumbar (low rotation/high compression) regions. Proper biomechanical synergy between the disc and facets is lost when degeneration reduces disc height and compliance (Niosi and Oxland 2004). The disc performs its mechanical function by synergistic interactions between the hydrophilic nucleus pulposus, fibrous annulus fibrosus, and cartilage/bone composite vertebral end plate. Each disc sub-tissue has a different composition of cells, matrix fibers (collagen, elastin, reticular), and ground substance (glycosaminoglycans (GAG), proteoglycans, glycoproteins) that define signature physical properties uniquely adapted for a specific role. Spinal loading is spatially filtered into regions of hydrostatic pressure and octahedral shear that correlate with variations in cell phenotype and extracellular matrix composition, consistent with current theories of tissue adaptation and homeostasis (Carter and Beaupre 2001). These interdependent functions are specified at development and regulated during growth (Hayes et al. 2001) and when disrupted can lead to degeneration and disease (Urban et al. 2000). As such, the disc represents a uniquely complex organ of the musculoskeletal system.

Based on how forces are distributed from organ to tissue levels, several mechanotransduction themes have emerged from the growing body of literature. The first is that the magnitude and distribution of loads within the nucleus pulposus and annulus fibrosus govern disc cell function. The second is that load frequency and duration significantly contribute to the disc's mechanical and mechanobiologic response. And the third is that age-related matrix changes may set off a vicious cycle of degeneration-promoting processes. In this section, we will examine the evidence that support these concepts.

Given the disc's complex matrix structure, mechanobiologic interactions are influenced at multiple hierarchical levels. Within each disc sub-tissue, a unique combination of extracellular matrix fibers and ground substance confer different physical properties, where the extracellular matrix molecules are adapted to manage and respond to mechanical stress. Consequently, the extracellular matrix physical properties are dynamic and regulated, and create a microenvironment that presents cells with physical and biochemical cues that are important for maintenance of a healthy tissue. Cues include chemical (hypoxia, pH), biochemical (growth factors, cytokines, neurotrophins, hormones), and physical (topography, fluid flow, stiffness) factors.

7.2.1 Physiologic Interplay in Mechanical Function in the Nucleus Pulposus and Annulus Fibrosus Is Critical for Tissue Homeostasis

Intervertebral disc loading depends on an individual's size, physical activity level, occupational demands, and degree of rest. In the human, spinal stability requires that the direction of the resultant force vectors at each vertebra passes through the centers of rotation of adjacent motion segments in the sagittal plane, a concept called follower load path (Patwardhan et al. 1999). The follower load strategy allows the spine to support static loads up to and significantly above typical physical demands (Patwardhan et al. 2000), without markedly sacrificing flexibility or range of motion (Rohlmann et al. 2001; Patwardhan et al. 2003). This suggests that during static conditions muscle activation patterns in vivo cause the disc to be primarily loaded in axial compression (Fig. 7.1), a loading mode that has been extensively studied in animal models.

In the healthy spine, the intervertebral disc responds to axial compression by nucleus pulposus pressurization facilitated by lateral annulus fibrosus constraint, which in turn generates circumferential and longitudinal annulus fibrosus tension. Preservation of this structural interrelationship is important for tissue maintenance. This is perhaps most clearly demonstrated in static compression of rodent discs. In such experiments, static loads induce fluid shifts that deplete nucleus pulposus volume, causing the annulus fibrosus to function more as a compression-bearing strut than a biaxially stretched membrane (Lotz et al. 1998). As fluid is expelled from the nucleus, the matrix and cells consolidate (Lotz 2004; Hsieh et al. 2005), ultimately leading to deregulated gene expression (Lotz et al. 1998), increased metalloproteinase (MMP) activation (Hsieh and Lotz 2003), and apoptosis (Chin et al. 1999; Lotz and Chin 2000). In both mice (Lotz et al. 1998) and rats (Iatridis et al. 1999), these cellular effects alter disc architecture and mechanics.

In contrast, beneficial effects of nucleus pulposus pressurization and annulus fibrosus tension are observed when the disc is subjected to cyclic loading. Low load magnitudes are most amenable to maintaining homeostatic stress environments in the nucleus pulposus and annulus fibrosus over extended loading durations. For example, under low cyclic loads comparable to normal activities, nucleus pulposus cells exhibit little alteration in expression of genes that would lead to matrix remodeling, regardless of loading frequency (Maclean et al. 2004). Similarly, annulus fibrosus cells undergo a low level of apoptosis and exhibit depressed expression of certain catabolic factors such as MMPs and ADAMTSs (Maclean et al. 2004; Walsh and Lotz 2004). High magnitudes of stress can be similarly accommodated for brief durations and frequencies, near 1 Hz. However, if applied at low frequency or long durations, high compression magnitudes lead to a shift in cell function and tissue morphology. Under these circumstances, nucleus pulposus cells respond via upregulation of genes associated with extracellular matrix remodeling (Maclean et al. 2004; MacLean et al. 2005; Wuertz et al. 2009), leading to decreases in disc height and mechanical stability (Ching et al. 2003, 2004). In the annulus fibrosus, lower loading frequencies also cause a shift in the balance of gene expression toward a more catabolic profile (Maclean et al. 2004).

Taken together, these studies demonstrate that physiologic load sharing between nucleus pulposus and annulus fibrosus (principally nucleus pulposus pressure and annulus fibrosus tension) promotes tissue homeostasis. This is underscored by experiments in which specific aspects of this interplay are selectively modulated. For instance, using mouse models, disc bending to induce tension and compression on opposing regions of the annulus stimulates apoptosis and altered gene expression only on the side of compression (Court et al. 2001, 2007). The restoration of annulus fibrosus tension has similarly been demonstrated to be potentially protective. Applying bending to discs that had previously been subjected to degeneration-inducing static compression was effective in preserving annulus fibrosus lamellar morphology, even though apoptosis could not be mitigated (Lotz et al. 2008). These effects can also be observed when needle stabs that reduce nucleus pulposus pressurization (and consequently annulus fibrosus tension) also trigger degenerative changes in the annulus with increased MMP-2 immunoreactivity, while those that are too small to affect disc pressurization do not (Rousseau et al. 2007; Hsieh et al. 2009; Rastogi et al. 2013).

7.2.2 Implications of Poroviscoelasticity in Nucleus Pulposus and Annulus Fibrosus Mechanobiology

Although the spine is dynamically loaded over the course of the day, trunk muscles stabilizing the spine generate resultant loads that subject discs to sustained, time-averaged compression. Due to the disc's poroviscoelastic nature, this sustained compression results in loss of stature, contributed in large part by decreases in spine length (Koeller et al. 1984; Leatt et al. 1986). Even low-impact activities, such as gentle walking, have been shown to decrease stature significantly (Hoe et al. 1994), although more strenuous exercise, work-related activities, and high body mass exacerbate this loss (Fig. 7.2, top) (Garbutt et al. 1990; McGill et al. 1996; Leivseth and Drerup 1997; Rodacki et al. 2005). These stature changes are primarily attributed to the redistribution of fluid as the applied stresses exceed the disc's swelling pressure (Adams and Hutton 1983; Koeller et al. 1984; Adams et al. 1990; Terahata et al. 1994; Ayotte et al. 2000; Hsieh et al. 2005; Schroeder et al. 2006).

As with other compressive load-bearing tissues such as articular cartilage, the disc's extracellular solid–fluid interactions define its viscoelastic behavior. Interstitial fluid in the hydrated extracellular matrix serves as a hydraulic cushion that helps distribute forces and absorb shock. Sustained intervertebral disc compression consolidates the disc extracellular matrix as there is an efflux of interstitial fluid and a decrease in water content (Fig. 7.2, bottom) (Adams et al. 1990). The importance of tissue hydration in intervertebral disc mechanics has been demonstrated in a number of studies that reveal a close relationship between hydration and disc mechanical properties (Bass et al. 1997; Pflaster et al. 1997; Race et al. 2000; Han et al. 2001; Costi et al. 2002). Of note, varying water content through load, by imposition of free swelling and creep compression boundary conditions, reveals the existence of an optimal hydration point at which the effective modulus reaches a peak value (Race et al. 2000). The principles behind this have not yet been elucidated, but likely involve both physical relationships among subregions, consolidation of the tissue, and transient solid–fluid interactions in the tissue. Nevertheless, these observations highlight the importance of water content in the disc's mechanical function.

Movement of moisture due to poroviscoelasticity is particularly relevant in nucleus pulposus mechanobiology. In human discs, the swelling properties of the nucleus

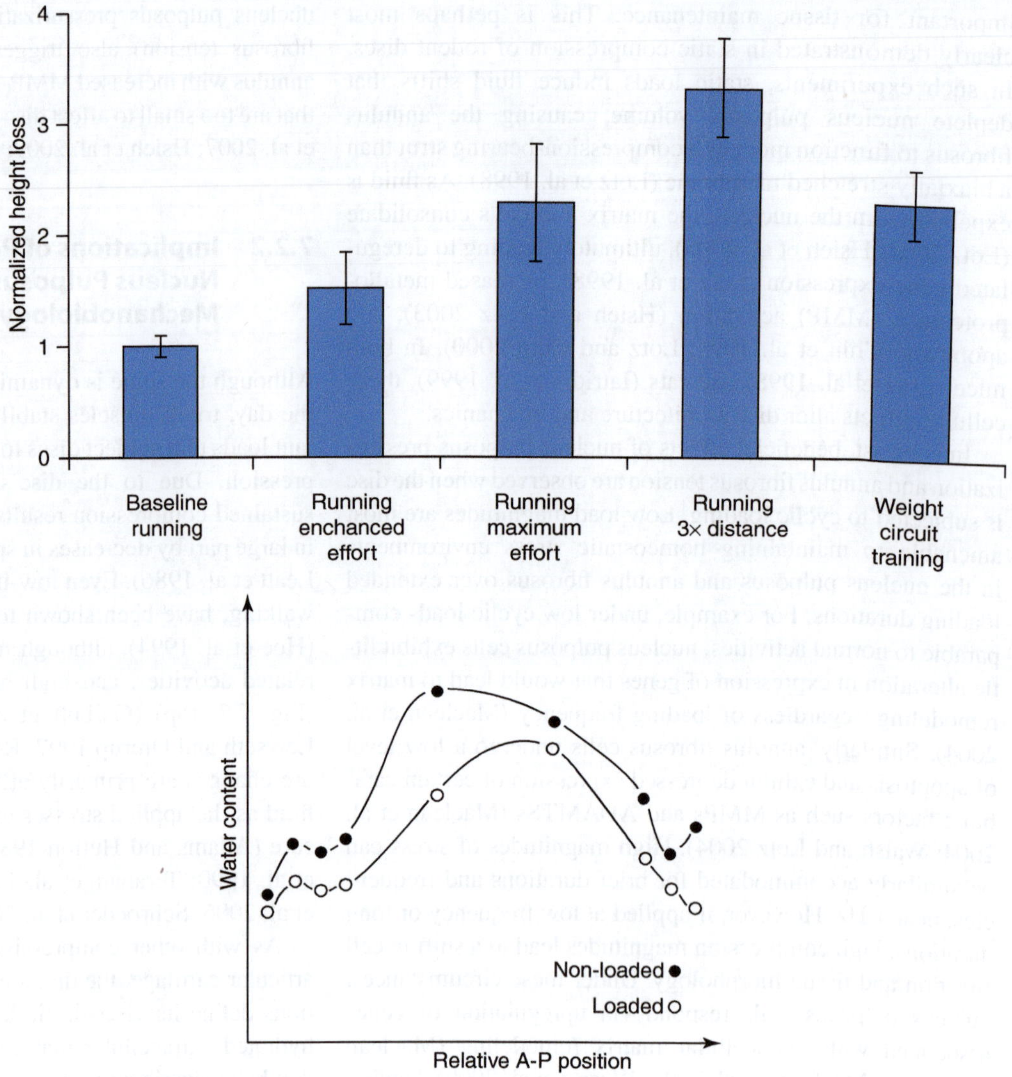

Fig. 7.2 *Top*: changes in stature due to various levels of activity (Adapted from Leatt et al. 1986; Garbutt et al. 1990; Hwang et al. 2012). *Bottom*: hydration profile of a human intervertebral disc before and after 4 h of sustained loading in a flexed position (Adapted from Adams et al. 1990)

pulposus are well recognized as a prominent contributor to intervertebral disc mechanics. As cut from the disc, the nucleus pulposus has a water content (WC = 1 − dry weight/wet weight) of approximately 0.85 in juvenile discs, and that decreases to approximately 0.75 in aged discs (Urban and McMullin 1988). Distribution of water also diminishes outwardly through annular lamellae, as a proportion of the nucleus pulposus water content, by 0.07, 0.11, and 0.22 from inner to mid to outer annulus fibrosus (Urban and Maroudas 1981). The marked spatial variation in fluid distribution is a unique hallmark of the intervertebral disc and plays a significant role in its function. In the nucleus pulposus, a high negative fixed charge density from concentrated localization of large aggregating proteoglycans produces increases in osmotic pressures that tend to promote tissue swelling and affects mechanically driven fluid exudation (Urban and Maroudas 1981; Urban and McMullin 1985, 1988). Studies have demonstrated that matrix alteration – particularly GAG degradation – adversely affects the poroviscoelastic behavior of nucleus pulposus tissues, intervertebral disc biomechanics, and degenerative changes in animal models (Boxberger et al. 2008).

Nucleus pulposus poroviscoelastic behavior, in turn, impacts the loading experienced by the annulus fibrosus, which itself is porous and viscoelastic. However, consistent with the similarities to ligament tissue in terms of function and microstructure, the contribution to viscoelastic properties in the annulus fibrosus is thought to be primarily flow independent. Specifically, it relies on collagen fiber bundles organized in parallel to resist tensile stresses (Broberg and von Essen 1980; Hickey and Hukins 1980; Stokes and Greenaple 1985; Cassidy et al. 1989; Holzapfel et al. 2005). The staggered discontinuous nature of the fibrillar collagen microstructure (Marchand and Ahmed 1990; Holzapfel et al. 2005) results in complex transmission of force along lamellae and has profound impact on mechanotransduction. As observed in the bovine annulus fibrosus (Bruehlmann et al. 2004a, b) and similarly in the rat tail tendon (Screen et al. 2004), tissue stretch does not uniformly propagate across the levels of collagen. Rather, straightening of collagen crimp and fibril-fibril sliding leads to nonuniformly, increasing fibril recruitment at different loads and appears to account for the majority of tissue-level deformations. These phenomena have been demonstrated both through intercellular measurements within and among collagen fibers (Bruehlmann et al. 2004a, b; Screen et al. 2004) and by measuring the deformation of photobleached lines across labeled collagen fibers (Bruehlmann et al. 2004b). The mechanisms and kinetics of recovery, whether passive or actively cell-mediated, are not yet clear. Thus, not only is cell stretch a mechanism of stimulation during annulus fibrosus deformation, but shear stress likely also serves as a robust determinant of cell function.

Poroviscoelastic interactions between the nucleus pulposus and annulus fibrosus cause nucleus pressurization and annulus tension to be time dependent, modulated by the nucleus pulposus hydration state and degree of annulus fibrosus stress relaxation (Fig. 7.3). Thus, for any spinal load applied over a finite duration, the micromechanical loading regime imposed on disc cells is defined both by the current stress to the motion segment and by the history of earlier experienced applied stresses. One demonstration of this dependence on the time history of loading is illustrated in the study of Hwang et al. (2012). This study showed that in rat discs, the effectiveness of the nucleus pulposus to pressurize varied according to the specific sequence of loading events and not just by the applied endpoint stress. Meanwhile, disc height was determined only by the endpoint stress and independent of temporal path of axial loads. This load history dependence of the internal pressure and shear could then have an impact on cellular mechanotransduction and differentiation.

As a corollary, there is also the implicit potential for restoring the homeostatic combination of nucleus pulposus pressure and annulus fibrosus shear. Introducing detours in the temporal path of spinal loading could have restorative effects on intervertebral disc hydration. Results from Gabai et al. (2007) using rat discs suggest that interspersing repeated axial compressive stresses with short, low-magnitude tensional loading allows intervertebral discs to preserve the pressure-shear balance between nucleus pulposus and annulus fibrosus. Thus, exploiting this phenomenon could be one strategy toward preventative maintenance.

While very pronounced in small animal discs, such load history effects in adult human intervertebral discs remain uncharacterized. It is possible that the temporal sequence of loading is more significant during early growth in juvenile discs and that the decreased baseline tissue hydration and calcification of end plates in aged discs reduce the impact of load history. If this is the case, the argument could be made for greater focus on spinal health in younger populations.

There are some parallels between the time load history effects and age-related changes in the intervertebral disc that are interesting to note. Similar to the expression of fluid out of the intervertebral disc with sustained compression, the aging disc possesses diminished swelling pressures and impaired capability to retain water. As such, the aged disc

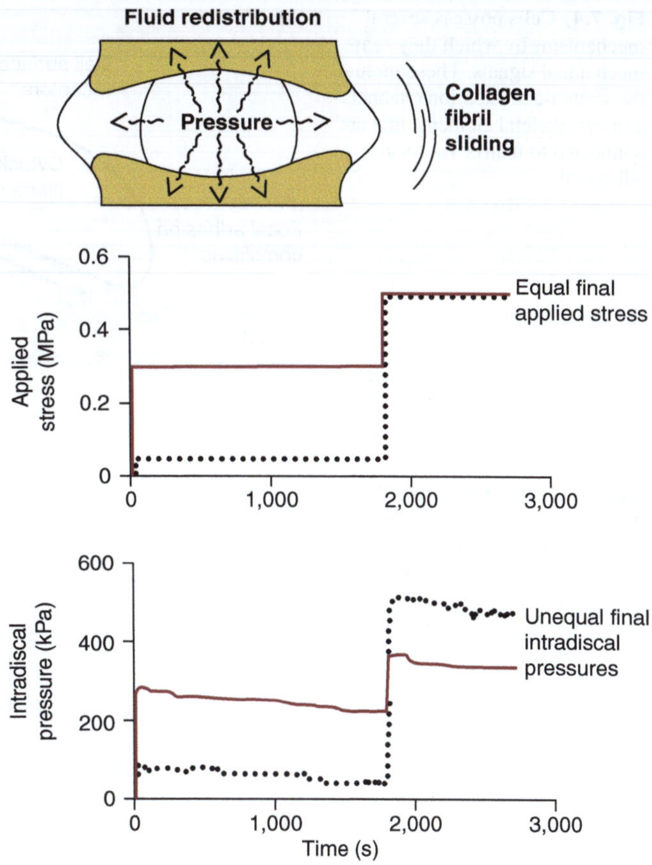

Fig. 7.3 Poroviscoelastic phenomena affect the internal mechanics of the disc (*top*). Graphs show that two temporal paths (*solid* and *dotted curves*) of applied stress (*middle*) lead to markedly different intradiscal pressures generated (*bottom*). Despite equivalent applied stresses at the end, the path with a higher intermediate load exhibited inferior final pressures (*solid, bottom*) than that with the lower intermediate load (*dotted, bottom*) (Adapted from Hwang et al. 2012)

may represent a state in which an adverse pressure-shear microenvironment is permanently maintained, resulting in a vicious cycle of matrix catabolism and abnormal matrix synthesis. Evidence in the literature demonstrating decreases in intradiscal pressure generation and increasing numbers of spikes in the stress profile with age and degeneration supports the notion that pressure and shear remain in a state of imbalance in the adult disc (Adams et al. 1996).

7.3 Cellular and Molecular Levels

7.3.1 Studies of Disc Cell Mechanical Responses In Vitro

Cells sense and respond to mechanical cues via a plethora of mechanisms that typically operate in four steps: mechanical coupling, mechanotransduction, signal transmission, and cell response. Mechanocoupling is facilitated by cellular load transducers that include integrins, ion channels,

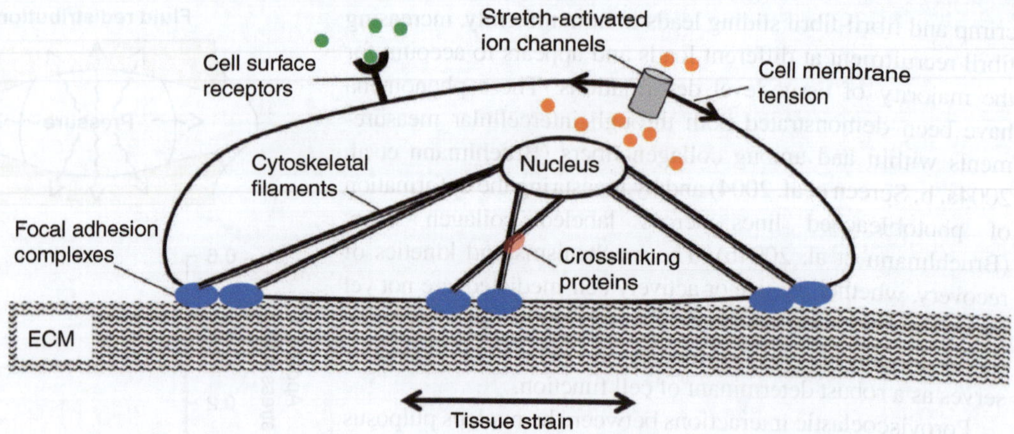

Fig. 7.4 Cells possess several mechanisms by which they sense mechanical signals. These include the stretch-activated ion channels and cytoskeletal elements that are connected to matrix via focal adhesions

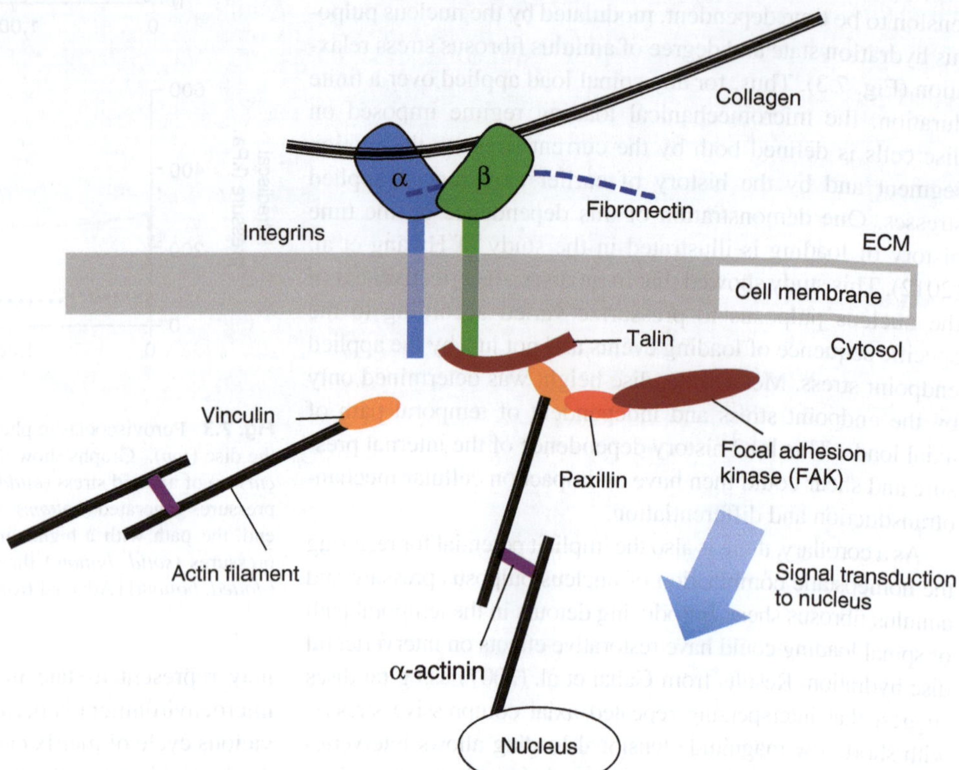

Fig. 7.5 Schematic of mechanism by which integrins interact with adhesion plaque proteins and cytoskeleton to activate specific downstream signaling

G protein-coupled receptors, and tyrosine kinase receptors (Fig. 7.4). These lead to cell-ECM adhesion assemblies that are sensitive to reciprocal tension between the cell and matrix.

Integrins are a class of cell membrane proteins that mediate adhesion of cells to substrates (Fig. 7.5). They consist of two transmembrane glycoprotein subunits with the extracellular domains interacting to form a functional heterodimer. Integrins functionally serve to connect the extracellular matrix with the cytoskeleton and have the capacity to bind collagen and fibronectin among other matrix constituents. This integrin/matrix bond may be influenced by tensile loading and matrix stiffness, with higher forces and stiffer matrices leading to enhanced attachment (Paszek et al. 2005). These types of load-dependent interactions are called catch bonds (Friedland et al. 2009). Mechanical reinforcement of "catch bonds" between the cell and matrix mediates integrin assembly and development of clusters to form focal adhesions. Focal adhesions elicit a reciprocal actomyosin-mediated cell contractility that is essential to amplify the mechanoresponse (Sniadecki and Chen 2007; Na et al. 2008; Wang et al. 2008). The affinity of integrins for extracellular matrix proteins can be modified by tissue deformation and molecular conformation force-dependent unfolding (such as with fibronectin) that can expose binding sites (Vogel and Baneyx 2003).

Disc cells express integrin receptors that vary by region and degree of degeneration. These include fibronectin-binding integrins ($\alpha_5\beta_1$ and $\alpha_v\beta_3$), collagen-binding integrins ($\alpha_1\beta_1$, $\alpha_2\beta_1$, and $\alpha_v\beta_1$), and laminin-binding integrins ($\alpha_6\beta_1$ and $\alpha_6\beta_4$) (Nettles et al. 2004; Xia and Zhu 2008; Chen et al. 2009); laminin-binding integrins are more prevalent in the nucleus (Gilchrist et al. 2007; Chen et al. 2009). Within the nucleus, fibronectin fragments are known to accumulate with disc degeneration (Oegema et al. 2000) and trigger upregulation of $\alpha_5\beta_1$ integrin expression and ERK signaling of catabolic processes (Xia and Zhu 2011).

Mechanotransduction occurs when extracellular matrix forces are coupled to the cytoskeleton and induce conformational changes of intracellular proteins that alter substrate availability leading to phosphorylation (Doyle and Yamada 2010; del Rio et al. 2009). Mechanosensing can also occur via mechanically gated calcium channels. Transmembrane ion channels influence the cell's lipid bilayer organization and tension (Fig. 7.6). When membrane tension increases (as observed during osmotic swelling), it can alter the channel cross section and protein configuration, leading to channel opening, even in the absence of direct activation by a specific chemical ligand (Janmey and Kinnunen 2006). Calcium modulates cell activity, growth and differentiation, motility, intercellular coupling, and apoptosis. Several studies demonstrate that disc cells can respond to mechanical loading via activation of calcium channels that cause intracellular calcium transients. This type of calcium signaling has been shown to be important in regulatory volume fluxes that are observed after hypo-osmotic or fluid-induced shear stress (Elfervig et al. 2001; Pritchard and Guilak 2004). Calcium transients can lead to F-actin remodeling that facilitates reestablishment of cell volume after an osmotic challenge.

Signals are propagated deep within the cell by the stiff cytoskeletal filaments (microfilaments (F-actin), intermediate filaments (vimentin, cytokeratin), and microtubules (tubulin)) that link the cell nucleus to the extracellular matrix via focal adhesion complexes and hemidesmosomes (Alenghat and Ingber 2002). Because cells contain a continuum of cytoskeletal elements, they display an integrated

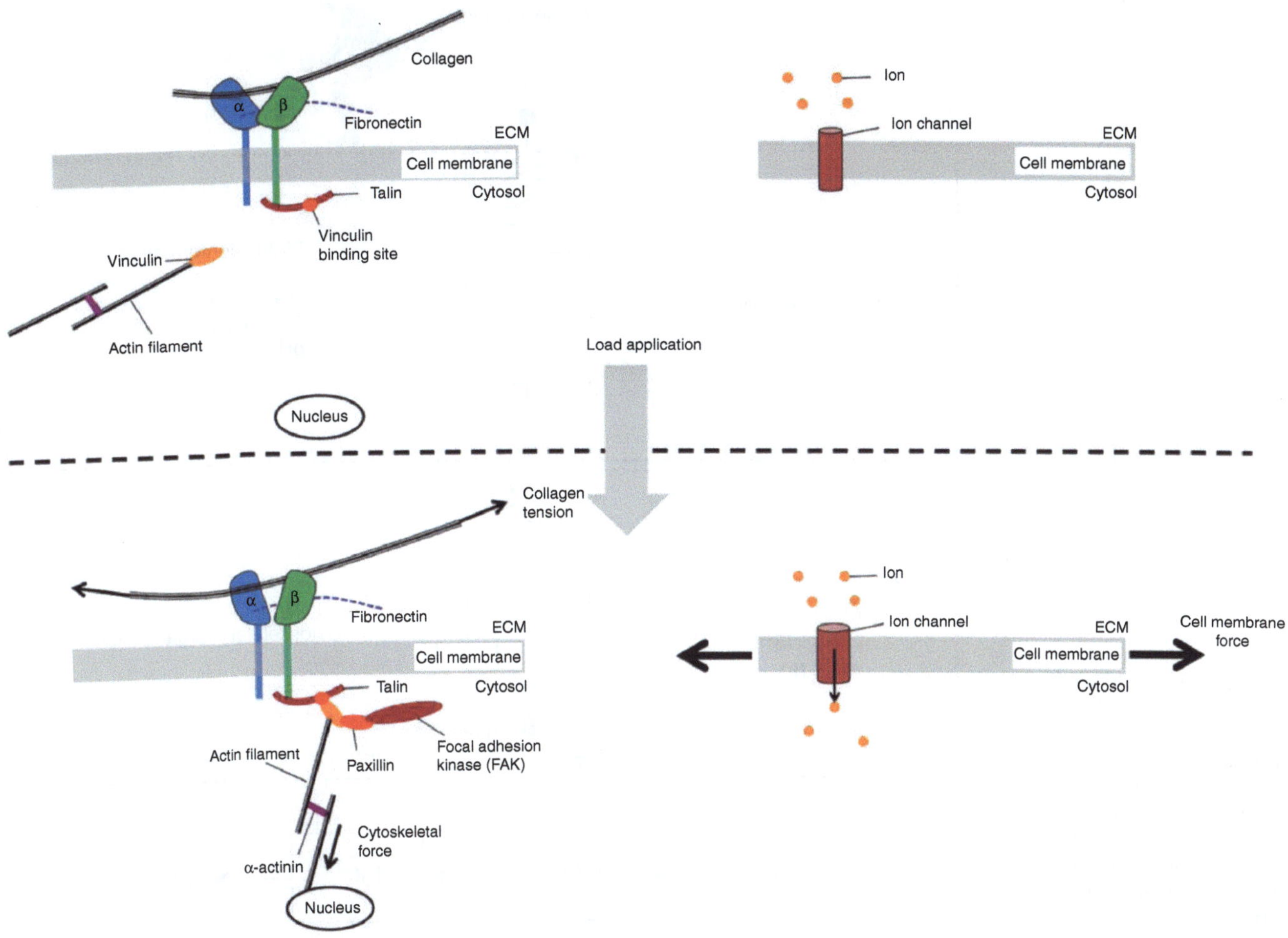

Fig. 7.6 Mechanotransduction can be viewed as a series of rapid switch-like events, activated in response to applications of force

mechanical behavior, whose properties depend on the composition and organization of the cytoskeleton, and extracellular matrix interactions via transmembrane proteins, cellular proteins, subcellular structures, and intracellular fluid volume and composition (Ingber 2003). Predictably, the mechanical properties of disc cells display zonal variations in cytoskeletal composition. While disc cells demonstrate an overall viscoelastic behavior, nucleus pulposus cells are three times stiffer and more viscous than annulus cells (Guilak et al. 1999).

Microtubules form an extensive mesh throughout the cytoplasm in both nucleus and annulus cells (Li et al. 2008). Likewise, vimentin filaments are densely distributed within the nucleus and annulus cells and extend into annular cell processes (Johnson and Roberts 2003; Li et al. 2008). Nucleus pulposus cells are also characterized by the presence of cytokeratin intermediate filaments. Pronounced differences exist in F-actin distribution between the nucleus and annulus cells. In the nucleus, F-actin is localized to punctate regions of the cell membrane, while in the annulus along with vimentin, it is more pronounced and extends into cell processes (Errington et al. 1998; Bruehlmann et al. 2002; Li et al. 2008).

Mechanoresponses involve downstream intracellular signaling and transcription networks. Intracellular signal transduction can occur via the cytoskeleton, small molecules (second messengers Ca^{2+}, 1,4,5-triphosphate (IP3), cAMP), protein kinases (focal adhesion kinase, cSrc, protein kinase C, mitogen-activated protein kinase), and transcription factors (c-fos, c-jun, c-myc, NF-kB).

Cellular response pathways function over different timescales that can define frequency-dependent cell behaviors (Fig. 7.7). For example, force can cause an immediate cell response (hundreds of milliseconds) through activation of ion channels or conformational changes in the cytoskeleton. In contrast, other signaling pathways require polymerization of cytoskeletal stress fibers and alterations of intracellular protein networks and act over minutes. Still others may take hours or days as they act by causing changes in gene expression that influence cytoskeletal or adhesion proteins and ultimately force-transmission pathways. Consequently,

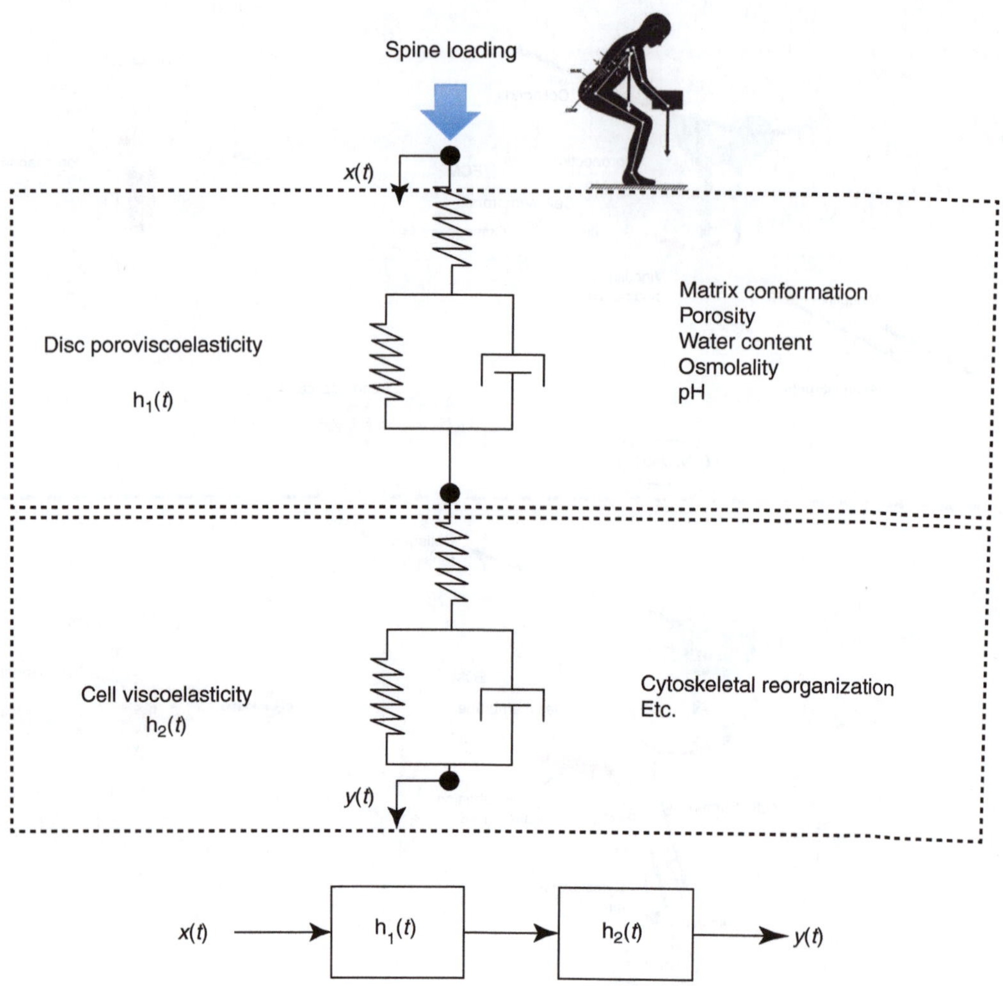

Fig. 7.7 A conceptual scheme of the multiscale, multifactorial influences on disc cell mechanobiology. The time-dependent cellular response ($y(t)$) resulting from spinal loading ($x(t)$) is dependent on dynamic tissue and cellular processes that may be quantified by transfer functions $h_1(t)$ and $h_2(t)$, respectively

these time-dependent behaviors lead to frequency-dependent signaling, where cells function as band-pass filters (Hoffman et al. 2011). To be stimulated, a particular signaling pathway needs to match the timescale of the applied forces.

7.3.2 Disc Cell Responses to Mechanical Perturbation

Disc cell phenotype varies between the annulus and nucleus, and accordingly, these cells are considered to have distinct repertoires of load-induced behaviors. These differences are likely due to spatially dependent adaptation to hydrostatic pressure (nucleus) and stretch (annulus) that are developed during spinal loading. To facilitate systematic study of cell mechanoresponsiveness, a number of in vitro test systems have been developed (Brown 2000). These allow the controlled application of known inputs (either stress or strain) so that dose–response functions can be established. Independent variables in these in vitro bioreactor studies include type, magnitude, frequency, and duration of mechanical stimulation.

7.3.3 Disc Cell Response to Pressure

The healthy disc nucleus is largely water and, consequently, is subjected to hydrostatic pressure during spinal loading. For that reason, both monolayer (2D) and hydrogel (3D) culture systems have been used to subject nucleus pulposus cells to hydrostatic pressure or compression. Nucleus cells are generally considered chondrocyte-like, while annulus fibrosus cells are fibroblastic. Accordingly, nucleus cells prefer the environment of inert hydrogels such as alginate or agarose that support a spherical configuration conducive to the assumption of a stable chondrocyte-like phenotype (Chen et al. 2002). In contrast, in monolayer culture, nucleus cells dedifferentiate as cell spreading leads to significant downregulation of Col2 gene expression and a change to a fibrotic phenotype with increased growth kinetics (Horner et al. 2002; Kluba et al. 2005; Rastogi et al. 2009; Wang et al. 2011). Conversely, annulus cells do less well in 3D culture in terms of cell morphology and survival (Horner et al. 2002).

Interpretation of published studies on disc cell mechanoresponsiveness is confounded by the fact that disc cells are isolated from many different tissue sources. These include human surgical samples and small and large animals. While human cells may be desirable to study disease pathogenesis, they are logistically difficult to acquire without close affiliation to high-volume surgical centers. Also, studies with human cells are complicated by individual-to-individual variability and degeneration-related phenotypic shifts (Kluba et al. 2005; Gruber et al. 2007). These factors will lead to experiment-to-experiment variability and require larger sample sizes for identifying statistically significant effects. In comparison, animal tissues are more readily available, but can be limited by the presence of persistent notochordal cells, which are lost in adolescence in humans but are maintained throughout life in mice, rats, rabbits, pigs, cats, and non-chondrodystrophic dogs (Risbud and Shapiro 2011; Hunter et al. 2003). The nucleus pulposus of several species has been observed to convert from notochordal to chondrocyte-like cells with age in a similar fashion to humans. These include cattle, horses, sheep, and chondrodystrophic dogs (beagles) (Miyazaki et al. 2009). Not surprisingly therefore, interspecies differences have been reported for disc cell responsiveness (Minogue et al. 2010; Miyazaki et al. 2009; Sakai et al. 2009), particularly when distinguishing notochordal from non-notochordal nucleus tissues (Miyazaki et al. 2009). Bovine tails may represent the best compromise for in vitro investigations, as they have a non-notochordal nucleus and are easy and inexpensive to procure in large numbers. For a full discussion of animal preferences in intervertebral disc research, see Chap. 18.

Hydrostatic pressure chambers are most commonly used to study disc cell responsiveness to compression loading (Hutton et al. 2001; Liu et al. 2001; Kasra et al. 2003; Wenger et al. 2005; Reza and Nicoll 2008). Alternatively, some use confined or unconfined compression of 3D gel/cell constructs. To simplify the latter tests, loading platens are often operated in displacement control, so that compressive strain, rather than compressive stress, becomes the independent test variable (Chen et al. 2004; Korecki et al. 2009; Fernando et al. 2011; Salvatierra et al. 2011; Wang et al. 2011). Note that, in Chap. 22, further details are provided on choices of bioreactors for disc research.

In vitro loading parameters are typically based on values obtained from human disc studies. For example, studies of human subjects suggest that due to the inherent resonant frequency of the torso, certain loading frequencies may be deleterious (between 4 and 6 Hz; Wilder and Pope 1996; Kumar et al. 1999). Due to upright posture, static or low-frequency (1 Hz) pressures from gravity loading and daily living activities are also of interest given the recognized differences in disc degeneration in humans when compared to quadrupeds (Lotz 2004). Accordingly, in vitro studies explore cell responses over a broad range of loading frequencies, from static to 20 Hz (Table 7.1).

The disc is one of the most highly loaded tissues in the body and routinely experiences compressive pressures in the 2 MPa range and as high as 3 MPa under extreme activities (Ranu 1990; Wilke et al. 1999). Diurnal fluctuations can be significant, for example, during sleep, pressures decrease to

Table 7.1 Experimental in vitro studies of pressure on disc cell function

Cell type	Cell source	Scaffold	Load	Frequency (Hz)	Duration	Reference
AF	Porcine	Alginate	1–3 MPa	0.5	3 h	Wenger et al. (2005)
NP	Rats	Alginate	10 kPa, 20 % strain	0.5	1 h	Wang et al. (2011)
AF, NP	Porcine	Agarose	15 % strain	2	4 h	Salvatierra et al. (2011)
IAF, OAF	Bovine	PGLA	5 MPa	0.5	4 h/day, 3–14 days	Reza and Nicoll (2008)
NP	Human, bovine	Col 1	0.25 and 2.5 MPa	0.1	1 h, 24 h	Neidlinger-Wilke et al. (2009)
NP	Human, bovine	Col 1	0.25, 2.5 MPa	0.1	24 h	Neidlinger-Wilke et al. (2006)
AF, NP	Human	Tissues	0.1, 0.3, 3 MPa	Static	2 h	Liu et al. (2001)
AF, NP	Human	Alginate	0.35–0.95 MPa	1	2 h	Le Maitre et al. (2009)
AF, NP	Porcine, bovine	Alginate	2–12 % strain	3	2 h/day, 7 days	Korecki et al. (2009)
AF, NP	Rabbit	Alginate (NP)	0–3 MPa	1–20	30 min/day, 3 days	Kasra et al. (2003)
AF, NP	Porcine	Alginate	1 MPa	1, 3, 5, 8, 10	30 min/day, 3 days	Kasra et al. (2006)
AF, NP	Canine	Alginate	0.35, 0.1 MPa	Static	9 days	Hutton et al. (2001)
IAF, OAF, NP	Human	Tissue	0.3, 3.0 MPa	Static	2 h	Handa et al. (1997)
NP	Rabbit	Alginate	0.7, 2, 4 MPa	Static	4, 24 h	Sowa et al. (2011a)
AF, NP	Porcine	Agarose	15 % strain	Static, 0.1 and 1	4 h	Fernando et al. (2011)
AF, NP	Porcine	Alginate	25 % strain	Static	2, 18, 30 h	Chen et al. (2004)

AF annulus fibrosus, *NP* nucleus pulposus, *IAF* inner annulus fibrosus, *OAF* outer annulus fibrosus

0.1 MPa and during quiet standing 0.5 MPa (Wilke et al. 1999). Pressures applied during in vitro tests, therefore, cover the range from atmospheric (free swelling control conditions) to as high as 5 MPa.

The disc cell's response to pressure is dependent on the magnitude, frequency, and duration of loading. In general, in vitro studies suggest that physiologic loading conditions (<1 MPa magnitude, <3 Hz frequency, and <24-h duration) are anabolic, whereas regimes outside this range are catabolic. For both nucleus and annulus cells, low pressure (0.2–1.0 MPa) tends to increase expression of anabolic matrix genes (collagen 1, aggrecan, biglycan, decorin, lumican, fibromodulin, fibronectin (Chen et al. 2004; Wenger et al. 2005; Sowa et al. 2011b; Wang et al. 2011)) and enzyme inhibitors (TIMP1) (Handa et al. 1997; Sowa et al. 2011a, b). In parallel, there is a reduction of catabolic factors (MMPs, iNOS, Cox2) (Sowa et al. 2011b). Conversely, high pressure (1–4 MPa) tends to reduce expression of anabolic genes (collagen and aggrecan) and increase catabolic (MMP-1, MMP-3, MMP-13) (Handa et al. 1997; Neidlinger-Wilke et al. 2006; Le Maitre et al. 2009) and inflammatory factors (Cox2, iNOS) (Sowa et al. 2011b).

With loading frequencies in the range of 3–5 Hz, nucleus pulposus cells reduce aggrecan and collagen synthesis and increase aggrecan degradation (Kasra et al. 2003, 2006; Korecki et al. 2009). This frequency effect may be age-related as young and mature disc cells show opposite trends at frequencies below 3 Hz (Korecki et al. 2009). Likewise, as the duration of static compressive loading approaches 24 h, catabolic and proinflammatory responses predominate (Sowa et al. 2011b).

A number of signaling mechanisms discussed above are implicated in these pressure-induced behaviors. Compressive stress can trigger cell volume regulatory mechanisms. For example, when disc cells are challenged by osmotic stress, calcium signaling and F-actin cytoskeletal elements play an important role in restoring homeostasis (Pritchard and Guilak 2004). The importance of the cytoskeleton is also implicated by observations that load-induced loss of proteoglycan expression can be inhibited by exposure to an RGD inhibitory peptide (Le Maitre et al. 2009). Given the role integrins play in connecting the cytoskeleton to extracellular matrix, this later observation further supports the importance of the cytoskeleton in the signaling cascade. Additionally, cell membrane water channels, aquaporins, have been identified in disc cells and are considered another important mechanism of cell volume regulatory control that may be stimulated by hydrostatic stress (Richardson et al. 2008; Haudenschild et al. 2009).

Other bioactive factors are also considered important to disc cell pressure responsiveness. Hydrostatic pressure regulates nitric oxide (NO) production by disc cells (Salvatierra et al. 2011). NO is a short-lived molecule that is produced from citrulline via the enzyme NO synthase (NOS) (Mitchell et al. 1997). NO production is known to inhibit aerobic oxidation of pyruvate after glycolysis and could regulate mitochondrial respiration (Fernando et al. 2011; Salvatierra et al. 2011). NO production by cells suppresses proteoglycan synthesis (Liu et al. 2001).

7.3.4 Disc Cell Response to Stretch

Generally speaking, the outer annulus fibrosus in the healthy disc is subjected to biaxial stretch as it acts to contain the pressurized nucleus (Shirazi-Adl et al. 1984). The extent of

Table 7.2 Experimental in vitro studies of stretch on disc cell function

Cell type	Cell source	Substrate	Stretch	Frequency (Hz)	Duration	Reference
AF	Rabbit	Col 1	3, 6, 8 %	0.1, 0.5, 1	4, 24 h	Sowa et al. (2011b)
AF, NP	Human		10 %	1	2 h/day, 7 days	Hee et al. (2010)
AF, NP	Rat	Col 1	20 %	0.05	48 h	Miyamoto et al. (2006)
AF	Rabbit, human		0.1 G vibration	6	up to 1 h	Yamazaki et al. (2003)
AF	Rat		6 %	0.05	4 h	Sowa and Agarwal (2008)
AF	Rabbit	Col 1	1, 5 %	1	0.5, 24 h	Rannou et al. (2003)
AF	Human		10 %	0.33, 1	0.3 h	Gilbert et al. (2010)
NP	Rabbit		10 %	0.5	8 days	Matsumoto et al. (1999)
AF	Human		10 %	1	0.3 h	Gilbert et al. (2011)

AF annulus fibrosus, *NP* nucleus pulposus

annular stretch generated in response to in vivo compression loading conditions is near 4 % strain and as high as 6 % during flexion and extension (Stokes 1987). The importance of stretch to annular homeostasis has been elegantly demonstrated by Hayes and colleagues who show that during development, pressures generated by the nucleus pulposus trigger stress fiber formation in annular fibroblasts and ultimately patterning of the complex lamellar architecture (Hayes et al. 1999). To mimic this process in a controlled fashion in vitro, several experimental systems have been described (Brown 2000). The most common system is the Flexercell (Vande Geest et al. 2004) that permits cells to be maintained in deformable culture plates. The strain pattern, magnitude, waveform, frequency, and duty cycle can be controlled thereby permitting a broad range of study parameters. Additionally, the dishes can be coated with matrix proteins such as collagen and laminin so as to better mimic in vivo cell/matrix interactions. Cell stretch is generated by vacuum pressures that deform the substrates over various sized posts and allow choice between uniaxial versus biaxial conditions. While the systems have been optimized for strain uniformity, variations in the strain field, particularly within the unsupported portion of the membranes, should be recognized (Gilbert et al. 1994; Vande Geest et al. 2004).

Disc cells are sensitive to stretch magnitude, duration, and duty cycle (Table 7.2). Continuous cyclic stretch (CCS) at low magnitude (1 %) and physiologic frequencies (1 Hz) is homeostatic (maintains proteoglycan production) for annulus cells over a 24-h period (Rannou et al. 2003). However, the response turns catabolic (decreased proteoglycan production, increased NO production, increased Cox2 and MMP-3 gene expression) with increasing strains (5–18 %) and time (beyond 4–6 h) (Rannou et al. 2003; Sowa et al. 2011a). For rabbit nuclear cells, CCS (10 % strain at 0.5 Hz) increases are evident in cell proliferation and collagen production during the first 1–2 days, but this anabolic effect is lost by 4 and 8 days (Matsumoto et al. 1999). The conversion from an anabolic to catabolic response to CCS with time may be due to fatigue: the cells' inability to sustain energy production necessary for biosynthetic processes. For example, Yamazaki and colleagues demonstrated that annulus cells initially increase their resting production of ATP in response to continuous vibration, but this is only transient and becomes suppressed after 15 min (Yamazaki et al. 2003). Consequently, when the duty cycle is limited to 2 h twice per day, 5 % strain maintains collagen and proteoglycan production for 2 weeks relative to unloaded controls (Hee et al. 2010) Increasing the strain magnitude to 10 % elevates cell proliferation and causes a 25 % increase in collagen production.

Loading frequency also influences the cellular response to stretch. Gilbert and coworkers subjected human annulus fibrosus cells to 10 % stretch for 20 min at either 0.33 or 1.0 Hz (Gilbert et al. 2010). For healthy disc cells, 1 Hz stimulation maintained collagen and aggrecan gene expression relative to control, whereas there was a shift toward catabolism when the frequency was changed to 0.33 Hz. A frequency-dependent response to stretch has also been reported for rabbit annular fibroblasts, where 1 Hz stimulation increased MMP-3 gene expression after 4 h of stimulation while TIMP-1 was downregulated with 0.1 and 0.5 Hz loading (Sowa et al. 2011a).

Because painful disc degeneration has been linked to elevated cytokine levels, several studies have questioned whether the cell's response to stretch is modulated by proinflammatory cytokines. Miyamoto and coworkers subjected rat nucleus pulposus and annulus fibrosus cells to CCS (20 % stretch at 0.05 Hz for 48 h) with and without inflammatory factors in the culture media (10 ng/mL IL-1β or TNF-α) (Miyamoto et al. 2006). Their data indicate that stretch and cytokines individually had comparable effect on inflammatory mediator production (prostaglandin E2, PGE2). Importantly, there was a significant synergistic increase when both stimuli were combined. The effect was more pronounced in annular cells and correlated with the gene expression of COX-2, a rate-limiting enzyme for the cellular production of PGE2. However, there is also evidence that CCS can be protective against inflammation-induced catabolic behaviors. When measuring alternate marker genes for proinflammatory cell responses, Sowa and colleagues reported that CCS (6 % stretch at 0.05 Hz for 4 h) decreased an IL-1-induced production of several inflammation markers (iNOS, TNF-alpha, MMP-3, and MMP-13) by 50 % (Sowa and Agarwal 2008). Consistent with this finding, Gilbert and co-investigators (Gilbert et al. 2010) report that the anti-catabolic effect of CCS (10 % stretch at 1 Hz for 1 h) on human annulus fibrosus cells (suppression of MMP-3 and ADAMTS4 gene expression) was lost by exposure to cytokine inhibitors (IL-1Ra or IL-4RAb).

7.4 Final Comments

Information is encoded in a time-dependent manner in conformational changes of cell membrane receptors and the cytoskeleton. These changes can be induced by relative differences in cell and matrix stiffness, matrix deformation, osmolality, with the responses tuned by inflammatory and other soluble molecules. Data from both organ- and cell-level studies suggest the existence of optimal loading regimens, where both excessive and negligible pressure/stretch responses are catabolic. This is consistent with clinical observations that show that disc injury rates are increased under situations of either chronic inactivity or extreme exposures, leading to the concept of a U-shaped distribution in the disc's response to load (Lotz 2011; Panel on Musculoskeletal Disorders and the Workplace 2001). Objectively, for both prevention and treatment, defining such boundaries would be very beneficial. Given that magnitude, frequency, and duration all contribute to cell responses, it would be valuable to combine these variables into a single-"dose" parameter (Gardner 2000). Dose–response relationships may be more easily compared between studies and ultimately extrapolated to humans.

It is hoped that this review clearly demonstrates the substantial effort that has been invested into elucidating tissue-level mechanobiologic principles and cellular mechanobiologic phenomena. Yet, relatively little is understood about how these two hierarchical levels are quantitatively linked. This knowledge gap exists because of complexities in matrix structure-function and in the nature by which the deforming matrix affects cells function (Bruehlmann et al. 2004a, b). For example, in situ visualization of whole-tissue preparations show that in highly ordered collagenous tissues, an 8 % applied strain results in displacements that approximate 1 % strain along a collagen fiber and approximately 4 % strain between fibers (Screen et al. 2004). This distribution suggests that cells may experience a smaller degree of elongation and a greater amount of shear than tissue-level strains might indicate. Moreover, pressure gradients in the disc result in interstitial fluid flux within and across tissue boundaries. Wang and colleagues (2011) have demonstrated that immature nucleus pulposus cells are sensitive to fluid shear stress. Fluid-induced shear stresses in tissues are not well characterized, but are likely also important determinants of cellular function. Thus, while extensive mechanobiology data are available at the tissue and cellular level, there remains a need to develop mathematical/computational models that link tissue/cellular dynamic responses so as to reconcile the phenomena observed at the two levels of scale.

More mechanistic studies are needed to define the activation of pathways that may underlie disease mechanisms and thereby inform pharmacologic interventions. In addition to those pathways discussed above, recent studies suggest alternate mechanisms by which disc cells transduce mechanical signals. For example, caveolae are plasma membrane invaginations that are highly enriched with cholesterol, with their main constituents being caveolin-1 and caveolin-2 (Sinha et al. 2011). Acute increases in cell volume or stretch lead to a rapid loss of caveolae, and as such they are implicated in a membrane-mediated mechanical response triggered by tyrosine phosphorylation (Alenghat and Ingber 2002). Caveolae are required to buffer fluctuations in cell membrane stress induced by acute membrane tension and osmotic shock, such that loss of caveolae compromises buffering of cell membrane tension (Parton and Simons 2007). Recently, caveolin-1 has been identified in nucleus pulposus cells, with its expression decreasing with age (Heathfield et al. 2008). These observations suggest caveolae may participate in nucleus pulposus cell responses to hydrostatic pressure.

Another potentially important component of the disc cell's mechanoregulatory machinery is the glycocalyx (Fuster and Esko 2005). Glycans can exist as cell membrane-bound glycoconjugates that mediate cell adhesion as well as other intracellular signaling events. The glycocalyx forms a portion of the pericellular matrix known as the chondron that has been observed both in chondrocytes and in nucleus pulposus cells (Roberts et al. 1991; Chang and Poole 1997). The presence of chondrons in the nucleus pulposus has been considered a phenotypical indicator of degeneration (Ciapetti et al. 2012). Recently, the glycocalyx has been shown to contribute to extracellular stiffness that mediates load-modulated fluctuations in integrin clustering and signaling (Paszek et al. 2009). Similarly to the glycocalyx pericellular stiffness, extracellular matrix stiffness can influence cell behaviors by modifying integrin-mediated TGF-β activation, heterodimerization and signaling between integrins and TGF-β receptors, or the activity of TAZ (transcriptional co-activator with PDZ-binding motif), a transcriptional co-regulator that is a common effector of stiffness sensing and TGF-β signaling (Dupont et al. 2011; Hinz 2009).

Ultimately, the translation of mechanobiologic understanding into clinical benefits for patients requires cooperative efforts of interdisciplinary teams that include clinicians, surgeons, bioengineers, and biologists. In this way, the necessarily diverse lines of evidence can be most efficiently stitched into testable theories and research programs that link basic and clinical studies.

7.5 Summary of Critical Concepts Discussed in the Chapter

- Spinal loading is filtered into intradiscal regions of hydrostatic pressure and octahedral shear.
- Disc matrix properties are poroviscoelastic, such that the extracellular environment is time varying.
- Coupled physical and biochemical cues in the tissue microenvironment signal cells to regulate the extracellular matrix dynamically.
- Microenvironment cues include pH, growth factor and nutrient concentration, osmolality, fluid flow, and extracellular matrix stiffness and conformation.
- Disc cells react to mechanical cues via four steps: mechanical coupling to matrix, mechanotransduction or conversion of mechanical to chemical signals, intracellular signal transmission, and the eventual cellular response.
- Matrix and cellular response pathways function over varying timescales, such that the disc/cell composite can function as a band-pass filter.
- Nucleus cells response to pressure is dependent on the magnitude, frequency, and duration. Physiologic pressure loading (<1 MPa magnitude, <3 Hz frequency, and <24-h duration) is anabolic, whereas pressures outside that range are catabolic.
- Annulus cell response to cyclic shear at low magnitude (<1 % strain) and at physiologic frequencies (1 Hz) is anabolic for up to 1–2 days.
- Cellular responses vary by species and are significantly altered by the presence of degenerated matrix fragments and proinflammatory cytokines.

Acknowledgements NIH AR049786 (JL), NIH AR049770 (JL), NIH AR063357 (JL), NIH AR059325 (AH), NSF CBET 0845754 (AH), NIST 70NANB11H191 (AH).

References

Adams M, Hutton W (1983) The effect of posture on the fluid content of lumbar intervertebral discs. Spine 8(6):665–671

Adams MA, Dolan P et al (1990) Diurnal changes in spinal mechanics and their clinical significance. J Bone Joint Surg Br 72-B(2):266–270

Adams MA, McNally DS et al (1996) 'Stress' distributions inside intervertebral discs. The effects of age and degeneration. J Bone Joint Surg Br 78(6):965–972

Alenghat FJ, Ingber DE (2002) Mechanotransduction: all signals point to cytoskeleton, matrix, and integrins. Sci STKE 2002(119):pe6

Ayotte DC, Ito K et al (2000) Direction-dependent constriction flow in a poroelastic solid: the intervertebral disc valve. J Biomech Eng 122(6):587–593

Bass EC, Duncan NA et al (1997) Frozen storage affects the compressive creep behavior of the porcine intervertebral disc. Spine 22(24):2867–2876

Boxberger JI, Auerbach JD et al (2008) An in vivo model of reduced nucleus pulposus glycosaminoglycan content in the rat lumbar intervertebral disc. Spine (Phila Pa 1976) 33(2):146–154

Broberg KB, von Essen HO (1980) Modeling of intervertebral discs. Spine 5(2):155–167

Brown TD (2000) Techniques for mechanical stimulation of cells in vitro: a review. J Biomech 33(1):3–14

Bruehlmann SB, Rattner JB et al (2002) Regional variations in the cellular matrix of the annulus fibrosus of the intervertebral disc. J Anat 201(2):159–171

Bruehlmann SB, Hulme PA et al (2004a) In situ intercellular mechanics of the bovine outer annulus fibrosus subjected to biaxial strains. J Biomech 37(2):223–231

Bruehlmann SB, Matyas JR et al (2004b) ISSLS prize winner: Collagen fibril sliding governs cell mechanics in the anulus fibrosus: an in situ confocal microscopy study of bovine discs. Spine (Phila Pa 1976) 29(23):2612–2620

Carter DR, Beaupre GS (2001) Skeletal function and form. Cambridge University Press, New York

Cassidy JJ, Hiltner A et al (1989) Hierarchical structure of the intervertebral disc. Connect Tissue Res 23(1):75–88

Chang J, Poole CA (1997) Confocal analysis of the molecular heterogeneity in the pericellular microenvironment produced by adult canine chondrocytes cultured in agarose gel. Histochem J 29(7):515–528

Chen J, Baer AE et al (2002) Matrix protein gene expression in intervertebral disc cells subjected to altered osmolarity. Biochem Biophys Res Commun 293(3):932–938

Chen J, Yan W et al (2004) Static compression induces zonal-specific changes in gene expression for extracellular matrix and cytoskeletal proteins in intervertebral disc cells in vitro. Matrix Biol 22(7): 573–583

Chen J, Jing L et al (2009) Expression of laminin isoforms, receptors, and binding proteins unique to nucleus pulposus cells of immature intervertebral disc. Connect Tissue Res 50(5):294–306

Chin JR, Court C et al (1999) Compression-induced apoptosis in the mouse intervertebral disc is time and stress dependent. 45th annual meeting, Orthopaedic Research Society, Anaheim

Ching CT, Chow DH et al (2003) The effect of cyclic compression on the mechanical properties of the inter-vertebral disc: an in vivo study in a rat tail model. Clin Biomech (Bristol, Avon) 18(3):182–189

Ching CT, Chow DH et al (2004) Changes in nuclear composition following cyclic compression of the intervertebral disc in an in vivo rat-tail model. Med Eng Phys 26(7):587–594

Ciapetti G, Granchi D et al (2012) Ex vivo observation of human intervertebral disc tissue and cells isolated from degenerated intervertebral discs. Eur Spine J 21(1):10–19

Costi JJ, Hearn TC et al (2002) The effect of hydration on the stiffness of intervertebral discs in an ovine model. Clin Biomech (Bristol, Avon) 17(6):446–455

Court C, Colliou OK et al (2001) The effect of static in vivo bending on the intervertebral disc. Spine J 1(4):239–245

Court C, Chin JR et al (2007) Biological and mechanical consequences of transient intervertebral disc bending. Eur Spine J 16(11):1899–1906

del Rio A, Perez-Jimenez R et al (2009) Stretching single talin rod molecules activates vinculin binding. Science 323(5914):638–641

Doyle AD, Yamada KM (2010) Cell biology: sensing tension. Nature 466(7303):192–193

Dupont S, Morsut L et al (2011) Role of YAP/TAZ in mechanotransduction. Nature 474(7350):179–183

Elfervig MK, Minchew JT et al (2001) IL-1beta sensitizes intervertebral disc annulus cells to fluid-induced shear stress. J Cell Biochem 82(2):290–298

Errington RJ, Puustjarvi K et al (1998) Characterisation of cytoplasm-filled processes in cells of the intervertebral disc. J Anat 192(Pt 3):369–378

Fernando HN, Czamanski J et al (2011) Mechanical loading affects the energy metabolism of intervertebral disc cells. J Orthop Res 29(11):1634–1641

Friedland JC, Lee MH et al (2009) Mechanically activated integrin switch controls alpha5beta1 function. Science 323(5914):642–644

Fuster MM, Esko JD (2005) The sweet and sour of cancer: glycans as novel therapeutic targets. Nat Rev Cancer 5(7):526–542

Gabai AS, YewAG et al (2007) Distraction helps maintain transient disc mechanical behavior before exertion. 34th annual meeting of the International Society for the Study of the Lumbar Spine, Hong Kong

Garbutt G, Boocock MG et al (1990) Running speed and spinal shrinkage in runners with and without low back pain. Med Sci Sports Exerc 22(6):769–772

Gardner SN (2000) A mechanistic, predictive model of dose–response curves for cell cycle phase-specific and -nonspecific drugs. Cancer Res 60(5):1417–1425

Gilbert JA, Weinhold PS et al (1994) Strain profiles for circular cell culture plates containing flexible surfaces employed to mechanically deform cells in vitro. J Biomech 27(9):1169–1177

Gilbert HT, Hoyland JA et al (2010) The response of human anulus fibrosus cells to cyclic tensile strain is frequency-dependent and altered with disc degeneration. Arthritis Rheum 62(11):3385–3394

Gilbert HT, Hoyland JA et al (2011) The involvement of interleukin-1 and interleukin-4 in the response of human annulus fibrosus cells to cyclic tensile strain: an altered mechanotransduction pathway with degeneration. Arthritis Res Ther 13(1):R8

Gilchrist CL, Chen J et al (2007) Functional integrin subunits regulating cell-matrix interactions in the intervertebral disc. J Orthop Res 25(6):829–840

Gruber HE, Ingram JA et al (2007) Senescence in cells of the aging and degenerating intervertebral disc: immunolocalization of senescence-associated beta-galactosidase in human and sand rat discs. Spine 32(3):321–327

Guilak F, Ting-Beall HP et al (1999) Viscoelastic properties of intervertebral disc cells. Identification of two biomechanically distinct cell populations. Spine (Phila Pa 1976) 24(23):2475–2483

Han SM, Lee SY et al (2001) Disc hydration measured by magnetic resonance imaging in relation to its compressive stiffness in rat models. Proc Inst Mech Eng H 215(5):497–501

Handa T, Ishihara H et al (1997) Effects of hydrostatic pressure on matrix synthesis and matrix metalloproteinase production in the human lumbar intervertebral disc. Spine 22(10):1085–1091

Haudenschild AK, Hsieh AH et al (2009) Pressure and distortion regulate human mesenchymal stem cell gene expression. Ann Biomed Eng 37(3):492–502

Hayes AJ, Benjamin M et al (1999) Role of actin stress fibres in the development of the intervertebral disc: cytoskeletal control of extracellular matrix assembly. Dev Dyn 215(3):179–189

Hayes AJ, Benjamin M et al (2001) Extracellular matrix in development of the intervertebral disc. Matrix Biol 20(2):107–121

Heathfield SK, Le Maitre CL et al (2008) Caveolin-1 expression and stress-induced premature senescence in human intervertebral disc degeneration. Arthritis Res Ther 10(4):R87

Hee HT, Zhang J et al (2010) Effects of cyclic dynamic tensile strain on previously compressed inner annulus fibrosus and nucleus pulposus cells of human intervertebral disc-an in vitro study. J Orthop Res 28(4):503–509

Hickey DS, Hukins DWL (1980) Relation between the structure of the annulus fibrosus and the function and failure of the intervertebral disc. Spine 5(2):106–116

Hinz B (2009) Tissue stiffness, latent TGF-beta1 activation, and mechanical signal transduction: implications for the pathogenesis and treatment of fibrosis. Curr Rheumatol Rep 11(2):120–126

Hoe A, Atha J et al (1994) Stature loss from sustained gentle body loading. Ann Hum Biol 21(2):171–178

Hoffman BD, Crocker JC (2009) Cell mechanics: dissecting the physical responses of cells to force. Annu Rev Biomed Eng 11:259–288

Hoffman BD, Grashoff C et al (2011) Dynamic molecular processes mediate cellular mechanotransduction. Nature 475(7356):316–323

Holzapfel GA, Schulze-Bauer CA et al (2005) Single lamellar mechanics of the human lumbar anulus fibrosus. Biomech Model Mechanobiol 3(3):125–140

Horner HA, Roberts S et al (2002) Cells from different regions of the intervertebral disc: effect of culture system on matrix expression and cell phenotype. Spine 27(10):1018–1028

Hsieh AH, Lotz JC (2003) Prolonged spinal loading induces matrix metalloproteinase-2 activation in intervertebral discs. Spine 28(16):1781–1788

Hsieh AH, Wagner DR et al (2005) Dependence of mechanical behavior of the murine tail disc on regional material properties: a parametric finite element study. J Biomech Eng 127(7):1158–1167

Hsieh AH, Hwang D et al (2009) Degenerative anular changes induced by puncture are associated with insufficiency of disc biomechanical function. Spine (Phila Pa 1976) 34(10):998–1005

Hunter CJ, Matyas JR et al (2003) The notochordal cell in the nucleus pulposus: a review in the context of tissue engineering. Tissue Eng 9(4):667–677

Hutton WC, Elmer WA et al (2001) Do the intervertebral disc cells respond to different levels of hydrostatic pressure? Clin Biomech (Bristol, Avon) 16(9):728–734

Hwang D, Gabai AS et al (2012) Role of load history in intervertebral disc mechanics and intradiscal pressure generation. Biomech Model Mechanobiol 11(1–2):95–106

Iatridis JC, Mente PL et al (1999) Compression-induced changes in intervertebral disc properties in a rat tail model. Spine 24(10):996–1002

Ingber DE (2003) Mechanobiology and diseases of mechanotransduction. Ann Med 35(8):564–577

Janmey PA, Kinnunen PK (2006) Biophysical properties of lipids and dynamic membranes. Trends Cell Biol 16(10):538–546

Johnson WE, Roberts S (2003) Human intervertebral disc cell morphology and cytoskeletal composition: a preliminary study of regional variations in health and disease. J Anat 203(6):605–612

Kasra M, Goel V et al (2003) Effect of dynamic hydrostatic pressure on rabbit intervertebral disc cells. J Orthop Res 21(4):597–603

Kasra M, Merryman WD et al (2006) Frequency response of pig intervertebral disc cells subjected to dynamic hydrostatic pressure. J Orthop Res 24(10):1967–1973

Kluba T, Niemeyer T et al (2005) Human anulus fibrosis and nucleus pulposus cells of the intervertebral disc: effect of degeneration and culture system on cell phenotype. Spine 30(24):2743–2748

Koeller W, Funke F et al (1984) Biomechanical behavior of human intervertebral discs subjected to long lasting axial loading. Biorheology 21(5):675–686

Korecki CL, Kuo CK et al (2009) Intervertebral disc cell response to dynamic compression is age and frequency dependent. J Orthop Res 27(6):800–806

Kumar A, Varghese M et al (1999) Effect of whole-body vibration on the low back. A study of tractor-driving farmers in north India. Spine (Phila Pa 1976) 24(23):2506–2515

Le Maitre CL, Frain J et al (2009) Altered integrin mechanotransduction in human nucleus pulposus cells derived from degenerated discs. Arthritis Rheum 60(2):460–469

Leatt P, Reilly T et al (1986) Spinal loading during circuit weight-training and running. Br J Sports Med 20(3):119–124

Leivseth G, Drerup B (1997) Spinal shrinkage during work in a sitting posture compared to work in a standing posture. Clin Biomech (Bristol, Avon) 12(7–8):409–418

Li S, Duance VC et al (2008) Zonal variations in cytoskeletal element organization, mRNA and protein expression in the intervertebral disc. J Anat 213(6):725–732

Liu GZ, Ishihara H et al (2001) Nitric oxide mediates the change of proteoglycan synthesis in the human lumbar intervertebral disc in response to hydrostatic pressure. Spine 26(2):134–141

Lotz JC (2004) Animal models of intervertebral disc degeneration: lessons learned. Spine 29(23):2742–2750

Lotz JC (2011) Load and the spine. How does the Goldilocks principle apply? Spine J 11(1):44–45

Lotz JC, Chin JR (2000) Intervertebral disc cell death is dependent on the magnitude and duration of spinal loading. Spine 25(12):1477–1483

Lotz JC, Colliou OK et al (1998) Compression-induced degeneration of the intervertebral disc: an in vivo mouse model and finite-element study. Spine 23(23):2493–2506

Lotz JC, Hadi T et al (2008) Anulus fibrosus tension inhibits degenerative structural changes in lamellar collagen. Eur Spine J 17(9):1149–1159

Maclean JJ, Lee CR et al (2004) Anabolic and catabolic mRNA levels of the intervertebral disc vary with the magnitude and frequency of in vivo dynamic compression. J Orthop Res 22(6):1193–1200

MacLean JJ, Lee CR et al (2005) The effects of short-term load duration on anabolic and catabolic gene expression in the rat tail intervertebral disc. J Orthop Res 23(5):1120–1127

Marchand F, Ahmed AM (1990) Investigation of the laminate structure of lumbar disc anulus fibrosus. Spine 15(5):402–410

Matsumoto T, Kawakami M et al (1999) Cyclic mechanical stretch stress increases the growth rate and collagen synthesis of nucleus pulposus cells in vitro. Spine 24(4):315–319

McGill SM, van Wijk MJ et al (1996) Studies of spinal shrinkage to evaluate low-back loading in the workplace. Ergonomics 39(1):92–102

Minogue BM, Richardson SM et al (2010) Transcriptional profiling of bovine intervertebral disc cells: implications for identification of normal and degenerate human intervertebral disc cell phenotypes. Arthritis Res Ther 12(1):R22

Mitchell JA, Williams FM et al (1997) Role of nitric oxide in the dilator actions of capsaicin-sensitive nerves in the rabbit coronary circulation. Neuropeptides 31(4):333–338

Miyamoto H, Doita M et al (2006) Effects of cyclic mechanical stress on the production of inflammatory agents by nucleus pulposus and anulus fibrosus derived cells in vitro. Spine (Phila Pa 1976) 31(1):4–9

Miyazaki T, Kobayashi S et al (2009) A phenotypic comparison of proteoglycan production of intervertebral disc cells isolated from rats, rabbits, and bovine tails; which animal model is most suitable to study tissue engineering and biological repair of human disc disorders? Tissue Eng Part A 15(12):3835–3846

Na S, Collin O et al (2008) Rapid signal transduction in living cells is a unique feature of mechanotransduction. Proc Natl Acad Sci U S A 105(18):6626–6631

Neidlinger-Wilke C, Wurtz K et al (2006) Regulation of gene expression in intervertebral disc cells by low and high hydrostatic pressure. Eur Spine J 15(Suppl 3):S372–S378

Neidlinger-Wilke C, Liedert A et al (2009) Mechanical stimulation alters pleiotrophin and aggrecan expression by human intervertebral disc cells and influences their capacity to stimulate endothelial migration. Spine (Phila Pa 1976) 34(7):663–669

Nelson CM, Jean RP et al (2005) Emergent patterns of growth controlled by multicellular form and mechanics. Proc Natl Acad Sci U S A 102(33):11594–11599

Nettles DL, Richardson WJ et al (2004) Integrin expression in cells of the intervertebral disc. J Anat 204(6):515–520

Niosi CA, Oxland TR (2004) Degenerative mechanics of the lumbar spine. Spine J 4(6 Suppl):202S–208S

Oegema TR Jr, Johnson SL et al (2000) Fibronectin and its fragments increase with degeneration in the human intervertebral disc. Spine 25(21):2742–2747

Panel on Musculoskeletal Disorders and the Workplace, C. o. B. a. S. S. a. E., National Research Council (2001) Musculoskeletal disorders and the workplace. National Academy Press, Washington, DC

Parton RG, Simons K (2007) The multiple faces of caveolae. Nat Rev Mol Cell Biol 8(3):185–194

Paszek MJ, Zahir N et al (2005) Tensional homeostasis and the malignant phenotype. Cancer Cell 8(3):241–254

Paszek MJ, Boettiger D et al (2009) Integrin clustering is driven by mechanical resistance from the glycocalyx and the substrate. PLoS Comput Biol 5(12):e1000604

Patwardhan AG, Havey RM et al (1999) A follower load increases the load-carrying capacity of the lumbar spine in compression. Spine (Phila Pa 1976) 24(10):1003–1009

Patwardhan AG, Havey RM et al (2000) Load-carrying capacity of the human cervical spine in compression is increased under a follower load. Spine (Phila Pa 1976) 25(12):1548–1554

Patwardhan AG, Havey RM et al (2003) Effect of compressive follower preload on the flexion-extension response of the human lumbar spine. J Orthop Res 21(3):540–546

Pflaster DS, Krag MH et al (1997) Effect of test environment on intervertebral disc hydration. Spine (Phila Pa 1976) 22(2):133–139

Pritchard S, Guilak F (2004) The role of F-actin in hypo-osmotically induced cell volume change and calcium signaling in anulus fibrosus cells. Ann Biomed Eng 32(1):103–111

Race A, Broom ND et al (2000) Effect of loading rate and hydration on the mechanical properties of the disc. Spine (Phila Pa 1976) 25(6):662–669

Rannou F, Richette P et al (2003) Cyclic tensile stretch modulates proteoglycan production by intervertebral disc annulus fibrosus cells through production of nitrite oxide. J Cell Biochem 90(1):148–157

Ranu HS (1990) Measurement of pressures in the nucleus and within the annulus of the human spinal disc: due to extreme loading. Proc Inst Mech Eng H 204(3):141–146

Rastogi A, Thakore P et al (2009) Environmental regulation of notochordal gene expression in nucleus pulposus cells. J Cell Physiol 220(3):698–705

Rastogi A, Kim H et al. (2013) MMP-2 mediates local degradation and remodeling of collagen by annulus fibrosus cells of the intervertebral disc. Arthritis Res Ther 15(2):R57

Reza AT, Nicoll SB (2008) Hydrostatic pressure differentially regulates outer and inner annulus fibrosus cell matrix production in 3D scaffolds. Ann Biomed Eng 36(2):204–213

Richardson SM, Knowles R et al (2008) Aquaporin expression in the human intervertebral disc. J Mol Histol 39(3):303–309

Risbud MV, Shapiro IM (2011) Notochordal cells in the adult intervertebral disc: new perspective on an old question. Crit Rev Eukaryot Gene Expr 21(1):29–41

Roberts S, Menage J et al (1991) Type III collagen in the intervertebral disc. Histochem J 23(11–12):503–508

Rodacki AL, Fowler NE et al (2005) Body mass as a factor in stature change. Clin Biomech (Bristol, Avon) 20(8):799–805

Rohlmann A, Neller S et al (2001) Influence of a follower load on intradiscal pressure and intersegmental rotation of the lumbar spine. Spine (Phila Pa 1976) 26(24):E557–E561

Rousseau MA, Ulrich JA et al (2007) Stab incision for inducing intervertebral disc degeneration in the rat. Spine (Phila Pa 1976) 32(1):17–24

Sakai D, Nakai T et al (2009) Differential phenotype of intervertebral disc cells: microarray and immunohistochemical analysis of canine nucleus pulposus and anulus fibrosus. Spine (Phila Pa 1976) 34(14):1448–1456

Salvatierra JC, Yuan TY et al (2011) Difference in energy metabolism of annulus fibrosus and nucleus pulposus cells of the intervertebral disc. Cell Mol Bioeng 4(2):302–310

Schroeder Y, Wilson W et al (2006) Osmoviscoelastic finite element model of the intervertebral disc. Eur Spine J 15(Suppl 3):S361–S371

Screen HR, Lee DA et al (2004) An investigation into the effects of the hierarchical structure of tendon fascicles on micromechanical properties. Proc Inst Mech Eng H 218(2):109–119

Shirazi-Adl A, Drouin G (1987) Load-bearing role of facets in a lumbar segment under sagittal plane loadings. J Biomech 20(6):601–613
Shirazi-Adl A, Shrivastava SC et al (1984) Stress analysis of the lumbar disc-body unit in compression: a three dimensional nonlinear finite element study. Spine 9(2):120–134
Sinha B, Koster D et al (2011) Cells respond to mechanical stress by rapid disassembly of caveolae. Cell 144(3):402–413
Sniadecki NJ, Chen CS (2007) Microfabricated silicone elastomeric post arrays for measuring traction forces of adherent cells. Methods Cell Biol 83:313–328
Sowa G, Agarwal S (2008) Cyclic tensile stress exerts a protective effect on intervertebral disc cells. Am J Phys Med Rehabil 87(7):537–544
Sowa G, Coelho P et al (2011a) Determination of annulus fibrosus cell response to tensile strain as a function of duration, magnitude, and frequency. J Orthop Res 29(8):1275–1283
Sowa GA, Coelho JP et al (2011b) Alterations in gene expression in response to compression of nucleus pulposus cells. Spine J 11(1):36–43
Stokes I (1987) Surface strain on human intervertebral discs. J Orthop Res 5(3):348–355
Stokes I, Greenaple D (1985) Measurement of surface deformation of soft tissue. J Biomech 18(1):1–7
Terahata N, Ishihara H et al (1994) Effects of axial traction stress on solute transport and proteoglycan synthesis in the porcine intervertebral disc in vitro. Eur Spine J 3(6):325–330
Urban JPG, Maroudas A (1981) Swelling of the intervertebral disc in vitro. Connect Tissue Res 9:1–10
Urban JPG, McMullin JF (1985) Swelling pressure of the intervertebral disc: influence of proteoglycan and collagen contents. Biorheology 22:145–157
Urban JP, McMullin JF (1988) Swelling pressure of the lumbar intervertebral discs: influence of age, spinal level, composition, and degeneration. Spine 13(2):179–187
Urban JP, Roberts S et al (2000) The nucleus of the intervertebral disc from development to degeneration. Am Zool 40:53–61
Vande Geest JP, Di Martino ES et al (2004) An analysis of the complete strain field within Flexercell membranes. J Biomech 37(12):1923–1928
Vogel V, Baneyx G (2003) The tissue engineering puzzle: a molecular perspective. Annu Rev Biomed Eng 5:441–463
Walsh AJ, Lotz JC (2004) Biological response of the intervertebral disc to dynamic loading. J Biomech 37(3):329–337
Wang Y, Shyy JY et al (2008) Fluorescence proteins, live-cell imaging, and mechanobiology: seeing is believing. Annu Rev Biomed Eng 10:1–38
Wang P, Yang L et al (2011) Nucleus pulposus cell response to confined and unconfined compression implicates mechanoregulation by fluid shear stress. Ann Biomed Eng 39(3):1101–1111
Wenger KH, Woods JA et al (2005) Matrix remodeling expression in anulus cells subjected to increased compressive load. Spine (Phila Pa 1976) 30(10):1122–1126
Wilder DG, Pope MH (1996) Epidemiological and aetiological aspects of low back pain in vibration environments - an update. Clin Biomech (Bristol, Avon) 11(2):61–73
Wilke HJ, Neef P et al (1999) New in vivo measurements of pressures in the intervertebral disc in daily life. Spine 24(8):755–762
Wuertz K, Godburn K et al (2009) In vivo remodeling of intervertebral discs in response to short- and long-term dynamic compression. J Orthop Res 27(9):1235–1242
Xia M, Zhu Y (2008) Expression of integrin subunits in the herniated intervertebral disc. Connect Tissue Res 49(6):464–469
Xia M, Zhu Y (2011) Fibronectin fragment activation of ERK increasing integrin alpha and beta subunit expression to degenerate nucleus pulposus cells. J Orthop Res 29(4):556–561
Yamazaki S, Weinhold PS et al (2003) Annulus cells release ATP in response to vibratory loading in vitro. J Cell Biochem 90(4):812–818

The Role of the ADAMTS Proteins in the Intervertebral Disc

8

Jason C. Ho, James Wylie, and Suneel S. Apte

Contents

J.C. Ho • J. Wylie
Department of Biomedical Engineering, Orthopedic and Rheumatologic Institute, Cleveland Clinic, Cleveland, OH, USA

S.S. Apte (✉)
Department of Biomedical Engineering, Orthopedic and Rheumatologic Institute, Cleveland Clinic, Cleveland, OH, USA

Department of Biomedical Engineering, Lerner Research Institute- ND20, Cleveland Clinic, 9500 Euclid Avenue, Cleveland, OH 44195, USA
e-mail: aptes@ccf.org

I.M. Shapiro, M.V. Risbud (eds.), *The Intervertebral Disc*,
DOI 10.1007/978-3-7091-1535-0_8, © Springer-Verlag Wien 2014

8.1 Overview

8.1.1 Biological Significance and General Features of Proteinases

Proteinases (often referred to as proteases) are enzymes that hydrolyze the peptide bonds that hold amino acids together within a polypeptide (protein) molecule. Secreted and cell-surface proteinases are indispensable in several processes, such as digestion, molecular maturation, or activation of precursor proteins (proproteins), and in the turnover of diverse cellular products such as cell-surface receptors and extracellular matrix (ECM) proteins and proteoglycans. These last two functions are highly relevant to the skeletal system, which comprises ECM proteins, including proproteins such as procollagens, as quantitatively major components having an indispensable structural role. In addition, the ECM is increasingly being recognized for its role in regulating cell behavior, such as in signaling through cell-matrix adhesion molecules, and proteolytic products of ECM (matrikines). Proteinases are required for and participate in all major phases of vertebrate life, e.g., during embryonic development, they are required for rapid tissue remodeling, whereas in the adult organism, they participate in essential homeostatic processes, such as coagulation, or adaptive responses to biomechanical fluxes, e.g., bone and connective tissue remodeling in response to mechanical stress. They are recognized to have diverse, complex roles in the origin and/or resolution of inflammatory, degenerative, and malignant disorders. Indeed, proteinases, including ADAMTS proteinases, are frequently targeted for drug development because of their pivotal role in diseases (Fosang and Little 2008).

The functional core of every proteinase is its catalytic domain, which is the effector domain for proteolysis, and it is usually conjoined with an ancillary domain, required for binding to the target protein that is cleaved (a *substrate*). Through the combination of binding properties of the ancillary domain and the lock and key fit of the protease active site with its substrate, a *substrate specificity* ranging from stringent to promiscuous is determined. Most proteinases contain an N-terminal regulatory peptide segment or domain (the *propeptide*) that is involved in maintaining the enzyme in an inactive or latent state (the *zymogen*) until its activity is required. An intriguing aspect of proteinase biology is existence of natural (endogenous) inhibitors, which bind to and inactivate proteinases and protect against indiscriminate, excess polypeptide destruction. The proteinase's activity is further restricted to specific substrates by its precise spatial localization. This is determined by information within the protease (such as a transmembrane domain or heparin-binding domain) that limits its activity to specific spatial domains, e.g., cell-surface or pericellular matrix, or binding sites in ECM, which favors cleavage of the accessible substrates. Additionally, spatial and temporal regulation of expression, such as by transcriptional and post-transcriptional mechanisms, is also crucial in proteinase regulation. Proteinases should be thought of as molecular scissors, usually cutting with precision, rather than indiscriminately destructive enzymes. Thus, the biology of a proteinase is closely linked to biology of its substrates, and it is the effect on the substrate that is the most relevant to biologic and disease processes.

8.1.2 Historical Perspective and Evolution of Metalloproteinases

Proteinases are grouped into distinct classes based on the chemical nature of their catalytic mechanism or their preferred pH optimum. Metalloproteinases (now known as matrix metalloproteinases or MMPs) comprise a very large and diverse group of proteinases whose catalytic mechanism requires a metal ion, most commonly zinc. In 1962, Gross and Lapiere identified the first metalloproteinase (an interstitial collagenase) physiologically responsible for turnover of collagen, which is a triple helical rodlike molecule otherwise resistant to cleavage by most proteinases. They used an elegant, yet simple model, i.e., digestion of collagen in vitro by the resorbing vestigial structures of tadpoles during morphogenesis, to identify this protease (Gross and Lapiere 1962). Starting with characterization of the tadpole collagenase, the study of MMPs expanded considerably over the past half century to encompass closely related families: A disintegrin and metalloproteinase (ADAMs) (Klein and Bischoff 2011), followed by A disintegrin-like and metalloproteinase with thrombospondin type 1 motif (ADAMTS) proteinases (Apte 2009). Collectively, these proteinases are referred to as metzincins. In general, MMPs have the most diverse substrate repertoire, being involved in processing of multiple ECM components, cytokines, and other soluble proteins, as well as shedding of cell-surface proteins. ADAMs appear to be almost exclusively involved in ectodomain shedding of cell-surface molecules and have little reported direct action on the ECM. ADAMTS proteinases appear thus far to have major roles related to proteolysis of the ECM rather than cell-surface substrates.

ADAMTS and ADAM proteinase catalytic domains are related to enzymes present in hemorrhagic snake venoms, such as those from rattlesnakes, since only these proteinases, but not MMPs, have the active-site zinc-binding sequence HEXXH + HD (single amino acid nomenclature, X is any amino acid). This sequence is referred to as the reprolysin signature. ADAMTS and ADAM proteinases also have a similar zymogen activation mechanism, since their propeptides are proteolytically excised within the secretory pathway, at the cell surface, or extracellularly by proprotein convertases such as furin. In contrast, only a handful of MMPs, such as the membrane-type (MT) MMPs, utilize this mechanism. Instead, most MMPs have a "cysteine-switch mechanism" that results in exposure of the active-site cleft during activation. In contrast to ADAMs, which are transmembrane proteins with an extracellular catalytic domain, the ADAMTS proteinases are secreted, but they may function as operational cell-surface or cell-proximate proteinases through their binding to cell-surface/pericellular molecules (Fig. 8.1). Furthermore, despite sharing propeptide and catalytic domain features, ADAMs and ADAMTSs have entirely different ancillary domains (Fig. 8.1).

Once genome sequencing of many organisms was completed, it became apparent that the repertoire of genes encoding for extracellular matrix had expanded substantially in vertebrates (Huxley-Jones et al. 2009), which intuitively suggests the reason for an observed concomitant expansion of genes encoding metzincins (Huxley-Jones et al. 2007). Furthermore, tissue inhibitors of metalloproteinases (TIMPs), the main endogenous inhibitors of metalloproteinases, evolved from a single gene in *Drosophila* into the four human TIMPs studied today (Brew and Nagase 2010), further substantiating the significance of proteolysis in advanced biologic systems.

MMPs have been extensively studied in orthopaedic biology (Pasternak and Aspenberg 2009). For the purpose of this chapter, we will focus only on ADAMTS metalloproteinases and summarize their emerging roles in the intervertebral disc. ADAMs are mentioned where relevant, since they are often wrongly thought to be the same as ADAMTS proteinases yet have been neglected in the context of the disc.

The first ADAMTS protease (ADAMTS1) was identified 15 years ago by Kuno et al. (1997), as an inflammation associated gene product and initially thought to be a variant ADAM since it had the reprolysin-type catalytic domain (Kuno et al. 1997). Subsequent molecular cloning of 18 structurally similar proteinases, facilitated greatly by rapid progress in the human genome project, demonstrated the existence of this hitherto unknown metalloproteinase

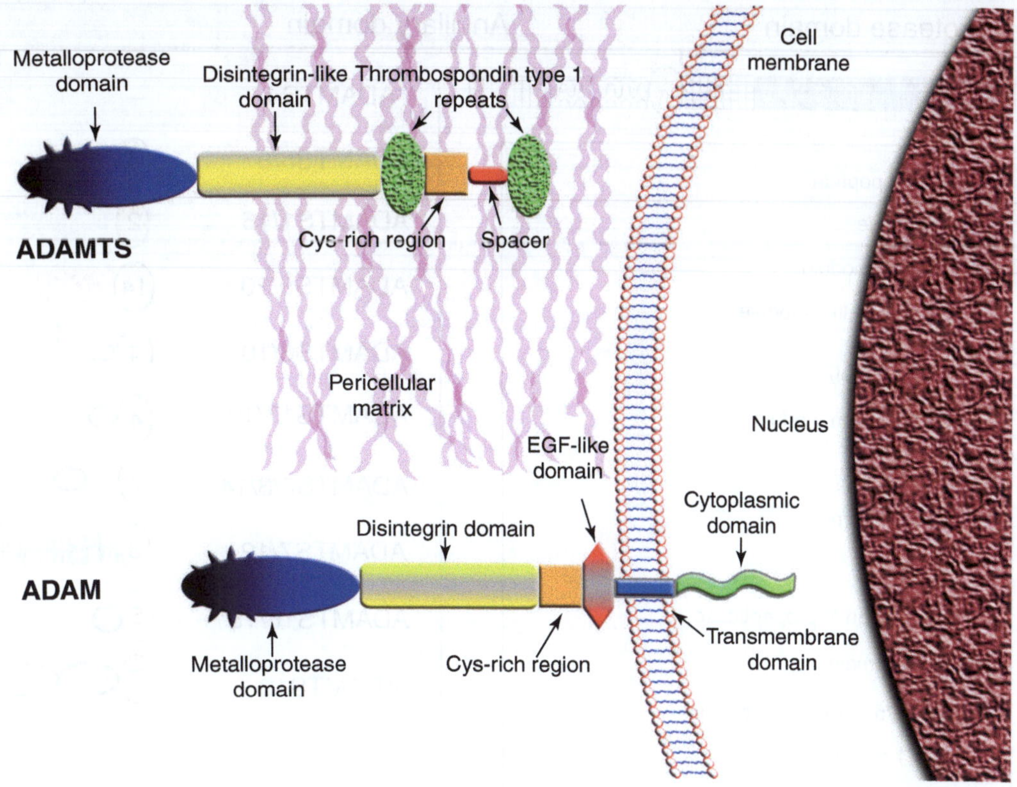

Fig. 8.1 Distinct domain structures and differential cell localization of ADAMTS and ADAM proteinases. The domain structures of ADAMTS5 and of a typical ADAM proteinase are shown in the context of the cell surface, with the various domains indicated. Note the transmembrane insertion of ADAMs. ADAMTS proteinases are secreted, but several bind near the cell surface, potentially through components of pericellular matrix or to cell-surface molecules

family as one that is distinct from ADAMs. It should be noted that the enzyme designated as ADAMTS11 (Abbaszade et al. 1999) is now referred to as ADAMTS5, and the designation ADAMTS11 is left vacant. Thus, although 20 ADAMTS numbers are assigned, there are 19 ADAMTS proteinases.

8.2 ADAMTS Structure and Function

Once the full repertoire of ADAMTS proteinases was determined, evolutionary analysis showed that they clustered into several distinct subgroups (Apte 2004; Huxley-Jones et al. 2005) (Fig. 8.2). Typically, ADAMTS proteinases within these subgroups have similar domain structures, high sequence similarity, and sufficient functional overlap that they work cooperatively in certain contexts. The ADAMTS ancillary domain consists of a disintegrin-like module, a thrombospondin type 1 repeat (TSR), a cysteine-rich region, a cysteine-free spacer region, one or more additional TSRs, as well as other modules (Apte 2009) (Fig. 8.2). The differences in the ancillary domains allow each proteinase to bind and act on distinct substrates, and with very few exceptions, ADAMTS catalytic domains without adjoining ancillary domains lack proteolytic activity. The detailed structure and posttranslational modification of ADAMTS proteases were previously reviewed (Apte 2009). Figure 8.1 contrasts the domain structure of a typical ADAMTS protease (ADAMTS5) with a prototypic ADAM, illustrating also the different localization with respect to cells.

A high degree of regulation of ADAMTS proteinases is a crucial aspect of their biology. Proprotein convertases such as furin cleave ADAMTS and ADAM proteinases after paired basic residues at the junction of the propeptide and catalytic domains. Furin processing of ADAMs mostly occurs within the secretory pathway, but some ADAMTS proteinases, such as ADAMTS5, ADAMTS7, and ADAMTS9, may be cleaved at the cell surface or extracellularly (Koo and Apte 2009; Longpré et al. 2009). Indeed, activation of stored zymogen in the ECM rather than de novo production of ADAMTS5 has been suggested as a potential mechanism for cartilage destruction in arthritis (Malfait et al. 2008; Wylie et al. 2012).

Of the four TIMPs, only TIMP3 is an ADAMTS/ADAM inhibitor; although all four TIMPs have inhibitory activity towards MMPs, certain TIMP-protease pairings (e.g., TIMP2-MMP2) show higher affinity. TIMP3 inhibitory activity towards ADAM17 and ADAMTS4 and ADAMTS5 implicates it as a key player in regulating inflammation and cartilage matrix breakdown (Kashiwagi et al. 2001; Sahebjam et al. 2007). As endogenous inhibitors of the metalloproteinases, TIMPs likely play an important role in ECM turnover of the intervertebral disc, although this has yet to be specifically investigated. The proteinase inhibitor α2-macroglobulin, which unlike TIMPs has an extremely broad spectrum of inhibition, is also capable of blocking ADAMTS

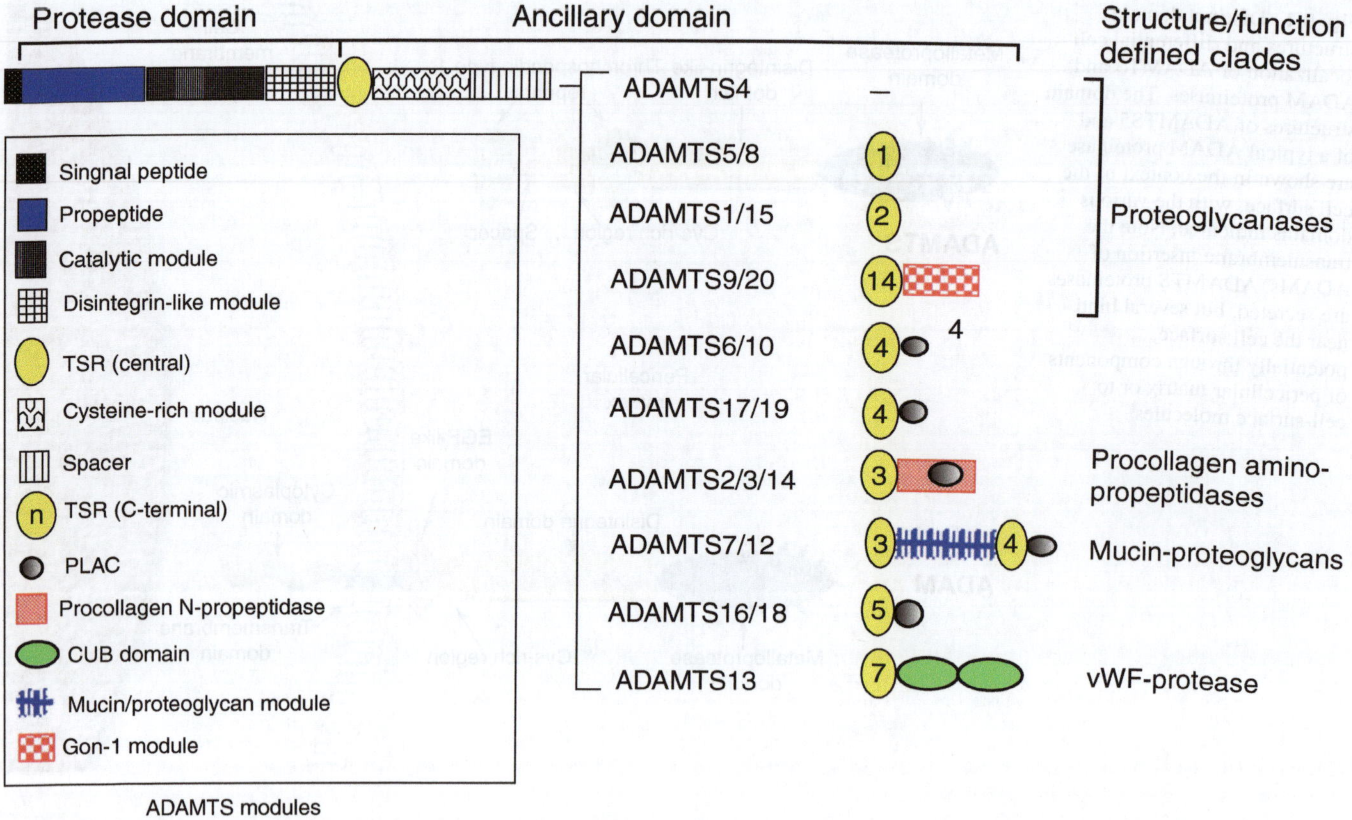

Fig. 8.2 Mammalian ADAMTS proteases. The domain backbone shared by each ADAMTS protease is shown at the *top*. The unique structure of each ADAMTS protease C-terminal to the backbone is indicated on the *right*, and the key to these modules is located at *left*. Some clades are named according to structural or functional characteristics that best define them; clades without a known function or a defining characteristic are not named. The proteoglycanases constitute a super-clade comprising ADAMTS proteases with different domain structures (The figure is based on reference sequences obtained from GenBank)

activity (Somerville et al. 2004; Tortorella et al. 2004) and presumably does so in the circulation.

Despite their brief history, functional contexts were rapidly established for several ADAMTS family members, aided by their clustering into functional family groups (Fig. 8.2), stringently established associations with hereditary and acquired diseases, and via several natural and engineered animal mutations. These are summarized in Table 8.1 and described in more detail in a previous review (Apte 2009). Since some of these molecular functions clearly have potential or established relevance to the intervertebral disc, they are discussed here and illustrated in Fig. 8.3. ADAMTS1 cleaves aggrecan, versican, thrombospondin-1 and thrombospondin-2, and the cell-surface proteoglycan syndecan-4 (Sandy et al. 2001; Lee et al. 2006; Rodríguez-Manzaneque et al. 2009). It is associated with inflammation, cancer cachexia, infertility, urinary tract anomalies, and bone metastasis and has potent antiangiogenic activity (Luque et al. 2003; Mittaz et al. 2004; Apte 2009; Lu et al. 2009). Thus, ADAMTS1 could be involved not only in matrix proteolysis but also in inflammatory disc disease. ADAMTS2, ADAMTS3, and ADAMTS14 are procollagen-processing enzymes involved in excision of the amino (N)-terminal propeptide of procollagens I, II, and III (Colige et al. 1999, 2002; Fernandes et al. 2001) but could also have additional properties unrelated to procollagens. Removal of the bulky procollagen N-propeptides is a prerequisite for proper collagen assembly. In the absence of ADAMTS2, an animal disorder named dermatosparaxis results, in which skin and other collagen-rich tissues show abnormal collagen fibrils (Lapière and Nusgens 1993), although the intervertebral disc was not one of the tissues specifically investigated. Dermatosparactic collagen forms branched and thin fibrils assuming a hieroglyphic or "cauliflower-like" pattern in electron microscopy, rather than highly ordered, broad, unbranched normal fibrils. These anomalous fibrils are structurally weak, a problem most strikingly evident in the exceedingly fragile skin of dermatosparactic cattle. A corresponding human-inherited connective tissue disorder, Ehlers-Danlos syndrome, dermatosparactic type, is similar in its clinical presentation (Colige et al. 1999). However, neither spine nor disc was specifically reported to be anomalous. In collagen II-rich tissues such as cartilage, ADAMTS3 is likely to have a more significant role than

Table 8.1 Functions of selected ADAMTS proteins and potential relevance to intervertebral disc biology

	Known functions	Potential function in IVD
ADAMTS1	Cleaves versican, thrombospondin-1 and thrombospondin-2, and syndecan-4; inhibits angiogenesis. Has a role in TGFβ activation. Null mice have impaired fertility, abnormal cardiac development, and hydronephrosis	Potentially involved in ECM turnover, TGFβ activation, and angiogenesis
ADAMTS2, ADAMTS3, ADAMTS14	Removal of amino-propeptide of procollagens I, II, and III. ADAMTS2 mutations lead to dermatosparaxis in animals and EDS dermatosparactic type in humans	Potential role in procollagen I and procollagen II processing, collagen assembly, and maintaining tensile strength of annulus fibrosus
ADAMTS4	Cleaves aggrecan and versican. Null mice are reported to be developmentally normal. Combinatorial null mice (with ADAMTS1) have a thin renal medulla	Potentially involved in proteoglycan turnover in nucleus pulposus, end plate, and perichondrium
ADAMTS5	Cleaves aggrecan, versican, and biglycan. ADAMTS5 null mice are resistant to induced cartilage degeneration. ADAMTS5 null mice lack embryonic sculpting of pulmonic valve leaflets and have reduced interdigital web regression. Cooperates with ADAMTS9 and ADAMTS20 in interdigital web regression	Potentially involved in proteoglycan turnover in nucleus pulposus, end plate, and perichondrium
ADAMTS7, ADAMTS12	Reported to bind to and cleave cartilage oligomeric protein (COMP, thrombospondin-5) and granulin-epithelin precursor. ADAMTS12 null mice are developmentally normal	Potentially involved in ECM turnover in annulus fibrosus
ADAMTS9	Cleaves aggrecan and versican. ADAMTS9 null mice die early during embryogenesis. ADAMTS9 haploinsufficient mice have cardiovascular defects. Cooperates with ADAMTS5 and ADAMTS20 in interdigital web regression and with ADAMTS20 in closure of the secondary palate in mice. ADAMTS9 is antiangiogenic	Potentially involved in proteoglycan turnover in nucleus pulposus, end plate, and perichondrium and regulation of angiogenesis
ADAMTS10	Binds to and possibly cleaves fibrillin-1. Promotes fibrillin microfibril assembly. ADAMTS10 is mutated in Weill-Marchesani syndrome in humans	Potential role in fibrillin microfibril assembly
ADAMTS13	ADAMTS13 is required for maturation of ultra-large forms of von Willebrand factor. ADAMTS13 mutations or autoantibodies lead to thrombotic thrombocytopenic purpura	
ADAMTS17	ADAMTS17 mutations lead to a Weill-Marchesani-like syndrome in humans and recessive isolated ectopia lentis in dogs	Potentially involved in fibrillin microfibril assembly
ADAMTS20	Cleaves versican. ADAMTS20 mutations in mice lead to a white spotting mutant named *belted* (*bt*)	Potentially involved in versican turnover
ADAMTSL2	ADAMTSL2 binds to fibrillin-1 and latent TGFβ-binding protein 1. ADAMTSL2 mutations lead to geleophysic dysplasia. In dogs, ADAMTSL2 mutations lead to Musladin-Lueke syndrome	Expressed in IVD. Potentially involved in regulating TGFβ binding and/or activation
ADAMTSL4	ADAMTSL4 binds to fibrillin-1 and enhances microfibril biogenesis in cultured fibroblasts. ADAMTSL4 mutations lead to recessive isolated ectopia lentis in the eye	Potentially involved in microfibril assembly
ADAMTSL6	ADAMTSL6 binds to fibrillin-1 and enhances microfibril biogenesis in cultured fibroblasts and transgenic mice when it is overexpressed	Potentially involved in microfibril assembly

ADAMTS2 because of its expression in cartilage and demonstrated ability to process procollagen II (Le Goff et al. 2006).

ADAMTS1, ADAMTS4, ADAMTS5, ADAMTS9, and ADAMTS20 have the ability to cleave the large aggregating chondroitin sulfate proteoglycans aggrecan and versican at specific sites in their core proteins (Apte 2009). ADAMTS9 is also an antiangiogenic protease that is widely distributed in microvascular endothelial cells of most organs as an apparently constitutive product (Koo et al. 2010). ADAMTS4 and ADAMTS5 seem to be the most important aggrecan-degrading proteinases (aggrecanases) in the articular cartilage degradation in arthritis (Fosang and Little 2008) and have thus been most extensively investigated in the intervertebral disc, although much on the published analysis is of gene expression and protein distribution rather than de novo functional analysis. ADAMTS7 and ADAMTS12 are unique proteinases in also being chondroitin sulfate proteoglycans (Somerville et al. 2004), the only known proteinases in mammalian genomes to have this property. They cleave cartilage oligomeric matrix protein (COMP) (Liu et al. 2006), which is an important component of cartilage ECM, as well as granulin-epithelin precursor (GEP) (Guo et al. 2010), a growth factor reported to be involved in tissue regeneration and inflammation (Bai et al. 2009). GEP was reported to act as a competitive inhibitor of ADAMTS7 and ADAMTS12 (Guo et al. 2010). Based on being a target of PTHrP and cleavage of GEP, ADAMTS7 was proposed as a negative regulator of endochondral bone formation, but this remains to be substantiated in genetic models (Bai et al. 2009; Liu 2009).

ADAMTS10 is mutated in a connective tissue disorder named recessive Weill-Marchesani syndrome (WMS). The identification of dominantly inherited fibrillin-1 mutations in WMS (Faivre et al. 2003; Sengle et al. 2012) suggested a functional link between ADAMTS10 and fibrillin-1. Such fibrillin-1 mutations typically lead to Marfan syndrome, yet WMS appears to constitute an "opposite of Marfan syndrome," featuring short stature, short digits, stiff skin and

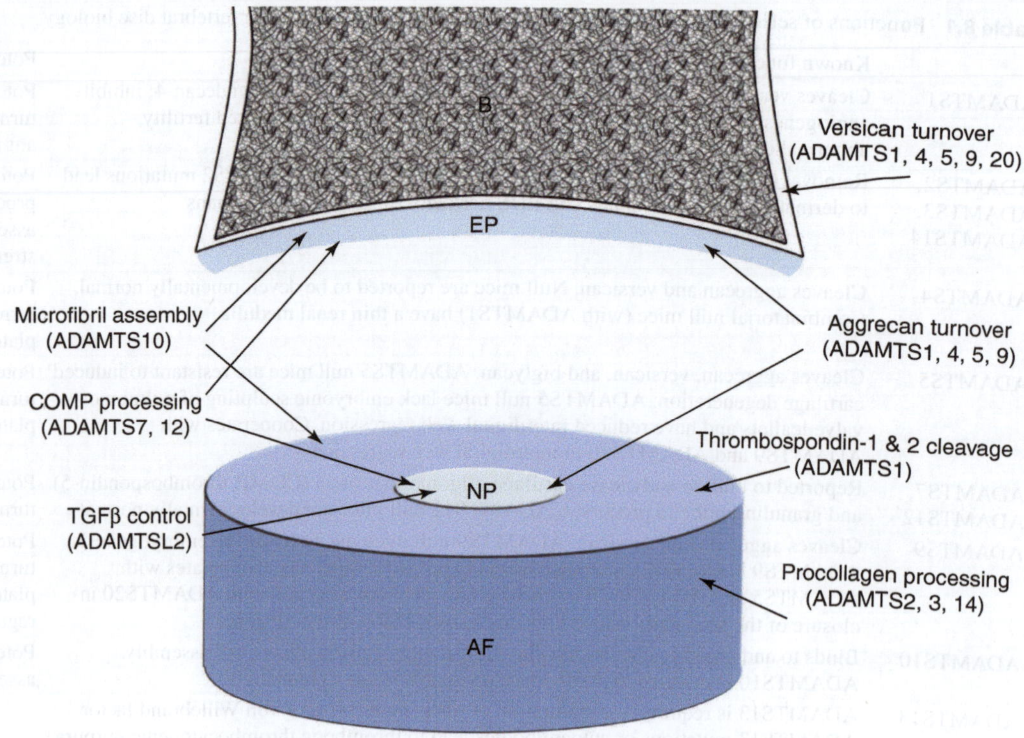

Fig. 8.3 Potential roles of ADAMTS proteinases in various processes within the context of intervertebral disc components. The nucleus pulposus (*NP*), annulus fibrosus (*AF*), cartilaginous end plate (*EP*), and vertebral bone (*B*) are indicated

joints, and in the eye, lens dislocation, and glaucoma. Recent work showed that ADAMTS10 bound to fibrillin-1 and fibrillin-2 was associated with fibrillin microfibrils in tissues and enhanced fibrillin-1 microfibrils formation in vitro (Kutz et al. 2011).

A unique aspect of ADAMTS proteases is the existence of a closely related family of seven independent gene products resembling ADAMTS ancillary domains (Apte 2009). These molecules, named ADAMTS-like proteins (ADAMTSL), lack catalytic domains and are therefore not proteinases; however, together with ADAMTS proteinases, they are thought to comprise a protein superfamily. Intriguingly, like ADAMTS10, the majority of ADAMTSLs, specifically, ADAMTSL2, ADAMTSL3, ADAMTSL4, and ADAMTSL6, also bind to or influence microfibril formation (Le Goff et al. 2011; Saito et al. 2011; Gabriel et al. 2012; Sengle et al. 2012) (Table 8.1). Human genetic disorders resulting from ADAMTSL2 or ADAMTSL4 mutations, i.e., geleophysic dysplasia (GD) and isolated ectopia lentis, respectively, are also caused by fibrillin-1 mutations, and both these proteins bind to fibrillin-1 (Hubmacher and Apte 2011; Le Goff et al. 2011). The mutations in GD lead to a short-stature, short-digit phenotype superficially resembling WMS (these conditions fall within a category named acromelic dysplasias), although GD is much more severe and frequently lethal in children because of cardiac involvement; however, unlike WMS, it lacks ocular involvement (Le Goff et al. 2008). ADAMTSL2 mutations in dogs also cause dwarfism and severe skin and joint stiffness, a connective tissue disorder named Musladin-Lueke syndrome (Bader et al. 2010). Analysis of cells from GD patients has suggested that there is profound TGFβ dysregulation, likely related to the pivotal role of fibrillin microfibrils in regulating TGFβ and bone morphogenetic proteins (Le Goff et al. 2008). Indeed, ADAMTSL2 also binds to latent TGFβ-binding protein-1 (LTBP1), which strongly supports a role in TGFβ sequestration in ECM or activation. We recently reviewed the strong functional involvement of ADAMTS proteinases in connective tissue regulation vis-à-vis fibrillins, specifically, in regulating the cellular microenvironment (Hubmacher and Apte 2011). ADAMTSL2 is expressed in the nucleus pulposus of the intervertebral disc (Koo et al. 2007; Sohn et al. 2010), and it could have a role in disc development because of the established role of TGFβ signaling in this process (Sohn et al. 2010).

Another cluster of ADAMTS proteinases highly relevant to IVD is the so-called proteoglycanase cluster, containing ADAMTS1, ADAMTS4, ADAMTS5, ADAMTS9, and ADAMTS20 (Apte 2004; Huxley-Jones et al. 2005). The major proteoglycan substrates of these proteinases are aggrecan, a cartilage-specific chondroitin sulfate proteoglycan, and its widely distributed relative in non-cartilaginous tissues, versican. The role of these proteinases in aggrecan destruction in osteoarthritis has been investigated by stringent analysis of null mice, biochemical assays, and association of mRNA, protein, and catabolic fragments with arthritic cartilage (Fosang and Little 2008). ADAMTS5-deficient mice are protected against either a mechanical instability-induced or cytokine-induced cartilage breakdown (Glasson et al. 2005; Stanton et al. 2005).

Although these five enzymes are potent aggrecanases, which of them has a role in physiological aggrecan breakdown, such as in skeletal development, is unclear. However, some of them were discovered to have a crucial role in turnover of versican in several developmental contexts, specifically, myocardial compaction, closure of the secondary palate, sculpting of heart valves, and resorption of interdigital webs (Stankunas et al. 2008; McCulloch et al. 2009; Enomoto et al. 2010; Dupuis et al. 2011). Two intriguing findings emerged from these discoveries: One, that proteoglycanases cooperated in versican proteolysis in the context of palate closure and web regression, and two, that a product of versican proteolysis was a matrikine with context-dependent function in cell proliferation or apoptosis in these processes (McCulloch et al. 2009; Enomoto et al. 2010). Further study of these families will no doubt find other important functions of these proteinases in normal development and disease pathogenesis.

In contrast to these functions of ADAMTS proteinases which are directly relevant to extracellular matrix maturation, assembly, and turnover, ADAMs are primarily involved in ectodomain shedding of cell-surface molecules. In particular they are identified to have a pivotal role in growth control through epidermal growth factor receptor signaling pathways, in cell adhesion, in Notch signaling, and in inflammation through processing of pro-TNF-α and cytokine receptors (Klein and Bischoff 2011; Saftig and Reiss 2011). Thus, ADAM proteinases may play a role in disc development and degeneration through modulation of these and several other pathways. Unfortunately direct effects of ADAM proteinases in the intervertebral disc have not been elucidated to any significant extent, and it remains an area of opportunity for future research.

8.3 ADAMTS Proteinases in Intervertebral Disc Biology and Disease

Three anatomic components of the intervertebral disc are relevant to its physiology and pathology in regard to metalloproteinases, namely the cartilaginous end plates, annulus fibrosus, and nucleus pulposus, which act together to fulfill the biological and mechanical functions of the disc but also differ in their matrix structure because each is mechanically specialized. The two major components of the ECM in the disc are the proteoglycan aggrecan and collagen, which are cleaved and modulated by ADAMTS proteinases. Collagen I, II, III, V, VI, IX, XI, XII, and XIV can be found in the disc at varying levels and will also change with age (Eyre et al. 2002). Of the collagens, I and II are most abundant, with I comprising the outer layers of the annulus fibrosus and II mainly located in the nucleus. Besides aggrecan in the nucleus pulposus, other proteoglycans found in lower amounts include versican, decorin, biglycan, fibromodulin, lumican, and perlecan (Roughley 2004). Aggrecan is found in both the nucleus pulposus and annulus fibrosus, mostly as aggregates complexed with hyaluronan and link protein, although it makes up a larger proportion of the nucleus pulposus (65 % dry weight) than the annulus fibrosus (15–20 % dry weight) (Le Maitre et al. 2007). The CEP of the vertebral bodies are similar in content and structure to articular cartilage found in other joints and are primarily comprised of collagen II fibers with aggrecan aggregates complexed to hyaluronan and link protein. Previous chapters in this book (Chaps. 4 and 5) provide further details regarding the roles of the proteoglycans and collagens in the intervertebral disc.

As the intervertebral disc ages, its ECM undergoes significant catabolic changes in which ADAMTS proteinases are likely to have a role. The majority of experimental studies to date have focused on the levels and localization of ADAMTS4, ADAMTS5, and catabolic products of aggrecan. Using immunohistochemistry, ADAMTS4 was detected in nondegrading disc cells from the nucleus pulposus and inner annulus fibrosus, with little immunoreactivity in the outer annulus fibrosus, suggesting a maintenance role, but in degenerated discs, the authors found an increase in ADAMTS4 that correlated with the severity of degeneration and increased TIMP1 and TIMP2 but not TIMP3 (Le Maitre et al. 2004). It was also found that the presence of inflammatory modulators such as TNF-α and IL-1 increased ADAMTS4 and ADAMTS5 expression and ADAMTS aggrecan degradation (Le Maitre et al. 2005; Séguin et al. 2005). Toll-like receptor adaptor signaling molecule MyD88 antagonized LPS or IL-1-mediated induction of ADAMTS4 and ADAMTS5 (Ellman et al. 2012). An immunohistochemical analysis of surgically resected discs showed ADAMTS4 primarily in CD68-positive mononuclear cells (monocyte/macrophages) in granulation tissue and adjacent disc, with a higher number of stained cells associated with specific herniation patterns (transligamentous extrusion and sequestration). A recent detailed analysis investigated the role of syndecan-4 in ADAMTS5 activity in nucleus pulposus cells. TNF-α and IL-1α increased ADAMTS4 and ADAMTS5 expression and promoted syndecan-4 interaction with ADAMTS5 (Wang et al. 2011). This was consistent with an association of aggrecan degradation with increased syndecan-4 and ADAMTS5 in the human intervertebral disc (Wang et al. 2011).

In addition to inflammatory modulators, studies have also shown that mechanical loading can alter proteinase expression (Maclean et al. 2004; MacLean et al. 2005). Long-term upright posture in rats demonstrated increased disc expression of *MMP13*, *ADAMTS5*, and *Col10a1* and decreased *Col2a1* and *Acan* (Liang et al. 2008). Static compression of rat disc led to upregulation of ADAMTS4, but not ADAMTS5, with concomitant increase of aggrecan catabolic fragments

(Yurube et al. 2012). Loading of rat caudal intervertebral discs was noted to increase expression of ADAMTS7 and ADAMTS12 mRNA (Yu and Zhu 2012). In human nucleus pulposus cells, a dynamic compressive load led to upregulation of ADAMTS1, ADAMTS4, and ADAMTS5 mRNA and the respective proteins (Huang et al. 2012), with the response to cyclic tensile stress being frequency dependent (Gilbert et al. 2010).

A comparative gene expression analysis of healthy and severely degenerated discs identified downregulation of ADAMTSL3 and ADAMTS10 mRNA in degenerated discs (Gruber et al. 2011). When comparing degenerated versus nondegenerated discs, it was found that *ADAMTS1*, *ADAMTS4*, *ADAMTS5*, and *ADAMTS15* expression were significantly increased in degenerated tissue and ADAMTS4, ADAMTS5, ADAMTS9, and ADAMTS15 immunohistochemical staining also increased (Pockert et al. 2009). A study of human discs suggested that ADAMTS5 was involved in intervertebral disc degeneration and that IL-1 induction of ADAMTS5 was mediated by nitric oxide (Zhao et al. 2011); another showed multiple positive correlations between MMPs and ADAMTS4 mRNA in herniated discs. In addition to defining the expression of proteinases in the disc itself, there appear to be significant differences among the cell types of the disc. It was found that nucleus pulposus cells express more ADAMTS1, ADAMTS2, ADAMTS17, and TIMP1, whereas ADAMTS4, ADAMTS5, ADAMTS6, ADAMTS14, ADAMTS18, ADAMTS19 and TIMP3 were lower in nucleus cells versus articular chondrocytes (Cui et al. 2010). A sheep annulus fibrosus transection model showed increased ADAMTS5 mRNA and ADAMTS4 mRNA in the annulus, but only ADAMTS5 mRNA increased in the nucleus pulposus, whereas ADAMTS4 mRNA decreased; however, there was no change in aggrecan neoepitopes (Melrose et al. 2012).

ADAMTS1 and ADAMTS5 were identified as candidate genes for lumbar disc disease in the Finnish population (Virtanen et al. 2007). A gene-profiling study comparing chondrocytes and nucleus pulposus cells found that NP cells expressed higher levels of ADAMTS1, ADAMTS2, and ADAMTS17, but lower levels of ADAMTS4, ADAMTS5, ADAMTS6, ADAMTS14, ADAMTS18, ADAMTS19, and TIMP3. Such analysis could be useful in identifying differences between the metabolic pathways of chondrocytes and nucleus pulposus cells. ADAMTS5 mRNA was increased in rat nucleus pulposus cells after inflammatory stimulation via a NO-dependent pathway, and the amount of ADAMTS5 protein appeared to increase with increasing age (Zhao et al. 2011). It was also found that ADAMTS4, but not ADAMTS5, content was higher in Grade 4 versus Grade 2 degenerative tissue, but there was no difference in the amount of fragments in each group, suggesting involvement of other proteases such as MMPs in turnover of aggrecan (Patel et al. 2007).

An intriguing study suggested that immunity to the versican G1 domain led to development of spondylitis in mice (Shi et al. 2003). Since one of the versican fragments released by ADAMTS proteases primarily comprises the G1 domain, it is an interesting possibility that humoral immunity to ADAMTS cleaved and released versican G1 domain could have a role in development of spinal pathology.

Figure 8.3 summarizes the various ways in which ADAMTS superfamily proteins, including ADAMTS proteinases and ADAMTSLs, could influence intervertebral disc biology and disease. Expectedly, analysis of aggrecan breakdown has seen the lion's share of attention, owing to its relevance for disc degeneration. The considerable evidence accumulated to date strongly associates ADAMTS4 and ADAMTS5 with aggrecan breakdown in the nucleus pulposus; however, definitive experiments using genetically deficient mice remain to be done. As shown in Fig. 8.3, the procollagen proteinases could have a crucial role in normal disc development and repair, since their function appears to be primarily anabolic. The evidence for expression of ADAMTS7 and ADAMTS12 in the intervertebral disc is compelling, but the precise functions of these proteinases remain unknown. The most intriguing possibilities, however, are related to the potential for microenvironmental regulation by ADAMTSLs and ADAMTS10. ADAMTSL2 and ADAMTS10 (authors unpublished data) are both expressed in the intervertebral disc, associated with inherited connective tissue disorders and functionally linked to fibrillins, which control both TGFβs and bone morphogenetic proteins. Their potential role is worthy of further investigation. A major challenge, however, is functional overlap (referred to as redundancy) between such functionally related proteins that requires complex combinatorial genetics to elucidate their true roles. Finally, the ADAMs have been substantially neglected in disc research, yet their function is highly relevant to tissue inflammation and repair.

8.4 Summary of Critical Concepts Discussed in the Chapter

- The proteolytic activities and regulatory mechanisms of ADAMTS and ADAM proteinases have considerable potential relevance for the intervertebral disc.
- ADAMTS proteinases have been studied in the disc primarily at the level of mRNA and protein expression. The published work has focused on a small number of proteases, namely, ADAMTS4, ADAMTS5, and ADAMTS7, yet the activities of many other family members as well as ADAMTSLs are worthy of deeper investigation.
- ADAM proteinases have not been extensively investigated in disc disease and are likely to be highly relevant to inflammation and cell-surface proteolysis.

- With further investigation into the roles of these proteinases into pathogenesis of intervertebral disc disease, future identification of potential disease-modifying targets is viable and could capitalize on availability of several well-characterized proteinase inhibitors.

Acknowledgment This work was supported by NIH award AR53890.

References

Abbaszade I, Liu RQ, Yang F, Rosenfeld SA, Ross OH, Link JR, Ellis DM, Tortorella MD, Pratta MA, Hollis JM, Wynn R, Duke JL, George HJ, Hillman MC Jr, Murphy K, Wiswall BH, Copeland RA, Decicco CP, Bruckner R, Nagase H, Itoh Y, Newton RC, Magolda RL, Trzaskos JM, Burn TC (1999) Cloning and characterization of ADAMTS11, an aggrecanase from the ADAMTS family. J Biol Chem 274:23443–23450

Apte SS (2004) A disintegrin-like and metalloprotease (reprolysin type) with thrombospondin type 1 motifs: the ADAMTS family. Int J Biochem Cell Biol 36:981–985

Apte SS (2009) A disintegrin-like and metalloprotease (reprolysin-type) with thrombospondin type 1 motif (ADAMTS) superfamily: functions and mechanisms. J Biol Chem 284:31493–31497

Bader HL, Ruhe AL, Wang LW, Wong AK, Walsh KF, Packer RA, Mitelman J, Robertson KR, O'Brien DP, Broman KW, Shelton GD, Apte SS, Neff MW (2010) An ADAMTSL2 founder mutation causes Musladin-Lueke Syndrome, a heritable disorder of beagle dogs, featuring stiff skin and joint contractures. PLoS One 5

Bai X-H, Wang D-W, Kong L, Zhang Y, Luan Y, Kobayashi T, Kronenberg HM, Yu X-P, Liu C-J (2009) ADAMTS-7, a direct target of PTHrP, adversely regulates endochondral bone growth by associating with and inactivating GEP growth factor. Mol Cell Biol 29:4201–4219

Brew K, Nagase H (2010) The tissue inhibitors of metalloproteinases (TIMPs): an ancient family with structural and functional diversity. Biochim Biophys Acta 1803:55–71

Colige A, Sieron AL, Li SW, Schwarze U, Petty E, Wertelecki W, Wilcox W, Krakow D, Cohn DH, Reardon W, Byers PH, Lapière CM, Prockop DJ, Nusgens BV (1999) Human Ehlers-Danlos syndrome type VII C and bovine dermatosparaxis are caused by mutations in the procollagen I N-proteinase gene. Am J Hum Genet 65:308–317

Colige A, Vandenberghe I, Thiry M, Lambert CA, Van Beeumen J, Li S-W, Prockop DJ, Lapiere CM, Nusgens BV (2002) Cloning and characterization of ADAMTS-14, a novel ADAMTS displaying high homology with ADAMTS-2 and ADAMTS-3. J Biol Chem 277:5756–5766

Cui Y, Yu J, Urban JPG, Young DA (2010) Differential gene expression profiling of metalloproteinases and their inhibitors: a comparison between bovine intervertebral disc nucleus pulposus cells and articular chondrocytes. Spine 35:1101–1108

Dupuis LE, McCulloch DR, McGarity JD, Bahan A, Wessels A, Weber D, Diminich AM, Nelson CM, Apte SS, Kern CB (2011) Altered versican cleavage in ADAMTS5 deficient mice; a novel etiology of myxomatous valve disease. Dev Biol 357:152–164

Ellman MB, Kim J-S, An HS, Chen D, Kc R, An J, Dittakavi T, van Wijnen AJ, Cs-Szabo G, Li X, Xiao G, An S, Kim S-G, Im H-J (2012) Toll-like receptor adaptor signaling molecule MyD88 on intervertebral disk homeostasis: in vitro, ex vivo studies. Gene 505:283–290

Enomoto H, Nelson CM, Somerville RPT, Mielke K, Dixon LJ, Powell K, Apte SS (2010) Cooperation of two ADAMTS metalloproteases in closure of the mouse palate identifies a requirement for versican proteolysis in regulating palatal mesenchyme proliferation. Development 137:4029–4038

Eyre DR, Matsui Y, Wu J-J (2002) Collagen polymorphisms of the intervertebral disc. Biochem Soc Trans 30:844–848

Faivre L, Gorlin RJ, Wirtz MK, Godfrey M, Dagoneau N, Samples JR, Le Merrer M, Collod-Beroud G, Boileau C, Munnich A, Cormier-Daire V (2003) In frame fibrillin-1 gene deletion in autosomal dominant Weill-Marchesani syndrome. J Med Genet 40: 34–36

Fernandes RJ, Hirohata S, Engle JM, Colige A, Cohn DH, Eyre DR, Apte SS (2001) Procollagen II amino propeptide processing by ADAMTS-3. Insights on dermatosparaxis. J Biol Chem 276: 31502–31509

Fosang AJ, Little CB (2008) Drug insight: aggrecanases as therapeutic targets for osteoarthritis. Nat Clin Pract Rheumatol 4:420–427

Gabriel LAR, Wang LW, Bader H, Ho JC, Majors AK, Hollyfield JG, Traboulsi EI, Apte SS (2012) ADAMTSL4, a secreted glycoprotein widely distributed in the eye, binds fibrillin-1 microfibrils and accelerates microfibril biogenesis. Invest Ophthalmol Vis Sci 53: 461–469

Gilbert HTJ, Hoyland JA, Millward-Sadler SJ (2010) The response of human annulus fibrosus cells to cyclic tensile strain is frequency-dependent and altered with disc degeneration. Arthritis Rheum 62:3385–3394

Glasson SS, Askew R, Sheppard B, Carito B, Blanchet T, Ma H-L, Flannery CR, Peluso D, Kanki K, Yang Z, Majumdar MK, Morris EA (2005) Deletion of active ADAMTS5 prevents cartilage degradation in a murine model of osteoarthritis. Nature 434:644–648

Gross J, Lapiere CM (1962) Collagenolytic activity in amphibian tissues: a tissue culture assay. Proc Natl Acad Sci U S A 48: 1014–1022

Gruber HE, Hoelscher GL, Ingram JA, Bethea S, Zinchenko N, Hanley EN Jr (2011) Variations in aggrecan localization and gene expression patterns characterize increasing stages of human intervertebral disk degeneration. Exp Mol Pathol 91:534–539

Guo F, Lai Y, Tian Q, Lin EA, Kong L, Liu C (2010) Granulin-epithelin precursor binds directly to ADAMTS-7 and ADAMTS-12 and inhibits their degradation of cartilage oligomeric matrix protein. Arthritis Rheum 62:2023–2036

Huang M, Wang H-Q, Zhang Q, Yan X-D, Hao M, Luo Z-J (2012) Alterations of ADAMTSs and TIMP-3 in human nucleus pulposus cells subjected to compressive load: implications in the pathogenesis of human intervertebral disc degeneration. J Orthop Res 30:267–273

Hubmacher D, Apte SS (2011) Genetic and functional linkage between ADAMTS superfamily proteins and fibrillin-1: a novel mechanism influencing microfibril assembly and function. Cell Mol Life Sci 68:3137–3148

Huxley-Jones J, Apte SS, Robertson DL, Boot-Handford RP (2005) The characterisation of six ADAMTS proteases in the basal chordate Ciona intestinalis provides new insights into the vertebrate ADAMTS family. Int J Biochem Cell Biol 37:1838–1845

Huxley-Jones J, Clarke T-K, Beck C, Toubaris G, Robertson DL, Boot-Handford RP (2007) The evolution of the vertebrate metzincins; insights from Ciona intestinalis and Danio rerio. BMC Evol Biol 7:63

Huxley-Jones J, Pinney JW, Archer J, Robertson DL, Boot-Handford RP (2009) Back to basics–how the evolution of the extracellular matrix underpinned vertebrate evolution. Int J Exp Pathol 90:95–100

Kashiwagi M, Tortorella M, Nagase H, Brew K (2001) TIMP-3 is a potent inhibitor of aggrecanase 1 (ADAM-TS4) and aggrecanase 2 (ADAM-TS5). J Biol Chem 276:12501–12504

Klein T, Bischoff R (2011) Active metalloproteases of the A Disintegrin and Metalloprotease (ADAM) family: biological function and structure. J Proteome Res 10:17–33

Koo B-H, Apte SS (2009) Cell-surface processing of the metalloprotease pro-ADAMTS9 is influenced by the chaperone GRP94/GP96. J Biol Chem 285(1):197–205

Koo B-H, Le Goff C, Jungers KA, Vasanji A, O'Flaherty J, Weyman CM, Apte SS (2007) ADAMTS-like 2 (ADAMTSL2) is a secreted glycoprotein that is widely expressed during mouse embryogenesis and is regulated during skeletal myogenesis. Matrix Biol 26:431–441

Koo B-H, Coe DM, Dixon LJ, Somerville RPT, Nelson CM, Wang LW, Young ME, Lindner DJ, Apte SS (2010) ADAMTS9 is a cell-autonomously acting, anti-angiogenic metalloprotease expressed by microvascular endothelial cells. Am J Pathol 176:1494–1504

Kuno K, Kanada N, Nakashima E, Fujiki F, Ichimura F, Matsushima K (1997) Molecular cloning of a gene encoding a new type of metalloproteinase-disintegrin family protein with thrombospondin motifs as an inflammation associated gene. J Biol Chem 272:556–562

Kutz WE, Wang LW, Bader HL, Majors AK, Iwata K, Traboulsi EI, Sakai LY, Keene DR, Apte SS (2011) ADAMTS10 protein interacts with fibrillin-1 and promotes its deposition in extracellular matrix of cultured fibroblasts. J Biol Chem 286:17156–17167

Lapière CM, Nusgens BV (1993) Ehlers-Danlos type VII-C, or human dermatosparaxis. The offspring of a union between basic and clinical research. Arch Dermatol 129:1316–1319

Le Goff C, Somerville RPT, Kesteloot F, Powell K, Birk DE, Colige AC, Apte SS (2006) Regulation of procollagen amino-propeptide processing during mouse embryogenesis by specialization of homologous ADAMTS proteases: insights on collagen biosynthesis and dermatosparaxis. Development 133:1587–1596

Le Goff C, Morice-Picard F, Dagoneau N, Wang LW, Perrot C, Crow YJ, Bauer F, Flori E, Prost-Squarcioni C, Krakow D, Ge G, Greenspan DS, Bonnet D, Le Merrer M, Munnich A, Apte SS, Cormier-Daire V (2008) ADAMTSL2 mutations in geleophysic dysplasia demonstrate a role for ADAMTS-like proteins in TGF-beta bioavailability regulation. Nat Genet 40:1119–1123

Le Goff C, Mahaut C, Wang LW, Allali S, Abhyankar A, Jensen S, Zylberberg L, Collod-Beroud G, Bonnet D, Alanay Y, Brady AF, Cordier M-P, Devriendt K, Genevieve D, Kiper PÖS, Kitoh H, Krakow D, Lynch SA, Le Merrer M, Mégarbane A, Mortier G, Odent S, Polak M, Rohrbach M, Sillence D, Stolte-Dijkstra I, Superti-Furga A, Rimoin DL, Topouchian V, Unger S, Zabel B, Bole-Feysot C, Nitschke P, Handford P, Casanova J-L, Boileau C, Apte SS, Munnich A, Cormier-Daire V (2011) Mutations in the TGFβ binding-protein-like domain 5 of FBN1 are responsible for acromicric and geleophysic dysplasias. Am J Hum Genet 89:7–14

Le Maitre CL, Freemont AJ, Hoyland JA (2004) Localization of degradative enzymes and their inhibitors in the degenerate human intervertebral disc. J Pathol 204:47–54

Le Maitre CL, Freemont AJ, Hoyland JA (2005) The role of interleukin-1 in the pathogenesis of human intervertebral disc degeneration. Arthritis Res Ther 7:R732–R745

Le Maitre CL, Pockert A, Buttle DJ, Freemont AJ, Hoyland JA (2007) Matrix synthesis and degradation in human intervertebral disc degeneration. Biochem Soc Trans 35:652–655

Lee NV, Sato M, Annis DS, Loo JA, Wu L, Mosher DF, Iruela-Arispe ML (2006) ADAMTS1 mediates the release of antiangiogenic polypeptides from TSP1 and 2. EMBO J 25:5270–5283

Liang Q-Q, Zhou Q, Zhang M, Hou W, Cui X-J, Li C-G, Li T-F, Shi Q, Wang Y-J (2008) Prolonged upright posture induces degenerative changes in intervertebral discs in rat lumbar spine. Spine 33:2052–2058

Liu C-J (2009) The role of ADAMTS-7 and ADAMTS-12 in the pathogenesis of arthritis. Nat Clin Pract Rheumatol 5:38–45

Liu C-J, Kong W, Ilalov K, Yu S, Xu K, Prazak L, Fajardo M, Sehgal B, Di Cesare PE (2006) ADAMTS-7: a metalloproteinase that directly binds to and degrades cartilage oligomeric matrix protein. FASEB J 20:988–990

Longpré J-M, McCulloch DR, Koo B-H, Alexander JP, Apte SS, Leduc R (2009) Characterization of proADAMTS5 processing by proprotein convertases. Int J Biochem Cell Biol 41:1116–1126

Lu X, Wang Q, Hu G, Van Poznak C, Fleisher M, Reiss M, Massagué J, Kang Y (2009) ADAMTS1 and MMP1 proteolytically engage EGF-like ligands in an osteolytic signaling cascade for bone metastasis. Genes Dev 23:1882–1894

Luque A, Carpizo DR, Iruela-Arispe ML (2003) ADAMTS1/METH1 inhibits endothelial cell proliferation by direct binding and sequestration of VEGF165. J Biol Chem 278:23656–23665

Maclean JJ, Lee CR, Alini M, Iatridis JC (2004) Anabolic and catabolic mRNA levels of the intervertebral disc vary with the magnitude and frequency of in vivo dynamic compression. J Orthop Res 22:1193–1200

MacLean JJ, Lee CR, Alini M, Iatridis JC (2005) The effects of short-term load duration on anabolic and catabolic gene expression in the rat tail intervertebral disc. J Orthop Res 23:1120–1127

Malfait A-M, Arner EC, Song R-H, Alston JT, Markosyan S, Staten N, Yang Z, Griggs DW, Tortorella MD (2008) Proprotein convertase activation of aggrecanases in cartilage in situ. Arch Biochem Biophys 478:43–51

McCulloch DR, Nelson CM, Dixon LJ, Silver DL, Wylie JD, Lindner V, Sasaki T, Cooley MA, Argraves WS, Apte SS (2009) ADAMTS metalloproteases generate active versican fragments that regulate interdigital web regression. Dev Cell 17:687–698

Melrose J, Shu C, Young C, Ho R, Smith M, Young A, Smith S, Gooden B, Dart A, Podadera J, Appleyard R, Little C (2012) Mechanical destabilisation induced by controlled annular incision of the intervertebral disc dysregulates metalloproteinase expression and induces disc degeneration. Spine (Phila Pa 1976) 37:18–25

Mittaz L, Russell DL, Wilson T, Brasted M, Tkalcevic J, Salamonsen LA, Hertzog PJ, Pritchard MA (2004) Adamts-1 is essential for the development and function of the urogenital system. Biol Reprod 70:1096–1105

Pasternak B, Aspenberg P (2009) Metalloproteinases and their inhibitors-diagnostic and therapeutic opportunities in orthopedics. Acta Orthop 80:693–703

Patel KP, Sandy JD, Akeda K, Miyamoto K, Chujo T, An HS, Masuda K (2007) Aggrecanases and aggrecanase-generated fragments in the human intervertebral disc at early and advanced stages of disc degeneration. Spine 32:2596–2603

Pockert AJ, Richardson SM, Le Maitre CL, Lyon M, Deakin JA, Buttle DJ, Freemont AJ, Hoyland JA (2009) Modified expression of the ADAMTS enzymes and tissue inhibitor of metalloproteinases 3 during human intervertebral disc degeneration. Arthritis Rheum 60:482–491

Rodríguez-Manzaneque JC, Carpizo D, Plaza-Calonge Mdel C, Torres-Collado AX, Thai SN-M, Simons M, Horowitz A, Iruela-Arispe ML (2009) Cleavage of syndecan-4 by ADAMTS1 provokes defects in adhesion. Int J Biochem Cell Biol 41:800–810

Roughley PJ (2004) Biology of intervertebral disc aging and degeneration: involvement of the extracellular matrix. Spine 29:2691–2699

Saftig P, Reiss K (2011) The "A Disintegrin and Metalloproteases" ADAM10 and ADAM17: novel drug targets with therapeutic potential? Eur J Cell Biol 90:527–535

Sahebjam S, Khokha R, Mort JS (2007) Increased collagen and aggrecan degradation with age in the joints of Timp3(–/–) mice. Arthritis Rheum 56:905–909

Saito M, Kurokawa M, Oda M, Oshima M, Tsutsui K, Kosaka K, Nakao K, Ogawa M, Manabe R, Suda N, Ganjargal G, Hada Y, Noguchi T, Teranaka T, Sekiguchi K, Yoneda T, Tsuji T (2011) ADAMTSL6β protein rescues fibrillin-1 microfibril disorder in a Marfan syndrome mouse model through the promotion of fibrillin-1 assembly. J Biol Chem 286:38602–38613

Sandy JD, Westling J, Kenagy RD, Iruela-Arispe ML, Verscharen C, Rodriguez-Mazaneque JC, Zimmermann DR, Lemire JM, Fischer JW, Wight TN, Clowes AW (2001) Versican V1 proteolysis in human aorta in vivo occurs at the Glu441-Ala442 bond, a site that is cleaved by recombinant ADAMTS-1 and ADAMTS-4. J Biol Chem 276:13372–13378

Séguin CA, Pilliar RM, Roughley PJ, Kandel RA (2005) Tumor necrosis factor-alpha modulates matrix production and catabolism in nucleus pulposus tissue. Spine 30:1940–1948

Sengle G, Tsutsui K, Keene DR, Tufa SF, Carlson EJ, Charbonneau NL, Ono RN, Sasaki T, Wirtz MK, Samples JR, Fessler LI, Fessler JH, Sekiguchi K, Hayflick SJ, Sakai LY (2012) Microenvironmental regulation by fibrillin-1. PLoS Genet 8:e1002425

Shi S, Ciurli C, Cartman A, Pidoux I, Poole AR, Zhang Y (2003) Experimental immunity to the G1 domain of the proteoglycan versican induces spondylitis and sacroiliitis, of a kind seen in human spondylarthropathies. Arthritis Rheum 48:2903–2915

Sohn P, Cox M, Chen D, Serra R (2010) Molecular profiling of the developing mouse axial skeleton: a role for Tgfbr2 in the development of the intervertebral disc. BMC Dev Biol 10:29

Somerville RPT, Longpré J-M, Apel ED, Lewis RM, Wang LW, Sanes JR, Leduc R, Apte SS (2004) ADAMTS7B, the full-length product of the ADAMTS7 gene, is a chondroitin sulfate proteoglycan containing a mucin domain. J Biol Chem 279:35159–35175

Stankunas K, Hang CT, Tsun Z-Y, Chen H, Lee NV, Wu JI, Shang C, Bayle JH, Shou W, Iruela-Arispe ML, Chang C-P (2008) Endocardial Brg1 represses ADAMTS1 to maintain the microenvironment for myocardial morphogenesis. Dev Cell 14:298–311

Stanton H, Rogerson FM, East CJ, Golub SB, Lawlor KE, Meeker CT, Little CB, Last K, Farmer PJ, Campbell IK, Fourie AM, Fosang AJ (2005) ADAMTS5 is the major aggrecanase in mouse cartilage in vivo and in vitro. Nature 434:648–652

Tortorella MD, Arner EC, Hills R, Easton A, Korte-Sarfaty J, Fok K, Wittwer AJ, Liu R-Q, Malfait A-M (2004) Alpha2-macroglobulin is a novel substrate for ADAMTS-4 and ADAMTS-5 and represents an endogenous inhibitor of these enzymes. J Biol Chem 279: 17554–17561

Virtanen IM, Noponen N, Barral S, Karppinen J, Li H, Vuoristo M, Niinimäki J, Ott J, Ala-Kokko L, Männikkö M (2007) Putative susceptibility locus on chromosome 21q for lumbar disc disease (LDD) in the Finnish population. J Bone Miner Res 22:701–707

Wang J, Markova D, Anderson DG, Zheng Z, Shapiro IM, Risbud MV (2011) TNF-α and IL-1β promote a disintegrin-like and metalloprotease with thrombospondin type I motif-5-mediated aggrecan degradation through syndecan-4 in intervertebral disc. J Biol Chem 286: 39738–39749

Wylie JD, Ho JC, Singh S, McCulloch DR, Apte SS (2012) Adamts5 (aggrecanase-2) is widely expressed in the mouse musculoskeletal system and is induced in specific regions of knee joint explants by inflammatory cytokines. J Orthop Res 30:226–233

Yu H, Zhu Y (2012) Expression of ADAMTS-7 and ADAMTS-12 in the nucleus pulposus during degeneration of rat caudal intervertebral disc. J Vet Med Sci 74:9–15

Yurube T, Takada T, Suzuki T, Kakutani K, Maeno K, Doita M, Kurosaka M, Nishida K (2012) Rat tail static compression model mimics extracellular matrix metabolic imbalances of matrix metalloproteinases, aggrecanases, and tissue inhibitors of metalloproteinases in intervertebral disc degeneration. Arthritis Res Ther 14:R51

Zhao C-Q, Zhang Y-H, Jiang S-D, Li H, Jiang L-S, Dai L-Y (2011) ADAMTS-5 and intervertebral disc degeneration: the results of tissue immunohistochemistry and in vitro cell culture. J Orthop Res 29:718–725

Part II

Intervertebral Disc Disease: Pathogenesis and Current Treatment Modalities

Epidemiology of Lumbar Disc Degeneration

9

Yue Wang and Michele C. Battié

Contents

9.1 Overview

The World Health Organization defines epidemiology as the study of the distribution and determinants of health-related states or events (WHO 2012). This chapter on the epidemiology of disc degeneration begins with a brief overview of the early observations of disc degeneration and growing interest in the phenomenon, including the introduction and evolution of the currently ambiguous term "degenerative disc disease." Attention is given to case definition, as it is a core concept in epidemiology and the study of occurrence rates. While definitions used for disc degeneration vary and depend greatly on the methods used to study or image the disc, the occurrence rates of degenerative findings reported in this chapter focus on population-based studies using MRI, which may provide a reference for clinical observations. Finally, we briefly discuss environmental, behavioral, and constitutional factors associated with accelerated disc degeneration, where there has been a recent dramatic shift in views.

9.2 Historical Perspective

9.2.1 Disc Degeneration

The description of degenerative changes can be traced back to 1824, when Wenzel first recorded pathological changes in discs of the lumbar spine (Wenzel 1824). Yet, the intervertebral disc received little attention over the following 100 years. During this time, degenerative findings of the disc were mentioned only sporadically by a few pathologists, including Luschka (Schmorl and Junghanns 1971) and Rokitanski (1855). In the 1920s, however, spine pathology and disc degeneration research substantially advanced, as did research in other medical disciplines.

Among the pioneers exploring the spine during this period, one of the most outstanding was Christian Georg Schmorl (1861–1932). The academic career and pioneering contributions of this legendary spine explorer were well

Y. Wang (✉)
Department of Orthopedic Surgery, The First Affiliated Hospital, College of Medicine, Zhejiang University, Hangzhou, People's Republic of China
e-mail: wangyuespine@gmail.com

M.C. Battié
Faculty of Rehabilitation Medicine, University of Alberta, 8205 114St, Edmonton, AB T6G 2G4, Canada
e-mail: mc.battie@ualberta.ca

I.M. Shapiro, M.V. Risbud (eds.), *The Intervertebral Disc*, DOI 10.1007/978-3-7091-1535-0_9, © Springer-Verlag Wien 2014

Box 9.1 Herbert Junghanns

Herbert Junghanns (1902–1986)

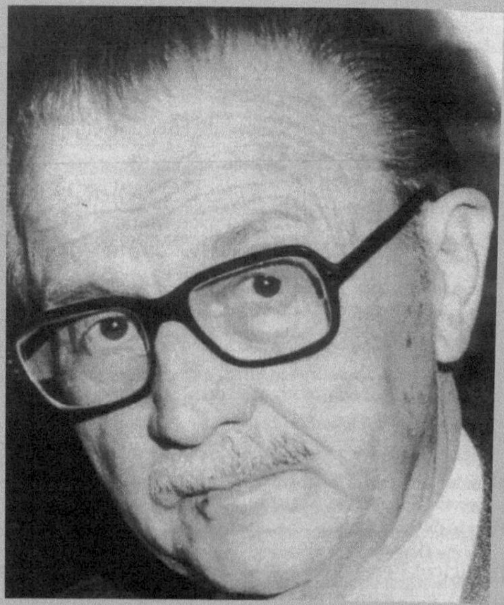

Herbert Junghanns was a German surgeon and a respected researcher who focused on the biomechanics of the spine. He was the head of the Institute for Spinal Column Research in Frankfurt, a president of the German Spine Society, and the founder of the Association of the Scientific Medical Societies in Germany, which consisted of 16 scientific medical professional societies and is now an umbrella organization for more than 150 German medical societies. He also served as the editor of the German book series *The Spine in Research and Practice.*

As one of Christian Georg Schmorl's outstanding students, Junghanns was responsible for bringing much of Schmorl's pioneering work on spinal pathology to light. It is this contribution for which he is perhaps best known. Junghanns produced a book compiling much of Schmorl's work on the spine, *The Human Spine in Health and Disease,* that was first published in 1937. After Schmorl's tremendous body of research on the spine contained in the 4th edition of the book was translated into English and printed in North America in 1959, it became widely known around the world and regarded as a landmark of modern spine research.

described previously (Vernon-Roberts 1994) and are only briefly noted here. Schmorl was a versatile German pathologist who creatively advanced a number of pathological techniques, including tissue processing and staining, photomicrography, and barium sulfate discography. While he substantially contributed to knowledge of the pathology associated with many nonskeletal diseases, in 1926 he focused his research on the spine and devoted the last 6 years of his career exclusively to spine pathology. By advancing pathological techniques used in spine autopsy, Schmorl's extensive work on spine pathology constituted the foundational knowledge of a number of spine conditions, including disc degeneration (Vernon-Roberts 1994). For example, based on autopsy examinations of over 4,000 spines, Schmorl systematically described the normal structure of the vertebrae and discs, including typical morphology of age-related disc degeneration, various types of annular tears, as well as posterior and vertical disc protrusions. The latter pathology was named after him as Schmorl's nodes (Schmorl and Junghanns 1971). Unfortunately, Schmorl's work was entirely written in German and did not obtain wide recognition until 1959 when his classic book was translated into English and published in North America as "The Human Spine in Health and Disease."

Schmorl's work on the intervertebral disc basically comprised postmortem autopsy descriptions and did not link pathological findings of the disc to clinical symptoms. In fact, Schmorl believed that such degenerative findings were too common to be clinically important (Parisien and Ball 1998). With the accumulation of pathological knowledge and clinical observations of the lumbar spine in the 1920s, surgeons began to suspect that a diseased intervertebral disc may cause sciatica. In 1929, Walter Dandy (1886–1946), a neurosurgeon from The Johns Hopkins Hospital, accurately described disc herniation in detail, including related surgical, pathological, and clinical findings (Dandy 1929; Weinstein and Burchiel 2009). Dandy's report on two such cases was a historical first. However, William Mixter's (1880–1958) 1934 paper on the relationship between disc herniation and sciatica (Mixter and Barr 1934) gained much more attention and is often credited with providing the foundation for the contemporary understanding of disc herniation and clinical symptoms. His work is also frequently credited or admonished for ushering in the so-called dynasty of the disc (Parisien and Ball 1998; Hadler et al. 2007). The intervertebral disc was thus pushed to the forefront of spine practice and research and remains there today as a primary target of spine-related activities.

9.2.2 Degenerative Disc Disease

Degenerative disc disease as a concept and a term has also flourished over recent decades. The word "disease" originated from "desaise" in the early fourteenth century, in which "des" means "without, away" and "aise" means "ease." Clearly, disease is related to symptoms. On the other hand, "degeneration" basically means the process of declining

Box 9.2 Alf Nachemson

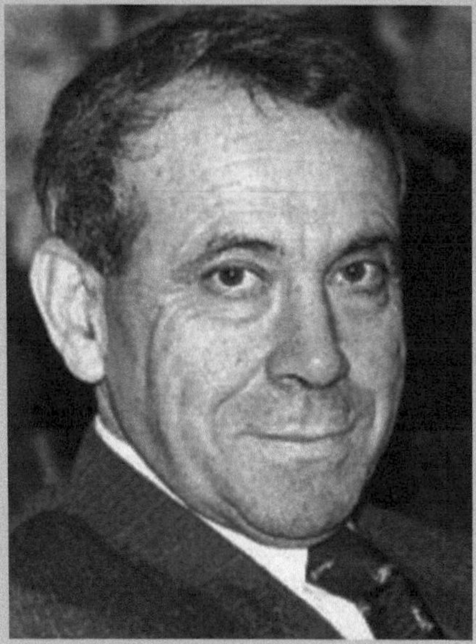

Alf Nachemson (1931–2006)

Alf Nachemson has been described as the most influential spinal researcher of the twentieth century. During more than 45 years as a clinician (orthopaedic surgeon)-scientist, his research on the spine had a broad span, ranging from basic science to population health. Before his work on macroscopic grading of disc degeneration and the disc's nutrient supply, noted in this chapter, he began his research career studying biomechanics. It was this early work in the 1950s that led him to intradiscal pressure measurements, which were the first in vivo measurements to directly determine loading conditions of the spine, the research for which he may be best known.

Above all, Nachemson was a passionate and outspoken advocate for research excellence and improved patient care, particularly in his discipline of orthopaedic surgery. He held innumerable related leadership positions in Sweden and internationally. Among them was founding member of the International Society for the Study of the Lumbar Spine (ISSLS), which became the premier research society on common spinal disorders. Through the ISSLS, he initiated the prestigious Volvo Award (now ISSLS Prize) in 1979, which is arguably the most well-recognized award in spine research. His genuine dedication to excellence, enthusiasm and humor, were an inspiration to all who had the good fortune to work with him.

from a former state, especially through loss of structure and function. Therefore, it is generally accepted that disc degeneration is one of the many progressive changes of the human body primarily attributable to natural aging (Adams and Roughley 2006), which surely is not a disease. The process of disc degeneration, however, may be dramatically accelerated by other etiological factors, such as severe trauma. This view, if generalized to lesser physical insults and more common loading of the spine through occupational and leisure activities, can lead in the notion that all disc degeneration is a result of injury or pathology and thus a "disease." While current research does not support the repetitive or cumulative trauma model of disc degeneration, this was once the dominant paradigm (Battie et al. 2004).

Also, as most degenerated discs are not symptomatic, the use of "degenerative disc disease" or "DDD" as a synonym of disc degeneration may be misleading. Such use may have contributed to the occasional clinical practice of labeling idiopathic low back pain, in the presence of disc degeneration, but no other clear pathology, as degenerative disc disease. Thus, the acronym of DDD has been translated humorously as "diagnostic deficiency disease."

To better understand the origin and evolution of the use of the term "degenerative disc disease," we traced it back to the early period of spine research in the 1940s and Captain Gilbert Fletcher, a military physician in Pennsylvania. In 1947, he studied a cohort of 600 veterans of World War II who were discharged from the army for back pain (Fletcher 1947). As is the case today, the pathologies underlying most spine disorders remained unclear. Based on radiographs, Captain Fletcher used signs of advanced disc degeneration of the lumbar spine, such as disc narrowing, sclerosis, hypertrophic changes (likely osteophytes), and "subluxation" of the facet joints, to diagnose "degenerative disc disease." Later he concluded that the degenerative findings were highly related to backward displacement of the lumbar vertebra. In retrospect, Captain Fletcher was describing radiographic manifestations of degenerative retrolisthesis.

Over the next two to three decades, the term "degenerative disc disease" was only occasionally used (Friedenberg and Miller 1963). When it was used, it was typically restricted to patients with symptomatic spinal disorders for which the disc was suspected as important, such as in nerve root impairment (Weiner and Macnab 1970), back and leg pain (Dilke et al. 1973; Macnab 1973), and disc herniation (Gertzbein et al. 1975). With growing interest in disc degeneration and back pain problems, use of the term "degenerative disc disease" also increased substantially in the 1970s. After 1975, however, use of the term was no longer reserved for symptomatic disc-related disorders and began to be used as a synonym of disc degeneration, as well. Among the dozen or so early papers we came across referring to findings of disc degeneration as "degenerative disc disease," a typical one was the well-cited paper published in the *Journal of Bone and Joint Surgery* (*Am*) (Torgerson and Dotter 1976). In this paper, disc degeneration was judged as disc space narrowing on lateral radiographs; it was later called "degenerative disc disease," a suggested cause of low back pain.

The term "degenerative disc disease" was widely used in medical and scientific literature in the 1980s, and its use has increased exponentially over subsequent years. Sometimes, the term refers to painful disorders that are suspected or known to be disc related. In fact, currently, degenerative disc disease is the most common reason for lumbar fusion in the USA (Rajaee et al. 2012). Yet, gradually "degenerative disc disease" has also become a commonly used synonym of disc degeneration, and unfortunately, its specificity for painful disc-related disorders has been lost. Adding to the confusion, this use of the term degenerative disc disease can also be seen in large-scale population-based epidemiologic studies of disc degeneration (Mok et al. 2010; Sambrook et al. 1999).

Imprecise case definitions and the interchangeable use of distinctly different terms, such as disc degeneration, degenerative disc disease, and back pain, so common in the epidemiological literature, continue to cloud the interpretation of available research (Battie et al. 2007a; Videman and Battie 2012). Clearer definitions and more uniform use of terms would help facilitate accurate communication in medicine and research, avoid unnecessary confusion, and allow clearer comparison of different studies. As the phenomenon of disc degeneration is also lacking a standard definition, the need to clarify concepts and terminology is of particular significance.

9.3 Case Definition: Measuring Disc Degeneration

No other human tissue or organ undergoes a process of such profound degeneration or starts so early (usually in the second decade of age) as the intervertebral disc (Schmorl and Junghanns 1971). Despite substantial clinical interest and extensive research, disc degeneration lacks a clear, standard definition. This may be due, in part, to the wide variation in methodologies used to interrogate the disc by researchers and clinicians from many different disciplines. Thus, one standard definition to address the pathogenesis and characteristics of disc degeneration is likely unrealistic. Other chapters in this book highlight what can be learned about the disc and its degeneration from histological, biochemical, biomechanical, radiological, and other perspectives, including clinical practice. In this chapter, taking an epidemiological perspective, we will focus on disc degeneration as defined primarily from imaging and, in particular, magnetic resonance imaging.

Measurement and case definition are fundamental to any study of occurrence, etiology, or clinical relevance of disc degeneration. According to a review (Kettler and Wilke 2006), there are at least 22 grading systems available to rate the degree of lumbar disc degeneration. These scales were classified into five groups based on materials and modalities used, including macroscopic anatomy, histology, plain radiography, discography, and magnetic resonance (MR) imaging. Due to technical limitations in detecting changes within the intervertebral discs, no grading system used computerized tomography.

Early descriptions of disc degeneration were based on autopsy examinations of cadaveric spines. Findings from macroscopic and histological observations primarily included desiccation of the nucleus pulposus, fibrous fraying, clefts, and a loss of disc height. Although degenerative changes of the lumbar intervertebral discs were described in detail by a number of scholars from the 1930s to the 1950s (Coventry et al. 1945b; Friberg and Hirsch 1948; Schmorl and Junghanns 1971; Virgin 1951), no grading system was proposed. In a 1960 study investigating the effects of disc degeneration on intradiscal pressure, Nachemson developed the first reliable macroscopic grading system to rate disc degeneration (Nachemson 1960). Grading disc degeneration using histological examination was introduced as late as the 1990s (Gunzburg et al. 1992). However, such macroscopic and histological measurements of the disc cannot be applied to nonsurgical patients and, thus, are of limited clinical value.

Plain radiography was extensively used in imaging the spine by Schmorl in the 1920s, in an attempt to correlate radiological features to pathological findings (Schmorl and Junghanns 1971). However, Schmorl realized that radiographs showed only bony signs that are secondary to disc degeneration, such as cortification of trabecular bone (Schmorl's nodes), endplate sclerosis, and narrowing of the intervertebral disc space. Schmorl clearly pointed out that "only with considerable degrees of degeneration of the disc tissue, a decrease in the height of the disc space takes place." Thus, he concluded that a loss of disc height cannot detect disc degeneration in the early stage. Yet, after 1950, the increasing clinical needs of investigating back pain demanded a noninvasive, feasible, and inexpensive modality to evaluate the lumbar spine and disc. Consequently, measuring disc degeneration by judging disc height and vertebral endplate sclerosis on plain radiographs of the spine was introduced in 1952 (Kellgren and Lawrence 1952). Since then, plain radiography has served as a primary approach to assess disc degeneration. Later, in the 1990s, osteophytes were added as another indicator of disc degeneration using the radiographic grading system (Mimura et al. 1994; Lane et al. 1993). Despite reasonable reliability (Kellgren and Lawrence 1952), measuring disc degeneration from plain radiography has inherent limitations, as previously mentioned. In addition to depicting primarily nonspecific bony degenerative findings of the lumbar spine and the inability to detect early degenerative changes, measuring disc height and surrounding osteophytes together may be questionable, as the measurement of one may bias the assessment of the other.

Another approach that gained popularity and was once regarded as a gold standard for evaluating disc degeneration is discography. Different from plain radiography, discography reflects the degree of morphological changes (annular disruption) within the disc by injecting opaque contrast into the disc and observing its distribution. The first discography using barium sulfate was performed in cadaveric spines by Schmorl in the 1920s to demonstrate various types of annular tears (Vernon-Roberts 1994). In 1948, Lindblom and Hirsch applied discography clinically to patients with back pain to image herniated lumbar discs (Hirsch 1948; Lindblom 1948). However, what impressed them most was that discography could provoke or replicate patients' back pain or sciatica. The enthusiasm for discography quickly grew, although it was later found to have a strikingly high false-positive rate (Guyer and Ohnmeiss 2003). For a long period, discography was used in clinics to diagnose so-called discogenic back pain, rather than to detect morphological changes of the disc.

The distribution of contrast in discography was used to assess disc degeneration as late as the 1980s (Adams et al. 1986; Videman et al. 1987, 1990). Before MR imaging was generally used in clinical practice, traditional discography was considered the best approach to evaluate disc degeneration. It can differentiate successive morphological changes inside the disc (Adams et al. 1986), beyond that possible with MRI (Schneiderman et al. 1987). Although discography may not be able to detect all annular lesions (e.g., those that do not connect to the nucleus), it was reported to be more sensitive in detecting annular tears than using MRI (Gunzburg et al. 1992). Yet, due to the invasive nature and the possibility of accelerating the progression of disc degeneration (Carragee et al. 2009), the application of discography clinically has fallen out of favor and may eventually fade from surgical practice.

The advent of MRI, and its widespread use since the beginning of the 1990s, was a major advance for clinical and research investigation of the disc. Capable of depicting disc morphology in multiple planes noninvasively and without ionizing radiation, it quickly became the clinical imaging modality of choice for the disc. MRI also allowed large-scale epidemiological studies of general population samples to investigate the prevalence, etiological factors, and clinical relevance of disc degeneration.

Traditionally, findings of disc degeneration on MR images have included decreased signal intensity (desiccation), disc bulging (anterior and posterior), disc height narrowing, annulus fissures, osteophytes, and endplate irregularities. Which one should be used to indicate the severity of disc degeneration remains a matter of controversy. Some investigators combine some or all of these findings and develop summary scores of overall disc degeneration, while others use individual findings (e.g., signal or bulging) to answer specific questions. In addition to the findings correlating to one another, the qualitative assessment of one finding may influence the assessment of another, such that summing of findings into a global score may exaggerate the degree of disc degeneration.

MR imaging of the disc depends largely on changes of water content (Modic et al. 1984), which is the first step in the process of disc degeneration. Therefore, MRI is able to detect disc degeneration in very early stages, even before morphological degenerative changes appear. Correspondingly, decreased signal intensity on T2-weighted MR imaging demonstrates the most marked change related to disc degeneration. There is evidence that digital signal measurements may provide the best MR depiction of degeneration available from standard imaging, as validated through association with age (Videman et al. 2008). Yet, these measurements require specialized software and do not have immediate clinical use. Thus, disc signal changes continue to be based primarily on visual impressions.

There are a number of visual rating systems used for disc degeneration (Kettler and Wilke 2006). The Pfirrmann classification of disc degeneration on MRI is one of the more commonly used grading protocols, with supporting evidence of reliability and validity (Pfirrmann et al. 2001). Based on the structure of the disc, distinction of the nucleus and annulus, signal intensity, and disc height, this system rates severity of disc degeneration using a five-grade ordinal scale. Due in part to its simplicity, the grading scheme is currently popular in both spine practice and research. However, the grading is more or less based on a subjective judgment of many perspectives of the disc, where it sometimes is difficult to distinguish one stage of disc degeneration from another (Haughton 2006). In addition, the ordinal nature of the scale also limits its sensitivity to detecting changes in disc degeneration in longitudinal studies. Yet, its current widespread use will likely aid comparisons between studies, which is needed to advance the field.

9.4 Prevalence of Disc Degeneration

Due to the wide variations in definitions, methodologies, and samples used, the prevalence rates of disc degeneration reported in the scientific literature vary substantially (Battie et al. 2004). Imaging approaches, such as radiography and discography, are currently less commonly used to evaluate disc degeneration and thus will not be fully discussed in this section. Instead, the focus will be on studies using MRI, the preferred clinical imaging modality, as results from such studies may provide a reference for clinical observations. Furthermore, while many studies of disc degeneration using MRI investigate various highly selected populations, such as patients with back or leg pain or workers of certain occupations, we restrict this chapter to studies of general population-based samples. In addition, in previous studies, some bony findings, such as osteophytes, Schmorl's nodes, and endplate irregularities, were included in the evaluation of disc degeneration. Although more or less associated with disc degeneration, they are not specific findings of the disc and, therefore, are not presented in this section. Instead, we will further discuss epidemiological studies of endplate findings in a later section and consider their relationship to disc degeneration.

A review of population-based studies of disc degeneration using MRI reveals that the prevalence rates vary considerably between different degenerative findings, spinal levels, and age groups. The most commonly studied degenerative finding of the lumbar disc, with the most consistent findings between studies, is reduced signal intensity, which reportedly is already present to some degree in approximately half of adolescents (Table 9.1). Perhaps the findings that vary most in prevalence between adolescence and later adulthood are annular tears and high-intensity zones, which are visualized in less than 10 % of adolescents and young adults and which increases to 30–50 % by middle adulthood. The prevalence of disc narrowing is relatively high in the young with nearly 40 % of adolescents having some degree of narrowing, but there is only one study on which to base this observation (Table 9.1).

As the prevalence of degenerative findings at different disc levels of the lumbar spine varies considerably, ideally

Table 9.1 Prevalence of disc degeneration findings on MR images in lumbar spines of general populations

Author and year	Sample size	Race	Age	Gender	Reduced signal intensity	Reduced disc height	Bulging	Annular tears	High-intensity zone
Videman (1995)[a]	232	Finnish	49.3 (35–69)	100 % M	L1/2 41.6 %	9.3 %	58.6 %	11.6 %	
					L2/3 48.7 %	13.6 %	74.7 %	17.5 %	
					L3/4 57.7 %	24.1 %	81.9 %	27.4 %	
					L4/5 80.4 %	51.3 %	92.8 %	53.1 %	
					L5/S1 86.0 %	55.6 %	78.5 %	49.8 %	
Kjaer (2005b)[a]	439	Danish	13.1 (12–14)	46.7 % M	L1/2 12 %	3 %	0 %	1 %	0 %
					L2/3 8 %	1 %	0.3 %	1 %	0 %
					L3/4 13 %	6 %	3 %	2 %	0 %
					L4/5 31 %	31 %	10 %	2 %	1 %
					L5/S1 50 %	17 %	12 %	3 %	4 %
					57.6 % of spine	38 %	16.1 %	7.3 %	5 %
Kjaer (2005a)[a]	412	Danish	40	48.2 % M	45.2 %	50.2 %	52.4 %	39.3 %	40.8 %
Takatalo (2009)[b]	558	Finnish	21 (20–22)	58 % M	L1/2 2 %				
					L2/3 3 %				
					L3/4 5 %				
					L4/5 22 %				
					L5/S1 35 %				
					47.2 % of spine		24.9 %	9.1 %	6.8 %
Cheung (2009)[c]	1,043	Chinese	(18–55)	–					
			18–29		42 %		27.3 %	3.4 %	
			30–39		48 %		20.6 %	8.2 %	
			40–49		70 %		27.3 %	16.1 %	
			≥50		88 %		43.1 %	29.0 %	
Mok (2010)[c]	2,449	Chinese	40.4 ± 10.9 (9.7–88.4)	40 % M	L1/2 9.5 %				
					L2/3 15.7 %				
					L3/4 27.2 %				
					L4/5 45.8 %				
					L5/S1 51.0 %				
Samartzis (2011)[c]	83	Chinese	18.3 ± 2.1 (13–20)	46 % M	34.9 %		22.9 %		3.6 %

[a]Signal intensity was judged using a 4-point scale, with 0 representing normal and 1–3 progressive signal loss

[b]A modified Pfirrmann scale was used to evaluate disc degeneration, which takes both signal and disc height into consideration. Discs with a Pfirrmann grade of 1 or 2 were classified as normal and discs with grades 3, 4, or 5 were defined as degenerated

[c]In these three studies, disc degeneration was rated using a 4-point Schneiderman scale, which assesses signal intensity and disc narrowing together

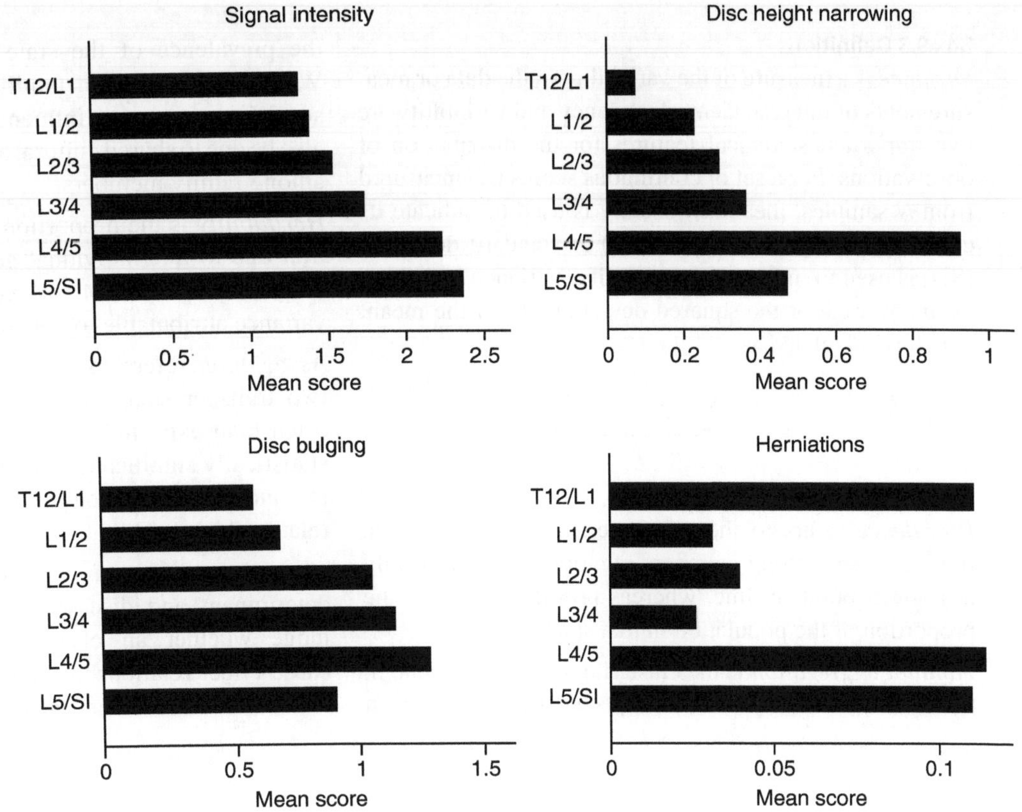

Fig. 9.1 Mean scores for specific manifestations of disc degeneration by disc level (Adapted from the paper by Battié et al. (2004), with permission)

prevalence would be presented level by level. Most disc-specific degenerative findings on MRI, such as bulging, herniation, disc space narrowing, and annular tears, are more common and more severe at the L4/5 and L5/S1 discs than the upper lumbar discs (Fig. 9.1) (Videman et al. 1995). This finding is also consistent between MR evaluation protocols of disc degeneration. In general, degenerative findings in the L1/2, L2/3, and L3/4 discs are more similar to each other, as compared to those in the L4/5 and L5/S1 discs (Table 9.1). Therefore, it may be advisable to, at least, divide the five lumbar intervertebral discs into upper (L1/2, L2/3, and L3/4 discs) and lower lumbar regions (L4/5 and L5/S1 discs) when investigating disc degeneration. There also appears to be a clear difference in genetic influences between upper and lower lumbar regions (Battie et al. 2008), further strengthening the case against using a summary score for degeneration across the entire lumbar spine.

9.5 Etiological Factors (Environmental, Behavioral, and Constitutional)

Before the mid- to late 1990s, the dominant model of the etiology of disc degeneration was one of repetitive loading or wear and tear. This paradigm generally viewed disc degeneration as a consequence of repeated loading and associated tissue insults and injuries. Correspondingly, behavioral and environmental factors, such as occupational materials handling, were viewed as the main causes of disc degeneration. Not surprisingly, these influences were the focus of research and prevention strategies. Based on knowledge of that time, Frymoyer summarized the findings of epidemiological studies on "degenerative disc disease" by stating "Among the factors associated with its occurrence are age, gender, occupation, cigarette smoking, and exposure to vehicular vibration. The contribution of other factors such as height, weight, and genetics is less certain" (Frymoyer 1992). A decade later, a major shift in views was underway. Taking into account new knowledge gained from the intervening decade, in 2002 Ala-Kokko concluded that "Even though several environmental and constitutional risk factors have been implicated in this disease, their effects are relatively minor, and recent family and twin studies have suggested that sciatica, disc herniation and disc degeneration may be explained to a large degree by genetic factors" (Ala-Kokko 2002). Disc degeneration is now considered a condition that is largely genetically influenced, with environmental factors, although elusive, also playing an important role (Battie et al. 2009). An overview of the main factors which have been of interest in the etiology of disc degeneration follows.

Box 9.3 Definitions

Variance is a measure of the variability in the data or measurements of interest. Central tendency and variability are two important statistical features for the distribution of observations. For a set of continuous scores (*X*) measured from *N* samples, mean (x) usually is used to indicate its central tendency and variance (S^2) or standard deviation (SD) is used to indicate its variability. Variance is defined as the average of the squared deviations from the mean, which is calculated as:

$$S^2 = \frac{\sum (X - \bar{X})^2}{n-1}$$

Prevalence refers to the existence of a particular state (e.g., disease) among members of a population, typically at a given point in time, whereas prevalence rate is the proportion of the population in that state.

Familial aggregation is the clustering of a trait or state in family members beyond that expected by chance given the prevalence of the state in the general population. While observations of familial aggregation often lead to suspicions of genetic influences, familial aggregation can also be due to shared cultural and environmental influences among family members.

Heritability is the proportion of population variance in a trait due to interindividual genetic variation or, in other words, the proportion of phenotypic (observable trait) variance attributable to genetic effects.

Association refers to an occurrence relation, such that two traits or states occur together either more or less often than expected by chance. However, an observed, statistically significant association between a risk indicator and a disease does not necessarily infer a causal relationship.

Causation infers a causal connection between a determinant and disease or outcome phenomenon. To judge whether an observed association represents a cause-effect relationship between exposure and disease, comprehensive inferences or criteria are needed.

9.5.1 Age

With the possible exception of genetics, which will be discussed later, age is perhaps the factor most strongly associated with disc degeneration. The clear relationship between age and disc degeneration has been observed since the time of the pioneering pathologists using autopsy studies in the early twentieth century. Some classic autopsy studies using large samples clearly documented that the occurrence of disc degeneration increased "linearly" with age. For example, in a study from 1926 based on 1,000 consecutive autopsies, Heine reported the prevalence rate of macroscopic disc degeneration (or so-called spondylitis deformans) increased from 0 to 72 % from the age of 39–70 years (Heine 1926). Schmorl and Coventry further confirmed that the occurrence rates of histological findings of disc degeneration, such as disc cell death, nucleus clefts, annular tears, and cartilage endplate fissures, increase consistently with greater age (Schmorl and Junghanns 1971; Coventry et al. 1945a). More recently, Miller reported that the prevalence of macroscopic disc degeneration increased from 16 % at 20 years of age to 98 % at 70 years (Miller et al. 1988). Later, in a systematic investigation of age-related changes in lumbar intervertebral discs, Boos et al. clearly depicted the association of increased prevalence rates of almost all histological degenerative findings in the disc with greater age in a sample spanning from fetal to 88 years (Boos et al. 2002).

On the other hand, some degenerative changes seen from histology can occur in early childhood, complicating the role of age in disc degeneration. For example, mucoid degeneration and mild clefts of the nucleus pulposus may present before the age of two (Boos et al. 2002). In the second decade of life, nucleus pulposus clefts and radial tears are often observed in the disc center, as are cartilage cracks (Boos et al. 2002). From 20 years old on, disc degenerative findings have been found to progressively increase in both frequency and severity. However, there is considerable variability in degenerative disc findings within age groups.

In general, use of MRI has provided a good opportunity to investigate the association between age and disc degeneration. Cerebrospinal fluid-adjusted disc signal intensity measurements, reflecting the water content of the nucleus pulposus, have been found to decrease from early childhood through late adulthood (Videman et al. 1994). In a study of 116 men ranging in age from 35 to 70 years, the associations of different degenerative findings on MRI were plotted in relation to age. Disc signal intensity measurement was more highly associated with age than other MR findings (Fig. 9.2). A further study reported that age could explain up to 31.7 % of the variation of signal-based digital measurements of disc degeneration, such as cerebrospinal fluid-adjusted disc signal, in the upper lumbar intervertebral discs and 11.5 % in the lower lumbar intervertebral discs (Videman et al. 2008). Another advantage of signal intensity measurements acquired through standard MRI, as opposed to qualitative assessments, is that they are continuous in nature, providing greater sensitivity to change and facilitating statistical analyses. However, such quantitative measurements can be influenced

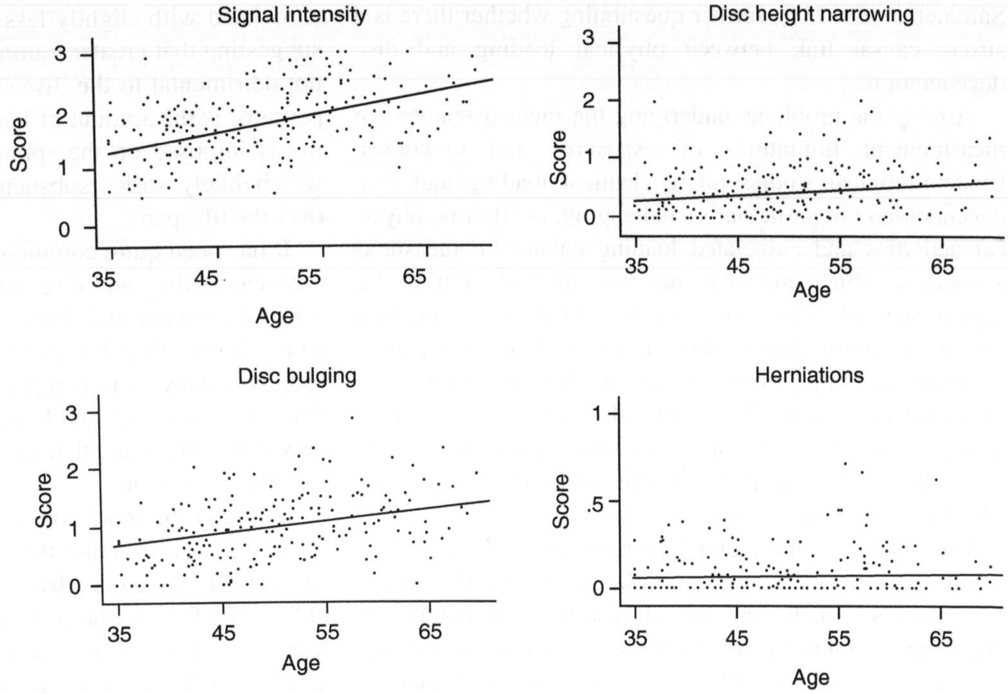

Fig. 9.2 Mean scores for specific manifestations of disc degeneration by age (Adapted from the paper by Battié el al. (2004), with permission)

by scanner variations and are currently only used for research purposes.

In epidemiological studies age is a more complicated factor than it may appear (Videman et al. 2008). Age is an intrinsic indicator of the natural process of aging, with a dose-response effect of greater age associated with more degenerative changes. It reflects, however, more than natural aging and can be a complex risk factor with respect to disc degeneration and other outcomes, as it represents not only natural aging but also associated factors. For example, age also reflects cumulative exposure to a variety of known or unknown etiological factors that generally increase with the passage of time. In fact, many factors suspected of accelerating disc degeneration, such as excessive mechanical loading or trauma to the spine, cannot be accurately measured, particularly when lifetime exposures are of interest. However, the exposure to such factors, more or less, is associated with age, with greater age generally associated with greater exposure to all risk factors.

9.5.2 Occupational and Leisure Physical Demands and Spinal Loading

Before genetic factors began to assume a leading role in disc degeneration in the middle to late 1990s (Battie et al. 1995a, b; Sambrook et al. 1999), a wear-and-tear model of disc degeneration prevailed. Various forms of physical demands and spinal loading conditions, particularly heavy material handling, were regarded as the main causes of disc degeneration. The natural assumption under such an injury or wear-and-tear model was that heavy work and greater physical demands would lead to greater disc degeneration. Yet, epidemiological evidence of this has always been conflicted.

In early studies using radiography, it was observed that disc degeneration, as judged from disc space narrowing and endplate sclerosis, was more common in miners and manual workers than in non-laborers (Lawrence 1955) and that the onset of disc degeneration was on average 10 years earlier in workers with heavy physical demands (Hult 1954). Conversely, in a study of 15,160 "back trouble" patients, disc degeneration, as judged from disc space narrowing and osteophytes, was not found to be associated with heavy physical work (Friberg and Hirsch 1949) nor was occupational lifting as reported by others (Frymoyer et al. 1984). More recent studies have continued to produce mixed results, with some suggesting a negative effect of greater physical demands (Seidler et al. 2009), while others fail to observe detrimental effects on the disc (Porter et al. 1989; Videman et al. 2007). In fact, Porter put forward the hypothesis that physical activity strengthens both the vertebrae and discs (Porter et al. 1989). Results of a recent study by Videman et al. suggest that greater loading of the discs during routine activities may even have some positive effects on the disc, as seen through higher disc signal (hydration) (Videman et al. 2010). Also, although occupational loading history, with a dose-response effect, was greater in patients with pain attributed to disc pathology than in controls (Seidler et al. 2009), most studies of the association between mechanical loading and disc degeneration have failed to uncover a clear relationship (Caplan et al. 1966; Riihimaki et al. 1990;

Sairanen et al. 1981), further questioning whether there is a strong causal link between physical loading and disc degeneration.

Among the problems underlying the inconsistencies are measurement limitations of exposures and outcomes. Epidemiological studies on mechanical loading and disc degeneration are particularly challenging, as lifetime physical activities and associated loading cannot be measured accurately, which invariably has the effect of diluting the appearance of true associations. Moreover, standard definitions of disc degeneration are also lacking. While most degenerative findings (e.g., signal loss, bulging, narrowing) are correlated to some degree, they do not necessarily represent the same phenomenon and important information may be lost by aggregating distinct findings into summary scores, which is a common practice.

Uncontrolled confounding factors are another major limitation of most epidemiological studies. Exposure-discordant twin studies, which may provide for the best control of known and unknown confounding factors while minimizing extraneous variability related to the substantial genetic influences, provide a particularly strong research design to investigate the effects of environmental exposures. Such studies have been employed to help clarify the effects of a number of suspected risk factors in disc degeneration, which are highlighted below.

It is well known that musculoskeletal tissues, such as bone, ligaments, cartilages, and muscles, are able to increase their physiological capacity and mechanical strength in response to repeated physical activities and greater physical loading. The adaptation to a changing mechanical environment is a rule in sport science and is typically the purpose of exercise and training. Yet, this rule is curiously often viewed as not "applicable" to the intervertebral disc. Instead, mechanical loading or repeated material handling, either from occupation or exercise, is viewed as a hazard that will accelerate disc degeneration. Herein is one of the great paradoxes in the relationship between physical loading and the lumbar spine as compared to other musculoskeletal structures.

Although doubts about the cumulative loading or wear-and-tear model of disc degeneration have long existed, substantial evidence to challenge this paradigm was forthcoming from exposure-discordant twin and heritability studies. Despite extreme exposure, discordance in monozygotic co-twins, very little variance in disc degeneration outcomes was explained by substantial, long-term occupational or sport physical demands and lumbar loading conditions (Battié et al. 2009).

Also, using monozygotic twins with similar lifestyle but substantially different body weights (average body weight difference of 30 lb), long-term physical loading in the form of additional body weight was not associated with increased disc degeneration. Instead, greater body weight within the range studied, which did not include extreme obesity, was associated with slightly less upper lumbar disc desiccation, suggesting that greater routine loading of the lumbar spine is not detrimental to the disc (Videman et al. 2010). The key, perhaps, is the amount of loading and the manner that loading is imposed on the spine in relation to tissue strength, which likely varies substantially between individuals and over the lifespan.

It has been quite common for epidemiological studies of physical loading and disc degeneration to focus on occupational exposures and ignore physical activities outside of work. Considering that activities outside of paid employment usually occupy more of a person's time than work hours and that combined work and leisure physical loading may give a very different picture than occupational loading alone, this is no small oversight.

In one of the more comprehensive epidemiological studies to date investigating the effects of lifetime exposures to suspected risk factors, physical loading exposures explained only 7 % of the variance in disc degeneration in the upper lumbar levels and 2 % in the lower lumbar levels, suggesting a modest role of commonly experienced occupational and leisure activities in disc degeneration (Battie et al. 1995b). Interestingly, it was exposures reported during leisure activities that accounted for the variance in lower lumbar disc degeneration explained by physical loading exposures.

9.5.3 Driving and Whole-Body Vibration

Whole-body vibration (WBV) resulting from operating or riding in motorized vehicles is a special form of physical loading that was long thought to be deleterious to the lumbar spine and disc, in particular. According to an extensive review conducted in the early 1990s during the height of research activity and interest in whole-body vibration and lumbar disc degeneration, degenerative findings tended to be more common in subjects with greater exposure (Kjellberg et al. 1994). However, the authors of the review also noted "uncontrolled confounding factors may have affected the results in all studies, and the conclusions about the causal role of WBV for the observed injuries and/or disorders therefore become uncertain."

Since that time, findings have been conflicting and effects uncertain. An exposure-discordant twin study, perhaps the most well-controlled epidemiological study of the association of lifetime exposure to motorized vehicles and related WBV, investigated 45 pairs of monozygotic twin siblings highly discordant for lifetime vehicular driving. No significant differences, nor trends, of greater disc degeneration (e.g., disc signal loss, bulging, herniation, narrowing) were found in drivers as compared to their lesser exposed twin brothers (Battie et al. 2002).

Whether or not WBV related to motorized vehicles exacerbates symptoms from lumbar degenerative conditions or affects other structures is unclear (Lings and Leboeuf-Yde 2000), but these are different issues. Interestingly, vibration has also been pursued more recently as a treatment for low back pain, using various frequencies (del Pozo-Cruz et al. 2011; Rittweger et al. 2002). With respect to deleterious effects of exposures to motorized vehicles and related WBV during work and leisure on disc degeneration in humans, findings have not been persuasive and, in any event, do not suggest a major effect. Yet, after more than 50 years of research on the topic, pleas for continued in-depth biomechanical studies of the effects of vibration on the disc, both good and bad, continue (Hill et al. 2009). This may signify the desire and need for rigorous scientific evaluation to clarify effects, better taking into account frequency, amplitude, and other aspects of vibration. On the other hand, it may also reflect the absence of clear environmental risk factors with substantial effects on which to focus etiological and intervention research.

9.5.4 Trauma

Evidence from both experimental and clinical observations support that clear trauma is a risk factor for disc degeneration. One animal model of disc degeneration involves surgically producing a peripheral annular lesion, which quickly leads to degenerative changes in the disc (Osti et al. 1990). A recent clinical study observed a similar, although less dramatic, causal association between injury to the annulus fibrosus and disc degeneration related to needle puncture in discography. Greater disc degeneration was observed in the non-degenerated or healthy discs following discography over a 10-year follow-up (Carragee et al. 2009). Direct trauma or injury to the disc may destroy the homeostasis of the disc, influence the metabolism of the disc cell, and alter biomechanics of the disc, leading to an accelerated degenerative process.

Trauma to tissues adjacent to the disc, including the vertebral body and endplate, may also accelerate disc degeneration. In animal models, endplate trauma directly induces disc cell apoptosis and promotes disc degeneration (Haschtmann et al. 2008). Clinical long-term follow-up of young people with previous vertebral compression fractures revealed greater amounts of disc degeneration than in healthy controls, also supporting an association of endplate trauma with accelerated disc degeneration (Kerttula et al. 2000).

The question is: how much trauma or force is needed to damage the human disc in vivo and accelerate disc degeneration? A recent autopsy study found that a history of lumbar injury, which referred to sudden onset back pain associated with a specific accident or unusual activity, was associated with the presence of lumbar endplate lesions, which were closely associated with more severe discographic disc degeneration (Wang et al. 2012a; Wang 2011) Endplate lesions may be one mechanism through which trauma or injury eventually leads to disc degeneration. Unfortunately, current clinical imaging modalities are unlikely to be capable of detecting endplate and annular lesions to the same degree, although the sensitivity of MRI to disc disruption may be improving.

Another study of recalled back "injuries" related to sport, leisure, or work activities, and episodes of sudden onset low back pain associated with an exceptional physical activity, used an exposure-discordant twin model. The study revealed that "back injury" based on recollection of such traumatic incidents was not associated with a subsequent increase in disc degeneration, as judged from disc height narrowing or reduced signal intensity (Hancock et al. 2010). The inconsistencies between studies could be explained by high variability in the degree of trauma experienced and reported and that pain was the indicator of "injury," which may not have been associated with substantial or consequential tissue change to the disc. Also, some painful injuries to the back may have been forgotten, resulting in recall bias.

9.5.5 Smoking

Cigarette smoking is the only chemical exposure known to associate with lumbar disc degeneration. While it is commonly accepted that smoking has deleterious effects on the disc and research has turned to understanding the mechanisms involved (Vo et al. 2011), it is important to keep in mind that the effects are likely to be very modest. Using identical twins grossly discordant for smoking exposure (over 32 pack-years), the overall disc degeneration across the entire lumbar spine was greater in smokers as compared to their nonsmoker siblings. Yet, the effect size was very small, explaining less than 2 % of the variance in degeneration scores (Battie et al. 1991).

9.5.6 Vertebral Endplate Morphology and Status

Although substantial progress has been made in understanding the pathogenesis of disc degeneration, the pathological mechanisms or pathways leading to degeneration are far from explicit. Recent research suggests that the endplate, an interface tissue between the vertebral body and the intervertebral disc, may be the structure through which a number of etiological factors lead to disc degeneration (Wang 2011).

The endplate is essential to maintaining the structural integrity and physiological function of the intervertebral disc (Moore 2006). It is the physical shield preventing the nucleus pulposus from "escaping" (Roberts et al. 1996) and the mechanical interface facilitating load distribution in the vertebra-disc complex (Brinckmann et al. 1983; Setton et al. 1993; Ferguson and Steffen 2003). In addition, it is the gateway for metabolite transport between the vertebral marrow and intervertebral disc (Benneker et al. 2005; Nachemson et al. 1970; Urban et al. 2004).

Given the multiple functions of the endplate, its morphometrics are generally thought to associate with disc degeneration. Yet, due to variations in study materials and limitations of inadequate measurements, the association between endplate morphometrics and disc degeneration remains largely unclear and controversial. In a series of studies to investigate the role of endplate morphometrics in disc degeneration (Wang 2011), a large sample of lumbar endplates was extensively measured in vitro using accurate technologies, such as laser scanning and micro-CT. Among the endplate morphometrics studied, including thickness, concavity, circularity, size, and bone mineral density, only endplate thickness (Wang et al. 2011) and size were found to associate with the degenerative disc (Wang 2011). However, the observed associations were relatively weak, suggesting their contribution may be relatively small.

A more interesting area in endplate research is endplate pathology or endplate lesions, which drew substantial attention in early spine research. Schmorl's nodes, one type of endplate lesion in which the nucleus pulposus protrudes through the endplate into the vertebral body, have been studied for over a century. To date the understanding of Schmorl's nodes remains limited. The reported prevalence of Schmorl's nodes varies dramatically from 9 to 75 % (Hamanishi et al. 1994; Hilton et al. 1976; Saluja et al. 1986; Williams et al. 2007), and the association between Schmorl's nodes and disc degeneration remains controversial (Hilton et al. 1976; Pfirrmann and Resnick 2001; Mok et al. 2010).

Using an archive of over 150 lumbar spines, endplate pathologies were systematically investigated to determine the prevalence rate and association with disc degeneration (Wang et al. 2012b). Strikingly, the study revealed that nearly half of the lumbar vertebral endplates examined had some sort of lesion, suggesting that the prevalence of endplate lesions has been substantially underestimated in clinical studies using MRI. Moreover, based on morphological characteristics, four types of endplate lesions were further identified, including Schmorl's nodes, fracture, erosion, and calcification. The various types of endplate lesions have different distribution patterns. For example, Schmorl's nodes usually involved the endplate center and were more common in the upper lumbar region, while calcification lesions tended to affect the whole endplate and were mainly located in the lower lumbar region (Wang 2011). Increasing age was found to associate with not only the presence of endplate lesions but also greater number and size of lesions, suggesting that age and other associated factors may play a critical role in the pathogenesis of endplate lesions. A further analysis suggested that various types of endplate lesions may have different pathological origins and varying degrees of association with adjacent disc degeneration (Wang et al. 2012a).

In summary, the endplate is important to the intervertebral disc. While the influence of endplate morphometrics on disc degeneration may be modest, endplate lesions may play an important role in the pathogenesis of disc degeneration. Endplate lesions are common findings in the spines of middle-aged men and appear to be grossly underestimated with standard clinical imaging approaches. In addition to Schmorl's nodes, there are various types of endplate lesions, which may have different effects on adjacent discs. Thus, it will be important to differentiate other types of endplate lesions from Schmorl's nodes to further understanding of their etiology and role in disc degeneration. Such research would greatly benefit from advances in imaging technologies for use in vivo.

9.5.7 Genetic Influences

This section will not deal with the specific genes associated with disc degeneration and the mechanisms through which they act, as this is the subject of another chapter (see Chap. 10). Instead, the focus here will be on the broad concept of genetic versus environmental influences on disc degeneration.

9.5.7.1 Familial Aggregation

Studies of genetic influences typically begin by determining whether familial aggregation of a disease or condition exists. If the condition is found to aggregate in family members beyond what would be expected by chance given its prevalence in the population, then distinguishing between genetic and other sources of familial similarity becomes of interest in better understanding the etiology of the condition.

There have been a number of studies of familial aggregation of disc pathology associated with painful conditions, particularly disc herniation with radiculopathy (Battié and Videman 2004). Yet, persons identified as having disc herniation are typically those who access and receive spine surgery for associated pain, and significant regional variations in rates of spine surgery demonstrate that this measure is likely to be significantly influenced by other factors than purely disc pathology (Cherkin et al. 1994).

There have been a number of case examples of strikingly similar histories within family members, both related to juvenile (Matsui et al. 1990; Varlotta et al. 1991) and adult disc herniation (Scapinelli 1993; Varughese and Quartey 1979; Scapinelli 1993). Such case reports demonstrate that familial aggregation occurs, but clarifying whether or not it occurs more often than might be expected by chance requires comparison to a control or reference group. When such studies were conducted, they, too, revealed a higher incidence of symptomatic disc herniation in the families of cases of juvenile disc herniation than in those without (Matsui et al. 1990; Varlotta et al. 1991), with one study providing a typical age-adjusted relative risk of herniation of 4.5 in family members of young patients who had undergone surgery for disc herniation as compared to control family members (Varlotta et al. 1991). Furthermore, when considering those 9 through 15, 16 through 19, and 20 through 25 years of age, younger patients who underwent discectomy were found to be significantly more likely to have a family history of back disorders than those of older age groups (Nelson et al. 1972). Such a finding is consistent with genetic epidemiological literature of stronger genetic effects associated with earlier onset. Case-control studies have also revealed familial aggregation of symptomatic lumbar disc herniation in adults (Matsui et al. 1998; Postacchini et al. 1988; Richardson et al. 1997; Simmons et al. 1996). Collectively, these studies make a convincing case that disc herniation for which care is sought in juveniles and adults is influenced by familial factors.

Evidence of substantial familial aggregation of type, extent, and location of degenerative changes was found in two earlier studies of monozygotic twins published in 1995 (Battie et al. 1995a, b). The first study of 20 pairs of adult male monozygotic (identical) twins assessed the degree of similarities in degenerative findings of qualitatively assessed disc desiccation, narrowing, and bulging or herniation in the upper and lower lumbar regions (Battie et al. 1995a). Concordance in findings between twins was compared to that which would have been expected by chance based on the prevalence of the findings among all 40 subjects. Depending on the specific disc degeneration phenotype and lumbar level, 0–15 % of the variance in disc degeneration was explained by age and smoking, but the explained variance rose to 26–72 % when familial aggregation (the twin sibling's findings) was also considered. Less variance in disc degeneration was explained at the lower than upper lumbar levels.

Subsequently, an investigation of the lumbar MRI of 115 pairs of adult male identical twins revealed even more substantial familial aggregation in terms of signal intensity, bulging, and height narrowing (Fig. 9.3) (Battie et al. 1995b). In the multivariable analysis of the T12–L4 region, history of physical loading explained 7 % of the variance in disc degeneration scores among the 230 subjects, which rose to 16 % with the addition of age and to 77 % with the addition of a variable representing familial aggregation. In the L4–5 and L5–S1 region, history of physical loading explained only 2 % of the variance in disc degeneration summary scores, which rose to 9 % with the addition of age and to 43 % with consideration of familial aggregation.

These studies revealing modest effects of suspected environmental risk factors and substantial familial influences suggested the possibility of a strong genetic influence on disc degeneration. Yet, the finding that significantly less variance in degeneration was explained in the lower lumbar region, as compared to the upper lumbar region, was puzzling. It was speculated that such a difference could be due to variations in spinal anthropometrics between upper and lower lumbar regions interacting with environmental conditions resulting in a disproportional effect at the lower lumbar levels (Battie et al. 1995b). Since that time, further study has suggested that while some genetic effects appear to act on all lumbar discs, there are also substantial genetic influences that are distinct for the upper and lower lumbar regions (Battie et al. 2007b).

9.5.7.2 Heritability

Once familial aggregation in a trait is established, interest shifts to disentangling genetic and shared environmental influences. Classic twin studies comparing concordance of findings in monozygotic and dizygotic twin pairs provide a methodology for doing this. Classic twin studies are based, in part, on the assumption that monozygotic (identical) twin siblings have 100 % of their genes in common, whereas dizygotic (nonidentical) same-sex twins share 50 % of their genes, on average, while co-twins of either zygosity share the same environment similarly. Such studies can provide overall estimates of genetic versus environmental influences. Specifically, heritability, which is the proportion of population variance in a trait, in this case disc degeneration, that is due to interindividual genetic variation, can be estimated.

Following the previous studies suggesting the strong possibility of substantial genetic influences, Sambrook et al. conducted a classic twin study to examine heritability of disc degeneration using spine MRI for 86 pairs of monozygotic and 77 dizygotic pairs, primarily women from Australia and the UK (Sambrook et al. 1999). A substantial genetic influence was found. For an overall disc degeneration score comprised of qualitative ratings of disc height, signal intensity, bulging and anterior osteophyte formation, heritability estimates were 74 % (95 % CI, 64–81 %) for the lumbar spine and 73 % (95 % CI, 64–80 %) for the cervical spine. Interestingly, when examining the components of the summary score, they reported that a genetic influence was not apparent for signal intensity, which is perhaps the most fundamental sign of disc degeneration on MRI, and that most highly associated with aging.

A later classic twin study of 600 Finnish men (300 twin pairs) further confirmed a substantial genetic influence on disc degeneration (Battie et al. 2008). In this case, the heritability estimates, ranging from 29 to 54 % (depending on the particular phenotype and lumbar level), were not as high as those reported in the earlier classic twin study of Australian and UK women. The substantial but more moderate genetic influences found for disc signal, height narrowing, and

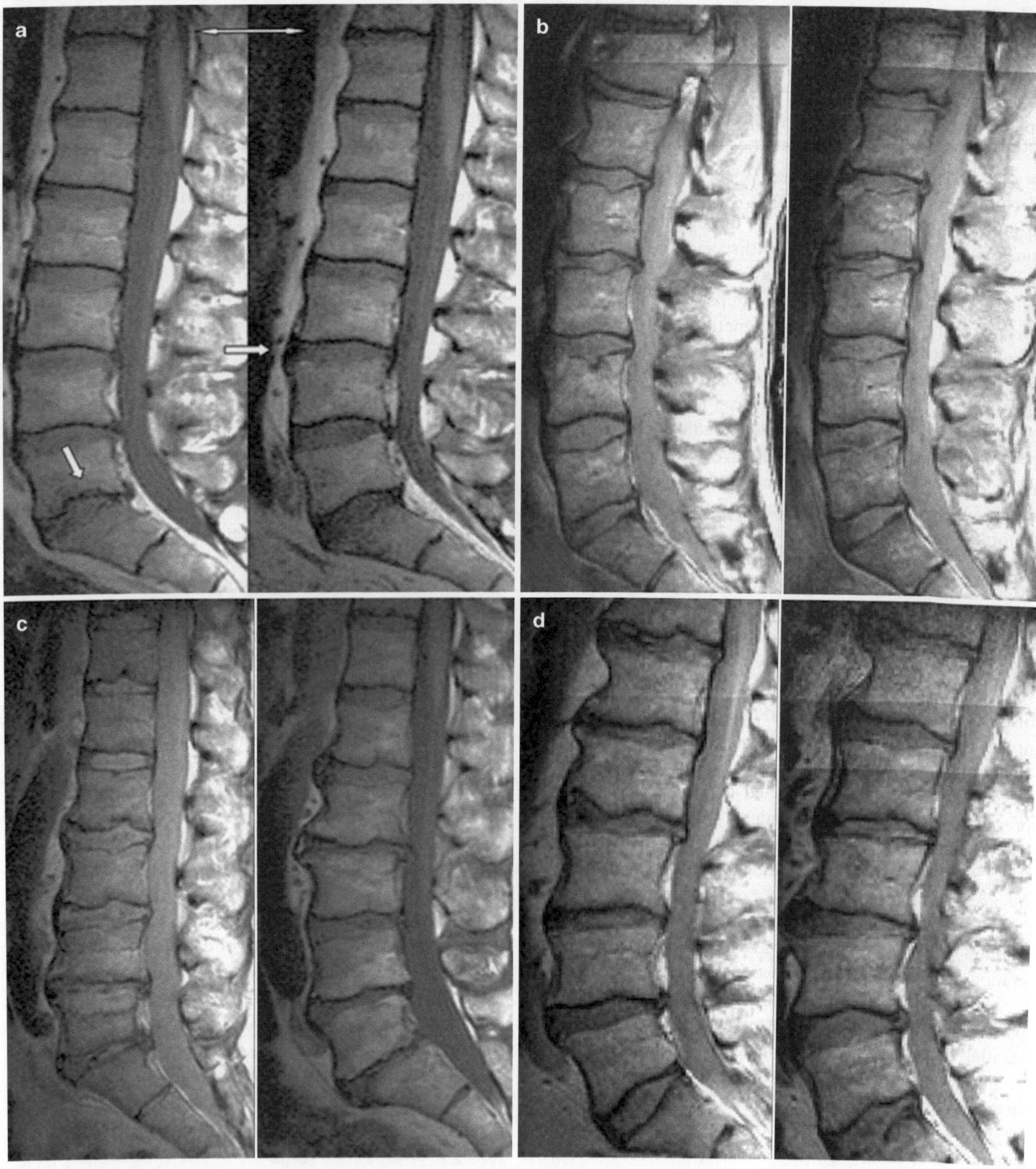

Fig. 9.3 Examples of monozygotic twin sibling MRIs demonstrating similarities in degenerative findings despite substantial lifelong differences in occupational physical loading. The twin siblings are 44 (**a**), 48 (**b**), 49 (**c**) and 61 years of age (**d**) (From the paper by Battié el al. (2004), with permission)

bulging in the study of Finnish twins were in line with what could have been expected from the earlier study of familial aggregation among male monozygotic twins. Among the strengths of the study of Finnish men were the examination of distinct disc degeneration phenotypes, the investigation of genetic influences by spinal level, and the use of multivariate genetic analyses to investigate shared genetic and environmental pathways between phenotypes.

The variance in heritability estimates between the classic twin studies may reflect differences in definitions of the phenotype of disc degeneration, sample characteristics, or true population differences. The disc degeneration phenotype used in the study by Sambrook et al. was a combination of individual qualitative ratings of disc narrowing, signal, bulging, and osteophytes, which were summed across all levels of the lumbar spine. Yet, as disc narrowing and bulging were credited with primarily being responsible for the heritability estimates, it seems unlikely that the difference in the estimates between studies would be mainly due to phenotypes used. The one dramatic exception, however, relates to the measurement of disc signal and related heritability estimates between studies. Heritability estimates for disc signal in Finnish men ranged from 30 to 54 %, depending on spinal level, whereas the study findings from the UK and Australia suggested that disc signal was not heritable. We suspect that this difference is largely due to the quality of the measures of signal used. A qualitative score of 0–3 was used in the study primarily of female twins, whereas the study of male twins used a quantitative measure with greater precision, based on the MRI digital data.

The most obvious difference in the classic twin studies samples was that one was comprised primarily of middle-aged women, and the other of men. Since heritability estimates are dependent on genotype and exposure to influential environmental factors, it may be that the adult men had greater exposure to environmental risk factors on average than the sample of women, such that the genetic contribution to total variance in disc degeneration was greater in women. Also, theoretically, sex-linked genetic differences may be influencing disc degeneration.

One potentially important finding from the study of Finnish twins was the surprisingly modest shared genetic and environmental influences between upper and lower lumbar regions. Although some genetic influences were shared, a large portion appeared to be unique to either the upper or lower lumbar discs. This finding has important implications for studying the effects of genes, environmental exposures, and biomechanical factors and strongly suggests that the upper and lower lumbar regions should be considered separately. It was speculated that in addition to genetic effects on the disc's structural components and their integrity, genes may also influence lumbar morphology, neuromuscular control, biomechanics, and other factors, which may have different or disproportionate effects on degeneration in upper and lower lumbar levels (Battie et al. 2008). Conversely, there was a high degree of shared genetic influences between the disc degeneration phenotypes of disc signal intensity, height narrowing, and bulging, suggesting that these phenotypes may have a common etiopathogenesis and represent different aspects or stages of the same degenerative process.

As might be expected from the strong genetic influence on disc degeneration based on cross-sectional data, there is also evidence of a strong familial and genetic influence on the rate of progression of disc degeneration in adulthood (Videman et al. 2006; Williams et al. 2011). It was suggested by one longitudinal study, however, that the heritability of progression of disc degeneration may be most apparent, at least in women, under the age of 50 years (Williams et al. 2011).

Several mechanisms have been suggested through which hereditary factors could influence disc degeneration and herniation. Turnover of the disc's biochemical and structural constituents could be genetically predetermined, in part, leading to varying susceptibility to degenerative changes in some persons relative to others. This has attracted the most attention in gene studies. Genes may also act through determining the size and shape of spinal structures, affecting the spine's mechanical properties and thus its vulnerability to internal and external forces. Given the far-reaching effects of genes, the heritability estimates of disc degeneration may come from a myriad of relevant, genetically influenced structural, functional, and behavioral factors.

In summary, the results of classic twin studies of disc degeneration reveal a substantial role for genetics but also emphasize that environmental factors are influential. Yet, the major suspected environmental risk factors of materials handling and physical demands, as indicated by occupation or regularly performed leisure and sports activities, explain little of the variation seen in disc degeneration. Progress in identifying important environmental influences will likely require new ideas and reconceptualizing influential environmental factors, as well as advances in their measurement.

9.6 Summary of Critical Concepts Discussed in the Chapter

- Although "degenerative disc disease" and disc degeneration have been used as synonyms in the scientific literature by many, disc degeneration does not equate to disc disease or necessarily result in back pain.
- Currently there is no universal case definition for disc degeneration. The presence and severity of disc degeneration are typically judged from MRI based on decreased signal intensity, disc bulging, disc height narrowing, annular fissures, and osteophytes, either separately or combined.
- Disc degeneration begins in youth and is ubiquitous in adulthood, with a higher prevalence and severity in the lower than upper lumbar region.
- Previously, disc degeneration was thought to be a consequence of mechanical wear and tear. Current research,

however, supports the view that disc degeneration is primarily a result of genetic influences, with environmental factors also being important.

- Age and age-associated factors also play a critical role in the pathogenesis of disc degeneration.
- The endplate may be the structure through which a number of etiological factors lead to disc degeneration.

Acknowledgements M.C. Battié receives support from the Canada Research Chairs Program.

References

Adams MA, Roughley PJ (2006) What is intervertebral disc degeneration, and what causes it? Spine 31:2151–2161

Adams MA, Dolan P, Hutton WC (1986) The stages of disc degeneration as revealed by discograms. J Bone Joint Surg Br 68:36–41

Ala-Kokko L (2002) Genetic risk factors for lumbar disc disease. Ann Med 34:42–47

Battié M, Videman T (2004) Genetic transmission of common spinal disorders. In: Herkowitz H (ed) The lumbar spine. Lippincott Williams &Wilkins, Philadelphia, pp 98–106

Battie MC, Videman T, Gill K, Moneta GB, Nyman R, Kaprio J, Koskenvuo M (1991) 1991 Volvo Award in clinical sciences. Smoking and lumbar intervertebral disc degeneration: an MRI study of identical twins. Spine (Phila Pa 1976) 16:1015–1021

Battie MC, Haynor DR, Fisher LD, Gill K, Gibbons LE, Videman T (1995a) Similarities in degenerative findings on magnetic resonance images of the lumbar spines of identical twins. J Bone Joint Surg Am 77:1662–1670

Battie MC, Videman T, Gibbons LE, Fisher LD, Manninen H, Gill K (1995b) 1995 Volvo Award in clinical sciences. Determinants of lumbar disc degeneration. A study relating lifetime exposures and magnetic resonance imaging findings in identical twins. Spine (Phila Pa 1976) 20:2601–2612

Battie MC, Videman T, Gibbons LE, Manninen H, Gill K, Pope M, Kaprio J (2002) Occupational driving and lumbar disc degeneration: a case-control study. Lancet 360:1369–1374

Battie MC, Videman T, Parent E (2004) Lumbar disc degeneration: epidemiology and genetic influences. Spine (Phila Pa 1976) 29: 2679–2690

Battie MC, Videman T, Carragee EJ (2007a) Re: Virtanen IM, Karppinen J, Taimela S, et al. Occupational and genetic risk factors associated with intervertebral disc disease. Spine 2007;32:1129–34. Spine (Phila Pa 1976) 32:2926–2927

Battie MC, Videman T, Levalahti E, Gill K, Kaprio J (2007b) Heritability of low back pain and the role of disc degeneration. Pain 131:272–280

Battie MC, Videman T, Levalahti E, Gill K, Kaprio J (2008) Genetic and environmental effects on disc degeneration by phenotype and spinal level: a multivariate twin study. Spine (Phila Pa 1976) 33:2801–2808

Battié MC, Videman T, Kaprio J, Gibbons LE, Gill K, Manninen H, Saarela J, Peltonen L (2009) The Twin Spine Study: contributions to a changing view of disc degeneration. Spine J 9:47–59

Benneker LM, Heini PF, Alini M, Anderson SE, Ito K (2005) 2004 Young Investigator Award Winner: vertebral endplate marrow contact channel occlusions and intervertebral disc degeneration. Spine (Phila Pa 1976) 30:167–173

Boos N, Weissbach S, Rohrbach H, Weiler C, Spratt KF, Nerlich AG (2002) Classification of age-related changes in lumbar intervertebral discs: 2002 Volvo Award in basic science. Spine (Phila Pa 1976) 27:2631–2644

Brinckmann P, Frobin W, Hierholzer E, Horst M (1983) Deformation of the vertebral end-plate under axial loading of the spine. Spine (Phila Pa 1976) 8:851–856

Caplan PS, Freedman LM, Connelly TP (1966) Degenerative joint disease of the lumbar spine in coal miners–a clinical and x-ray study. Arthritis Rheum 9:693–702

Carragee EJ, Don AS, Hurwitz EL, Cuellar JM, Carrino JA, Herzog R (2009) 2009 ISSLS Prize Winner: does discography cause accelerated progression of degeneration changes in the lumbar disc: a ten-year matched cohort study. Spine (Phila Pa 1976) 34:2338–2345

Cherkin DC, Deyo RA, Loeser JD, Bush T, Waddell G (1994) An international comparison of back surgery rates. Spine (Phila Pa 1976) 19:1201–1206

Cheung KM, Karppinen J, Chan D, Ho DW, Song YQ, Sham P, Cheah KS, Leong JC, Luk KD (2009) Prevalence and pattern of lumbar magnetic resonance imaging changes in a population study of one thousand forty-three individuals. Spine (Phila Pa 1976) 34:934–940

Coventry M, Ghormley R, Kernohan JW (1945a) The intervertebral disc: its microscopic anatomy and pathology. Part II. Changes in the intervertebral disc concomitant with age. J Bone Joint Surg Am 27:233–247

Coventry M, Ghormley R, Kernohan JW (1945b) The intervertebral disc: its microscopic anatomy and pathology. Part III, Pathological changes in the intervertebral disc. J Bone Joint Surg Am 27:460–474

Dandy W (1929) Loose cartilage from intervertebral disc simulating tumor of the spinal cord. Arch Surg 660–672

del Pozo-Cruz B, Hernandez Mocholi MA, Adsuar JC, Parraca JA, Muro I, Gusi N (2011) Effects of whole body vibration therapy on main outcome measures for chronic non-specific low back pain: a single-blind randomized controlled trial. J Rehabil Med 43: 689–694

Dilke TF, Burry HC, Grahame R (1973) Extradural corticosteroid injection in management of lumbar nerve root compression. Br Med J 2:635–637

Ferguson SJ, Steffen T (2003) Biomechanics of the aging spine. Eur Spine J 12:S97–S103

Fletcher GH (1947) Backward displacement of fifth lumbar vertebra in degenerative disc disease; the significance of the difference in anteroposterior diameters of the fifth lumbar and first sacral vertebrae. J Bone Joint Surg Am 29:1019–1026

Friberg S, Hirsch C (1948) Anatomical studies on lumbar disc degeneration. Acta Orthop Scand 17:224–230

Friberg S, Hirsch C (1949) Anatomical and clinical studies on lumbar disc degeneration. Acta Orthop Scand 19:222–242

Friedenberg Z, Miller W (1963) Degenerative disc disease of the cervical spine. J Bone Joint Surg Am 45:1171–1178

Frymoyer JW (1992) Lumbar disk disease: epidemiology. Instr Course Lect 41:217–223

Frymoyer JW, Newberg A, Pope MH, Wilder DG, Clements J, MacPherson B (1984) Spine radiographs in patients with low-back pain. An epidemiological study in men. J Bone Joint Surg Am 66:1048–1055

Gertzbein SD, Tile M, Gross A, Falk R (1975) Autoimmunity in degenerative disc disease of the lumbar spine. Orthop Clin North Am 6:67–73

Gunzburg R, Parkinson R, Moore R, Cantraine F, Hutton W, Vernon-Roberts B, Fraser R (1992) A cadaveric study comparing discography, magnetic resonance imaging, histology, and mechanical behavior of the human lumbar disc. Spine (Phila Pa 1976) 17:417–426

Guyer RD, Ohnmeiss DD (2003) Lumbar discography. Spine J 3: 11S–27S

Hadler NM, Tait RC, Chibnall JT (2007) Back pain in the workplace. JAMA 297:1594–1596

Hamanishi C, Kawabata T, Yosii T, Tanaka S (1994) Schmorl's nodes on magnetic resonance imaging. Their incidence and clinical relevance. Spine (Phila Pa 1976) 19:450–453

Hancock MJ, Battie MC, Videman T, Gibbons L (2010) The role of back injury or trauma in lumbar disc degeneration: an exposure-discordant twin study. Spine (Phila Pa 1976) 35:1925–1929

Haschtmann D, Stoyanov JV, Gedet P, Ferguson SJ (2008) Vertebral endplate trauma induces disc cell apoptosis and promotes organ degeneration in vitro. Eur Spine J 17:289–299

Haughton V (2006) Imaging intervertebral disc degeneration. J Bone Joint Surg Am 88(Suppl 2):15–20

Heine J (1926) Ûber die Arthritis deformans. Virch Arch Pathol Anat 521–663

Hill TE, Desmoulin GT, Hunter CJ (2009) Is vibration truly an injurious stimulus in the human spine? J Biomech 42:2631–2635

Hilton RC, Ball J, Benn RT (1976) Vertebral end-plate lesions (Schmorl's nodes) in the dorsolumbar spine. Ann Rheum Dis 35:127–132

Hirsch C (1948) On lumbar facetectomies. Acta Orthop Scand 17: 240–252

Hult L (1954) The Munkfors investigation; a study of the frequency and causes of the stiff neck-brachialgia and lumbago-sciatica syndromes, as well as observations on certain signs and symptoms from the dorsal spine and the joints of the extremities in industrial and forest workers. Acta Orthop Scand Suppl 16:1–76

Kellgren JH, Lawrence JS (1952) Rheumatism in miners. II. X-ray study. Br J Ind Med 9:197–207

Kerttula LI, Serlo WS, Tervonen OA, Paakko EL, Vanharanta HV (2000) Post-traumatic findings of the spine after earlier vertebral fracture in young patients: clinical and MRI study. Spine (Phila Pa 1976) 25:1104–1108

Kettler A, Wilke HJ (2006) Review of existing grading systems for cervical or lumbar disc and facet joint degeneration. Eur Spine J 15:705–718

Kjaer P, Leboeuf-Yde C, Korsholm L, Sorensen JS, Bendix T (2005a) Magnetic resonance imaging and low back pain in adults: a diagnostic imaging study of 40-year-old men and women. Spine 30: 1173–1180

Kjaer P, Leboeuf-Yde C, Sorensen JS, Bendix T (2005b) An epidemiologic study of MRI and low back pain in 13-year-old children. Spine (Phila Pa 1976) 30:798–806

Kjellberg A, WikstrÕm B-Q, LandstrÕm U (1994) Injuries and other adverse effects of occupational exposure to whole-body vibration: a review for criteria documentation. Arbete Och Hãlsa vetenskaplig skriftserie 41:1–74

Lane NE, Nevitt MC, Genant HK, Hochberg MC (1993) Reliability of new indices of radiographic osteoarthritis of the hand and hip and lumbar disc degeneration. J Rheumatol 20:1911–1918

Lawrence JS (1955) Rheumatism in coal miners. III. Occupational factors. Br J Ind Med 12:249–261

Lindblom K (1948) Diagnostic puncture of intervertebral disks in sciatica. Acta Orthop Scand 17:231–239

Lings S, Leboeuf-Yde C (2000) Whole-body vibration and low back pain: a systematic, critical review of the epidemiological literature 1992-1999. Int Arch Occup Environ Health 73:290–297

Macnab I (1973) Chapter 14. Pain and disability in degenerative disc disease. Clin Neurosurg 20:193–196

Matsui H, Tsuji H, Terahata N (1990) Juvenile lumbar herniated nucleus pulposus in monozygotic twins. Spine (Phila Pa 1976) 15:1228–1230

Matsui H, Kanamori M, Ishihara H, Yudoh K, Naruse Y, Tsuji H (1998) Familial predisposition for lumbar degenerative disc disease. A case-control study. Spine (Phila Pa 1976) 23:1029–1034

Miller JA, Schmatz C, Schultz AB (1988) Lumbar disc degeneration: correlation with age, sex, and spine level in 600 autopsy specimens. Spine (Phila Pa 1976) 13:173–178

Mimura M, Panjabi MM, Oxland TR, Crisco JJ, Yamamoto I, Vasavada A (1994) Disc degeneration affects the multidirectional flexibility of the lumbar spine. Spine (Phila Pa 1976) 19:1371–1380

Mixter W, Barr J (1934) Rupture of the intervertebral disc with involvement of the spinal canal. N Engl J Med 210–215

Modic MT, Pavlicek W, Weinstein MA, Boumphrey F, Ngo F, Hardy R, Duchesneau PM (1984) Magnetic resonance imaging of intervertebral disk disease. Clinical and pulse sequence considerations. Radiology 152:103–111

Mok FP, Samartzis D, Karppinen J, Luk KD, Fong DY, Cheung KM (2010) ISSLS prize winner: Prevalence, determinants, and association of Schmorl nodes of the lumbar spine with disc degeneration: a population-based study of 2449 individuals. Spine (Phila Pa 1976) 35:1944–1952

Moore RJ (2006) The vertebral endplate: disc degeneration, disc regeneration. Eur Spine J 15:S333–S337

Nachemson A (1960) Lumbar intradiscal pressure. Experimental studies on post-mortem material. Acta Orthop Scand Suppl 43:1–104

Nachemson A, Lewin T, Maroudas A, Freeman MA (1970) In vitro diffusion of dye through the end-plates and the annulus fibrosus of human lumbar inter-vertebral discs. Acta Orthop Scand 41: 589–607

Nelson CL, Janecki CJ, Gildenberg PL, Sava G (1972) Disk protrusions in the young. Clin Orthop Relat Res 88:142–150

Osti OL, Vernon-Roberts B, Fraser RD (1990) 1990 Volvo Award in experimental studies. Anulus tears and intervertebral disc degeneration. An experimental study using an animal model. Spine (Phila Pa 1976) 15:762–767

Parisien RC, Ball PA (1998) William Jason Mixter (1880-1958). Ushering in the "dynasty of the disc". Spine (Phila Pa 1976) 23: 2363–2366

Pfirrmann CW, Resnick D (2001) Schmorl nodes of the thoracic and lumbar spine: radiographic-pathologic study of prevalence, characterization, and correlation with degenerative changes of 1,650 spinal levels in 100 cadavers. Radiology 219:368–374

Pfirrmann CW, Metzdorf A, Zanetti M, Hodler J, Boos N (2001) Magnetic resonance classification of lumbar intervertebral disc degeneration. Spine (Phila Pa 1976) 26:1873–1878

Porter RW, Adams MA, Hutton WC (1989) Physical activity and the strength of the lumbar spine. Spine (Phila Pa 1976) 14:201–203

Postacchini F, Lami R, Pugliese O (1988) Familial predisposition to discogenic low-back pain. An epidemiologic and immunogenetic study. Spine (Phila Pa 1976) 13:1403–1406

Rajaee SS, Bae HW, Kanim LE, Delamarter RB (2012) Spinal fusion in the United States: analysis of trends from 1998 to 2008. Spine (Phila Pa 1976) 37:67–76

Richardson JK, Chung T, Schultz JS, Hurvitz E (1997) A familial predisposition toward lumbar disc injury. Spine (Phila Pa 1976) 22:1487–1492

Riihimaki H, Mattsson T, Zitting A, Wickstrom G, Hanninen K, Waris P (1990) Radiographically detectable degenerative changes of the lumbar spine among concrete reinforcement workers and house painters. Spine (Phila Pa 1976) 15:114–119

Rittweger J, Just K, Kautzsch K, Reeg P, Felsenberg D (2002) Treatment of chronic lower back pain with lumbar extension and whole-body vibration exercise: a randomized controlled trial. Spine (Phila Pa 1976) 27:1829–1834

Roberts S, Urban JP, Evans H, Eisenstein SM (1996) Transport properties of the human cartilage endplate in relation to its composition and calcification. Spine (Phila Pa 1976) 21:415–420

Rokitansky C (1855) Lehrbuch der patholoqische Anatomie. Braumüller, Wien

Sairanen E, Brushaber L, Kaskinen M (1981) Felling work, low-back pain and osteoarthritis. Scand J Work Environ Health 7:18–30

Saluja G, Fitzpatrick K, Bruce M, Cross J (1986) Schmorl's nodes (intravertebral herniations of intervertebral disc tissue) in two historic British populations. J Anat 145:87–96

Samartzis D, Karppinen J, Mok F, Fong DY, Luk KD, Cheung KM (2011) A population-based study of juvenile disc degeneration and its association with overweight and obesity, low back pain, and diminished functional status. J Bone Joint Surg Am 93:662–670

Sambrook PN, MacGregor AJ, Spector TD (1999) Genetic influences on cervical and lumbar disc degeneration: a magnetic resonance imaging study in twins. Arthritis Rheum 42:366–372

Scapinelli R (1993) Lumbar disc herniation in eight siblings with a positive family history for disc disease. Acta Orthop Belg 59:371–376

Schmorl G, Junghanns H (1971) The human spine in health and disease. Grune and Stratton, New York

Schneiderman G, Flannigan B, Kingston S, Thomas J, Dillin WH, Watkins RG (1987) Magnetic resonance imaging in the diagnosis of disc degeneration: correlation with discography. Spine (Phila Pa 1976) 12:276–281

Seidler A, Bergmann A, Jager M, Ellegast R, Ditchen D, Elsner G, Grifka J, Haerting J, Hofmann F, Linhardt O, Luttmann A, Michaelis M, Petereit-Haack G, Schumann B, Bolm-Audorff U (2009) Cumulative occupational lumbar load and lumbar disc disease–results of a German multi-center case-control study (EPILIFT). BMC Musculoskelet Disord 10:48

Setton LA, Zhu W, Weidenbaum M, Ratcliffe A, Mow VC (1993) Compressive properties of the cartilaginous end-plate of the baboon lumbar spine. J Orthop Res 11:228–239

Simmons ED Jr, Guntupalli M, Kowalski JM, Braun F, Seidel T (1996) Familial predisposition for degenerative disc disease. A case-control study. Spine (Phila Pa 1976) 21:1527–1529

Takatalo J, Karppinen J, Niinimaki J, Taimela S, Nayha S, Jarvelin MR, Kyllonen E, Tervonen O (2009) Prevalence of degenerative imaging findings in lumbar magnetic resonance imaging among young adults. Spine (Phila Pa 1976) 34:1716–1721

Torgerson WR, Dotter WE (1976) Comparative roentgenographic study of the asymptomatic and symptomatic lumbar spine. J Bone Joint Surg Am 58:850–853

Urban JP, Smith S, Fairbank JC (2004) Nutrition of the intervertebral disc. Spine (Phila Pa 1976) 29:2700–2709

Varlotta GP, Brown MD, Kelsey JL, Golden AL (1991) Familial predisposition for herniation of a lumbar disc in patients who are less than twenty-one years old. J Bone Joint Surg Am 73:124–128

Varughese G, Quartey GR (1979) Familial lumbar spinal stenosis with acute disc herniations. Case reports of four brothers. J Neurosurg 51:234–236

Vernon-Roberts B (1994) Christian Georg Schmorl. Pioneer of spinal pathology and radiology. Spine (Phila Pa 1976) 19:2724–2727

Videman T, Battie MC (2012) Commentary: back pain epidemiology-the challenge of case definition and developing new ideas. Spine J 12:71–72

Videman T, Malmivaara A, Mooney V (1987) The value of the axial view in assessing discograms. An experimental study with cadavers. Spine 12:299–304

Videman T, Nurminen M, Troup JD (1990) 1990 Volvo Award in clinical sciences. Lumbar spinal pathology in cadaveric material in relation to history of back pain, occupation, and physical loading. Spine 15:728–740

Videman T, Nummi P, Battie MC, Gill K (1994) Digital assessment of MRI for lumbar disc desiccation. A comparison of digital versus subjective assessments and digital intensity profiles versus discogram and macroanatomic findings. Spine (Phila Pa 1976) 19:192–198

Videman T, Battie MC, Gill K, Manninen H, Gibbons LE, Fisher LD (1995) Magnetic resonance imaging findings and their relationships in the thoracic and lumbar spine. Insights into the etiopathogenesis of spinal degeneration. Spine (Phila Pa 1976) 20:928–935

Videman T, Battie MC, Ripatti S, Gill K, Manninen H, Kaprio J (2006) Determinants of the progression in lumbar degeneration: a 5-year follow-up study of adult male monozygotic twins. Spine (Phila Pa 1976) 31:671–678

Videman T, Levalahti E, Battie MC (2007) The effects of anthropometrics, lifting strength, and physical activities in disc degeneration. Spine 32:1406–1413

Videman T, Gibbons LE, Battie MC (2008) Age- and pathology-specific measures of disc degeneration. Spine (Phila Pa 1976) 33: 2781–2788

Videman T, Gibbons LE, Kaprio J, Battie MC (2010) Challenging the cumulative injury model: positive effects of greater body mass on disc degeneration. Spine J 10:26–31

Virgin W (1951) Experimental investigations into the physical properties of the intervertebral disc. J Bone Joint Surg Br 33-B: 607–611

Vo N, Wang D, Sowa G, Witt W, Ngo K, Coelho P, Bedison R, Byer B, Studer R, Lee J, Di YP, Kang J (2011) Differential effects of nicotine and tobacco smoke condensate on human annulus fibrosus cell metabolism. J Orthop Res 29:1585–1591

Wang Y (2011) The roles of vertebra and vertebral endplate in lumbar disc degeneration. Doctoral Thesis, University of Alberta

Wang Y, Battie MC, Boyd SK, Videman T (2011) The osseous endplates in lumbar vertebrae: thickness, bone mineral density and their associations with age and disk degeneration. Bone 48:804–809

Wang Y, Videman T, Battie M (2012a) ISSLS prize winner: Lumbar vertebral endplate lesions: associations with disc degeneration and back pain history. Spine (Phila Pa 1976) 37:1490–1496

Wang Y, Videman T, Battie MC (2012b) Lumbar vertebral endplate lesions: prevalence, classification and association with age. Spine (Phila Pa 1976) 37:1432–1439

Weiner DS, Macnab I (1970) The use of chymopapain in degenerative disc disease: a preliminary report. Can Med Assoc J 102:1252–1256

Weinstein JS, Burchiel KJ (2009) Dandy'S disc. Neurosurgery 65: 201–205

Wenzel C (1824) Uber die Krankbeiten am Ruckgrate. Wesche, Bamberg

WHO (2012) World Health Organization website. www.who.int/topics/epidemiology/en/. Access date Feb 2012

Williams FM, Manek NJ, Sambrook PN, Spector TD, MacGregor AJ (2007) Schmorl's nodes: common, highly heritable, and related to lumbar disc disease. Arthritis Rheum 57:855–860

Williams FM, Popham M, Sambrook PN, Jones AF, Spector TD, MacGregor AJ (2011) Progression of lumbar disc degeneration over a decade: a heritability study. Ann Rheum Dis 70:1203–1207

Genetic Basis of Intervertebral Disc Degeneration

10

Anita Yee and Danny Chan

Contents

10.1 Understanding Disease Mechanism Through Genetic Studies

Genetics is an area of study that connects genes with functions, variations with phenotypes, and, of most interest to scientists and clinicians, mutations with diseases. According to the Online Mendelian Inheritance in Man (OMIM), an online catalog for human genes and Mendelian disorders, over 3,000 known "genotype-phenotype" pairs have been recorded. A direct application of such knowledge is *diagnosis*, of which prenatal testing and newborn screening of rare conditions are common nowadays; ideally, this would be extended in future for disease prevention or the development of personalized medicine. It is clear that our understanding of disease mechanism of rare skeletal disorders such as osteogenesis imperfecta (OI), spondyloepiphyseal dysplasia (SED), achondroplasia, and Ehlers-Danlos syndrome (EDS) has come directly from knowing the genes involved, allowing detailed in vitro and in vivo functional studies. While more difficult for common disorders such as intervertebral disc degeneration, the same principle can be applied, bearing in mind the effect size, the number of genes involved, and contributions from environment factors. These are the issues that this chapter will address systematically, namely, to provide the basic concepts of what genetic studies can

A. Yee • D. Chan (✉)
Department of Biochemistry,
The University of Hong Kong,
3/F Laboratory Block, LKS Faculty of Medicine,
21 Sassoon Road, Pokfulam, Hong Kong
e-mail: chand@hku.hk

I.M. Shapiro, M.V. Risbud (eds.), *The Intervertebral Disc*,
DOI 10.1007/978-3-7091-1535-0_10, © Springer-Verlag Wien 2014

achieve and with the benefit of hindsight from studies of similar disorders such as osteoarthritis (OA) to generate a road map for studies of intervertebral disc degeneration.

10.2 Applying Genetic Studies to Intervertebral Disc Degeneration

10.2.1 Classical Approaches in Human Genetic Studies

Gregor Mendel, regarded as the "Father of Genetics," laid the foundation of modern genetics with his work in the nineteenth century, *Versuche über Pflanzen-Hybriden* (Experiments in Plant Hybridization).

10.2.1.1 Mendelian Genetics: Single Gene Defects

The genetic materials in human, except those in sex chromosomes, exist in pairs which are called alleles (Box 10.1). The two alleles at a certain position can be the same or different. In a simple scenario of genetic diseases, they represent normal and disease-causing alleles. Disease-causing alleles (often regarded as mutations) connect to phenotypes; however, whether or not one would develop the phenotype depends on the number of disease-causing allele being carried and whether the allele exerts a dominant or recessive trait. For dominant alleles, a single copy is sufficient to show an effect or phenotype, while for recessive alleles, two copies are required. To pass on the alleles to next generation, Mendelian genetics state that the parental alleles would segregate, and an individual would obtain one allele from each parent randomly. In dominant inheritance, one parent would be carrying a disease-causing allele, and the offspring who receive this allele will have the phenotype (Fig. 10.1a). For recessive inheritance, both parents must carry at least one copy of the disease-causing allele, and only the offspring who obtain both copies would show the phenotype (Fig. 10.1b).

Box 10.1: Glossary

Allele: An alternative form of the genetic material at a certain position (locus), which may or may not lead to a difference in observable traits (phenotype).

Mutation: A change in the genetic material which can involve a single nucleotide (point mutation) or a segment of genomic sequence (insertion, deletion, duplication, inversion, and translocation). The outcome of a mutation can be harmful leading to diseases, while neutral or beneficial effects are also possible.

Phenotype: An observable trait as a result of the genotypic composition but at the same time can be affected by environmental factors and their interactions with the genetic components.

Dominance: The relationship of the two alleles at a certain locus where one allele can mask the effect of the other to demonstrate the phenotype.

Recessive: The relationship of the two alleles at a certain locus where the effect of one allele is masked by the other and thus two copies of such allele are required to demonstrate the phenotype.

Linkage disequilibrium (*LD*): A situation when genotypes at two or more loci are not independent of each other and that there would be a difference between the observed and expected frequencies of certain combinations of alleles (haplotype) in a population.

Restriction fragment length polymorphism (*RFLP*): Genetic variation leading to the creation or destruction of restriction enzyme site and therefore generating different DNA fragments after enzymatic digestion. The variation can be identified simply by detecting the resultant fragment lengths using gel electrophoresis. This is an inexpensive technique for genotyping.

Variable number of tandem repeat (*VNTR*): A type of genetic variation in which a short nucleotide sequence repeats consecutively. The number of repeats can be variable, and thus in a population, more than two alleles can be present for a particular locus.

Single nucleotide polymorphism (*SNP*): The most common type of genetic variation which involves only a single nucleotide difference. It occurs throughout the whole genome. Unlike VNTR, each SNP typically contains only two alleles.

Genome-wide association study (*GWAS*): Examination of a huge number of genetic variants that are distributed all over the genome in multiple individuals to identify whether any of them are associated with a trait. The focuses are generally placed on the common SNPs and traits such as common diseases.

Epigenome-wide association study (*EWAS*): A new concept similar to GWAS – examination of a large number of epigenetic variations, such as DNA methylation, over the genome in multiple individuals to identify their associations with a trait.

There are a number of skeletal abnormalities that follow Mendelian inheritance. Classic examples included osteogenesis imperfecta (OI), a fragile bone condition due to mutations in one of the two α-chains of the collagen I genes (*COL1A1* and *COL1A2*), and spondyloepiphyseal dysplasia (SED), which is characterized by dwarfism and shortened limbs, caused by mutations in the gene encoding collagen II (*COL2A1*), affecting the spine and epiphyses of long bones. These are rare disorders

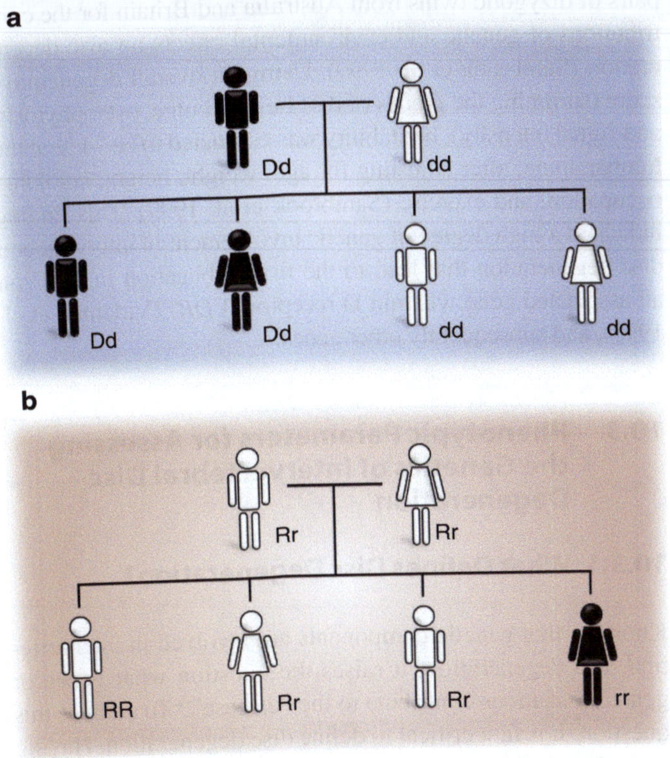

Fig. 10.1 Concepts of Mendelian inheritance. (**a**) In dominant inheritance, one parent carries the disease-causing allele *D*, with one copy sufficient to show the phenotype. Offspring who inherited the *D* allele from this parent would show the phenotype. Based on Mendelian genetics, the ratio of inheriting to not inheriting the *D* allele would be 1:1. (**b**) In recessive inheritance, both parents have to be carriers of the disease-causing allele *r*. Only the offspring who inherited two *r* alleles from both parents would show the phenotype. The Mendelian ratio of non-carrier to carrier to diseased offspring in this example would be 1:2:1

resulting from a single rare mutation which seriously affects the proper functioning of the gene products. On the other hand, common genetic variants in these genes can give rise to milder conditions. For example, genetic variations in *COL1A1* are associated with reduced bone density and osteoporosis (Grant et al. 1996), while the *COL2A1* gene is linked to osteoarthritis (OA) (Vikkula et al. 1993). These conditions, in general, are caused by multiple factors rather than a single genetic mutation, leading to the concept of complex diseases.

10.2.1.2 Complex Diseases

Complex diseases are dependent on multiple factors, which can be due to genes alone, or genes in combination with environmental factors. Taking osteoporosis as an example, apart from *COL1A1*, genes associated with bone loss include apolipoprotein E (*APOE*), vitamin D receptor (*VDR*), and interleukin 6 (*IL6*); identified environmental risk factor are age, gender, body mass index, smoking, and medications. Moreover, the association with *APOE* and *COL1A1* being restricted to a subgroup of postmenopausal women not using hormone replacement therapy suggests that environmental

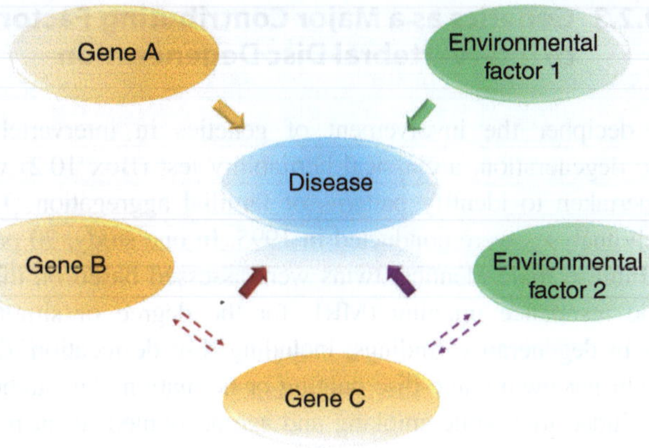

Fig. 10.2 Concept of complex diseases. Multiple genetic and environmental factors can be involved in a complex disease. They can act independently (e.g., *gene A* and *environmental factor 1*). Genetic factors can interact (e.g., *gene B* and *gene C*), or they can interact with environmental factor (e.g., *environmental factor 2* and *gene C*) contributing to the disease

factor could modulate the genetic effect on the disease (Mitchell and Yerges-Armstrong 2011). Similarly for OA, multiple genes including *COL2A1*, *SMAD3*, growth differentiation factor 5 (*GDF5*), and type II iodothyronine deiodinase (*DIO2*) also showed association with age, gender, and body mass index as known risk factors (Valdes and Spector 2011). In these cases, the allelic variations associated with the diseases are common, and individuals with these alleles may only increase their risk of developing the diseases. Therefore, in complex diseases, multiple genetic susceptibility and environmental factors contribute to disease outcome; they may act independently, or they modify the effect of each other through gene-gene interaction and/or gene-environment interaction (Fig. 10.2). Such effects can be additive, synergistic, or suppressive. Thus, complex diseases no longer present as simple Mendelian inheritance, and intervertebral disc degeneration is another such an example.

10.2.2 Intervertebral Disc Degeneration Is a Complex Trait

Prior to the involvement of genetic studies, age, gender, cigarette smoking, and mechanical loading related to occupation and sport activities have been reported to influence disc degeneration (this topic is discussed in more detail in Chap. 9). These findings place disc degeneration within the category of a complex trait. However, there is no consensus on the contribution of these environment factors to the degenerative process and hence this begs the question: what is the contribution of genetics to the intervertebral disc disease?

10.2.3 Genetics as a Major Contributing Factor to Intervertebral Disc Degeneration

To decipher the involvement of genetics in intervertebral disc degeneration, a classical heritability test (Box 10.2) was undertaken to identify patterns of familial aggregation. Two such analyses were conducted in 1995. In one study, 20 pairs of Finnish male identical twins were assessed based on magnetic resonance imaging (MRI) for the degree of similarities in degenerative findings, including disc desiccation, disc height narrowing, and disc bulging or herniation. The authors concluded that while smoking and age accounted for at most 15 % of the variability in the degenerative findings, 26–72 % of the variability was explained when the co-twin status was included (Battie et al. 1995a). In another study, 115 pairs of male identical twins with discordant exposures to suspected environmental risks were assessed for degenerative changes of the spine and symptomology. For changes in the upper lumbar region, occupational physical loading explained only 7 % of the variability in the summary score for degeneration; this increased to 16 % when age was included and to 77 % when twin status was added. In the lower lumbar region, leisure physical loading explained only 2 % of the variability in the degeneration scores; this increased to 9 % with the addition of age as a factor and to 43 % with the addition of the twin status (Battie et al. 1995b). These studies provide quantitative evidence for the existence of familial aggregation and potential genetic influences in intervertebral disc degeneration. These findings were later consolidated in a study comparing 86 pairs of monozygotic twins and 77 pairs of dizygotic twins from Australia and Britain for the contributions of genetic and environmental effects on disc degeneration (Sambrook et al. 1999). Using an overall degenerative score (summing the grades of disc height, bulge, osteophytosis, and signal intensity), heritability was estimated to be 74 % at the lumbar spine, after adjusting for age, weight, height, smoking, occupation, and exercise (Sambrook et al. 1999). This finding indicated a high degree of genetic involvement in intervertebral disc degeneration that lead to the first publication in 1997 on an associated gene, vitamin D receptor (*VDR*) (Videman et al. 1998), and subsequently other genes.

Box 10.2: Heritability Test

Heritability refers to the proportion of phenotypic variance attributed to genetic variance. It involves observing and statistically analyzing the patterns of phenotypes with varying levels of genetic or environmental background in close kin, such as parent-offspring, siblings, and twins (Visscher et al. 2008). More often, heritability can be estimated from identical twins grown up in separate environment (adoption studies). Under this situation, the genotype would be identical but the environmental factors vary, and thus the effects of the two factors can be separated. However, such twins are not easy to gather, and the age when they are separated may affect the findings. Another design would be to compare monozygotic and dizygotic twin pairs. In this scenario, the twin pairs would experience similar environmental factors, and thus comparing the phenotypic concordance of these two types of twins allows an estimation of the impact of genetic factors

10.3 Phenotypic Parameters for Assessing the Genetics of Intervertebral Disc Degeneration

10.3.1 What Defines Disc Degeneration?

Knowing that genetic components are involved in intervertebral disc degeneration, it raises the question what genes or genetic variations contribute to the "disease"? To address this question, it is first critical to define disc degeneration. Having a precise phenotype definition is essential for genetic studies in that the phenotype should be a distinguishable trait and preferably quantifiable (Wagner and Zhang 2011). Disc degeneration is a continuous process throughout life: predictable macroscopic changes include disruption of the highly organized lamellae structure, formation of tears and fissures in the annulus fibrosus, leakage of the nucleus pulposus through the fissures leading to disc bulge and herniation, damage of the end plate, an overall reduction in disc height, dehydration, increased cell death, and cell cluster formation. From a biochemical perspective, the major biochemical alterations include the loss and breakdown of collagens and aggrecan, resulting in reduced tensile strength and impaired hydration, respectively. Thus, while ample observations have been made to assess the alterations in disc degeneration, its definition remains indistinct, and there is a poor understanding of the relationship between these changes and their representation in the degenerative process.

10.3.2 Parameter Currently Used to Define Disc Degeneration

Theoretically, all the features mentioned above, and in other chapters of this book, could be used as measurable parameters for the study of disc degeneration; however, only a few can be assessed in vivo. Current assessments of disc degeneration rely on radiography and MRI. Radiographs display the density and composition of an object based on the proportion of X-rays being absorbed, providing information such as disc height and osteophyte formation. In contrast, MRI detects the rotating magnetic field of photons, an obvious advantage for the intervertebral disc as the nucleus pulposus is a hydrated tissue. Therefore, MRI can provide information on the hydration status, bulging and herniation, as well as irregularities of the end plates. In particular, the MRI images of a disc which is bright and bloated represent a highly hydrated tissue, and with the progressive loss of water, the image becomes dark. As indicated in Chap. 12, MRI can also assess proteoglycan contents in the disc, although improvements in accuracy are still required (Benneker et al. 2005; Marinelli et al. 2009).

There are multiple ways to evaluate the degenerative changes in the intervertebral disc. The first one would be to provide a definitive notation on the presence or absence of disc degeneration. This method is simple but the shortcoming is loss of information on the progressive changes during the degenerative process. Another method is to classify the severity of degeneration based on a scaling system. This is the most widely used method, and a number of classification systems have been developed. For example, Kellgren scale (Kellgren et al. 1963) combines the features of osteophytes and joint space narrowing based on radiographs and summarizes using a four-point score, ranging from score of 1 indicating no or very small osteophytes to score of 4 representing large osteophytes and pronounced disc space narrowing; Schneiderman's grading (Schneiderman et al. 1987) focuses on the signal intensity of the nucleus pulposus from MRI images and classifies them into four grades, with the lowest grade indicating hyperintense signal to the highest grade illustrating hypointense signal with disc space narrowing; Pfirrmann's classification (Pfirrmann et al. 2001) also utilizes the MRI images to evaluate the homogeneity of disc structure, signal intensity, distinction of nucleus pulposus and annulus fibrosus, as well as disc height. The information is converted into five grades, the lowest grade being homogeneous disc structure, hyperintense bright signal intensity, and normal disc height and the highest grade being inhomogeneous disc structure, hypointense black signal, loss of distinction between nucleus pulposus and annulus fibrosus, as well as collapsed disc space. While these grading systems maintain information regarding the severity of disc degeneration and provide semiquantitative evaluation of the degenerative status, interpretation of the MRI images is subjective and thus requires multiple experienced observers to perform the grading. The third method for assessing disc degeneration is by computational evaluation of the absolute signal intensity values of the MRI images (Videman et al. 1994). This approach can circumvent the potential bias arising from observers' judgment, but the data generated would likely be composed of a spectrum of values complicating subsequent data analyses.

The methods mentioned above evaluate the status of a single disc, whereas there are multiple disc levels and each may display a different stage of degeneration. This raises the question, should the grades of various levels be combined and a summation score obtained representative of the degree of proneness of an individual to disc degeneration? Alternatively, should each level be treated separately and reported as multilevel disc degeneration? Moreover, should other parameters such as disc bulging, herniation, and end-plate irregularities from the MRI images be treated independently or considered as a part of the degenerative process? This is still uncertain, again due to the limited understanding of disc degeneration.

The variability of phenotypic parameters that define the degenerative status of the intervertebral disc confounds genetic studies. This is especially true for many situations, where replication and meta-analysis studies are required to substantiate the research findings, particularly, when the effect size is small. Replication provides credibility to initial findings of association, while meta-analysis increases the statistical power to detect associated genes. Both require comparable phenotypes among studies to produce meaningful results (Chanock et al. 2007; Nakaoka and Inoue 2009). Therefore, a unified phenotypic definition for disc degeneration is an absolute requirement for the successful identification of the involved genetic components.

10.3.3 Aging and Intervertebral Disc Degeneration

Disc degeneration is part of the normal aging process. With age, an increasing prevalence and severity of disc degeneration have been observed (Cheung et al. 2009). However, an understanding of what constitutes "normal progression" remains unclear, as many factors can participate and modify the degenerative process. Genetics is one of the components that can alter this "normality" by accelerating or decelerating the degenerative process. This change is reviewed elsewhere in the book and includes changes in cell function such as expression levels of genes, the stability of mRNA transcripts or proteins, or the binding affinity of proteins interacting partners, caused by the genetic variations in or near participating genes. In establishing a cohort for genetic study of disc degeneration, the effect of age must be taken into consideration in terms of subject recruitment and data analyses. Statistically, if sufficient population information is available, then appropriate adjustments can be established. An example would be a sliding window method, in which the degenerative score was logarithmic transformed to reduce skewness and standardized to a mean of 0 and a variance of 1 in each decade of age of the samples (Virtanen et al. 2007). The idea behind such adjustment is to identify the "normality" within the age band of a certain cohort, such that samples showing "accelerated" or "retarded" degeneration can be highlighted during analysis.

10.4 Moving from Phenotype Information to Identification of Genes Causing or Contributing to Disease

10.4.1 Candidate Genes

This approach utilizes the biological knowledge and etiology of the disease to identify genes of interest and to determine correlations between variants within the genes and the phenotype. The phenotype can provide clues to potential candidate genes, while information gathered from expression studies and animal models can enhance the selection process (Tabor et al. 2002). This method has been successful in identifying the genetic components of several skeletal diseases. For example, although over 90 % of the osteogenesis imperfecta cases are due to mutations in *COL1A1* and *COL1A2* genes, the causes of the remaining cases remained unknown. Until recently, candidate gene approach helped identify mutations in genes involved in posttranslational modifications required for collagen folding and stability. One of the modifying complexes, prolyl 3-hydroxylase 1 (*LEPRE1*) coupled with cartilage-associated protein (*CRTAP*) and cyclophilin B (*PPIB*), converts specific proline to 3-hydroxyproline, which is important in the formation of collagen triple helix. Also, since *Crtap*-null mice demonstrated skeletal abnormalities resembling a subtype of OI (Morello et al. 2006), mutation analysis of *CRTAP* in this subtype of OI (Barnes et al. 2006) identified mutations associated with the disease. Similarly, mutations in *LEPRE1* and *PPIB* were also detected in OI patients (Cabral et al. 2007; van Dijk et al. 2009).

Apart from rare diseases, candidate gene approach also aids the identification of risk factors in common skeletal diseases, with osteoarthritis being an excellent example. There have been many genes reported to be associated with OA (Valdes and Spector 2011), among which *GDF5* is one of the promising candidates as it survived testing in multiple populations and showed high significance in a meta-analysis (Miyamoto et al. 2007). It was selected as a candidate since it is involved in joint formation (Francis-West et al. 1999), and thus, a common variant in *GDF5* could play a role in the disease (Miyamoto et al. 2007). Similarly, genes related to cartilage homeostasis have been studied as candidates, including extracellular matrix components, matrix degrading enzymes, and genes involved in TGF-β and Wnt signaling pathways, inflammation, and apoptosis. A careful selection of candidates with high biological relevance to the diseases of interest is often the key to success. Moreover, the results and downstream functional studies can provide new understanding in connecting molecular mechanisms with the disease state.

10.4.2 Family Linkage Analysis

Unlike the candidate gene approach, classical linkage analysis relies less on biological knowledge of the disease being studied; rather, it utilizes the principle of co-segregation where the disease-causing alleles, together with nearby markers, are passed on to the next generation within a family. These markers are linked to the disease because recombination events are infrequent within a short stretch of DNA. They can be in the form of restriction fragment length polymorphisms (RFLP) of a candidate gene, where specific patterns of DNA fragments are linked to disease. If there is no clue to any candidate genes, whole-genome scans using microsatellite markers can be used to locate disease susceptible loci, while further genotyping or sequencing can identify the causative variants. More recently, initial mapping has used high-density whole-genome SNP arrays and was successful in locating several new OI loci for downstream investigation (Alanay et al. 2010; Lapunzina et al. 2010; Martinez-Glez et al. 2011). In general, detection is most successful with large families with multiple generations of affected members evidencing a clearly defined phenotype. As such, the traditional family linkage approach is more commonly used to identify affected genetic regions of rare disorders.

10.4.3 Case-Control Association Studies

This is the method of choice for common diseases with a complex trait. It does not rely on family data, but rather on a large cohort selected from the general population or recruitment of patients with a defined phenotype. The allele or genotype frequencies between the case and control groups are compared, with statistical tests being applied to objectively discern if there are differences (Daly 2009). Chi-square test is commonly used for this purpose, while Fisher's exact test should be used when sample sizes are small. On the other hand, regression analysis can be used if it is presumed that there is varying degree of effects, such as an additive influence between different genotypes. A disadvantage of this approach is that if the effect size is small, statistical significance is usually achieved only with very large cohorts (in the thousands) or if meta-analysis is performed using different cohort collected from multiple centers, regional and international.

10.5 Genes Associated with Intervertebral Disc Degeneration

While different strategies can be used to find genetic risk factors for intervertebral disc degeneration, the predominant approach is through case-control studies and the selection of

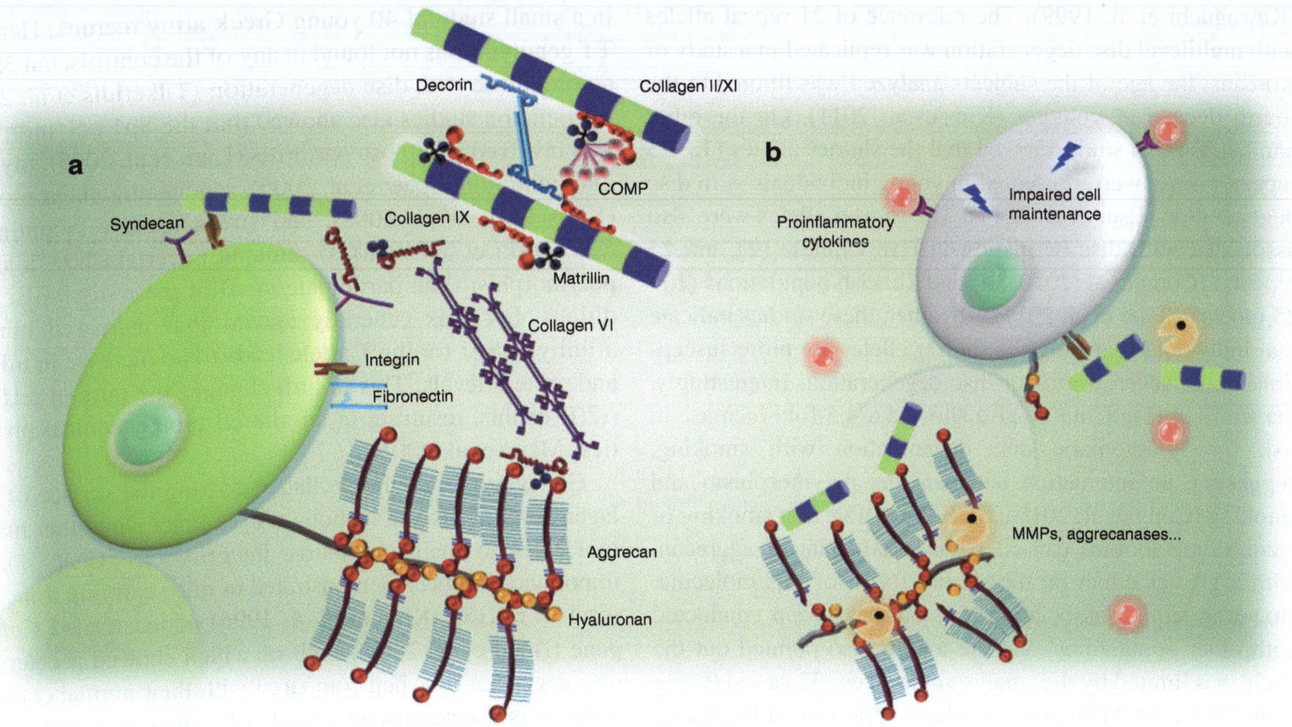

Fig. 10.3 Current concepts of candidate gene selection. Candidate gene selection is closely related to the biology of normal disc and involvement in disc degeneration. (**a**) The extracellular matrix molecules form an integral part of the disc, providing mechanical strength, water absorption properties, as well as proper environment for cells. Their functional importance and high abundance make them the major genetic candidates. (**b**) During degeneration, increased matrix degradation is caused by enzymes such as MMPs and aggrecanases, while the presence of proinflammatory cytokines can accelerate such a process; moreover, cell maintenance is affected. These are the current understanding of the degeneration mechanisms, in which the involved molecules serve as important candidates to be studied

appropriate candidate genes. These genes are usually chosen based on our current knowledge of the biology of the disc in health and disease, and the logic behind the selection is centered on the integrity of the disc tissue (Fig. 10.3). Collagens and aggrecan, together with other structural proteins, form the basis of the extracellular matrix which is an integral part of the disc. Not only are they the most abundant molecules, their role in providing tensile strength and osmotic pressure is essential for proper disc function. Therefore, it is not surprising that the extracellular matrix genes were prime candidates for study. In addition, tissue homeostasis – a balance between synthesis and degradation – would be equally important, and there are a number of studies focusing on catabolic genes, namely, the aggrecanases and matrix metalloproteinases (MMPs). In fact, a number of these genes are found to have elevated expression levels as well as increased enzymatic activity during disc degeneration (Roberts et al. 2000; Le Maitre et al. 2004). Such changes can be triggered by the proinflammatory cytokines, such as interleukins (Millward-Sadler et al. 2009), which are also expressed at elevated levels in the degenerative process (Le Maitre et al. 2005, 2007), resulting in overall accelerated degradation and posing an adverse effect on matrix integrity. Ultimately, it is the disc cells that are responsible for producing and maintaining the extracellular matrix; thus, genes that affect cell function and survival have also been studied for their associations with disc degeneration. In this section, specific genes will be highlighted, enhancing our understanding of their functions in the disc as well as their roles in the degenerative process.

10.5.1 Extracellular Matrix Proteins

Aggrecan is the major proteoglycan in the disc, responsible for water absorption and retention through its highly negative charged chondroitin sulfate (CS) side chains. A variable number of tandem repeat (VNTR), located at exon 12 encoding the CS attachment domain, have been identified, which dictate the length of the aggrecan core protein as well as the potential number of attached CS chains (Doege et al. 1997). The first study showed an association between this VNTR of aggrecan with lumbar disc degeneration in a group of 64 young Japanese women aged 20–29 (Kawaguchi et al. 1999). There was an overrepresentation of the shorter alleles of 18 and 21 repeats in multilevel disc degeneration as well as an association with the severity of disc degeneration

(Kawaguchi et al. 1999). The relevance of 21 repeat alleles with multilevel disc degeneration was replicated in a study of Koreans; the age of the subjects analyzed was limited to the fourth decade or younger (Kim et al. 2011). On the other hand, a Turkish study showed that the shorter alleles (13–25 repeats) were overrepresented in young individuals with disc degeneration (Eser et al. 2011). The shorter alleles were also associated with disc herniation in Han Chinese (21 and 25 repeats) (Cong et al. 2010a, b) and Turkish populations (13–25 repeats) (Eser et al. 2011). Together, these studies indicate that individuals carrying the shorter alleles are more susceptible to the severe forms of disc degeneration. Interestingly, the study in Han Chinese also showed a 4.5-fold increase in risk for symptomatic disc degeneration with smoking, suggesting an interaction between this polymorphism and smoking (Cong et al. 2010a, b). It is possible that smoking or nicotine metabolites can alter the metabolism of aggrecan, with a greater effect on the shorter forms of this molecule. However, similar association tests have not been conducted with other populations, and the author also pointed out the study was limited by the small sample size (132 cases) (Cong et al. 2010a, b). While most studies support the influence of the shorter alleles, 25 repeats or less, with disc degeneration, a study conducted with a Finnish cohort of 132 males, 40–45 years of age, showed that only the allele with 26 repeats was significantly associated among individuals with a dark nucleus pulposus (Solovieva et al. 2007). The differences could be due to ethnic variations, as well as the relatively small sample size. Nevertheless, as these studies provided supportive evidence for aggrecan as a genetic risk factor for disc degeneration, it would be worthwhile to perform a meta-analysis.

Collagen I is the predominant collagen in the annulus fibrosus and responsible for the highly organized lamellae structure that provides the tissue with its tensile strength. It is encoded by two genes, *COL1A1* and *COL1A2*. An SNP located at the binding site of the transcription factor Sp1 (rs1800012) in the first intron of *COL1A1* was initially identified and found to be associated with reduced bone mineral density and an increased risk of fracture and turnover (Grant et al. 1996; Garnero et al. 1998; Uitterlinden et al. 1998). Since it was suggested that there was an inverse relationship between osteoporosis and disc degeneration, the Sp1 binding site polymorphism in the *COL1A1* gene was investigated in a Dutch cohort of 517 individuals who are at least 65 years of age (Pluijm et al. 2004). Individuals with the TT genotype were shown to have a 3.6 times higher risk of disc degeneration when compared with those having GT or GG genotype, after adjusting for age, sex, and body weight (Pluijm et al. 2004). It should be noted that disc degeneration in this study was defined by the presence of osteophytes and articular joint space narrowing based on radiographs, as opposed to the reduced signal intensity seen on MRI images. Despite this limitation, the Sp1 polymorphism was replicated in a small study of 40 young Greek army recruits. Here, the TT genotype was not found in any of the controls, but 33.3 % among those with disc degeneration (Tilkeridis et al. 2005). Association studies also showed that the Sp1 polymorphism was involved in hip osteoarthritis (Lian et al. 2005), myocardial infarction (Speer et al. 2006), cruciate ligament ruptures (Khoschnau et al. 2008), and stress urinary incontinence (Skorupski et al. 2006). It remains uncertain how a single polymorphism can participate in all of these dissimilar conditions, but it is generally agreed that increased binding affinity of Sp1 for the T allele leads to an increase in mRNA and protein levels. This in turn changes the ratio of $\alpha1(I)$ to $\alpha2(I)$ chains, resulting in an altered biomechanical properties (Mann et al. 2001).

Collagen IX is minor collagen coating the surface of collagen II/XI fibrils and is thought to interact with other matrix molecules to maintain matrix integrity (see Chap. 5). Its importance has been demonstrated in mice carrying truncated form of $\alpha1(IX)$ (Kimura et al. 1996) or inactivated *Col9a1* gene (Boyd et al. 2008), both of which showed accelerated disc degeneration when compared with their normal counterparts. It is a heterotrimer encoded by three different genes, namely, *COL9A1*, *COL9A2*, and *COL9A3*. Analysis of the *COL9A2* gene identified two consecutive SNP polymorphisms (rs12077871 and rs2228564) in exon 19, leading to a substitution of tryptophan for either glutamine or arginine at residue 326 (Annunen et al. 1999). Interestingly, this tryptophan allele was present in 6 out of 157 Finnish individuals with disc degeneration and associated sciatica, but none among the 174 controls (Annunen et al. 1999). Since this polymorphism involves a tryptophan (Trp) substitution in the $\alpha2(IX)$ chain, it is named the Trp2 allele. An age-stratified analysis of a group of 804 Southern Chinese (40–49 years) showed a 2.4-fold increase in risk of developing disc degeneration and end-plate herniation in those carrying the Trp2 allele (Jim et al. 2005). Moreover, affected Trp2 individuals were found to have more severe disc degeneration (Jim et al. 2005). This was confirmed in a study of 84 Japanese patients (under 40 years) undergoing lumbar disc nucleotomy (Higashino et al. 2007). However, another larger-scale Japanese study of 658 controls and 470 cases could not replicate the findings (Seki et al. 2006).

In addition to the Trp2 allele, a similar arginine to tryptophan substitution at residue 103 was detected in exon 5 of the *COL9A3* gene (rs61734651) (Paassilta et al. 2001). This Trp3 allele was found in a Finnish cohort of patients at a significantly higher frequency of 12.2 % among 171 cases when compared to 4.7 % among the 321 controls, with a threefold increase in the risk of disc degeneration (Paassilta et al. 2001). A higher proportion of the Trp3 allele was also detected among people with disc degeneration than controls in a Greek study, but the difference did not reach statistical significance (Kales et al. 2004). There was also the possibility that the Trp3 allele might act synergistically with persistent obesity, an interaction that would serve to increase the risk of disc degeneration (Solovieva et al. 2002). In addition, interaction of Trp3 with another polymorphism, interleukin-1β (C(3954)-T), was examined. It was noted that carrying this allele in the absence of the interleukin-1β 3954T allele resulted in an increase in the risk of a "dark nucleus pulposus" (Solovieva et al. 2006). These results indicated the potential of the Trp3 allele interacting with environmental and genetic factors modifying its effect. There were other studies testing the association of Trp2 and Trp3 alleles, but the Trp2 allele was absent in Greek (Kales et al. 2004) and only present at a low frequency of 1.2 % in German (Wrocklage et al. 2000), while Trp3 was absent in Southern Chinese (Jim et al. 2005) and Japanese (Higashino et al. 2007), suggesting substantial ethnic variations.

An association for the *COL9A1* gene with disc degeneration was also suggested in a study of 25 selected candidate genes in a cohort of 588 Finnish male monozygotic and dizygotic twins (Videman et al. 2009). A particular SNP (rs696990) located at the 5′ of the gene was associated with the disc signal intensity, which survived an empirical threshold value for global significance.

The Trp2 and Trp3 allelic products are incorporated into the cross-linked fibrillar network of developing human cartilage (Matsui et al. 2003). Thus, any pathological consequences are likely to be long term and cause alterations in the tissues mechanical properties (Matsui et al. 2003). Indeed, among human disc samples carrying the Trp2 allele, altered or comprised swelling pressure and compressive modulus was detected (Aladin et al. 2007). Although, the precise mechanism is still unclear, a hypothesis is the bulk side chain of Trp residue may interfere with the interaction of collagen IX with other matrix molecules including collagen II. This would destabilize the matrix and thus affect the biomechanical properties of the disc.

Type XI collagen forms the core of collagen II/XI/XI fibrils and functions to control the diameter of the fibril. It is composed of three α-chains encoded by the *COL11A1*, *COL11A2*, and *COL2A1* genes (see Chap. 5). An initial screening of these genes identified an SNP c.4603C T (rs1676486) in the coding region of *COL11A1* to be associated with lumbar disc herniation among Japanese (Mio et al. 2007). The association was confirmed by testing all the sequence variations in *COL11A1*, among which this SNP remained the most significant, as well as by increasing the cohort size to a total of 823 cases and 838 controls. It was suggested that this SNP affected mRNA stability since the expression level of the T allele is significantly lower than that of the C allele (Mio et al. 2007).

Cartilage intermediate layer protein (CILP) is a non-collagenous matrix component initially found in the middle zone of human articular cartilage (Lorenzo et al. 1998). An SNP 1184T→C (rs2073711) in the encoded region of the gene was identified to be significantly associated with disc degeneration in a cohort of 467 cases and 654 controls of a Japanese population (Seki et al. 2005). This SNP is non-synonymous, resulting in an amino acid substitution of isoleucine at residue 395 to threonine. The authors demonstrated in vitro that CILP could inhibit TGF-β-induced transcription, and the effect of inhibition was increased in the presence of C allelic product (Seki et al. 2005). This SNP might also exhibit a differential gender effect since a small study in Japanese collegiate athletes showed an association in male, but not female athletes (Min et al. 2010). On the other hand, a recent study in a Finnish cohort found an association only in females (Kelempisioti et al. 2011), while replication in Chinese population cohort failed (Virtanen et al. 2007), suggesting that other factors such as ethnicity, sex, and environment may be modulating the effect of this polymorphism.

Asporin (ASPN) belongs to the family of small leucine-rich proteoglycans (SLRP), members of which include decorin and biglycan (see Chap. 4) (Lorenzo et al. 2001). It contains a stretch of aspartic acid residues at the amino-terminal, which are variable in number (Lorenzo et al. 2001). While a repeat of 13 aspartic acid residues (D13) was the most common variant, a repeat of 14 residues (D14) was overrepresented among patients with osteoarthritis in a Japanese population (Kizawa et al. 2005). Since both osteoarthritis and disc degeneration are degenerative "cartilage diseases," *ASPN* was hypothesized as a candidate gene for disc degeneration (Song et al. 2008a). The aspartic acid repeats were tested in Chinese and Japanese cohorts of 1,055 and 1,353 individuals, respectively, and the D14 allele was overrepresented in the case groups. Meta-analysis showed that individuals carrying this allele were at higher risk with an overall odds ratio of 1.7 (Song et al. 2008a). Increased asporin expression was detected among degenerated discs (Song et al. 2008a; Gruber et al. 2009); in addition, the D14 allelic product showed a greater suppression of TGF-β-mediated transcription than that of the D13 allelic product in vitro (Kizawa et al. 2005). As discussed elsewhere in this book, TGF-β signaling regulates the expression of key matrix proteins such as collagen II and aggrecan. Indeed, in vitro studies support the notion that the risk allele would have a negative effect on the synthesis of matrix molecules (Kizawa et al. 2005).

Matrilins are a four-member family of multi-subunit extracellular matrix proteins (see Chap. 5). They function as adaptors in the assembly of various matrix molecules including aggrecan, collagen type II, SLRPs, and cartilage oligomeric matrix protein (COMP) (Klatt et al. 2011). In a Rotterdam study, it was found that a non-synonymous SNP (rs28939676) of matrilin-3, in which threonine at position 303 was substituted by methionine, was associated with disc degeneration at two or more levels based on radiographs, leading to an increased risk of 2.9 among individuals carrying the T allele (Min et al. 2006). On the other hand, this association was not confirmed in another cohort study of sibling pairs of Dutch origin (Min et al. 2006). While the effect of this polymorphism during disc degeneration remained unknown, it was postulated that the polymorphism weakened the role of matrilin-3 in stabilizing the extracellular matrix molecules (Min et al. 2006). Related to this finding, recent studies demonstrated that in primary human chondrocytes, the presence of matrilin-3 can induce the expression a number of proinflammatory cytokines including IL6, IL8, and TNFα, as well as degradative enzymes MMP1, MMP3, and MMP13 (Klatt et al. 2009). These molecules are known to be triggered during disc degeneration, suggesting a possible relationship between matrilin-3 and inflammation.

Thrombospondin-2 (THBS2) belongs to a family of extracellular matrix proteins, thrombospondins, with multi-subunit. The protein is thought to be involved in cell-matrix interaction, antiangiogenesis, regulation of collagen fibrillogenesis, and the effective levels of MMP2 and MMP9 (Bornstein et al. 2004). An intronic SNP, IVS10-8C$\rightarrow$T (rs9406328) in *THBS2* was shown to be significantly associated with lumbar disc herniation in two independent Japanese populations, composed of 847 cases and 896 controls (Hirose et al. 2008). The TT genotype caused a significantly higher rate of exon 11 skipping when compared to the CC genotype, with a reduction of MMP2 and MMP9 binding. These data suggested that THBS2 could be involved in regulating MMP expression in the disc, which in turn participate in the pathogenesis of disc herniation. Moreover, the authors also identified a combinatorial effect with a non-synonymous SNP (rs17576) in *MMP9*, with an odds ratio of 3.03, indicating a potential gene-gene interaction (Hirose et al. 2008).

10.5.2 Matrix Metalloproteinases and Other Proteases

Matrix metalloproteinases (MMPs) are a large protein family with a wide spectrum of substrates including extracellular matrix components. Based on their specificity, they can be broadly categorized into subgroups such as collagenases (MMP1, MMP8, and MMP13), gelatinases (MMP2 and MMP9), and stromelysins (MMP3) (Goupille et al. 1998). Details of these enzymes are presented in Chap. 8. A polymorphism for G insertion/deletion (G/D) at the −1607 promoter region of *MMP1* was assessed in a Southern Chinese cohort of 691 individuals. The identified deletion (D) allele was found to be significantly associated with disc degeneration; this was particularly evident among individuals aged 40 or above (Song et al. 2008b). In another Chinese cohort of 162 cases and 318 controls, an SNP in the promoter region of *MMP2*, −1306C$\rightarrow$T, was shown to be associated with disc degeneration, with the CC genotype being more prevalent in cases of severe degeneration (Dong et al. 2007). This polymorphism was previously found to disrupt an Sp1 binding site that can lead to a reduction in transcriptional activity (Price et al. 2001).

A polymorphic site for either six continuous adenosines (6A) or five adenosines (5A) in the promoter region of *MMP3* was assessed for an association with disc degeneration in 49 elderly Japanese (Takahashi et al. 2001). When compared with individuals having only the 6A allele, the 5A allele was associated with disc degeneration as well as severity of degeneration; however, this association was not detected in a group of 54 young subjects (Takahashi et al. 2001). For *MMP9*, in addition to the interacting *THBS2* SNP described earlier, an SNP at the promoter region, −1562C$\rightarrow$T, was shown to be associated with disc degeneration in a Northern Chinese cohort of 408 cases and 451 controls. Those individuals carrying the TT or CT genotype had an increased risk of developing and having more severe grades of disc degeneration (Sun et al. 2009). One explanation for this observation was that the T allele may have a higher transcriptional activity than the C allele (Sun et al. 2009). These studies, while limited, have focused on polymorphic sites within the promoter region of MMP genes that functionally influence transcriptional activity, thus providing a functional support for the genetic findings. It is likely that variations at promoters or cis-regulatory elements of genes could have a more significant role in disc degeneration, and hence, a more thorough investigation of the genome is warranted.

10.5.3 Proinflammatory Cytokines

Genes within the interleukin 1 (IL1) cluster are among the proinflammatory cytokines that have been associated with disc degeneration; from a functional viewpoint, elevated expression could enhance the expression of MMPs, an initiation factor in the degenerative process. A number of common variants in the *IL1* gene cluster were evaluated in a group of 133 Finnish males, and *IL1α* 889C$\rightarrow$T and *IL1β* 3954C$\rightarrow$T were found to be associated with disc bulges, with odds ratio of 2.4 and 1.9 for individuals carrying the respective T alleles (Solovieva et al. 2004). Interestingly, a genetic interaction between the *IL1β* 3954T and the *COL9A3* Trp3 allele was identified; its implication however is not clear.

Two SNPs at the promoter region, −592C$\rightarrow$A and −1082G$\rightarrow$A, of interleukin 10 (*IL10*) were studied for an association in a Chinese cohort of 320 cases and 269 controls (Lin et al. 2011). The AA genotypes for both SNPs were found to be more frequent in the cases. An effect on transcriptional level is suggested as lower IL10 mRNA levels were detected in disc samples from individuals with the AA genotypes, when compared to the CC genotype at −592 and GG genotype at −1082 (Lin et al. 2011).

A number of other specific polymorphic sites in genes of the inflammatory pathways have been studied in relationship to disc degeneration. These included a GGG haplotype from three respective SNPs rs1800797, rs1800796, and rs1800795 of interleukin 6 (*IL6*) (Kelempisioti et al. 2011), the SNP rs1420100 in intron 2 and rs917997 downstream of interleukin 18 receptor accessory protein (*IL18RAP*) (Videman et al. 2009), and a synonymous substitution of Val at position 102 (rs5277) in cyclooxygenase 2 (*COX2*) (Valdes et al. 2005). How these variations may affect the respective genes in disc degeneration is not clear.

10.5.4 Genes Affecting Cell Function and Survival

Vitamin D receptor (VDR) is an intracellular receptor for 1,25-dihydroxyvitamin D3, the metabolite involved in mineral metabolism. VDR was the first gene to be found associated with disc degeneration in a Finnish population (Videman et al. 1998). Two variants of *VDR*, namely, the FokI polymorphism at exon 2 and the TaqI polymorphism at exon 9, were initially studied in 85 pairs of monozygotic twins. The TaqI tt genotype (with restriction enzyme site) was found to be associated with individuals with significantly lower disc MRI signal intensities when compared with the other two genotypes; similar findings were noted when FokI polymorphism was evaluated (Videman et al. 1998). The association of the TaqI polymorphism with disc degeneration was replicated in a Japanese cohort of 205 individuals (Kawaguchi et al. 2002). The tt genotype was absent, while the Tt genotype was associated with multilevel and severe disc degeneration, as well as disc herniation (Kawaguchi et al. 2002). In a study of a Southern Chinese cohort, individuals carrying the t allele were 2.6 times more likely to develop disc degeneration and disc bulge. Moreover, the association was highly significant for a subgroup of individuals age 40 or below (Cheung et al. 2006). The TaqI polymorphism represents a synonymous substitution, which is believed, in conjunction with other nearby polymorphisms, to affect mRNA stability (Uitterlinden et al. 2004).

Insulin-like growth factor 1 receptor (IGF1R) acts as a signal transducer for insulin-like growth factor 1 (IGF1), an anabolic protein that stimulates matrix synthesis and cell proliferation in the disc. An intronic SNP, IVS1 + 14488C → G (rs11247361) in *IGF1R* was found to be associated with radiographic disc narrowing in a cohort of 434 postmenopausal Japanese women (Urano et al. 2008). However, the effect of this polymorphism remained unknown.

Sickle tail (*SKT*) is a gene recently identified through gene-trap mutagenesis in mice. *SKT*-null mice showed developmental spinal abnormalities including dislocation and defects of the nucleus pulposus at E17.5, leading to a kinky tail phenotype in the adult (Semba et al. 2006). As these observations suggested that SKT has an important role in the development and maintenance of the intervertebral disc, it thus served as a candidate gene. In a study of two independent Japanese populations with a total of 862 cases and 896 controls, out of the 68 selected tag SNPs in *SKT*, two SNPs located at intron 2 (rs16924573 and 2285592) were found to be significantly associated with disc herniation. Moreover, rs16924573 was further replicated in Finnish cohorts (Karasugi et al. 2009; Kelempisioti et al. 2011). The function of SKT is unknown and further studies are needed to evaluate the effect of this SNP on disc herniation.

As mentioned earlier, growth and differentiation factor 5 (*GDF5*) is required for joint formation (Francis-West et al. 1999) (see Chap. 3). An SNP (rs143383) located at the 5′ untranslated region of the gene was identified as a key risk factor for OA, and in vitro studies suggested that the risk allele T led to a reduced promoter activity (Miyamoto et al. 2007). In five independent European cohorts with a total sample size of 5,259, this SNP was recently tested for association with disc degeneration. Meta-analysis showed significant association between the SNP and the combination of disc space narrowing plus osteophytes in women (Williams et al. 2011). The result suggested that in addition to *ASPN*, *GDF5* is another shared genetic risk factor for both disc degeneration and OA, further implicating similarities in "disease" mechanisms.

10.6 Making Sense of Risk Factors and Intervertebral Disc Degeneration

At present, over 20 genes have been reported to be associated with intervertebral disc degeneration. Since these are selected candidates, they are not difficult to assign an individual biological function while grouping of these genes can be easily linked to molecular processes leading to disc degeneration. However, many of the findings need to be critically scrutinized for the "quality" of the genetic data: interim guidelines proposed by the HuGENet working group in 2008 provide an excellent assessment based on three criteria: amount of evidence, replication, and protection from bias (Ioannidis et al. 2008). Under each criterion, a classification of strong (A), moderate (B), or weak (C) can be assigned to the gene study or studies. The degree of credibility can then be estimated from standardized 3×3 tables as illustrated in Fig. 10.4: a score of AAA represents the highest credibility and CCC is the lowest. Additional validation is provided by biological data and functional studies. Leaving the complex issue of the phenotype aside, none of the studies of disc degeneration genes reach the level of strong credibility, and few are within the level of moderate support. Reasons for this include relatively small cohort size and lack of replication.

VDR represents the best replicated gene linked to disc degeneration across three different populations. In contrast,

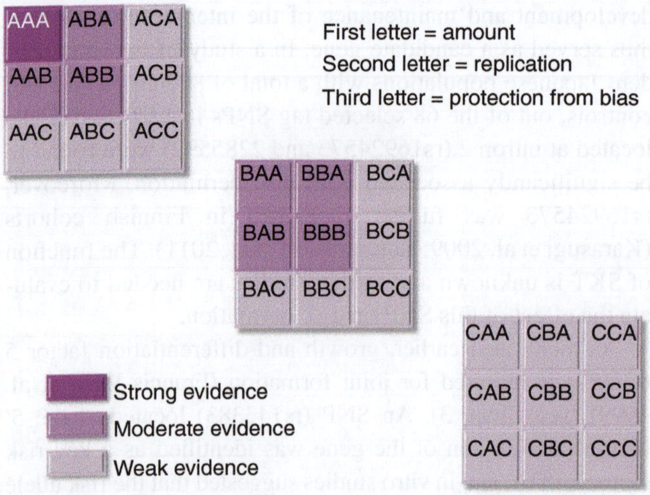

Fig. 10.4 Categories for the credibility of cumulative epidemiology evidence. The three letters, *A*, *B*, and *C* correspond (in order) to the "amount" of evidence, replication, and protection from bias. Evidence is categorized as strong when there is *A* for all three items and is categorized as weak when there is a *C* for any of the three items. All other combinations are categorized as moderate (Permission obtained from Springer for the reproduction of this figure from Ioannidis et al. 2008; License number 2938180337505)

ASPN (OR 1.70 [95 % CI 1.35–2.20], *P*=0.000013), *CILP* (OR 1.61 [95 % CI 1.31–1.98], *P*=0.0000068), *COL11A1* (OR 1.42 [95 % CI 1.23–1.65], *P*=0.0000033), *GDF5* (OR 1.72 [95 % CI 1.15–2.57], *P*=0.008), *SKT* (OR 1.34 [95 % CI 1.14–1.58], *P*=0.0004), *THBS2* (OR 1.43 [95 % CI 1.20–1.70], *P*=0.00004), and *MMP9* (OR 1.29 [95 % CI 1.12–1.48], *P*=0.00049) could be considered as potential risk factors with moderate genetic evidence. Based on this limited set of genes, it is clear that the effect size of these genes is very modest with odd ratios between 1.3 and 1.7. With the estimated heritability of 74 %, there is likely to be many more genes associated with disc degeneration yet to be discovered. Whether there are genes with strong effects remains to be seen and perhaps such genes will be identified from a more unbiased genome-wide approach.

In general, increasing emphasis should be placed on replication of association studies in cohorts with comparable phenotypes; this is important when evaluating the initial findings and minimizing false positives (Neale and Sham 2004; Chanock et al. 2007). False positives may easily arise when the sample size is small, leading to insufficient power and imprecise statistical estimation. It can also occur when the experimental design is inappropriate. Heterogeneity in the genetic background, environmental exposures, and population stratification between cases and controls will result in bias. Technical and genotyping artifacts can also be another source of false positives. Ideally, functional studies should be performed to provide an understanding of the biological relevance of the associated polymorphisms with the disease.

10.7 Technologies in Genetic Studies and Intervertebral Disc Degeneration

Advances in both the knowledge of genetic variants and in genotyping technologies provide a useful platform for understanding how genes influence disc degeneration. The International HapMap Project aims to capture common variants across the genome, as well as frequencies and correlations in different populations (International HapMap Consortium 2003; Altshuler et al. 2010) (Box 10.3). SNPs were the initial focus of study as they represented major types of variations in populations. From the data generated, the variants and their frequencies provide useful reference information and allow identification of regions of SNPs with strong associations where alleles are co-inherited or in linkage disequilibrium (LD). An LD map can be produced allowing the visualization of the relative co-inheritance of the SNPs. A practical application of this information is that by careful selection, genotyping of only a few SNPs (tag SNPs) can be informative as they cover a large region of interest. Information concerning the remaining common SNPs in that region can be predicted, thus significantly reducing genotyping costs. More recently, the 1000 Genomes Project has been launched, which is aimed at providing a more profound characterization of genetic variations in multiple populations (1000 Genomes Project Consortium 2010). Through high-throughput sequencing technologies, its target is to identify over 95 % of variants, with the ability to detect low-frequency variants down to 1 %. The types of variants being detected are also broadened to cover short insertions and deletions (indels) and structural variations.

Box 10.3: The International HapMap Project

The International HapMap Project is a large-scale collaborative program involving multiple research centers from Japan, UK, Canada, China, USA, and Nigeria, aiming to determine the common genetic variants in human genome, their frequencies and correlations between them, in populations with ancestry from Africa, Asia, and Europe (International HapMap Consortium 2003). The idea for initiation of this project is as follows. Common diseases are believed to be caused by common variants, each having a modest effect. Although one can genotype all the variants for testing their association with the traits of interest, it is impractical due to the cost. An alternative method is to identify a subset of these variants that can serve as genetic markers to refine the regions for association, which can then be further analyzed in details. However, how can the suitable markers be selected?

The probability of recombination events reduces with genetic distance, and therefore, alleles in close proximity are likely to be co-inherited together. Such group of alleles is known as a haplotype. A stronger association among the nearby variants represents a higher level of linkage disequilibrium (LD) and that there would only be a few haplotypes in that region accounting for most of the variations in a population. By choosing and genotyping a few key variants within the haplotype ("tags"), the identity of remaining variants can be predicted. Unfortunately, the extent of association of nearby variants varies across the genome. Neither a random nor an evenly spaced selection of variants is ideal for recognizing good "tags." The International HapMap Project assists this important step in association studies by developing a haplotype map ("HapMap") of the human genome which contains comprehensive information of the common SNPs and the association between them. "Tag SNPs" that best represent the regions of interest can be generated based on this information.

For genotyping platforms, there are now more options than the traditional, labor-intensive approach of RFLP. For SNP genotyping, the multiplexing Sequenom MassARRAY system can process up to 40 SNPs with a maximum of 384 DNA samples in a single assay. Illumina VeraCode technology is similar multiplexing system. They are efficient and cost-effective when there are well-selected candidate genes or specific regions for fine-mapping with a considerable number of SNPs to be genotyped in a large cohort. On the other hand, the whole-genome approach can also be used to identify new candidates. Predesigned genotyping arrays of genetic markers of SNPs and copy number variations are commercially available. The Illumina Omni array is able to detect more than 4.3 million markers, while the Affymetrix SNP array can assess 1.8 million markers. The objective of both systems is to cover variants with at least 1% of frequency. Huge amount of data can thus be generated using these arrays and tested directly for genotype-phenotype association; this type of whole-genome association is termed as genome-wide association study (GWAS).

As common diseases usually require large sample size for statistical power, a major drawback is cost. To address this problem, studies can be designed in which smaller representative sets of cases and controls are used for GWAS. The results can then be validated in larger cohorts or other GWAS in order to achieve desirable sample size for meta-analysis. Another issue is the limited flexibility of predesigned arrays, which are restricted to relatively common variants and ethnicity. These limitations can be overcome by next-generation sequencing (NGS), an emerging technology which provides the most comprehensive genetic information with low frequency and simultaneously identifies rare SNPs, indels, and structural variants (Metzker 2010). Its application is not only restricted to genotyping but also includes genome-wide marker and variant discovery (Davey et al. 2011). Despite a continuous reduction in NGS costs and improvement in throughput, sequencing the whole genome of every individual in a large cohort would appear to be ideal, but not practical. Depending on the purpose of the study, various methods for restricting the specified region and reducing the number of samples to be sequenced have been proposed so as to maximize the data yield at reasonable price (Davey et al. 2011).

The dramatic increase in genetic information and improvements in genotyping technology over this past decade has changed the usual practice of studying the genetics of human disease. The comprehensive resources of the International HapMap Project can be used to select variants for association studies, while the 1000 Genomes Project has the potential of providing information on the relationship between low-frequency variants and diseases. Various genotyping platforms provide opportunities for study of large number of variants or samples in a short period of time. At present, genetic studies of disc degeneration are based on the candidate gene approach, analyzing specific variants within the genes. It is clear that GWAS analysis is the direction that the spine community needs to consider as it is lagging behind genetic studies of other common disorders such as diabetes, neural degenerative disorder, cardiovascular diseases, and osteoarthritis (Bertram et al. 2010; Loughlin 2011; Visscher et al. 2012; Zeller et al. 2012). However, as we enter into yet another new era of genetic data acquisition and building on important lessons learnt from other GWAS, we should be able to custom design a new approach to evaluate genes associated with disc degeneration.

10.8 The Moving Goals in Modern-Day Genetic Studies

Large-scale genetic studies of a plethora of many common diseases provide an excellent baseline on which to refine study designs and anticipate potential problems that may arise. Indeed, over 1,100 GWAS for various human traits and diseases have been published, with the identification of over 2,700 SNP associations ($P < 10^{-8}$) (Hindorff et al. 2012). Large-scale GWAS has also been conducted for osteoarthritis in populations that include Dutch (Rotterdam study) (Kerkhof et al. 2010), Japanese (Nakajima et al. 2010), and British (arcOGEN) (Panoutsopoulou et al. 2011), which sums to a total sample size of over 17,000. Despite regions such as chromosome 7q22, human leukocyte antigen (HLA) locus on chromosome 6p, and other SNPs being identified that influence osteoarthritis susceptibility, the effect sizes are small and appear to explain only a small portion of the genetic variance of the disease. Since this is similar to other diseases that include type 2 diabetes, coronary artery disease, and schizophrenia (So et al. 2011), this begs the question: what contributes to the "missing heritability"? There are intense discussions on this topic and a number of possibilities have been raised (Manolio et al. 2009; Eichler et al. 2010). GWAS focuses on mainly common SNPs, whereas the human genome contains many more low-frequency SNPs and structural variants, including deletions, duplication, and inversion. These variants, although individually rare, are collectively common, and their impact on common diseases has not been widely studied. Moreover, interactions among genes and to what extent they shape phenotypic, epigenetic, and transgenerational genetic effects may introduce another level of complexity. Genetic variants may also influence noncoding microRNA, involving translational regulation and therefore, in turn, influencing mRNA and protein expression and interactions. The contribution of these variables may explain missing heritability and, more importantly, shed light on future research strategies.

Rare variants are generally not in linkage disequilibrium with common variants, as they are likely to occur in more recent generations of the population, and therefore may not be detectable in GWAS (Bodmer and Bonilla 2008). However, collectively, these variants can be numerous. There is increasing evidences that rare variants do play a role in common diseases, contributing to intermediate effect sizes. Examples include three rare deletions associated with schizophrenia, with one demonstrating an odds ratio of 14.8 (Stefansson et al. 2008); four rare SNPs in *IFIH1* independently reduced the risk of type 1 diabetes, with one of the SNPs having an odds ratio of 0.5 (Nejentsev et al. 2009); as well as 36 very rare non-synonymous variants associated with type 2 diabetes with odds ratio of 3.3 (Bonnefond et al. 2012). These findings suggest that rare variants contribution to susceptibility of common diseases is not an unusual event. Even though the 1000 Genomes Project can serve as a reference panel for the less common variants, it has a limitation in terms of identifying variants with frequency of at least 1 %. Genetic variants with lower frequencies are unlikely to be revealed in this database. Moreover, rare variants are generally population specific, and that information generated from a certain population may not be applicable to another. To uncover the rare variants in a specific cohort study, sequencing is currently the best, but expensive, method. Strategies to reduce costs have been proposed; whole-exome sequencing is useful when the variants contributing to the diseases are expected to be located in exons; or sequencing the regions where potential associations have been indicated by GWAS, or with relevance to disease etiology. Alternatively, sequencing can be performed on co-affected members in families to determine co-segregated variants or on a small number of selected individuals with extreme phenotypes to identify shared rare variants. The resultant candidates can then be genotyped in a large cohort for validation (Cirulli and Goldstein 2010). Apart from the sequencing study design, other challenges for studying rare variants that need to be overcome include selection of appropriate controls and performing proper statistical analysis.

So far the discussion has focused on the presence and identification of genetic variants leading to disease. However, there are numerous potential "modifiers" that can alter the impact on the penetrance of genetic susceptibility, and epigenetics is one good example. Epigenetics refers to the heritable changes of gene expression that are due to mechanisms other than the underlying DNA sequences (Box 10.4). These mechanisms can be DNA methylation and histone modification, which remodel chromatin and modify the accessibility of transcription factors to gene promoters. The involvement of epigenetic factors in common diseases has been demonstrated in a recent study of schizophrenia and bipolar disorder, in which genome-wide DNA methylation patterns between monozygotic twins discordant for the phenotypes were analyzed. Substantial differences were identified, indicating that epigenetic variations contribute to phenotypic differences (Dempster et al. 2011). These observations have culminated in a new hypothesis, common disease genetic and epigenetic (CDGE), which argues that epigenetic variations can interplay with genetic variations, thus serving as a potential heritable determinant and modulating the outcome of a disease (Bjornsson et al. 2004;

Box 10.4: Epigenetics

Epigenetics refers to the heritable changes of gene expression that are due to mechanisms other than the underlying DNA sequences, such as DNA methylation and histone modifications. DNA methylation generally occurs at GC-rich regions; however, in certain special areas named CpG islands, the proportion of methylation is much lower. CpG islands are mainly located near the promoter regions of human genes. Their methylation patterns, which may change during development, are believed to affect the transcriptional activity of the associated genes. Histones are molecules that allow DNA to wrap around to form a highly ordered chromatin structure. Various types of modifications such as methylation, acetylation, and phosphorylation can occur on the histone molecules. The chromatin structure would be opened up or tightened depending on the positions and types of modification acquires, thus, changing the accessibility of transcription factors to the DNA and, in turn, the expression level of corresponding genes.

Epigenetics can be stable as well as plastic (Petronis 2010). It can be transmitted to the next generation (transgenerational epigenetic heritability) while at the same time reprogrammed during fertilization and gametogenesis. This can be used to interpret the situations of sporadic and familial diseases, when pathological epigenetic marks are reprogrammed or failed to reset, respectively. Epigenetic changes can be induced by environmental stimuli, but these events can be stochastic as well. The fidelity of epigenetic pattern transmission during mitosis is much lower than that of DNA replication, leading to high variability which can account for the differences observed in monozygotic twins. All these properties of epigenetics fit in with the understanding of complex diseases, and therefore, there are increasing emphasis of investigating the roles of epigenetics in the etiology of complex diseases.

Feinberg 2007). Attempt has been made to integrate genetic and epigenetic data, in which increased DNA methylation was noted in the *FTO* locus, a region previously shown to be susceptible to type 2 diabetes and obesity. While the methylation difference was driven by several SNPs creating CpG sites, the resultant effects on the diseases still require further elucidation (Bell et al. 2010). This study provides a hint concerning the potential genetic and epigenetic interactions in shaping common diseases; from this perspective there is a need to further global investigation of epigenetics. "Epigenome-wide association studies" (EWAS), similar to the notion of GWAS, is a new concept directed at studying epigenetic variations in relationship to disease in a genome-wide manner (Rakyan et al. 2011b). This has been made possible by array-based profiling or whole-genome bisulphite sequencing with appropriate experimental design and statistical analysis. Despite these approaches, currently the only target to detect is DNA methylation. An initial EWAS study has already been conducted in type 1 diabetes (Rakyan et al. 2011a), which has provided insights on its application to common human diseases.

Due to the ability to regulate gene expression, microRNAs, a class of small noncoding RNAs of approximately 22 nucleotides, also contribute to genetic outcomes. Depending on the degree of complementarity between microRNAs and mRNAs, they repress translation processes through mRNA degradation, or by inhibiting translation initiation. Differential expression of microRNAs has been reported for many common diseases, such as osteoarthritis (Jones et al. 2009), schizophrenia (Perkins et al. 2007), and bipolar disorder (Moreau et al. 2011). Another level of regulation complexity arises when the genetic variants occur at microRNA binding sites of mRNA. This can alter the binding affinity and differentially regulate the mRNA allelic products (Sethupathy et al. 2007; Brest et al. 2011); moreover, variance can also exist at the level of the microRNA transcripts themselves (Ripke et al. 2011), potentially affecting multiple mRNAs.

Currently, there is no gold standard for identification of genetic components causing or promoting disc degeneration. Based on what was discussed earlier in this and other chapters of the book, it is unlikely that its genetic architecture would be too different from the many other common diseases. The ample examples of large-scale GWAS would suggest that a more comprehensive whole-genome approach should be used to identify new susceptible loci that may not be obvious from the current understanding of the biology of disc degeneration. Successful studies of rare variants, epigenetics, and noncoding RNAs are important references to consider, thus broadening the scope of investigation. Given that there are many advances in DNA sequencing technology, we should not be confined to candidate gene case-control analysis. Instead, every possibility should be explored to achieve the best understanding of the genetic components of disc degeneration.

10.9 Genetic Studies of Intervertebral Disc Degeneration: The Way Forward

It is difficult to recommend a specific direction for future investigations of the genetics of disc degeneration. Nevertheless, from the authors' experience, there are several points that hopefully can make the most of the studies already performed and maximize the chance of identifying new risk factors. A unified phenotypic definition is required such that there is a consensus of what constitutes the disease status, so that the same group of underlying genetic factors can be identified. Careful selection of cases and controls can avoid biases and hidden population stratifications leading to false positive results. Larger sample sizes always provide a more accurate evaluation of variants under study. All these criteria form the important basis of genetic studies; when fulfilled, they can make each individual study more reliable and relevant. Moreover, the new information can be easily integrated for replication in other populations and for confirmation through meta-analysis. Regions previously showing (marginal) significance should be considered for reanalysis. For example, partially linked common variants with weak associations may actually reflect causal and neighboring rare alleles. As we now know, since rare variants can affect common diseases with moderate effect sizes, revisiting these studies can help to provide a more comprehensive evaluation of these regions. In parallel, functional analyses of the associated variants are required as they provide biological insights while at the same time further consolidating the initial findings.

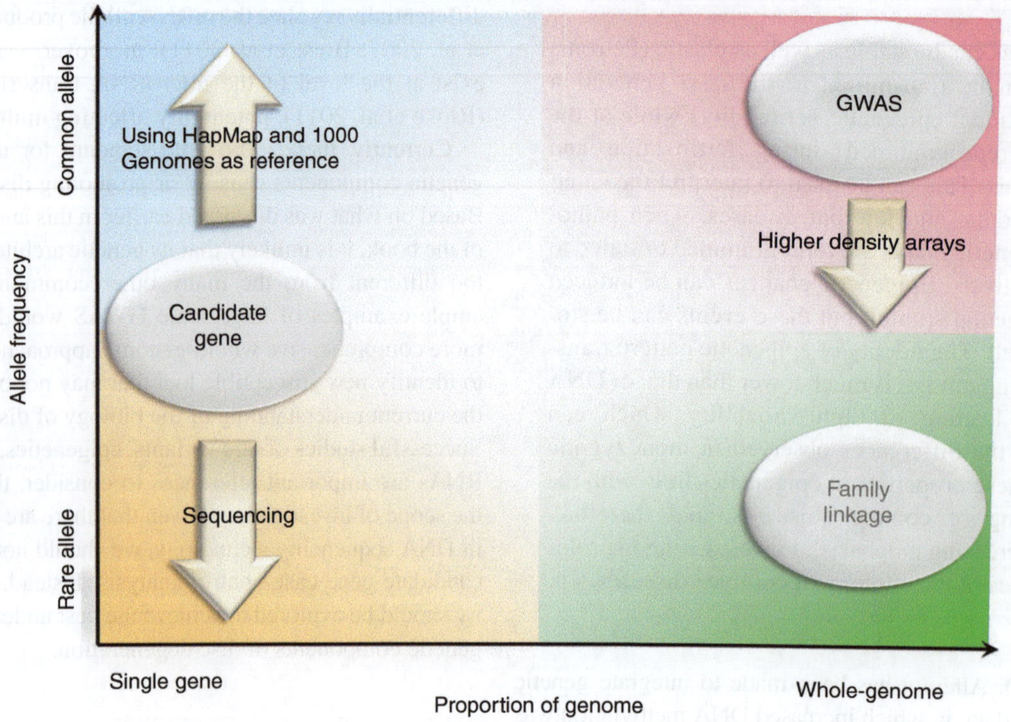

Fig. 10.5 Summary on the approaches for genetic studies. Candidate gene approach is a primarily gene-by-gene investigation. Common alleles (or lower frequency alleles) can be studied easily using databases such as HapMap and 1000 Genomes as reference. On the other hand, if rare alleles are of interest, one would need to adopt the sequencing method. GWAS approach, as its name suggested, looks into the whole genome. In general, it is designed to accommodate common alleles, but now, lower frequency alleles are also incorporated in the higher density arrays as well. Family linkage is also a whole-genome approach. Its detection of susceptible loci relies on large families with multiple affected members and, more importantly, variants with high penetrance and large effect sizes. Therefore, its application in detecting common disease variants is limited

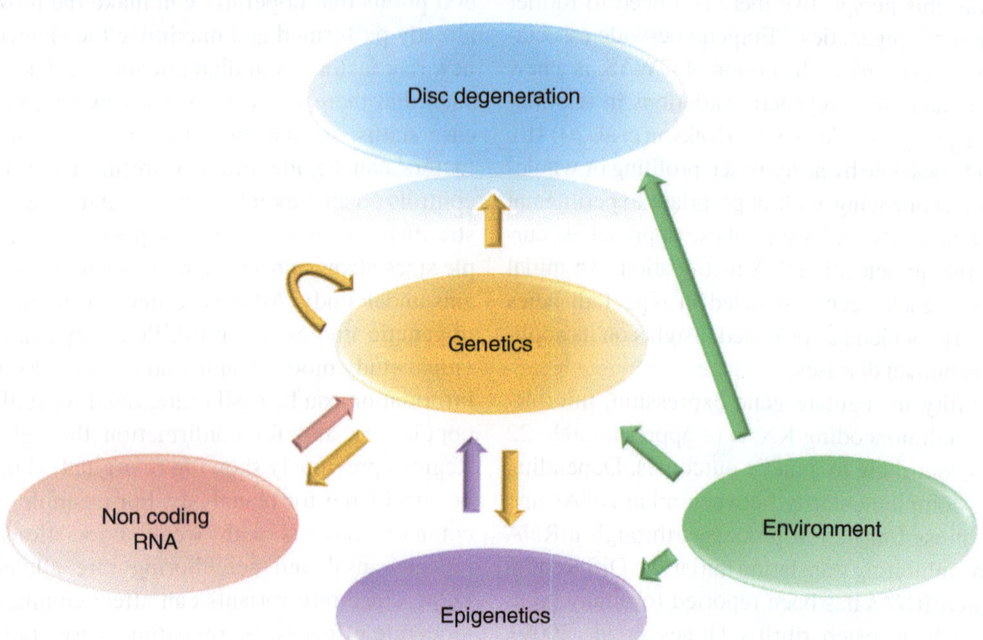

Fig. 10.6 Current and future genetics studies of disc degeneration. Based on the studies of other common diseases, we understand that genetics, while by itself is one of the major contributor to disc degeneration, can also interact with a number of other factors leading to altered effects. Both noncoding RNA and epigenetics can modulate the expression outcome. On the other hand, noncoding RNAs can be affected by the genetic variants at their expression levels, binding sites, or even their own sequence, while epigenetic patterns may be modified by genetic variants. Environmental factors can interact with genes and epigenetics, and at the same time, they can directly contribute to disc degeneration. Last but not least, gene-gene interactions also exist, which leads to variable consequences. Together, these represent a complicated network that needs to be investigated for a better understanding of disc degeneration and that genetics is not independent but should be studied in conjunction with other factors

Technology for providing genetic information is rapidly developing. Its success with other common diseases leads to the following questions: is it necessary to catch up with the latest technology in studying the genetics of disc degeneration, and if so, how should that be achieved? Obviously, each of the current technologies has its own strength: GWAS allows SNP analysis on the whole genome and is advantageous for identifying new susceptible loci, while sequencing is favorable for discovering new variants (Fig. 10.5). Both are promising tools; however, instead of blindly chasing after a new technology, it is more important to consider carefully which aspects of genetics is being studied and the type of information desired. Based on these considerations, the optimum technology can be chosen or various strategies can be combined to maximize data generation while minimizing costs. Factors modifying expression outcome such as epigenetics and noncoding RNA and interactions between genes, genes and proteins, as well as genes and environment should not be neglected (Fig. 10.6). The overall information can then be fed back to the investigators to provide a more complete understanding of the biology of the intervertebral disc and mechanisms of degeneration.

10.10 Summary of Critical Concepts Discussed in the Chapter

- Intervertebral disc degeneration is a complex trait contributed by genetics and multiple environmental factors such as age, gender, smoking, and mechanical loading.
- Heritability for disc degeneration at the lumbar region is approximately 70 %, suggesting a high degree of genetic involvement.
- Over 20 genes are reported to be associated with disc degeneration by case-control studies of selected candidates.
- *VDR* is the best replicated gene, while *ASPN*, *CILP*, *COL11A1*, *GDF5*, *SKT*, *THBS2*, and *MMP9* can be considered as potential risk factors with moderate genetic evidence based on interim guidelines propose by HuGENet to assess the "quality" of genetic data.
- The International HapMap Project and 1000 Genomes Project, as well as the latest high-throughput genotyping technologies, are valuable resources that can be integrated with current approaches to push forward genetics studies of disc degeneration.
- Factors such as epigenetics and noncoding RNA and interactions between genes, genes and proteins, as well as genes and environment should not be neglected as they may affect the final outcome of the genetic components.

Acknowledgements This work is supported by the University Grants Committee of Hong Kong (AoE/M-04/04) and AOSPINE (AOSBRC-07-2).

References

1000 Genomes Project Consortium GP (2010) A map of human genome variation from population-scale sequencing. Nature 467(7319):1061–1073

Aladin DM, Cheung KM et al (2007) Expression of the Trp2 allele of COL9A2 is associated with alterations in the mechanical properties of human intervertebral discs. Spine 32(25):2820–2826

Alanay Y, Avaygan H et al (2010) Mutations in the gene encoding the RER protein FKBP65 cause autosomal-recessive osteogenesis imperfecta. Am J Hum Genet 86(4):551–559

Altshuler DM, Gibbs RA et al (2010) Integrating common and rare genetic variation in diverse human populations. Nature 467(7311):52–58

Annunen S, Paassilta P et al (1999) An allele of COL9A2 associated with intervertebral disc disease. Science 285(5426):409–412

Barnes AM, Chang W et al (2006) Deficiency of cartilage-associated protein in recessive lethal osteogenesis imperfecta. N Engl J Med 355(26):2757–2764

Battie MC, Haynor DR et al (1995a) Similarities in degenerative findings on magnetic resonance images of the lumbar spines of identical twins. J Bone Joint Surg Am 77(11):1662–1670

Battie MC, Videman T et al (1995b) 1995 Volvo Award in clinical sciences. Determinants of lumbar disc degeneration. A study relating lifetime exposures and magnetic resonance imaging findings in identical twins. Spine 20(24):2601–2612

Bell CG, Finer S et al (2010) Integrated genetic and epigenetic analysis identifies haplotype-specific methylation in the FTO type 2 diabetes and obesity susceptibility locus. PLoS One 5(11):e14040

Benneker LM, Heini PF et al (2005) Correlation of radiographic and MRI parameters to morphological and biochemical assessment of intervertebral disc degeneration. Eur Spine J 14(1):27–35

Bertram L, Lill CM et al (2010) The genetics of Alzheimer disease: back to the future. Neuron 68(2):270–281

Bjornsson HT, Fallin MD et al (2004) An integrated epigenetic and genetic approach to common human disease. Trends Genet 20(8):350–358

Bodmer W, Bonilla C (2008) Common and rare variants in multifactorial susceptibility to common diseases. Nat Genet 40(6):695–701

Bonnefond A, Clement N et al (2012) Rare MTNR1B variants impairing melatonin receptor 1B function contribute to type 2 diabetes. Nat Genet 44(3):297–301

Bornstein P, Agah A et al (2004) The role of thrombospondins 1 and 2 in the regulation of cell-matrix interactions, collagen fibril formation, and the response to injury. Int J Biochem Cell Biol 36(6):1115–1125

Boyd LM, Richardson WJ et al (2008) Early-onset degeneration of the intervertebral disc and vertebral end plate in mice deficient in type IX collagen. Arthritis Rheum 58(1):164–171

Brest P, Lapaquette P et al (2011) A synonymous variant in IRGM alters a binding site for miR-196 and causes deregulation of IRGM-dependent xenophagy in Crohn's disease. Nat Genet 43(3):242–245

Cabral WA, Chang W et al (2007) Prolyl 3-hydroxylase 1 deficiency causes a recessive metabolic bone disorder resembling lethal/severe osteogenesis imperfecta. Nat Genet 39(3):359–365

Chanock SJ, Manolio T et al (2007) Replicating genotype-phenotype associations. Nature 447(7145):655–660

Cheung KM, Chan D et al (2006) Association of the Taq I allele in vitamin D receptor with degenerative disc disease and disc bulge in a Chinese population. Spine 31(10):1143–1148

Cheung KM, Karppinen J et al (2009) Prevalence and pattern of lumbar MRI changes in a population study of 1043 individuals. Spine 34(9):934–940

Cirulli ET, Goldstein DB (2010) Uncovering the roles of rare variants in common disease through whole-genome sequencing. Nat Rev Genet 11(6):415–425

Cong L, Pang H et al (2010a) The interaction between aggrecan gene VNTR polymorphism and cigarette smoking in predicting incident symptomatic intervertebral disc degeneration. Connect Tissue Res 51(5):397–403

Cong L, Pang H et al (2010b) Association between the expression of aggrecan and the distribution of aggrecan gene variable number of tandem repeats with symptomatic lumbar disc herniation in Chinese Han of Northern China. Spine 35(14):1371–1376

Daly MJ (2009) Assessing significance in genetic association studies. Cold Spring Harb Protoc 2009(8):pdb top58

Davey JW, Hohenlohe PA et al (2011) Genome-wide genetic marker discovery and genotyping using next-generation sequencing. Nat Rev Genet 12(7):499–510

Dempster EL, Pidsley R et al (2011) Disease-associated epigenetic changes in monozygotic twins discordant for schizophrenia and bipolar disorder. Hum Mol Genet 20(24):4786–4796

Doege KJ, Coulter SN et al (1997) A human-specific polymorphism in the coding region of the aggrecan gene. Variable number of tandem repeats produce a range of core protein sizes in the general population. J Biol Chem 272(21):13974–13979

Dong DM, Yao M et al (2007) Association between the -1306C/T polymorphism of matrix metalloproteinase-2 gene and lumbar disc disease in Chinese young adults. Eur Spine J 16(11):1958–1961

Eichler EE, Flint J et al (2010) Missing heritability and strategies for finding the underlying causes of complex disease. Nat Rev Genet 11(6):446–450

Eser O, Eser B et al (2011) Short aggrecan gene repetitive alleles associated with lumbar degenerative disc disease in Turkish patients. Genet Mol Res 10(3):1923–1930

Feinberg AP (2007) Phenotypic plasticity and the epigenetics of human disease. Nature 447(7143):433–440

Francis-West PH, Abdelfattah A et al (1999) Mechanisms of GDF-5 action during skeletal development. Development 126(6):1305–1315

Garnero P, Borel O et al (1998) Collagen Ialpha1 Sp1 polymorphism, bone mass, and bone turnover in healthy French premenopausal women: the OFELY study. J Bone Miner Res 13(5):813–817

Goupille P, Jayson MI et al (1998) Matrix metalloproteinases: the clue to intervertebral disc degeneration? Spine 23(14):1612–1626

Grant SF, Reid DM et al (1996) Reduced bone density and osteoporosis associated with a polymorphic Sp1 binding site in the collagen type I alpha 1 gene. Nat Genet 14(2):203–205

Gruber HE, Ingram JA et al (2009) Asporin, a susceptibility gene in osteoarthritis, is expressed at higher levels in the more degenerate human intervertebral disc. Arthritis Res Ther 11(2):R47

Higashino K, Matsui Y et al (2007) The alpha2 type IX collagen tryptophan polymorphism is associated with the severity of disc degeneration in younger patients with herniated nucleus pulposus of the lumbar spine. Int Orthop 31(1):107–111

Hindorff LA, MacArthur J et al (2012) A catalog of published genome-wide association studies. Available at www.genome.gov/gwastudies. Accessed 24 Feb 2012

Hirose Y, Chiba K et al (2008) A functional polymorphism in THBS2 that affects alternative splicing and MMP binding is associated with lumbar-disc herniation. Am J Hum Genet 82(5):1122–1129

Internation HapMap Consortium (2003) The International HapMap Project. Nature 426(6968):789–796

Ioannidis JP, Boffetta P et al (2008) Assessment of cumulative evidence on genetic associations: interim guidelines. Int J Epidemiol 37(1): 120–132

Jim JJ, Noponen-Hietala N et al (2005) The TRP2 allele of COL9A2 is an age-dependent risk factor for the development and severity of intervertebral disc degeneration. Spine 30(24):2735–2742

Jones SW, Watkins G et al (2009) The identification of differentially expressed microRNA in osteoarthritic tissue that modulate the production of TNF-alpha and MMP13. Osteoarthritis Cartilage 17(4): 464–472

Kales SN, Linos A et al (2004) The role of collagen IX tryptophan polymorphisms in symptomatic intervertebral disc disease in Southern European patients. Spine 29(11):1266–1270

Karasugi T, Semba K et al (2009) Association of the tag SNPs in the human SKT gene (KIAA1217) with lumbar disc herniation. J Bone Miner Res 24(9):1537–1543

Kawaguchi Y, Osada R et al (1999) Association between an aggrecan gene polymorphism and lumbar disc degeneration. Spine 24(23):2456–2460

Kawaguchi Y, Kanamori M et al (2002) The association of lumbar disc disease with vitamin-D receptor gene polymorphism. J Bone Joint Surg Am 84-A(11):2022–2028

Kelempisioti A, Eskola PJ et al (2011) Genetic susceptibility of intervertebral disc degeneration among young Finnish adults. BMC Med Genet 12(1):153

Kellgren JH, Jeffrey MR et al (1963) The epidemiology of chronic rheumatism: atlas of standard radiographs. Blackwell Scientific, Oxford

Kerkhof HJ, Lories RJ et al (2010) A genome-wide association study identifies an osteoarthritis susceptibility locus on chromosome 7q22. Arthritis Rheum 62(2):499–510

Khoschnau S, Melhus H et al (2008) Type I collagen alpha1 Sp1 polymorphism and the risk of cruciate ligament ruptures or shoulder dislocations. Am J Sports Med 36(12):2432–2436

Kim NK, Shin DA et al (2011) The association of aggrecan gene polymorphism with the risk of intervertebral disc degeneration. Acta Neurochir (Wien) 153(1):129–133

Kimura T, Nakata K et al (1996) Progressive degeneration of articular cartilage and intervertebral discs. An experimental study in transgenic mice bearing a type IX collagen mutation. Int Orthop 20(3):177–181

Kizawa H, Kou I et al (2005) An aspartic acid repeat polymorphism in asporin inhibits chondrogenesis and increases susceptibility to osteoarthritis. Nat Genet 37(2):138–144

Klatt AR, Klinger G et al (2009) Matrilin-3 activates the expression of osteoarthritis-associated genes in primary human chondrocytes. FEBS Lett 583(22):3611–3617

Klatt AR, Becker AK et al (2011) The matrilins: modulators of extracellular matrix assembly. Int J Biochem Cell Biol 43(3): 320–330

Lapunzina P, Aglan M et al (2010) Identification of a frameshift mutation in Osterix in a patient with recessive osteogenesis imperfecta. Am J Hum Genet 87(1):110–114

Le Maitre CL, Freemont AJ et al (2004) Localization of degradative enzymes and their inhibitors in the degenerate human intervertebral disc. J Pathol 204(1):47–54

Le Maitre CL, Freemont AJ et al (2005) The role of interleukin-1 in the pathogenesis of human intervertebral disc degeneration. Arthritis Res Ther 7(4):R732–R745

Le Maitre CL, Hoyland JA et al (2007) Catabolic cytokine expression in degenerate and herniated human intervertebral discs: IL-1beta and TNFalpha expression profile. Arthritis Res Ther 9(4):R77

Lian K, Zmuda JM et al (2005) Type I collagen alpha1 Sp1 transcription factor binding site polymorphism is associated with reduced risk of hip osteoarthritis defined by severe joint space narrowing in elderly women. Arthritis Rheum 52(5):1431–1436

Lin WP, Lin JH et al (2011) Interleukin-10 promoter polymorphisms associated with susceptibility to lumbar disc degeneration in a Chinese cohort. Genet Mol Res 10(3):1719–1727

Lorenzo P, Bayliss MT et al (1998) A novel cartilage protein (CILP) present in the mid-zone of human articular cartilage increases with age. J Biol Chem 273(36):23463–23468

Lorenzo P, Aspberg A et al (2001) Identification and characterization of asporin. A novel member of the leucine-rich repeat protein family closely related to decorin and biglycan. J Biol Chem 276(15): 12201–12211

Loughlin J (2011) Osteoarthritis year 2010 in review: genetics. Osteoarthritis Cartilage 19(4):342–345

Mann V, Hobson EE et al (2001) A COL1A1 Sp1 binding site polymorphism predisposes to osteoporotic fracture by affecting bone density and quality. J Clin Invest 107(7):899–907

Manolio TA, Collins FS et al (2009) Finding the missing heritability of complex diseases. Nature 461(7265):747–753
Marinelli NL, Haughton VM et al (2009) T2 relaxation times of intervertebral disc tissue correlated with water content and proteoglycan content. Spine 34(5):520–524
Martinez-Glez V, Valencia M et al (2011) Identification of a mutation causing deficient BMP1/mTLD proteolytic activity in autosomal recessive osteogenesis imperfecta. Hum Mutat 33(2):343–350
Matsui Y, Wu JJ et al (2003) Matrix deposition of tryptophan-containing allelic variants of type IX collagen in developing human cartilage. Matrix Biol 22(2):123–129
Metzker ML (2010) Sequencing technologies – the next generation. Nat Rev Genet 11(1):31–46
Millward-Sadler SJ, Costello PW et al (2009) Regulation of catabolic gene expression in normal and degenerate human intervertebral disc cells: implications for the pathogenesis of intervertebral disc degeneration. Arthritis Res Ther 11(3):R65
Min JL, Meulenbelt I et al (2006) Association of matrilin-3 polymorphisms with spinal disc degeneration and osteoarthritis of the first carpometacarpal joint of the hand. Ann Rheum Dis 65(8):1060–1066
Min SK, Nakazato K et al (2010) Cartilage intermediate layer protein gene is associated with lumbar disc degeneration in male, but not female, collegiate athletes. Am J Sports Med 38(12):2552–2557
Mio F, Chiba K et al (2007) A functional polymorphism in COL11A1, which encodes the alpha 1 chain of type XI collagen, is associated with susceptibility to lumbar disc herniation. Am J Hum Genet 81(6):1271–1277
Mitchell BD, Yerges-Armstrong LM (2011) The genetics of bone loss: challenges and prospects. J Clin Endocrinol Metab 96(5):1258–1268
Miyamoto Y, Mabuchi A et al (2007) A functional polymorphism in the 5′ UTR of GDF5 is associated with susceptibility to osteoarthritis. Nat Genet 39(4):529–533
Moreau MP, Bruse SE et al (2011) Altered microRNA expression profiles in postmortem brain samples from individuals with schizophrenia and bipolar disorder. Biol Psychiatry 69(2):188–193
Morello R, Bertin TK et al (2006) CRTAP is required for prolyl 3-hydroxylation and mutations cause recessive osteogenesis imperfecta. Cell 127(2):291–304
Nakajima M, Takahashi A et al (2010) New sequence variants in HLA class II/III region associated with susceptibility to knee osteoarthritis identified by genome-wide association study. PLoS One 5(3): e9723
Nakaoka H, Inoue I (2009) Meta-analysis of genetic association studies: methodologies, between-study heterogeneity and winner's curse. J Hum Genet 54(11):615–623
Neale BM, Sham PC (2004) The future of association studies: gene-based analysis and replication. Am J Hum Genet 75(3):353–362
Nejentsev S, Walker N et al (2009) Rare variants of IFIH1, a gene implicated in antiviral responses, protect against type 1 diabetes. Science 324(5925):387–389
Paassilta P, Lohiniva J et al (2001) Identification of a novel common genetic risk factor for lumbar disk disease. JAMA 285(14): 1843–1849
Panoutsopoulou K, Southam L et al (2011) Insights into the genetic architecture of osteoarthritis from stage 1 of the arcOGEN study. Ann Rheum Dis 70(5):864–867
Perkins DO, Jeffries CD et al (2007) microRNA expression in the prefrontal cortex of individuals with schizophrenia and schizoaffective disorder. Genome Biol 8(2):R27
Petronis A (2010) Epigenetics as a unifying principle in the aetiology of complex traits and diseases. Nature 465(7299):721–727
Pfirrmann CW, Metzdorf A et al (2001) Magnetic resonance classification of lumbar intervertebral disc degeneration. Spine 26(17):1873–1878
Pluijm SM, van Essen HW et al (2004) Collagen type I alpha1 Sp1 polymorphism, osteoporosis, and intervertebral disc degeneration in older men and women. Ann Rheum Dis 63(1):71–77
Price SJ, Greaves DR et al (2001) Identification of novel, functional genetic variants in the human matrix metalloproteinase-2 gene: role of Sp1 in allele-specific transcriptional regulation. J Biol Chem 276(10):7549–7558
Rakyan VK, Beyan H et al (2011a) Identification of type 1 diabetes-associated DNA methylation variable positions that precede disease diagnosis. PLoS Genet 7(9):e1002300
Rakyan VK, Down TA et al (2011b) Epigenome-wide association studies for common human diseases. Nat Rev Genet 12(8):529–541
Ripke S, Sanders AR et al (2011) Genome-wide association study identifies five new schizophrenia loci. Nat Genet 43(10): 969–976
Roberts S, Caterson B et al (2000) Matrix metalloproteinases and aggrecanase: their role in disorders of the human intervertebral disc. Spine 25(23):3005–3013
Sambrook PN, MacGregor AJ et al (1999) Genetic influences on cervical and lumbar disc degeneration: a magnetic resonance imaging study in twins. Arthritis Rheum 42(2):366–372
Schneiderman G, Flannigan B et al (1987) Magnetic resonance imaging in the diagnosis of disc degeneration: correlation with discography. Spine 12(3):276–281
Seki S, Kawaguchi Y et al (2005) A functional SNP in CILP, encoding cartilage intermediate layer protein, is associated with susceptibility to lumbar disc disease. Nat Genet 37(6):607–612
Seki S, Kawaguchi Y et al (2006) Association study of COL9A2 with lumbar disc disease in the Japanese population. J Hum Genet 51(12): 1063–1067
Semba K, Araki K et al (2006) A novel murine gene, Sickle tail, linked to the Danforth's short tail locus, is required for normal development of the intervertebral disc. Genetics 172(1):445–456
Sethupathy P, Borel C et al (2007) Human microRNA-155 on chromosome 21 differentially interacts with its polymorphic target in the AGTR1 3′ untranslated region: a mechanism for functional single-nucleotide polymorphisms related to phenotypes. Am J Hum Genet 81(2):405–413
Skorupski P, Krol J et al (2006) An alpha-1 chain of type I collagen Sp1-binding site polymorphism in women suffering from stress urinary incontinence. Am J Obstet Gynecol 194(2):346–350
So HC, Gui AH et al (2011) Evaluating the heritability explained by known susceptibility variants: a survey of ten complex diseases. Genet Epidemiol 35(5):310–317
Solovieva S, Lohiniva J et al (2002) COL9A3 gene polymorphism and obesity in intervertebral disc degeneration of the lumbar spine: evidence of gene-environment interaction. Spine 27(23):2691–2696
Solovieva S, Kouhia S et al (2004) Interleukin 1 polymorphisms and intervertebral disc degeneration. Epidemiology 15(5):626–633
Solovieva S, Lohiniva J et al (2006) Intervertebral disc degeneration in relation to the COL9A3 and the IL-1ss gene polymorphisms. Eur Spine J 15(5):613–619
Solovieva S, Noponen N et al (2007) Association between the aggrecan gene variable number of tandem repeats polymorphism and intervertebral disc degeneration. Spine 32(16):1700–1705
Song YQ, Cheung KM et al (2008a) Association of the asporin D14 allele with lumbar-disc degeneration in Asians. Am J Hum Genet 82(3):744–747
Song YQ, Ho DW et al (2008b) Association between promoter -1607 polymorphism of MMP1 and lumbar disc disease in Southern Chinese. BMC Med Genet 9:38
Speer G, Szenthe P et al (2006) Myocardial infarction is associated with Spl binding site polymorphism of collagen type 1A1 gene. Acta Cardiol 61(3):321–325
Stefansson H, Rujescu D et al (2008) Large recurrent microdeletions associated with schizophrenia. Nature 455(7210):232–236
Sun ZM, Miao L et al (2009) Association between the -1562 C/T polymorphism of matrix metalloproteinase-9 gene and lumbar disc disease in the young adult population in North China. Connect Tissue Res 50(3):181–185

Tabor HK, Risch NJ et al (2002) Candidate-gene approaches for studying complex genetic traits: practical considerations. Nat Rev Genet 3(5):391–397

Takahashi M, Haro H et al (2001) The association of degeneration of the intervertebral disc with 5a/6a polymorphism in the promoter of the human matrix metalloproteinase-3 gene. J Bone Joint Surg Br 83(4):491–495

Tilkeridis C, Bei T et al (2005) Association of a COL1A1 polymorphism with lumbar disc disease in young military recruits. J Med Genet 42(7):e44

Uitterlinden AG, Burger H et al (1998) Relation of alleles of the collagen type Ialpha1 gene to bone density and the risk of osteoporotic fractures in postmenopausal women. N Engl J Med 338(15): 1016–1021

Uitterlinden AG, Fang Y et al (2004) Genetics and biology of vitamin D receptor polymorphisms. Gene 338(2):143–156

Urano T, Narusawa K et al (2008) Association of a single nucleotide polymorphism in the insulin-like growth factor-1 receptor gene with spinal disc degeneration in postmenopausal Japanese women. Spine 33(11):1256–1261

Valdes AM, Spector TD (2011) Genetic epidemiology of hip and knee osteoarthritis. Nat Rev Rheumatol 7(1):23–32

Valdes AM, Hassett G et al (2005) Radiographic progression of lumbar spine disc degeneration is influenced by variation at inflammatory genes: a candidate SNP association study in the Chingford cohort. Spine 30(21):2445–2451

van Dijk FS, Nesbitt IM et al (2009) PPIB mutations cause severe osteogenesis imperfecta. Am J Hum Genet 85(4):521–527

Videman T, Nummi P et al (1994) Digital assessment of MRI for lumbar disc desiccation. A comparison of digital versus subjective assessments and digital intensity profiles versus discogram and macroanatomic findings. Spine 19(2):192–198

Videman T, Leppavuori J et al (1998) Intragenic polymorphisms of the vitamin D receptor gene associated with intervertebral disc degeneration. Spine 23(23):2477–2485

Videman T, Saarela J et al (2009) Associations of 25 structural, degradative, and inflammatory candidate genes with lumbar disc desiccation, bulging, and height narrowing. Arthritis Rheum 60(2):470–481

Vikkula M, Palotie A et al (1993) Early-onset osteoarthritis linked to the type II procollagen gene. Detailed clinical phenotype and further analyses of the gene. Arthritis Rheum 36(3):401–409

Virtanen IM, Song YQ et al (2007) Phenotypic and population differences in the association between CILP and lumbar disc disease. J Med Genet 44(4):285–288

Visscher PM, Hill WG et al (2008) Heritability in the genomics era – concepts and misconceptions. Nat Rev Genet 9(4):255–266

Visscher PM, Brown MA et al (2012) Five years of GWAS discovery. Am J Hum Genet 90(1):7–24

Wagner GP, Zhang J (2011) The pleiotropic structure of the genotype-phenotype map: the evolvability of complex organisms. Nat Rev Genet 12(3):204–213

Williams FM, Popham M et al (2011) GDF5 single-nucleotide polymorphism rs143383 is associated with lumbar disc degeneration in Northern European women. Arthritis Rheum 63(3): 708–712

Wrocklage C, Wassmann H et al (2000) COL9A2 allelotypes in intervertebral disc disease. Biochem Biophys Res Commun 279(2):398–400

Zeller T, Blankenberg S et al (2012) Genomewide association studies in cardiovascular disease – an update 2011. Clin Chem 58(1):92–103

Pathogenesis of Intervertebral Disc Degeneration

11

Stephen M. Richardson, Anthony J. Freemont, and Judith A. Hoyland

Contents

11.1 Introduction

It is estimated that as much as 84 % of the population will suffer from low back pain (LBP) at some point in their lifetime (Walker 2000), with around 10 % of sufferers being chronically disabled. As such LBP is one of the most prevalent musculoskeletal conditions affecting Western society (Stewart et al. 2003), and its prevalence has increased over recent decades (Harkness et al. 2005). The socio-economic cost of LBP is also huge, with associated costs, in terms of lost productivity, disability benefits and direct and indirect health-care costs, estimated in the UK to be around £12 billion annually (Maniadakis and Gray 2000) and in the USA to be over $85 billion per annum (Martin et al. 2008). Importantly, increases in both the size and average age of the population both suggest that the prevalence and costs associated with LBP will continue to rise over future decades, unless novel therapies can be developed to alleviate pain and restore long-term function and mobility to the spine. However, in order to develop such therapies, a more thorough understanding of the underlying aetiology is required.

While it is acknowledged that LBP is a multifactorial condition, a strong correlation with degeneration of the intervertebral disc has been shown in 40 % of cases (Cheung et al. 2009). However, until recently, the pathogenesis of disc degeneration and its role in LBP were poorly understood.

S.M. Richardson • J.A. Hoyland (✉)
Centre for Regenerative Medicine,
Institute of Inflammation and Repair,
Faculty of Medical and Human Sciences,
The University of Manchester,
Stopford Building Oxford Road,
Manchester M13 9PT, UK
e-mail: s.ricahrdson@manchester.ac.uk;
judith.hoyland@manchester.ac.uk

A.J. Freemont
Centre for Regenerative Medicine,
Institute of Inflammation and Repair,
Faculty of Medical and Human Sciences,
The University of Manchester,
Stopford Building Oxford Road,
Manchester M13 9PT, UK

School of Medicine, The University of Manchester,
Stopford Building Oxford Road,
Manchester M13 9PT, UK
e-mail: tony.freemont@manchester.ac.uk

I.M. Shapiro, M.V. Risbud (eds.), *The Intervertebral Disc*,
DOI 10.1007/978-3-7091-1535-0_11, © Springer-Verlag Wien 2014

This chapter will describe the normal intervertebral disc and the changes which occur during degeneration at a molecular, cellular and tissue level and review the clinical implications of these pathological changes in the context of LBP.

11.2 The Cell Biology of the Normal Human Intervertebral Disc

The intervertebral disc is located between the vertebrae of the spine and is comprised of three morphologically distinct regions. The central core of the disc, the nucleus pulposus, is a highly hydrated, gelatinous tissue containing small rounded nucleus pulposus cells embedded within a dense extracellular matrix. These cells are routinely described as being chondrocyte-like (Sive et al. 2002), due in part to similarities in both their morphology and composition of the matrix that they synthesise and secrete. Noteworthy, recent microarray studies have shed new light on the exact phenotype of nucleus pulposus and annulus fibrosus cells, illustrating distinct differences in gene expression profiles between these cells and articular chondrocytes (Lee et al. 2007; Sakai et al. 2009; Minogue et al. 2010a, b). The extracellular matrix of the nucleus pulposus is rich in proteoglycans, particularly the large aggregating proteoglycans aggrecan and versican which possess a large number of negatively charged glycosaminoglycan (GAG) side chains. The GAGs attract positively charged ions, which gives the nucleus pulposus a high osmotic potential, which in turn acts to draw in water resulting in a tissue with a water content between 70 and 90 % (Antoniou et al. 1996). A range of other smaller PGs are also present, including biglycan, decorin and fibromodulin, which are thought to play a number of structural and physiological roles, including growth factor binding and mediation of signalling between cells and the extracellular matrix (Roughley 2004; Feng et al. 2006). Further details of the proteoglycans of the disc are presented in Chap. 4. The nucleus pulposus also contains a range of collagens, predominantly collagen II, although III, V, VI, IX and XI have also been described (Nerlich et al. 1998; Roughley 2004). The collagen II fibrils appear randomly distributed within the matrix, meaning the extracellular matrix lacks the structural architecture noted in similar tissues such as articular cartilage (see Chap. 5). While the extracellular matrix possesses many of the same component molecules as articular cartilage, the ratio of PGs/collagens in the nucleus pulposus is substantially higher, at around 27:1, compared to only around 2:1 in cartilage (Mwale et al. 2004). The elevated proteoglycans content of the nucleus pulposus, in conjunction with the associated high water content, results in a high swelling pressure giving it the ability to effectively act as a 'shock absorber' and withstand the high compressive forces experienced within the spine (see Chap. 2).

The nucleus pulposus is constrained circumferentially by the outer region of the disc, the annulus fibrosus, a fibrous ring of tissue with highly ordered collagen I fibrils orientated in 60° oblique lamellae (Marchand and Ahmed 1990). Collagens II and III are also present in the annulus fibrosus and the total collagen content is around 80 %, compared to only around 20 % in the nucleus pulposus (Roughley 2004; Le Maitre et al. 2007d). While the extracellular matrix of the annulus fibrosus does contain proteoglycans, predominantly versican, they are mainly located between the lamellae, along with elastin fibres which are thought to allow flexion or extension during movement (Yu et al. 2002; Melrose et al. 2008; Smith et al. 2009). Morphologically and phenotypically, fibroblastic annulus fibrosus cells appear to orientate with the collagen fibres in each lamella ring. Although the cell and matrix biology differs between the nucleus pulposus and annulus fibrosus, there is no distinct demarcation between the tissues. Instead, the inner annulus fibrosus, sometimes referred to as a 'transition zone', demonstrates a mix of cell types with both rounded nucleus pulposus and flattened annulus fibrosus cells present. The matrix changes are also gradual, with collagens I and II contents being inversely correlated (Eyre and Muir 1976). This integration of tissues allows the disc to bulge in a constrained manner under loading, allowing distribution and dissipation of the mechanical forces, including flexion, tension, compression and torsion, experienced during everyday motion. These concepts are further developed in Chap. 7.

The inferior and superior faces on the disc, where they meet adjacent vertebral bodies, are covered by a thin layer of hyaline cartilage, the cartilaginous end plates. This is a thin layer of hyaline cartilage containing a population of chondrocytic cells. Collagen fibres from the annulus fibrosus embed directly into the vertebral bodies and into the cartilaginous end plates, which prevent the nucleus pulposus bulging into the vertebral bodies (Humzah and Soames 1988). The cartilaginous end plates are also thought to play a crucial role in regulating disc nutrition (Nachemson et al. 1970; Roberts et al. 1996).

The adult human intervertebral disc is both avascular and aneural, with blood vessels and associated nerves found only in the very outer regions of the annulus fibrosus and in the vertebral bodies adjacent to the cartilaginous end plates (Yasuma et al. 1993; Repanti et al. 1998; Roughley 2004). It is these capillaries that provide nutrients to cells within the disc, through a process of diffusion facilitated by fluid transport that occurs during normal movement. Under compressive loading, water is extruded from the nucleus pulposus, taking metabolic waste products such as lactic acid away from cells towards the blood vessels. As load is briefly alleviated, the osmotic potential of the nucleus draws water back in, supplying the cells with nutrients such as glucose and oxygen. However, as cells in the core of the nucleus pulposus can be as much as 8 mm from the nearest blood vessel, this results in a tissue which is both nutrient and oxygen poor and with a relatively low pH, primarily due to an accumulation of lactic acid (Urban et al. 1982; Katz et al. 1986). This hostile environment is reflected in the cell densities of the tissue which are considerably less than in other cartilaginous tissues. In early life, cellularity decreases to approximately 4,000 cells/mm^3 in the normal adult nucleus pulposus and 9,000 cells/mm^3 in the annulus fibrosus by the time skeletal maturity is achieved (Maroudas et al. 1975). There is also a reduction in the proportion of large, vacuolated, morphologically distinct notochordal cells within the nucleus pulposus and an increase in or transition to smaller mature nucleus cells, which are thought to have a lower metabolic activity than notochordal cells (Guehring et al. 2008). Cell metabolism within the disc is also thought to be relatively low, due in part to the low pH and oxygen concentration, with cells generating ATP predominantly through glycolysis (Urban et al. 2004).

However, while cell number and metabolic activity are both low, the resident cells are responsible for homeostatic turnover of the extracellular matrix, producing catabolic factors and degradative enzymes, as well as anabolic growth factors and new matrix proteins. This process is tightly controlled and any imbalance in degradative and synthetic processes can lead to a matrix breakdown and loss of tissue integrity. While the exact reasons for this imbalance are not fully understood, research over recent years has shed light on the processes which contribute to, or are potentially responsible for, the tissue breakdown observed during intervertebral disc degeneration.

11.3 Intervertebral Disc Degeneration

Disc degeneration is characterised by an overall breakdown of extracellular matrix, combined with altered matrix synthesis and changes in resident cell number, cell phenotype and behaviour. While many of these features are evident during normal ageing, changes are accelerated in degeneration and are associated with discogenic pain or pain caused by spinal instability and impingement of nerve roots in the spine.

11.3.1 Morphological Features of Degeneration

Degeneration is routinely characterised radiographically (Antoniou et al. 1998; Pfirrmann et al. 2001), with the Thompson grading system used to classify gross morphological changes (Thompson et al. 1990). This system describes the decreasing water content within the nucleus pulposus, combined with disc narrowing and bulging and eventually osteophyte formation and end-plate sclerosis. Histologically, degeneration can be characterised using a range of features (Sive et al. 2002). There is progressive loss of demarcation between the nucleus pulposus and annulus fibrosus with loss of the transition zone. This is due, in part, to a change in collagen synthesis by the nucleus cells from collagen II to collagen I; a loss of proteoglycan, which results in dehydration of the nucleus pulposus; presence and extent of fissuring within the nucleus pulposus, which radiate eventually into the annulus fibrosus; and formation of cell clusters due to abnormal cell turnover. Changes also occur in the annulus fibrosus, with disruption of the collagen lamellae as fissures extend, and there is a change in collagen fibre organisation with fibres bifurcating and interdigitating (Lyons et al. 1981). The poor repair capacity of the disc means that in the late stages of degeneration, the nucleus pulposus is replaced by disorganised scar and granulation tissue, and repair of the annulus fibrosus results in scaring and neovascularisation (Peng et al. 2006). Vascular ingrowth extends eventually into the nucleus pulposus and is associated with innervation into the disc causing discogenic pain (Freemont et al. 1997, 2002). The decrease in water content and increasing fibrous nature of the nucleus pulposus cause the disc narrowing observed radiographically. There is also an increase in collagen cross-linking with tissue sugars, making the disc stiffer, more difficult to repair and more easily injured (Hormel and Eyre 1991; Duance et al. 1998; Pokharna and Phillips 1998; Wagner et al. 2006). Importantly, this reduced disc height significantly alters the biomechanics of the spinal motion segment, with decompression of the nucleus pulposus and removal of stress within fibres of the annulus fibrosus that ultimately causes spinal instability and leaves the disc less able to resist forces experienced during motions such as bending (Zhao et al. 2005; Adams and Roughley 2006). Increased pressure is also placed on the neural arch and this can result in non-discogenic nerve pain during movement (Pollintine et al. 2004).

Although the anatomical and morphological features of degeneration have been well documented, the underlying cellular and pathophysiological changes occurring during degeneration have not been thoroughly described. However, in an attempt to identify novel therapies, recent widespread interest in the elucidating mechanisms underlying degeneration has resulted in a more thorough understanding of the pathogenesis of degenerative disc disease.

11.3.2 Genetic Influences

Age and environmental factors, such as smoking, vibration, excessive heavy loading and localised injury, have all been proposed as risk factors (Holm and Nachemson 1988; Hirano et al. 1988; Deyo and Bass 1989; Wilder et al. 1996; Adams et al. 1999, 2000). Genetic and hereditary factors are considered to play a dominant role in predisposing individuals to disc degeneration and back pain. A familial survey by Postacchini et al. found that in the group of individuals with discogenic LBP, 35 % had at least 1 family member with a history of discogenic LBP and 5 % had one or two members who had undergone disc surgery (Postacchini et al. 1988). This compared to 12 and 1 % respectively in the asymptomatic cohort. Further studies, including identical and nonidentical twin studies, have also shown strong familial links in discogenic LBP predisposition (Richardson et al. 1997; MacGregor et al. 2004; Frino et al. 2006).

In addition to familial studies, a growing body of research has investigated genetic associations with degeneration. The genes for collagen I (COL1A1), IX (COL9A2 and COL9A3), XI (COL11A2), aggrecan, MMP-3, IL-1, IL-6, vitamin D receptor (VDR), cartilage intermediate layer protein (CILP) and hyaluronan and proteoglycan link protein 1 (HAPLN1) have all been associated with disc degeneration (Videman et al. 1998; Annunen et al. 1999; Takahashi et al. 2001; Kawaguchi et al. 2002; Pluijm et al. 2004; Solovieva et al. 2004, 2006; Seki et al. 2005; Kawakami et al. 2005; Roughley et al. 2006). However, to date, in different ethnic groups, only COL1A1, COL9A2, MMP-3 and VDR polymorphisms have been shown reproducibly to be disease associated. This topic is developed further in Chap. 10. In order to prove links between gene polymorphisms and disc degeneration, then more detailed and large-scale linkage studies on families with members who are predisposed to early onset degeneration are required. If genetic predisposition and association with single gene polymorphisms can be established, this may lead to the development of diagnostic tools to screen disc degeneration predisposition. However, these studies may also reveal that disc degeneration is a complex, multifactorial, oliogenic disorder for which a clear predisposition is difficult to detect.

11.3.3 Alterations in Extracellular Matrix Composition

While many of the matrix changes evident during degeneration are due to increased matrix catabolism by degradative enzymes (as will be discussed in the next section), there are also alterations in the synthesis and distribution of matrix components. In the early stages of degeneration, there is an increase in expression of collagen II, thought to be an attempted repair mechanism (Takaishi et al. 1997). However, with advancing degeneration, there is a general decrease in collagen II synthesis and a shift to collagen I production by nucleus pulposus and inner annulus fibrosus cells (Buckwalter 1995; Schollmeier et al. 2000; Le Maitre et al. 2007d). Collagen X has been identified in the disc during advanced degeneration, particularly around clefts and cell clusters (Boos et al. 1997). The induction of collagen X during late-stage degeneration is suggested to be a cellular response to enhance oxidative stress and is thought to signify nucleus pulposus cell hypertrophy as it is often accompanied by increased expression of Runt-related transcription factor 2 (Runx2), osteoprotegerin and alkaline phosphatase in areas of calcification (Boos et al. 1997; Nerlich et al. 1997; Rutges et al. 2010).

Collagen cross-linking also changes during degeneration, with a decrease in pyridinoline cross-links which give stability to collagen fibrils, especially in the nucleus pulposus where the collagen fibres are less densely packed than the annulus fibrosus. There is also an increase in nonenzymatic glycosylation, which causes cross-linking of matrix proteins, with an increase in pentosidine during degeneration being one marker of this process. This increase in advanced glycation end products (AGEs) within the disc during both natural ageing and degeneration has been demonstrated to cause tissue stiffness, particularly in the annulus fibrosus, and may make the disc more susceptible to mechanical damage during degeneration (Hormel and Eyre 1991; Duance et al. 1998; Pokharna and Phillips 1998; Wagner et al. 2006; Adams et al. 2010).

Combined with the changes in collagen expression, there is a decrease in the proteoglycans content of the disc (Pearce et al. 1987; Inkinen et al. 1998; Cs-Szabo et al. 2002; Sztrolovics et al. 2002). While degenerate nucleus pulposus cells are capable of synthesising aggrecan, versican synthesis increases, as does production of biglycan and decorin (Lyons et al. 1981; Buckwalter 1995; Inkinen et al. 1998; Le Maitre et al. 2007d). In contrast, there is increased degradation of aggrecan and versican fragmentation thereby reducing disc overall proteoglycans content. Several versican isoforms have been identified in the disc with varying molecular weights (Sztrolovics et al. 2002). However, one of the key features of all isoforms is that they contain fewer chondroitin sulphate side chains than aggrecan and hence have a lower negative charge which reduces the osmotic potential of versican-containing aggregates. Therefore, the overall loss of aggrecan, combined with the shift to versican production, reduces the water content in the disc, and the shift in collagen production to collagen I results in a more fibrous tissue, less capable of withstanding load.

There are other changes evident in the disc, caused either as a result of degeneration or as an attempt at repair. One example is the increase in fibronectin and importantly fibronectin fragments during degeneration (Oegema et al. 2000). Fibronectin is a large extracellular glycoprotein that contains binding sites for several cell membrane and matrix proteins, including integrins and collagens, respectively, and is thought to play a role in extracellular matrix organisation. Its expression increases in degeneration, although there is also an increase in fibronectin fragments which have been demonstrated in vitro to stimulate matrix metalloprotein

(MMP) production and suppress aggrecan synthesis (Anderson et al. 2005; Aota et al. 2005) and in vivo to stimulate disc degeneration (Greg et al. 2003). One mechanism for this change may be the stimulation of catabolic cytokine expression, which has been demonstrated to occur following the addition of fibronectin fragments to cartilage explants in vitro (Homandberg et al. 1997).

11.3.4 Matrix Degradation

A range of proteolytic enzymes are responsible for breakdown of the extracellular matrix, including members of the MMP and 'a disintegrin and metalloproteinase with thrombospondin motifs' (ADAMTS) families (for details of these enzymes, see Chap. 8). MMPs are capable of cleaving the majority of constituents of the disc extracellular matrix. Most notably, MMPs 1, 8 and 13 degrade intact triple-helical collagens including collagens I and II, while 2 and 9 are gelatinases cleaving partially degraded triple-helical domains (Nagase and Woessner 1999).

MMPs 1, 2, 3, 7, 8, 9, 10, 13, 19 and 28 have all been identified within the disc, with levels of many increasing during degeneration (Roberts et al. 2000; Weiler et al. 2002; Le Maitre et al. 2004, 2006b; Gruber et al. 2005; Richardson et al. 2009; Bachmeier et al. 2009; Klawitter et al. 2011). In particular, the number of cells immunopositive for MMPs 1, 3, 7 and 13 was shown to be increased in degeneration (Le Maitre et al. 2004, 2006b). We have also demonstrated a significant increase in the expression of MMP-10 in symptomatic (painful) degenerate discs and shown a correlation between expression of MMP-10 and IL-1 and NGF, but not TNF-α, suggesting a possible role for MMP-10 in the initiation of nociception during degeneration (Richardson et al. 2009). MMP-10 is also capable of activating proMMPs, including MMPs 1, 7, 8, 9 and 13, and has been shown to be capable of 'superactivating' proMMPs 1, 8 and 13, giving them a higher-than-normal specific activity and potentially shifting the homeostatic balance of activity towards catabolism (Barksby et al. 2006).

In addition to their activity against collagens, members of the MMP family also have the ability to degrade aggrecan at discrete sites within the G1-G2 and G2-G3 interglobular domains, although their activity against this substrate is significantly lower than that of the aggrecanase members of the ADAMTS family. The ADAMTS family includes the aggrecanases ADAMTSs 1, 4, 5, 8, 9 and 15, which are all capable of degrading aggrecan at sites distinct from those of the MMPs and at an activity substantially higher than that of the MMPs (Tortorella et al. 1999; Abbaszade et al. 1999; Cal et al. 2002; Nagase and Kashiwagi 2003; Somerville et al. 2003; Collins-Racie et al. 2004). An increase in aggrecanase-generated aggrecan fragments has been identified in both aged and diseased discs, with a correlation being shown between increasing grade of degeneration and an increase in the presence of aggrecanase-generated fragments (Sztrolovics et al. 1997; Roberts et al. 2000). Studies initially identified ADAMTS 4 (aggrecanase 1) in the disc (Le Maitre et al. 2004; Hatano et al. 2006), with a correlation noted between ADAMTS 4, but not ADAMTS 5 (aggrecanase 2), expression with degeneration (Patel et al. 2007). Subsequently, we have shown that the expression of ADAMTSs 1, 4, 5, 9 and 15 are all increased with intervertebral disc degeneration (Pockert et al. 2009), with their expression potentially being regulated by IL-1β (Demircan et al. 2005). Building on this finding, in vitro stimulation experiments demonstrated increased expression of both ADAMTSs 4 and 5 following IL-1β stimulation, with nitric oxide being the mediating factor (Le Maitre et al. 2005a; Zhao et al. 2011). More recently, ADAMTSs 7 and 12, enzymes which are capable of degrading cartilage oligomeric matrix protein (COMP), were both shown to be upregulated in a rat model of degeneration; however, their presence in human discs or role in degeneration is yet to be elucidated (Yu and Zhu 2012).

Those molecules discussed above, along with a broad spectrum of other proteolytic enzymes including cathepsins D, G, K and L (Konttinen et al. 1999; Ariga et al. 2001), are responsible for the homeostatic turnover of disc extracellular matrix. Their expression and activity are closely controlled by soluble mediators, such as catabolic (pro-inflammatory) cytokines and anabolic growth factors, and through blocking cognate inhibitors, the tissue inhibitors of metalloproteinases (TIMPs). The TIMP family consists of four members (TIMPs 1, 2, 3 and 4) which play various roles, including MMP activation and inhibition and induction of angiogenesis (Brew et al. 2000). However, their main role is the inhibition of MMPs and ADAMTSs, which is achieved primarily through irreversible non-covalent coupling to active MMPs in a 1:1 stoichiometric fashion (Cooper et al. 1985; Stetler-Stevenson et al. 1989). TIMPs 1, 2 and 3 have been identified in the disc, with TIMPs 1 and 2 exhibiting broad specificity of inhibition of members of the MMP family, while TIMP 3 appears to selectively inhibit aggrecanases (Kashiwagi et al. 2001). Both TIMP 1 and 2 are upregulated in degeneration (Le Maitre et al. 2004), although they have higher specificity for certain MMPs than others, suggesting those MMPs (e.g. MMP 7) that are resistant to TIMP inhibition may play a greater role in degeneration (Le Maitre et al. 2006b). Conversely, while TIMP 3 expression levels in nondegenerate human nucleus pulposus cells have been shown to be higher than that of any of the ADAMTSs (Pockert et al. 2009), its expression does not change in degeneration (Le Maitre et al. 2004; Pockert et al. 2009), suggesting a potential imbalance between active ADAMTSs and TIMP 3 that could lead to the matrix, particularly aggrecan, degradation, a characteristic of the degenerate disc.

11.4 Vascular and Nerve Ingrowth

At birth, both the end plates and annulus fibrosus possess blood vessels, although these soon recede, meaning that, with the exception of the external lamellae of the annulus, the normal adult intervertebral disc is both avascular and aneural (Yasuma et al. 1993; Repanti et al. 1998; Roughley 2004; Roberts et al. 2006b). However, during degeneration, both neovascularisation and innervation occur, with blood vessels and nerve fibres infiltrating the annulus fibrosus and eventually the nucleus pulposus (Freemont et al. 1997, 2002; Coppes et al. 1997; Nerlich et al. 2007). Matrix alterations, particularly vascular ingrowth, and increasing angiogenesis have been correlated with decreasing proteoglycan content in an ovine annular lesion model (Melrose et al. 2002a). Indeed, aggrecan has been shown to be inhibitory to endothelial cell adhesion and migration in a concentration-dependant manner (Johnson et al. 2005), a finding that provides a possible mechanism for accelerating the degenerative process. Extensive capillary networks have also been found to be associated with annular clefts and tears (Nerlich et al. 2007), suggesting the breakdown of the normal disc extracellular matrix is permissive for neovascularisation. However, the mechanisms or the factors underlying initiation of angiogenesis have not yet been clearly elucidated. Pleiotrophin, a growth factor reported to be involved in cell migration and differentiation in various cellular processes, has been implicated as an angiogenic factor in the disc as it has been shown that the frequency of pleiotrophin-positive disc cells was significantly correlated with the amount of vascularisation (Johnson et al. 2007). Additionally, other angiogenic factors have also been implicated including vascular endothelial growth factor (VEGF) (Ohba et al. 2009), basic fibroblast growth factor (FGF-2), TGF-β and osteonectin (Melrose et al. 2002b). More recently, it has also been suggested that IL-1β is capable of inducing angiogenesis through stimulation of the growth factors VEGF, NGF and BDNF, although these results were based on immunohistochemical correlation studies rather than direct stimulation with IL-1β (Lee et al. 2011). While the mechanisms underlying vascular ingrowth are still unclear, neovascularisation is thought to provide a route for various cytokines and growth factors to reach the inner disc regions at an accelerated rate than through the usual route of diffusion (Nerlich et al. 2007), which may be one of the driving forces behind the increased nucleus pulposus cell-derived degradative enzyme production and accelerated proteoglycan loss in the inner annulus fibrosus and nucleus pulposus.

During degeneration, there is also an increase in nerve fibres both physically associated with, and distant from, infiltrating blood vessels. In the majority of these cases, nerve fibres are found alongside blood vessels, and during angiogenesis, endothelial cells from infiltrating vessels secrete NGF. Since nerves possess the high-affinity NGF receptor TrkA, it is likely that there is a vasoregulatory role for the nerve fibres (Freemont et al. 2002). These nerve fibres have been shown to be positive for protein gene product 9.5 (PGP9.5), acetylcholinesterase, neurofilament protein (NFP), substance P (SP) and calcitonin gene-related peptide (CGRP), amongst other proteins. On this basis, it has been suggested that these nerve fibres originate from the dorsal root ganglion (Ashton et al. 1994; Brown et al. 1997; Ohtori et al. 2002; Takahashi et al. 2009; Garcia-Cosamalon et al. 2010) and are nociceptive. Studies on degenerate intervertebral disc tissues have demonstrated a similar protein expression profile for nerves infiltrating the inner annulus fibrosus and nucleus pulposus, suggesting a quantitative increase in nociceptive neurite number, rather than a change in type of neurite (Ashton et al. 1994; Freemont et al. 1997; Brown et al. 1997; Johnson et al. 2002; Melrose et al. 2002a; Takahashi et al. 2009). On the other hand, there is evidence that suggests there is an increase in sympathetic afferents in degenerate tissue, which are hypothesised to play a significant role in low back pain (Takebayashi et al. 2006). In vitro studies demonstrated a concentration-dependant inhibition in nerve fibre outgrowth by human aggrecan, suggesting the decreases in proteoglycans content in the disc during degeneration may permit neural ingrowth (Johnson et al. 2002). The same study also indicates that deglycosylation of aggrecan may also be important as enzymatic removal of keratan and chondroitin sulphate from aggrecan abrogated the inhibitory effect of intact aggrecan. As the effect was greater following chondroitinase ABC than keratanase treatment, it was inferred that there was a greater role for chondroitin sulphate than keratan sulphate in inhibiting nerve outgrowth. Since there is an increase in the ratio of keratin sulphate/chondroitin sulphate, the authors also hypothesised that this change may also be important in terms of allowing nerve infiltration into the disc.

Importantly, however, a complex interplay between catabolic cytokines, neurotrophins, neurotrophin receptors and chemorepellant molecules may be responsible for guiding nerve ingrowth during degeneration, in particular semaphorins, a large family of secreted and membrane-bound axonal guidance molecules (Kolodkin et al. 1993). Gene and protein expression studies of the class 3 semaphorin family member Sema3A, which can cause axonal collapse when found in high concentrations, identified high levels of cell immunopositivity in the outer annulus fibrosus of normal tissue (Tolofari et al. 2010). The percentage of semaphorin-positive cells was found to decrease with increasing grades of degeneration, particularly in individuals with symptomatic (painful) degeneration, suggesting an important role for Sema3A in inhibiting nerve ingrowth into normal disc tissue.

Both nucleus pulposus and annulus fibrosus cells from normal discs have been shown to express low levels of the neurotrophin nerve growth factor (NGF) and brain-derived neurotrophic factor (BDNF), and expression levels increase in degeneration, particularly in individuals with symptomatic (painful) disc degeneration (Abe et al. 2007; Purmessur et al. 2008; Gruber et al. 2008). Interestingly, these disc cells also express the high-affinity NGF receptor TrkA, the high-affinity BDNF receptor TrkB and the low-affinity NGF/BDNF receptor $p75^{NTR}$, as well as SP, suggesting possible autocrine signalling by the disc cells themselves (Purmessur et al. 2008). However, the predominant role for NGF and BDNF may be to act in a paracrine manner on dorsal root ganglion neurons to stimulate nerve ingrowth. We have recently demonstrated that coculture of human nucleus pulposus cells, derived from the degenerate intervertebral disc, with the neural cell line SH-SY5Y cells caused an increase in both percentage of neurite-expressing cells and mean neurite length (Richardson et al. 2011). This finding supports earlier work by Johnson and colleagues who showed that normal inhibition of neurite outgrowth by aggrecan could be prevented by cells derived from degenerate disc, suggesting that such cells release neurotrophins (Johnson et al. 2006). Indeed, our own studies show that these increases in neurite-expressing cells and neurite length could be inhibited by the addition of anti-BDNF antibodies. In contrast, when inhibition was activated by anti-NGF antibodies, there was only a decrease in the percentage number of neurite-expressing cells (Richardson et al. 2011).

Interestingly, both NGF and BDNF expression can be stimulated by addition of recombinant IL-1β and TNF-α (cytokines shown to be increased in intervertebral disc degeneration) to cultured human nucleus pulposus cells in vitro, while TNF-α stimulation also induces expression of substance P (Purmessur et al. 2008). Such in vitro results suggest that these pro-inflammatory cytokines stimulate the production of neurotrophins which promotes the growth of sensory nerve fibres into the intervertebral disc and induce substance P related with pain transmission. Noteworthy, signalling of NGF and BDNF through their receptors initiates activation of a number of pathways, including the NF-κB pathway; activation induces a range of pro-inflammatory cytokines which may then perpetuate the cycle leading to innervation (Wallach et al. 2002). The expression of NGF also correlates with expression of specific MMPs (Richardson et al. 2009), suggesting a potential role for neurotrophins in driving matrix catabolism, possibly to ease nerve ingrowth through the disc. Importantly, this interaction between cytokines and neurotrophins is complex and requires further extensive study before a clear pathway can be elucidated. Unfortunately, however, this is hindered by the inability to study nerve ingrowth in humans and the potential differences between humans and the model animal systems routinely used in disc degeneration research.

11.5 Alterations in Disc Cell Biology in Degeneration

A wide range of factors are thought to be involved in the initiation and progression of degeneration (Fig. 11.1). While individuals may experience discogenic back pain for different reasons, correlation studies and detailed molecular and cellular biology studies suggest that there are four main categories of factors influencing cell function and hence drive intervertebral disc degeneration. These include soluble regulators of disc cell function (mainly cytokines and growth factors), nutritional status, cell ageing and death and response to mechanical load.

11.5.1 Soluble Regulators of Cellular Function

During degeneration, a range of pro-inflammatory cytokines and inflammatory mediators are increased. These include members of the interleukin family, including IL-1, IL-2, IL-6, IL-12 and IL-17, as well as interferon gamma (IFN-γ), TNF-α and the inflammatory mediators prostaglandin E2 (PGE2) and nitric oxide (NOx) (Kang et al. 1996; Olmarker and Larsson 1998; Le Maitre et al. 2005a, 2007b; Bachmeier et al. 2007; Akyol et al. 2010; Gabr et al. 2011; Studer et al. 2011). The pro-inflammatory cytokines are all thought to play independent roles in matrix catabolism, although interplays between the molecules have been identified. For example, IL-6 is thought to potentiate the response of nucleus pulposus cells to both IL-1 and TNF-α (Studer et al. 2011), while IL-17 synergises with both TNF-α and IFN-γ, increasing the catabolic activities of human nucleus pulposus and annulus fibrosus cells and possibly serving as a key regulator of inflammation in the degenerating disc (Gabr et al. 2011).

However, although there is evidence for the involvement of multiple pro-inflammatory cytokines in the pathogenesis of disc degeneration, the predominant catabolic cytokines appear to be interleukin-1 (IL-1) and tumour necrosis factor-alpha (TNF-α). While there is no clear consensus on which molecule mediates degeneration, research suggests both are fundamentally important in controlling the observed cellular and matrix changes.

11.5.1.1 Interleukin-1

Both isoforms of IL-1 (IL-1α and IL-1β) have been identified within the disc, along with their receptor (IL-1R1), the exported decoy receptor (IL-1RII) and their natural inhibitor (IL-1 receptor antagonist or IL-1Ra) (Le Maitre et al. 2005a). During degeneration, expression of IL-1α and β and IL1RI increases significantly in both the nucleus pulposus and inner annulus fibrosus. However, IL-1Ra expression does not increase and this imbalance leads to an excess of IL-1 isoforms in degenerate tissues. Importantly, in vitro studies have

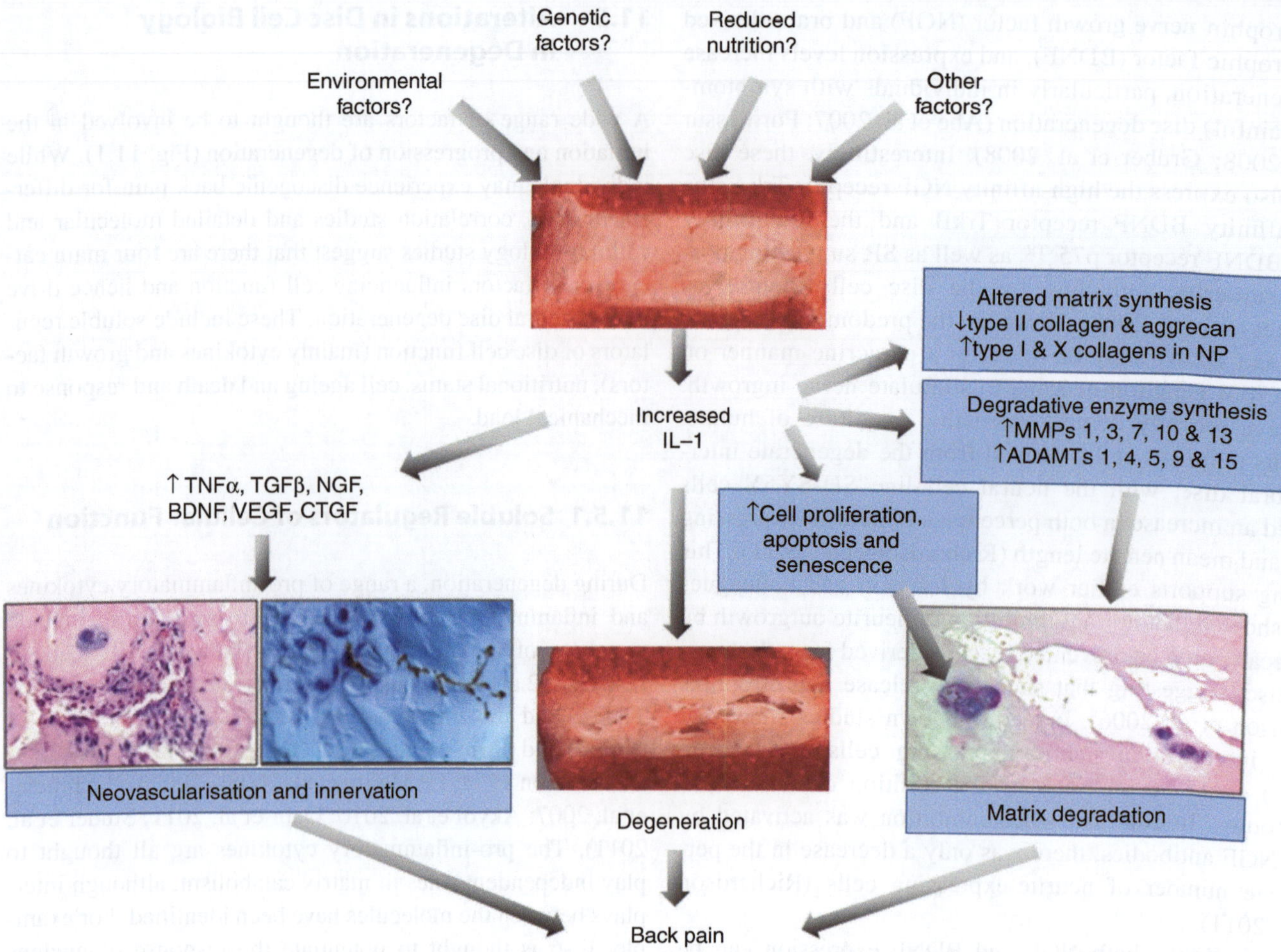

Fig. 11.1 A schematic overview of the pathogenesis of intervertebral disc degeneration demonstrating the involvement of IL-1 in driving the aberrant cell biology and processes involved in matrix catabolism and generation of back pain

shown that IL-1 induces a number of cellular and molecular changes associated with disc degeneration. Stimulation of human nucleus pulposus cells with recombinant IL-1 has been shown to induce an upregulation of both MMPs, including MMPs 3 and 13, and ADAMTSs, including ADAMTS 4, a shift in collagen expression from II to I and reduction in aggrecan expression (Le Maitre et al. 2005a). There appear to be differences in the responses of normal and degenerate disc cells to IL-1 stimulation, with a more catabolic response in degenerate nucleus pulposus cells compared to normal. IL-1 stimulation also resulted in significant increases in both IL-1 isoforms by degenerate nucleus pulposus cells and a decrease in expression by normal nucleus pulposus cells, suggesting a homeostatic response in nondegenerate cells and an aberrant catabolic response once degeneration has been activated. IL-1 has also been shown to induce both angiogenesis (by inducing expression of VEGF) and neuronogenesis (via the stimulation of neurotrophic factors) into disc tissue (Lee et al. 2011) and stimulation of apoptosis (Cui et al. 2007; Zhao et al. 2007a). Conversely an inhibition or reversal of these processes has been demonstrated through the addition of exogenous IL-1Ra, and application of IL-1Ra has been proposed as a potential therapeutic intervention to inhibit intervertebral disc degeneration (Le Maitre et al. 2006a, 2007c; Box 11.1).

Box 11.1: Interleukin-1 as the Driving Force Behind the Pathogenesis of Disc Degeneration

While for some TNF-α has been the focus of investigation as the molecular regulator of disc degeneration, our research has focussed on the involvement of IL-1. These studies have demonstrated an increase in the expression of both isoforms (α and β) of IL-1, along with its receptor (IL-1RI) during degeneration. However, no such increase was demonstrated for its natural inhibitor, IL-1Ra, suggesting an imbalance that may be responsible for driving the cellular and matrix changes evident during degeneration. These roles include inducing expression of both MMPs and ADAMTSs, which are known to catabolise the extracellular matrix; reducing matrix component molecule expression, most notably aggrecan; inducing apoptosis and senescence of disc cells; and inducing both angiogenesis and innervation into the disc. However, the key question at present is: what initiates the upregulation of IL-1 that then induces the degenerative cascade? Elucidation of this mechanism may lead to the development of novel therapies or allow disc degeneration to be prevented.

11.5.1.2 TNF-α

TNF-α, like IL-1, has been shown to be capable of inducing neural ingrowths into the degenerate intervertebral disc. TNF-α has also been implicated in causing nerve root damage and sciatic pain, with blocking studies supporting this theory (Igarashi et al. 2000; Olmarker and Rydevik 2001). While evidence for a role for TNF-α in nerve ingrowth is compelling, evidence supporting its role in driving matrix catabolism during degeneration is less clear. Although expression of TNF-α is increased in degenerate tissues (Weiler et al. 2005; Bachmeier et al. 2007), other studies have either failed to identify TNF receptor I in degenerate samples or shown that there is no increase in the receptor gene expression in degenerate samples. The result suggests that native disc cells in vivo may not be able to respond to TNF-α (Le Maitre et al. 2007b). However, in studies where recombinant TNF-α was used to stimulate cultured nucleus pulposus cells, there were increases in expression of MMPs 1, 3, 9 and 13, as well as ADAMTSs 4 and 5, although induction of expression of a number of these enzymes was greater following stimulation with IL-1 than with TNF-α (Hoyland et al. 2008). Conversely, in situ zymography studies of normal and degenerate human nucleus pulposus tissue treated with either IL-1 or TNF-α indicated there was only an increase in enzyme activity in the IL-1 group and not the TNF-α group. In this study, addition of IL-1Ra caused a decrease in enzyme activity that was not evident following addition of anti-TNF. While demonstrating an increase in TNF-α in degeneration, the documented low expression of its receptor on disc cells together with differences in findings from the other studies begs the question: what is the target of nucleus pulposus cell secreted TNF-α? Does it play a more fundamental role in innervation and development of discogenic pain, than in matrix catabolism and tissue breakdown?

11.5.1.3 Anabolic Growth Factors

Growth factors have a number of effects on cells, most notably the shift in metabolic balance towards anabolism, promotion of cell proliferation and prevention of cell death. A range of growth factors, including many members of the TGF-β superfamily, are known to be present in the normal intervertebral disc, while evidence for their involvement in disease comes from both in vitro cell stimulation studies and studies of in vivo models of disc degeneration. Many workers have focussed on the ability of growth factors to stimulate proteoglycans synthesis by nucleus pulposus and annulus fibrosus cells and shown positive results following stimulation with transforming growth factor-β (TGF-β), epidermal growth factor (EGF), insulin-like growth factor-1 (IGF-1), connective tissue growth factor (CTGF) and the bone morphogenetic proteins (BMPs) 2, 7 (also known as osteogenic protein-1 or OP-1), 12, 13 (also known as growth and differentiation factor 6 (GDF-6) or cartilage-derived morphogenetic protein-2 (CDMP-2)) and 14 (also known as growth and differentiation factor 5 (GDF-5) or cartilage-derived morphogenetic protein-1 (CDMP-1)) either alone or in combination (Thompson et al. 1991; Osada et al. 1996; Gruber et al. 1997; Masuda et al. 2003; Tim et al. 2003; Imai et al. 2007a; Gilbertson et al. 2008; Le Maitre et al. 2009). Cell proliferation has also been demonstrated in vitro following stimulation with TGF-β and IGF-1, while the same growth factors and platelet-derived growth factor (PDGF) are all capable of reducing disc cell apoptosis and secretion of catabolic cytokines (Gruber et al. 1997, 2000).

In vivo studies also show positive effects of TGF-β, IGF-1, BMPs 2 and 5, fibroblast growth factor-2 (FGF-2) and OP-1 on cell proliferation, matrix synthesis and restoration of disc height in models of disc degeneration (Walsh et al. 2004; An et al. 2005; Masuda et al. 2006; Miyamoto et al. 2006). Of these, the most widely studied is OP-1, with positive effects noted both in vitro and in vivo. Indeed, OP-1 was capable of stimulating proteoglycans and collagen synthesis by human nucleus pulposus cells following IL-1 and chondroitinase ABC treatment in vitro (Takegami et al. 2005; Imai et al. 2007a) and restoring disc height and matrix degradation caused by annular needle injury or chemonucleolysis with chondroitinase ABC (Miyamoto et al. 2006; Imai et al. 2007b). OP-1 also reduced the production of aggrecanase, MMP-13, substance P, TNF-α and IL-1β, suggesting that it may have both anabolic and anti-catabolic effects (Chubinskaya et al. 2007). The effect of OP-1 on substance P expression, combined with the interplay between catabolic cytokines and pain markers or pain modulators, has led to the hypothesis that application of recombinant growth factors may have beneficial effects in terms of pain reduction, as well as matrix restoration during degeneration (Kawakami et al. 2005). However, the clinical translation of growth factor therapies is complicated by their diverse and sometimes biphasic roles. While growth factors such as TGF-β and CTGF are known to promote extracellular matrix synthesis, studies on clinical human samples have linked their overexpression to fibrosis and angiogenesis (Ali et al. 2008; Peng et al. 2009). The application of growth factor therapies is further complicated by possible changes in receptor distribution. While data in this area is limited, studies suggest that there is no change in the expression levels of major growth factor receptors, including TGFβRII, BMPRII, FGFR3 and IGFRI (Le Maitre et al. 2005b; Peng et al. 2006). However, expression of growth factor receptors, including TGFRII, FGFR3, IGFRI and VEGF receptors I and II, on ingrowing blood vessels (Haro et al. 2002; Le Maitre et al. 2005b) and in granulation tissue in painful degenerate discs (Peng et al. 2006) suggests that the use of growth factors should carefully be controlled to avoid stimulation of unwanted events such as angiogenesis. Therefore, a more detailed understanding of their expression profiles and roles in both disc degeneration and repair are currently required.

Another area where growth factors show potential is in the stimulation of adult mesenchymal stem cell (MSC) differentiation. Previous studies have shown that TGF-β, along with members of the BMP family, most notably BMPs 2 and 14, can stimulate MSC differentiation towards nucleus pulposus-like cells in vitro (Stoyanov et al. 2011; McCanless et al. 2011). Given the increasing information on the nucleus pulposus phenotype, further studies will no doubt shed light on the role that growth factors play in MSC differentiation and may lead to combined regenerative cell/growth factor therapies for treatment of disc degeneration.

11.6 Changes in Disc Nutrition and Oxygen Tension

As mentioned previously, nutrient supply to the disc is predominantly from blood vessels in the vertebral bodies and occurs via diffusion through the cartilaginous end plates. This theory has been well studied and confirmed using a range of tracer diffusion experiments, including MRI contrast media, fluorescent and radioactive tracers and gaseous tracers such as nitrous oxide (Brodin 1955; Holm and Nachemson 1982, 1983; Adams and Hutton 1986; Urban et al. 2001). Exposure to cigarette smoke has also been shown to inhibit transport of oxygen into, and lactic acid out of, the disc in animal experiments due to constriction of the microvasculature in the vertebrae (Holm and Nachemson 1988); this finding supports epidemiological evidence linking smoking to disc degeneration in humans. The size and charge of solutes also affect their penetration into the disc, with anions showing lower rates of diffusion than cations due to the polyanionic nature of the disc (Urban et al. 2004), while larger molecules such as albumin are effectively prevented from diffusing through the cartilaginous end plate (Urban et al. 2004). Compared to uni- or bivalent electrolytes, and the fact that glucose is a relatively large molecule, Urban et al. opined that diffusion into and through the disc may be slow (Urban et al. 2004). This lack of nutrient supply to the core of the nucleus pulposus is reflected in the non-uniform cell distribution throughout the disc: cell number in the outer annulus (which is closer to capillaries surrounding the tissue) is substantially higher than that of the nucleus which can be as far as 8 mm from the nearest capillary.

With age, the nutrient supply to the disc is reduced in part due to reductions in both the density and integrity of capillaries in the vertebral bodies and in part due to calcification of the cartilaginous end plates (Bernick and Cailliet 1982; Roberts et al. 1996). While it is currently unclear whether cartilaginous end-plate calcification is causative of, or the result of, disc degeneration, it is thought to play an important role in disease progression by posing a significant barrier to diffusion of solutes into and out of the disc. However, recent μCT studies on graded normal and degenerate human samples have suggested that, contrary to popular belief, porosity in vertebral end plates increases in degeneration by as much as 130 %, while trabecular thickness decreases by as much as 50 % (Rodriguez et al. 2011, 2012). One result of these changes appeared to be an increase in cell proliferation and decrease in proteoglycan content in the nucleus pulposus. While solute transport was not assessed in this study, the authors proposed that ischemic cell changes in degeneration may reflect capillary transport activity rather than a decrease in end-plate permeability.

Whatever its cause, a reduction in essential nutrients is thought to drive the progression of degeneration. Given that the main energy-generating pathway in disc cells, even in the presence of oxygen, is glycolysis (Holm et al. 1981; Ishihara and Urban 1999), which requires principally glucose and produces lactic acid, free diffusion of solutes to and from the cells is essential. Evidence suggests that reduction in glucose concentration below 0.5 mmol/L, even for a relatively short period, can cause cell death. Likewise, reduction in the pH to below 6.4 can also promote death (Horner and Urban 2001; Bibby and Urban 2004), while less severe reductions in pH can impact cell metabolism (Ohshima and Urban 1992). Evidence from a range of assays, including biochemical assays and microelectrode measurements, shows that this drop in glucose concentration and pH is similar to that observed in degenerate discs. Therefore, while cell activity and even viability may be impaired by a decrease in nutrient supply, enzyme activity is not reduced. In this case, there would be an imbalance between matrix anabolism and catabolism which may contribute to an elevation in matrix degradation in degenerate discs.

The other key metabolite in the disc is oxygen, although its role is less clear than that of glucose. Oxygen levels vary widely in human discs, with no clear correlation between a change in oxygen tension and disc degeneration. However, there exists a steep oxygen gradient within discs – studies in dogs demonstrating a decrease from 8 to 10 % O_2 at the disc-vertebral body interface to 0.3–0.5 % in the centre of the nucleus pulposus (Holm et al. 1981). Human discs show similar trends, with readings as low as 0.7 % O_2 in the core of the degenerate human nucleus (Bartels et al. 1998). While oxygen is consumed by disc cells, relatively little CO_2 is produced and disc cells can survive for at least 2 weeks without oxygen (Horner and Urban 2001), suggesting oxidative phosphorylation is not the primary mechanism for energy metabolism. Further studies on both canine and bovine disc cells demonstrated that as O_2 concentration decreases from 21 to 1 %, there was a decrease in oxygen consumption of around 75 % and a sharp increase in lactate production (Ishihara and Urban 1999). This suggests a positive Pasteur effect since glycolysis is stimulated under hypoxic conditions. However, studies on the effect of hypoxia on disc cells have also demonstrated cellular inactivity (Horner and Urban 2001) and a loss of matrix synthesis (Ishihara and Urban 1999) below an oxygen concentration of around 5 %. As the increase in lactate production under hypoxic conditions is likely to reduce the pH, this in turn would reduce matrix synthesis (Ohshima and Urban 1992) and eventually cause cell death (Horner and Urban 2001; Bibby and Urban 2004). Hence, the effects of low oxygen and low pH are likely to be cumulative and a destructive influence of disc cell survival. The mechanism by which cells sense oxygen and accommodate to the oxemic state is discussed in exhaustive detail in Chap. 6.

Confounding the problem of evaluating the consequences of oxygen and nutrient limitation is the fact that human tissues are different from those of animal models. Therefore, investigators have increasingly turned to mathematical finite element modelling to elucidate the effect of nutrient limitation on the disc microenvironment and cellular metabolism. However, since all of the variables involved in disc nutrition are poorly understood, the studies published in this area are relatively simple, dealing with only one or two aspects of nutrient supply. Nevertheless, they all suggest that limited nutrient supply affects disc cell viability and metabolic activity (Selard et al. 2003; Yao and Gu 2006; Mokhbi et al. 2009; Malandrino et al. 2011; Jackson et al. 2011).

As with findings from finite element modelling, in vitro studies appear to confirm that during degeneration, glucose limitation and decrease in pH are the predominant factors affecting cell metabolism. While nucleus pulposus cells have mechanisms to regulate intracellular pH, such as the expression of the carbonic anhydrases 9 and 12 (Minogue et al. 2010a), our preliminary data indicates that the expression of these molecules decreases with degeneration, suggesting that cells may not be capable of withstanding the low pH over extended periods (Fig. 11.2). Likewise, changes in the nucleus pulposus membrane glucose transporters (GLUTs), present in degenerative tissues, suggest that there are molecular adaptations to compensate for the reduced glucose concentrations (Richardson et al. 2008b). However, the harsh environment of the degenerate disc is likely to be detrimental not just to resident cells but also to cells that are introduced into the disc. Accordingly, for future cell-based therapies, the introduction of too many cells, or cells which are unable to withstand the conditions of the microenvironmental niche, may exacerbate the degenerative problem rather than provide a cure.

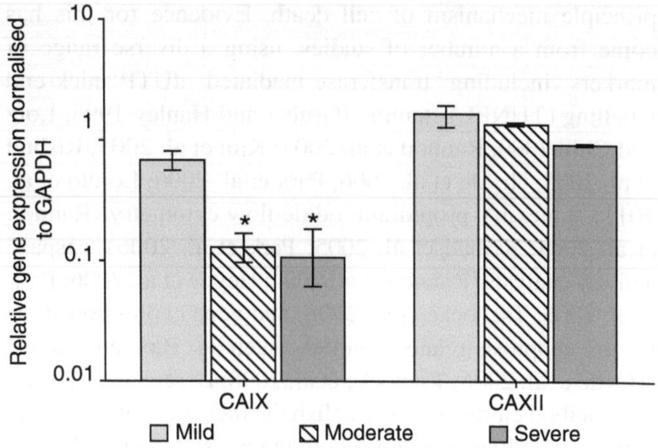

Fig. 11.2 Histogram illustrating real-time quantitative PCR data demonstrating a decrease in expression of carbonic anhydrase 9 (CAIX) and 12 (CAXII) in nucleus pulposus cells during disc degeneration. The expression of CAIX is significantly decreased with disease progression, while a decrease is also seen for CAXII. The carbonic anhydrases play a role in regulating intracellular pH, and a downregulation in their expression may result in cells being incapable of withstanding the harsh physicochemical environment of the degenerate intervertebral disc

11.7 Cell Ageing and Death

During development, the nucleus pulposus is populated by large, vacuolated, metabolically active and morphologically distinct notochordal cells which produce high levels of proteoglycans (Boos et al. 2002; Cappello et al. 2006). However, by the age of 10, this population has been replaced by smaller, chondrocyte-like nucleus pulposus cells which are less metabolically active (Wolfe et al. 1965; Pazzaglia et al. 1989; Boos et al. 2002; Guehring et al. 2008). The period between 3 and 10 years of age, during which identifiable notochordal cells disappear, is also the time during which there is a high level of cell death (Boos et al. 2002). These changes appear to signal the initiation of a transition from a highly hydrated, gelatinous extracellular matrix to a more fibrous, cartilaginous nucleus pulposus seen in adults. It also coincides with the earliest identifiable signs of degeneration seen in MRI studies. In addition, histological studies have identified matrix changes in this age group, which progress throughout adult life (Boos et al. 2002). Although these changes may be considered to be part of the normal ageing process, as discussed previously, the accelerated matrix degradation suggests that in disc degeneration, there is premature ageing.

Several studies have identified necrotic cells within the disc which increase both with age and degeneration; however, more recently, apoptosis has been identified as the principle mechanism of cell death. Evidence for this has come from a number of studies, using a diverse range of markers including transferase-mediated dUTP nick-end labelling (TUNEL) staining (Gruber and Hanley 1998; Lotz and Chin 2000; Rannou et al. 2004; Kim et al. 2005; Risbud et al. 2005; Heyde et al. 2006; Park et al. 2006; Loreto et al. 2011), annexinV-propidium iodide flow cytometry (Rannou et al. 2004; Risbud et al. 2005; Park et al. 2006), caspase activity analysis (Rannou et al. 2004; Heyde et al. 2006; Park et al. 2006; Tschoeke et al. 2008) and gene expression studies of apoptosis-related markers such as Bax and Bcl-2 (Heyde et al. 2006; Tschoeke et al. 2008; Loreto et al. 2011). The method employed to establish the incidence of apoptosis appears to influence findings both in vivo and in vitro. Serum deprivation resulted in only 1 % cell apoptosis when studied using TUNEL staining (Gruber et al. 2000); in contrast, similar conditions increased in the incidence of apoptosis in rat annulus fibrosus cells to 56 % when annexinV-propidium iodide flow cytometry was used (Risbud et al. 2005). Other studies have also suggested that incidence of apoptosis in disc cells can be as high as 73–74 % (Gruber and Hanley 1998; Ha et al. 2006), although this would be an overestimate since it would result in the de-cellularisation of the disc within days (Alvarez and Ortiz 1999). Conversely, studies using fluorescent cell viability assays on fresh disc tissue have repeatedly demonstrated 60 % to over 90 % cell viability even in degenerate and scoliotic discs, further suggesting that the apoptosis measurements are an overestimation (Bibby et al. 2002; Johnson and Roberts 2007). However, while no causative link has been found between apoptosis and increased extracellular matrix degradation, it is probable that programmed cell death plays an essential role in the pathogenesis of disc disease.

Autophagy, a pathway that may lead to programmed cell death, has recently been identified in the rat nucleus pulposus (Ye et al. 2011) and annulus fibrosus (Shen et al. 2011). We have also demonstrated evidence of autophagy in tissues of the degenerate human intervertebral disc, through immunostaining for the key markers LC-3 and beclin-1 (Fig. 11.3). While autophagy can lead to cell death, it can also maintain cell viability during periods of environmental or nutritional stress by catabolism of intracellular

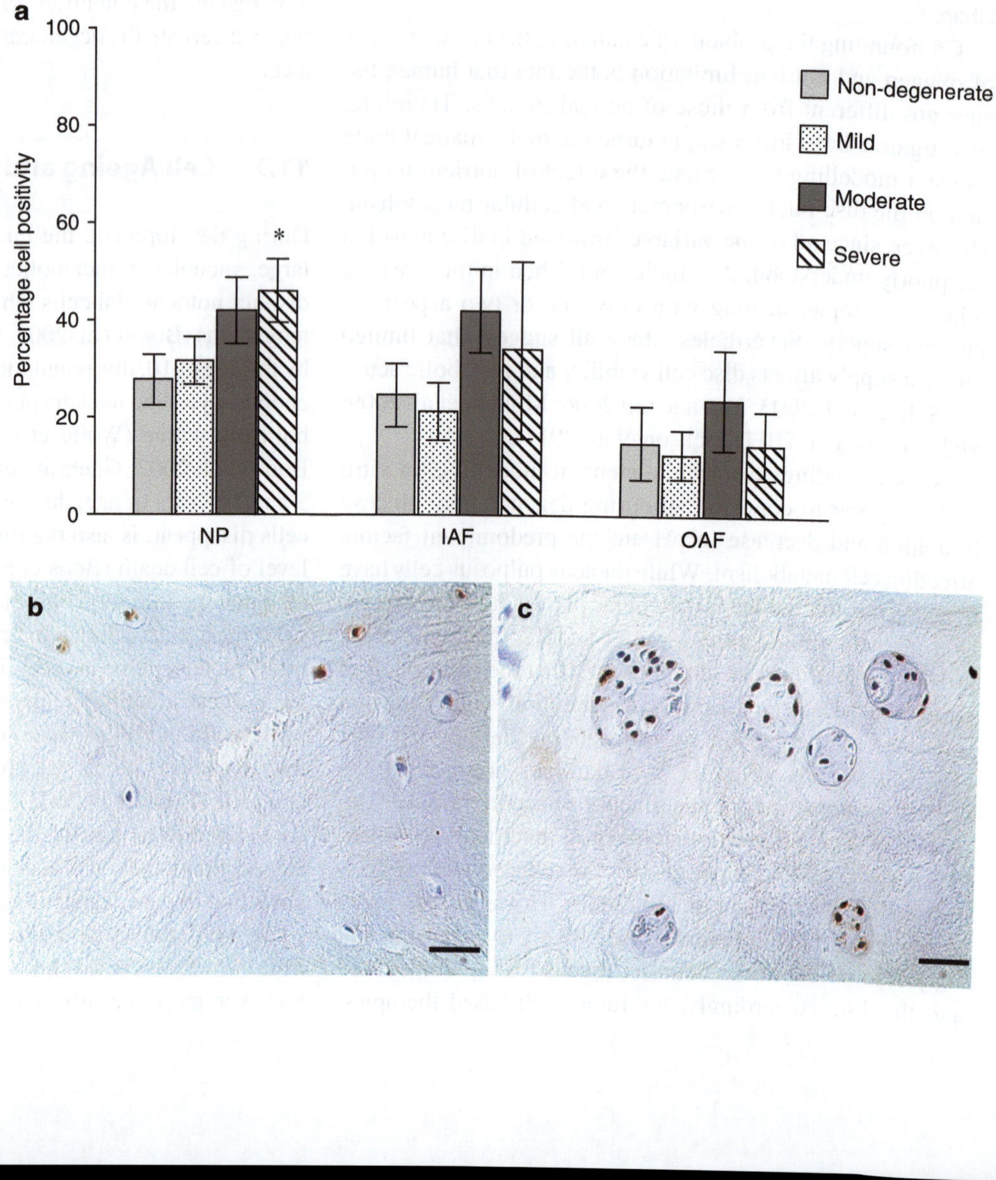

Fig. 11.3 Evidence for the presence of autophagy markers in normal and degenerate human IVD cells. Immunohistochemistry for LC-3 (**a–c**) and beclin-1 (**d–f**) demonstrated staining for both markers in normal (**b, e**) and degenerate (**c, f**) nucleus pulposus cells, with strong immunopositivity in degenerate cell clusters. Semi-quantitative analysis of cell positivity demonstrated significant increases in both LC-3 and beclin-1 in the nucleus pulposus with progression of degeneration (**a, d**) and in the inner annulus fibrosus (*IAF*), but not outer annulus fibrosus (*OAF*), for beclin-1. Although preliminary data, these findings suggest a role for autophagy in disc cells and that there may be an increase in the number of autophagic cells in intervertebral disc degeneration

Fig. 11.3 (continued)

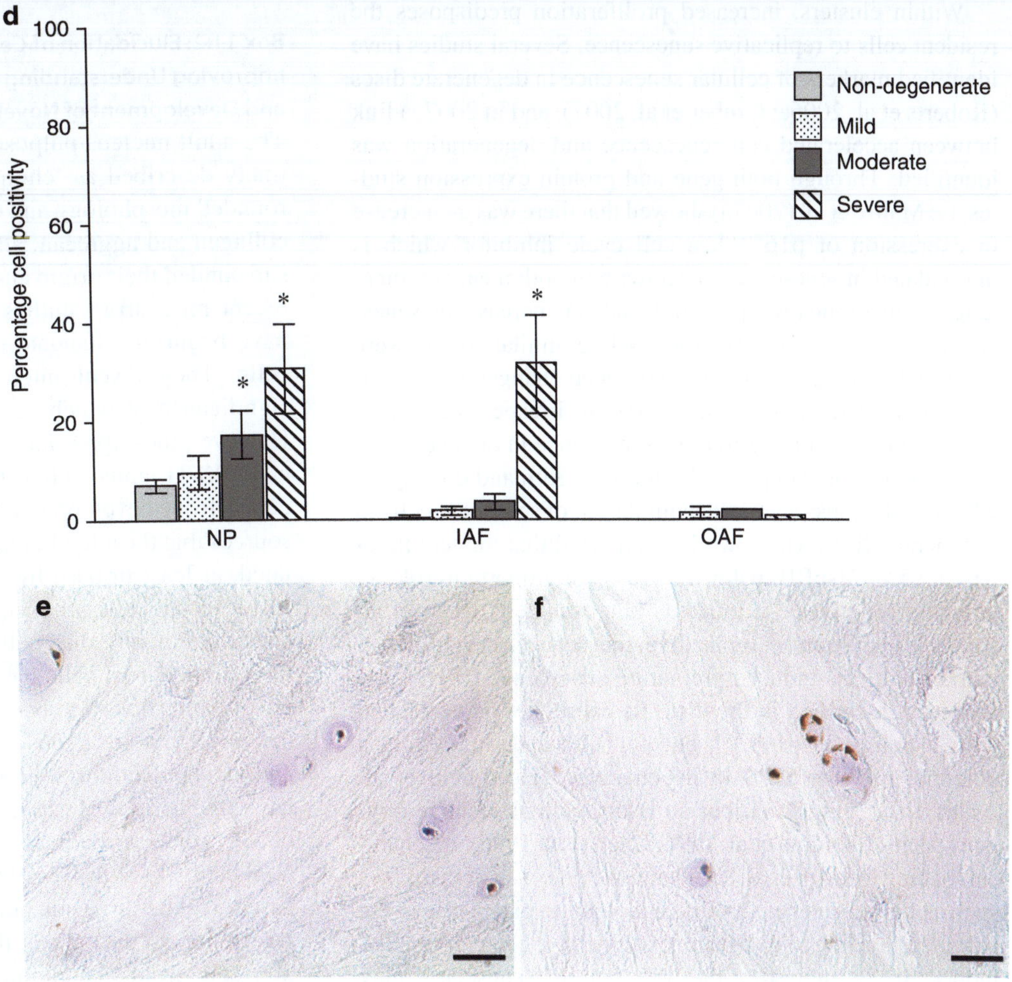

organelles and unfolded or damaged proteins. Therefore, more work is required to establish the role of autophagy in disc degeneration.

Studies on intervertebral disc cell number suggest that rather than a steady decline in cell numbers over time, there is a cyclical pattern of cell death followed by a period of proliferation. Indeed between 11 and 16 years, following the extensive cell death noted between 3 and 10 years, there is notable cell proliferation. The authors hypothesise that this is a compensatory mechanism in response to the early matrix changes seen during this time period (Boos et al. 2002). Cell clustering and proliferation, a characteristic phenomenon of degenerating tissue, is seen in the nucleus pulposus; both parameters increase both with age and with stage of degeneration (Boos et al. 2002). Both histological parameters are routinely identified adjacent to clefts and tears within the tissue, possibly due to a localised increase in the local nutrient supply in these regions (compared to an overall decrease in nutrients within the disc) rather than as a reparative mechanism (Beard et al. 1981; Boos et al. 2002; Zhao et al. 2007b). This hypothesis is further supported by evidence obtained from scoliotic discs which exhibit an increase in cell population in the inner annulus fibrosus in association with regional neovascularisation (Beard et al. 1981). Although signs of cell death are seldom seen, markers of cell proliferation, most notably proliferating cell nuclear antigen (PCNA) and the proliferation-associated Ki-67, have been identified within these cell clusters (Johnson et al. 2001; Zhao et al. 2007b).

A number of potential theories have been proposed to explain this finding. The increased local nutrition may enable cells within clusters to resist apoptosis, or possibly dead cells may be cleared more quickly from clusters than from the rest of the disc. In this respect, other workers have identified morphologically nucleus pulposus-like but CD68-positive cells within cells cluster in the nucleus pulposus of degenerate discs (Nerlich et al. 2002). These cells have the ability to phagocytose apoptotic bodies and are thought to be transformed nucleus pulposus cells, rather than infiltrating cells. In vitro studies have also demonstrated the ability of bovine nucleus pulposus cells to phagocytose apoptotic cells, suggesting that cell clearance from the disc may be undertaken by resident disc cells rather than infiltrating macrophages or monocytes (Jones et al. 2008).

Within clusters, increased proliferation predisposes the resident cells to replicative senescence. Several studies have identified markers of cellular senescence in degenerate discs (Roberts et al. 2006a; Gruber et al. 2007), and in 2007, a link between accelerated cell senescence and degeneration was identified. Through both gene and protein expression studies, Le Maitre et al. (2007a) showed that there was an increase in expression of p16^{INK4A}, a cell cycle inhibitor which is upregulated in senescence, a decrease in both mean telomere length and replicative potential and an increase in senescence-associated β-gal staining. While similar trends were identified with ageing, these senescence changes were positively related to stage of degeneration, irrespective of age, clearly demonstrating a role for senescence in degeneration. Such findings are supported by those of Kim and colleagues who also demonstrated an accumulation of senescent cells in degenerate discs. These workers reported that the telomere-based p53-p21-pRB pathway plays an important role in inducing senescence in nucleus pulposus cells (Kim et al. 2009). In addition to replicative senescence, caveolin-1, a marker of stress-induced premature senescence (SIPS), has also been identified in the disc. Its expression is correlated with increases in p16^{INK4A}, but not with age, suggesting a potential role for SIPS in degeneration (Heathfield et al. 2008). Interestingly, various stressors such as reactive oxygen species (Homma et al. 1994; Chen et al. 1995), mechanical loading (Martin et al. 2004) and the presence of cytokines such as IL-1 (Dai et al. 2006), all thought to play a role in the processes leading to disc degeneration, have been reported to induce SIPS, suggesting that this type of senescence may contribute to disc degeneration. However, more work is required to confirm these links.

Expression of cell senescence markers in the study by Le Maitre et al. was also shown to be correlated with changes in expression of two proteolytic enzymes, MMP 13 and ADAMTS 5, which are known to be upregulated in degenerate tissue. This finding indicated that a link may exist between senescence and induction of matrix catabolism (Le Maitre et al. 2007a). As well as inhibiting proliferation, studies in other tissues show that senescent cells adopt an altered phenotype, described as the senescence-associated secretory phenotype (SASP) (Freund et al. 2011). Such cells secrete a range of pro-ageing and catabolic factors, most notably IL-1, which are found to be elevated in the degenerate intervertebral disc. Studies on senescent chondrocytes show similar increases in cytokines, as well as MMPs (including MMP 13) and other proteolytic enzymes. Likewise, these cells exhibit a decreased response to anabolic stimuli that is characteristic of cells from degenerate discs. While more work is clearly needed to elucidate a potential causative link between senescence and disc degeneration, it is clear that the increase in senescence in degeneration and the phenotype adopted by the senescent cell suggest that this process may be important in disease progression.

Box 11.2: Elucidation of Cellular Phenotype Is Central to Improving Understanding of the Degenerative Process and Development of Novel Therapies

The adult nucleus pulposus is populated by cells routinely described as 'chondrocyte-like' based on their rounded morphology and expression of SOX-9, type II collagen and aggrecan, although controversy has long surrounded their origin and exact phenotype. However, recent microarray studies from our group and others have begun to elucidate the true phenotype of these cells. They reveal interesting gene signatures, the significance of which are yet to be fully understood. However, the expression of some of these genes (such as FOXF1) lends weight to the growing body of evidence from developmental biology studies and other sources that the adult human nucleus pulposus is populated, at least in part, by notochordally derived cells. Notochordal cells produce higher levels of proteoglycans than mature disc cells and animals which retain their notochordal cells have a gelatinous nucleus pulposus which does not show signs of degeneration. How the novel marker genes change during degeneration and their potential role in the pathogenesis of disease has yet to be fully elucidated. However, the elucidation of the nucleus pulposus phenotype has important implications for the development of novel stem cell-based regenerative medicine therapies as it allows researchers to understand the end point of differentiation and avoid generation of chondrocyte-like cells which may not produce a correctly functioning extracellular matrix.

11.8 Response to Mechanical Load

The human intervertebral disc is exposed to a number of physical stresses, including compressive loading, which predominantly affects the nucleus pulposus, and stretch, shear and torsion which mainly affect the annulus fibrosus. Using pressure-sensitive needles inserted into the nucleus pulposus, Nachemson et al. demonstrated that loads experienced within the human disc ranged from 250N when lying down to 1900N when lifting a 10 kg weight with a bent spine (Nachemson 1981). However, further analysis of this data, taking into consideration the tensile forces exerted by muscles in the back, suggests that loading may be as high as 9000N when lifting. It has been suggested that this combination of compression and flexion is responsible for disc prolapse, with over-flexion combined with moderate load being more detrimental than excessive load with moderate flexion (Hutton and Adams 1982). Following on from Nachemsons research, Wilke et al. demonstrated a load of between 0.1 MPa when lying prone and 2.3 MPa when lifting a 20 kg weight with a flexed spine (Wilke et al. 1999); however, this study again did not take into consideration the tensile forces exerted by the musculature in the back.

The investigations mentioned above indicate that cells in the disc experience substantial loads, and predictably, these loads are thought to have a profound effect on cell behaviour. Indeed, mechanical-loading studies using in vivo animal models and in vitro cell culture techniques have demonstrated that the type, magnitude, frequency and duration of loading are paramount in determining cell response (MacLean et al. 2004, 2005; Wang et al. 2007; Wuertz et al. 2009; Korecki et al. 2009; Sowa et al. 2011). In particular, while moderate loads and low-frequency loading both promote anabolic responses, high-magnitude, high-frequency as well as sustained static loads all elicit a catabolic or anti-anabolic response in disc cells. Using human intervertebral disc cells, Neidlinger-Wilke et al. reported increased matrix protein expression (type I collagen and aggrecan), but no change in the expression of matrix-degrading enzymes (MMPs 1, 2, 3 and 13) after low-magnitude compressive loading; high-magnitude loads led to decreased matrix protein expression with increased matrix-degrading enzyme expression (mainly MMP 3) (Neidlinger-Wilke et al. 2006). Similarly, Handa et al. found that load influenced proteoglycan synthesis and MMP gene expression in human nucleus explants, with low loads promoting matrix anabolism and high loads leading to matrix catabolism (Handa et al. 1997).

While the effect of mechanical load on nondegenerate disc cells has been well documented, studies into the response of degenerate nucleus pulposus cells remain limited. To address this need, recent investigations have compared loading responses of nondegenerate and degenerate human nucleus pulposus. With physiological loads, Le Maitre et al. showed that nondegenerate nucleus pulposus cells produced an anabolic response, while degenerate cells remained unresponsive (Le Maitre et al. 2008). This finding suggests an alteration in mechanotransduction pathways between normal and degenerate cells. In support of this notion, Gilbert et al. showed differences in response to cyclic tensile strain between nondegenerate and degenerate human annulus fibrosus cells (Gilbert et al. 2010, 2011). Accordingly, while cyclic tensile strain applied at 1 Hz to nondegenerate annulus fibrosus cells resulted in a decrease in catabolic gene expression, the same strain caused a decrease in anabolic gene expression by degenerate annulus fibrosus cells. In the latter cells, there was evidence of an altered mechanotransduction pathway which appeared to be independent of cytokine involvement (Gilbert et al. 2010, 2011). While the implications of these changes require further elucidation, the profound effects of mechanical forces on cell behaviour cannot be ignored, and the possibility exists that force plays a fundamental role in the initiation or progression of disc degeneration. For a further discussion of the effects of force on cells, see Chap.7.

11.9 Clinical Implications: Relevance of Understanding the Cell Biology and Pathogenesis of Intervertebral Disc Degeneration for Development of Novel Therapeutic Agents

Current clinical interventions for back pain are predominantly aimed at relieving symptoms rather than treating the underlying disorder. In many cases, this involves regular administration of pain-relieving pharmaceuticals, e.g. nonsteroidal anti-inflammatories, or application of more novel therapies, such as transcutaneous electrical nerve stimulation, physical manipulation, exercise therapy or behavioural therapies (Bogduk 2004). However, despite widespread use, the efficacy of these interventions is still questionable (van der Roer et al. 2005). In patients who are unresponsive to conservative therapies, but have identifiable imaging deficits and clinical symptoms of back pain, fusion surgery is the ultimate end point (Errico 2005). This approach removes the source of pain, but due to alterations in spinal biomechanics, it reduces mobility and can cause problems at adjacent motion segments (Hilibrand and Robbins 2004). One alternative to spinal fusion is whole intervertebral disc or nucleus pulposus transplantation, using either autologous or allogeneic tissues (Katsuura and Hukuda 1994; Luk et al. 1997). These procedures have been successfully performed, but require complicated surgery, and issues have arisen regarding loss of tissue integrity, tissue instability and immunogenicity (Alini et al. 2002). While tissue transplantation does not seem a feasible alternative, an increasing range of disc replacement devices are currently being investigated. These include devices such as the prosthetic disc nucleus (PDN) device or whole-disc replacements such as Charite and ProDisc (Jin et al. 2003; Guyer et al. 2009; Delamarter et al. 2011). Large-scale trials are ongoing with these devices, and with the whole-disc replacement, a significant reduction in pain score has been demonstrated. However, complications including device migration, extrusion and failure are all issues and studies have so far failed to show improved outcomes compared to fusion (Errico 2005; Di et al. 2005; Lindley et al. 2010). For a more detailed discussion of these devices, see Chaps. 13 and 14.

This lack of clinically successful long-term treatment for discogenic back pain has led researchers to investigate both biological modulators of disc cell function and novel cell-based tissue engineering and regenerative medicine therapies.

In line with the increase in knowledge surrounding the control of disc matrix anabolism and tissue degradation during degeneration, the utility of a number of biologically active agents has been evaluated. These modulators include cytokine inhibitors, such as IL-1Ra, to inhibit matrix degradation (Le Maitre et al. 2006a) and growth factors, such as OP-1, to promote matrix restoration (Masuda et al. 2006). Given the growing understanding of nerve ingrowth into the degenerate disc, it should also be possible to use biological modulators to prevent or inhibit migration of nerves into the disc and thereby block transmission of discogenic pain. Of course, while biological agents provide a mechanism to inhibit the progression of early-stage degeneration, they may not be sufficient to regenerate tissue at later stages of degeneration. At this late stage, pain is the driver behind an individual seeking clinical help, and thus, identification of a suitable cohort of early-stage patients may be difficult. However, a clearer understanding of genetic predisposition may enable individuals to be screened and interventions targeted prior to the development of symptomatic back pain.

The other area where biological modulators may be beneficial is in combination with cell-based tissue engineering therapies, where they may be used to stimulate cell differentiation or matrix formation. For intervertebral disc tissue engineering, the use of nucleus pulposus cells would initially appear to be the obvious choice, with disc cell reimplantation showing promising results in both animal models and small-scale human safety trials (Meisel et al. 2006). However, the alterations in disc cell phenotype and function during degeneration raises questions about the applicability of using autologous cells, isolated from degenerate discs, for such therapies. Problems also surround the acquisition of autologous cells from discs adjacent to the degenerate level, as the local damage caused by removing tissue from those regions has been shown to lead to degeneration at an accelerated rate (Nomura et al. 2001). The use of allogeneic cells from young, healthy donors also poses immunogenicity risks. For these reasons, the focus has shifted to the use of autologous adult stem cells, derived from either bone marrow or adipose tissue, which have been shown to be capable of differentiating into nucleus pulposus-like cells and producing an nucleus pulposus-like extracellular matrix both in vitro and in vivo (Sakai et al. 2005; Richardson et al. 2006a, b, 2008a; Box 11.2). The potential value of these therapies is that they may be able to regenerate disc tissue and restore long-term functionality. However, for the therapy to be successful, it is important to take into account the environment into which these cells will be implanted. Thus, these studies must be conducted under conditions which closely mimic the complex microenvironment of the degenerate disc. This microenvironment includes increased levels of catabolic cytokines, with low levels of nutrients and a low pH, all factors which are known to affect cell function and may have a profound effect on the ability of stem cells to survive, differentiate or secrete matrix.

To aid cell survival and function following implantation, advanced biomaterials are required which can be implanted using minimally invasive procedures. These materials must be deformable and able to withstand the loads experienced by the spine; they must be able to support or promote cell survival, differentiation and matrix formation; and finally, they can biodegrade over a suitable timescale to non-toxic by-products. At present, no 'ideal' biomaterials exist, but the field is developing rapidly and cell-based regenerative medicine therapies appear likely to revolutionise the treatment of discogenic back pain over the coming decades.

11.10 Summary of Critical Concepts Discussed in the Chapter

- Disc degeneration is a complex, multifactorial process, in which disc cells themselves play a fundamental role. While there are strong genetic predeterminants, a clear predisposition is difficult to detect.
- During degeneration, there is a cell-driven loss of proteoglycans from the extracellular matrix, which results in gross morphological, biological and biomechanical changes within the spine and the development of clinical back pain.
- Members of the MMP and ADAMTS families are responsible for breakdown of the extracellular matrix, including an imbalance between ADAMTSs and TIMP that could lead to aggrecan degradation.
- In the disease state, the loss of aggrecan, with the shift to versican production, reduces the disc water content and the shift to collagen type I production results in a more fibrous tissue, less capable of withstanding load.
- Expression levels of NGF and BDNF are increased in individuals with symptomatic disc degeneration. The disc cells express the high-affinity NGF and BDNF receptors and the low-affinity NGF/BDNF receptor $p75^{NTR}$, as well as SP, suggesting autocrine signalling.
- Interplay between catabolic cytokines and neurotrophins, neurotrophin receptors and chemorepellant molecules may guide nerve ingrowth during degeneration.
- The predominant catabolic cytokines are IL-1 and TNF-α. During degeneration, interleukin family members, interferon gamma (IFN-γ), TNF-α, PGE2 and NOx are increased.
- TGF-β, along with BMPs 2 and 14, can stimulate MSC differentiation towards nucleus pulposus-like cells in vitro.
- A reduction in essential nutrients drives degeneration. With tissue hypoxia, an increase in lactate production reduces the pH, which in turn reduces matrix synthesis and can cause cell death. The effects of low oxygen and low pH may be cumulative and promote disc cell death.

- During 3 and 10 years of age, identifiable notochordal cells disappear, and the highly hydrated, gelatinous extracellular matrix converts to a more fibrous, cartilaginous nucleus pulposus.
- It is probable that apoptosis plays a critical role in the pathogenesis of disc disease. Autophagic changes have also been identified in the degenerate disc. While autophagy can lead to cell death, it can also maintain cell viability during periods of stress.
- Senescent cells are present in the disc, adopt a senescence-associated secretory phenotype and secrete pro-ageing and catabolic factors.
- Disc loading has a profound effect on cell behaviour. Moderate loads and low-frequency loading promote anabolic responses; high-magnitude, high-frequency and static loads elicit a catabolic response.

The increasing understanding of the processes involved in degeneration is leading to the development of novel strategies which have the potential to revolutionise medical intervention in discogenic back pain.

Acknowledgments Supported by grants from the Biotechnology and Biological Sciences Research Council (BBSRC), Arthritis Research UK (ARUK) and Research Councils UK (RCUK).

References

Abbaszade I, Liu RQ, Yang F, Rosenfeld SA, Ross OH, Link JR, Ellis DM, Tortorella MD, Pratta MA, Hollis JM, Wynn R, Duke JL, George HJ, Hillman MC Jr, Murphy K, Wiswall BH, Copeland RA, Decicco CP, Bruckner R, Nagase H, Itoh Y, Newton RC, Magolda RL, Trzaskos JM, Burn TC et al (1999) Cloning and characterization of ADAMTS11, an aggrecanase from the ADAMTS family. J Biol Chem 274:23443–23450

Abe Y, Akeda K, An HS, Aoki Y, Pichika R, Muehleman C, Kimura T, Masuda K (2007) Proinflammatory cytokines stimulate the expression of nerve growth factor by human intervertebral disc cells. Spine (Phila Pa 1976) 32:635–642

Adams MA, Hutton WC (1986) The effect of posture on diffusion into lumbar intervertebral discs. J Anat 147:121–134

Adams MA, Roughley PJ (2006) What is intervertebral disc degeneration, and what causes it? Spine (Phila Pa 1976) 31:2151–2161

Adams MA, Mannion AF, Dolan P (1999) Personal risk factors for first-time low back pain. Spine (Phila Pa 1976) 24:2497–2505

Adams MA, Freeman BJ, Morrison HP, Nelson IW, Dolan P (2000) Mechanical initiation of intervertebral disc degeneration. Spine (Phila Pa 1976) 25:1625–1636

Adams MA, Stefanakis M, Dolan P (2010) Healing of a painful intervertebral disc should not be confused with reversing disc degeneration: implications for physical therapies for discogenic back pain. Clin Biomech (Bristol, Avon) 25:961–971

Akyol S, Eraslan BS, Etyemez H, Tanriverdi T, Hanci M (2010) Catabolic cytokine expressions in patients with degenerative disc disease. Turk Neurosurg 20:492–499

Ali R, Le Maitre CL, Richardson SM, Hoyland JA, Freemont AJ (2008) Connective tissue growth factor expression in human intervertebral disc: implications for angiogenesis in intervertebral disc degeneration. Biotech Histochem 83:239–245

Alini M, Roughley PJ, Antoniou J, Stoll T, Aebi M (2002) A biological approach to treating disc degeneration: not for today, but maybe for tomorrow. Eur Spine J 11(Suppl 2):S215–S220

Alvarez L, Ortiz A (1999) The study of apoptosis in spine pathology. Spine (Phila Pa 1976) 24:500

An HS, Takegami K, Kamada H, Nguyen CM, Thonar EJ, Singh K, Andersson GB, Masuda K (2005) Intradiscal administration of osteogenic protein-1 increases intervertebral disc height and proteoglycan content in the nucleus pulposus in normal adolescent rabbits. Spine (Phila Pa 1976) 30:25–31

Anderson DG, Li X, Balian G (2005) A fibronectin fragment alters the metabolism by rabbit intervertebral disc cells in vitro. Spine (Phila Pa 1976) 30:1242–1246

Annunen S, Paassilta P, Lohiniva J, Perala M, Pihlajamaa T, Karppinen J, Tervonen O, Kroger H, Lahde S, Vanharanta H, Ryhanen L, Goring HH, Ott J, Prockop DJ, la-Kokko L (1999) An allele of COL9A2 associated with intervertebral disc disease. Science 285: 409–412

Antoniou J, Steffen T, Nelson F, Winterbottom N, Hollander AP, Poole RA, Aebi M, Alini M (1996) The human lumbar intervertebral disc: evidence for changes in the biosynthesis and denaturation of the extracellular matrix with growth, maturation, ageing, and degeneration. J Clin Invest 98:996–1003

Antoniou J, Pike GB, Steffen T, Baramki H, Poole AR, Aebi M, Alini M (1998) Quantitative magnetic resonance imaging in the assessment of degenerative disc disease. Magn Reson Med 40:900–907

Aota Y, An HS, Homandberg G, Thonar EJ, Andersson GB, Pichika R, Masuda K (2005) Differential effects of fibronectin fragment on proteoglycan metabolism by intervertebral disc cells: a comparison with articular chondrocytes. Spine (Phila Pa 1976) 30:722–728

Ariga K, Yonenobu K, Nakase T, Kaneko M, Okuda S, Uchiyama Y, Yoshikawa H (2001) Localization of cathepsins D, K, and L in degenerated human intervertebral discs. Spine (Phila Pa 1976) 26: 2666–2672

Ashton IK, Roberts S, Jaffray DC, Polak JM, Eisenstein SM (1994) Neuropeptides in the human intervertebral disc. J Orthop Res 12: 186–192

Bachmeier BE, Nerlich AG, Weiler C, Paesold G, Jochum M, Boos N (2007) Analysis of tissue distribution of TNF-alpha, TNF-alpha-receptors, and the activating TNF-alpha-converting enzyme suggests activation of the TNF-alpha system in the aging intervertebral disc. Ann N Y Acad Sci 1096:44–54

Bachmeier BE, Nerlich A, Mittermaier N, Weiler C, Lumenta C, Wuertz K, Boos N (2009) Matrix metalloproteinase expression levels suggest distinct enzyme roles during lumbar disc herniation and degeneration. Eur Spine J 18:1573–1586

Barksby HE, Milner JM, Patterson AM, Peake NJ, Hui W, Robson T, Lakey R, Middleton J, Cawston TE, Richards CD, Rowan AD (2006) Matrix metalloproteinase 10 promotion of collagenolysis via procollagenase activation: implications for cartilage degradation in arthritis. Arthritis Rheum 54:3244–3253

Bartels EM, Fairbank JC, Winlove CP, Urban JP (1998) Oxygen and lactate concentrations measured in vivo in the intervertebral discs of patients with scoliosis and back pain. Spine (Phila Pa 1976) 23:1–7

Beard HK, Roberts S, O'Brien JP (1981) Immunofluorescent staining for collagen and proteoglycan in normal and scoliotic intervertebral discs. J Bone Joint Surg Br 63B:529–534

Bernick S, Cailliet R (1982) Vertebral end-plate changes with aging of human vertebrae. Spine (Phila Pa 1976) 7:97–102

Bibby SR, Urban JP (2004) Effect of nutrient deprivation on the viability of intervertebral disc cells. Eur Spine J 13:695–701

Bibby SR, Fairbank JC, Urban MR, Urban JP (2002) Cell viability in scoliotic discs in relation to disc deformity and nutrient levels. Spine (Phila Pa 1976) 27:2220–2228

Bogduk N (2004) Management of chronic low back pain. Med J Aust 180:79–83

Boos N, Nerlich AG, Wiest I, von der Mark K, Aebi M (1997) Immunolocalization of type X collagen in human lumbar intervertebral discs during ageing and degeneration. Histochem Cell Biol 108:471–480

Boos N, Weissbach S, Rohrbach H, Weiler C, Spratt KF, Nerlich AG (2002) Classification of age-related changes in lumbar intervertebral discs: 2002 Volvo Award in basic science. Spine (Phila Pa 1976) 27:2631–2644

Brew K, Dinakarpandian D, Nagase H (2000) Tissue inhibitors of metalloproteinases: evolution, structure and function. Biochim Biophys Acta 1477:267–283

Brodin H (1955) Paths of nutrition in articular cartilage and intervertebral discs. Acta Orthop Scand 24:177–183

Brown MF, Hukkanen MV, McCarthy ID, Redfern DR, Batten JJ, Crock HV, Hughes SP, Polak JM (1997) Sensory and sympathetic innervation of the vertebral endplate in patients with degenerative disc disease. J Bone Joint Surg Br 79:147–153

Buckwalter JA (1995) Aging and degeneration of the human intervertebral disc. Spine (Phila Pa 1976) 20:1307–1314

Cal S, Obaya AJ, Llamazares M, Garabaya C, Quesada V, Lopez-Otin C (2002) Cloning, expression analysis, and structural characterization of seven novel human ADAMTSs, a family of metalloproteinases with disintegrin and thrombospondin-1 domains. Gene 283: 49–62

Cappello R, Bird JL, Pfeiffer D, Bayliss MT, Dudhia J (2006) Notochordal cell produce and assemble extracellular matrix in a distinct manner, which may be responsible for the maintenance of healthy nucleus pulposus. Spine (Phila Pa 1976) 31:873–882

Chen Q, Fischer A, Reagan JD, Yan LJ, Ames BN (1995) Oxidative DNA damage and senescence of human diploid fibroblast cells. Proc Natl Acad Sci U S A 92:4337–4341

Cheung KM, Karppinen J, Chan D, Ho DW, Song YQ, Sham P, Cheah KS, Leong JC, Luk KD (2009) Prevalence and pattern of lumbar magnetic resonance imaging changes in a population study of one thousand forty-three individuals. Spine (Phila Pa 1976) 34: 934–940

Chubinskaya S, Kawakami M, Rappoport L, Matsumoto T, Migita N, Rueger DC (2007) Anti-catabolic effect of OP-1 in chronically compressed intervertebral discs. J Orthop Res 25:517–530

Collins-Racie LA, Flannery CR, Zeng W, Corcoran C, Annis-Freeman B, Agostino MJ, Arai M, DiBlasio-Smith E, Dorner AJ, Georgiadis KE, Jin M, Tan XY, Morris EA, LaVallie ER (2004) ADAMTS-8 exhibits aggrecanase activity and is expressed in human articular cartilage. Matrix Biol 23:219–230

Cooper TW, Eisen AZ, Stricklin GP, Welgus HG (1985) Platelet-derived collagenase inhibitor: characterization and subcellular localization. Proc Natl Acad Sci U S A 82:2779–2783

Coppes MH, Marani E, Thomeer RT, Groen GJ (1997) Innervation of "painful" lumbar discs. Spine (Phila Pa 1976) 22:2342–2349

Cs-Szabo G, Ragasa-San JD, Turumella V, Masuda K, Thonar EJ, An HS (2002) Changes in mRNA and protein levels of proteoglycans of the anulus fibrosus and nucleus pulposus during intervertebral disc degeneration. Spine (Phila Pa 1976) 27:2212–2219

Cui LY, Liu SL, Ding Y, Huang DS, Ma RF, Huang WG, Hu BS, Pan QH (2007) IL-1beta sensitizes rat intervertebral disc cells to Fas ligand mediated apoptosis in vitro. Acta Pharmacol Sin 28:1671–1676

Dai SM, Shan ZZ, Nakamura H, Masuko-Hongo K, Kato T, Nishioka K, Yudoh K (2006) Catabolic stress induces features of chondrocyte senescence through overexpression of caveolin 1: possible involvement of caveolin 1-induced down-regulation of articular chondrocytes in the pathogenesis of osteoarthritis. Arthritis Rheum 54:818–831

Delamarter R, Zigler JE, Balderston RA, Cammisa FP, Goldstein JA, Spivak JM (2011) Prospective, randomized, multicenter Food and Drug Administration investigational device exemption study of the ProDisc-L total disc replacement compared with circumferential arthrodesis for the treatment of two-level lumbar degenerative disc disease: results at twenty-four months. J Bone Joint Surg Am 93: 705–715

Demircan K, Hirohata S, Nishida K, Hatipoglu OF, Oohashi T, Yonezawa T, Apte SS, Ninomiya Y (2005) ADAMTS-9 is synergistically induced by interleukin-1beta and tumor necrosis factor alpha in OUMS-27 chondrosarcoma cells and in human chondrocytes. Arthritis Rheum 52:1451–1460

Deyo RA, Bass JE (1989) Lifestyle and low-back pain. The influence of smoking and obesity. Spine (Phila Pa 1976) 14:501–506

Di MA, Vaccaro AR, Lee JY, Denaro V, Lim MR (2005) Nucleus pulposus replacement: basic science and indications for clinical use. Spine 30:S16–S22

Duance VC, Crean JK, Sims TJ, Avery N, Smith S, Menage J, Eisenstein SM, Roberts S (1998) Changes in collagen cross-linking in degenerative disc disease and scoliosis. Spine (Phila Pa 1976) 23:2545–2551

Errico TJ (2005) Lumbar disc arthroplasty. Clin Orthop Relat Res 435:106–117

Eyre DR, Muir H (1976) Types I and II collagens in intervertebral disc. Interchanging radial distributions in annulus fibrosus. Biochem J 157:267–270

Feng H, Danfelter M, Stromqvist B, Heinegard D (2006) Extracellular matrix in disc degeneration. J Bone Joint Surg Am 88(Suppl 2):25–29

Freemont AJ, Peacock TE, Goupille P, Hoyland JA, O'Brien J, Jayson MI (1997) Nerve ingrowth into diseased intervertebral disc in chronic back pain. Lancet 350:178–181

Freemont AJ, Watkins A, Le MC, Baird P, Jeziorska M, Knight MT, Ross ER, O'Brien JP, Hoyland JA (2002) Nerve growth factor expression and innervation of the painful intervertebral disc. J Pathol 197:286–292

Freund A, Patil CK, Campisi J (2011) p38MAPK is a novel DNA damage response-independent regulator of the senescence-associated secretory phenotype. EMBO J 30:1536–1548

Frino J, McCarthy RE, Sparks CY, McCullough FL (2006) Trends in adolescent lumbar disk herniation. J Pediatr Orthop 26: 579–581

Gabr MA, Jing L, Helbling AR, Sinclair SM, Allen KD, Shamji MF, Richardson WJ, Fitch RD, Setton LA, Chen J (2011) Interleukin-17 synergizes with IFNgamma or TNFalpha to promote inflammatory mediator release and intercellular adhesion molecule-1 (ICAM-1) expression in human intervertebral disc cells. J Orthop Res 29:1–7

Garcia-Cosamalon J, del Valle ME, Calavia MG, Garcia-Suarez O, Lopez-Muniz A, Otero J, Vega JA (2010) Intervertebral disc, sensory nerves and neurotrophins: who is who in discogenic pain? J Anat 217:1–15

Gilbert HT, Hoyland JA, Millward-Sadler SJ (2010) The response of human anulus fibrosus cells to cyclic tensile strain is frequency-dependent and altered with disc degeneration. Arthritis Rheum 62:3385–3394

Gilbert HT, Hoyland JA, Freemont AJ, Millward-Sadler SJ (2011) The involvement of interleukin-1 and interleukin-4 in the response of human annulus fibrosus cells to cyclic tensile strain: an altered mechanotransduction pathway with degeneration. Arthritis Res Ther 13:R8

Gilbertson L, Ahn SH, Teng PN, Studer RK, Niyibizi C, Kang JD (2008) The effects of recombinant human bone morphogenetic protein-2, recombinant human bone morphogenetic protein-12, and adenoviral bone morphogenetic protein-12 on matrix synthesis in human annulus fibrosis and nucleus pulposus cells. Spine J 8: 449–456

Greg AD, Li X, Tannoury T, Beck G, Balian G (2003) A fibronectin fragment stimulates intervertebral disc degeneration in vivo. Spine (Phila Pa 1976) 28:2338–2345

Gruber HE, Hanley EN Jr (1998) Analysis of aging and degeneration of the human intervertebral disc. Comparison of surgical specimens with normal controls. Spine (Phila Pa 1976) 23:751–757

Gruber HE, Fisher EC Jr, Desai B, Stasky AA, Hoelscher G, Hanley EN Jr (1997) Human intervertebral disc cells from the annulus: three-dimensional culture in agarose or alginate and responsiveness to TGF-beta1. Exp Cell Res 235:13–21

Gruber HE, Norton HJ, Hanley EN Jr (2000) Anti-apoptotic effects of IGF-1 and PDGF on human intervertebral disc cells in vitro. Spine (Phila Pa 1976) 25:2153–2157

Gruber HE, Ingram JA, Hanley EN Jr (2005) Immunolocalization of MMP-19 in the human intervertebral disc: implications for disc aging and degeneration. Biotech Histochem 80:157–162

Gruber HE, Ingram JA, Norton HJ, Hanley EN Jr (2007) Senescence in cells of the aging and degenerating intervertebral disc: immunolocalization of senescence-associated beta-galactosidase in human and sand rat discs. Spine (Phila Pa 1976) 32:321–327

Gruber HE, Ingram JA, Hoelscher G, Zinchenko N, Norton HJ, Hanley EN Jr (2008) Brain-derived neurotrophic factor and its receptor in the human and the sand rat intervertebral disc. Arthritis Res Ther 10:R82

Guehring T, Urban JP, Cui Z, Tirlapur UK (2008) Noninvasive 3D vital imaging and characterization of notochordal cells of the intervertebral disc by femtosecond near-infrared two-photon laser scanning microscopy and spatial-volume rendering. Microsc Res Tech 71:298–304

Guyer RD, McAfee PC, Banco RJ, Bitan FD, Cappuccino A, Geisler FH, Hochschuler SH, Holt RT, Jenis LG, Majd ME, Regan JJ, Tromanhauser SG, Wong DC, Blumenthal SL (2009) Prospective, randomized, multicenter Food and Drug Administration investigational device exemption study of lumbar total disc replacement with the CHARITE artificial disc versus lumbar fusion: five-year follow-up. Spine J 9:374–386

Ha KY, Koh IJ, Kirpalani PA, Kim YY, Cho YK, Khang GS, Han CW (2006) The expression of hypoxia inducible factor-1alpha and apoptosis in herniated discs. Spine (Phila Pa 1976) 31:1309–1313

Handa T, Ishihara H, Ohshima H, Osada R, Tsuji H, Obata K (1997) Effects of hydrostatic pressure on matrix synthesis and matrix metalloproteinase production in the human lumbar intervertebral disc. Spine (Phila Pa 1976) 22:1085–1091

Harkness EF, Macfarlane GJ, Silman AJ, McBeth J (2005) Is musculoskeletal pain more common now than 40 years ago?: Two population-based cross-sectional studies. Rheumatology (Oxford) 44:890–895

Haro H, Kato T, Komori H, Osada M, Shinomiya K (2002) Vascular endothelial growth factor (VEGF)-induced angiogenesis in herniated disc resorption. J Orthop Res 20:409–415

Hatano E, Fujita T, Ueda Y, Okuda T, Katsuda S, Okada Y, Matsumoto T (2006) Expression of ADAMTS-4 (aggrecanase-1) and possible involvement in regression of lumbar disc herniation. Spine (Phila Pa 1976) 31:1426–1432

Heathfield SK, Le Maitre CL, Hoyland JA (2008) Caveolin-1 expression and stress-induced premature senescence in human intervertebral disc degeneration. Arthritis Res Ther 10:R87

Heyde CE, Tschoeke SK, Hellmuth M, Hostmann A, Ertel W, Oberholzer A (2006) Trauma induces apoptosis in human thoracolumbar intervertebral discs. BMC Clin Pathol 6:5

Hilibrand AS, Robbins M (2004) Adjacent segment degeneration and adjacent segment disease: the consequences of spinal fusion? Spine J 4:190S–194S

Hirano N, Tsuji H, Ohshima H, Kitano S, Itoh T, Sano A (1988) Analysis of rabbit intervertebral disc physiology based on water metabolism. II. Changes in normal intervertebral discs under axial vibratory load. Spine (Phila Pa 1976) 13:1297–1302

Holm S, Nachemson A (1982) Nutritional changes in the canine intervertebral disc after spinal fusion. Clin Orthop Relat Res 169: 243–258

Holm S, Nachemson A (1983) Variations in the nutrition of the canine intervertebral disc induced by motion. Spine (Phila Pa 1976) 8:866–874

Holm S, Nachemson A (1988) Nutrition of the intervertebral disc: acute effects of cigarette smoking. An experimental animal study. Ups J Med Sci 93:91–99

Holm S, Maroudas A, Urban JP, Selstam G, Nachemson A (1981) Nutrition of the intervertebral disc: solute transport and metabolism. Connect Tissue Res 8:101–119

Homandberg GA, Hui F, Wen C, Purple C, Bewsey K, Koepp H, Huch K, Harris A (1997) Fibronectin-fragment-induced cartilage chondrolysis is associated with release of catabolic cytokines. Biochem J 321(Pt 3):751–757

Homma Y, Tsunoda M, Kasai H (1994) Evidence for the accumulation of oxidative stress during cellular ageing of human diploid fibroblasts. Biochem Biophys Res Commun 203:1063–1068

Hormel SE, Eyre DR (1991) Collagen in the ageing human intervertebral disc: an increase in covalently bound fluorophores and chromophores. Biochim Biophys Acta 1078:243–250

Horner HA, Urban JP (2001) 2001 Volvo Award Winner in Basic Science Studies: effect of nutrient supply on the viability of cells from the nucleus pulposus of the intervertebral disc. Spine (Phila Pa 1976) 26:2543–2549

Hoyland JA, Le MC, Freemont AJ (2008) Investigation of the role of IL-1 and TNF in matrix degradation in the intervertebral disc. Rheumatology (Oxford) 47:809–814

Humzah MD, Soames RW (1988) Human intervertebral disc: structure and function. Anat Rec 220:337–356

Hutton WC, Adams MA (1982) Can the lumbar spine be crushed in heavy lifting? Spine (Phila Pa 1976) 7:586–590

Igarashi T, Kikuchi S, Shubayev V, Myers RR (2000) 2000 Volvo Award winner in basic science studies: exogenous tumor necrosis factor-alpha mimics nucleus pulposus-induced neuropathology. Molecular, histologic, and behavioral comparisons in rats. Spine (Phila Pa 1976) 25:2975–2980

Imai Y, Miyamoto K, An HS, Thonar EJ, Andersson GB, Masuda K (2007a) Recombinant human osteogenic protein-1 upregulates proteoglycan metabolism of human anulus fibrosus and nucleus pulposus cells. Spine (Phila Pa 1976) 32:1303–1309

Imai Y, Okuma M, An HS, Nakagawa K, Yamada M, Muehleman C, Thonar E, Masuda K (2007b) Restoration of disc height loss by recombinant human osteogenic protein-1 injection into intervertebral discs undergoing degeneration induced by an intradiscal injection of chondroitinase ABC. Spine (Phila Pa 1976) 32: 1197–1205

Inkinen RI, Lammi MJ, Lehmonen S, Puustjarvi K, Kaapa E, Tammi MI (1998) Relative increase of biglycan and decorin and altered chondroitin sulfate epitopes in the degenerating human intervertebral disc. J Rheumatol 25:506–514

Ishihara H, Urban JP (1999) Effects of low oxygen concentrations and metabolic inhibitors on proteoglycan and protein synthesis rates in the intervertebral disc. J Orthop Res 17:829–835

Jackson AR, Huang CY, Gu WY (2011) Effect of endplate calcification and mechanical deformation on the distribution of glucose in intervertebral disc: a 3D finite element study. Comput Methods Biomech Biomed Engin 14:195–204

Jin D, Qu D, Zhao L, Chen J, Jiang J (2003) Prosthetic disc nucleus (PDN) replacement for lumbar disc herniation: preliminary report with six months' follow-up. J Spinal Disord Tech 16:331–337

Johnson WE, Roberts S (2007) 'Rumours of my death may have been greatly exaggerated': a brief review of cell death in human intervertebral disc disease and implications for cell transplantation therapy. Biochem Soc Trans 35:680–682

Johnson WE, Eisenstein SM, Roberts S (2001) Cell cluster formation in degenerate lumbar intervertebral discs is associated with increased disc cell proliferation. Connect Tissue Res 42:197–207

Johnson WE, Caterson B, Eisenstein SM, Hynds DL, Snow DM, Roberts S (2002) Human intervertebral disc aggrecan inhibits nerve growth in vitro. Arthritis Rheum 46:2658–2664

Johnson WE, Caterson B, Eisenstein SM, Roberts S (2005) Human intervertebral disc aggrecan inhibits endothelial cell adhesion and cell migration in vitro. Spine (Phila Pa 1976) 30:1139–1147

Johnson WE, Sivan S, Wright KT, Eisenstein SM, Maroudas A, Roberts S (2006) Human intervertebral disc cells promote nerve growth over substrata of human intervertebral disc aggrecan. Spine (Phila Pa 1976) 31:1187–1193

Johnson WE, Patterson AM, Eisenstein SM, Roberts S (2007) The presence of pleiotrophin in the human intervertebral disc is associated with increased vascularization: an immunohistologic study. Spine (Phila Pa 1976) 32:1295–1302

Jones P, Gardner L, Menage J, Williams GT, Roberts S (2008) Intervertebral disc cells as competent phagocytes in vitro: implications for cell death in disc degeneration. Arthritis Res Ther 10:R86

Kang JD, Georgescu HI, Intyre-Larkin L, Stefanovic-Racic M, Donaldson WF III, Evans CH (1996) Herniated lumbar intervertebral discs spontaneously produce matrix metalloproteinases, nitric oxide, interleukin-6, and prostaglandin E2. Spine (Phila Pa 1976) 21:271–277

Kashiwagi M, Tortorella M, Nagase H, Brew K (2001) TIMP-3 is a potent inhibitor of aggrecanase 1 (ADAM-TS4) and aggrecanase 2 (ADAM-TS5). J Biol Chem 276:12501–12504

Katsuura A, Hukuda S (1994) Experimental study of intervertebral disc allografting in the dog. Spine 19:2426–2432

Katz MM, Hargens AR, Garfin SR (1986) Intervertebral disc nutrition. Diffusion versus convection. Clin Orthop Relat Res (210):243–245

Kawaguchi Y, Kanamori M, Ishihara H, Ohmori K, Matsui H, Kimura T (2002) The association of lumbar disc disease with vitamin-D receptor gene polymorphism. J Bone Joint Surg Am 84-A:2022–2028

Kawakami M, Matsumoto T, Hashizume H, Kuribayashi K, Chubinskaya S, Yoshida M (2005) Osteogenic protein-1 (osteogenic protein-1/bone morphogenetic protein-7) inhibits degeneration and pain-related behavior induced by chronically compressed nucleus pulposus in the rat. Spine (Phila Pa 1976) 30:1933–1939

Kim KW, Kim YS, Ha KY, Woo YK, Park JB, Park WS, An HS (2005) An autocrine or paracrine Fas-mediated counterattack: a potential mechanism for apoptosis of notochordal cells in intact rat nucleus pulposus. Spine (Phila Pa 1976) 30:1247–1251

Kim KW, Chung HN, Ha KY, Lee JS, Kim YY (2009) Senescence mechanisms of nucleus pulposus chondrocytes in human intervertebral discs. Spine J 9:658–666

Klawitter M, Quero L, Bertolo A, Mehr M, Stoyanov J, Nerlich AG, Klasen J, Aebli N, Boos N, Wuertz K (2011) Human MMP28 expression is unresponsive to inflammatory stimuli and does not correlate to the grade of intervertebral disc degeneration. J Negat Results Biomed 10:9

Kolodkin AL, Matthes DJ, Goodman CS (1993) The semaphorin genes encode a family of transmembrane and secreted growth cone guidance molecules. Cell 75:1389–1399

Konttinen YT, Kaapa E, Hukkanen M, Gu XH, Takagi M, Santavirta S, Alaranta H, Li TF, Suda A (1999) Cathepsin G in degenerating and healthy discal tissue. Clin Exp Rheumatol 17:197–204

Korecki CL, Kuo CK, Tuan RS, Iatridis JC (2009) Intervertebral disc cell response to dynamic compression is age and frequency dependent. J Orthop Res 27:800–806

Le Maitre CL, Freemont AJ, Hoyland JA (2004) Localization of degradative enzymes and their inhibitors in the degenerate human intervertebral disc. J Pathol 204:47–54

Le Maitre CL, Freemont AJ, Hoyland JA (2005a) The role of interleukin-1 in the pathogenesis of human intervertebral disc degeneration. Arthritis Res Ther 7:R732–R745

Le Maitre CL, Richardson SM, Baird P, Freemont AJ, Hoyland JA (2005b) Expression of receptors for putative anabolic growth factors in human intervertebral disc: implications for repair and regeneration of the disc. J Pathol 207:445–452

Le Maitre CL, Freemont AJ, Hoyland JA (2006a) A preliminary in vitro study into the use of IL-1Ra gene therapy for the inhibition of intervertebral disc degeneration. Int J Exp Pathol 87:17–28

Le Maitre CL, Freemont AJ, Hoyland JA (2006b) Human disc degeneration is associated with increased MMP 7 expression. Biotech Histochem 81:125–131

Le Maitre CL, Freemont AJ, Hoyland JA (2007a) Accelerated cellular senescence in degenerate intervertebral discs: a possible role in the pathogenesis of intervertebral disc degeneration. Arthritis Res Ther 9:R45

Le Maitre CL, Hoyland JA, Freemont AJ (2007b) Catabolic cytokine expression in degenerate and herniated human intervertebral discs: IL-1beta and TNFalpha expression profile. Arthritis Res Ther 9:R77

Le Maitre CL, Hoyland JA, Freemont AJ (2007c) Interleukin-1 receptor antagonist delivered directly and by gene therapy inhibits matrix degradation in the intact degenerate human intervertebral disc: an in situ zymographic and gene therapy study. Arthritis Res Ther 9:R83

Le Maitre CL, Pockert A, Buttle DJ, Freemont AJ, Hoyland JA (2007d) Matrix synthesis and degradation in human intervertebral disc degeneration. Biochem Soc Trans 35:652–655

Le Maitre CL, Frain J, Fotheringham AP, Freemont AJ, Hoyland JA (2008) Human cells derived from degenerate intervertebral discs respond differently to those derived from non-degenerate intervertebral discs following application of dynamic hydrostatic pressure. Biorheology 45:563–575

Le Maitre CL, Freemont AJ, Hoyland JA (2009) Expression of cartilage-derived morphogenetic protein in human intervertebral discs and its effect on matrix synthesis in degenerate human nucleus pulposus cells. Arthritis Res Ther 11:R137

Lee CR, Sakai D, Nakai T, Toyama K, Mochida J, Alini M, Grad S (2007) A phenotypic comparison of intervertebral disc and articular cartilage cells in the rat. Eur Spine J 16:2174–2185

Lee JM, Song JY, Baek M, Jung HY, Kang H, Han IB, Kwon YD, Shin DE (2011) Interleukin-1beta induces angiogenesis and innervation in human intervertebral disc degeneration. J Orthop Res 29:265–269

Lindley EM, Jaafar S, Noshchenko A, Baldini T, Nair DP, Shandas R, Burger EL, Patel VV (2010) Nucleus replacement device failure: a case report and biomechanical study. Spine (Phila Pa 1976) 35:E1241–E1247

Loreto C, Musumeci G, Castorina A, Loreto C, Martinez G (2011) Degenerative disc disease of herniated intervertebral discs is associated with extracellular matrix remodeling, vimentin-positive cells and cell death. Ann Anat 193:156–162

Lotz JC, Chin JR (2000) Intervertebral disc cell death is dependent on the magnitude and duration of spinal loading. Spine (Phila Pa 1976) 25:1477–1483

Luk KD, Ruan DK, Chow DH, Leong JC (1997) Intervertebral disc autografting in a bipedal animal model. Clin Orthop Relat Res 337:13–26

Lyons G, Eisenstein SM, Sweet MB (1981) Biochemical changes in intervertebral disc degeneration. Biochim Biophys Acta 673:443–453

MacGregor AJ, Andrew T, Sambrook PN, Spector TD (2004) Structural, psychological, and genetic influences on low back and neck pain: a study of adult female twins. Arthritis Rheum 51:160–167

MacLean JJ, Lee CR, Alini M, Iatridis JC (2004) Anabolic and catabolic mRNA levels of the intervertebral disc vary with the magnitude and frequency of in vivo dynamic compression. J Orthop Res 22:1193–1200

MacLean JJ, Lee CR, Alini M, Iatridis JC (2005) The effects of short-term load duration on anabolic and catabolic gene expression in the rat tail intervertebral disc. J Orthop Res 23:1120–1127

Malandrino A, Noailly J, Lacroix D (2011) The effect of sustained compression on oxygen metabolic transport in the intervertebral

disc decreases with degenerative changes. PLoS Comput Biol 7:e1002112
Maniadakis N, Gray A (2000) The economic burden of back pain in the UK. Pain 84:95–103
Marchand F, Ahmed AM (1990) Investigation of the laminate structure of lumbar disc anulus fibrosus. Spine 15:402–410
Maroudas A, Stockwell RA, Nachemson A, Urban J (1975) Factors involved in the nutrition of the human lumbar intervertebral disc: cellularity and diffusion of glucose in vitro. J Anat 120:113–130
Martin JA, Brown TD, Heiner AD, Buckwalter JA (2004) Chondrocyte senescence, joint loading and osteoarthritis. Clin Orthop Relat Res (427 Suppl):S96–103
Martin BI, Deyo RA, Mirza SK, Turner JA, Comstock BA, Hollingworth W, Sullivan SD (2008) Expenditures and health status among adults with back and neck problems. JAMA 299:656–664
Masuda K, Takegami K, An H, Kumano F, Chiba K, Andersson GB, Schmid T, Thonar E (2003) Recombinant osteogenic protein-1 upregulates extracellular matrix metabolism by rabbit annulus fibrosus and nucleus pulposus cells cultured in alginate beads. J Orthop Res 21:922–930
Masuda K, Imai Y, Okuma M, Muehleman C, Nakagawa K, Akeda K, Thonar E, Andersson G, An HS (2006) Osteogenic protein-1 injection into a degenerated disc induces the restoration of disc height and structural changes in the rabbit anular puncture model. Spine (Phila Pa 1976) 31:742–754
McCanless JD, Cole JA, Slack SM, Bumgardner JD, Zamora PO, Haggard WO (2011) Modeling nucleus pulposus regeneration in vitro: mesenchymal stem cells, alginate beads, hypoxia, BMP-2, and synthetic peptide B2A. Spine (Phila Pa 1976) 36:2275–2285
Meisel HJ, Ganey T, Hutton WC, Libera J, Minkus Y, Alasevic O (2006) Clinical experience in cell-based therapeutics: intervention and outcome. Eur Spine J 15(Suppl 3):S397–S405
Melrose J, Roberts S, Smith S, Menage J, Ghosh P (2002a) Increased nerve and blood vessel ingrowth associated with proteoglycan depletion in an ovine anular lesion model of experimental disc degeneration. Spine (Phila Pa 1976) 27:1278–1285
Melrose J, Smith S, Little CB, Kitson J, Hwa SY, Ghosh P (2002b) Spatial and temporal localization of transforming growth factor-beta, fibroblast growth factor-2, and osteonectin, and identification of cells expressing alpha-smooth muscle actin in the injured anulus fibrosus: implications for extracellular matrix repair. Spine (Phila Pa 1976) 27:1756–1764
Melrose J, Smith SM, Appleyard RC, Little CB (2008) Aggrecan, versican and type VI collagen are components of annular translamellar crossbridges in the intervertebral disc. Eur Spine J 17:314–324
Minogue BM, Richardson SM, Zeef LA, Freemont AJ, Hoyland JA (2010a) Characterization of the human nucleus pulposus cell phenotype and evaluation of novel marker gene expression to define adult stem cell differentiation. Arthritis Rheum 62:3695–3705
Minogue BM, Richardson SM, Zeef LA, Freemont AJ, Hoyland JA (2010b) Transcriptional profiling of bovine intervertebral disc cells: implications for identification of normal and degenerate human intervertebral disc cell phenotypes. Arthritis Res Ther 12:R22
Miyamoto K, Masuda K, Kim JG, Inoue N, Akeda K, Andersson GB, An HS (2006) Intradiscal injections of osteogenic protein-1 restore the viscoelastic properties of degenerated intervertebral discs. Spine J 6:692–703
Mokhbi SD, Shirazi-Adl A, Urban JP (2009) Investigation of solute concentrations in a 3D model of intervertebral disc. Eur Spine J 18:254–262
Mwale F, Roughley P, Antoniou J (2004) Distinction between the extracellular matrix of the nucleus pulposus and hyaline cartilage: a requisite for tissue engineering of intervertebral disc. Eur Cell Mater 8:58–63
Nachemson AL (1981) Disc pressure measurements. Spine (Phila Pa 1976) 6:93–97
Nachemson A, Lewin T, Maroudas A, Freeman MA (1970) In vitro diffusion of dye through the end-plates and the annulus fibrosus of human lumbar inter-vertebral discs. Acta Orthop Scand 41:589–607
Nagase H, Kashiwagi M (2003) Aggrecanases and cartilage matrix degradation. Arthritis Res Ther 5:94–103
Nagase H, Woessner JF Jr (1999) Matrix metalloproteinases. J Biol Chem 274:21491–21494
Neidlinger-Wilke C, Wurtz K, Urban JP, Borm W, Arand M, Ignatius A, Wilke HJ, Claes LE (2006) Regulation of gene expression in intervertebral disc cells by low and high hydrostatic pressure. Eur Spine J 15(Suppl 3):S372–S378
Nerlich AG, Schleicher ED, Boos N (1997) 1997 Volvo Award winner in basic science studies. Immunohistologic markers for age-related changes of human lumbar intervertebral discs. Spine (Phila Pa 1976) 22:2781–2795
Nerlich AG, Boos N, Wiest I, Aebi M (1998) Immunolocalization of major interstitial collagen types in human lumbar intervertebral discs of various ages. Virchows Arch 432:67–76
Nerlich AG, Weiler C, Zipperer J, Narozny M, Boos N (2002) Immunolocalization of phagocytic cells in normal and degenerated intervertebral discs. Spine (Phila Pa 1976) 27:2484–2490
Nerlich AG, Schaaf R, Walchli B, Boos N (2007) Temporo-spatial distribution of blood vessels in human lumbar intervertebral discs. Eur Spine J 16:547–555
Nomura T, Mochida J, Okuma M, Nishimura K, Sakabe K (2001) Nucleus pulposus allograft retards intervertebral disc degeneration. Clin Orthop Relat Res 389:94–101
Oegema TR Jr, Johnson SL, Aguiar DJ, Ogilvie JW (2000) Fibronectin and its fragments increase with degeneration in the human intervertebral disc. Spine (Phila Pa 1976) 25:2742–2747
Ohba T, Haro H, Ando T, Wako M, Suenaga F, Aso Y, Koyama K, Hamada Y, Nakao A (2009) TNF-alpha-induced NF-kappaB signaling reverses age-related declines in VEGF induction and angiogenic activity in intervertebral disc tissues. J Orthop Res 27:229–235
Ohshima H, Urban JP (1992) The effect of lactate and pH on proteoglycan and protein synthesis rates in the intervertebral disc. Spine (Phila Pa 1976) 17:1079–1082
Ohtori S, Takahashi K, Chiba T, Yamagata M, Sameda H, Moriya H (2002) Substance P and calcitonin gene-related peptide immunoreactive sensory DRG neurons innervating the lumbar intervertebral discs in rats. Ann Anat 184:235–240
Olmarker K, Larsson K (1998) Tumor necrosis factor alpha and nucleus-pulposus-induced nerve root injury. Spine (Phila Pa 1976) 23: 2538–2544
Olmarker K, Rydevik B (2001) Selective inhibition of tumor necrosis factor-alpha prevents nucleus pulposus-induced thrombus formation, intraneural edema, and reduction of nerve conduction velocity: possible implications for future pharmacologic treatment strategies of sciatica. Spine (Phila Pa 1976) 26:863–869
Osada R, Ohshima H, Ishihara H, Yudoh K, Sakai K, Matsui H, Tsuji H (1996) Autocrine/paracrine mechanism of insulin-like growth factor-1 secretion, and the effect of insulin-like growth factor-1 on proteoglycan synthesis in bovine intervertebral discs. J Orthop Res 14:690–699
Park JB, Park IC, Park SJ, Jin HO, Lee JK, Riew KD (2006) Anti-apoptotic effects of caspase inhibitors on rat intervertebral disc cells. J Bone Joint Surg Am 88:771–779
Patel KP, Sandy JD, Akeda K, Miyamoto K, Chujo T, An HS, Masuda K (2007) Aggrecanases and aggrecanase-generated fragments in the human intervertebral disc at early and advanced stages of disc degeneration. Spine (Phila Pa 1976) 32:2596–2603
Pazzaglia UE, Salisbury JR, Byers PD (1989) Development and involution of the notochord in the human spine. J R Soc Med 82:413–415
Pearce RH, Grimmer BJ, Adams ME (1987) Degeneration and the chemical composition of the human lumbar intervertebral disc. J Orthop Res 5:198–205

Peng B, Hao J, Hou S, Wu W, Jiang D, Fu X, Yang Y (2006) Possible pathogenesis of painful intervertebral disc degeneration. Spine (Phila Pa 1976) 31:560–566

Peng B, Chen J, Kuang Z, Li D, Pang X, Zhang X (2009) Expression and role of connective tissue growth factor in painful disc fibrosis and degeneration. Spine (Phila Pa 1976) 34:E178–E182

Pfirrmann CW, Metzdorf A, Zanetti M, Hodler J, Boos N (2001) Magnetic resonance classification of lumbar intervertebral disc degeneration. Spine (Phila Pa 1976) 26:1873–1878

Pluijm SM, van Essen HW, Bravenboer N, Uitterlinden AG, Smit JH, Pols HA, Lips P (2004) Collagen type I alpha1 Sp1 polymorphism, osteoporosis, and intervertebral disc degeneration in older men and women. Ann Rheum Dis 63:71–77

Pockert AJ, Richardson SM, Le Maitre CL, Lyon M, Deakin JA, Buttle DJ, Freemont AJ, Hoyland JA (2009) Modified expression of the ADAMTS enzymes and tissue inhibitor of metalloproteinases 3 during human intervertebral disc degeneration. Arthritis Rheum 60: 482–491

Pokharna HK, Phillips FM (1998) Collagen crosslinks in human lumbar intervertebral disc aging. Spine (Phila Pa 1976) 23: 1645–1648

Pollintine P, Przybyla AS, Dolan P, Adams MA (2004) Neural arch load-bearing in old and degenerated spines. J Biomech 37:197–204

Postacchini F, Lami R, Pugliese O (1988) Familial predisposition to discogenic low-back pain. An epidemiologic and immunogenetic study. Spine (Phila Pa 1976) 13:1403–1406

Purmessur D, Freemont AJ, Hoyland JA (2008) Expression and regulation of neurotrophins in the nondegenerate and degenerate human intervertebral disc. Arthritis Res Ther 10:R99

Rannou F, Lee TS, Zhou RH, Chin J, Lotz JC, Mayoux-Benhamou MA, Barbet JP, Chevrot A, Shyy JY (2004) Intervertebral disc degeneration: the role of the mitochondrial pathway in annulus fibrosus cell apoptosis induced by overload. Am J Pathol 164:915–924

Repanti M, Korovessis PG, Stamatakis MV, Spastris P, Kosti P (1998) Evolution of disc degeneration in lumbar spine: a comparative histological study between herniated and postmortem retrieved disc specimens. J Spinal Disord 11:41–45

Richardson JK, Chung T, Schultz JS, Hurvitz E (1997) A familial predisposition toward lumbar disc injury. Spine (Phila Pa 1976) 22:1487–1492

Richardson SM, Curran JM, Chen R, Vaughan-Thomas A, Hunt JA, Freemont AJ, Hoyland JA (2006a) The differentiation of bone marrow mesenchymal stem cells into chondrocyte-like cells on poly-L-lactic acid (PLLA) scaffolds. Biomaterials 27:4069–4078

Richardson SM, Walker RV, Parker S, Rhodes NP, Hunt JA, Freemont AJ, Hoyland JA (2006b) Intervertebral disc cell-mediated mesenchymal stem cell differentiation. Stem Cells 24:707–716

Richardson SM, Hughes N, Hunt JA, Freemont AJ, Hoyland JA (2008a) Human mesenchymal stem cell differentiation to NP-like cells in chitosan-glycerophosphate hydrogels. Biomaterials 29:85–93

Richardson SM, Knowles R, Tyler J, Mobasheri A, Hoyland JA (2008b) Expression of glucose transporters GLUT-1, GLUT-3, GLUT-9 and HIF-1alpha in normal and degenerate human intervertebral disc. Histochem Cell Biol 129:503–511

Richardson SM, Doyle P, Minogue BM, Gnanalingham K, Hoyland JA (2009) Increased expression of matrix metalloproteinase-10, nerve growth factor and substance P in the painful degenerate intervertebral disc. Arthritis Res Ther 11:R126

Richardson SM, Purmessur D, Baird P, Probyn B, Freemont AJ, Hoyland JA (2012) Degenerate human nucleus pulposus cells promote neurite outgrowth in neural cells. PLoS One 7(10):e47735. PubMed PMID: 23091643

Risbud MV, Fertala J, Vresilovic EJ, Albert TJ, Shapiro IM (2005) Nucleus pulposus cells upregulate PI3K/Akt and MEK/ERK signaling pathways under hypoxic conditions and resist apoptosis induced by serum withdrawal. Spine (Phila Pa 1976) 30:882–889

Roberts S, Urban JP, Evans H, Eisenstein SM (1996) Transport properties of the human cartilage endplate in relation to its composition and calcification. Spine (Phila Pa 1976) 21:415–420

Roberts S, Caterson B, Menage J, Evans EH, Jaffray DC, Eisenstein SM (2000) Matrix metalloproteinases and aggrecanase: their role in disorders of the human intervertebral disc. Spine (Phila Pa 1976) 25:3005–3013

Roberts S, Evans EH, Kletsas D, Jaffray DC, Eisenstein SM (2006a) Senescence in human intervertebral discs. Eur Spine J 15(Suppl 3): S312–S316

Roberts S, Evans H, Trivedi J, Menage J (2006b) Histology and pathology of the human intervertebral disc. J Bone Joint Surg Am 88(Suppl 2):10–14

Rodriguez AG, Slichter CK, Acosta FL, Rodriguez-Soto AE, Burghardt AJ, Majumdar S, Lotz JC (2011) Human disc nucleus properties and vertebral endplate permeability. Spine (Phila Pa 1976) 36: 512–520

Rodriguez AG, Rodriguez-Soto AE, Burghardt AJ, Berven S, Majumdar S, Lotz JC (2012) Morphology of the human vertebral endplate. J Orthop Res 30:280–287

Roughley PJ (2004) Biology of intervertebral disc aging and degeneration: involvement of the extracellular matrix. Spine 29: 2691–2699

Roughley P, Martens D, Rantakokko J, Alini M, Mwale F, Antoniou J (2006) The involvement of aggrecan polymorphism in degeneration of human intervertebral disc and articular cartilage. Eur Cell Mater 11:1–7

Rutges JP, Duit RA, Kummer JA, Oner FC, van Rijen MH, Verbout AJ, Castelein RM, Dhert WJ, Creemers LB (2010) Hypertrophic differentiation and calcification during intervertebral disc degeneration. Osteoarthritis Cartilage 18:1487–1495

Sakai D, Mochida J, Iwashina T, Watanabe T, Nakai T, Ando K, Hotta T (2005) Differentiation of mesenchymal stem cells transplanted to a rabbit degenerative disc model: potential and limitations for stem cell therapy in disc regeneration. Spine (Phila Pa 1976) 30: 2379–2387

Sakai D, Nakai T, Mochida J, Alini M, Grad S (2009) Differential phenotype of intervertebral disc cells: microarray and immunohistochemical analysis of canine nucleus pulposus and anulus fibrosus. Spine (Phila Pa 1976) 34:1448–1456

Schollmeier G, Lahr-Eigen R, Lewandrowski KU (2000) Observations on fiber-forming collagens in the anulus fibrosus. Spine (Phila Pa 1976) 25:2736–2741

Seki S, Kawaguchi Y, Chiba K, Mikami Y, Kizawa H, Oya T, Mio F, Mori M, Miyamoto Y, Masuda I, Tsunoda T, Kamata M, Kubo T, Toyama Y, Kimura T, Nakamura Y, Ikegawa S (2005) A functional SNP in CILP, encoding cartilage intermediate layer protein, is associated with susceptibility to lumbar disc disease. Nat Genet 37:607–612

Selard E, Shirazi-Adl A, Urban JP (2003) Finite element study of nutrient diffusion in the human intervertebral disc. Spine (Phila Pa 1976) 28:1945–1953

Shen C, Yan J, Jiang LS, Dai LY (2011) Autophagy in rat annulus fibrosus cells: evidence and possible implications. Arthritis Res Ther 13:R132

Sive JI, Baird P, Jeziorsk M, Watkins A, Hoyland JA, Freemont AJ (2002) Expression of chondrocyte markers by cells of normal and degenerate intervertebral discs. Mol Pathol 55:91–97

Smith SM, Whitelock JM, Iozzo RV, Little CB, Melrose J (2009) Topographical variation in the distributions of versican, aggrecan and perlecan in the foetal human spine reflects their diverse functional roles in spinal development. Histochem Cell Biol 132: 491–503

Solovieva S, Kouhia S, Leino-Arjas P, la-Kokko L, Luoma K, Raininko R, Saarela J, Riihimaki H (2004) Interleukin 1 polymorphisms and intervertebral disc degeneration. Epidemiology 15:626–633

Solovieva S, Lohiniva J, Leino-Arjas P, Raininko R, Luoma K, la-Kokko L, Riihimaki H (2006) Intervertebral disc degeneration in relation to the COL9A3 and the IL-1ss gene polymorphisms. Eur Spine J 15:613–619

Somerville RP, Longpre JM, Jungers KA, Engle JM, Ross M, Evanko S, Wight TN, Leduc R, Apte SS (2003) Characterization of ADAMTS-9 and ADAMTS-20 as a distinct ADAMTS subfamily related to Caenorhabditis elegans GON-1. J Biol Chem 278:9503–9513

Sowa GA, Coelho JP, Bell KM, Zorn AS, Vo NV, Smolinski P, Niyonkuru C, Hartman R, Studer RK, Kang JD (2011) Alterations in gene expression in response to compression of nucleus pulposus cells. Spine J 11:36–43

Stetler-Stevenson WG, Krutzsch HC, Liotta LA (1989) Tissue inhibitor of metalloproteinase (TIMP-2). A new member of the metalloproteinase inhibitor family. J Biol Chem 264:17374–17378

Stewart WF, Ricci JA, Chee E, Morganstein D, Lipton R (2003) Lost productive time and cost due to common pain conditions in the US workforce. JAMA 290:2443–2454

Stoyanov JV, Gantenbein-Ritter B, Bertolo A, Aebli N, Baur M, Alini M, Grad S (2011) Role of hypoxia and growth and differentiation factor-5 on differentiation of human mesenchymal stem cells towards intervertebral nucleus pulposus-like cells. Eur Cell Mater 21:533–547

Studer RK, Vo N, Sowa G, Ondeck C, Kang J (2011) Human nucleus pulposus cells react to IL-6: independent actions and amplification of response to IL-1 and TNF-alpha. Spine (Phila Pa 1976) 36:593–599

Sztrolovics R, Alini M, Roughley PJ, Mort JS (1997) Aggrecan degradation in human intervertebral disc and articular cartilage. Biochem J 326(Pt 1):235–241

Sztrolovics R, Grover J, Cs-Szabo G, Shi SL, Zhang Y, Mort JS, Roughley PJ (2002) The characterization of versican and its message in human articular cartilage and intervertebral disc. J Orthop Res 20:257–266

Takahashi M, Haro H, Wakabayashi Y, Kawa-uchi T, Komori H, Shinomiya K (2001) The association of degeneration of the intervertebral disc with 5a/6a polymorphism in the promoter of the human matrix metalloproteinase-3 gene. J Bone Joint Surg Br 83:491–495

Takahashi Y, Ohtori S, Takahashi K (2009) Peripheral nerve pathways of afferent fibers innervating the lumbar spine in rats. J Pain 10:416–425

Takaishi H, Nemoto O, Shiota M, Kikuchi T, Yamada H, Yamagishi M, Yabe Y (1997) Type-II collagen gene expression is transiently upregulated in experimentally induced degeneration of rabbit intervertebral disc. J Orthop Res 15:528–538

Takebayashi T, Cavanaugh JM, Kallakuri S, Chen C, Yamashita T (2006) Sympathetic afferent units from lumbar intervertebral discs. J Bone Joint Surg Br 88:554–557

Takegami K, An HS, Kumano F, Chiba K, Thonar EJ, Singh K, Masuda K (2005) Osteogenic protein-1 is most effective in stimulating nucleus pulposus and annulus fibrosus cells to repair their matrix after chondroitinase ABC-induced in vitro chemonucleolysis. Spine J 5:231–238

Thompson JP, Pearce RH, Schechter MT, Adams ME, Tsang IK, Bishop PB (1990) Preliminary evaluation of a scheme for grading the gross morphology of the human intervertebral disc. Spine (Phila Pa 1976) 15:411–415

Thompson JP, Oegema TR Jr, Bradford DS (1991) Stimulation of mature canine intervertebral disc by growth factors. Spine (Phila Pa 1976) 16:253–260

Tim YS, Su KK, Li J, Soo PJ, Akamaru T, Elmer WA, Hutton WC (2003) The effect of bone morphogenetic protein-2 on rat intervertebral disc cells in vitro. Spine (Phila Pa 1976) 28:1773–1780

Tolofari SK, Richardson SM, Freemont AJ, Hoyland JA (2010) Expression of semaphorin 3A and its receptors in the human intervertebral disc: potential role in regulating neural ingrowth in the degenerate intervertebral disc. Arthritis Res Ther 12:R1

Tortorella MD, Burn TC, Pratta MA, Abbaszade I, Hollis JM, Liu R, Rosenfeld SA, Copeland RA, Decicco CP, Wynn R, Rockwell A, Yang F, Duke JL, Solomon K, George H, Bruckner R, Nagase H, Itoh Y, Ellis DM, Ross H, Wiswall BH, Murphy K, Hillman MC Jr, Hollis GF, Newton RC, Magolda RL, Trzaskos JM, Arner EC (1999) Purification and cloning of aggrecanase-1: a member of the ADAMTS family of proteins. Science 284:1664–1666

Tschoeke SK, Hellmuth M, Hostmann A, Robinson Y, Ertel W, Oberholzer A, Heyde CE (2008) Apoptosis of human intervertebral discs after trauma compares to degenerated discs involving both receptor-mediated and mitochondrial-dependent pathways. J Orthop Res 26:999–1006

Urban JP, Holm S, Maroudas A, Nachemson A (1982) Nutrition of the intervertebral disc: effect of fluid flow on solute transport. Clin Orthop Relat Res (170):296–302

Urban MR, Fairbank JC, Etherington PJ, Loh FL, Winlove CP, Urban JP (2001) Electrochemical measurement of transport into scoliotic intervertebral discs in vivo using nitrous oxide as a tracer. Spine (Phila Pa 1976) 26:984–990

Urban JP, Smith S, Fairbank JC (2004) Nutrition of the intervertebral disc. Spine (Phila Pa 1976) 29:2700–2709

van der Roer N, Goossens ME, Evers SM, van Tulder MW (2005) What is the most cost-effective treatment for patients with low back pain? A systematic review. Best Pract Res Clin Rheumatol 19:671–684

Videman T, Leppavuori J, Kaprio J, Battie MC, Gibbons LE, Peltonen L, Koskenvuo M (1998) Intragenic polymorphisms of the vitamin D receptor gene associated with intervertebral disc degeneration. Spine (Phila Pa 1976) 23:2477–2485

Wagner DR, Reiser KM, Lotz JC (2006) Glycation increases human annulus fibrosus stiffness in both experimental measurements and theoretical predictions. J Biomech 39:1021–1029

Walker BF (2000) The prevalence of low back pain: a systematic review of the literature from 1966 to 1998. J Spinal Disord 13:205–217

Wallach D, Arumugam TU, Boldin MP, Cantarella G, Ganesh KA, Goltsev Y, Goncharov TM, Kovalenko AV, Rajput A, Varfolomeev EE, Zhang SQ (2002) How are the regulators regulated? The search for mechanisms that impose specificity on induction of cell death and NF-kappaB activation by members of the TNF/NGF receptor family. Arthritis Res 4(Suppl 3):S189–S196

Walsh AJ, Bradford DS, Lotz JC (2004) In vivo growth factor treatment of degenerated intervertebral discs. Spine (Phila Pa 1976) 29:156–163

Wang DL, Jiang SD, Dai LY (2007) Biologic response of the intervertebral disc to static and dynamic compression in vitro. Spine (Phila Pa 1976) 32:2521–2528

Weiler C, Nerlich AG, Zipperer J, Bachmeier BE, Boos N (2002) 2002 SSE Award Competition in Basic Science: expression of major matrix metalloproteinases is associated with intervertebral disc degradation and resorption. Eur Spine J 11:308–320

Weiler C, Nerlich AG, Bachmeier BE, Boos N (2005) Expression and distribution of tumor necrosis factor alpha in human lumbar intervertebral discs: a study in surgical specimen and autopsy controls. Spine (Phila Pa 1976) 30:44–53

Wilder DG, Pope MH, Magnusson M (1996) Mechanical stress reduction during seated jolt/vibration exposure. Semin Perinatol 20:54–60

Wilke HJ, Neef P, Caimi M, Hoogland T, Claes LE (1999) New in vivo measurements of pressures in the intervertebral disc in daily life. Spine (Phila Pa 1976) 24:755–762

Wolfe HJ, Putschar WG, Vickery AL (1965) Role of the notochord in human intervetebral disk. I. Fetus and infant. Clin Orthop Relat Res 39:205–212

Wuertz K, Godburn K, MacLean JJ, Barbir A, Donnelly JS, Roughley PJ, Alini M, Iatridis JC (2009) In vivo remodeling of intervertebral discs in response to short- and long-term dynamic compression. J Orthop Res 27:1235–1242

Yao H, Gu WY (2006) Physical signals and solute transport in human intervertebral disc during compressive stress relaxation: 3D finite element analysis. Biorheology 43:323–335

Yasuma T, Arai K, Yamauchi Y (1993) The histology of lumbar intervertebral disc herniation. The significance of small blood vessels in the extruded tissue. Spine (Phila Pa 1976) 18:1761–1765

Ye W, Xu K, Huang D, Liang A, Peng Y, Zhu W, Li C (2011) Age-related increases of macroautophagy and chaperone-mediated autophagy in rat nucleus pulposus. Connect Tissue Res 52:472–478

Yu H, Zhu Y (2012) Expression of ADAMTS-7 and ADAMTS-12 in nucleus pulposus during degeneration of rat caudal intervertebral disc. J Vet Med Sci 74:9–15

Yu J, Winlove PC, Roberts S, Urban JP (2002) Elastic fibre organization in the intervertebral discs of the bovine tail. J Anat 201:465–475

Zhao F, Pollintine P, Hole BD, Dolan P, Adams MA (2005) Discogenic origins of spinal instability. Spine (Phila Pa 1976) 30:2621–2630

Zhao CQ, Liu D, Li H, Jiang LS, Dai LY (2007a) Interleukin-1beta enhances the effect of serum deprivation on rat annular cell apoptosis. Apoptosis 12:2155–2161

Zhao CQ, Wang LM, Jiang LS, Dai LY (2007b) The cell biology of intervertebral disc aging and degeneration. Ageing Res Rev 6:247–261

Zhao CQ, Zhang YH, Jiang SD, Li H, Jiang LS, Dai LY (2011) ADAMTS-5 and intervertebral disc degeneration: the results of tissue immunohistochemistry and in vitro cell culture. J Orthop Res 29:718–725

Imaging Modalities for Studying Disc Pathology

12

Ari Borthakur and Ravinder Reddy

Contents

A. Borthakur, PhD (✉) • R. Reddy, PhD
Department of Radiology,
Center for Magnetic Resonance and Optical Imaging,
Perelman School of Medicine at the
University of Pennsylvania,
B1 Stellar-Chance Laboratories,
422 Curie Boulevard, Philadelphia, PA 19104-6100, USA
e-mail: borthaku@upenn.edu; URL: http://med.cmroi.upenn.edu,
krr@upenn.edu

I.M. Shapiro, M.V. Risbud (eds.), *The Intervertebral Disc*,
DOI 10.1007/978-3-7091-1535-0_12, © Springer-Verlag Wien 2014

12.1 Introduction

Low back pain is the second most frequent reason for a physician visit and permanently disables more than 5 million Americans with annual costs of $100 billion in the USA (Sheehan 2010; Chou et al. 2007). While not well understood, it is widely accepted that degenerative disc disease of the intervertebral disc contributes directly to axial back pain (Deyo 2002). With degeneration, alterations in matrix composition, structure, and mechanical loading occur in a progressive cascade that leads to tissue breakdown and pain. It would not be unreasonable to surmise that (1) aging alone does not account for degenerative disc disease since that would imply that all older people have painful discs and (2) success of treatment strategies aimed at halting the progression of degenerative disc disease-related chronic back pain will benefit from noninvasive methods to detect early changes in discs undergoing transition down the cascade.

New imaging technologies (Sheehan 2010) have proven useful for surgical planning and to categorize patients into those with radiculopathy (nerve root pain) and stenosis (spinal pathology). However, the majority of chronic low back pain patients fall into a third category, nonspecific low back pain, where no specific pathology can be identified, and consequently, the use of advanced imaging has not been shown to improve outcomes (Chou et al. 2007). In some cases, imaging can increase the identification of incidental findings that can trigger a cascade of diagnostic procedures or treatments that can be costly and may be riskier to the patient (Deyo 2002; Lurie et al. 2000). Consequently, current consensus recommends against the routine use of advanced imaging except in cases of suspected serious pathology and when conservative care is unsuccessful (Rubinstein and van Tulder 2008; Koes et al. 2010).

Mixed pathologies are common in degenerative disc disease, challenging the clinician's ability to identify the single or dominant pathology responsible for the patient's pain. Hence, reducing the chances for unnecessary and unsuccessful treatment will require a shift from the traditional approach of detecting and diagnosing specific types of late-stage disc pathology based on the clinical phenotype of back pain to one that includes the detection of the responsible pathology as part of the diagnostic inclusion criteria. To this end, noninvasive imaging methods have the potential to increase diagnostic certainty, particularly during the initial stage of disc degeneration, and to provide information about disease activity that can be used to measure treatment efficacy in clinical trials.

What follows are highlights of novel MRI-based imaging tools that may localize functional attributes specific to pathological disc degeneration rather than simply anatomical features readily visualized in conventional MRI, X-ray, or CT imaging. The novel approaches not only would detect painful spinal levels but also could sensitively monitor new and experimental therapies aimed at preventing or repairing diseased disc tissue. We begin with a description of the degenerative changes amenable to targeting with imaging biomarkers.

12.2 Targeting Degenerative Disc Disease

The early stage of degenerative disc disease is characterized by loss of proteoglycan in the nucleus pulposus resulting in reduced capacity to bind water and a loss of hydration and pressure in the disc (Antoniou et al. 1996; Sieber and Kostuik 2004). In its late stages, degenerative disc disease is characterized by a loss of disc height, annular tears and rim lesions, and osteophyte formation (Andersson 1998). It has been implicated as a potential source of low back pain (Erkintalo et al. 1995; Luoma et al. 2000; Urban and Maroudas 1979). Marked compositional changes also occur with degeneration: water and proteoglycan content decrease, proteoglycan distribution changes, total collagen content increases, and the distribution of collagen types changes (Eyre 1979; Roberts et al. 1991; Antoniou et al. 1996; Nerlich et al. 1998). The earliest structural degenerative changes occur in the nucleus pulposus and the endplate (Buckwalter et al. 2000; Boos et al. 2002). As early as the teenage years, the nucleus pulposus exhibits granular changes, clefts, tears, and cell death (Boos et al. 2002). The moderately fibrous nucleus pulposus during this time period is intact with no tears (Yu et al. 1989). At this same early age, proteoglycan of the nucleus pulposus begins to form clusters of short aggregated and non-aggregated molecules, the glycosaminoglycan content decreases, and the water content falls (Antoniou et al. 1996; Buckwalter et al. 2000). Mechanically, the nucleus pulposus is the first substructure to exhibit degenerative changes. Its increased modulus and decreased hydrostatic pressure result in a phase change from a fluidlike gel to a more solid-like material (Urban and McMullin 1988; Iatridis et al. 1997; Johannessen and Elliott 2005). With increasing age and degeneration, the granular changes, mucoid degeneration, clefts and tears, and decaying cells are seen with increasing frequency throughout the disc (Boos et al. 2002). Mechanical function of degenerated motion segments is compromised in all loading categories (Goel 1996; Pope 1992). However, predicting mechanical changes with degeneration is complicated because motion segment stiffness tends to decrease with moderate degeneration and increase with advanced degeneration under all loading conditions (Berkson et al. 1979; Fujiwara et al. 2000; Haughton et al. 2000; Reuber et al. 1982).

Pathologic, painful degeneration can occur when matrix damage at disc margins exceeds the body's ability to heal, thereby inciting a wound reaction. Increased production of growth factors such as fibroblast growth factor, insulin-like growth factor, and platelet-derived growth factor within annular fissures can encourage granulation tissue formation (Pratsinis and Kletsas 2008). Inflammatory stimulation of disc cells causes secretion of neurotrophic factors, such as nerve growth factor and brain-derived neurotrophic factor that, along with decreases in proteoglycan, encourage neoinnervation and neovascularization at the vertebral endplate and peripheral annulus (Purmessur et al. 2008). Inflammatory and neurotrophic factors may diffuse into the adjacent vertebra through endplate fissures leading to bone marrow edema (Ulrich et al. 2007; Crock 1986; Brown et al. 1997; Ohtori et al. 2006). Endplate and annular nociceptors can be further sensitized by release of pro-inflammatory cell products, such as TNF-alpha or lactic acid (Olmarker et al. 1995).

12.3 Radiographic Imaging

The main objective of imaging the intervertebral disc is to provide the physician with a classification scheme that provides information concerning treatment options. The ideal classification system for disc degeneration is quantitative, permits region-specific evaluation within the disc substructures, avoids observer bias, can detect early subtle changes, and correlates with clinical symptoms. X-ray radiographic detection of disc degeneration via the Thompson grading scale (Thompson et al. 1990) is the most common clinical method in use but can only detect gross morphological deformities. Moreover, it does not depict soft tissues clearly and requires the injection of contrast agents to detect subtle disc abnormalities such as fissures.

12.4 Computed Tomography

Computed tomography (CT) discography has been used to improve surgical outcome (Tehranzadeh 1998). However, it is an invasive technique due to its use of radiation and some cases require the placement of needle and injection of a contrast agent through the annular fibers; a further drawback to its use is the high incidence of false positives (An and Haughton 1993). While CT can accurately visualize disc morphology, it fails to distinguish findings that are symptomatic from those that are incidental. Related to these problems, CT fails to demonstrate the cause of pain in patients without obvious nerve root compression. "Dynamic" CT can be employed to accurately measure ranges of motion of vertebrae when a load or torque is applied, in vivo. This technique is made possible due to the advent of high-speed capability and image processing tools in CT scanners (Haughton 2004).

12.5 MRI Methods to Investigate Spinal Morphology

MRI with its exquisite soft tissue contrast has tremendous potential for characterizing disc quality through morphological and functional parameters. In conventional (T_2-weighted) MR images, the nucleus pulposus appears bright and the annulus fibrosus is invisible due to its short T_2 in the normal disc. Degeneration can be qualitatively graded by quantifying the reduction in signal intensity of the nucleus pulposus (Modic et al. 1984), while in advance stages of degeneration, there is no clear distinction between nucleus and annulus. The widely used classification system of Pfirrmann (Pfirrmann et al. 2001) is based on T_2-weighted MR images. An integer grade (between I and V) is assigned to the disc, based on structural morphology (e.g., homogeneity within the nucleus pulposus, distinction between the nucleus and annulus, signal intensity, and disc height). Although this classification system is among the most widely accepted and used (Kettler and Wilke 2005) and provides excellent detection of advanced stage degeneration, integer-based classification systems cannot discriminate among early degenerative changes (Bertagnoli and Kumar 2002; Luoma et al. 2001). Moreover, these classification systems are qualitative, are susceptible to observer bias, and are not specific for disc substructures. As there is little correlation with presence or severity of clinical symptoms, its usefulness in clinical decision-making is dependent on correlating Pfirrmann grades with other clinical and radiographic findings.

To improve the capability of MRI-based methods to objectively quantify disc degeneration, several studies have measured T_1 and T_2 relaxation times and the diffusion coefficient of water. In *ex vivo* disc specimens (Chatani et al. 1993; Weidenbaum et al. 1992; Chiu et al. 2001), correlations were observed between T_2 and water content and significant differences noted in relaxation rates between the human nucleus and annulus fibrosus (Marinelli et al. 2009). And although an in vivo study (Jenkins et al. 1985) found no correlation between proton density and age, there were significant differences in T_1 and T_2 between normal and degenerated discs. However, a later study (Boos et al. 1994) showed that the differences were only 196 ms for T_1 and 15 ms for T_2 and reproducibility for the measurements were low, at 16.4 and 13.4 %, respectively. Diurnal variations in T_2 due to changing water content from morning to evening in the same individual would further confound the T_2 measurements. However, quantitative T_2 measurements may have a clinical relevance, for example, if diurnal differences were present between cohorts of patients with back pain and asymptomatic controls (Roberts et al. 1998). Indeed, significant decreases in these parameters were observed in both human nucleus and annulus fibrosus compartments with increase in Thompson grade and loading in disc specimens (Chiu et al. 2001). A decrease in the diffusion of water in the nucleus was detected by diffusion-weighted MRI with reduction of proteoglycan *ex vivo* (Antoniou et al. 2004) and with degeneration in vivo compared to healthy controls (Kerttula et al. 2001; Kealey et al. 2005). However, diffusion-weighted MR images suffer from low SNR and resolution and are susceptible to motion artifacts and difficult to reproduce measurements in vivo.

Box 12.1 What Is MRI?

Magnetic resonance imaging is a diagnostic imaging method that uses radiofrequency (RF) waves to excite and detect a magnetic signal from the human body. The MRI system consists of a scanner that produces a strong magnetic field in order to magnetize hydrogen nuclei of water in tissues. The MRI scanner is typically cylindrical shaped and also contains magnetic gradient coils that can be electronically controlled to alter the main magnetic field. A computer-controlled console has several "pulse sequence" software to dynamically manipulate the RF and gradient fields so that the subsequently detected MRI signal can be spatially encoded. The MR "image" is simply a computer-processed "map" of hydrogen nuclei in tissues. The 2003 Nobel Prize in physiology or medicine was awarded to Paul Lauterbur, of the University of Illinois, and Sir Peter Mansfield, of the University of Nottingham, for their invention of MRI.

Unlike other imaging modalities like X-rays, computed tomography (CT), and positron emission tomography (PET), MRI uses no ionizing radiation and, hence, is ideally suited for clinical research.

MRI scanners differ in field strength, shape, dimensions, and bore size. Clinical scanners found in hospitals are typically 1.5T or 3T, in units of magnetic field strength (tesla), while a few research centers now have 7T whole-body scanners. The higher field strength produces more magnetization and could potentially generate higher quality images. There are open-bore scanners that are more comfortable for some patients but come at the cost of lower field strength. Smaller bore scanners used for small animal imaging typically attain higher field strengths (4.7T and 9.4T) and are a more cost-effective option than clinical scanners.

Variations in T_1, T_2, T_2*, and $T_1\rho$ *relaxation time constants* produce different MRI signal decay and recovery characteristics in different tissues. A MRI technician will utilize predefined *protocols* to generate several images during a single scan session. The protocols manipulate parameters in the MRI pulse sequence in order to create images with different contrasts to fulfill the clinical diagnostic or research study requirements.

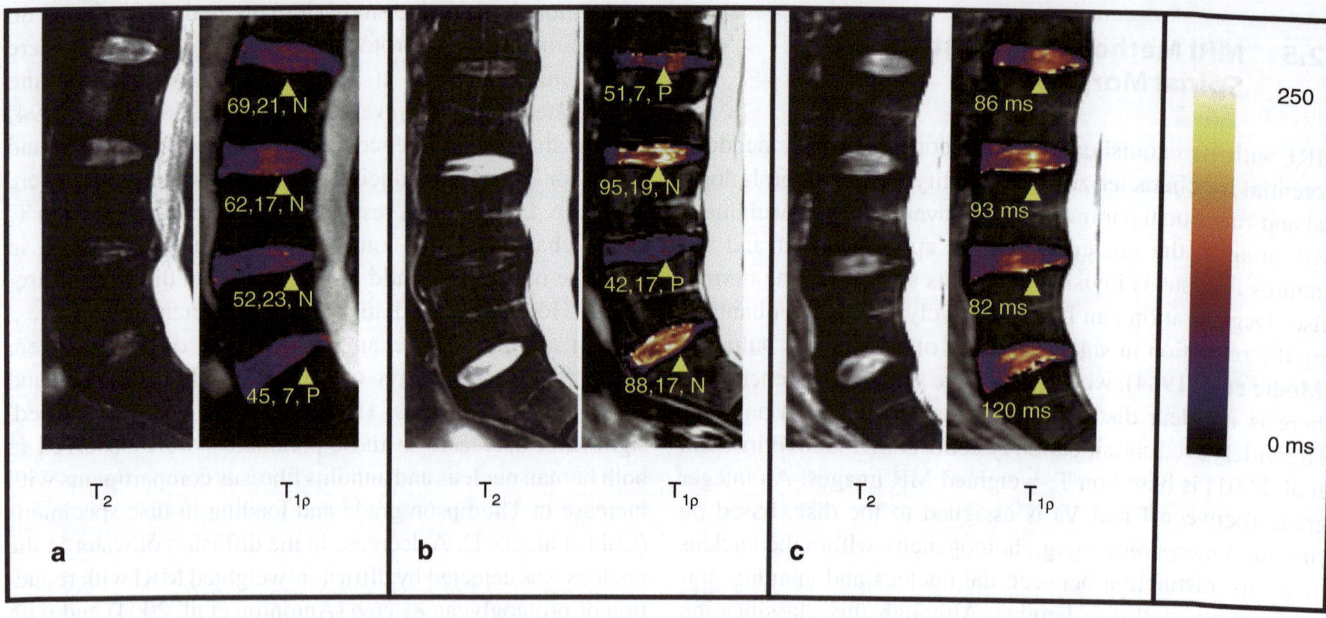

Fig. 12.1 Representative proton T2 MRI (grayscale) and corresponding T1ρ maps (in color overlaid on grayscale T1ρ-weighted image) of the lumbar discs from a 52-year-old female (**a**) and a 35-year-old male (**b**) patients diagnosed with low back pain and from an asymptomatic 38-year-old male (**c**). Average T1ρ (in ms) was measured in the disc nucleus and is displayed below each disc, followed by the opening pressure (in psi) and whether discs were painful (*P*) or non-painful (*N*), both determined by discography are indicated in the lower back pain patients (Borthakur et al. 2011). This data demonstrates the potential for noninvasive $T_{1\rho}$ measurements as a surrogate measure of disc pressure in the clinics

12.6 Biochemistry-Based MRI Techniques

A major drawback of the MRI methods discussed above is that while they effectively detect morphological changes in the disc, they lack sensitivity at the early stages of disc degeneration. Since changes in nucleus pulposus and annulus fibrosus composition and structure are the earliest changes in degenerative disc disease, the newer MRI-based methods have approached the diagnostic process by attempting to detect and quantify the biochemical composition of the extracellular matrix of the disc. The following techniques have evolved over the last few years by several research groups for eventual clinical application.

12.6.1 T_{1P} MRI

Tumors, muscle, myocardium, blood flow, and cartilage have been imaged using $T_{1\rho}$("T-1-rho") (Santyr et al. 1989; Lamminen et al. 1993; Dixon et al. 1996; Markkola et al. 1997; Charagundla et al. 1998; Mlynarik et al. 1999; Grohn et al. 2000; Poptani et al. 2001; Duvvuri et al. 2001; Borthakur et al. 2004; Wheaton et al. 2004; Hulvershorn et al. 2005). $T_{1\rho}$ MRI is an alternative to conventional T_1 and T_2 MRI (Borthakur et al. 2006) in which a long-duration, low-power radiofrequency (RF) referred to as "spin-lock" (SL) pulse is applied to the magnetization in the transverse plane (Fig. 12.1). The spin-locked magnetization undergoes

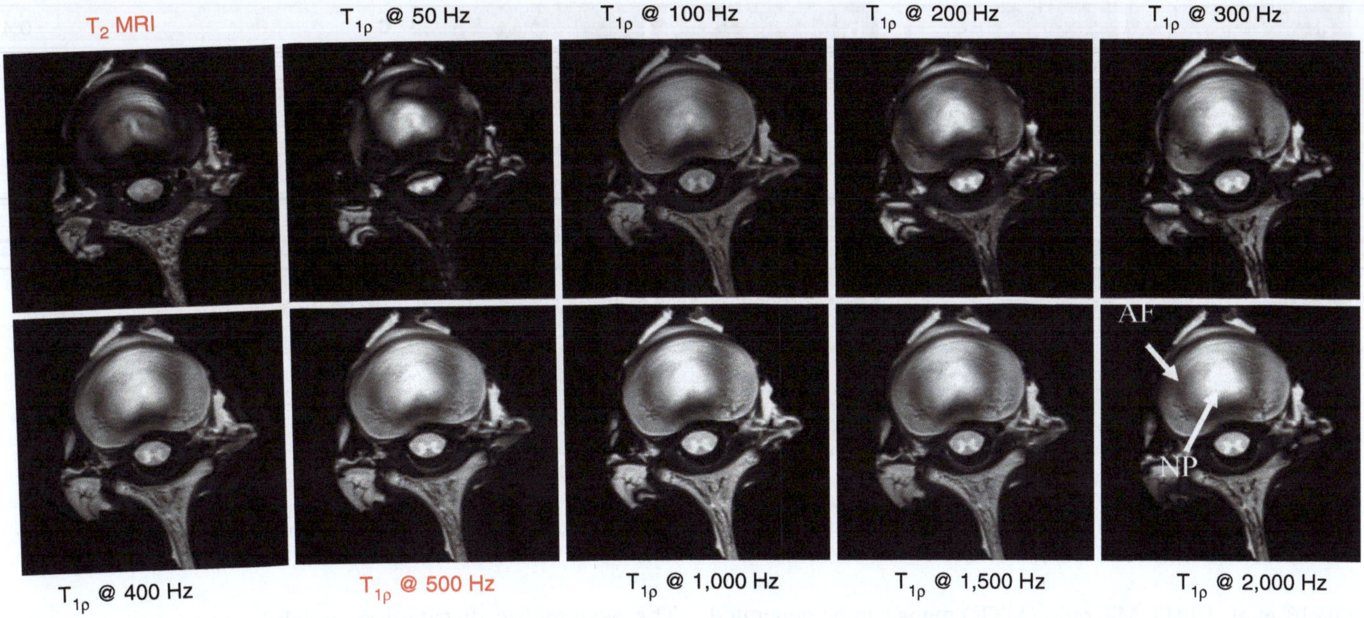

Fig. 12.2 Increased MRI signal was observed in the annulus fibrosus region in bovine disc specimens compared to T2 MRI (image in the *top left*) by increasing the spin-lock frequency of the T1ρ MRI pulse sequence. The qualitative difference between T2 and T1ρ images, especially in the annulus fibrosus, at the standard operating frequency of 500 Hz for clinical T1ρ MRI protocol is clearly visible. T1ρ MRI provides a twofold higher signal in the nucleus pulposus and fourfold higher in the annulus fibrosus compared to T2 MRI

relaxation in the presence of a RF field (B_1) in the rotating frame, a situation similar to that of the longitudinal magnetization in the main magnetic (B_0) field. The spin-locked magnetization will relax with a time constant $T_{1\rho}$, called the spin–lattice relaxation in the rotating frame, during the B_1 field which attenuates the effect of signal loss mechanisms (i.e., dipolar relaxation, static dipolar coupling, chemical exchange, and background gradients) on the MRI signal (Borthakur et al. 2006). For this reason, $T_{1\rho}$ is always greater than T_2. In a typical $T_{1\rho}$ mapping experiment, the duration of the SL pulse is incremented while the amplitude of SL pulse ($\gamma B_1 \sim 0.1$-few kHz) is fixed. $T_{1\rho}$ MRI has recently been used as a biomarker for degenerative disc disease with low values correlating with higher degeneration, low proteoglycan content, and reduced swelling pressure in the nucleus pulposus (Johannessen et al. 2006; Auerbach et al. 2006; Nguyen et al. 2008; Wang et al. 2010b; Borthakur et al. 2011).

Since annular fissures can be innervated, degeneration of the annulus fibrosus may be the source of back pain in patients with degenerative disc disease (Peng et al. 2006). Unfortunately, due to the non-averaged dipolar interaction of water bound to highly oriented collagen fibers, which shorten T_2, the annulus appears dark in conventional MRI. The effect of spin-locking on the laminar appearance of cartilage in MRI, using orientation-dependent studies, indicated that when the normal to the surface of cartilage was parallel to B_0, a typical laminar appearance was present in T_2-weighted images but was absent in $T_{1\rho}$-weighted images of the same specimen (Akella et al. 2004). At the "magic angle" orientation (when the surface normal was 54.7° with respect to B_0), neither T_2 nor $T_{1\rho}$ images demonstrated laminae. However, $T_{1\rho}$ values were greater than T_2 at both orientations throughout the cartilage layers.

In experiments on a bovine disc specimen (Fig. 12.2), we noted that the annulus signal could be enhanced by simply increasing the spin-lock frequency of the $T_{1\rho}$ MRI pulse sequence compared to T_2 MRI (image in the top left). The qualitative difference between T_2 and $T_{1\rho}$ images, especially in the annulus fibrosus, at the standard operating frequency of 500 Hz for clinical $T_{1\rho}$ MRI protocol is obvious. $T_{1\rho}$ MRI provides 2-fold higher signal in the nucleus and 4-fold higher in the annulus compared to T_2 MRI. This approach serves as a method to overcome MRI signal loss mechanisms. The measurement of $T_{1\rho}$ as a function of the B_1 amplitude is known as "$T_{1\rho}$-dispersion" and contrast is governed by the spectral density components of the sample that are in the neighborhood of γB_1. While the literature on the contributors to $T_{1\rho}$ dispersion in cartilage is sparse, the data in Fig. 12.2 clearly supports the notion that the non-averaged dipolar interaction between water protons associated with collagen is the predominant contributor.

12.6.2 Magnetization Transfer (MT) MRI

The MT pulse sequence employs a pulse to selectively saturate magnetization, and hence the MRI signal, from water bound to macromolecules such as collagen

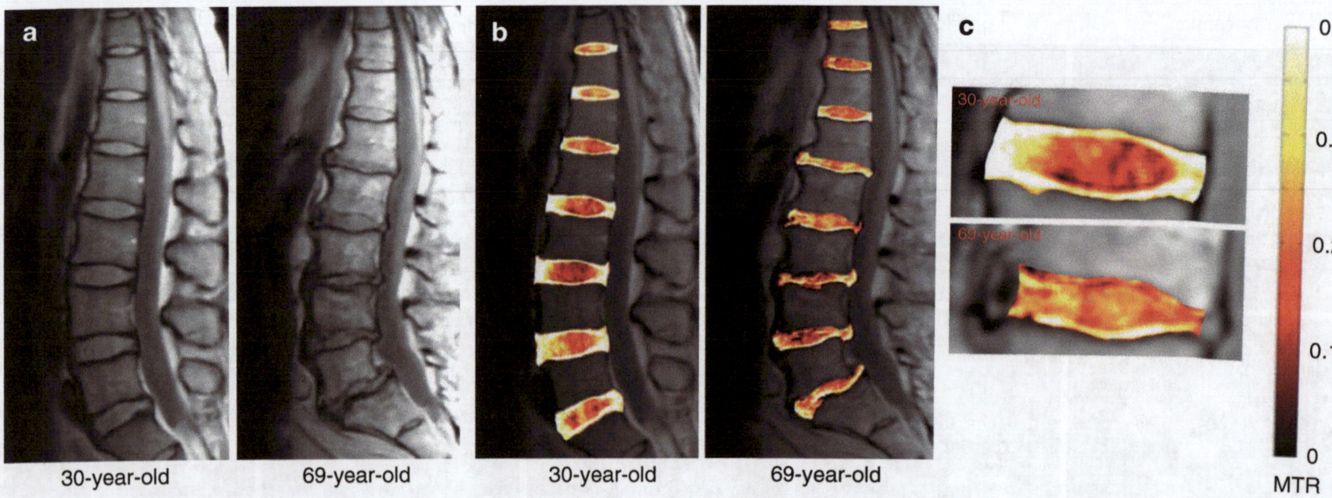

Fig. 12.3 (**a**) Proton-density MRI of a 30-year-old healthy and a 69-year-old asymptomatic subject. (**b**) MTR map (in color), (**c**) MTR maps of the L3/L2 disc (Wang et al. 2010c)

(Wolff et al. 1991). MT ratio (MTR) maps can be generated from two images that are collected, with MT preparation (M_s) and without (M_0). These maps are generated by setting the off-resonance saturation pulse at 6.4 kHz down field of the free water proton resonance frequency (Fig. 12.3). Differences in lumbar discs can be seen in the proton-density MRI of a 30-year-old healthy individual and a 69-year-old asymptomatic subject who exhibits decreased disc height, loss of nucleus pulposus hydration, as well as herniation in the lower lumbar discs. The corresponding MTR maps (in color) showed increased values in the nucleus pulposus of the 69-year-old subject, while there is a clear delineation of the annulus fibrosus-nucleus pulposus boundary in the 30-year-old subject. High MTR values (in white) indicate intact collagen in the annulus fibrosus of the younger individual. A closer look at the MTR maps of the L3/L2 disc, for example, demonstrates a distinct boundary between MTR values within the nucleus pulposus and annulus fibrosus of the 30-year-old subject, while it is diffuse in the 69-year-old subject, indicating a loss of collagen architecture in the annulus and deposition of collagen into the nucleus (Wang et al. 2010c).

12.6.3 Chemical Exchange Saturation Transfer (CEST) MRI

Chemical exchange saturation transfer (CEST) is a method to directly detect exchangeable solute protons in tissues by constant irradiation and saturation of their chemically shifted magnetization (Ward et al. 2000; Ward and Balaban 2000). The CEST signal is detected as a reduction in the water signal after the saturated spins undergo chemical exchange with water (Forsen and Hoffman 1963), provided that the exchange is more rapid than the T_1 of either site. The asymmetric distribution of labile protons around the central water peak in cartilage is readily detected in the difference image obtained after saturating symmetrically on either side of the water. A very homogeneous B_0 is necessary for a robust estimation of the difference signal. Furthermore, care must also be taken to avoid the direct saturation of the water peak due to the close resonances of labile species of interest.

In spite of these stringent requirements, solutes in the nanomolar to millimolar range have been reliably detected using this approach in vitro (Aime et al. 1988; Zhang et al. 2001; Goffeney et al. 2001; Gilad et al. 2007) and in vivo (Zhou et al. 2003; van Zijl et al. 2007). The feasibility of CEST MRI to reliably detect glycosaminoglycan (GAG) in vivo was recently demonstrated in the cartilage of the knee joint (Schmitt et al. 2011) by comparing it with sodium MRI of the same joint and in the disc by Kim et al. (Fig. 12.4) utilizing a new water frequency mapping approach called "water saturation shift referencing" (WASSR), which provides a more accurate quantification of CEST effects (Kim et al. 2011). However, the "gagCEST" approach (Ling et al. 2008) should be limited to high-field scanners such as 7T since –OH protons in cartilage are only 1 ppm downfield from the water resonance and exchange at a rate of ~1,000 s^{-1} (Schiller et al. 2001). Hence, the –OH chemical shift is only 129 Hz at 3FT and CEST MRI would introduce a substantial direct water saturation. Further, the slow to intermediate exchange limit (i.e., chemical shift between exchanging site and water, $\Delta\omega >$ exchange rate, k), required for optimal CEST effect, is not fulfilled in the case of –OH protons at 3T. However, at 7T and higher fields, the larger frequency separation of –OH resonance from water fulfills both the ($\Delta\omega > k$) condition and also reduces the direct water saturation effect enabling a more reliable quantification of GAG at 7T using the gagCEST approach (Schmitt et al. 2011).

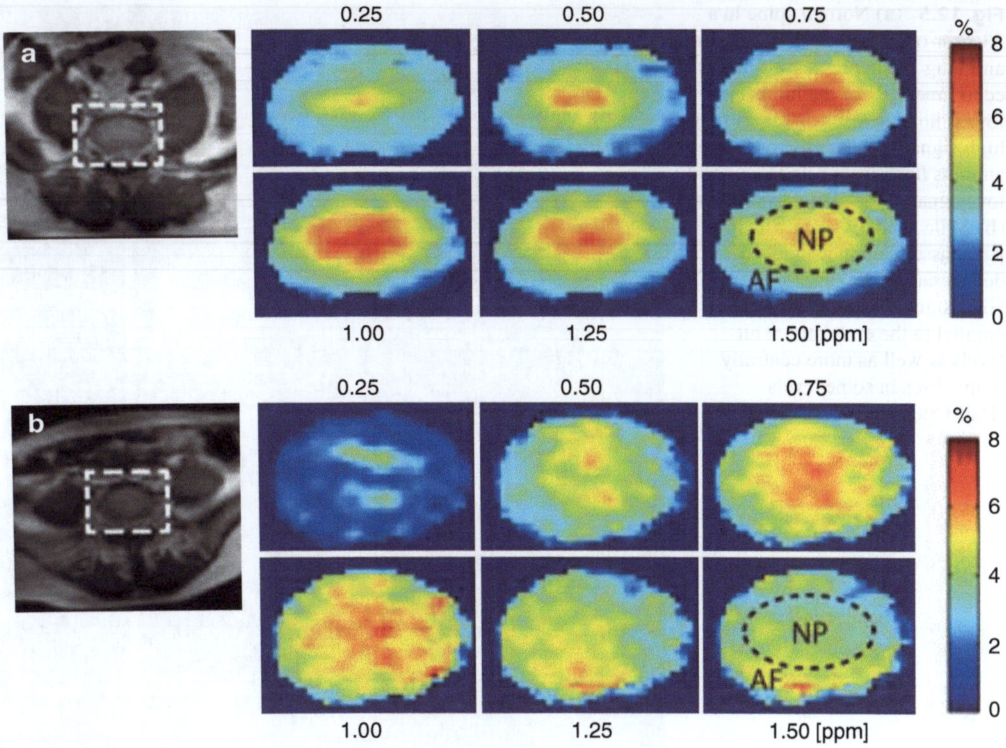

Fig. 12.4 Representative water saturation shift referencing (WASSR)-corrected glycosaminoglycan chemical exchange saturation transfer (gagCEST) maps of intervertebral disc (IVD) (*zoomed*) in two subjects: (**a**) 25-year-old woman at L5/S1 and (**b**) 54-year-old man at L5/S1. The gagCEST maps are shown at 0.25, 0.5, 0.75, 1, 1.25, and 1.5 ppm. The broken circle inside the map at 1.5 ppm shows an approximation of the nucleus pulposus (*NP*) and annulus fibrosus (*AF*) regions. In both subjects, the gagCEST effect is highest in the 0.75–1 ppm frequency range (Kim et al. 2011)

12.6.4 Ultrashort Echo Time (UTE) MRI

The vertebral endplate is composed of an inner bony and outer cartilaginous endplates. This endplate is the route for nutrient and metabolite supply to the avascular disc and is involved in metabolism, exchange of waste products, and biomechanics of the disc (Urban and Winlove 2007). It has previously been hypothesized that changes in disc mechanics may be initiated by damage to the endplate (Adams and Roughley 2006). Hence, visualizing morphological defects in the endplate could facilitate diagnosis of the cause of disc degeneration.

However, it appears dark on T_2, endplate integrity is not discernable by conventional T_2 MRI. This is due to a strong dipolar interaction experienced by protons in water bound to collagen resulting in short T_2s (~1–10 ms). The UTE MRI pulse sequence overcomes this impediment by one of the two methods, selecting the short T_2 components with RF pulses or combining images acquired at different echo times effectively producing a MRI of only the short T_2 species (Robson et al. 2003). There are several methods to perform UTE MRI on clinical scanners. Some employ a narrow bandwidth excitation RF pulse to selectively nutate long T_2 components into the transverse plane, where they are nominally de-phased by gradients, leaving the short T_2 components largely unaffected (Sussman et al. 1998; Larson et al. 2006). Other methods combine pairs of images such as those obtained by a half RF excitation, with and without gradient reversal, followed by radial imaging (Gatehouse and Bydder 2003). The later method has been employed to visualize the collagen-rich annulus fibrosus in human discs (Hall-Craggs et al. 2004) in which patients with the most severe degeneration show irregular signal from the endplates compared to normal; however, the reason for this observation is not clear (Fig. 12.5).

12.6.5 Sodium MRI

Based on the fact that Donnan equilibrium holds for cartilage equilibrated in very dilute solutions, Maroudas et al. have shown that the fixed charge density of cartilage is correlated with the proteoglycan content of the extracellular matrix of cartilage (Maroudas et al. 1969). In addition, Gu et al. reported that there was a reduction in the streaming potential (a measurement directly related to the fixed charge density) with intervertebral disc degeneration in tissue specimens (Gu et al. 1999a, b). As the charge density is counterbalanced by Na^+ activity, the loss of the negatively charged PG due to degeneration lowers the fixed charge density in the tissue. Hence, there is a reduction in the concentration of positively charged sodium ions and a lowering tissue osmotic pressure.

Sodium (^{23}Na) is one of the most "NMR-visible" nuclei in living systems. As a spin-3/2 nucleus with a nonzero quadrupolar moment, ^{23}Na exhibits bi-exponential relaxation in tissues, i.e., fast and slow components of T_2 and T_2*. While nonquantitative sodium MRI of the spine has been performed (Insko et al. 2002), Wang et al. (2010a) recently imaged

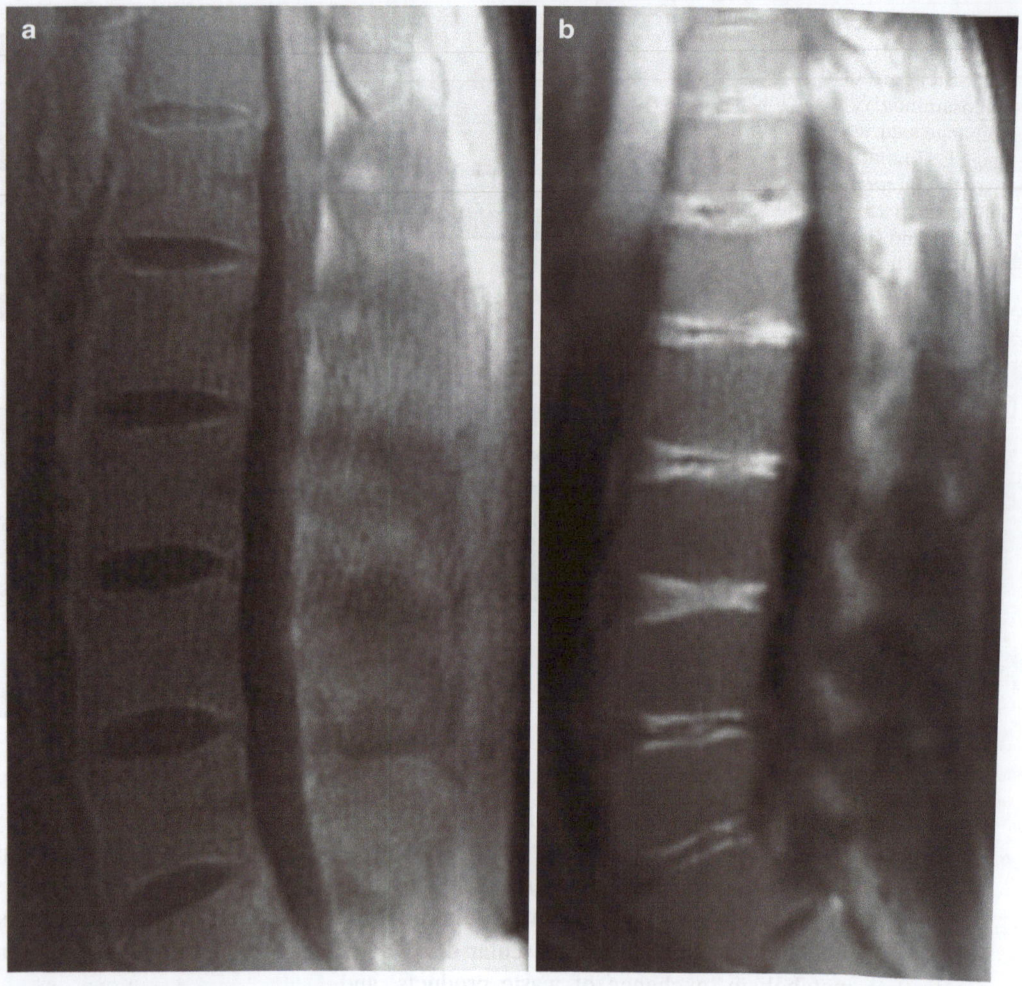

Fig. 12.5 (**a**) Normal spine in a 33-year-old volunteer. Sagittal fat and long T_2-suppressed ultrashort echo time MRI of the lumbar and lower thoracic discs display a faint high signal in the region of the annulus fibrosus and endplates and low signal in the nucleus pulposus. (**b**) Male aged 29 years with β-thalassemia major-induced degenerative disc disease. High-signal bands are observed parallel to the endplates at all levels as well as more centrally in the discs in some levels (Hall-Craggs et al. 2004)

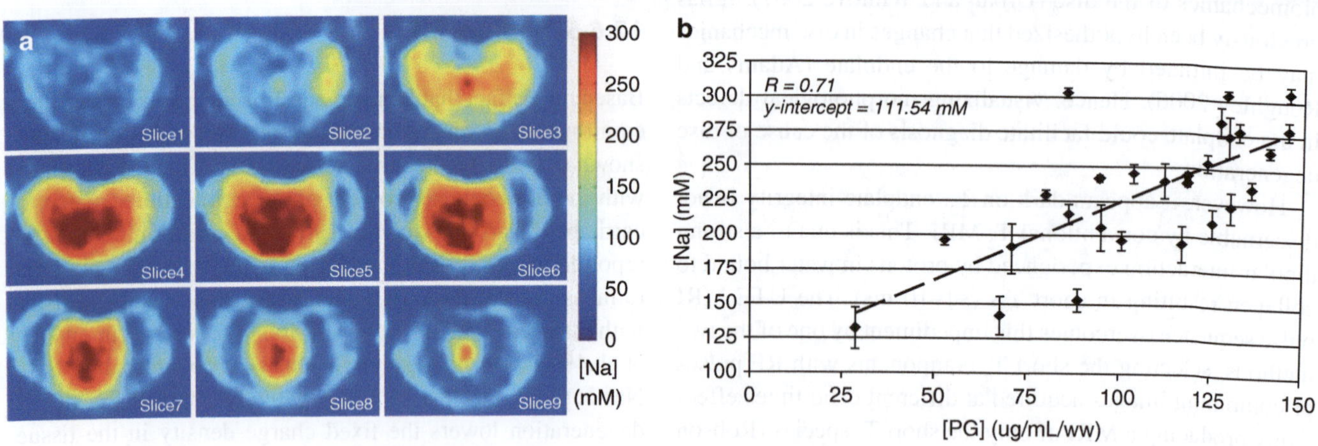

Fig. 12.6 Nine consecutive axial slices of a bovine disc specimen with [Na] ranging from 150 to 300 mM as calculated from sodium MRI (**a**). A plot of [Na] from the nucleus pulposus (NP) correlated well ($r=0.7$) with PG measured by DMMB blue assay (**b**) (Wang et al. 2010a)

sodium in the bovine intervertebral disc and noted a significant correlation with proteoglycans measured by DMMB assay (Fig. 12.6). Subsequent imaging of the human disc in vivo revealed differences in the sodium MRI between an asymptomatic subject and a subject with lower back pain (Fig. 12.7). The lower sodium concentration in both L3–L4 and L4–L5 discs in the patient with back pain indicated a loss of proteoglycan, perhaps an early sign of disc disease.

Due to its low gyromagnetic ratio (γ) and concentrations in tissues, sodium MRI requires field strengths ≥3T to obtain quality images to enable accurate quantification of fixed charge density and proteoglycan. The short T_2 of

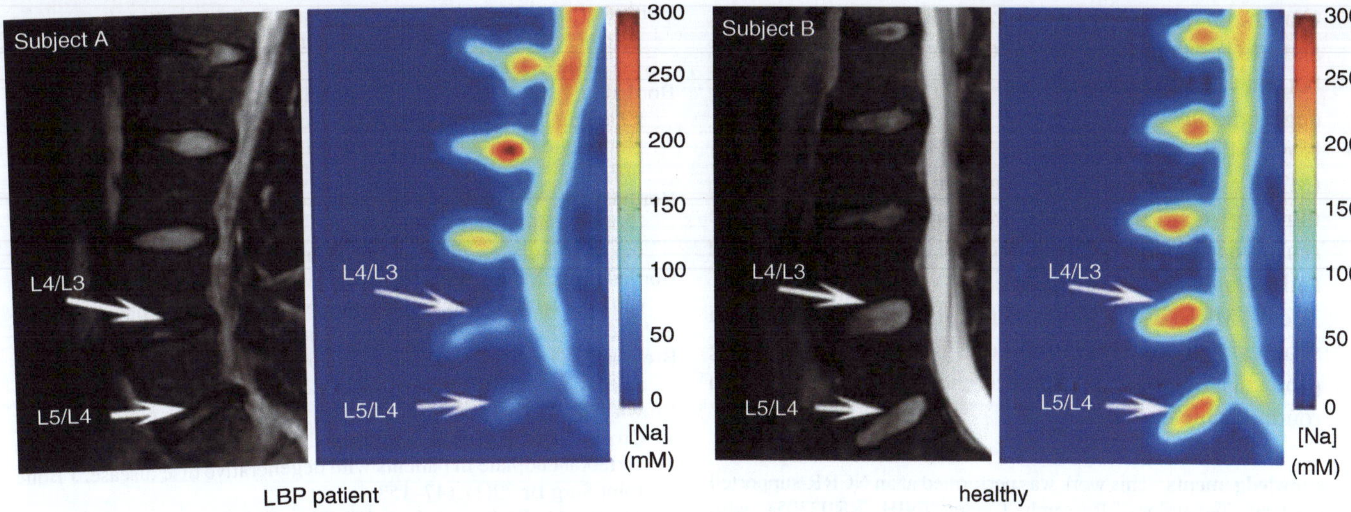

Fig. 12.7 Representative proton T2 MRI (grayscale) and corresponding [Na] maps (color) obtained in vivo on a 22-year-old male with lower lumbar trauma that resulted in chronic lower back pain and a 26-year-old healthy male (Wang et al. 2010a)

^{23}Na (~few ms) indicates that sodium MRI has to be performed with MRI pulse sequences with ultrashort echo times. Since ^{23}Na γ is 1/4 of that of proton, sodium MRI requires 4 times stronger gradients to obtain images with identical resolution to that of proton MRI. Consequently, sodium MRI pulse sequences are forced to image at a long echo time (TE) of ≥2 ms, but again because of the short T_2, substantial MRI signal is lost before acquisition. Recent advances in the development of high-field 7-tesla MRI scanners and gradient technology (with a gradient strength of >4 G/cm) should allow an ultrashort TE (<200 μs) that can significantly improve resolution and signal and provide hope for clinical sodium MRI. Radiofrequency coil technology (multiple channel capability) and parallel imaging approaches such as SENSE (Pruessmann et al. 1999) and SMASH (Sodickson and Manning 1997) and tuned preamplifiers could further contribute to make clinical sodium MRI feasible.

12.7 Path to Clinical Utility

The biochemical-based MRI biomarker technologies discussed here detect subtle molecular events that occur with disc degeneration, and therefore, they are of considerable clinical value. However, there remain some conflicts concerning their use (Lurie et al. 2000), while the natural history of the subtle findings revealed by the new technologies needs careful consideration and study (Deyo 2010). Further, image biomarkers are considerably more complex than biochemical biomarkers, and even if a composite biomarker can be delineated in the future, it is not clear how this would impact disease diagnosis. One potential answer is to utilize statistical and machine-learning algorithms to combine biomarkers to build a classifier suitable for diagnosis (Breiman 1996; Guyon et al. 2002) to answer the question: which approach gives the most timely, reliable, and accurate measurement of the pathological changes due to degenerative disc disease?

The experimental MRI CEST, MT, and $T_{1\rho}$ pulse sequences represent small modification to routine clinical imaging sequences and carry a potential risk of local tissue heating from the RF pulses. A previously validated method has been used to determine that the heat generated both theoretically and experimentally (Borthakur et al. 2003) by these pulse sequences is not in violation of FDA guidelines (Borthakur et al. 2004). Additional safeguards are also built into the scanner software, such that during MRI, the scanner continuously monitors the RF power automatically stopping the scan when FDA-allowed limits are exceeded. This safeguard eliminates the risk associated with any inadvertent errors during the scan. In addition, MRI near metallic implants remains a challenge because of severe image artifacts mainly stemming from large metal-induced field inhomogeneities causing local gradient-induced eddy currents (Guermazi et al. 2003). This is an impediment to routine MRI in back pain patients who have implants, such as pedicle screws, from prior surgery. To meet this challenge, new methods of MRI artifact reduction (Glover 1999; Lu et al. 2009) may need to be incorporated into existing protocols in order to advance these MRI-based biomarker technologies into routine clinical use.

12.8 Summary of Critical Concepts Discussed in the Chapter

- Noninvasive imaging methods have the potential to increase diagnostic certainty and to provide information about disease activity that can be used to measure treatment efficacy in clinical trials.

- Current imaging methods (X-ray, computed tomography, and MRI) can detect morphological changes in the disc, but they lack sensitivity at the early stages of disc degeneration.
- Novel MRI techniques such as $T_{1\rho}$, magnetization transfer (MT), chemical exchange saturation transfer (CEST), ultrashort echo time (UTE) MRI, and sodium MRI are sensitive to matrix macromolecules such as proteoglycan and collagen to varying degrees.
- These MRI-based biomarkers of IVD degeneration should be incorporated into existing research imaging protocols in order to advance these technologies into routine clinical use.

Acknowledgements This work was performed at an NCRR-supported Biomedical Technology Research Center (NIH RR02305) with additional funding from an AOSpine research grant (AOSBRC-07-05).

References

Adams MA, Roughley PJ (2006) What is intervertebral disc degeneration, and what causes it? Spine 31:2151–2161

Aime S, Nano R, Grandi M (1988) A new class of contrast agents for magnetic resonance imaging based on selective reduction of water-T2 by chemical exchange. Invest Radiol 23(Suppl 1):S267–S270

Akella SV, Regatte RR, Wheaton AJ, Borthakur A, Reddy R (2004) Reduction of residual dipolar interaction in cartilage by spin-lock technique. Magn Reson Med 52(5):1103–1109

An HS, Haughton VM (1993) Nondiscogenic lumbar radiculopathy: imaging considerations. Semin Ultrasound CT MR 14(6):414–424

Andersson GB (1998) What are the age-related changes in the spine? Baillieres Clin Rheumatol 12(1):161–173

Antoniou J, Goudsouzian NM, Heathfield TF, Winterbottom N, Steffen T, Poole AR et al (1996) The human lumbar endplate. Evidence of changes in biosynthesis and denaturation of the extracellular matrix with growth, maturation, aging, and degeneration. Spine 21(10):1153–1161

Antoniou J, Demers CN, Beaudoin G, Goswami T, Mwale F, Aebi M et al (2004) Apparent diffusion coefficient of intervertebral discs related to matrix composition and integrity. Magn Reson Imaging 22(7):963–972

Auerbach JD, Johannessen W, Borthakur A, Wheaton AJ, Dolinskas CA, Balderston RA et al (2006) In vivo quantification of human lumbar disc degeneration using T(1rho)-weighted magnetic resonance imaging. Eur Spine J 15(Suppl 3):S338–S344

Berkson MH, Nachemson A, Schultz AB (1979) Mechanical properties of human lumbar spine motion segments – part II: responses in compression and shear; influence of gross morphology. J Biomech Eng 101:53–57

Bertagnoli R, Kumar S (2002) Indications for full prosthetic disc arthroplasty: a correlation of clinical outcome against a variety of indications. Eur Spine J 11(Suppl 2):S131–S136

Boos N, Wallin A, Schmucker T, Aebi M, Boesch C (1994) Quantitative MR imaging of lumbar intervertebral disc and vertebral bodies: methodology, reproducibility, and preliminary results. Magn Reson Imaging 12(4):577–587

Boos N, Weissbach S, Rohrbach H, Weiler C, Spratt KF, Nerlich AG (2002) Classification of age-related changes in lumbar intervertebral discs (2002 Volvo Award in basic science). Spine 27(23): 2631–2644

Borthakur A, Wheaton A, Charagundla SR, Shapiro EM, Regatte RR, Akella SV et al (2003) Three-dimensional T1rho-weighted MRI at 1.5 Tesla. J Magn Reson Imaging 17(6):730–736

Borthakur A, Wheaton AJ, Gougoutas AJ, Akella SV, Regatte RR, Charagundla SR et al (2004) In vivo measurement of T1rho dispersion in the human brain at 1.5 tesla. J Magn Reson Imaging 19(4): 403–409

Borthakur A, Mellon E, Niyogi S, Witschey W, Kneeland JB, Reddy R (2006) Sodium and T1rho MRI for molecular and diagnostic imaging of articular cartilage. NMR Biomed 19(7):781–821

Borthakur A, Maurer PM, Fenty M, Wang C, Berger R, Yoder J et al (2011) T1ρ MRI and discography pressure as novel biomarkers for disc degeneration and low back pain. Spine 36:2190–2196

Breiman L (1996) Heuristics of instability and stabilization in model selection. Ann Statist 24(6):2350–2383

Brown MF, Hukkanen MV, McCarthy ID, Redfern DR, Batten JJ, Crock HV et al (1997) Sensory and sympathetic innervation of the vertebral endplate in patients with degenerative disc disease. J Bone Joint Surg Br 79(1):147–153

Buckwalter JA, Boden SD, Eyre DR, Mow VC, Weidenbaum M (2000) Intervertebral disk aging, degeneration, and herniation. In: Buckwalter JA, Einhorn TA, Simon SR (eds) Orthopaedic basic science. American Academy of Orthopaedic Surgeons, Rosemont

Charagundla SR, Stolpen AH, Leigh JS, Reddy R (1998) Off-resonance proton T1r dispersion imaging of 17O-enriched tissue phantoms. Magn Reson Med 39(4):588–595

Chatani K, Kusaka Y, Mifune T, Nishikawa H (1993) Topographic differences of 1H-NMR relaxation times (T1, T2) in the normal intervertebral disc and its relationship to water content. Spine 18(15):2271–2275

Chiu EJ, Newitt DC, Segal MR, Hu SS, Lotz JC, Majumdar S (2001) Magnetic resonance imaging measurement of relaxation and water diffusion in the human lumbar intervertebral disc under compression in vitro. Spine 26(19):E437–E444

Chou R, Qaseem A, Snow V, Casey D, Cross JT, Shekelle P, Clinical Efficacy Assessment Subcommittee of the American College of Physicians, American College of Physicians, and American Pain Society Low Back Pain Guidelines Panel (2007) Diagnosis and treatment of low back pain: a joint clinical practice guideline from the American College of Physicians and the American Pain Society. Ann Intern Med 147(7):478–491

Crock HV (1986) Internal disc disruption. A challenge to disc prolapse fifty years on. Spine 11(6):650–653

Deyo RA (2002) Cascade effects of medical technology. Annu Rev Public Health 23:23–44

Deyo RA (2010) Treatment of lumbar spinal stenosis: a balancing act. Spine J 10(7):625–627

Dixon WT, Oshinski JN, Trudeau JD, Arnold BC, Pettigrew RI (1996) Myocardial suppression in vivo by spin locking with composite pulses. Magn Reson Med 36(1):90–94

Duvvuri U, Charagundla SR, Kudchodkar SB, Kaufman JH, Kneeland JB, Rizi R et al (2001) Human knee: in vivo T1(rho)-weighted MR imaging at 1.5 T–preliminary experience. Radiology 220(3):822–826

Erkintalo MO, Salminen JJ, Alanen AM, Paajanen HE, Kormano MJ (1995) Development of degenerative changes in the lumbar intervertebral disk: results of a prospective MR imaging study in adolescents with and without low-back pain. Radiology 196(2):529–533

Eyre DR (1979) Biochemistry of the intervertebral disc. Int Rev Connect Tissue Res 8:227–291

Forsen S, Hoffman RA (1963) Study of moderately rapid chemical exchange reactions by means of nuclear magnetic double resonance. J Chem Phys 39:2892–2901

Fujiwara A, Lim TH, An HS, Tanaka N, Jeon CH, Andersson GB et al (2000) The effect of disc degeneration and facet joint osteoarthritis on the segmental flexibility of the lumbar spine. Spine 25(23): 3036–3044

Gatehouse PD, Bydder GM (2003) Magnetic resonance imaging of short T2 components in tissue. Clin Radiol 58(1):1–19

Gilad AA, McMahon MT, Walczak P, Winnard PT, Raman V, van Laarhoven HW et al (2007) Artificial reporter gene providing MRI contrast based on proton exchange. Nat Biotechnol 25(2):217–219

Glover GH (1999) 3D z-shim method for reduction of susceptibility effects in BOLD fMRI. Magn Reson Med 42(2):290–299

Goel VK (1996) Biomechanics of disk herniation and related issues. In: Weinstein JN, Gordon SL (eds) Low back pain: a scientific and clinical overview. American Academy of Orthopaedic Surgeons, Rosemont

Goffeney N, Bulte JW, Duyn J, Bryant LH, van Zijl PC (2001) Sensitive NMR detection of cationic-polymer-based gene delivery systems using saturation transfer via proton exchange. J Am Chem Soc 123(35):8628–8629

Grohn OHJ, Kettunen MI, Makela HI, Penttonen M, Pitkanen A et al (2000) Early detection of irreversible cerebral ischemia in the rat using dispersion of the magnetic resonance imaging relaxation time, T1rho. J Cereb Blood Flow Metab 20(10):1457–1466

Gu WY, Mao XG, Foster RJ, Weidenbaum M, Mow VC, Rawlins BA (1999a) The anisotropic hydraulic permeability of human lumbar anulus fibrosus. Influence of age, degeneration, direction, and water content. Spine 24(23):2449–2455

Gu WY, Mao XG, Rawlins BA, Iatridis JC, Foster RJ, Sun DN et al (1999b) Streaming potential of human lumbar anulus fibrosus is anisotropic and affected by disc degeneration. J Biomech 32(11): 1177–1182

Guermazi A, Miaux Y, Zaim S, Peterfy CG, White D, Genant HK (2003) Metallic artefacts in MR imaging: effects of main field orientation and strength. Clin Radiol 58(4):322–328

Guyon I, Weston J, Barnhill S, Vapnik V (2002) Gene selection for cancer classification using support vector machines. Mach Learn 46(1):389–422

Hall-Craggs MA, Porter J, Gatehouse PD, Bydder GM (2004) Ultrashort echo time (UTE) MRI of the spine in thalassaemia. Br J Radiol 77(914):104–110

Haughton V (2004) Medical imaging of intervertebral disc degeneration: current status of imaging. Spine (Phila Pa 1976) 29(23):2751–2756

Haughton VM, Schmidt TA, Keele K, An HS, Lim TH (2000) Flexibility of lumbar spinal motion segments correlated to type of tears in the annulus fibrosus. J Neurosurg 92(1 Suppl):81–86

Hulvershorn J, Borthakur A, Bloy L, Gualtieri EE, Reddy R, Leigh JS, Elliott MA (2005) T1rho contrast in functional magnetic resonance imaging. Magn Reson Med 54(5):1155–1162

Iatridis JC, Setton LA, Weidenbaum M, Mow VC (1997) Alterations in the mechanical behavior of the human lumbar nucleus pulposus with degeneration and aging. J Orthop Res 15:318–322

Insko EK, Clayton DB, Elliott MA (2002) In vivo sodium MR imaging of the intervertebral disk at 4 T. Acad Radiol 9(7):800–804

Jenkins JP, Hickey DS, Zhu XP, Machin M, Isherwood I (1985) MR imaging of the intervertebral disc: a quantitative study. Br J Radiol 58(692):705–709

Johannessen W, Elliott DM (2005) Effects of degeneration on the biphasic material properties of human nucleus pulposus in confined compression. Spine 30(24):E724–E729

Johannessen W, Auerbach JD, Wheaton AJ, Kurji A, Borthakur A, Reddy R et al (2006) Assessment of human disc degeneration and proteoglycan content using T1rho-weighted magnetic resonance imaging. Spine 31(11):1253–1257

Kealey SM, Aho T, Delong D, Barboriak DP, Provenzale JM, Eastwood JD (2005) Assessment of apparent diffusion coefficient in normal and degenerated intervertebral lumbar disks: initial experience. Radiology 235(2):569–574

Kerttula L, Kurunlahti M, Jauhiainen J, Koivula A, Oikarinen J, Tervonen O (2001) Apparent diffusion coefficients and T2 relaxation time measurements to evaluate disc degeneration. A quantitative MR study of young patients with previous vertebral fracture. Acta Radiol 42(6):585–591

Kettler A, Wilke HJ (2005) Review of existing grading systems for cervical or lumbar disc and facet joint degeneration. Eur Spine J 15:705–718

Kim M, Chan Q, Anthony MP, Cheung KM, Samartzis D, Khong PL (2011) Assessment of glycosaminoglycan distribution in human lumbar intervertebral discs using chemical exchange saturation transfer at 3 T: feasibility and initial experience. NMR Biomed 24:1137–1144

Koes BW, van Tulder M, Lin CW, Macedo LG, McAuley J, Maher C (2010) An updated overview of clinical guidelines for the management of non-specific low back pain in primary care. Eur Spine J 19(12):2075–2094

Lamminen AE, Tanttu JI, Sepponen RE, Pihko H, Korhola OA (1993) T1rho dispersion imaging of diseased muscle tissue. Br J Radiol 66(789):783–787

Larson PE, Gurney PT, Nayak K, Gold GE, Pauly JM, Nishimura DG (2006) Designing long-T2 suppression pulses for ultrashort echo time imaging. Magn Reson Med 56(1):94–103

Ling W, Regatte RR, Navon G, Jerschow A (2008) Assessment of glycosaminoglycan concentration in vivo by chemical exchange-dependent saturation transfer (gagCEST). Proc Natl Acad Sci U S A 105(7):2266–2270

Lu W, Pauly KB, Gold GE, Pauly JM, Hargreaves BA (2009) SEMAC: slice encoding for metal artifact correction in MRI. Magn Reson Med 62(1):66–76

Luoma K, Riihimaki H, Luukkonen R, Raininko R, Viikari-Juntura E, Lamminen A (2000) Low back pain in relation to lumbar disc degeneration. Spine 25(4):487–492

Luoma K, Vehmas T, Riihimaki H, Raininko R (2001) Disc height and signal intensity of the nucleus pulposus on magnetic resonance imaging as indicators of lumbar disc degeneration. Spine 26(6): 680–686

Lurie JD, Gerber PD, Sox HC (2000) Clinical problem-solving. A pain in the back. N Engl J Med 343(10):723–726

Marinelli NL, Haughton VM, Muñoz A, Anderson PA (2009) T2 relaxation times of intervertebral disc tissue correlated with water content and proteoglycan content. Spine (Phila Pa 1976) 34(5):520–524

Markkola AT, Aronen HJ, Paavonen T, Hopsu E, Sipila LM, Tanttu JI, Sepponen RE (1997) T1rho dispersion imaging of head and neck tumors: a comparison to spin lock and magnetization transfer techniques. J Magn Reson Imaging 7(5):873–879

Maroudas A, Muir H, Wingham J (1969) The correlation of fixed negative charge with glycosaminoglycan content of human articular cartilage. Biochim Biophys Acta 177(3):492–500

Mlynarik V, Trattnig S, Huber M, Zembsch A, Imhof H (1999) The role of relaxation times in monitoring proteoglycan depletion in articular cartilage. J Magn Reson Imaging 10(4):497–502

Modic MT, Pavlicek W, Weinstein MA, Boumphrey F, Ngo F, Hardy R et al (1984) Magnetic resonance imaging of intervertebral disk disease. Clinical and pulse sequence considerations. Radiology 152(1):103–111

Nerlich AG, Boos N, Wiest I, Aebi M (1998) Immunolocalization of major interstitial collagen types in human lumbar intervertebral discs of various ages. Virchows Arch 432(1):67–76

Nguyen AM, Johannessen W, Yoder JH, Wheaton AJ, Vresilovic EJ, Borthakur A et al (2008) Noninvasive quantification of human nucleus pulposus pressure with use of T1rho-weighted magnetic resonance imaging. J Bone Joint Surg Am 90(4):796–802

Ohtori S, Inoue G, Ito T, Koshi T, Ozawa T, Doya H et al (2006) Tumor necrosis factor-immunoreactive cells and PGP 9.5-immunoreactive nerve fibers in vertebral endplates of patients with discogenic low back Pain and Modic Type 1 or Type 2 changes on MRI. Spine 31(9):1026–1031

Olmarker K, Blomquist J, Strömberg J, Nannmark U, Thomsen P, Rydevik B (1995) Inflammatogenic properties of nucleus pulposus. Spine 20(6):665–669

Peng B, Hao J, Hou S, Wu W, Jiang D, Fu X et al (2006) Possible pathogenesis of painful intervertebral disc degeneration. Spine 31(5):560–566

Pfirrmann CW, Metzdorf A, Zanetti M, Hodler J, Boos N (2001) Magnetic resonance classification of lumbar intervertebral disc degeneration. Spine 26(17):1873–1878

Pope MH (1992) Intervertebral disk: mechanical changes that occur with age. In: Buckwalter JA, Goldberg VM, Woo SLY (eds) Musculoskeletal soft-tissue aging: impact on mobility. American Academy of Orthopaedic Surgeons, Rosemont

Poptani H, Duvvuri U, Miller CG, Mancuso A, Charagundla S, Fraser NW et al (2001) T1rho imaging of murine brain tumors at 4 T. Acad Radiol 8(1):42–47

Pratsinis H, Kletsas D (2008) Growth factors in intervertebral disc homeostasis. Connect Tissue Res 49(3):273–276

Pruessmann KP, Weiger M, Scheidegger MB, Boesiger P (1999) SENSE: sensitivity encoding for fast MRI. Magn Reson Med 42(5):952–962

Purmessur D, Freemont AJ, Hoyland JA (2008) Expression and regulation of neurotrophins in the nondegenerate and degenerate human intervertebral disc. Arthritis Res Ther 10(4):R99

Reuber M, Schultz A, Denis F, Spencer D (1982) Bulging of lumbar intervertebral discs. J Biomech Eng 104:187–192

Roberts S, Menage J, Duance V, Wotton S, Ayad S (1991) Collagen types around the cells of the intervertebral disc and cartilage end plate: an immunolocalization study (1991 Volvo Award in basic sciences). Spine 16(9):1030–1038

Roberts N, Hogg D, Whitehouse GH, Dangerfield P (1998) Quantitative analysis of diurnal variation in volume and water content of lumbar intervertebral discs. Clin Anat 11(1):1–8

Robson MD, Gatehouse PD, Bydder M, Bydder GM (2003) Magnetic resonance: an introduction to ultrashort TE (UTE) imaging. J Comput Assist Tomogr 27(6):825–846

Rubinstein SM, van Tulder M (2008) A best-evidence review of diagnostic procedures for neck and low-back pain. Best Pract Res Clin Rheumatol 22(3):471–482

Santyr GE, Henkelman RM, Bronskill MJ (1989) Spin locking for magnetic resonance imaging with application to human breast. Magn Reson Med 12(1):25–37

Schiller J, Naji L, Huster D, Kaufmann J, Arnold K (2001) 1H and 13C HR-MAS NMR investigations on native and enzymatically digested bovine nasal cartilage. MAGMA 13(1):19–27

Schmitt B, Zbyn S, Stelzeneder D, Jellus V, Paul D, Lauer L et al (2011) Cartilage quality assessment by using glycosaminoglycan chemical exchange saturation transfer and Na MR imaging at 7 T. Radiology 260:257–264

Sheehan NJ (2010) Magnetic resonance imaging for low back pain: indications and limitations. Ann Rheum Dis 69(1):7–11

Sieber AN, Kostuik JP (2004) Concepts in nuclear replacement. Spine J 4(6 Suppl):322S–324S

Sodickson DK, Manning WJ (1997) Simultaneous acquisition of spatial harmonics (SMASH): fast imaging with radiofrequency coil arrays. Magn Reson Med 38(4):591–603

Sussman MS, Pauly JM, Wright GA (1998) Design of practical T2-selective RF excitation (TELEX) pulses. Magn Reson Med 40(6):890–899

Tehranzadeh J (1998) Discography 2000. Radiol Clin North Am 36(3):463–495

Thompson JP, Pearce RH, Schechter MT, Adams ME, Tsang IK, Bishop PB (1990) Preliminary evaluation of a scheme for grading the gross morphology of the human intervertebral disc. Spine 15(5):411–415

Ulrich JA, Liebenberg EC, Thuillier DU, Lotz JC (2007) ISSLS prize winner: repeated disc injury causes persistent inflammation. Spine 32(25):2812–2819

Urban JPG, Maroudas A (1979) The measurement of fixed charged density in the intervertebral disc. Biochimica et Biophysica Acta (BBA) – General Subjects 586(1):166–178

Urban JP, McMullin JF (1988) Swelling pressure of the lumbar intervertebral discs: influence of age, spinal level, composition, and degeneration. Spine 13(2):179–187

Urban JP, Winlove CP (2007) Pathophysiology of the intervertebral disc and the challenges for MRI. J Magn Reson Imaging 25(2):419–432

van Zijl PC, Jones CK, Ren J, Malloy CR, Sherry AD (2007) MRI detection of glycogen in vivo by using chemical exchange saturation transfer imaging (glycoCEST). Proc Natl Acad Sci U S A 104(11):4359–4364

Wang C, McArdle E, Fenty M, Witschey W, Elliott M, Sochor M, Reddy R, Borthakur A (2010a) Validation of sodium magnetic resonance imaging of intervertebral disc. Spine 35(5):505–510

Wang C, Witschey W, Elliott MA, Borthakur A, Reddy R (2010b) Measurement of intervertebral disc pressure with T 1ρ MRI. Magn Reson Med 64(6):1721–1727

Wang C, Witschey W, Goldberg A, Elliott M, Borthakur A, Reddy R (2010c) Magnetization transfer ratio mapping of intervertebral disc degeneration. Magn Reson Med 64(5):1520–1528

Ward KM, Balaban RS (2000) Determination of pH using water protons and chemical exchange dependent saturation transfer (CEST). Magn Reson Med 44(5):799–802

Ward KM, Aletras AH, Balaban RS (2000) A new class of contrast agents for MRI based on proton chemical exchange dependent saturation transfer (CEST). J Magn Reson 143(1):79–87

Weidenbaum M, Foster RJ, Best BA, Saed-Nejad F, Nickoloff E, Newhouse J et al (1992) Correlating magnetic resonance imaging with the biochemical content of the normal human intervertebral disc. J Orthop Res 10(4):552–561

Wheaton AJ, Casey FL, Gougoutas AJ, Dodge GR, Borthakur A, Lonner JH et al (2004) Correlation of T1rho with fixed charge density in cartilage. J Magn Reson Imaging 20(3):519–525

Wolff SD, Chesnick S, Frank JA, Lim KO, Balaban RS (1991) Magnetization transfer contrast: MR imaging of the knee. Radiology 179(3):623–628

Yu S, Haughton VM, Sether LA, Ho KC, Wagner M (1989) Criteria for classifying normal and degenerated lumbar intervertebral disks. Radiology 170(2):523–526

Zhang S, Winter P, Wu K, Sherry AD (2001) A novel europium(III)-based MRI contrast agent. J Am Chem Soc 123(7):1517–1518

Zhou J, Lal B, Wilson DA, Laterra J, van Zijl PC (2003) Amide proton transfer (APT) contrast for imaging of brain tumors. Magn Reson Med 50(6):1120–1126

Surgical Indications for Lumbar Degenerative Disease

13

Ravi R. Patel, Jeffrey A. Rihn, Ravi K. Ponnoppan, and Todd J. Albert

Contents

R.R. Patel, MD
Department of Orthopaedic Surgery,
Emory University School of Medicine,
49 Jesse Hill Jr. Drive, #307, Atlanta, GA 30303, USA
e-mail: ravi.r.patel@gmail.com

J.A. Rihn, MD (✉) • T.J. Albert, MD
Department of Orthopaedic Surgery,
Thomas Jefferson University Hospital, The Rothman Institute,
925 Chestnut Street, 5th Floor, Philadelphia, PA 19107, USA
e-mail: jrihno16@yahoo.com; tjsurg@aol.com

R.K. Ponnoppan, MD
Private Orthopaedic Practice, Jersey Spine Associates,
110 Roosevelt Blvd #2w, Marmora, NJ 08223, USA
e-mail:rkp500@gmail.com

I.M. Shapiro, M.V. Risbud (eds.), *The Intervertebral Disc*,
DOI 10.1007/978-3-7091-1535-0_13, © Springer-Verlag Wien 2014

13.1 Introduction

Lumbar degenerative disease is a common and debilitating condition that describes the age-dependent pathologic changes that occur in the spine. Degenerative disease of the lumbar spine accounts for a relatively large proportion of the annual health-care expenditures in the USA and is responsible for considerable indirect losses due to time-off of work (Luo et al. 2008). A study by Hanson et al. assessed the health status of patients with musculoskeletal pathology requiring surgical treatment and found that patients with lumbar spinal conditions (i.e., chronic low back pain, stenosis, and spondylolisthesis) suffered from considerable disability when compared to patients with other orthopedic conditions, such as hip and knee arthritis (Hansson et al. 2008).

Degenerative changes that occur in the lumbar spine with aging include intervertebral disc degeneration, facet arthropathy and hypertrophy, and ligamentum flavum hypertrophy. This process may manifest as discogenic low back pain, disc herniation, spinal stenosis, and/or spondylolisthesis. It can cause a variety of symptoms including low back pain, neurogenic claudication, or radicular symptoms, including pain, numbness, tingling, and weakness in the affected nerve root distribution. The pathophysiology producing these symptoms is multifactorial and often a specific pain generator cannot be identified. Each component of the functional spinal unit undergoes changes with aging and degeneration. It is not clear, however, why some people become symptomatic and others do not. Boden et al. reviewed the lumbar spine MRI studies in patients who had never experienced back pain or sciatica and noted that in patients under age 60, 22 % had a disc herniation, 54 % had a disc bulge, and 46 % had disc degeneration. In patients over age 60, the percentages increased to 36, 79 and 93 %, respectively (Boden et al. 1999a, b). The purpose of this chapter is to provide an overview of the most common manifestations of lumbar degeneration and the indications for surgical management of these conditions.

13.2 Discogenic Low Back Pain

13.2.1 Epidemiology of Low Back Pain

Disc degeneration and low back pain is a difficult condition to evaluate. Chronic low back pain is the most common cause of morbidity and chronic pain in the USA (Deyo et al. 2006). It is estimated that up to 80 % of individuals will experience low back pain at one time in their lives (Walker 2000). For a detailed discussion of the epidemiology of back pain, see Chaps. 9 and 16. The majority of mechanical nonspecific low back pain requires little or no formal medical treatment and should be an infrequent indication for surgical intervention. Surgery for chronic low back pain in the absence of deformity or instability is generally reserved for when a degenerated disc is thought to be the primary generator of non-radicular discogenic pain.

13.2.2 Pathogenesis of Disc Disease

Discogenic low back pain is the result of a complex cascade of degenerative changes. The intervertebral discs lie between each vertebral segment and they provide motion and flexibility to the spine. They are approximately 7–10 mm thick and 4 cm in diameter in the lumbar section (Twomey and Taylor 1987; Roberts et al. 1989). The disc consists of two distinct anatomic regions: the outer annulus fibrosus and the inner nucleus pulposus. The annulus fibrosus in the lumbar spine has upwards of 25 layers containing mostly collagen I arranged in a dense parallel pattern (Roberts 2002). The intricate cross-linked configuration of the collagen fibrils allows the intervertebral disc to resist the tensile forces that occur in the lumbar spine during bending and torsional movements. The central nucleus pulposus consists of predominantly collagen II fibrils within a rich proteoglycan matrix. This composition produces a highly viscoelastic core that allows resistance to axial loads (Buckwalter et al. 2002). A third morphologically distinct region that is often described is the cartilaginous end plate. The end plate is a thin horizontal layer of hyaline cartilage measuring less than 1 mm in thickness. Its collagen fibers interface the disc and the vertebral body (Johnson et al. 2001). For more detailed information on the structure of the intervertebral disc, see Chaps. 4 and 5.

Kirkaldy-Willis described a widely accepted pathway that divided lumbar disc degeneration into three stages based on the amount of damage that has occurred (Johnson et al. 2001; Yong-Hing and Kirkaldy-Willis 1983). These stages were dysfunction, instability, and stabilization (Yong-Hing and Kirkaldy-Willis 1983). However, it is important to note that this cascade of individual motion segment degeneration is a continuum rather than as three definable and separate stages. Most commonly, the L4–5 and L5–S1 discs typically are the first two lumbar levels to undergo degenerative changes. The initial change that occurs during disc degeneration is circumferential fissuring of the outer annulus fibrosus. This is thought to be the result of repetitive microtrauma and subsequent disruption in the intervertebral vascular supply and impairment of the normal disc metabolism (Yong-Hing and Kirkaldy-Willis 1983). Over time, there is delamination of the annular layers and the circumferential tears coalesce to form larger radial tears. There is a decrease in the amount and organization of proteoglycans in the nucleus pulposus (Yong-Hing and Kirkaldy-Willis 1983). Vertebral segment instability occurs, and this results in a decline in the amount of nuclear proteoglycan composition with a resulting fall in osmotic pressure and of water content (Yong-Hing and Kirkaldy-Willis 1983). Over time, there are continued end-stage tissue damage and unsuccessful attempts at repair. The end result is intervertebral disc space narrowing, fibrosis, end plate irregularities, and osteophyte formation. The pathophysiology of the degenerative process is described in considerable detail in Chap. 11.

The changes that occur with intervertebral disc degeneration have a major effect on disc function and its load-bearing capacity. With matrix disorganization and the fragmentation and loss of proteoglycan, the osmotic pressure of the disc is reduced and it is subsequently less able to maintain hydration under load (Yong-Hing and Kirkaldy-Willis 1983; Lyons et al. 1981). Inappropriate stress develops along the end plate and in the annulus.

The relationship between disc degeneration and low back pain is incompletely understood. Some patients with pronounced degenerative changes will have low back pain while others with a similar degree of pathology are pain-free. Indeed, approximately one third of asymptomatic individuals will have degenerative changes apparent on a lumbar MRI scan (Boden et al. 1999a, b). Factors that may contribute to the generation of pain include altered spine biomechanics, neural hypersensitivity, and neurovascular ingrowth into the disc.

13.2.3 Clinical Presentation of Discogenic Disease

Discogenic disease of the lumbar spine may produce low back pain. Acute low back pain is defined as pain lasting less than 3 months and chronic pain as greater than 3 months. Patient complaints are often of nonspecific back symptoms. Typically, discogenic pain is associated with activities that increase the pressure within the intervertebral disc such as sitting and trunk flexion. Most episodes of acute low back pain are self-limiting. It is important for the clinician to maintain an awareness of the so-called red flags that may signify a serious underlying pathology such as fracture, infection, or malignancy.

13.2.4 Evaluation of the Spine by Imaging Technologies

AP and lateral radiographs should be the first study in the evaluation of the lumbar spine. These views should be reserved for patients who have had low back pain for 6 weeks. However, earlier imaging is warranted if there is a concern for serious pathology ("red flags"). MRI should be performed if back pain is unresponsive to conservative management for 3 months. Plain radiographs, magnetic resonance imaging (MRI), and computed tomography (CT) are sensitive to degenerative changes but clinically are nonspecific (Boden et al. 1999a, b; Wiesel et al. 1984), as indicated by the relatively high incidence of degenerative changes noted by the MRI study by Boden et al. in asymptomatic patients (Boden et al. 1999a, b) (Fig. 13.1).

Discography can be a useful tool to differentiate the source in discogenic low back pain. The test involves pressurizing the disc with contrast dye in an attempt to stimulate nerve endings in injured discs. Discography can provide information regarding the morphology of the degenerated disc and can assist with identifying the pain generator (Fig. 13.2). Precise reproduction of the patients presenting pain symptoms, or concordance, makes the test clinically useful. Some studies have identified a high level of sensitivity and specificity, whereas others have disputed this claim (Mooney et al. 1988; Walsh et al. 1990; Simmons et al. 1988; Carragee et al. 2000; Guyer and Ohnmeiss 1995). Carragee et al. showed discography to have a best-case positive predictive value of 50–60 % (Carragee et al. 2006). The subjective nature of the test can never completely be overcome, but it is arguably the only study whereby a painful degenerated disc can potentially be identified. However, the use of discography should be carefully considered in terms of risks and benefits because accelerated disc degeneration, disc herniation, and loss of disc height have been reported in comparison to matched controls at a 7–10-year follow-up (Carragee et al. 2009).

13.2.5 Treatment of Discogenic Pain

The initial treatment of discogenic pain is nonsurgical. It is important to note, however, that the evidence available supporting various nonsurgical treatment options is limited (Ostelo et al. 2009; Thomas et al. 2006). For non-radicular low

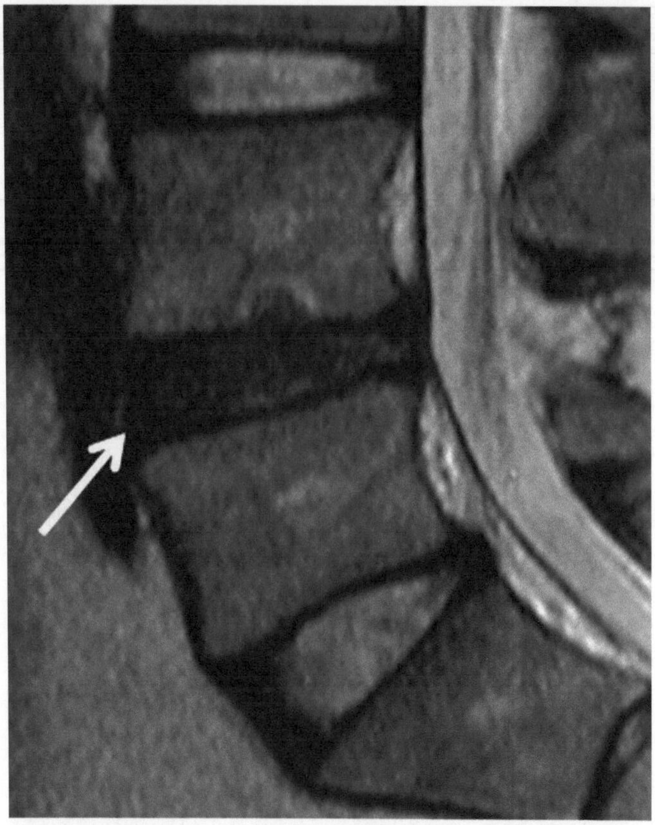

Fig. 13.1 Sagittal T2-weighted lumbar MRI image demonstrating degeneration of the L4–5 intervertebral disc (*white arrow*). Water has high signal intensity on T2-weighted MRI imaging. As the disc degenerates, it loses its water content and, as such, loses its high signal intensity compared to the healthy disc. The degenerative disc becomes grey or black and is often referred to as a "dark disc." Note that the L3–4 and L5–S1 discs above and below the L4–5 level still have high signal intensity

back pain, systematic review has shown no or insufficient evidence to support the use of botulinum toxin injections, local injections, prolotherapy, intraspinal steroid injections, epidural injections, facet joint or intradiscal steroid injections, sacroiliac injections or medial branch blocks, intradiscal electrothermic therapy, radiofrequency denervation, or spinal cord stimulation (Chou et al. 2007, 2009). There are "weak recommendations" from the American Pain Society for exercise, spinal manipulation, and interdisciplinary rehabilitation for chronic LBP or subacute LBP, as well as acupuncture, massage therapy, and yoga (Chou et al. 2007, 2009).

Despite these limitations, the initial treatment of discogenic LBP is nonsurgical and includes medication and physical therapy. Acetaminophen is effective for pain relief but has minimal anti-inflammatory effects. Hepatotoxicity may be encountered at high doses. Nonsteroidal anti-inflammatory drugs (NSAIDs) and COX-2 inhibitors are a mainstay in treatment as well. Opiate analgesics are more useful in treating chronic nociceptive pain and are rarely necessary in the treatment of acute pain. Muscle relaxants and antidepressants, particularly those that block norepinephrine, may

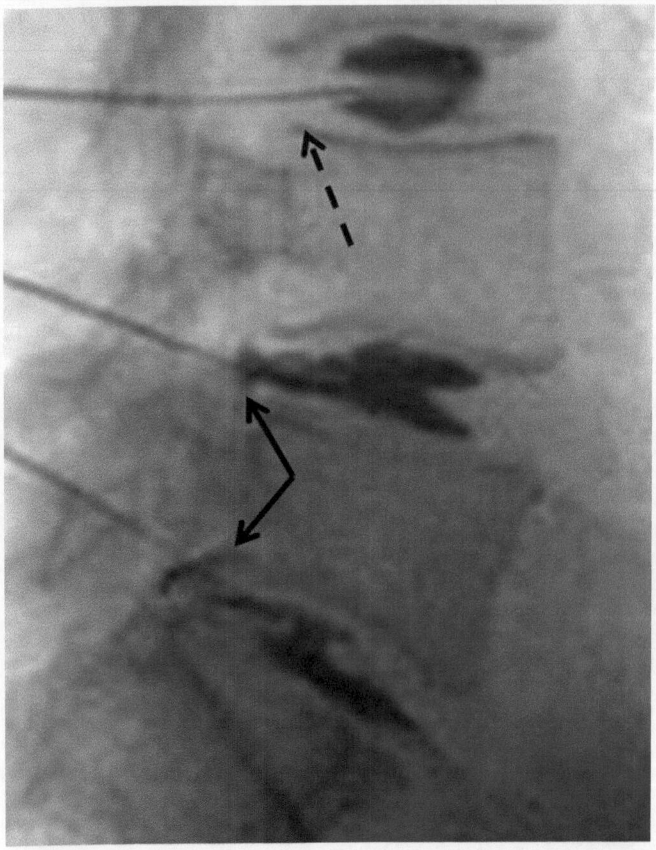

Fig. 13.2 A lateral lumbar fluoroscopic image obtained during a discogram. Needles are inserted into the L3–4, L4–5, and L5–S1 discs (in this specific case), and contrast dye is inserted under pressure into each of the discs. The L4–5 and L5–S1 levels (*solid black arrows*) demonstrate posterior leakage of the dye, indicating the presence of an annular tear at each of these levels. There is no dye leakage at L3–4 level (*broken black arrow*) as it all remains contained within the disc space, thus indicating the absence of a significant annular tear. If, while injecting the dye into a certain disc, the patient complains of pain similar to that which he/she experiences clinically, the disc that triggers such pain is said to cause concordant pain. This study is largely used in patients who are considering a surgical fusion for low back pain and is used to help decide which levels need to be fused, i.e., those levels which produce concordant pain on discography

provide analgesia. Physical therapy relies on mobilization, stretching, conditioning, and aerobic training. For discogenic low back pain, McKenzie extension-based exercise programs are the most beneficial. It is believed that these exercises will unload the disc by restoring lumbar lordosis and decreasing mechanical strain. Other recommendations include smoking cessation, weight loss, and activity alteration. The topic of nonsurgical treatment of low back pain is discussed in detail in Chap. 15.

Surgical interventions for discogenic disc disease are controversial and the results of high-level randomized studies are conflicting (Ostelo et al. 2009; Thomas et al. 2006; Chou et al. 2007, 2009). Surgery should not be considered until a structured 6-month regimen of physical therapy, NSAIDs, and activity modification has failed to improve the patient's symptoms. In addition, it is important to rule out serious underlying pathology as the source of pain – it is necessary to screen for secondary pain, localize the pain to a specific region, and characterize the type of pain as mechanical versus myofascial. Brox et al. performed a single-blind randomized study to compare the effectiveness of lumbar instrumented fusion with cognitive intervention and exercises in patients with chronic low back pain and disc degeneration (Brox et al. 2003). At 1-year follow-up, there was equal improvement in patients with chronic low back pain and disc degeneration randomized to cognitive intervention and exercises, or lumbar fusion (Brox et al. 2003). Fairbanks et al. performed a randomized control trial to assess the effectiveness of spinal fusion versus intensive rehabilitation in patients with chronic low back pain. Over the 2-year follow-up, both groups reported statistically similar reductions in disability (Fairbank et al. 2005). A randomized controlled study was carried out to determine whether lumbar fusion could reduce pain and diminish disability more effectively than nonsurgical treatment in patients with severe chronic low back pain (Fritzell et al. 2001). Patients in the nonsurgical group were treated with different kinds of physical therapy. At 2 years, back pain was reduced in the surgical group by 33 % compared with 7 % (63 to 58) in the nonsurgical group (Fritzell et al. 2001).

Surgical options are largely limited to lumbar arthrodesis through an anterior, posterior, or combined approach. More recent options that are still under investigation include dynamic stabilization and total disc arthroplasty. Surgery is considered if the patient has failed a prolonged course of conservative management and there exists a strong correlation between clinical presentation and radiographic findings, and possibly discography. Posterolateral fusion has been shown to successfully manage chronic discogenic back pain in a highly selected subset of patients receiving worker's compensation and those chronically disabled (Parker et al. 1996).

13.3 Intervertebral Disc Herniation

13.3.1 Epidemiology of Disc Herniation

Disc herniation is one of the most common intervertebral disc pathologies presented to spinal surgeons. Lumbar disc herniation has a peak incidence in the fourth decade of life, and men are more likely to be affected than women (Weinstein et al. 2008a, b). However, it is reported that only 4–6 % of lumbar herniations will become symptomatic (Weinstein et al. 2008a, b).

13.3.2 Pathoetiology of Disc Herniation

A cascade of degenerative changes occurs in the lumbar spine with age. The nucleus pulposus desiccates and loses its ability to recover from compressive deformation. In the annulus fibrosis, there are fissures that form between the collagen fibrils of the lamellae. With continued torsional, axial, and flexion strains across the disc, the nucleus pulposus can herniate through the fissures in the weakened outer annulus. The loss of nucleus pulposus containment alters the biomechanics of the entire disc. The annular fibrils become exposed to higher forces, which may lead to chondro-osseous changes at the disc–vertebral body junction. Details of these changes are presented in greater detail in Chaps. 7 and 19. A herniated nucleus pulposus can cause mechanical and/or chemical irritation of the affected nerve root and lead to severe radicular symptoms.

Disc herniation may have one of three morphological characteristics. A disc protrusion is defined as an eccentric bulging of the nucleus pulposus into an intact but thinned annulus. Disc extrusion occurs when disc material crosses through an annular defect but remains continuous with the disc space. A sequestered disc refers to one that is not continuous with the disc space and is a free fragment. Disc herniation can also be classified according to the location of the disc herniation in relation to the spinal canal, i.e., central, paracentral, foraminal, or far lateral. The most common location of disc herniation is paracentral, in which the herniated disc compresses the traversing nerve root (e.g., the L5 nerve root at the L4–5 disc level). A foraminal or far lateral disc will compress the exiting nerve root of the involved level (e.g., the L4 nerve root at the L4–5 disc level).

13.3.3 Clinical Presentation of Herniation

Most disc herniations are characterized by back and leg pain of varying severity and duration. Onset may be insidious or proceeded by a traumatic event. The L4–5 and L5–S1 discs are most commonly affected. Leg pain commonly occurs in the dermatome supplied by the compressed nerve root. Low back pain may subside after herniation because of the depressurization of the intervertebral space and relief of annular tension. Radiculopathy can present as pain, paresthesias, motor deficits, sensory deficits, and/or depressed reflexes. The distribution of symptoms (i.e., specific dermatome and myotome) often provides information as to the level of disc herniation than can then be correlated with the findings on MRI. Symptoms from a disc herniation are typically worse with sitting and improved with standing and walking. Sitting with the waist flexed not only causes an increase in the disc pressure but also causes the involved nerve to be stretched over the herniated disc. Often, paracentral and foraminal herniations will present with a predominance of leg pain, whereas central herniations often present with a predominance of back pain, as the central herniation, unless very large, does not directly compress the exiting or traversing nerve root.

A thorough evaluation and examination is needed for a patient with suspected disc disease. A detailed medical history includes investigation of possible serious underlying pathology, such as tumor, infection, fracture, or critical neurologic compromise. "Red flags" such as fever, chills, night pain, unrelenting pain, unexplained weight loss, progressive lower extremity weakness, and bowel or bladder dysfunction are indicative of a more severe and potentially emergent condition. These symptoms should prompt an expedited workup, including advanced imaging, such as an MRI. Family history may be informative as well as reports exist of a familiar and genetic predisposition to lumbar disc herniation. A full neurologic evaluation of muscle strength, sensation, proprioception, vibration, and deep tendon reflexes should be performed. Examination of patient standing position and gait may also provide useful information. A variety of maneuvers exist, such as the straight leg raise, to help diagnose a herniated disc.

13.3.4 Imaging of Herniation

Imaging studies are useful to confirm clinical diagnosis. Plain lumbar radiographs are of little benefit in the direct evaluation of a disc herniation, as they do not show soft tissue. However, they are indicated in patients with longer than 6 weeks of low back pain and in patients with medical history of serious underlying pathology, such as cancer or infection. Furthermore, radiographs (anteroposterior, lateral, flexion, and extension views) are helpful in evaluating a patient with lumbar degenerative disease for evidence of instability, disc collapse, and deformity (i.e., scoliosis). MRI is the diagnostic test of choice for evaluating a patient for a disc herniation (Fig. 13.3a, b). However, relatively high rates of lumbar disc herniations are found on MRI in asymptomatic patients (Boden et al. 1999a, b). Therefore, clinical correlation is of great importance. Dynamic MRI performed with patients in a variety of patients has begun to gain popularity. CT scan may be useful in specific situations, such as to assess bony anatomy in a patient who has had prior fusion surgery. CT myelogram is the study of choice in patients who cannot have an MRI. It is important to keep in mind when treating a patient with a symptomatic lumbar disc herniation that up to 90 % of patients will have gradual resolution of symptoms within 3 months of onset. For this reason, unless "red flags"

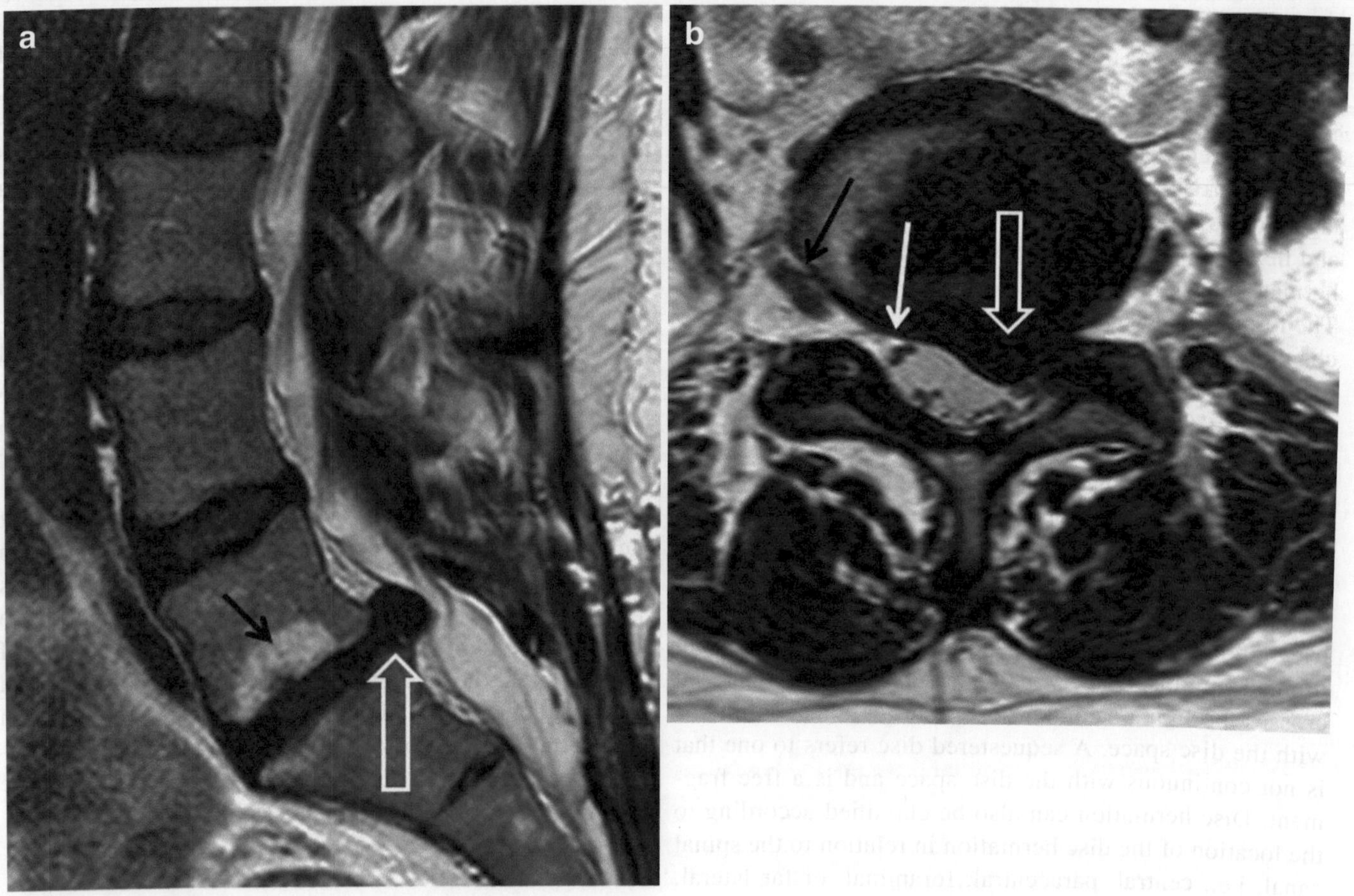

Fig. 13.3 Sagittal (**a**) and axial (**b**) T2-weighted lumbar MRI images demonstrating a left-sided L5–S1 paracentral disc herniation. On the sagittal image (**a**) the disc herniation is demonstrated by the open white arrow. The herniated disc can be seen protruding posteriorly into the spinal canal. The L5–S1 disc itself is considerably degenerated, and bone marrow edema (*black arrow*) is noted within this L5 vertebral body, adjacent to the inferior end plate, and, to a lesser extent, in the S1 vertebral body, adjacent to the superior end plate. This edema likely represents the bone response to abnormal load distribution that results from the degenerative disc. The axial image (**b**) demonstrates the location of the disc in the left paracentral region, extending somewhat into the left L5–S1 intervertebral foramen (*open white arrow*). The right exiting L5 nerve root (*black arrow*) and right traversing S1 nerve root (*closed white arrow*) are demonstrated. The exiting L5 and traversing S1 nerve roots on the left side are significantly compressed by the disc herniation

exist, imaging is not indicated for at least 6 weeks following the onset of radiculopathy and low back pain.

13.3.5 Herniation Treatment

Initial treatment for patients presenting with acute radicular symptoms is conservative. It involves a short period of rest, activity modification, and anti-inflammatory analgesia. Muscle relaxants and a short course of oral steroids have also proven beneficial. Physical therapy and spinal manipulation are used frequently as well. Fluoroscopic epidural steroid injections can be administered to reduce nerve root inflammation and significantly improve symptoms. Generally, conservative management is performed for at least 6 weeks.

Radicular symptoms not relieved by nonoperative methods are often treated by surgery to remove the herniated disc. Relative indications for surgery include intractable radicular pain, pseudoclaudication, neurologic deficit that does not improve with conservative treatment, recurrent symptoms following a successful trial of nonsurgical care, and significant motor deficit. Absolute indications include cauda equina disease or a progressive neurologic deficit.

The Spine Patient Outcomes Research Trial (SPORT) prospectively evaluated the outcomes of surgical versus nonsurgical intervention in patients with symptomatic lumbar disc herniation. Candidates with image-confirmed herniation meeting eligibility criteria were enrolled and randomized to standard open discectomy versus nonoperative care. At 4 years, patients who underwent surgery achieved greater improvement than nonoperatively treated patients (Weinstein et al. 2008a, b). Furthermore, it has also been demonstrated that with appropriate patient selection (i.e., symptoms and physical examination correlate to the findings on MRI), surgery provides faster resolution of symptoms and perceived quicker recovery than nonoperative management at 1–2 years (Weinstein et al. 2006; Peul et al. 2007).

Microdiscectomy is the gold standard surgical procedure for lumbar disc herniation. This procedure can be performed through a small incision in an outpatient setting. Complications of surgical intervention include inadvertent durotomy, nerve root injury, and infection. Later complications can include postoperative instability and recurrent disc herniation, which can occur up to 7 % of cases (Weinstein et al. 2008a, b). It is often difficult to discern recurrent disc herniation from epidural fibrosis on standard MRI imaging. Therefore, when evaluating for recurrent disc herniation, gadolinium-enhanced MRI should be used to differentiate between disc herniation and fibrosis.

13.4 Lumbar Stenosis

13.4.1 Epidemiology of Lumbar Stenosis

Lumbar stenosis refers to the narrowing of the neural canal and neuroforaminal spaces of the lumbar spine. It is the most common end-stage consequence of disc degeneration often resulting from adaptive changes of the facet joints and end plates. Most patients with symptomatic lumbar stenosis present between the ages of 60 and 80 (Johnson et al. 1992; Arbit and Pannullo 2001). Women are slightly more likely to have lumbar stenosis than men, and the majority of patients with lumbar stenosis are of Caucasian descent (Johnson et al. 1992; Arbit and Pannullo 2001). Degenerative spinal stenosis most commonly affects the L3–4 and L4–5 (Arbit and Pannullo 2001). Clinically, adults with radiographic evidence of lumbar stenosis may be asymptomatic; however, as age increases, a higher percentage becomes symptomatic (Johnson et al. 1992; Arbit and Pannullo 2001).

13.4.2 Etiology of Lumbar Stenosis

The most common cause of lumbar stenosis is age-related degenerative changes of the spine (Arbit and Pannullo 2001). End-stage lumbar disc degeneration alters facet and disc biomechanics and may induce hypertrophy and overgrowth of the facet joints and vertebral end plates, respectively. The resultant encroachment and the narrowing of the neuroforamina from osteophyte formation, loss of disc space height, and hypertrophy of the ligamentum flavum can cause marked reduction in space available for the spinal nerve roots.

Another cause of spinal stenosis is congenital lumbar spinal stenosis, which is associated with shorter pedicle lengths and innately narrowed spaces for neural elements in patients from birth. Instability associated with spinal stenosis most commonly occurs due to lumbar disc and/or facet degeneration and translation (spondylolisthesis) of the vertebra relative to each other. Instability can also result from the structural incompetence of the pars interarticularis (isthmic spondylolisthesis) or scoliosis. The shift forward, backward, or laterally can further reduce space in the spinal column centrally and/or foraminal spaces. Less common causes of lumbar spinal stenosis include epidural lipomatosis, tumors, infections, and metabolic bone disorders such as Paget's disease. The main anatomic regions of lumbar stenosis include the central canal, lateral recess (subarticular), foraminal, and extraforaminal (Arbit and Pannullo 2001).

13.4.3 Clinical Presentation of Lumbar Stenosis

Lumbar spinal stenosis symptoms are often reflective of the severity and the anatomic region of the narrowed spaces. Often insidious due to the gradual narrowing over many years, spinal stenosis can be asymptomatic for long periods of time (Arbit and Pannullo 2001). Early symptoms may include intermittent low back pain without radiculopathy, signaling the onset of early disc degeneration. As the narrowing of the spaces continues to compress nerves and limit normal nerve gliding and excursion, radiculopathy or claudication symptoms may become more apparent. Patients often complain of leg pain that is activity related, associated with upright posture and/or prolonged walking (Paine 1976; Wilson 1969). The symptoms are often distributed along dermatomes or myotomes corresponding to the areas of affected neural compression. Pain symptoms may also be associated with weakness, paresthesias, or numbness.

The classic clinical presentation of lumbar stenosis is neurogenic claudication (Paine 1976; Wilson 1969). Claudication refers to the gradual increase in symptoms with prolonged or repetitive activity (i.e., walking), which often is associated with upright posture. The patients often relieve this pain by changing posture such as sitting or leaning forward (lumbar flexion) which results in neuroforaminal and spinal canal opening. Patients presenting with spinal stenosis may note symptoms gradually worsening over time or acute onset radiculopathy. Aggravation of severe stenosis can sometimes lead to cauda equina syndrome (loss of bowel or bladder control). There are no specific physical exam tests or signs associated with lumbar stenosis. Patients often have normal strength and sensation. Confirmation of posture-related improvement of pain (i.e., sitting or lumbar flexion) may further assist in clinical diagnosis. Nerve tension signs may be present in patients with severe radiculopathy.

13.4.4 Imaging of Lumbar Stenosis

Lumbar stenosis is a radiological finding as well as a clinical diagnosis. Imaging studies are often used to correlate clinical symptoms and quantify severity. Initial evaluation is performed using plain lumbar radiographs to assess spinal alignment and rule out instability or metabolic bone disease.

CT scans are useful to view bony anatomy in detail and rule out fractures or detect other bone defects. Plain CT is not often employed for the diagnosis of lumbar stenosis. CT scan combined with myelography is extremely useful to visualize neural element compression and confirm areas of bony impingement and is often used to evaluate patients who cannot undergo MRI. The most common test used to confirm lumbar stenosis is MRI, which can show disc degeneration, end plate morphology, facet and ligamentum hypertrophy, neural elements, and available neural spaces (Fig. 13.4). Analysis of sequential images of the lumbar spine in sagittal and axial planes can allow localization of specific areas of stenosis in all four anatomic regions (central, lateral recess, foraminal, and extraforaminal). Relative stenosis is defined as a central canal diameter of 10–13 mm, whereas absolute spinal stenosis describes a canal diameter of less than 10 mm (Verbiest 1979).

It is important to note that there is very little correlation between radiological findings and patient symptoms (Sirvanci et al. 2008). Severe stenosis radiologically can be asymptomatic in some patients, while low-grade stenosis may cause

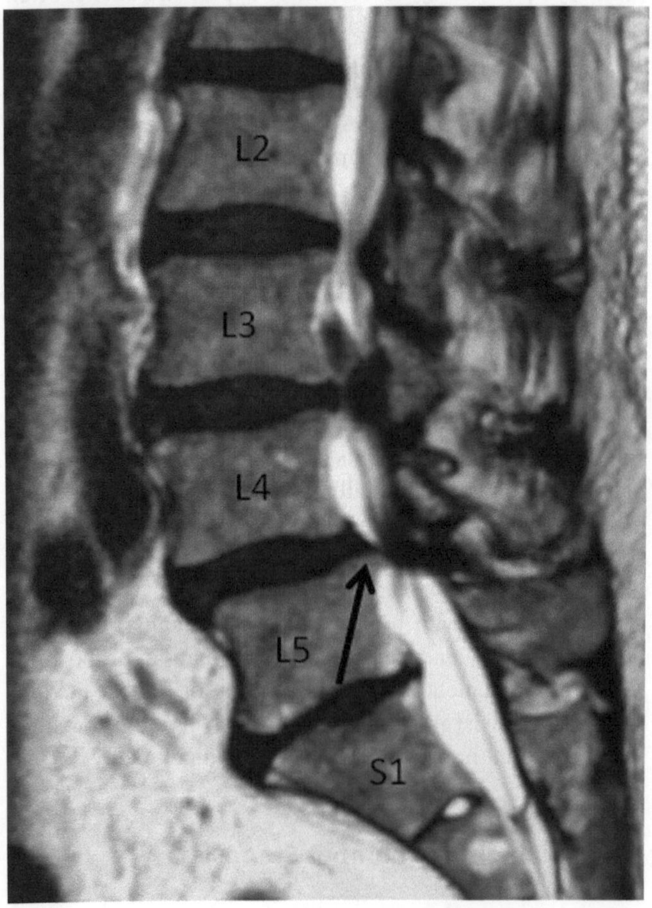

Fig. 13.4 Sagittal T2-weighted lumbar MRI image demonstrating moderate L2–3 and severe L3–4 and L4–5 stenosis. In addition, there is a slight degenerative spondylolisthesis at L4–5, where the L4 vertebral body is located slightly anterior to the L5 vertebral body (*black arrow*)

severe pain in others (Sirvanci et al. 2008). In patients whose radiological findings confirm their clinical symptoms, appropriate treatment plans can be employed and predictable outcomes can be anticipated.

13.4.5 Treatment of Lumbar Stenosis

The first-line treatment in lumbar spinal stenosis is nonoperative. These measures may include NSAIDs, analgesics, and activity modification. Oral steroids may also be given to help reduce acute inflammatory symptoms and minimize radicular pain. Physical therapy can also be attempted, with the main exercises being low impact, core strengthening, aerobic conditioning, and stretching. Alternative exercise modalities include Tai chi, water therapy, chiropractic care, and stationary biking.

Epidural steroid injections can reduce inflammation around the nerve roots and may help treat radiculopathy. Selective nerve root block can be very effective for pain relief in the short term and can also be useful as a diagnostic tool. Recent level 1 evidence confirms their effectiveness for short-term relief of radicular pain (Weinstein et al. 2008a, b). Unlike injections for radiculopathy associated with a herniated disc where the natural history is spontaneous resolution, injections for stenosis do not resolve the underlying compression of the nerve root(s) associated with bony stenosis, and symptoms may recur.

Definitive management of symptomatic lumbar stenosis involves surgery. Surgery is indicated for patients who fail nonoperative management. The standard surgical procedure for degenerative lumbar stenosis is a decompressive laminectomy. Neural decompression is achieved by removing the central bony elements of the posterior spine (spinous process and lamina). This allows the restoration of adequate central canal space, whereas medial facetectomy and foraminotomy allow for lateral recess and foraminal decompression, respectively. Surgical outcomes for decompressive laminectomy are cost effective, reliable, and superior to nonoperative management in functional restoration (Weinstein et al. 2008a, b; Tosteson et al. 2008). Complications of lumbar laminectomy include incidental dural tears, postoperative instability, persistent back pain, persistent radiculopathy, and recurrence of stenosis.

13.5 Degenerative Spondylolisthesis

13.5.1 Epidemiology of Spondylolisthesis

Degenerative spondylolisthesis refers to spinal instability and translation resulting from lumbar degenerative conditions. Most commonly, patients initially present after 50 years of age; however, more severe symptoms are often noted with increasing age and in patients over 65 years of age (Valkenburg and Haanen 1982; Frymoyer 1994). Females are affected more, with a 3:1 ratio over men (Frymoyer 1994). Body mass index, age, and angle of lordosis were significantly associated with degenerative spondylolisthesis in women. In men, no individual risk factors for degenerative spondylolisthesis were found, save increased age (Jacobsen et al. 2007).

13.5.2 Etiology of Spondylolisthesis

Degenerative spondylolisthesis is most commonly brought on by facet joint degeneration and intervertebral disc degeneration. This occurs most commonly at level L4–5 (Frymoyer 1994). Degenerative changes of the facet joints result in associated morphological changes that allow vertebral body translation and secondary neuroforaminal compression. Loss of disc height contributes to the magnitude of translation and subsequent neural compression. In degenerative spondylolisthesis, slippage of the vertebral body is typically less than 50 % of the anterior–posterior vertebral body diameter (Frymoyer 1994). Facet joints tend to enlarge in degenerative spondylolisthesis, which further encroaches into the spinal canal and can cause lateral recess stenosis and radicular symptoms.

13.5.3 Clinical Presentation of Spondylolisthesis

It should be noted that the degree of slippage is not always directly correlated with the severity of clinical findings or pain. Symptomatic patients most often present with aching back pain that travels into the buttocks and back of the thighs (radiculopathy). Concomitant neurogenic claudication may also be noted. Neuroforaminal stenosis is often associated with radicular pain along the affected nerve root.

Physical exam findings are similar to lumbar spinal stenosis and may include point tenderness at the lumbosacral junction and a restricted trunk range of motion. Neurological examination is usually normal in terms of strength and sensation; however, paresthesias and weakness may be noted in patients with a significant radiculopathy component. Mechanical back pain may be present more in patients with spinal stenosis associated with spondylolisthesis. Patients often report more pain with extremes of flexion and extension.

13.5.4 Imaging of Spondylolisthesis

Standing orthogonal radiographs with dynamic views are very useful to diagnose disc degeneration and instability. The lateral views will show slippage of one vertebra in relation to the vertebra below it, and grading is often done based on the percentage of slip as measured by the posterior vertebral body wall translation (Meyerding Grading System) (Fig. 13.5). Oblique radiographs can be used to diagnose pars defects. Advanced imaging such as MRI or CT myelography can further delineate areas of neural compression and severity of stenosis (Fig. 13.6). Evaluation of fluid in the facet joints on axial cuts may also indicate instability or spondylolisthesis when x-rays are unavailable (Rihn et al. 2007).

13.5.5 Treatment of Spondylolisthesis

Conservative treatment should be employed initially. This may include activity modification, NSAIDs, and low-impact exercise programs. A weight loss regimen can aid in the alleviation of symptoms, but this will not cure or reverse the problem. Increased activity can cause aggravation of pain

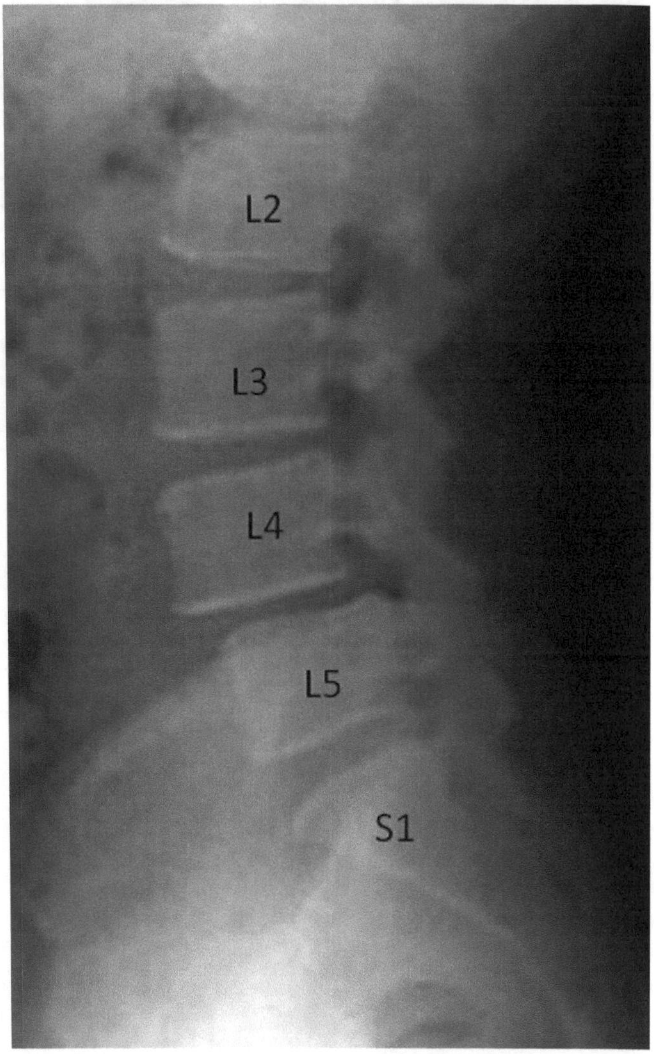

Fig. 13.5 Lateral lumbar plain radiograph demonstrating a degenerative spondylolisthesis at L4–5, where the L4 vertebral body is located slightly anterior to the L5 vertebral body. There is also multilevel lumbar disc collapse, most significant at L4–5

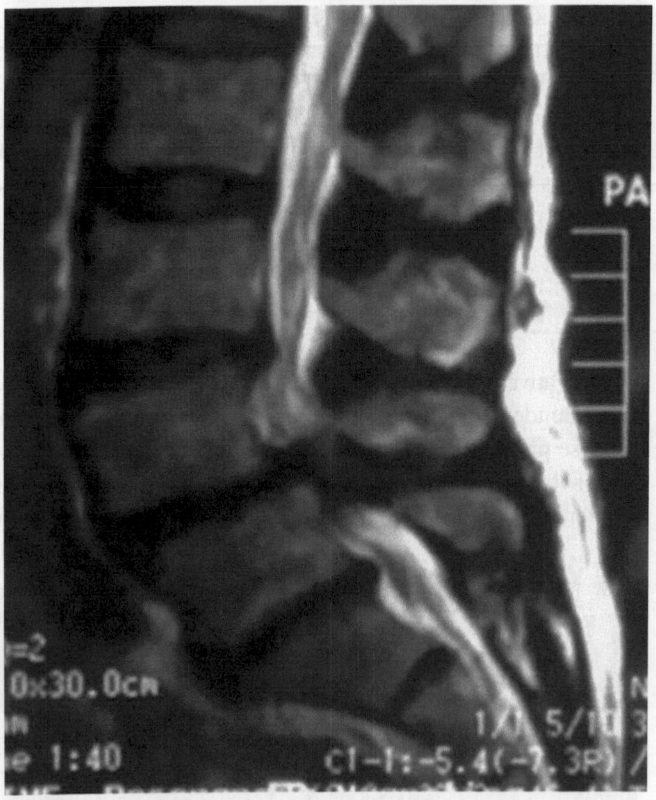

Fig. 13.6 Sagittal T2-weighted lumbar MRI image demonstrating degenerative spondylolisthesis and severe stenosis at the L4–5 level

symptoms; however, physical therapy may help improve mechanical back pain associated with a slipping vertebral body, but may not improve nerve compression and neurogenic symptoms. Focal epidural steroid injections may help reduce inflammation and alleviate radicular pain.

If nonoperative measures fail, surgical options should be considered. Indicated procedures should include neural decompression with laminectomy and foraminotomy. Often times, fusion is also performed to reduce risk of slippage progression and recurrence of symptoms and optimize long-term outcomes. Decompressive laminectomy with successful fusion has been shown to result in improved outcomes when compared to decompression alone (Herkowitz and Kurz 1991; Fischgrund et al. 1997; Kornblum et al. 2004) (Fig. 13.7a, b). Clinical outcomes of lumbar decompression and fusion for degenerative spondylolisthesis indicate high success rates and better outcomes than nonoperative management alone (Weinstein et al. 2009). Complications unique to spinal fusion include failure to achieve solid fusion, stiffness, and/or persistent back pain.

13.6 Concluding Comments

Degenerative changes of lumbar spine produce a spectrum of potentially disabling conditions that affect patients

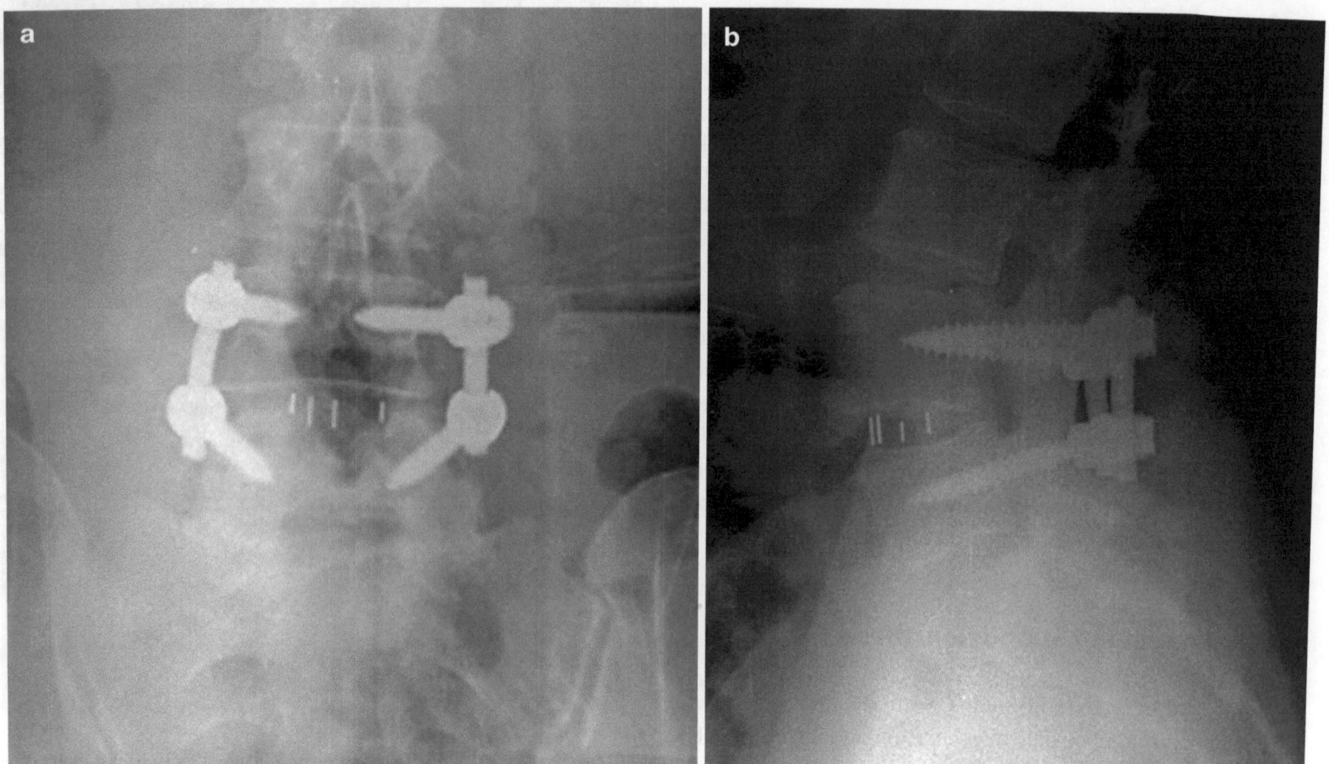

Fig. 13.7 Postoperative anteroposterior (**a**) and lateral (**b**) lumbar plain radiographs in the patient from Fig. 13.6 who underwent a lumbar laminectomy and a posterior and transforaminal lumbar interbody fusion with the use of a posterior pedicle screw-rod construct and an interbody cage with bone grafting

across a wide age range, including discogenic low back pain, lumbar disc herniation, lumbar stenosis, and degenerative spondylolisthesis. In the absence of "red flags" such as progressive neurological deficits, loss of bowel and/or bladder function, and constitutional symptoms, these conditions should initially be managed conservatively with a combination of medication, physical therapy, patient education, and possibly epidural injections. In patients who have persistent, disabling symptoms despite a dedicated conservative treatment program, surgery may offer significant benefit over a continued nonoperative approach.

13.7 Summary of Critical Concepts Discussed in the Chapter

- Degenerative disease of the lumbar spine accounts for a relatively large proportion of the annual health-care expenditures in the USA and is responsible for considerable indirect losses due to time-off of work.
- Chronic low back pain is the most common cause of morbidity and chronic pain in the USA. It is estimated that up to 80 % of individuals will experience low back pain at one time in their lives.
- Kirkaldy-Willis described a widely accepted pathway that divided lumbar disc degeneration into three stages based on the amount of damage that has occurred; these stages are dysfunction, instability, and stabilization.
- The relationship between disc degeneration and low back pain is incompletely understood.
- Most episodes of acute low back pain are self-limiting. It is important for the clinician to maintain an awareness of the so-called red flags that may signify a serious underlying pathology such as fracture, infection, or malignancy.
- Surgical intervention for discogenic disc disease is controversial, and the results of high-level randomized studies are conflicting.
- Patients who underwent surgery for disc herniation achieved greater improvement than nonoperatively treated patients at 4 years. Furthermore, it has been demonstrated that with appropriate patient selection (i.e., symptoms and physical examination correlate to the findings on MRI), surgery provides faster resolution of symptoms and perceived quicker recovery than nonoperative management at one to two years.
- There may be poor correlation between radiological findings in patients with lumbar stenosis and their symptoms.
- For degenerative lumbar spondylolisthesis, clinical outcomes of decompression and fusion indicate high success rates and better outcomes than nonoperative management alone.

References

Arbit E, Pannullo S (2001) Lumbar stenosis: a clinical review. Clin Orthop Relat Res 384:137–143

Boden SD, Davis DO, Dina TS, Patronas NJ, Wiesel SW (1999a) Abnormal magnetic-resonance scans of the lumbar spine in asymptomatic subjects: a prospective investigation. J Bone Joint Surg Am 72(3):403–408

Boden SD, McCowin PR, Davis DO, Dina TS, Mark AS, Wiesel S (1999b) Abnormal magnetic-resonance scans of the cervical spine in asymptomatic patients: a prospective investigation. J Bone Joint Surg Am 72:1178–1184

Brox JI, Sorenson R, Friis A et al (2003) Randomized clinical trial of lumbar instrumented fusion and cognitive intervention and exercises in patients with chronic low back pain and disc degeneration. Spine 28:1913–1921

Buckwalter JA, Mow VC, Boden SD, Eyre DR, Weidenbaum M (2002) Intervertebral disc structure, composition, and mechanical function. In: Buckwalter JA, Einhorn TA, Simon SR (eds) Orthopaedic basic science-biology and biomechanics for the musculoskeletal system, 2nd edn. American Academy of Orthopaedic Surgeons, Rosemont, pp 548–555

Carragee EJ, Chen Y, Tanner CM, Hayward C, Rossi M, Hagle C (2000) Can discography cause long-term back symptoms in previously asymptomatic subjects? Spine 25:1803–1808

Carragee EJ, Lincoln T, Parmar VS, Alamin T (2006) A gold standard evaluation of the "discogenic pain" diagnosis as determined by provocative discography. Spine 31(18):2115–2123

Carragee EJ, Don AS, Hurwitz EL, Cuellar JM, Carrino J, Herzog R (2009) Does discography cause accelerated progression of degeneration changes in the lumbar disc: a ten-year matched cohort study. Spine 34(21):2338–2345

Chou R, Qaseem A, Snow V et al (2007) Diagnosis and treatment of low back pain: a joint clinical practice guideline from the American College of Physicians and the American Pain Society. Ann Intern Med 147:478–491

Chou R, Loeser JD, Owens DK et al (2009) Interventional therapies, surgery, and interdisciplinary rehabilitation for low back pain. An evidence-based clinical practice guideline from the American Pain Society. Spine 34:1066–1077

Deyo RA, Mirza SK, Martin BL (2006) Back pain prevalence and visit rates: estimates from U.S. national surveys 2002. Spine 31(23): 2724–2727

Fairbank J, Frost H, Wilson-MacDonald J, Yu LM, Barker K, Collins R (2005) Randomized controlled trial to compare surgical stabilization of the lumbar spine with an intensive rehabilitation programme for patients with chronic low back pain: the MRC spine stabilization trial. BMJ 330:1233

Fischgrund JS, Mackay M et al (1997) 1997 Volvo Award winner in clinical studies. Degenerative lumbar spondylolisthesis with spinal stenosis: a prospective, randomized study comparing decompressive laminectomy and arthrodesis with and without spinal instrumentation. Spine 22(24):2807–2812

Fritzell P, Hagg O, Wessberg P, Nordwall A, Swedish Lumbar Spine Study Group (2001) 2001 Volvo Award winner in clinical studies: lumbar fusion versus nonsurgical treatment for chronic low back pain: a multicenter randomized controlled trial from the Swedish Lumbar Spine Study Group. Spine 26:2521–2532

Frymoyer J (1994) Degenerative spondylolisthesis: diagnosis and treatment. J Am Acad Orthop Surg 2:9–15

Guyer RD, Ohnmeiss DD (1995) Lumbar discography: position statement from the North American Spine Society Diagnostic and Therapeutic Committee. Spine 20:2048–2059

Hansson T, Hansson E, Malchau H (2008) Utility of spine surgery: a comparison of common elective orthopaedic surgical procedures. Spine 33(25):2819–2830

Herkowitz HN, Kurz LT (1991) Degenerative lumbar spondylolisthesis with spinal stenosis. A prospective study comparing decompression with decompression and intertransverse process arthrodesis. J Bone Joint Surg Am 73(6):802–808

Jacobsen S, Sonne-Holm S, Rovsing H, Monrad H, Gebuhr P (2007) Degenerative lumbar spondylolisthesis: an epidemiological perspective: the Copenhagen Osteoarthritis Study. Spine 1(32):120–125

Johnson KE, Rosean I, Udean A (1992) The natural course of lumbar spinal stenosis. Clin Orthop Relat Res 279:82–86

Johnson WE, Evans H, Menage J, Eisenstein SM, El Haj A, Roberts S (2001) Immunohistochemical detection of Schwann cells in innervated and vascularized human intervertebral discs. Spine 26:2550–2557

Kornblum MB, Fischgrund JS et al (2004) Degenerative lumbar spondylolisthesis with spinal stenosis: a prospective long-term study comparing fusion and pseudarthrosis. Spine 29:726–733; discussion 733–724

Luo X, Pietrobon R, Sun SX, Liu GG, Hey L (2004) Estimates and patterns of direct health care expenditures among individuals with back pain in the United States. Spine 29(1):79–86

Lyons G, Eisenstein SM, Sweet MB (1981) Biochemical changes in intervertebral disc degeneration. Biochim Biophys Acta 673:443–453

Mooney V, Haldeman S, Nasca RJ et al (1988) Position statement on discography: the executive committee of the North American Spine Society. Spine 13:1343

Ostelo RWJG, van Tulder MW, Vlaeyen JWS, Linton SJ, Morley S, Assendelft WJJ (2009) Behavioral treatment for chronic low-back pain (Review). Cochrane Collab 2:1–49

Paine KWE (1976) Clinical features of lumbar spinal stenosis. Clin Orthop Relat Res 115:77–82

Parker LM, Murrell SE, Boden S, Horton WC (1996) The outcome of posterolateral fusion in highly selected patients with discogenic low back pain. Spine 21(16):1909–1916

Peul WC, van Houwelingen HC, van den Hout WB et al (2007) Surgery versus prolonged conservative treatment for sciatica. N Engl J Med 356:2245–2256

Rihn JA et al (2007) Does lumbar facet fluid detected on magnetic resonance imaging correlate with radiographic instability in patients with degenerative lumbar disease? Spine 32(14):1555–1560

Roberts S (2002) Disc morphology in health and disease. Biochem Soc Trans 30:864–869

Roberts S, Menage J, Urban JPG (1989) Biochemical and structural properties of the cartilage end-plate and its relation to the intervertebral disc. Spine 14:166–174

Simmons JW, Aprill CN, Dwyer AP, Brodsky AE (1988) A reassessment of Holt's data on: "the question of lumbar discography". Clin Orthop Relat Res 237:120–124

Sirvanci M, Bhatia M, Ganiyusufoglu KA, Duran C, Tezer M, Ozturk C, Aydogan M, Hamzaoglu A (2008) Degenerative lumbar spinal stenosis: correlation with Oswestry Disability Index and MR imaging. Spine J 17:679–685

Thomas KJ, MacPherson H, Thorpe L et al (2006) Randomised controlled trial of a short course of traditional acupuncture compared with usual care for persistent non-specific low back pain. BMJ 333:623

Tosteson AN, Lurie JD et al (2008) Surgical treatment of spinal stenosis with and without degenerative spondylolisthesis: cost-effectiveness after 2 years. Ann Intern Med 149(12):845–853

Twomey LT, Taylor JR (1987) Age changes in lumbar vertebrae and intervertebral discs. Clin Orthop Relat Res 224:97–104

Valkenburg HA, Haanen HCM (1982) The epidemiology of low back pain. In: White AA III, Gordon SL (eds) AAOS symposium on idiopathic low back pain. CV Mosby, St. Louis, pp 9–22

Verbiest H (1979) The significance and principles of computed axial tomography in idiopathic developmental stenosis of the bony lumbar vertebral canal. Spine 4:369–378

Walker BF (2000) The prevalence of low back pain: a systematic review of the literature from 1966 to 1998. J Spinal Disord 13(3):205–217

Walsh TR, Weinstein JN, Spratt KF, Lehmann TR, April C, Sayre H (1990) Lumbar discography in normal subjects: a controlled, prospective study. J Bone Joint Surg Am 72:1081–1088

Weinstein JN, Lurie JD, Tosteson TD, Skinner JS, Hanscom B, Tosteson AN, Herkowitz H, Fischgrund J, Cammisa FB, Albert T, Devo RA (2006) Surgical vs nonoperative treatment for lumbar disk herniation: the Spine Patient Outcomes Research Trial (SPORT) observational cohort. JAMA 296(20):2441–2459

Weinstein JN, Tosteson TD et al (2008a) Surgical versus nonsurgical therapy for lumbar spinal stenosis. N Engl J Med 358(8):794–810

Weinstein JN, Lurie JD, Tosteson TD et al (2008b) Surgical versus nonoperative treatment for lumbar disk herniation: four-year results for the Spine Patient Outcomes Research Trial (SPORT). Spine 33(25): 2789–2800

Weinstein JN, Lurie JD et al (2009) Surgical compared with nonoperative treatment for lumbar degenerative spondylolisthesis. Four-year results in the Spine Patient Outcomes Research Trial (SPORT) randomized and observational cohorts. J Bone Joint Surg Am 91:1295–1304

Wiesel SW, Tsoursmas N, Feffer HL, Citrin CM, Patronas N (1984) A study of computer-assisted tomography. Part I: the incidence of positive CAT scans in an asymptomatic group of patients. Spine 9:549–551

Wilson CB (1969) Significance of the small lumbar spinal canal: cauda equina compression syndromes due to spondylosis, 3: intermittent claudication. J Neurosurg 31:499–506. http://www.ncbi.nlm.nih.gov/pubmed/5351760

Yong-Hing K, Kirkaldy-Willis WH (1983) The pathophysiology of degenerative disease of the lumbar spine. Orthop Clin North Am 14:491–504

Spinal Motion Restoration Devices for the Degenerative Disc

14

Daniel G. Kang, Melvin D. Helgeson, and Alexander R. Vaccaro

Contents

The opinions or assertions contained herein are the private views of the authors and are not to be construed as official or as reflecting the views of the United States Army or the Department of Defense. Two authors are employees of the United States government. This work was prepared as part of their official duties and as such, there is no copyright to be transferred.

D.G. Kang, MD (✉) • M.D. Helgeson, MD
Department of Orthopaedic Surgery and Rehabilitation,
Walter Reed National Military Medical Center,
8901 Wisconsin Avenue, Bethesda, MD 20889, USA
e-mail: daniel.g.kang@gmail.com; mel_helgeson@yahoo.com

A.R. Vaccaro, MD, PhD
Department of Orthopaedic Surgery,
Rothman Institute/Thomas Jefferson University,
925 Chestnut Street, 5th Floor, Philadelphia, PA 19107, USA
e-mail: alexvaccaro3@aol.com

I.M. Shapiro, M.V. Risbud (eds.), *The Intervertebral Disc*,
DOI 10.1007/978-3-7091-1535-0_14, © Springer-Verlag Wien 2014

14.1 Introduction

Cervical and lumbar degenerative disc disease is common in today's society and can be associated with significant pain and disability (Taksali et al. 2004). Spinal fusion continues to be the most common surgical treatment for degenerative conditions in the neck and low back (Davis 1994; Lee and Langrana 2004). While fusion has been similarly used for the treatment of degenerative arthritis of the hip and knee joints, it has been replaced by revolutionary joint arthroplasty techniques with excellent outcomes in terms of relieving pain and restoring function (Santos et al. 2004). In contrast, disc arthroplasty has only recently been considered an alternative to spinal arthrodesis and has not replaced fusion as the "gold standard" treatment. Studies regarding spinal fusion for degenerative disc disease have demonstrated inconsistent clinical results even in properly selected patients, and despite advances in spinal fusion technique and instrumentation, patient outcomes have not been significantly altered (Barrick et al. 2000; Kleeman et al. 2001; Madan and Boeree 2003; Bono and Lee 2004; Lee and Langrana 2004; Santos et al. 2004).

A particular concern following spinal arthrodesis has been the failure to restore normal physiologic motion, possibly leading to an increase in adjacent segment degeneration and disease (Lehmann et al. 1987; Lee 1988; Eck et al. 1999; Akamaru et al. 2003; Gillet 2003; Lee and Langrana 2004; Santos et al. 2004). Alterations in spine biomechanics following arthrodesis include loss of motion and shock absorption; these changes have been shown to cause a compensatory increase in motion, abnormal stress flow, and elevated intradiscal pressure at adjacent segments (Lee and Langrana 1984, 2004; Shono et al. 1998; Akamaru et al. 2003; Chang et al. 2007; Gao et al. 2011). Although adjacent segment degeneration and disease may be due to natural disease progression, rather than a consequence of spinal fusion, there has been continued enthusiasm and advancement of motion restoration surgery for the degenerative disc (Santos et al. 2004). With the basic premise that motion preservation at the treated symptomatic degenerative disc may slow progression or even prevent symptomatic degeneration at adjacent segments, the change represents a potential paradigm shift in approach: from motion-elimination surgery to motion-preserving surgery (Santos et al. 2004; Madigan et al. 2009).

Spinal motion restoration devices encompass various new technologies and surgical procedures, including total disc arthroplasty (TDA), posterior soft tissue stabilization, posterior dynamic screw and rod systems, nucleus pulposus replacement, and even injection of the degenerative disc with polymeric agents (Madan and Boeree 2003). However, most of these spinal motion restoration devices remain experimental with limited clinical use. However, TDA has been routinely performed in Europe since the early 1990s, although a few devices have been recently approved in the USA by the Food and Drug Administration (FDA) following prospective, randomized clinical trials (Santos et al. 2004; Mummaneni et al. 2007; Sasso et al. 2007; Zigler et al. 2007; Guyer et al. 2009; Murrey et al. 2009; Burkus et al. 2010; Garrido et al. 2010; Delamarter et al. 2011). While total disc arthroplasty continues to gain popularity as an alternative to spinal fusion, the ideal device design, as well as the appropriate indications for arthroplasty in the cervical spine and lumbar spine, remains unknown. Further experience and long-term follow-up studies will determine if TDA provides acceptable clinical outcomes, as well as influencing the rate of adjacent segment disease (Hilibrand and Robbins 2004). Clinical success of total disc arthroplasty will require a combination of appropriate patient selection, good implant materials and design, and proper implantation technique. The following discussion will address the evolving history and principles of TDA; describe the biomechanical, biomaterial, and design concepts behind TDA; and then detail the surgical indications and techniques for TDA in both the cervical and lumbar spines. In addition, other emerging spinal motion restoration devices for the lumbar spine will be briefly considered.

14.2 Adjacent Segment Disease: Does There Need to Be an Alternative to Spinal Fusion?

Spinal fusion has evolved over the past 100 years for treatment of numerous pathologic conditions, throughout the human spine, involving spinal segments from the occiput to pelvis (Hilibrand and Robbins 2004). Spinal segment arthrodesis was first described in 1911 by Hibbs (1911) for treatment of spinal deformity and Albee (1911) for the treatment of Pott's disease. While spinal fusion has also been used for other spinal conditions such as spinal trauma, spondylolisthesis, spinal stenosis, or tumors, it is most commonly used for the treatment of symptomatic degenerative disc disease causing neck or low back pain (Davis 1994; Hilibrand and Robbins 2004). Treatment goals, not unlike those for fusion of arthritic appendicular joints, are to eliminate pain, maintain or restore stability, and correct deformity/height loss (Orr et al. 2007).

Chandler first reported the use of spinal fusion for the treatment of low back pain in 1929 (Chandler 1929), while Robinson and Smith described anterior cervical discectomy and fusion (ACDF) in 1955 (Robinson and Smith 1955) for treatment of degenerative spondylotic conditions (Lee and Langrana 2004). In fact, ACDF is considered by many to be one of the most successful spine procedures performed in the last several decades (Murrey et al. 2009). Following ACDF, patients have reported greater than 90 % rate of relief of radicular complaints and stabilization/improvement of myelopathic symptoms (Hilibrand and Robbins 2004; Riew et al. 2008; Murrey et al. 2009). On the other hand, use of spinal fusion for treatment of discogenic low back pain has been a controversial subject, with often conflicting findings (Frymoyer et al. 1978; Lee and Langrana 2004). In a landmark study, Fritzell et al. (2003) found that patients with discogenic low back pain have better outcomes after successful spinal fusion compared with continued conservative treatment (McAfee 2004). The study was a randomized controlled trial of 294 patients with a 2-year follow-up by an independent observer. It was reported that disability assessed by the Oswestry Disability Index (ODI) was reduced to 25 % in the surgical group compared with 6 % in the nonsurgical group (Fritzell et al. 2003). Despite these findings, because of the published variable success rates ranging from 32 to 99 % and because of the wide variety of study methods, it is difficult to draw definitive conclusions concerning the indications for fusion and surgical techniques (Jackson et al. 1985; Lehmann et al. 1987; O'Beirne et al. 1992; Bono and Lee 2004; Lee and Langrana 2004; Lin and Wang 2006).

Although symptomatic degenerative disc disease continues to be treated surgically, there is debate concerning the long-term consequences of spinal fusion. Of particular concern has been adjacent segment degeneration and adjacent segment disease. The term "adjacent segment degeneration" is used to describe radiographic changes without symptoms evident at a level adjacent to a previous fusion, while "adjacent segment disease" refers to radiographic findings that correlate with new clinical symptoms (Hilibrand et al. 1999; Hilibrand and Robbins 2004; Lee and Langrana 2004). The current scientific literature fails to clearly demonstrate if adjacent segment disease is the result of altered biomechanics due to an iatrogenic rigid motion segment, a consequence of surgical technique, progression of the natural history of degenerative disease, or more likely a combination of all of these factors (Hilibrand et al. 1999; Hilibrand and Robbins 2004; Ishihara et al. 2004; Robertson et al. 2005; Yue et al. 2005; Lin and Wang 2006). However, biomechanical studies have shown increased motion, strain, and intradiscal pressures at a spine segment adjacent to a spinal fusion, which may explain the occurrence of adjacent segment disease (Lee and Langrana 1984; Weinhoffer et al. 1995; Matsunaga et al. 1999; Reitman et al. 2004; Murrey et al. 2009). These consequences have been inconsistently experienced in the clinical setting, and there have been conflicting findings in the cervical and lumbar spines due to dissimilar biomechanical environments.

Following cervical spine fusion, the prevalence of adjacent segment disease requiring additional surgery ranges from 9 to 17 %, with an annual incidence of 1.5 to 4 % (Williams et al. 1968; Gore and Sepic 1984; Bohlman et al. 1993; Hilibrand and Robbins 2004). In a landmark study, Hilibrand et al. (1999) reported that following anterior cervical fusion, the annual incidence of adjacent segment disease was approximately 3 % and predicted prevalence of 25.6 % at 10 years. Interestingly, it was noted that when anterior cervical fusion was performed at more than one level, adjacent segment disease was at a significantly lower rate than when performed at a single level. The authors therefore concluded that adjacent segment disease is a common problem following anterior cervical fusions but may also be related to the natural history of cervical spondylosis (Hilibrand et al. 1999). The argument for natural disease progression is also supported by Herkowitz et al. (1990). Thus, following posterior foraminotomy without fusion, 41 % of patients randomized to anterior cervical fusion developed adjacent segment degeneration compared to 50 % of patients.

In the lumbar spine, studies of adjacent segment disease following spinal fusion have also elicited conflicting results. Although one-third to one-half of patients develop adjacent segment degeneration following lumbar fusion, the radiographic findings did not correlate with clinical symptoms (Lehmann et al. 1987; Luk et al. 1987; Hilibrand and Robbins 2004). Regarding the argument for natural disease progression, Penta et al. (1995) compared patients with greater than 10-year follow-up treated nonoperatively with those treated by anterior lumbar interbody fusion. These workers found no difference in the rate of adjacent segment degeneration (approximately one-third of patients) between the two groups. However, a study by Ghiselli et al. (2004) found a significantly higher incidence (27.4 %) of adjacent segment disease requiring further surgery at 6.7 years.

The inconsistent clinical results and conflicting opinions on the efficacy of spinal fusion lend strength to the notion that cervical and lumbar degenerative disc disease is exceedingly complex, and a complete understanding of its etiology continues to be elusive. Even in carefully selected patient populations, a successful clinical result can be difficult to achieve even when radiographic fusion is successful. Since pain is a critical measure of success, fusion may fail due to generation of pain from the degenerative nucleus pulposus, nociceptive nerve endings within the annulus fibrosus, dorsal root ganglion, facet joints, and joint capsules, or even the surrounding ligamentous and muscular structures at a single or multiple levels (Bono and Garfin 2004). Incomplete pain relief due to failure to address a specific pain generator may lead to treatment failure and may be further impacted by factors such as psychosocial dysfunction, pseudarthrosis, adjacent segment disease, as well as morbidity arising from surgery (Kumar et al. 2001; Lin and Wang 2006; Orr et al. 2007). Given the uncertainties and potential complications following spinal fusion for treatment of degenerative disc disease, there has been increasing enthusiasm for total disc arthroplasty.

14.3 History and Evolution of Disc Arthroplasty Devices

Disc arthroplasty devices are an emerging technology for the treatment of spinal disc degeneration. With recent advances in our understanding of this technology, an appreciation of its origins, history, and evolution provides a useful perspective on its role in the treatment of spinal disorders (Bono and Garfin 2004). The earliest disc replacement procedure was reported in the late 1950s by Fernstrom, at approximately the time of Charnley's initial reports on total hip arthroplasty (Fernstrom 1966; Bono and Garfin 2004). Following nucleus pulposus removal, Fernstrom implanted a rudimentary intervertebral disc (a metallic ball) prosthesis into the annulus fibrosus, in both the cervical and lumbar spines of human patients (Fernstrom 1966). Although simplistic in design, Fernstrom's metallic ball achieved the intended goal: pain relief through removal of the painful nucleus, along with maintaining intervertebral height and motion. Despite good short-term results, there was long-term failure from subsidence of the implant through the vertebral end plates, resulting in loss of intervertebral height in about 88 % of cases at 4- to 7-year follow-up (Fernstrom 1966; Bono and Garfin 2004). In hindsight and with continued understanding of total disc requirements, this failure was predictable given the very limited contact of the steel ball with the flat vertebral end plate. In addition to the problem of excessive stress concentration, there was also a mismatch in the modulus of elasticity of the steel ball and bone, especially as the device was placed in the soft, central portion of the vertebral end plate (Bono and Garfin 2004). Despite the shortcomings of the technique, the surgeons were thoughtful in their approach: similar to contemporary disc arthroplasty designs, the steel ball was positioned along the spinal motion segments sagittal arc of angular rotation at the junction of the middle and posterior thirds of the disc space (Bono and Garfin 2004).

To address these biologic failures, Fassio developed a disc arthroplasty device consisting of a central silastic compressible ball with intrinsic shock-absorbing properties and with a larger noncompressible footprint (Fassio and Ginestie 1978). The authors implanted the device into three patients; however, the overall contact surface area of the implant failed to prevent subsidence. In all patients, at 4-year follow-up, there was implant migration and subsidence into the vertebral body (Fassio and Ginestie 1978). Kostuik also developed a device with intrinsic shock-absorption properties; however, it was never implanted in humans and is thus of only historical importance (Kostuik 1997). The device consisted of an articulating hinge in the posterior third of the disc space, with a spring interposed between the two metallic end plates. Despite promising biomechanical cyclical testing, the device failed when implanted in animals and was never made available for clinical use (Kostuik 1997).

An important design concept was the development of the SB Charité (DePuy Spine, Raynham, MA) lumbar disc arthroplasty device by Büttner-Janz and Schellnack in the 1980s. The initial first-generation design consisted of a small bottle-cap-like end-plate interface with a polyethylene core and used a synthetic-on-synthetic articulating surface (Link 2002). However, this design also exhibited insufficient contact area and high stress concentrations, leading to subsidence into the vertebral bodies (Lin and Wang 2006). In an attempt to address this complication, the second-generation device used thin lateral extensions to augment the surface area; however, failure occurred with fatigue fracture of the lateral extensions. This led to a third-generation device, engineered with a broad end-plate interface and manufactured from cobalt-chromium-molybdenum (CoCrMo): (Lin and Wang 2006).

Important lessons were learned from these early design concepts which have provided a base for development of current arthroplasty systems. The most common impediment of the early designs was implant subsidence, and several general principles were adopted to prevent this complication including maximizing vertebral end-plate contact area as well as using a synthetic-on-synthetic articulating surface to avoid direct articulation with the bone. From these principles, there have been continued efforts to develop and improve total disc arthroplasty devices, although none have fully replicated the healthy intervertebral disc.

14.4 Total Disc Arthroplasty Design: Concepts and Biomechanics

Since their inception, the primary clinical objectives of contemporary disc arthroplasty devices have been pain relief and successful functional recovery (Bono and Garfin 2004). Despite continued advancements in understanding, much work needs to be done to optimize disc arthroplasty design and material properties so as to replicate the functional spinal unit.

14.4.1 Biomechanics of the Functional Spinal Unit

Consisting of three components – the intervertebral disc and two facet joints – the functional spinal unit, also termed the spinal motion segment, is a complex articulation, which is significantly different from most other joints (Lee and Goel 2004; Lee and Langrana 2004). As has been discussed in other chapters of the book, the intervertebral disc is also made of three tissues, including the nucleus pulposus, annulus fibrosus, and the vertebral end plates. The three components of the functional spinal unit together with the three tissues of the intervertebral disc are interdependent in terms of their contributions to spinal motion and function. As was discussed in Chaps. 2 and 8, the healthy functional spinal unit plays a significant role in resisting or transmitting loads across the intervertebral disc, maintaining disc height, and segmental stability (Lee and Goel 2004; Lee and Langrana 2004). From a functional viewpoint, the spine cycles between 100,000 and 1 million times per year and experiences load up to three times its body weight (Silva et al. 2002; Polly 2003; Santos et al. 2004). Under axial compression, with a small contribution by the facet joints, the intervertebral disc supports most of the load (Lee and Goel 2004; Lee and Langrana 2004). However, at higher axial compression loads and greater extension, there may be an increased biomechanical role of the facet joints through contact of the inferior facets with the lamina of the vertebra below (Lee and Langrana 1984, 2004; Luk et al. 1987; Weinhoffer et al. 1995). This distribution of load is also reflected in intradiscal pressure, which is proportional to the external load under axial compression; it is significantly increased with flexion and minimal with pure extension and torsion (Weinhoffer et al. 1995; Lee and Goel 2004; Lee and Langrana 2004). In the degenerative disc, this complex biomechanical environment is altered, placing an extra burden on the facet joints, ligamentous structures, and adjacent motion segments (Lee and Langrana 1984, 2004; Lee and Goel 2004).

Total disc arthroplasty is intended to replace the dysfunctional nucleus pulposus and annulus fibrosus and restore the biomechanical environment of a healthy functional spinal

Table 14.1 Properties of total disc arthroplasty prostheses

Implant (year of FDA approval)	Material	Bearing surface	Articulations	Constraint	COR	Fixation
Cervical						
ProDisc-C (2007)	CoCrMo UHMWPE	Metal on polymer	1	Semiconstrained	Fixed	Midline keel bone ingrowth
Prestige (2007)	Stainless steel	Metal on metal	1	Semiconstrained	Mobile	Anterior screws
Bryan (2009)	Titanium Polyurethane	Metal on polymer	2	Unconstrained	Mobile	Milled cavities bone ingrowth
Lumbar						
SB Charité III (2004)	CoCrMo UHMWPE	Metal on polymer	2	Unconstrained	Mobile	Small fins/teeth bone ingrowth
ProDisc-L (2006)	CoCrMo UHMWPE	Metal on polymer	1	Semiconstrained	Fixed	Midline keel bone ingrowth

Adapted from Lin and Wang (2006)
COR center of rotation, *CoCrMo* cobalt-chromium-molybdenum alloy, *UHMWPE* ultrahigh molecular weight polyethylene

unit. However, as with disc degeneration, any significant deviation in implant design or placement can cause abnormal and detrimental effects on the facet joints within the same segment and on adjacent levels (Lee and Goel 2004; Lee and Langrana 2004). Biomechanical cadaveric studies indicate that a properly placed total disc arthroplasty device maintains motion within physiologic range at the treated level and decreases stresses and intradiscal pressure on adjacent segments (Cunningham et al. 2003b; DiAngelo et al. 2004; Puttlitz et al. 2004; Dmitriev et al. 2005).

14.4.2 Biomechanical Objectives of Disc Arthroplasty

As our understanding of cervical and lumbar spine function has continued to increase, several biomechanical objectives of total disc arthroplasty have been defined: preservation of motion, restoration of intervertebral height, maintenance of stability, and conversion of shock-absorption properties. Preservation of motion involves coupled motion patterns in compression-bending and compression-torsion, as well as the instantaneous axis of rotation (Lee and Goel 2004; Lee and Langrana 2004). Restoration of intervertebral height is required for indirect neuroforaminal decompression, to adequately restore spinal alignment, and to unload abnormal stresses on the facet joints. Immediate implant stability prevents displacement or migration, maintains the stability of the spinal motion segment, and prevents abnormal motion and wear events which can lead to early device failure (Lee and Goel 2004; Lee and Langrana 2004). Finally, shock absorption incorporates load transmission with shock attenuation and ultimately prevents abnormal stress concentration on surrounding structures and adjacent motion segments. These biomechanical objectives have been used to develop many different arthroplasty devices; however, each has specific differences with respect to material, bearing surface, number of articulations, constraint, mobility of the center of rotation, and fixation to bone (Table 14.1). The biomechanical significance of each of these design variations on the surrounding structures such as the facet joints of the same segment and on adjacent segments has received limited study, and different arthroplasty devices have not been compared to each other in clinical trials. Notwithstanding, it is important to recognize that lumbar disc arthroplasty devices prompted advancements in cervical disc devices. The design concepts and biomechanical objectives were similar; however, specific differences exist which will be further discussed.

14.4.3 Disc Arthroplasty: Material Considerations and Bearing Surfaces

The development of a successful total disc arthroplasty device with acceptable long-term survival has relied on the immense clinical and technical experience of surgeons and engineers. The lessons learned from this field of study have helped to better understand and improve motion-preserving devices in the spine while avoiding some of the intrinsic pitfalls and complications especially in relation to the properties of materials and the mechanics of the system (Santos et al. 2004). The material properties necessary for any prosthesis must be determined based on the requirements expected of the implant (Taksali et al. 2004). For example, the lumbar spine sustains significantly greater loads than the cervical spine, whereas the cervical spine has a different kinematic pattern and greater range of motion. From this perspective, materials that perform well in the cervical spine may perform poorly in the lumbar spine.

Modern disc arthroplasty devices have a prosthesis-bone interface consisting of a broad rigid end plate made of metal; most devices are flat or slightly convex (dome) shaped. Not surprisingly, implant geometry is an important factor in disc arthroplasty, the goal being to maximize prosthesis-bone contact for bony ingrowths and to prevent subsidence. The primary alloys used in disc arthroplasty devices are stainless steel, cobalt chrome and titanium alloys. Cobalt chrome alloys have the greatest wear resistance, whereas titanium alloys have poor wear characteristics and surface hardness, making them unacceptable as an articulating surface. Titanium alloys demonstrate excellent biocompatibility with less susceptibility to bacterial surface colonization. Also, they generate a significantly less artifact during computed tomography or magnetic resonance imaging (Arens et al. 1996; Hallab et al. 2003a; Santos et al. 2004). They are most commonly used as a coating of the end-plate interface to facilitate bony ingrowth (Santos et al. 2004).

In terms of a bearing surface, the basic requirements is that the articular surface must allow for mobility, load distribution, low friction, and high wear resistance, as well as being biologically compatible with adequate longevity (Taksali et al. 2004; Lin and Wang 2006). Like total joint arthroplasty, the principal bearing surfaces of disc arthroplasty devices are metal-on-polymer or metal-on-metal articulations. Although ceramic-bearing surfaces have gained some popularity due to excellent wear characteristic, the brittle material properties and concerns for catastrophic failure in proximity to neural elements have precluded significant development (Garino 2000; Santos et al. 2004). In fact, a recent case report has demonstrated catastrophic failure of an experimental ceramic-bearing surface disc device implanted in a human patient (Nguyen et al. 2011).

The two primary polymers used for arthroplasty devices have been polyethylene and polyurethane. Ultrahigh molecular weight polyethylene has a good track record for several decades in extremity arthroplasty and has avoided complications associated with poor wear properties due to polyethylene sterilization techniques (Kurtz et al. 1999a, b; Hallab et al. 2003a; Taksali et al. 2004). Polyurethane has been used for decades for cardiovascular devices but has had limited use in spine surgery. Recently, the importance of its shock-absorbing properties has been recognized and incorporated into a disc arthroplasty device, in particular the Bryan cervical disc replacement (Medtronic Sofamor Danek, Memphis, TN). However, there are few studies evaluating axial motion and load transfer properties. This is unfortunate because one of the functions of the normal, healthy intervertebral disc is to provide shock absorption, and if absent may produce abnormal stress concentrations on surrounding structures within the segment and at the adjacent segment (Dahl et al. 2006). Dahl evaluated axial stiffness, energy absorption, and viscous damping of metal-on-polyurethane cervical disc arthroplasty with both a fusion construct and an intact intervertebral disc. The investigators found the dynamic stiffness of metal-on-polyurethane was similar to that of the intact disc, and energy absorption and viscous damping exceeded both the intact disc and fusion construct. In another study, Dahl et al. (2011) compared the shock-absorbing properties of polyurethane, polyethylene, and titanium alloy bearing surface materials. These workers demonstrated that polyurethane provides significantly lower stiffness and greater energy absorption and damping characteristics than polyethylene and titanium alloy. Of note, titanium alloy is currently not available as a bearing surface due to its poor wear characteristics. A concern with the use of polyurethane is the biologic durability or wear resistance. However, polyurethane has compared favorably to polyethylene and has been found to have excellent wear properties, with wear particles that do not incite a significant inflammatory response (Anderson et al. 2003, 2004; Taksali et al. 2004; Pitzen et al. 2007). While these reports acknowledged that shock absorption remains a theoretical benefit of disc arthroplasty devices, no clinical study has compared outcomes of shock- versus non-shock-absorbing devices (LeHuec et al. 2003).

Also of importance is the polymer core design, which predominately exists as either a single-gliding surface with a securely fixed polymer core or one with a metal end plate (ProDisc; Synthes Spine, Paoli, PA) or a double-gliding surface with a mobile polymer core sandwiched between two metal end plates (Bryan Cervical Disc; Medtronic Sofamor Danek, Memphis, TN). Concerns with the fixed polymer core are the presence of another point of implant failure due to constant micromotion, stress concentration, and a large difference in elastic properties at the metal-polymer interface. Problems associated with a mobile polymer core include concerns for polymer extrusion as well as increased debris from wear of the two articulating surfaces. Not surprisingly, there are continued research efforts to maximize the design properties and wear characteristics of metal-on-polymer bearing surfaces. Questions remain regarding wear debris and subsequent osteolysis with late implant failure, although the amount of debris from disc arthroplasty devices may be insignificant when compared to hip and knee joints due to the low range of motion and cyclic rate (Santos et al. 2004).

Despite concerns for systemic metal deposition (Wagner and Wagner 2000; Bisseling et al. 2011), adverse soft tissue reactions (i.e., pseudotumor) (Williams et al. 2011), and higher rates of early failure for some total hip replacement implants, metal-on-metal articulations have been used in total hip arthroplasty devices (Bernthal et al. 2012; Langton et al. 2011). The advantage of a metal-on-metal articulation compared to metal-on-polymer bearing surface is the significantly lower (approximately 10 times) wear rate (Goldsmith et al. 2000; Santos et al. 2004; Taksali et al. 2004). However, there have been reports of elevated systemic metal ion levels in patients following lumbar metal-on-metal total disc replacement (Wagner and Wagner 2000; Bisseling et al. 2011). A recent review of complications in metal-on-metal disc arthroplasty devices reported abnormal inflammatory reactions and soft tissue masses with lymphocyte or macrophage infiltration, similar to those found in patients following metal-on-metal bearing surface total hip arthroplasty (Golish and Anderson 2012). Because of this paucity of information, the surgical community awaits information on the long-term outcomes and complication profile concerning the use of metal-on-metal disc arthroplasty devices.

14.4.4 Semiconstrained Versus Unconstrained Devices

Similar to total joint arthroplasty implants, the amount of constraint is an important factor in disc arthroplasty design. With increasing constraint in total joint arthroplasty, the trade-off is greater stability for greater stress on the implant-bone interface. For disc arthroplasty, there are both semiconstrained and unconstrained designs, with each having advantages and disadvantages (Huang et al. 2003; Santos et al. 2004). The unconstrained design provides a mobile instantaneous axis of rotation and is more representative of the physiologic axis, which was demonstrated by Gertzbein et al. (1986) to be an ellipse rather than a single point. Theoretically, an unconstrained device would provide a greater range of motion and may be more tolerant of small errors in implant placement (Hallab et al. 2003a; Huang et al. 2003). However, an unconstrained articulation subjects the facets and posterior ligaments to increased shear and torsional loads, whereas semiconstrained devices unload the facet joints and ligaments (Cunningham et al. 2003a; Huang et al. 2003; Polly 2003; Santos et al. 2004). Semiconstrained disc arthroplasty devices have increased stability, but similar to joint arthroplasty there is higher load transfer to the implant-bone interface. Currently, the ideal amount of constraint remains unknown and will eventually be determined by long-term clinical studies.

14.4.5 Implant Fixation

Fixation of the disc arthroplasty device to host bone is another important factor to consider, taking into account both initial and long-term implant stability (Santos et al. 2004). Unlike total joint arthroplasty which has successfully used cemented knee arthroplasty implants and cemented femoral stem implants as originally advocated by Charnley (Schulte et al. 1993), disc arthroplasty has not been performed with cement fixation because of the proximity to neural elements (Santos et al. 2004). Another reason cement fixation may be inappropriate for disc arthroplasty is because of the younger patient population compared to extremity arthroplasty, which may potentially increase the incidence of cement fatigue and aseptic loosening due to greater activity levels and physical demands (MacWilliam et al. 1996; McLaughlin and Lee 2000; Santos et al. 2004).

Therefore, immediate stability is obtained by screw fixation of metal end plates to the anterior vertebral body in some devices, whereas others have end-plate designs with a midline fin/keel, or spikes that project perpendicular to the end plate (Lee and Goel 2004). There have been some concerns regarding screw fixation, particularly in the lumbar spine which presents a greater risk for major vascular complications. In the cervical spine, due to the increased anterior profile, there is the possibility of causing dysphagia; due to fixation on the anterior cervical body, difficulties may be experienced in revision surgery in the setting of adjacent segment disease (Kulkarni et al. 2003; van Ooij et al. 2003; Bertagnoli et al. 2005b; Patel et al. 2008).

Long-term stability requires osseointegration achieved through porous ingrowth surfaces or on-growth surface coatings (Taksali et al. 2004). The basic requirements of successful bone ingrowth include implant stability, optimal pore size, and optimal surface geometry/surface area (Kienapfel et al. 1999; Santos et al. 2004). Surface coatings to improve bone on-growth include roughened titanium, titanium wire mesh, plasma-sprayed titanium, and bioactive materials such as hydroxyapatite and calcium phosphate (Taksali et al. 2004). Animal studies have shown successful bone integration with titanium- or hydroxyapatite-coated surfaces (Cunningham et al. 2002, 2003a; Santos et al. 2004). In fact, Cunningham et al. (2002) reported that a lumbar disc arthroplasty device with porous-coated titanium end plates in a nonhuman primate model evidenced bone ingrowth into 56 % of the end-plate surface at 12 months. This is comparable to total joint replacement components, which have found cementless femoral and acetabular implant ingrowth of 9.7–33 % (Sumner et al. 1990; Harvey et al. 1999) and 12 % (Pidhorz et al. 1993), respectively. However, these coatings should continue to be carefully evaluated to ensure acceptable tensile strength, shear strength, and fatigue strength. The potential concern is that inadequate surface coating integrity may cause migration of coating material debris in between the articular surface, leading to accelerated third-body wear (Taksali et al. 2004).

14.5 Comparison of Total Disc Arthroplasty Devices

Cervical and lumbar disc replacements have been categorized as "significant risk devices" by the United States Food and Drug Administration (FDA) and require both preclinical and clinical evaluations to determine their safety and effectiveness (Orr et al. 2007). As noted previously, many of these devices have been used in Europe for decades, and only recent interest in the United States has resulted in several ongoing FDA-sponsored clinical trials, comparing the outcomes and safety of disc arthroplasty devices, using fusion procedures as the control. Although there have been over 100 disc arthroplasty designs and patents, to date there have been two lumbar disc replacement devices (SB Charité III, DePuy Spine, Raynham, MA; and ProDisc-L, Synthes Spine, Paoli, PA) and three cervical disc replacement devices cleared for marketing (Prestige, Medtronic Sofamor Danek, Memphis, TN; ProDisc-C, Synthes Spine, Paoli, PA; Bryan, Medtronic Sofamor Danek, Memphis, TN) by the FDA (Orr et al. 2007). All devices have demonstrated that human use for one-level degenerative disc disease is "non-inferior" to the fusion control group (Orr et al. 2007). We will further discuss the specific design considerations for each FDA-approved device.

Box 14.1 FDA Investigational Device Exemption (IDE), Premarket Approval, and 510(k) Notification

Cervical and lumbar disc replacements are categorized as "significant risk devices" (Class III) by the US Food and Drug Administration (FDA) and have required both preclinical and clinical evaluations to determine their safety and effectiveness prior to marketing. The FDA authorizes an investigational device exemption (IDE), which allows a device to be used for the purpose of a clinical study to collect safety and effectiveness data to support a premarket approval or premarket notification 510(k). When under IDE status, the device remains unapproved by the FDA and typically can only be used on human subjects when it is under clinical investigation and used by investigators participating in the clinical trial. However, the FDA also allows the use of an unapproved device before premarket approval for "emergency use" to save the life of a patient or prevent irreversible morbidity, for "compassionate use" to help a patient suffering from a serious disease or condition for which there exists no other alternative therapy, and after an IDE clinical trial for "continued access" if there is a public health need, and preliminary evidence suggests the device will be effective with no significant safety concerns.

There have been only a few total disc arthroplasty devices which have received FDA premarket approval, which is a rigorous process of scientific and regulatory review to evaluate the safety and effectiveness of Class III medical devices. The completion of a premarket approval for a device usually requires the manufacturer to dedicate a significant amount of time, energy, and funding. However, the FDA allows certain modified devices to undergo the 510(k) notification process which relies on comparisons with an already-approved and similar device and provides an expedited review, usually within 90 days. The 510(k) notification does not require the modified device to undergo extensive clinical testing, thereby avoiding the rigorous premarket approval process. Many manufacturers attempt 510(k) notifications for their devices because of the ability to rapidly market their product; however, this process may permit a modified device to be used in a widespread fashion without a full understanding of the risks, failure rate, and complications.

14.5.1 Lumbar TDA Devices

The SB Charité III (DePuy Spine, Raynham, MA) (Fig. 14.1) was the first total disc arthroplasty device to be implanted in the USA in 2000 as part of a controlled randomized study and was subsequently the first FDA-approved disc arthroplasty device in 2004. SB Charité has evolved from its initial design (SB Charité I and II) designed by Shellnack and Büttner-Janz in the early 1980s, which consisted of small, shell-like end plates made of stainless steel, which resulted in implant subsidence and migration (Buttner-Janz et al. 2002; Link 2002). The Charité II attempted to address this problem by adding thin lateral wings to increase the surface area of the end plates; however, these wings developed early fatigue fractures (Lin and Wang 2006). The device is now in its third and current version and was developed in 1987 with broad flat end plates manufactured from cobalt-chromium-molybdenum (CoCrMo) alloy with small teeth projecting into the vertebral end plates (Lin and Wang 2006). There is also the new InMotion design, which retains the essential characteristics of the Charité III, with the modifications involving the teeth orientation and the addition of a central rail portion allowing the prosthesis to glide onto a ramp inserter (Serhan et al. 2011). The device end plates are porous-coated with

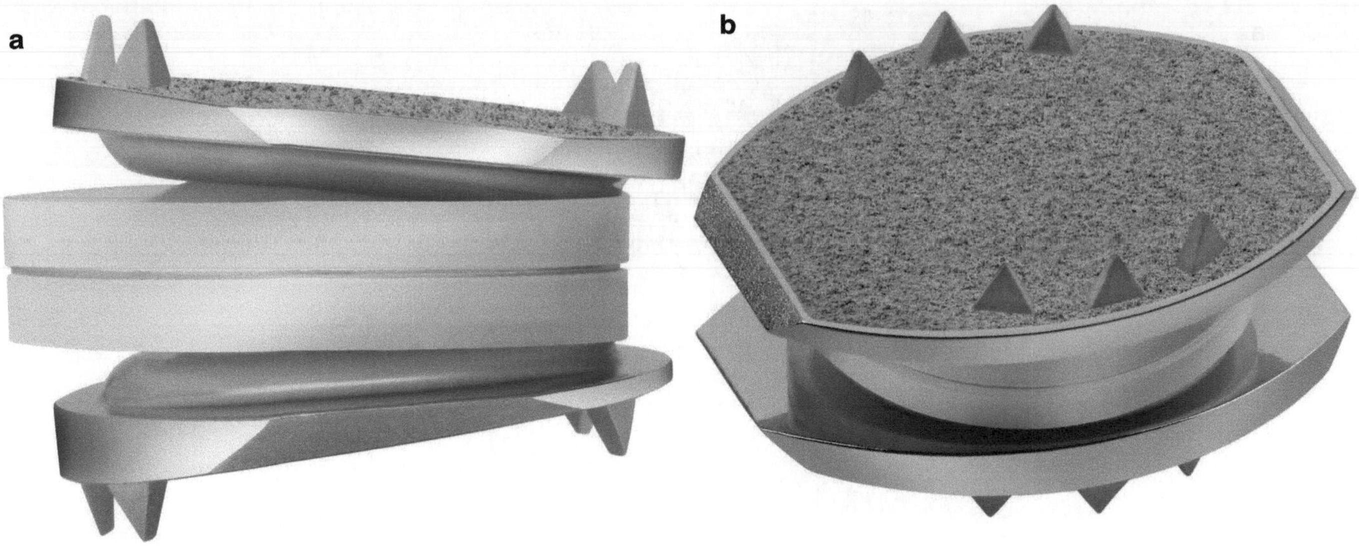

Fig. 14.1 (a, b) SB Charité III lumbar disc arthroplasty device (Images provided by DePuy Spine, Raynham, MA)

plasma-sprayed titanium and calcium phosphate (TiCaP) to assist with bony ingrowth. The polyethylene core is a sliding, unconstrained biconvex design to allow for an instantaneous axis of rotation (IAR) that permits anterior and posterior movement to the midpoint of the disc during flexion and extension, respectively, which is believed to more closely replicate normal segmental motion (Lin and Wang 2006). However, the IAR of the arthroplasty device has been found to be more anterior than normal, in both flexion and extension, and may detract from its presumed advantage (Bono and Garfin 2004). Cunningham showed that the motion of the Charité III prosthesis closely resembles normal motion in cadaveric testing, with disc motion similar to the intact segment in flexion-extension and lateral bending; however, normal limits of axial rotation were exceeded (Cunningham 2004). Another disadvantage is that there are two articulating surfaces which theoretically may increase polyethylene wear and debris formation, compared to only one gliding surface. Also, the polyethylene core is unconstrained with the potentially catastrophic complication of core extrusion.

ProDisc-L (Synthes Spine, Paoli, PA) (Fig. 14.2) was designed and developed by Marnay in the 1980s and first implanted in France in 1990. The device received FDA approval in 2006 after undergoing several design modifications, including a change of end-plate material from titanium to CoCrMo and the addition of ultrahigh molecular weight polyethylene (UHMWPE) bearing surface as a separate modular piece which is snap-locked to the inferior end plate (Lin and Wang 2006). A single, titanium plasma spray-coated midline sagittal fin is used to improve immediate and long-term end-plate fixation, as opposed to the six small teeth of the SB Charité III. The semiconstrained interface between the polyethylene core fixed to the inferior end plate articulating with a polished superior metallic end plate is thought to decrease the risk of polymer extrusion. However, the rotational axis lies within the anterosuperior aspect of the lower vertebral body, and the fixed axis of rotation does not allow for an anatomic coupled anteroposterior translation with flexion and extension (Lin and Wang 2006). In patients with a degenerative spinal motion segment with abnormally increased range of motion, the semiconstrained design is thought to be beneficial by allowing stability through a more controlled arc of motion and protecting the facet joints from shear forces. However, some authorities believe that increased constraint may cause abnormal force transfer to the bone-end plate interface resulting in premature loosening, abnormal forces within the facet joints, and anteroposterior dimensional changes of the neuroforamina during motion (Huang et al. 2003; Bono and Garfin 2004).

14.5.2 Cervical TDA Devices

ProDisc-C (Synthes Spine, Paoli, PA) (Figs. 14.3 and 14.4) is similar in design to its lumbar counterpart and received FDA approval in 2007. The device is also made up of three components, which include an inferior and superior CoCrMo alloy end plate with a midline keel-oriented anteroposterior anchoring into the end plate of the respective vertebral body. In addition there is a highly polished concave bearing surface from the superior alloy end plate which articulates with a convex (spherical dome) UHMWPE

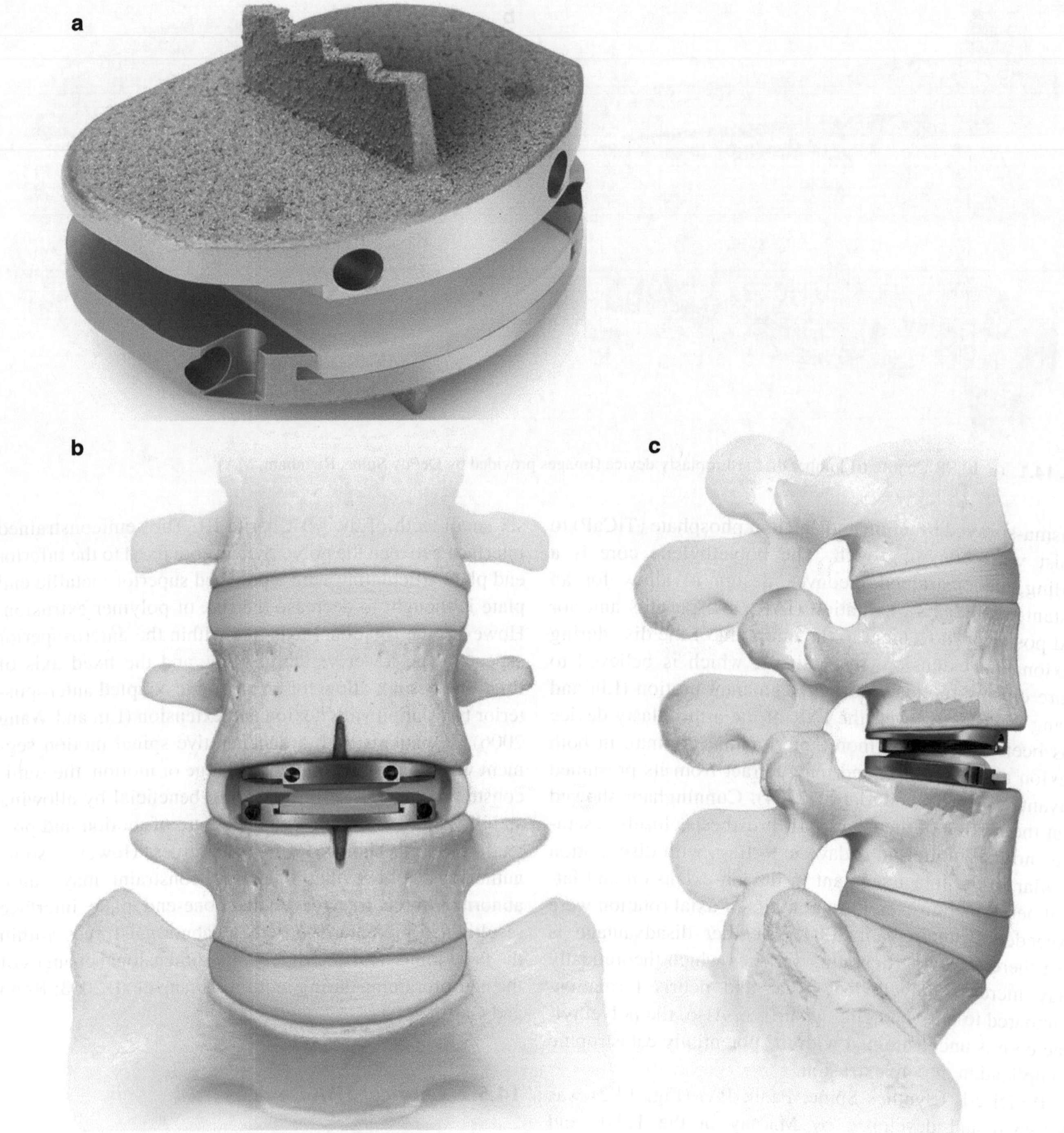

Fig. 14.2 (a–c) ProDisc-L lumbar disc arthroplasty device (Images provided by Synthes Spine, Paoli, PA)

insert that is preassembled and snap-locked into the inferior alloy end plate (Lin and Wang 2006). Similar concerns exist regarding the semiconstrained articulation and may be of greater concern in the cervical spine due to the inherent greater range of motion; however, this has yet to be evaluated.

The Prestige ST (Medtronic Sofamor Danek, Memphis, TN) (Figs. 14.5 and 14.6) was developed by Gill and colleagues in 2002 and was approved by the FDA in 2007. The Prestige ST is a modification of the original Prestige I (1989) and II (1999) initially designed and developed by Bristol-Cummins at Frenchay Hospital in 1989 (Traynelis 2004).

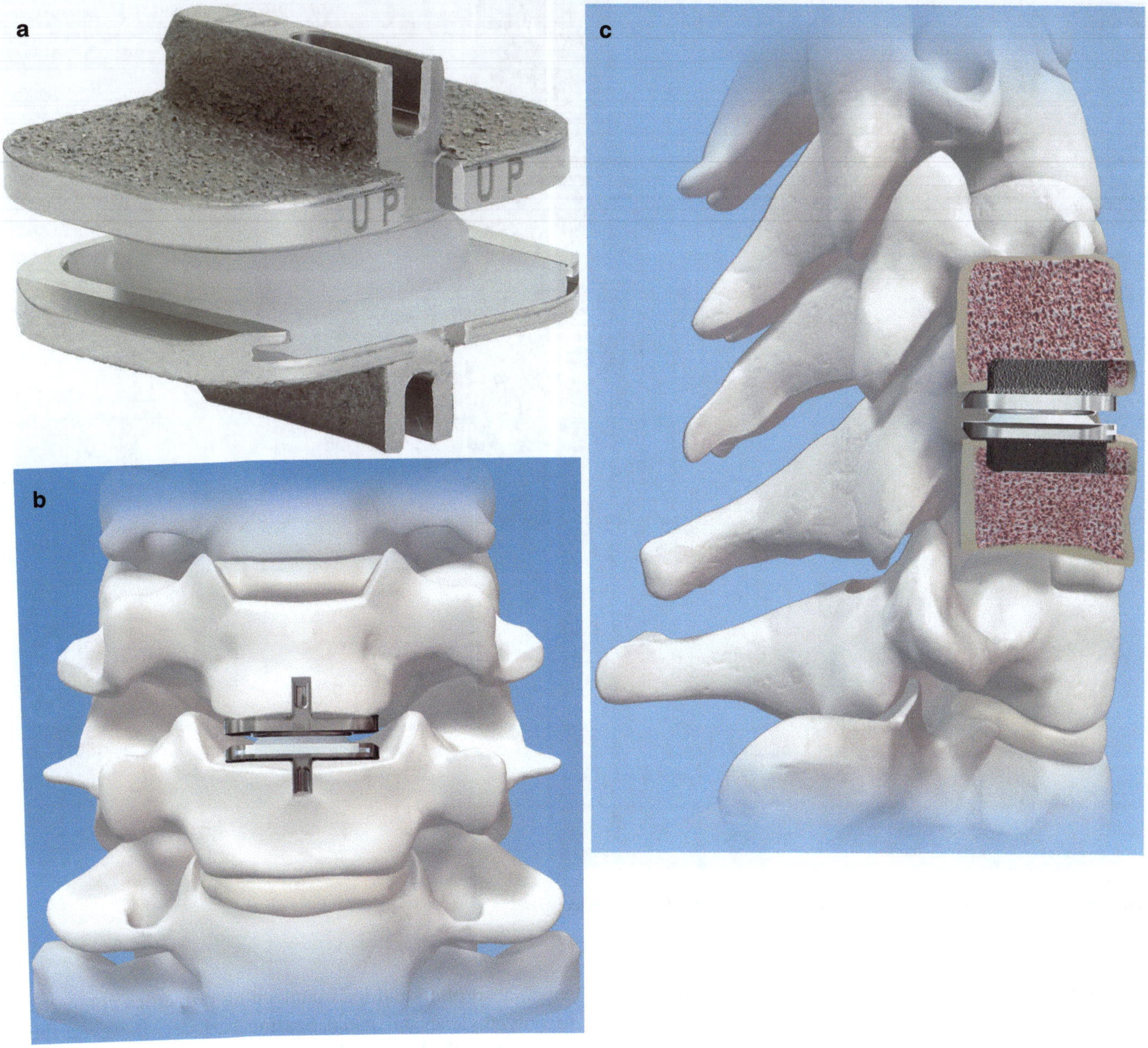

Fig. 14.3 (**a-c**) ProDisc-C cervical disc arthroplasty device (Images provided by Synthes Spine, Paoli, PA)

The key improvements between Prestige I and Prestige II were a more anatomic end-plate design, which was roughened/grit-blasted to promote bony ingrowth; an improvement from Prestige II to Prestige ST was a 2-mm reduction in the height of each anterior flange. The device is a semiconstrained metal-on-metal prosthesis (stainless steels), with a ball-in-trough design which is postulated to replicate physiologic segmental motion (Traynelis 2004). To provide immediate stability, and unique to other designs, screws are placed through plate-like extensions on the superior and inferior, anterior vertebral bodies (Bono and Garfin 2004). The ball-in-trough design provides semiconstrained motion; however, unlike the ProDisc ball-in-socket design, there is some coupled translation with flexion-extension. Again, the consequences of this added translation are unknown, and further long-term follow-up is necessary to determine if there are detrimental effects on the facets joints from shear forces.

The Bryan Cervical Disc (Medtronic Sofamor Danek, Memphis, TN) (Figs. 14.7 and 14.8) was developed in the

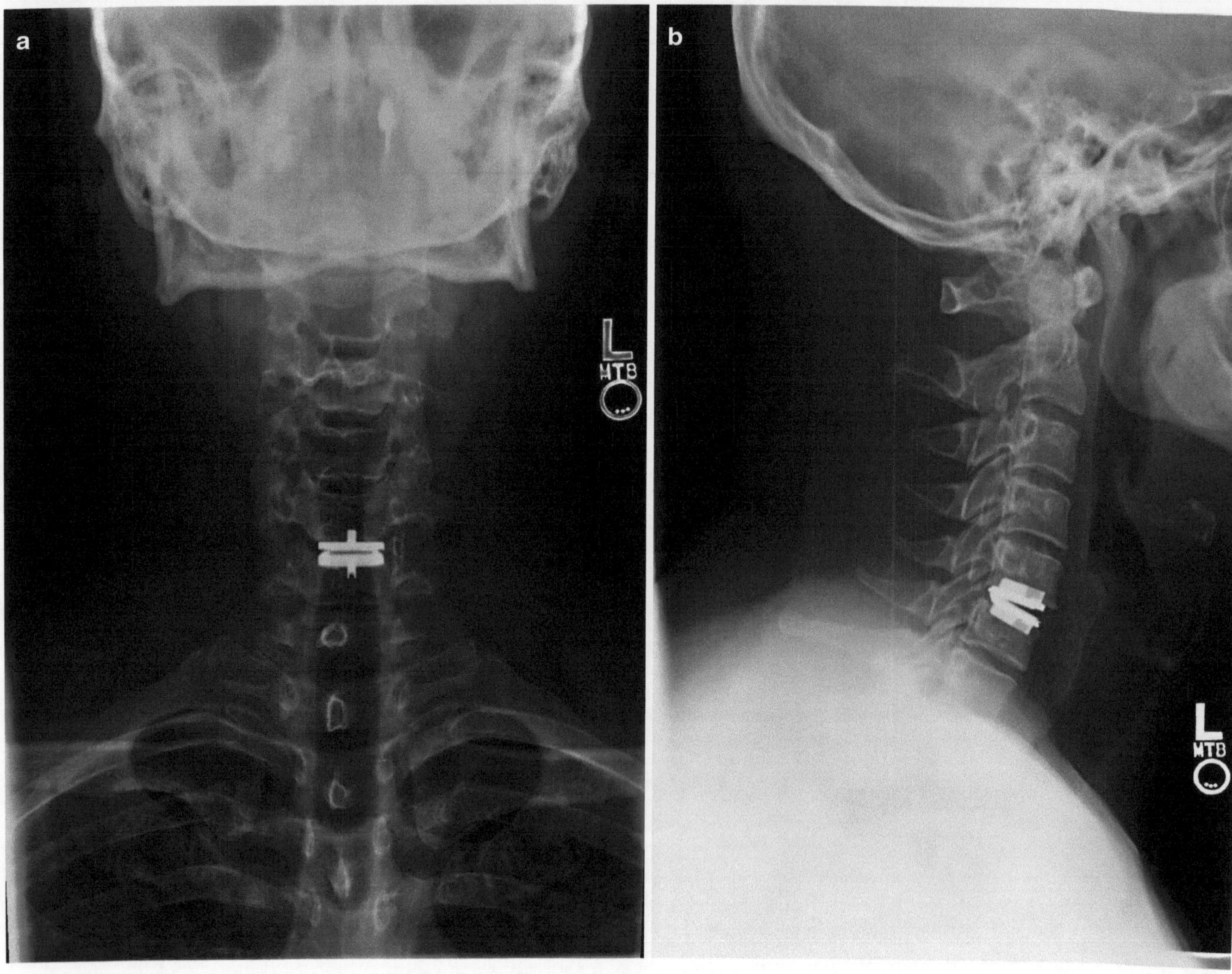

Fig. 14.4 (**a**, **b**) Radiographs of patient with single-level ProDisc-C device

late 1990s and received FDA approval in 2009. The device is an unconstrained, biarticulating metal-on-polyurethane prosthesis. It is composed of two titanium alloy shells, a polycarbonate polyurethane nucleus, and a polyether polyurethane sheath with titanium-retaining wires. The polyurethane sheath spans between the metal end plates and surrounds the nucleus, forming a cavity that is filled with saline, acting as synovial fluid or lubricant (Bono and Garfin 2004). This is thought to keep potential wear debris within the cavity while also preventing soft tissue ingrowth between the articulating surfaces (Lin and Wang 2006). The device also has a unique method of fixation to the bone, sitting in a pocket milled into the vertebral end plate; long-term stability is provided by bone incorporation with a beaded titanium coating on the device end plates – it is not screwed or secured by teeth to the vertebra. As previously discussed, the polyurethane nucleus provides greater shock-absorption and load-dampening properties compared to polyethylene and metal bearing surfaces; however, the clinical benefits have not been established.

Box 14.2 Spinal Device Registry

The development of a spinal device registry within the USA remains a necessity, particularly with the real and potential benefits demonstrated by registries for other medical devices. Registries for hip and knee replacement devices have become a worldwide reality with preeminent registries in Sweden, Finland, Norway, Australia, Denmark, and New Zealand, approaching 15 years of experience. A device registry allows a real-time assessment of the current clinical practice and associated outcomes, providing

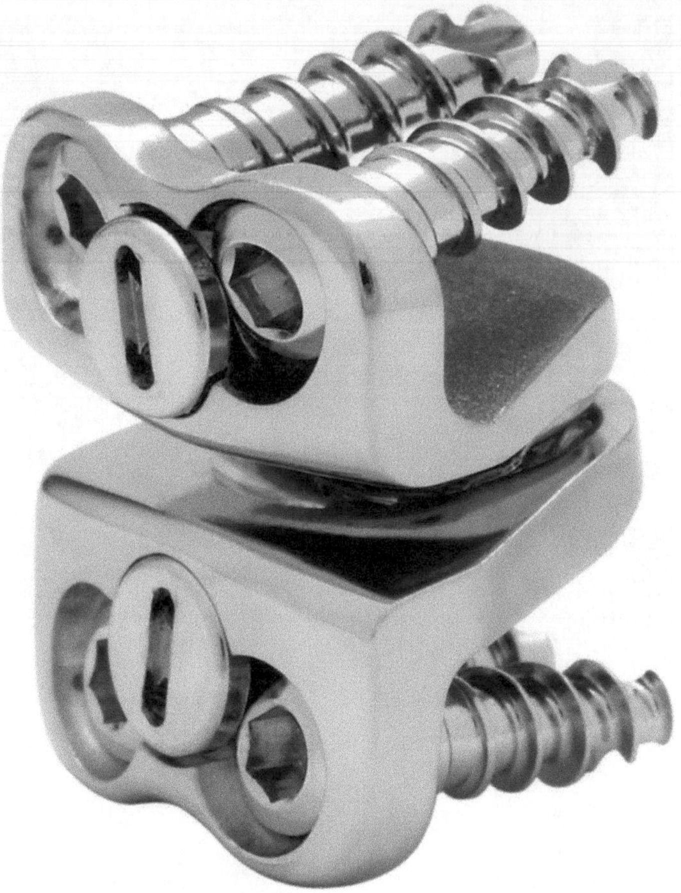

Fig. 14.5 Prestige ST cervical disc arthroplasty device (Images provided by Medtronic Sofamor Danek USA, Inc.)

timely feedback, and permits healthcare organizations to significantly influence physician behavior. Most importantly, to avoid unnecessary complications for patients, device registries provide an early warning system for early implant failure. Device registries also validate the value and cost-effectiveness for the use of healthcare resources and promote improved clarity and evidence in the development of clinical practice guidelines.

The Swiss Spine Registry is the first national spine device registry started in March 2005 to gather data on patient outcomes, cost, and performance information for cervical and lumbar total disc arthroplasty and balloon kyphoplasty procedures. A 3-year pilot study with 135 participating Swiss surgeons demonstrated an 80 % data capture rate for total disc arthroplasty cases performed (925 cervical and 497 lumbar disc replacements), and analysis of registry data generated sufficient evidence to validate continued federal health insurance reimbursement. The success of the Swiss spine registry should serve as an example for the development of a US spinal device registry and collection of observational data in a nationwide framework to enhance the quality of patient care and tracking the performance of spinal implants.

Box 14.3 Evolution of Total Disc Arthroplasty Devices: Timeline

1950s Fernstrom ball, considered the first rudimentary intervertebral disc prosthesis

1978 Fassio develops disc arthroplasty device with a central silastic compressible ball

1997 Kostuik develops a device with an articulating hinge and springs between two metallic end plates; however, it was never implanted in humans

SB Charite Lumbar Disc Arthroplasty

Early 1980s SB Charité I lumbar disc arthroplasty device developed by Büttner-Janz and Schellnack

1987 SB Charité III, third generation and current version was developed

2000 SB Charité III, first total disc arthroplasty device implanted in the USA

2004 SB Charité III, approved by US FDA for marketing

2011 SB Charité III, removed from market by manufacturer

ProDisc-L and ProDisc-C Disc Arthroplasty

1980s ProDisc-L, developed by Marnay

1990 ProDisc-L, first implanted in France

2006 ProDisc-L, approved by US FDA for marketing

2007 ProDisc-C, approved by US FDA for marketing

Prestige Cervical Disc Arthroplasty

1989 Prestige I, developed by Bristol-Cummins at Frenchay Hospital

1999 Prestige II, modified with a more anatomic end-plate design

2002 Prestige ST, developed by Gill and colleagues, modified with a 2-mm reduction in the height of each anterior flange

2007 Prestige ST, approved by US FDA for marketing

Bryan Cervical Disc Arthroplasty

Late 1990s Bryan Disc, developed by Medtronic

2009 Bryan Disc, approved by US FDA for marketing

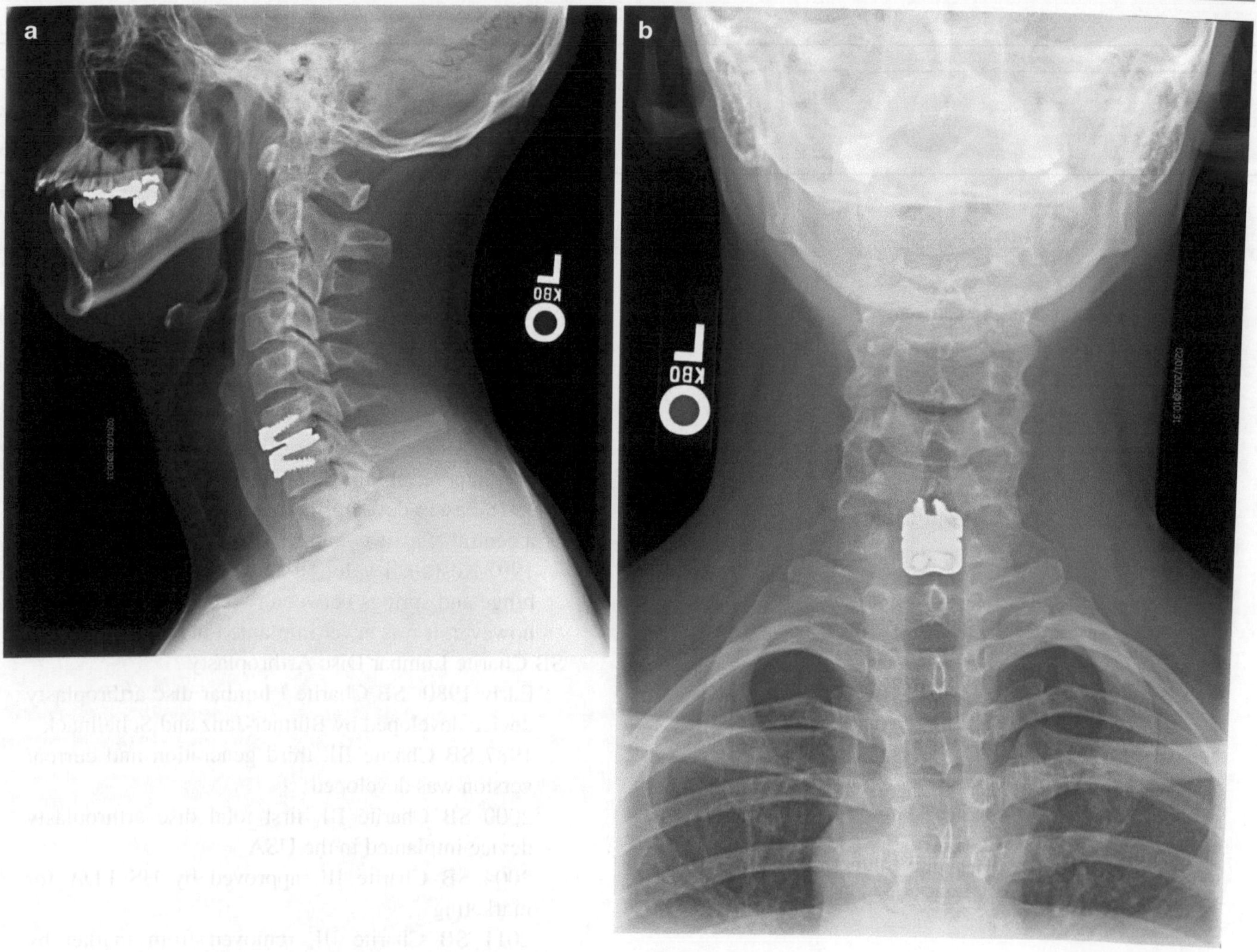

Fig. 14.6 (**a**, **b**) Radiographs of patient with single-level Prestige ST cervical disc device

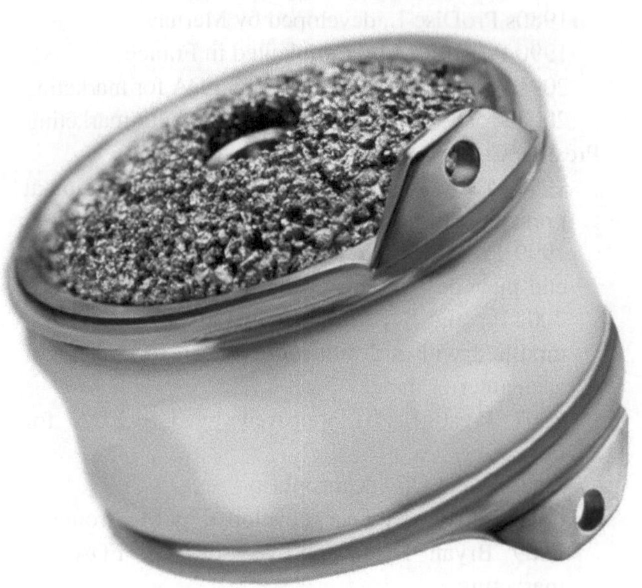

Fig. 14.7 Bryan cervical disc arthroplasty device (Images provided by Medtronic Sofamor Danek USA, Inc.)

14.6 Operative Technique

Careful preoperative planning is required for each patient, and although there is currently no method to template for implant size/positioning, the surgeon should be fully familiar with implant-specific instructions, instrumentation, and sizing options. Additional equipment and implants for a fusion procedure should also be readily available in the rare instance the arthroplasty procedure must be aborted. The operative techniques for both lumbar and cervical disc replacements use an anterior approach. In the lumbar spine, an anterior retroperitoneal dissection is performed to access the desired disc space, and assistance may be provided by a general or vascular surgeon. In the cervical spine, a standard Smith-Robinson anterior approach is used to access the diseased level. Once adequate exposure is obtained, the diseased intervertebral disc is removed, and the end plates of the vertebral bodies are prepared based on device-specific requirements. Some require arduous end-plate preparation,

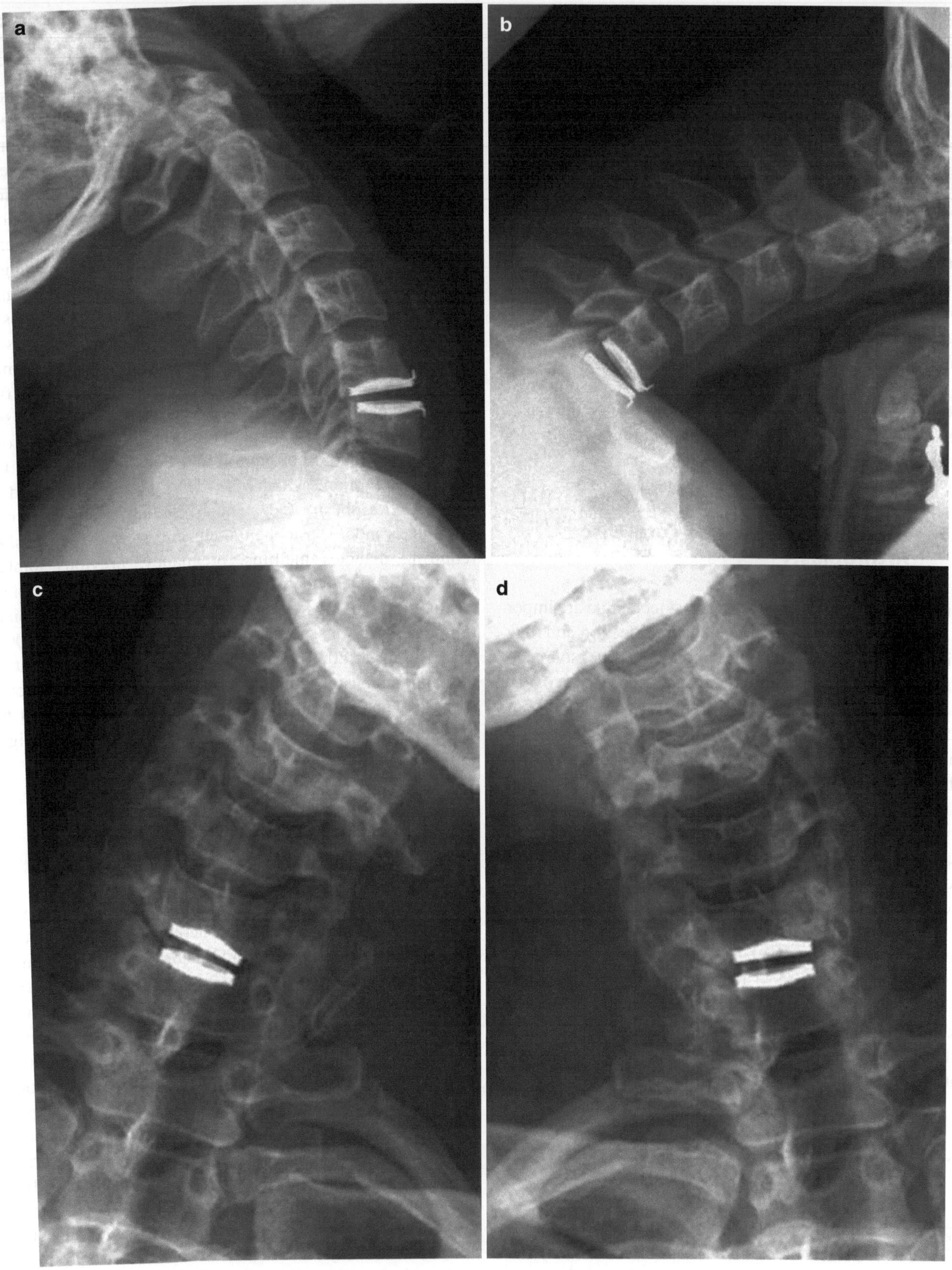

Fig. 14.8 (**a–d**) Radiographs of patient with single-level Bryan cervical disc arthroplasty device (Images provided by Medtronic Sofamor Danek USA, Inc.)

whereas others recommend limited end-plate disruption to reduce the risk of implant subsidence. An important step for most devices is to adequately release the posterior longitudinal ligament to allow correct positioning and function of the prosthesis. At this step, each arthroplasty device varies in specific technique, instrumentation, and implant positioning/sizing, and for lumbar TDA the lordotic angle should be verified using biplanar fluoroscopic imaging (Lin and Wang 2006). In positioning most prostheses, the axis of rotation should be posteriorly located in the disc space, but caution should be taken due to the risk of encroachment of the neural elements (Santos et al. 2004). Appropriately sizing the implant is also important to restore intervertebral disc space height and provide indirect decompression, and to allow normal soft tissue and ligamentous tension, thereby providing additional stability to the implant. Also, a prosthesis covering a large surface area is desired to reduce the risk of subsidence as well as allowing greater range of motion (Cinotti et al. 1996; Santos et al. 2004).

14.7 Deciding When to Use Total Disc Arthroplasty

While ideal implant design and surgical technique are important, more critical are appropriate patient selection and diagnosis. The importance of determining the true source of symptoms cannot be overemphasized, as failure to recognize and treat all sources of pain will result in a suboptimal outcome. History and physical examination are vital in determining the true source of symptoms and may be complemented with radiologic investigations such as plain radiographs, computed tomography (CT), myelography, and magnetic resonance imaging (MRI), when indicated. For degenerative disc disease, the ideal surgical candidate is one who has severe, functionally debilitating symptoms and has exhausted all conservative treatment modalities for a minimum of 6 months in the lumbar spine and 6 weeks in the cervical spine (McAfee 2004; Santos et al. 2004). Conservative management may include physical therapy, facet joint injections, epidural steroids, acupuncture, back school, behavior modification, ultrasound, anti-inflammatory medications, analgesic medications, muscle relaxants, lumbosacral stabilization therapy, and orthotic management (McAfee 2004).

14.7.1 Indications for Lumbar Total Disc Arthroplasty

Appropriate patient selection requires an understanding of the indications and contraindications for lumbar total disc arthroplasty, which have been established from the enrollment criteria of FDA IDE trials (Mummaneni et al. 2007; Sasso et al. 2007; Zigler et al. 2007; Guyer et al. 2009; Murrey et al. 2009). The primary indication for lumbar TDA is isolated mechanical discogenic back pain without radiculopathy or instability at L3–L4, L4–L5, or L5–S1 intervertebral levels. Degenerative disc disease as the primary symptom source is corroborated on CT or MRI studies with one or more of the following findings: vacuum disc sign, contained nucleus pulposus, absence of lateral recess stenosis, paucity of facet joint degeneration changes, decrease of intervertebral disc height of greater than 4 mm, scarring/thickening of the annulus fibrosus, formation of degenerative cyst, or marginal vertebral body osteophytes. Controversy continues to exist regarding the utility and validity of discography as an investigative tool (Sandhu et al. 2000; Carragee and Alamin 2001). However, a provocative discogram can be used to further delineate the symptomatic levels, with a positive result demonstrating concordant pain reproduction and at least one control level that is not painful and does not reproduce the patient's symptoms. Otherwise, TDA is contraindicated in patients with obesity (>1 standard deviation above normal body mass index), osteopenia, chronic steroid use, insulin-requiring diabetes mellitus, pregnancy, previous lumbar fusion, objective evidence of nerve root compression, spinal fracture, spondylolysis, spondylolisthesis, scoliosis, spinal tumor, stenosis, or severe facet joint arthrosis (McAfee 2004; Madigan et al. 2009). The only exception for treatment of radicular pain using a lumbar TDA may be carefully selected cases of neuroforaminal stenosis that can be corrected by restoring intervertebral disc and neuroforaminal height through TDA placement (Table 14.2).

14.7.2 Indications for Cervical Total Disc Arthroplasty

The primary indication for cervical TDA is radiculopathy and/or myelopathy due to disc herniation or spondylosis without instability, requiring discectomy/decompression at intervertebral levels between C3 and T1 (Orr et al. 2007). The patient must have an abnormal neurologic examination indicative of radiculopathy or myelopathy, which may include abnormal reflexes or decrease in sensation or motor strength in a correlating dermatome/myotome. Also, a focal compressive lesion must be observed by CT, myelography, or MRI (McAfee 2004). Cervical TDA should be avoided in patients with ankylosing spondylitis, rheumatoid arthritis, ossification of the posterior longitudinal ligament, or diffuse idiopathic skeletal hyperostosis, as well as a relative contraindication in patients with obesity (>1 standard deviation above normal body mass index), osteopenia, chronic steroid use, insulin-requiring diabetes mellitus, pregnancy, previous

Table 14.2 Current indications for lumbar disc arthroplasty

Indications	Relative contraindication
Symptomatic 1- to 2-level discogenic back pain without radiculopathy or instability at L3–L4, L–L5, or L5–S1 levels	Central or lateral recess stenosis
Concordant degenerative disc disease on CT or MRI studies or discograms	Facet arthroplasty
Failure of >6 months of conservative treatment	Obesity (>1 standard deviation above normal body mass index)
Specific radiographic findings include vacuum disc sign, contained nucleus pulposus, absence of lateral recess stenosis, paucity of facet joint degeneration changes, decrease of intervertebral disc height of greater than 4 mm, scarring/thickening of the annulus fibrosus, formation of degenerative cyst, or marginal vertebral body osteophytes	Osteopenia
Treatment of radicular pain may be performed in carefully selected cases of neuroforaminal stenosis	Chronic steroid use Insulin-requiring diabetes mellitus Pregnancy Previous lumbar fusion/infection/fracture Objective evidence of nerve root compression Spondylolysis/spondylolisthesis Scoliosis Spinal tumor Spinal stenosis

cervical spinal infection, spinal fracture, or severe facet joint arthrosis. Axial neck pain as a solitary symptom is also a contraindication for cervical TDA, which is in contrast to lumbar TDA where an ideal candidate has isolated mechanical back pain with no radicular symptoms (McAfee 2004). A potential complication of cervical arthroplasty is the potential for recurrent radiculopathy resulting from spondylotic progression and/or ossification (Albert and Eichenbaum 2004). Because motion preservation may lead to recurrence of spondylosis when compared to fusion procedures, patients with spondylotic radiculopathy or myelopathy may require wider uncinate resection and decompression. Although not studied in the FDA IDE trials, there are reports of implanting cervical TDA for adjacent-level disease next to an established fusion (Kim et al. 2003); these have been performed in multilevel TDA constructs (Cardoso and Rosner 2010) and in hybrid constructs with TDA above a primary fusion (Cardoso et al. 2011). There have been few reported complications and adverse implant-related events (Table 14.3).

Table 14.3 Current indications for cervical disc arthroplasty

Indications	Relative contraindication
Radiculopathy and/or myelopathy due to disc herniation or spondylosis without instability, requiring discectomy, or decompression at intervertebral levels between C3 to T1, with 1- to 3-level disc disease	Isolated axial neck pain
Concordant focal compressive lesion on CT, myelography, or MRI	Ankylosing spondylitis
Failure >6 weeks of conservative treatment	Rheumatoid arthritis Ossification of the posterior longitudinal ligament Diffuse idiopathic skeletal hyperostosis Cervical instability Previous spinal fusion/infection/fracture Obesity (>1 standard deviation above normal body mass index) Osteopenia Chronic steroid use Insulin-requiring diabetes mellitus Pregnancy Spinal tumor Severe facet joint arthrosis

14.8 Total Disc Arthroplasty Revision Strategies

Total disc arthroplasty failure and complications may require revision or removal of the prosthesis; however, the long-term failure rate and all potential complications remain unknown. Moreover, there are currently no known specific considerations or protocols for revision or replacement surgery (Lee and Goel 2004). Failure of disc arthroplasty can be due to many different factors, including suboptimal surgical technique, implant malpositioning, and poor patient selection; others include mechanical implant and biologic failure (Kostuik 2004; Bertagnoli et al. 2005b; Patel et al. 2008). In fact, the Charité FDA IDE study evaluating 304 patients found 17 % had suboptimal or poor placement of the prosthesis, which was significantly correlated with ODI and VAS scores (McAfee et al. 2005). Van Ooji et al. (2003) reported on 27 patients with failed SB Charité devices, with all index procedures performed at other institutions. The failures occurred 53 months (range 11–127 months) after initial surgery. All replacements were either at L4–L5 or at L5–S1 levels, and the most common causes of failure were adjacent-level spinal disease, subsidence, and facet joint arthrosis. Two patients experienced anterior dislocation of the implant, and 11 patients required additional salvage surgery (Kostuik 2004). Other authors of ongoing clinical trials with short-term follow-up have reported a low incidence of infection, vertebral body fracture, implant malposition, subsidence, mechanical failure, and paravertebral heterotopic ossification (Delamarter et al. 2003; Lin and Wang 2006; Guyer et al. 2009).

Indications for revision surgery of a failed total disc arthroplasty may include, but are not limited to, implant loosening, malposition, displacement, early wear, and infection (Kostuik 2004). There is currently limited understanding of the effects of wear debris and osteolysis on spinal arthroplasty devices, and the long-term effects, such as aseptic loosening seen in extremity joint replacements, remain unknown. With metal-on-metal disc arthroplasty, patients experience an inflammatory response similar to that seen in total joint arthroplasty (Hallab et al. 2003b; Golish and Anderson 2012).

A comprehensive strategy for treating failed disc arthroplasty begins by defining patient symptoms and the radiographic status of the arthroplasty device (Patel et al. 2008). Asymptomatic patients with implant subsidence or migration without extrusion can be treated nonsurgically with frequent serial examinations. Symptomatic patients may present with (1) continued pain secondary to implant failure, (2) pain due to symptomatic disease at an adjacent level, (3) pain due to late surgical site infection, or may be categorized as (4) continued pain of unknown etiology (Kostuik 2004). Although differentiating between these states may be difficult, it is important to determine whether the new pain resembles or is significantly different from the pain/symptoms originally treated by the disc replacement. A diagnostic algorithm for patients with new pain after a period of relief or continued pain of unknown etiology may include careful attention to history and physical examination, the use of radiographs with flexion-extension views, and a CT scan to ensure adequate prosthesis placement, stability, and incorporation. If imaging fails to reveal an underlying pathology, further investigations may include injection of local anesthetic and radiosensitive dye into the periprosthetic area, a facet block at the level of arthroplasty, or discography at adjacent levels (Kostuik 2004). These modalities can provide additional information and identify a potential source of pain which may have not been recognized prior to the arthroplasty procedure. If the pain is relieved after periprosthetic injection, the assumed diagnosis would be implant loosening, malposition, or displacement (Kostuik 2004).

Periprosthetic loosening from infection may be more difficult to differentiate, and laboratory tests associated with infection such as leukocytosis, elevated erythrocyte sedimentation rate, and high C-reactive protein levels may be a helpful starting point. Also, bacterial culture after aspiration of periprosthetic fluid, with saline lavage, can provide additional information regarding the presence of infection, as well as sensitivity analysis for antibiotic treatment (Kostuik 2004). Evidence of bone resorption on CT scan may be another indicator of infection, but it is not specifically diagnostic (Kostuik 2004). However, in the presence of a metal and/or plastic prosthesis, nonsurgical management with targeted antibiotics may be insufficient to eradicate infection. Use of long-term suppressive antibiotics may be indicated if the patient is unable to undergo revision surgery. Otherwise, the surgical technique for management of infection would consist of implant removal, meticulous debridement, and irrigation, followed by fusion and an extended course of targeted antibiotics. Fusion may be best achieved in the setting of infection, with structural autograft rather than allograft, and consideration should be given to a staged posterior fusion procedure with instrumentation (Kostuik 2004).

Surgical options for disc arthroplasty failure include revision arthroplasty, anterior interbody fusion, or instrumented posterior fusion. A particular problem with removal or revision arthroplasty for devices in current use is the surgery through previous scar tissue. This may be difficult for revision cervical arthroplasty, but for lumbar exposure, this is a challenge even for a technically advanced vascular surgeon (McAfee 2004; Patel et al. 2008). For lumbar revision surgery through an anterior approach, preventative measures can reduce the incidence of life-threatening adverse events. The ureter must be carefully identified and ureteral stents may be placed before reexposure to prevent iatrogenic injury (Wagner et al. 2006; Patel et al. 2008). Also, angiography and venography can define the location and distortions of the great vessels due to scar tissue, and catheterization of the iliac vessels with inflatable balloon catheters can prevent catastrophic blood loss (Patel et al. 2008).

Noteworthy, removal of the arthroplasty device may create a significant bone loss that would preclude revision arthroplasty (Kostuik 2004). If there is infection and prosthesis failure due to displacement, loosening, or malposition, anterior interbody fusion will be required. In the absence of infection, after removal of the failed arthroplasty device and preparation of the interbody space, the use of allograft should enhance fusion; however, some cases may warrant same-day posterior fusion and/or instrumentation at the level of the revision surgery (Kostuik 2004). The use of instrumented posterior fusion or dynamic stabilization alone at the level of the failed arthroplasty has been suggested, but its role has not been defined and may be insufficient to alleviate symptoms. It should be stated that because there are no significant reports or experience with failed arthroplasty devices, protocols and strategies for revision arthroplasty remain speculative and unclear. Continued long-term follow-up, of at least 5–10 years, will likely further elucidate the best management strategies for patients with continued pain after disc arthroplasty surgery (Kostuik 2004).

14.9 Other Spinal Motion-Preserving Devices

14.9.1 Nuclear Replacements

There have been continued efforts to develop a prosthetic nuclear replacement device (Bono and Garfin 2004). In essence, the previously discussed Fernstrom ball is the predecessor for modern nuclear replacement devices. It differs from the current total disc arthroplasty system in that it lacks an end-plate component (Bono and Garfin 2004). The prosthesis replaces the nucleus pulposus and serves to restore load transfer through the spinal segment, particularly the annulus fibrosus and facet joints. Therefore, the prerequisite for nuclear replacement is an intact or minimally disrupted annulus structure and vertebral end plates (Lee and Goel 2004). There are currently four nucleus prosthesis designs which aim to reproduce the biomechanical environment of the intact intervertebral disc. The first design is an impermeable balloon or bladder, filled with gas, fluid, gel, oil, or a soft polymer. The second is a solid body such as a metal ball or spacer that is placed in the nuclear cavity (Fernstrom 1966). The third approach is to implant a dehydrated or partially hydrated hydrophilic polymer material into a permeable cavity or fibrous jacket, which becomes hydrated within the nuclear cavity (Ray 2002). The final approach is nucleus augmentation, which involves injection of a biomaterial into the nuclear cavity for in situ polymerization.

Nuclear replacements remain in the experimental phase, mostly evaluated in vitro and by animal implant studies. Limited clinical trials in humans have reported clinical improvement and restoration of disc function. Other preliminary studies indicate problems with migration, extrusion, vertebral end-plate changes, or subsidence (Bertagnoli and Schonmayr 2002; Klara and Ray 2002; Ray 2002; Lee and Goel 2004; Bertagnoli et al. 2005b; Ahrens et al. 2009). Design criteria which may predispose to these complications include a small contact surface area at the interface between the nucleus replacement device and the vertebral end plates, causing abnormal stress concentration and subsidence. Also, abnormal movement of the implanted prosthesis within the disc during motion could cause harmful effects on the annulus. To overcome this problem, some devices allow fit and/or interlocking at the interface (Lee and Goel 2004). At this time, it is unclear which patients would benefit from total disc arthroplasty versus nuclear replacement. Contraindications to nuclear replacement may include advanced disc space collapse (<5 mm of residual disc height), end-plate defects, and obesity (BMI >30) (Ray 2002).

14.9.2 Lumbar Dynamic Posterior Stabilization/Facet Replacement

Other motion-preserving devices for the lumbar spine include posterior dynamic devices and facet replacements. The only approved interspinous device is the X-stop (Kyphon, Sunnyvale, CA), achieving FDA approval in 2005 (Zucherman et al. 2005). The device is made of titanium and PEEK components with side wings surrounding the lateral aspects of the spinous processes. It is inserted between the spinous processes of a spinal segment and holds the spine in a position of slight flexion to decompress the spinal cord or spinal nerve roots. The rationale for the use of the interspinous device for spinal stenosis is reasonable; however, their role in the treatment of the degenerative disc remains unknown (Anderson et al. 2006).

The role of facet replacement continues to grow, and it has been proposed as an adjunct total disc arthroplasty: as a method of reconstruction after laminectomy and for treatment of facet joint pain. As previously mentioned, as disc degeneration progresses, facet loads increase significantly (Yang and King 1984) and may lead to additional pain due to facet arthrosis. In fact, as continued motion across an arthritic and painful facet joint is thought to be a cause of arthroplasty failure, a common contraindication for total disc arthroplasty is facet arthrosis (Wong et al. 2007). To date, there are no FDA-approved devices, and a substantial amount of clinical data will be needed before facet replacements can be considered as a viable treatment option.

14.10 Summary of Critical Concepts Discussed in the Chapter

- Despite the enthusiasm and excitement surrounding total disc arthroplasty, the long-term clinical results, durability, and complications remain unknown.
- No studies have conclusively demonstrated any difference in patient outcomes when compared to fusion in both the lumbar and cervical spine.
- Short-term clinical results through FDA IDE trials appear to be promising, with acceptable complication rates, and all demonstrating non-inferior results compared to fusion. However, many questions remain regarding the true place of total disc arthroplasty in spine surgery, and only well-performed, prospective studies with long-term outcomes data and cost analysis will provide the answer.

- The indications and role of other motion-preserving devices such as posterior stabilization and facet replacements remain unproven.
- Efforts must continue to understand the origins of pain within the lumbar and cervical spine, as surgical treatment of neck or back pain in the absence of radiculopathy or myelopathy has demonstrated inconsistent results with the potential for failure.

References

Ahrens M, Tsantrizos A et al (2009) Nucleus replacement with the DASCOR disc arthroplasty device: interim two-year efficacy and safety results from two prospective, non-randomized multicenter European studies. Spine (Phila Pa 1976) 34(13):1376–1384

Akamaru T, Kawahara N et al (2003) Adjacent segment motion after a simulated lumbar fusion in different sagittal alignments: a biomechanical analysis. Spine (Phila Pa 1976) 28(14):1560–1566

Albee FH (1911) Transplantation of a portion of the tibia into the spine for Pott's disease. JAMA 57:885

Albert TJ, Eichenbaum MD (2004) Goals of cervical disc replacement. Spine J 4(6 Suppl):292S–293S

Anderson PA, Rouleau JP et al (2003) Wear analysis of the Bryan Cervical Disc prosthesis. Spine (Phila Pa 1976) 28(20):S186–S194

Anderson PA, Sasso RC et al (2004) The Bryan Cervical Disc: wear properties and early clinical results. Spine J 4(6 Suppl):303S–309S

Anderson PA, Tribus CB et al (2006) Treatment of neurogenic claudication by interspinous decompression: application of the X STOP device in patients with lumbar degenerative spondylolisthesis. J Neurosurg Spine 4(6):463–471

Arens S, Schlegel U et al (1996) Influence of materials for fixation implants on local infection. An experimental study of steel versus titanium DCP in rabbits. J Bone Joint Surg Br 78(4):647–651

Barrick WT, Schofferman JA et al (2000) Anterior lumbar fusion improves discogenic pain at levels of prior posterolateral fusion. Spine (Phila Pa 1976) 25(7):853–857

Bernthal NM, Celestre PC et al (2012) Disappointing short-term results with the DePuy ASR XL metal-on-metal total hip arthroplasty. J Arthroplasty 27:539–544

Bertagnoli R, Schonmayr R (2002) Surgical and clinical results with the PDN prosthetic disc-nucleus device. Eur Spine J 11(Suppl 2): S143–S148

Bertagnoli R, Sabatino CT et al (2005a) Mechanical testing of a novel hydrogel nucleus replacement implant. Spine J 5(6):672–681

Bertagnoli R, Zigler J et al (2005b) Complications and strategies for revision surgery in total disc replacement. Orthop Clin North Am 36(3):389–395

Bisseling P, Zeilstra DJ et al (2011) Metal ion levels in patients with a lumbar metal-on-metal total disc replacement: should we be concerned? J Bone Joint Surg Br 93(7):949–954

Bohlman HH, Emery SE et al (1993) Robinson anterior cervical discectomy and arthrodesis for cervical radiculopathy. Long-term follow-up of one hundred and twenty-two patients. J Bone Joint Surg Am 75(9):1298–1307

Bono CM, Garfin SR (2004) History and evolution of disc replacement. Spine J 4(6 Suppl):145S–150S

Bono CM, Lee CK (2004) Critical analysis of trends in fusion for degenerative disc disease over the past 20 years: influence of technique on fusion rate and clinical outcome. Spine (Phila Pa 1976) 29(4):455–463; discussion Z455

Burkus JK, Haid RW et al (2010) Long-term clinical and radiographic outcomes of cervical disc replacement with the Prestige disc: results from a prospective randomized controlled clinical trial. J Neurosurg Spine 13(3):308–318

Buttner-Janz K, Hahn S et al (2002) Basic principles of successful implantation of the SB Charité model LINK intervertebral disk endoprosthesis. Orthopade 31(5):441–453

Cardoso MJ, Rosner MK (2010) Multilevel cervical arthroplasty with artificial disc replacement. Neurosurg Focus 28(5):E19

Cardoso MJ, Mendelsohn A et al (2011) Cervical hybrid arthroplasty with 2 unique fusion techniques. J Neurosurg Spine 15(1):48–54

Carragee EJ, Alamin TF (2001) Discography. A review. Spine J 1(5): 364–372

Chandler FA (1929) Spinal fusion operations in the treatment of low back and sciatic pain. JAMA 93:1447

Chang UK, Kim DH et al (2007) Changes in adjacent-level disc pressure and facet joint force after cervical arthroplasty compared with cervical discectomy and fusion. J Neurosurg Spine 7(1):33–39

Cinotti G, David T et al (1996) Results of disc prosthesis after a minimum follow-up period of 2 years. Spine (Phila Pa 1976) 21(8): 995–1000

Cunningham BW (2004) Basic scientific considerations in total disc arthroplasty. Spine J 4(6 Suppl):219S–230S

Cunningham BW, Lowery GL et al (2002) Total disc replacement arthroplasty using the AcroFlex lumbar disc: a non-human primate model. Eur Spine J 11(Suppl 2):S115–S123

Cunningham BW, Dmitriev AE et al (2003a) General principles of total disc replacement arthroplasty: seventeen cases in a nonhuman primate model. Spine (Phila Pa 1976) 28(20):S118–S124

Cunningham BW, Gordon JD et al (2003b) Biomechanical evaluation of total disc replacement arthroplasty: an in vitro human cadaveric model. Spine (Phila Pa 1976) 28(20):S110–S117

Dahl MC, Rouleau JP et al (2006) Dynamic characteristics of the intact, fused, and prosthetic-replaced cervical disk. J Biomech Eng 128(6): 809–814

Dahl MC, Jacobsen S, Metcalf N, Sasso R, Ching RP (2011) A comparison of the shock-absorbing properties of cervical disc prosthesis bearing materials. SAS J 5:48–54

Davis H (1994) Increasing rates of cervical and lumbar spine surgery in the United States, 1979–1990. Spine (Phila Pa 1976) 19(10): 1117–1123; discussion 1123–1114

Delamarter RB, Fribourg DM et al (2003) ProDisc artificial total lumbar disc replacement: introduction and early results from the United States clinical trial. Spine (Phila Pa 1976) 28(20):S167–S175

Delamarter R, Zigler JE et al (2011) Prospective, randomized, multicenter Food and Drug Administration investigational device exemption study of the ProDisc-L total disc replacement compared with circumferential arthrodesis for the treatment of two-level lumbar degenerative disc disease: results at twenty-four months. J Bone Joint Surg Am 93(8):705–715

DiAngelo DJ, Foley KT et al (2004) In vitro biomechanics of cervical disc arthroplasty with the ProDisc-C total disc implant. Neurosurg Focus 17(3):E7

Dmitriev AE, Cunningham BW et al (2005) Adjacent level intradiscal pressure and segmental kinematics following a cervical total disc arthroplasty: an in vitro human cadaveric model. Spine (Phila Pa 1976) 30(10):1165–1172

Eck JC, Humphreys SC et al (1999) Adjacent-segment degeneration after lumbar fusion: a review of clinical, biomechanical, and radiologic studies. Am J Orthop (Belle Mead NJ) 28(6):336–340

Fassio B, Ginestie JF (1978) Discal prosthesis made of silicone: experimental study and 1st clinical cases. Nouv Presse Med 7(3):207

Fernstrom U (1966) Arthroplasty with intercorporal endoprosthesis in herniated disc and in painful disc. Acta Chir Scand Suppl 357:154–159

Fritzell P, Hagg O et al (2003) Complications in lumbar fusion surgery for chronic low back pain: comparison of three surgical techniques used in a prospective randomized study. A report from the Swedish Lumbar Spine Study Group. Eur Spine J 12(2):178–189

Frymoyer JW, Hanley E et al (1978) Disc excision and spine fusion in the management of lumbar disc disease. A minimum ten-year followup. Spine (Phila Pa 1976) 3(1):1–6

Gao SG, Lei GH et al (2011) Biomechanical comparison of lumbar total disc arthroplasty, discectomy, and fusion: effect on adjacent-level disc pressure and facet joint force. J Neurosurg Spine 15(5): 507–514

Garino JP (2000) Modern ceramic-on-ceramic total hip systems in the United States: early results. Clin Orthop Relat Res (379):41–47

Garrido BJ, Taha TA et al (2010) Clinical outcomes of Bryan cervical disc arthroplasty a prospective, randomized, controlled, single site trial with 48-month follow-up. J Spinal Disord Tech 23(6):367–371

Gertzbein SD, Seligman J et al (1986) Centrode characteristics of the lumbar spine as a function of segmental instability. Clin Orthop Relat Res (208):48–51

Ghiselli G, Wang JC et al (2004) Adjacent segment degeneration in the lumbar spine. J Bone Joint Surg Am 86-A(7):1497–1503

Gillet P (2003) The fate of the adjacent motion segments after lumbar fusion. J Spinal Disord Tech 16(4):338–345

Goldsmith AA, Dowson D et al (2000) A comparative joint simulator study of the wear of metal-on-metal and alternative material combinations in hip replacements. Proc Inst Mech Eng H 214(1):39–47

Golish SR, Anderson PA (2012) Bearing surfaces for total disc arthroplasty: metal-on-metal versus metal-on-polyethylene and other biomaterials. Spine J 12:693–701

Gore DR, Sepic SB (1984) Anterior cervical fusion for degenerated or protruded discs. A review of one hundred forty-six patients. Spine (Phila Pa 1976) 9(7):667–671

Guyer RD, McAfee PC et al (2009) Prospective, randomized, multicenter Food and Drug Administration investigational device exemption study of lumbar total disc replacement with the CHARITE artificial disc versus lumbar fusion: five-year follow-up. Spine J 9(5):374–386

Hallab N, Link HD et al (2003a) Biomaterial optimization in total disc arthroplasty. Spine (Phila Pa 1976) 28(20):S139–S152

Hallab NJ, Cunningham BW et al (2003b) Spinal implant debris-induced osteolysis. Spine (Phila Pa 1976) 28(20):S125–S138

Harvey EJ, Bobyn JD et al (1999) Effect of flexibility of the femoral stem on bone-remodeling and fixation of the stem in a canine total hip arthroplasty model without cement. J Bone Joint Surg Am 81(1): 93–107

Herkowitz HN, Kurz LT et al (1990) Surgical management of cervical soft disc herniation. A comparison between the anterior and posterior approach. Spine (Phila Pa 1976) 15(10):1026–1030

Hibbs RA (1911) An operation for progressive spinal deformities. NY Med J 93:1013

Hilibrand AS, Robbins M (2004) Adjacent segment degeneration and adjacent segment disease: the consequences of spinal fusion? Spine J 4(6 Suppl):190S–194S

Hilibrand AS, Carlson GD et al (1999) Radiculopathy and myelopathy at segments adjacent to the site of a previous anterior cervical arthrodesis. J Bone Joint Surg Am 81(4):519–528

Huang RC, Girardi FP et al (2003) The implications of constraint in lumbar total disc replacement. J Spinal Disord Tech 16(4):412–417

Ishihara H, Kanamori M et al (2004) Adjacent segment disease after anterior cervical interbody fusion. Spine J 4(6):624–628

Jackson RK, Boston DA et al (1985) Lateral mass fusion. A prospective study of a consecutive series with long-term follow-up. Spine (Phila Pa 1976) 10(9):828–832

Kienapfel H, Sprey C et al (1999) Implant fixation by bone ingrowth. J Arthroplasty 14(3):355–368

Kim WJ, Lee SH et al (2003) Treatment of juxtafusional degeneration with artificial disc replacement (ADR): preliminary results of an ongoing prospective study. J Spinal Disord Tech 16(4):390–397

Klara PM, Ray CD (2002) Artificial nucleus replacement: clinical experience. Spine (Phila Pa 1976) 27(12):1374–1377

Kleeman TJ, Ahn UM et al (2001) Laparoscopic anterior lumbar interbody fusion with rhBMP-2: a prospective study of clinical and radiographic outcomes. Spine (Phila Pa 1976) 26(24):2751–2756

Kostuik JP (1997) Intervertebral disc replacement. Experimental study. Clin Orthop Relat Res (337):27–41

Kostuik JP (2004) Complications and surgical revision for failed disc arthroplasty. Spine J 4(6 Suppl):289S–291S

Kulkarni SS, Lowery GL et al (2003) Arterial complications following anterior lumbar interbody fusion: report of eight cases. Eur Spine J 12(1):48–54

Kumar MN, Jacquot F et al (2001) Long-term follow-up of functional outcomes and radiographic changes at adjacent levels following lumbar spine fusion for degenerative disc disease. Eur Spine J 10(4):309–313

Kurtz SM, Muratoglu OK et al (1999a) Advances in the processing, sterilization, and crosslinking of ultra-high molecular weight polyethylene for total joint arthroplasty. Biomaterials 20(18): 1659–1688

Kurtz SM, Pruitt LA et al (1999b) Radiation and chemical crosslinking promote strain hardening behavior and molecular alignment in ultra high molecular weight polyethylene during multi-axial loading conditions. Biomaterials 20(16):1449–1462

Langton DJ, Jameson SS et al (2011) Accelerating failure rate of the ASR total hip replacement. J Bone Joint Surg Br 93(8):1011–1016

Lee CK (1988) Accelerated degeneration of the segment adjacent to a lumbar fusion. Spine (Phila Pa 1976) 13(3):375–377

Lee CK, Goel VK (2004) Artificial disc prosthesis: design concepts and criteria. Spine J 4(6 Suppl):209S–218S

Lee CK, Langrana NA (1984) Lumbosacral spinal fusion. A biomechanical study. Spine (Phila Pa 1976) 9(6):574–581

Lee CK, Langrana NA (2004) A review of spinal fusion for degenerative disc disease: need for alternative treatment approach of disc arthroplasty? Spine J 4(6 Suppl):173S–176S

Lehmann TR, Spratt KF et al (1987) Long-term follow-up of lower lumbar fusion patients. Spine (Phila Pa 1976) 12(2):97–104

LeHuec JC, Kiaer T et al (2003) Shock absorption in lumbar disc prosthesis: a preliminary mechanical study. J Spinal Disord Tech 16(4): 346–351

Lin EL, Wang JC (2006) Total disk arthroplasty. J Am Acad Orthop Surg 14(13):705–714

Link HD (2002) History, design and biomechanics of the LINK SB Charité artificial disc. Eur Spine J 11(Suppl 2):S98–S105

Luk KD, Lee FB et al (1987) The effect on the lumbosacral spine of long spinal fusion for idiopathic scoliosis. A minimum 10-year follow-up. Spine (Phila Pa 1976) 12(10):996–1000

MacWilliam CH, Yood MU et al (1996) Patient-related risk factors that predict poor outcome after total hip replacement. Health Serv Res 31(5):623–638

Madan SS, Boeree NR (2003) Comparison of instrumented anterior interbody fusion with instrumented circumferential lumbar fusion. Eur Spine J 12(6):567–575

Madigan L, Vaccaro AR et al (2009) Management of symptomatic lumbar degenerative disk disease. J Am Acad Orthop Surg 17(2): 102–111

Matsunaga S, Kabayama S et al (1999) Strain on intervertebral discs after anterior cervical decompression and fusion. Spine (Phila Pa 1976) 24(7):670–675

McAfee PC (2004) The indications for lumbar and cervical disc replacement. Spine J 4(6 Suppl):177S–181S

McAfee PC, Cunningham B et al (2005) A prospective, randomized, multicenter Food and Drug Administration investigational device exemption study of lumbar total disc replacement with the CHARITE artificial disc versus lumbar fusion: part II: evaluation of radiographic outcomes and correlation of surgical technique accuracy with clinical outcomes. Spine (Phila Pa 1976) 30(14):1576–1583; discussion E1388–E1590

McLaughlin JR, Lee KR (2000) Total hip arthroplasty in young patients. 8- to 13-year results using an uncemented stem. Clin Orthop Relat Res (373):153–163

Mummaneni PV, Burkus JK et al (2007) Clinical and radiographic analysis of cervical disc arthroplasty compared with allograft fusion: a randomized controlled clinical trial. J Neurosurg Spine 6(3): 198–209

Murrey D, Janssen M et al (2009) Results of the prospective, randomized, controlled multicenter Food and Drug Administration investigational device exemption study of the ProDisc-C total disc replacement versus anterior discectomy and fusion for the treatment of 1-level symptomatic cervical disc disease. Spine J 9(4):275–286

Nguyen NQ, Kafle D et al (2011) Ceramic fracture following cervical disc arthroplasty: a case report. J Bone Joint Surg Am 93(22): e1321–e1324

O'Beirne J, O'Neill D et al (1992) Spinal fusion for back pain: a clinical and radiological review. J Spinal Disord 5(1):32–38

Orr RD, Postak PD et al (2007) The current state of cervical and lumbar spinal disc arthroplasty. J Bone Joint Surg Am 89(Suppl 3):70–75

Patel AA, Brodke DS et al (2008) Revision strategies in lumbar total disc arthroplasty. Spine (Phila Pa 1976) 33(11):1276–1283

Penta M, Sandhu A et al (1995) Magnetic resonance imaging assessment of disc degeneration 10 years after anterior lumbar interbody fusion. Spine (Phila Pa 1976) 20(6):743–747

Pidhorz LE, Urban RM et al (1993) A quantitative study of bone and soft tissues in cementless porous-coated acetabular components retrieved at autopsy. J Arthroplasty 8(2):213–225

Pitzen T, Kettler A et al (2007) Cervical spine disc prosthesis: radiographic, biomechanical and morphological post mortal findings 12 weeks after implantation. A retrieval example. Eur Spine J 16(7): 1015–1020

Polly DW Jr (2003) Adapting innovative motion-preserving technology to spinal surgical practice: what should we expect to happen? Spine (Phila Pa 1976) 28(20):S104–S109

Puttlitz CM, Rousseau MA et al (2004) Intervertebral disc replacement maintains cervical spine kinetics. Spine (Phila Pa 1976) 29(24): 2809–2814

Ray CD (2002) The PDN prosthetic disc-nucleus device. Eur Spine J 11(Suppl 2):S137–S142

Reitman CA, Hipp JA et al (2004) Changes in segmental intervertebral motion adjacent to cervical arthrodesis: a prospective study. Spine (Phila Pa 1976) 29(11):E221–E226

Riew KD, Buchowski JM et al (2008) Cervical disc arthroplasty compared with arthrodesis for the treatment of myelopathy. J Bone Joint Surg Am 90(11):2354–2364

Robertson JT, Papadopoulos SM et al (2005) Assessment of adjacent-segment disease in patients treated with cervical fusion or arthroplasty: a prospective 2-year study. J Neurosurg Spine 3(6):417–423

Robinson RA, Smith GW (1955) Anterolateral cervical disc removal and interbody fusion for cervical disc syndrome. Bull Johns Hopkins Hosp 96:223–224

Sandhu HS, Sanchez-Caso LP et al (2000) Association between findings of provocative discography and vertebral endplate signal changes as seen on MRI. J Spinal Disord 13(5):438–443

Santos EG, Polly DW Jr et al (2004) Disc arthroplasty: lessons learned from total joint arthroplasty. Spine J 4(6 Suppl):182S–189S

Sasso RC, Smucker JD et al (2007) Clinical outcomes of BRYAN cervical disc arthroplasty: a prospective, randomized, controlled, multicenter trial with 24-month follow-up. J Spinal Disord Tech 20(7): 481–491

Schulte KR, Callaghan JJ et al (1993) The outcome of Charnley total hip arthroplasty with cement after a minimum twenty-year follow-up. The results of one surgeon. J Bone Joint Surg Am 75(7): 961–975

Serhan H, Mhatre D, Defossez H, Bono CM (2011) Motion-preserving technologies for degenerative lumbar spine: the past, present, and future horizons. SAS J 5:75–89

Shono Y, Kaneda K et al (1998) Stability of posterior spinal instrumentation and its effects on adjacent motion segments in the lumbosacral spine. Spine (Phila Pa 1976) 23(14):1550–1558

Silva M, Shepherd EF et al (2002) Average patient walking activity approaches 2 million cycles per year: pedometers under-record walking activity. J Arthroplasty 17(6):693–697

Sumner DR, Bryan JM et al (1990) Measuring the volume fraction of bone ingrowth: a comparison of three techniques. J Orthop Res 8(3):448–452

Taksali S, Grauer JN et al (2004) Material considerations for intervertebral disc replacement implants. Spine J 4(6 Suppl):231S–238S

Traynelis VC (2004) The Prestige cervical disc replacement. Spine J 4(6 Suppl):310S–314S

van Ooij A, Oner FC et al (2003) Complications of artificial disc replacement: a report of 27 patients with the SB Charité disc. J Spinal Disord Tech 16(4):369–383

Wagner M, Wagner H (2000) Medium-term results of a modern metal-on-metal system in total hip replacement. Clin Orthop Relat Res (379):123–133

Wagner WH, Regan JJ et al (2006) Access strategies for revision or explantation of the Charite lumbar artificial disc replacement. J Vasc Surg 44(6):1266–1272

Weinhoffer SL, Guyer RD et al (1995) Intradiscal pressure measurements above an instrumented fusion. A cadaveric study. Spine (Phila Pa 1976) 20(5):526–531

Williams JL, Allen MB Jr et al (1968) Late results of cervical discectomy and interbody fusion: some factors influencing the results. J Bone Joint Surg Am 50(2):277–286

Williams DH, Greidanus NV et al (2011) Prevalence of pseudotumor in asymptomatic patients after metal-on-metal hip arthroplasty. J Bone Joint Surg Am 93(23):2164–2171

Wong DA, Annesser B et al (2007) Incidence of contraindications to total disc arthroplasty: a retrospective review of 100 consecutive fusion patients with a specific analysis of facet arthrosis. Spine J 7(1):5–11

Yang KH, King AI (1984) Mechanism of facet load transmission as a hypothesis for low-back pain. Spine (Phila Pa 1976) 9(6): 557–565

Yue WM, Brodner W et al (2005) Long-term results after anterior cervical discectomy and fusion with allograft and plating: a 5- to 11-year radiologic and clinical follow-up study. Spine (Phila Pa 1976) 30(19):2138–2144

Zigler J, Delamarter R et al (2007) Results of the prospective, randomized, multicenter Food and Drug Administration investigational device exemption study of the ProDisc-L total disc replacement versus circumferential fusion for the treatment of 1-level degenerative disc disease. Spine (Phila Pa 1976) 32(11):1155–1162; discussion 1163

Zucherman JF, Hsu KY et al (2005) A multicenter, prospective, randomized trial evaluating the X STOP interspinous process decompression system for the treatment of neurogenic intermittent claudication: two-year follow-up results. Spine (Phila Pa 1976) 30(12):1351–1358

The Nonsurgical Treatment of Back Pain 15

Isaac L. Moss, Howard S. An, Francis H. Shen, Zemin Li,
Gunnar B.J. Andersson, and Yejia Zhang

The single most striking chaos in the whole field of medicine in a disease that is the most common

Kochs (1925)

Contents

I.L. Moss, MD
Comprehensive Spine Center,
New England Musculoskeletal Institute,
University of Connecticut Health Center,
263 Farmington Avenue, Farmington, CT 06030-5353, USA
e-mail: imoss@uchc.edu

H.S. An, MD • G.B.J. Andersson, MD, PhD
Y. Zhang, MD, PhD (✉)
Department of Orthopaedic Surgery,
Rush University Medical Center,
1735 W. Harrison St., Chicago, IL 60612, USA
e-mail: howard.an@rushortho.com;
gunnar_andersson@rush.edu; yejia_zhang@rush.edu

F.H. Shen, MD
Department of Orthopaedic Surgery,
University of Virginia,
Charlottesville, VA, USA
e-mail: fhs2g@hscmail.mcc.virginia.edu

Z. Li, MD
Department of Spine Surgery,
The First Affiliated Hospital of Sun Yat-sen University,
58 Zhongshan 2nd Road, #74, Guangzhou
510080, People's Republic of China
e-mail: sdlizemin@gmail.com

I.M. Shapiro, M.V. Risbud (eds.), *The Intervertebral Disc*,
DOI 10.1007/978-3-7091-1535-0_15, © Springer-Verlag Wien 2014

15.1 Etiology of Back Pain

Each spinal motion segment is a three-joint complex comprised of the intervertebral disc, two facet joints, and a host of ligamentous and muscular attachments. This complex allows for multiaxial movement and loading of the spine while maintaining an upright posture and protection of the neural elements. The anatomic complexity of this articulation has complicated the search for a specific pathoanatomic cause for low back pain. The most common etiologies can be broadly categorized as neural, muscular, osseous, disc-related, and facet-related and have been the subject of much debate (Lutz et al. 2003). In the early decades of the twentieth century, nerve dysfunction, including neuritis and neuralgia, as well as muscular dysfunction were proposed as the leading causes of back pain. As the use of radiographs became more widespread, the classic bony changes associated with disc degeneration and spondylosis were found in many patients complaining of low back pain; hence, osseous etiologies became a popular theory. Initially, an inflammatory etiology for these bony changes was assumed; however, when no consistent marker of inflammation was found, it was then seen as a degenerative disorder. In the late 1930s and early 1940s, intervertebral disc pathology began to be recognized as a major low back pain generator (Barr 1938; Key 1945) and became the dominant theory for several decades. This resulted in an increase in the number and variety of surgical procedures directed at the intervertebral disc. By the end of the twentieth century, evidence emerged that anatomic abnormalities, as visualized by diagnostic imaging tests, often did not correlate with clinical symptoms (Boden et al. 1990). As a result, most modern treatments for low back pain are pragmatic in approach rather than searching for a specific anatomic directed cause (Lutz et al. 2003), with nonsurgical intervention taking center stage.

However, several indications for prompt surgery exist. While they only account for a small percentage of all patients receiving surgery, unless they are diagnosed and treated, they can lead to significant morbidity or mortality. These conditions are flagged from the patient's history and physical examination and require further investigation. The presence of neurologic deficits, including saddle anesthesia, urinary retention or incontinence, and progressive lower extremity weakness, should prompt rapid evaluation for cauda equina syndrome. A history of significant trauma in a young individual or minor trauma in an individual with osteoporosis should prompt the clinician to rule out a fracture of the spinal column. Nonmechanical back pain, which wakes patients from their sleep, can be associated with spinal neoplasm or infection, especially if associated with constitutional symptoms, history of cancer, or disseminated infection.

It is important to recognize nonorganic etiologies of low back pain as treatment can be difficult, requiring specialized expertise (Waddell et al. 1980). Symptoms include pain, numbness, or weakness in a nonanatomic distribution. Common physical examination findings are nonspecific and include widespread tenderness, lumbar pain with axial loading, improvement in straight leg raise with distraction, and inconsistent motor or sensory exam. Evaluation of the psychosocial context of the pain with the rehabilitation team that includes a psychologist and a social worker is often necessary.

15.2 Epidemiology and Natural History

Back pain is an extremely common public health problem with significant social and economic ramifications. It is estimated that 70–85 % of people in developed countries will experience back pain at some point in their life (Andersson 1999). In a US national survey, 26.4 % of the population had back pain lasting at least 1 day in the past 3 months (Deyo et al. 2006). Prevalence was found to be highest in Native Americans and Alaska Natives and lowest in Asian Americans. Back pain was more common in adults over the age of 45 and was slightly more prevalent in women as compared to men. The annual prevalence of significant back pain is approximately 15 % (Andersson 1999). These statistics have remained relatively stable over the past 30 years. The health-care resource utilization and cost of care for patients with back pain are extraordinarily high. Back pain is responsible for approximately 12–15 % of all physician visits (Deyo et al. 2006). In 2005, the treatment of back and neck disorders accounted for $86 billion in health-care expenditure (Martin et al. 2008). It affects approximately 2 % of the workforce, and back pain is the largest single cause of absence from work (12.5 % of all sick days) (Andersson 1999). For more details of the epidemiology of low back pain, see Chaps. 9 and 16.

Most acute back pain is self-limited, with the majority of patients recovering quickly with no residual loss of function. Of individuals with symptoms severe enough to miss work, 60–70 % will return to work within 6 weeks and 80–90 % will return within 12 weeks (Andersson et al. 1983). Unfortunately, recurrence of back pain is common affecting 20–72 % of individuals (Andersson 1999).

Chronic low back pain has been variably defined as back pain which lasts longer than 3 months, reoccurs frequently, or lasts longer than the expected healing time for this type of malady. The course of chronic back pain can be variable and unpredictable (Von Korff and Saunders 1996). In many cases, mild pain may persist for long periods of time with little impact on overall function. Therefore, when evaluating treatment strategies, activity limitation may be a better measure of outcome than level or presence of pain.

15.3 Nonoperative Treatment

Despite the extremely high prevalence of back pain in society, a streamlined and successful treatment strategy still eludes physicians. While rates of operative intervention have steadily and dramatically increased over the past 20 years (Deyo et al. 2009), treatment outcomes for back pain without radicular symptoms remain unpredictable with success rates in the 50–70 % range depending on the measures used (Chou et al. 2009b; Mirza and Deyo 2007). Given the limited benefit, high cost, and significant risk, surgery is reserved as a last resort in a carefully selected population. Nonsurgical measure is, therefore, the mainstay of treatment for both acute and chronic back pain (Table 15.1).

15.3.1 Education, Activity Modification, Behavioral Therapy, and Exercise Therapy

15.3.1.1 Patient Education

Patient education, including information about correct spine biomechanics during regular activity and posture, and simple methods for reducing symptom are key elements in the management of both acute and chronic back pain. Ensuring that patients understand the favorable natural history of the disorder can empower them to take an active role in the treatment. As past incidences are the strongest predictor for future episodes of back pain, the importance of a lifelong commitment to active treatment must be conveyed to the symptomatic individuals. Several studies have demonstrated that brief education can be more effective than conventional care on reducing sick leave and disability (Brox et al. 2008).

More formal educational interventions have been the subject of investigation since the introduction of the Swedish back school in 1980 (Forssell 1980). The original program was designed to teach patients how to protect the spine during daily activities and involved four educational sessions on spine anatomy, biomechanics, ergonomics, optimal posture, and back exercises in a group setting. The specific format and content of back schools have varied over the years;

Table 15.1 Nonsurgical management options for back pain and recommended stages for interventions based on currently available evidence

Treatment	Therapy	Stage of symptoms
Nonsurgical therapies	Patient education	Acute
	Activity modification	Acute
	Behavioral therapy	Acute and chronic
	Exercise therapy	Subacute and chronic
Oral medication	Non-narcotic analgesic	Acute
	Narcotic analgesic	Acute
	Nonsteroidal anti-inflammatory drugs	Acute and chronic
	Muscle relaxants	Acute
	Oral corticosteroids	Acute, only with radiculopathy
	Antidepressants	Chronic
	Topical treatment	Acute and chronic
Injection therapy	Epidural corticosteroids	Acute, only with radiculopathy
	Soft tissue	Subacute and chronic
	Facet joint	Subacute and chronic
	Sacroiliac joint	Chronic
Modalities	Manipulation	Acute and chronic
	Traction	Unknown
	Acupuncture	Chronic
	Transcutaneous electrical nerve stimulation	Unknown
	Orthoses	Not recommended

however, the general concept has been the subject of several investigations and systematic reviews (Airaksinen et al. 2006; Cohen et al. 1994; Koes et al. 1994; Maier-Riehle and Härter 2001; Tveito et al. 2004). In comparison to other interventions or no treatment at all, the results of these studies conflict with the claims for success of back schools in reducing pain, improving function, and accelerating return to work. The most recent systematic reviews (Airaksinen et al. 2006; Brox et al. 2008; Heymans et al. 2005) conclude that forms of group back education can be effective for short-term improvements in pain and disability, especially as part of a multidisciplinary program. In addition, within an occupational setting, back school can have a positive effect on return to work and function.

15.3.1.2 Activity Modification

Most patients with acute back pain naturally modify their activities to avoid exacerbation of symptoms. This subconscious protective mechanism is likely helpful when bounded with appropriate education. It is generally accepted that, while activity may worsen symptoms, it is unlikely to cause physical injury to the spine or the surrounding soft tissues (Indahl et al. 1995). Therefore, the common recommendation is to limit activity for a short period of time (2–3 days). There is, however, strong evidence against the historically common recommendation for bed rest as a treatment for acute low back pain, which can negatively affect outcomes (Atlas and Volinn 1997; Waddell et al. 1997). Results of investigations support the view that after the acute symptoms subside, timely return to modified activities avoids the deleterious effects associated with prolonged immobilization and bed rest. Patients who continue moderate levels of activities during episodes of acute back pain generally have a more rapid recovery, quicker return to work, and a lower risk of chronic disability (Mäkelä et al. 2011; Waddell et al. 1997).

15.3.1.3 Behavioral Therapy

The concept of fear avoidance was introduced as a model of exaggerated pain perception in 1983 (Lethem et al. 1983) and has subsequently been applied to chronic back and musculoskeletal pain (Vlaeyen and Linton 2000; Waddell et al. 1993). Central to this model is the concept that the fear of increased pain, as a result of a movement or activity, may lead to a phobic state and result in inferior physical performance and increased disability. Conversely, confrontation of the fear of pain via exposure to an activity or movement can lead overtime to a reduction in fear. The application of this concept, by including fear-reducing techniques, in the treatment of low back pain in the primary care setting has been shown to produce an increase in activity, but not impact return to employment (Von Korff et al. 2005). Furthermore, when this type of cognitive intervention is combined with an exercise program, the effect on back pain, disability, and sick leave has been shown to be equivalent to that of spinal fusion (Brox et al. 2003; Brox et al. 2006).

15.3.1.4 Exercise Therapy

Exercise therapy, including trunk or core stabilization, restoring normal lumbosacral motion, and low-impact aerobic activity, is among the most commonly prescribed noninvasive interventions for patients with back pain. Based on the current literature, exercise therapy is no more effective for pain relief or functional improvement when compared to no treatment or other nonoperative interventions for acute low back pain (Chou et al. 2007b; Hayden et al. 2005). There is, however, a general acceptance that low-impact cardiovascular and aerobic fitness programs are beneficial in that they can reduce fatigue, improve mood, and prevent general deconditioning (Anshel and Russell 1994; Casazza et al. 1998). Trunk stabilization and muscle strengthening exercises are not tolerated by patients; thus, they are not recommended during acute episodes of back pain. Low-impact aerobic exercise can be commenced as early as tolerated, often by 2 weeks after the onset of acute low back pain, and activity can progress in a graded fashion.

In contrast to the acute situation, for chronic pain, low back pain exercise therapy has been shown to have a beneficial effect (Chou et al. 2007b). When compared to no treatment, usual care, or other noninvasive treatments, exercise therapy has been associated with a small but significant improvement in pain and function (Hayden et al. 2005; Team 2004). Exercise therapy has also been linked with reduced sick leave and a higher rate of return to work within 1 year of treatment in patients with subacute (<90 days of sick leave) low back pain who were not already severely disabled (Oesch et al. 2010). Core strengthening exercises are routinely recommended to improve performance and prevent future injuries (McGill 2010).

15.3.2 Medications

Most patients with both acute and chronic low back pain will include medication in the management of their condition. While the oral route of administration is most common, injections also play a role. The most common classes of oral drugs include analgesics, nonsteroidal anti-inflammatory drugs (NSAIDs), muscle relaxants, and antidepressants. Injection therapy employs the use of corticosteroids and often local anesthetics. As the choices are numerous, it is important to distinguish specific indications, doses, durations, and potential side effects. Patient education with regard to use of safe and effective medication so as to avoid dependence, particularly when prescribing narcotic analgesics, is an important consideration and should be included in the treatment goals.

15.3.2.1 Analgesics

Analgesic medications can be divided into narcotic and nonnarcotic. Few patients require narcotics and most have adequate pain relief from over-the-counter analgesics.

Non-narcotic Analgesics

Acetaminophen is effective for mild to moderate pain. Although prolonged use of high-dose acetaminophen is contraindicated and may result in hepatotoxicity, acetaminophen is generally safe, affordable, and available over the counter thus making it a common choice for most patients with acute low back pain (Malanga and Nadler 1999). Acetaminophen use in patients with chronic low back pain and with known liver sensitivities due to disease or alcohol abuse is generally not recommended. In patients with renal impairment, acetaminophen is recommended over NSAIDs as the risk of renal toxicity due to acetaminophen is low. Acetaminophen does not have any muscle-relaxing or anti-inflammatory properties.

In patients with more severe pain, the centrally acting non-opiate analgesic tramadol is an attractive alternative as it has a more favorable side effect profile and lower potential for abuse than narcotics. Based on a meta-analysis, which included 908 patients being treated for chronic lower back pain, tramadol was shown to be superior to placebo in reducing pain and improving function (Deshpande et al. 2007). Tramadol inhibits uptake of serotonin and norepinephrine and should therefore be used with caution in patients on monoamine oxidase inhibitors. Dosage should be reduced in patients over the age of 75 years old or in those with renal or hepatic function impairment.

Box 15.1 Robin McKenzie, CNZM, O.B.E., FCSP (Hon), FNZSP (Hon), NZCP (HLM), Dip. MT, Dip.MDT

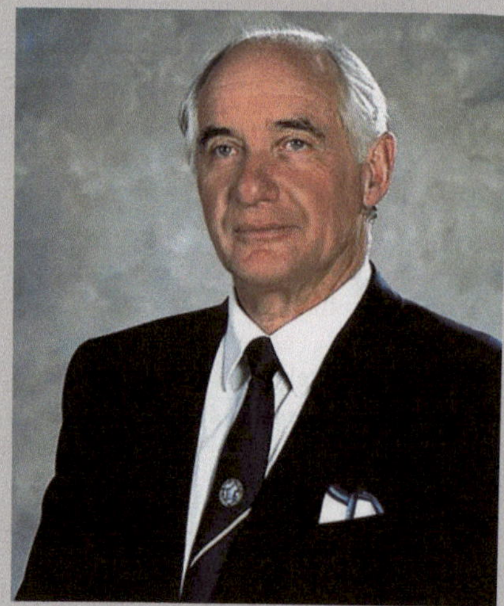

Robin McKenzie is a New Zealand-born physical therapist that revolutionized the nonoperative treatment of back pain. As is the case with many important advancements in science and medicine, McKenzie discovered the "centralization" phenomenon by accident in 1956 when he asked a patient to lie down in a prone position in a treatment room while finishing up with another patient. The end of the treatment table had been elevated, forcing the patient's lumbar spine into a hyperextension, a position previously thought to be harmful. When McKenzie returned to the room and saw the patient's position, he was surprised to find that the patient's leg pain had completely resolved, that residual pain was mild and "centralized" to the middle of the low back, and that after getting up, the pain relief was sustained. As he worked with subsequent patients, McKenzie discovered that based on an assessment of a patient in various positions, an effective patient-specific exercise treatment program could be developed. This has come to be known as Mechanical Diagnosis and Therapy and is the centerpiece of the McKenzie Method which is practiced worldwide. Once the appropriate exercises are found, patients are instructed to perform the program on their own and thus can take ownership over their disorder. McKenzie spent much of his life disseminating his methods to practitioners throughout the world and has published many articles and books on the subject. He is now retired and lives in New Zealand.

Box 15.2 Prostaglandins (PG) Biosynthesis

The starting molecule for PG biosynthesis is the fatty acid of the phospholipid phosphatidylinositol. PG and related molecules are eicosanoids, the term derived from "eicosa" meaning "twenty," referring to the 20 carbons of the fatty acid. Most PGs are synthesized from arachidonic acid, released by phospholipase A2. PG biosynthesis has two control points. The first control point is the release of the fatty acid from the phospholipid. The second is prostaglandin synthase, also known as cyclooxygenase (COX). The eicosanoids generally act locally due to their short half-lives.

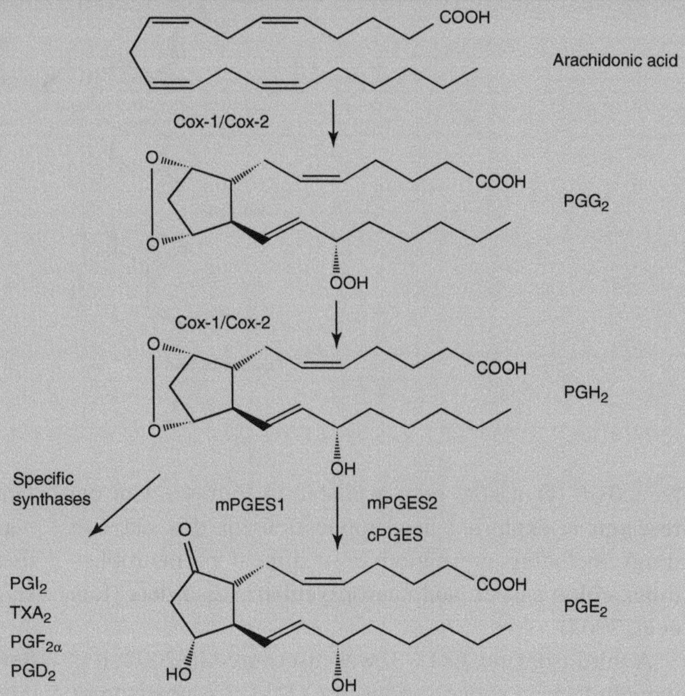

Prostaglandins (PG) biosynthesis. *Cox* cyclooxygenase, *PG* prostaglandin, *TX* thromboxane

Box 15.3 Cyclooxygenase (COX) Inhibitors

The mechanism of action of NSAIDs is based on their ability to block the synthesis of prostaglandin (PG) by inhibiting COX, an enzyme responsible for catalyzing the conversion of arachidonic acid to prostaglandin, PGH_2. In 1991, Daniel Simmons of Brigham Young University discovered a second isoform of the COX enzymes, now known as COX-2 (Xie et al. 1991). Research has since clarified that the COX-1 isoform is a constitutive enzyme responsible for the maintenance of renal and gastric functions. The COX-2 isoform, however, is an inducible enzyme which drives the inflammatory process. The classical NSAIDs (e.g., aspirin, ibuprofen, naproxen) nonspecifically inhibit both COX isoforms and are thus associated with side effects, mostly notable a risk of gastric injury and bleeding. Therefore, since its discovery, there has been a push to develop medications which selectively inhibit the COX-2 isoform and potentially increase the safety profile of these important drugs, primarily by limiting gastrointestinal side effects. The use of computer-aided drug design, where a computer modeling is used to synthesize a drug based on the structure of a particular target, was instrumental in the development of this new drug class. The introduction of COX-2 inhibitors was met with significant enthusiasm, and they became among the most widely prescribed medications. This enthusiasm was tempered when a somewhat controversial study demonstrated a fourfold increased risk of myocardial infarction in patients taking rofecoxib (Vioxx), one of the more commonly prescribed COX-2 inhibitors, when compared to patients taking naproxen, a classical NSAID. Rofecoxib was voluntarily removed from the market by Merck, the drug's manufacturer, in 2004. Since 2005, no new COX-2 inhibitors have been approved for use in the USA. Other COX-2 inhibitors remain on the market and are still widely prescribed including celecoxib (Celebrex) and

Chemical structure of common cyclooxygenase (COX) inhibitors

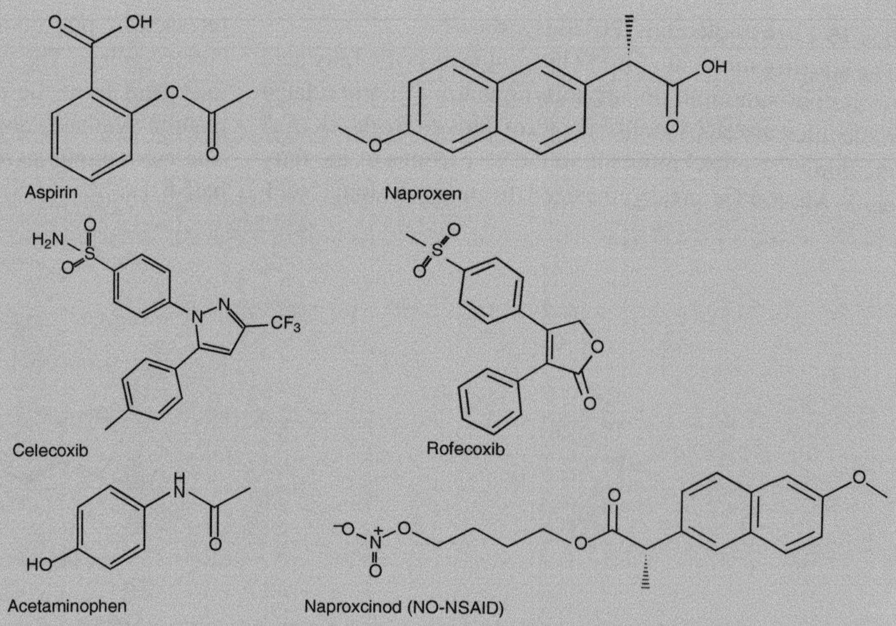

parecoxib (Dynastat, only available in Europe). Current research is exploring new application for this class of drugs including prevention or treatment of neuroblastoma, colon cancer, and neuropsychiatric disorders (Lau et al. 2007).

A third isozyme, COX-3, was discovered in 2002; it is thought to be a splice variant of COX-1. Comparison of canine COX-3 activity with murine COX-1 and COX-2 demonstrated that this enzyme is selectively inhibited by analgesic/antipyretic drugs such as acetaminophen and is potently inhibited by some nonsteroidal anti-inflammatory drugs.

COX-inhibiting nitric oxide (NO) donors (aka NO-NSAIDs) are another novel class of drugs developed to further improve the safety profile of the traditional NSAIDs by taking advantage of some of the known effects of NO (Wallace et al. 1994). These are produced by chemically fusing existing NSAIDs to a nitric oxide-donating moiety and are intended to provide the COX-inhibiting benefits in addition to vasorelaxation, and inhibition of white blood cell adhesion and caspase activity (Keeble and Moore 2002). No NO-NSAIDs have been approved for use at this time; however, several are in clinical trials.

Lipoxygenase (LOX)/COX inhibitors are a final novel class of NSAIDs. These drugs inhibit not only COX and prostaglandin formation but also inhibition of 5-lipoxygenase (LOX) and prevent formation of leukotrienes, another family of molecules involved in the inflammatory pathway. LOX/COX inhibitors have been shown to be effective and have a tolerable safety profile in pre-market studies (Alvaro-Gracia 2004).

References

Alvaro-Gracia JM (2004) Licofelone – clinical update on a novel LOX/COX inhibitor for the treatment of osteoarthritis. Rheumatology (Oxford) 43(Suppl 1):i21–i25

Keeble JE, Moore PK (2002) Pharmacology and potential therapeutic applications of nitric oxide-releasing nonsteroidal anti-inflammatory and related nitric oxide-donating drugs. Br J Pharmacol 137(3):295–310

Lau L, Hansford LM, Cheng LS, Hang M, Baruchel S, Kaplan DR, Irwin MS (2007) Cyclooxygenase inhibitors modulate the p53/HDM2 pathway and enhance chemotherapy-induced apoptosis in neuroblastoma. Oncogene 26(13):1920–1931

Wallace JL, Reuter B, Cicala C, McKnight W, Grisham MB, Cirino G (1994) Novel nonsteroidal anti-inflammatory drug derivatives with markedly reduced ulcerogenic properties in the rat. Gastroenterology 107(1):173–179

Xie WL, Chipman JG, Robertson DL, Erikson RL, Simmons DL (1991) Expression of a mitogen-responsive gene encoding prostaglandin synthase is regulated by mRNA splicing. Proc Natl Acad Sci U S A 88(7):2692–2696

Narcotic Analgesics

Despite ongoing controversies concerning the use of narcotic (also known as opioid) analgesics for the treatment of chronic low back pain, there has been a steady rise in prescription rates of both long- and short-acting varieties of these medications (Deyo et al. 2011). Concerns with opioid analgesics center around the high risk of dependency and the complications related to overdose, which have risen in parallel to prescription rates (Edlund et al. 2010). The use of narcotics to treat chronic low back pain has been associated with age, psychiatric and personality disorders, and substance abuse as opposed to severity of the underlying pathology (Breckenridge and Clark 2003). With regard to efficacy, there is some evidence to suggest that short-term use of narcotic analgesics may be efficacious; however, long-term use has little or no benefit in reduction of pain (Martell et al. 2007) or improvement of function (Deshpande et al. 2007). When chronic narcotics are prescribed, aberrant medication-taking behavior can be found in as high as 24 % of patients (Martell et al. 2007). Therefore, use of these medications requires regular follow-up to evaluate efficacy, overuse, and complications.

15.3.2.2 Nonsteroidal Anti-inflammatory Drugs (NSAIDs)

NSAIDs are among the most widely prescribed groups of medications for the treatment of back pain. Their mechanism of actions involves inhibition of cyclooxygenase (COX), an essential enzyme for the synthesis of the pro-inflammatory prostaglandins. Two types of COX enzymes exist, with COX-1 implicated in the protection of the gastric and intestinal lining and COX-2 involved in the pathways that produce pain, fever, and inflammation. The first-generation NSAIDs (e.g., ibuprofen, naproxen) nonspecifically inhibit both COX enzymes. The second-generation NSAIDs (e.g., celecoxib, meloxicam) are more selectively directed at COX-2 inhibition. In an effort to reduce gastrointestinal side effects associated with the first-generation NSAID, several randomized controlled studies have demonstrated a significant effect on the improvement of pain and possibly function for the treatment of both acute and chronic back pain (Chou et al. 2007a; White et al. 2011). COX-2-selective NSAIDs are probably as effective as non-selective NSAIDs. Remarkably, there have been few studies that directly compare the two drugs (Pohjolainen et al. 2000). However, both prescription and over-the-counter NSAIDs are associated with adverse effect, including gastrointestinal upset, bleeding, and exacerbation of preexisting renal dysfunction. Patients should therefore be closely monitored, especially with long-term usage.

15.3.2.3 Muscle Relaxants

Acute back pain is often accompanied by muscle spasm, but the association with pain is not well understood. Nonetheless, both benzodiazepine (e.g., diazepam) and non-benzodiazepine (e.g., cyclobenzaprine, methocarbamol) muscle relaxants are often prescribed as part of the treatment regimen. Systematic reviews of clinical trials have found that muscle relaxants are superior to placebo for the treatment of acute and chronic low back pain (Chou et al. 2007a; Van Tulder et al. 2003). There are no well-controlled studies that directly compare the efficacy of muscle relaxants to that of NSAIDs. Muscle relaxants are likely to be most beneficial as an adjunct to pharmacologic therapies with other drug classes, specifically NSAIDs and analgesics (Chou et al. 2007a; Van Tulder et al. 2003). There is little evidence to aid with the selection of one muscle relaxant over the others. Carisoprodol was found to be superior to diazepam in one study (Van Tulder et al. 2003). However, due to issues with dependency and abuse when combined with narcotics, the use of carisoprodol is generally limited. Muscle relaxants have been shown to lead to a number of central nervous system adverse effects, including somnolence and dizziness. These are increased when used in conjunction with other medications and should be closely monitored by the treating physician.

15.3.2.4 Oral Corticosteroids

The systemic administration of corticosteroids can be an effective treatment for patients with acute radiculopathy. However, when back pain is not accompanied by radiculopathy, studies have shown no clinically significant benefit over placebo (Chou et al. 2007a). Systemic corticosteroids can have a significant side effect when administered over the long term or in high doses in the short term. Thus, this class of medications is only recommended for the treatment of low back pain with radiculopathy.

15.3.2.5 Antidepressants

There is an intimate association between pain and mood, especially in chronic pain disorders (Fishbain et al. 1997). While the mechanism is unknown, there is some evidence that tricyclic antidepressants (TCAs) can effectively alleviate neuropathic pain, independent of mood or depression status (McQuay et al. 1996). Serotonin reuptake inhibitors (SSRIs) are less effective than TCAs; however, they are prescribed for neuropathic pain (Jung et al. 1997). The utility of antidepressants in the treatment of low back pain is not as clear. The efficacy of both tricyclic antidepressants and selective SSRIs has been the subject of several studies and recent systematic reviews. There is no generally accepted role for antidepressants in the treatment of acute back pain. For chronic back pain, TCAs have been demonstrated to be moderately effective in pain reduction when compared to placebo (Chou et al. 2007a; Staiger et al. 2003; White et al. 2011). As with neuropathic pain, SSRIs are not as effective as TCAs and offer no benefit over placebo. The effect of antidepressants on function is not clear (Staiger et al. 2003).

Antidepressants can have significant side effects, including drowsiness, dry mouth, dizziness, and constipation. Some of these adverse events can be mitigated with low starting doses that are slowly titrated up for efficacy. Due to the sedative properties of TCAs, these drugs should be administered at night and may in fact improve the sleep disturbance often associated with chronic back pain (Harman et al. 2002).

15.3.2.6 Topical Treatments

Both topical NSAIDs and local anesthetics in the form of patches, creams, or gels are used to treat low back pain. Topical application of NSAIDs is attractive as it can theoretically reduce the adverse events associated with their systemic administration. It should be noted, however, that with all topical formulations, systemic NSAID absorption occurs to variable degrees and adverse effects have been documented (Zimmerman et al. 1995). There is evidence to suggest that topical NSAIDs are effective for the treatment of musculoskeletal pain, although there is no evidence with regard to their efficacy specifically for acute or chronic back pain (Haroutiunian et al. 2010). Adhesive local anesthetic lidocaine patches are also often used to treat back pain. Again, their efficacy is unknown. Thus, topical treatments should be used with discretion and caution as adjuvants to other treatment modalities.

15.3.3 Injection Therapy

Therapeutic injections are often incorporated into back pain treatment regimens, particularly after less invasive methods, including exercise and oral medications, have failed. Injections can be directed at anatomic location both within and around the axial skeleton. Injection therapy should only be considered when a reasonable etiologic diagnosis has been made and should not be used for nonspecific low back pain.

15.3.3.1 Epidural Corticosteroid Injections and Medial Branch Blocks

Injection of corticosteroid, often with local anesthetic, is commonly administered for treatment of acute and chronic spine pathology. The medication can be delivered via an interlaminar, caudal, or transforaminal approach, depending on the pathoanatomy and specific patient symptoms. The potent anti-inflammatory effects of the corticosteroids coupled with the analgesic effects of local anesthetics are thought to interrupt the pain and spasm cycle as well as nociceptive transmission. Preclinical experiments suggest that corticosteroids can reduce cell membrane permeability, diminish neural peptide synthesis and neuronal discharge, and moderate sensitization of dorsal horn neurons (Byröd et al. 2000; Devor et al. 1985; Lee et al. 1998). While specialized training is required for all epidural injections, caudal injection is the least technically demanding and has a lower risk of dural puncture when compared to the other approaches. Transforaminal injections must be directed at specific pathologies, while interlaminar injections can result in more broad distribution of medication. Fluoroscopy is routinely used to improve the accuracy of injection needle placement, although an improvement in efficacy has not been proven (Chou et al. 2009a).

The efficacy of epidural corticosteroid injections has been the subject of multiple studies and reviews. In patients with back pain accompanied by radiculopathy, there is some, albeit weak, evidence to suggest the epidural corticosteroid injection provides short-term (up to 6 weeks) pain relief (Carette et al. 1997; Karppinen et al. 2001; Ng et al. 2005). There is, however, no evidence that epidural corticosteroid injections are effective in patients with back pain *without* radicular symptoms and they are, therefore, not a recommended treatment option (Chou et al. 2009a, b). When epidural injection therapy is pursued, a series of two to three injections is often recommended. Generally, no more than three injections are administered over a 6–12-month period, and if there is no response to the first injection, there is some evidence to suggest that further injections within the acute period are unlikely to be of significant benefit (Arden et al. 2005). Complications from epidural injections are rare; however, dural puncture, epidural hematoma, spinal cord injury, infection, and nerve damage have been reported (Chou et al. 2009a).

15.3.3.2 Soft Tissue Injections

Injections for back pain outside of the spine, the most common being trigger point injections, are targeted at soft tissue structures believed to be significant pain generators. These treatments involve the injection of local anesthetic and/or corticosteroid into specific myofascial trigger points, which are thought to result from irritable foci of taut muscle bands. Focal pressure on these points should produce a local twitch response with distally referred pain (Kraus and Fischer 1991). This so-called myofascial syndrome generally responds to a regimen of exercise or manual therapy, with injections considered as an adjuvant. The evidence to support local trigger point injection therapy alone is weak, showing short-term relief for subacute or chronic back pain (Chou et al. 2009a, b). However, some studies showed no difference when compared to placebo, and the addition of corticosteroid to local anesthetic does not appear to exert a significant effect. Therefore, the number of intramuscular injections should be limited, as there is concern for development of muscle damage, scar tissue, and altered function after multiple injections.

Injection of botulinum toxin A has been studied to treat chronic low back pain (Foster et al. 2001). Results demonstrated reduction in pain and patient reported disability in the short term, with cessation of benefits after 3–4 months in 60 % of patients.

Prolotherapy utilizes injection of sclerosing agents into the back and pelvic ligaments. Studies on this controversial intervention have not shown any consistent benefit in the improvement of pain or disability (Chou et al. 2009a, b).

15.3.3.3 Facet Joint Injections

The facet joints are richly innervated synovial articulations that frequently develop osteoarthritic degenerative changes. These joints are thus implicated as significant pain generator in patients with low back pain, especially when symptoms are exacerbated by lumbar extension maneuvers. Intra-articular facet injections as well as medial branch blocks and ablation are often incorporated into a back pain treatment strategy. However, despite their common use, there is no clear evidence as to their efficacy. One systematic review found facet joint injections were associated with short-term improvement (Boswell et al. 2007); conversely, other reviews found no benefit when compared to placebo injection especially over the long term (Slipman et al. 2003; Staal et al. 2009). Thus, facet joint-directed therapy is rarely indicated in cases of acute back pain.

The literature, with regard to medial branch block and ablations (also known as rhizotomy), is scant, although there may be some degree of short-term pain relief when treating chronic back pain (Leclaire et al. 2001; Niemistö et al. 2003; Slipman et al. 2003).

15.3.3.4 Sacroiliac Joint Injections

The sacroiliac is generally not considered a primary pain generator in patients with low back pain; however, it can be a common area of referred pain (Fortin et al. 1994). Based on history and physical examination, difficulties are experienced in diagnosing sacroiliac joint dysfunction (Dreyfuss et al. 1996), and it is thus regarded as a diagnosis of exclusion after other sources of pain have been ruled out. When dysfunction is evident, diagnostic and therapeutic injections of corticosteroids and local anesthetics can be considered; however, there is no convicting evidence with regard to efficacy (Chou et al. 2009a, b).

15.3.4 Physical Modalities

15.3.4.1 Manipulation

Spinal manipulation is among the most popular non-pharmaceutical alternative treatments for low back pain (Carey et al. 1995). Chiropractors, osteopaths, physical therapists, and other practitioners perform various types of manual therapy, which usually include a combination of massage and joint mobilization. Evidence with regard to the efficacy of spinal manipulation is unclear, with contradictory findings in two recent systematic reviews (Assendelft et al. 2004; Bronfort et al. 2004). There is some evidence to suggest that spinal manipulation can provide short-term relief of acute low back pain. In cases of chronic low back pain, spinal manipulation has an effect comparable to that of NSAIDs and superior to placebo in the short term and an effect comparable to that of physical therapy in the long term. Efficacy can likely be improved when spinal manipulation is combined with other nonoperative treatment modalities including an exercise program, medication, and lifestyle changes, but this has not been rigorously documented.

If patients choose to pursue spinal manipulation therapy, defined treatment goals should be established. If symptoms do abate, there is no evidence to suggest a need for ongoing "maintenance" therapy. However, if back pain persists or if radicular symptoms develop, treatment should be discontinued and the patient should be reassessed. The risk of significant injury with manipulation in the alert patient without significant spinal stenosis is considered to be low. However, manipulation under general anesthesia is thought to carry significant risk of injury (Koes et al. 1996). Manipulation is contraindicated in patients with progressive neurologic deficits.

15.3.4.2 Traction

Another physical treatment modality often sought by patients for relief of both radicular and non-radicular back pain is spinal traction. Traction is thought to distract the disc space and widen the neural foramen. In order to achieve distraction, the traction force must be sufficient to overcome muscle contraction, ligamentous resistance, and friction from the table surface and machinery and is estimated to be 35–50 % of total body weight (Beurskens et al. 1997). Based on several published reviews of the literature, there is currently no evidence that traction is an effective treatment for low back pain (Beurskens et al. 1997; Borman et al. 2003; Malanga and Nadler 1999; van der Heijden et al. 1995; van Middelkoop et al. 2011).

15.3.4.3 Acupuncture

Acupuncture is a traditional Chinese medicine technique, which has been practiced for over 2,000 years and has gained popularity in the Western world. Acupuncture is used to treat a wide variety of ailments and involves insertion and manipulation of thin, solid metal needles at specific points throughout the body. It has been difficult to produce high-quality evidence with regard to the efficacy of acupuncture as the treatment involves close patient-practitioner interaction, which may have a positive effect in and of itself, and the historical lack of an appropriate sham procedure to serve as a control (Madsen et al. 2009). There is currently no strong evidence to support the use of acupuncture for acute low back pain. For chronic low back pain, there is evidence from a systematic review of the literature to suggest that it can provide some degree of pain relief and improvement in function in the short term (Furlan et al. 2005). In the same review, it is suggested that acupuncture has a small effect in improving outcomes as an adjunct to conventional therapies. Acupuncture is therefore not generally recommended as a first-line treatment for back pain, but is often considered as a part of a comprehensive chronic pain management program.

15.3.4.4 Transcutaneous Electrical Nerve Stimulation

Transcutaneous electrical nerve stimulation therapy applies electrical stimulation to the skin in an effort to achieve pain relief. The common high-frequency (>50 Hz) low-intensity stimulation results in sensory stimulation without motor contraction and is thought to disturb neural pathway conduction and thus modulate pain. There is no convincing evidence that transcutaneous electrical nerve stimulation therapy provides significant relief of acute or chronic low back pain; however, there is a lack of high-quality investigations on the subject (van Middelkoop et al. 2011).

15.3.4.5 Other Modalities

Cold packs, superficial heat, short-wave diathermy, massage, and ultrasound are often part of physical therapy and chiropractic treatment. Further, many patients use cold or heat to relieve symptoms. The choice between the two depends on the stage of injury. Cold provides pain relief and reduces the inflammatory response following an acute injury by vasoconstriction. Heat relaxes muscles and improves tolerance to exercise, and may be a reasonable modality when the acute phase is over. Apart from the short-term relief, there is no documented value to the use of these modalities.

Magnets have been used for centuries to "cure" a variety of ailments, including back pain. Magnets sold for pain are weak and have no effect on circulation or tissue temperature. Controlled trials have found no benefit of magnet therapy for chronic low back pain (Collacott et al. 2000).

15.3.4.6 Orthoses

There is no evidence to support the effectiveness of orthoses in the treatment of acute and chronic low back pain (Million et al. 1981). There is some, but quite weak, evidence that they may decrease absence in the workplace (van Poppel et al. 1997, 1998; Walsh and Schwartz 1990). The mechanism of action of orthoses is debated because they do not improve lumbosacral biomechanics or enhance dynamic lifting capacity. Their effectiveness may be attributed to their capacity as proprioceptive reminders to use correct spine mechanics during lifting and bending activities (Reyna et al. 1995; Woodhouse et al. 1995).

15.4 Future Directions

The pathologic changes associated with intervertebral disc degeneration are well described. With aging, there is a reduction in disc cell concentration and an imbalance in extracellular matrix homeostasis resulting in molecular and biomechanical alteration in intervertebral disc structure and function. The precise mechanism linking these changes to symptomatic back pain remains elusive. Present research hopes to better delineate the link between pathology and symptoms, thus leading to more accurate diagnoses and treatments. The eventual goal of this research is to allow for a paradigm shift to more biological and mechanistic treatment strategies for discogenic pain that are less invasive, yet more effective than current regimens. Biological treatment strategies involve the application of three principal components: application of therapeutic molecules, delivery of cells to repopulate the disc, and supplementation of the matrix (Yoon 2005).

15.5 Summary of Critical Concepts Discussed in the Chapter

- The most common etiologies can be broadly categorized as neural, muscular, osseous, facet related, and disc related and have been the subject of much debate.
- Back pain is an extremely common public health problem, with a relatively benign natural history.
- After a thorough physical examination and imaging studies, education, activity modification, behavioral therapy, and exercise therapy may help the patients recover.
- Medications include analgesics, anti-inflammatories, muscle relaxants, antidepressants, and topical remedies.
- Steroids injected into the epidural space, facet joints, soft tissues, and sacroiliac joints may help to alleviate symptoms and promote recovery.
- Physical modalities that are commonly used such as manipulations, traction, orthoses, acupuncture, and transcutaneous electrical nerve stimulation (TENS) have limited value in treating back pain.
- Investments in research may result in a new generation of biological nonoperative therapies to provide reliable, safe, and efficacious relief of spinal pain.

Acknowledgment Yejia Zhang, MD, PhD, is supported by the Eunice Kennedy Shriver National Institute of Child Health and Human Development (NICHD, 1K08 HD049598-01).

References

Airaksinen O, Brox J, Cedraschi C, Hildebrandt J, Klaber-Moffett J, Kovacs F, Mannion A, Reis S, Staal J, Ursin H, Zanoli G (2006) Chapter 4 European guidelines for the management of chronic nonspecific low back pain. Eur Spine J 15(S2): s192–s300

Andersson GB (1999) Epidemiological features of chronic low-back pain. Lancet 354(9178):581–585

Andersson GB, Svensson HO, Odén A (1983) The intensity of work recovery in low back pain. Spine 8(8):880–884

Anshel MH, Russell KG (1994) Effect of aerobic and strength training on pain tolerance, pain appraisal and mood of unfit males as a function of pain location. J Sports Sci 12(6): 535–547

Arden NK, Price C, Reading I, Stubbing J, Hazelgrove J, Dunne C, Michel M, Rogers P, Cooper C (2005) A multicentre randomized controlled trial of epidural corticosteroid injections for sciatica: the WEST study. Rheumatology (Oxford) 44(11):1399–1406

Assendelft WJ, Morton SC, Yu EI, Suttorp MJ, Shekelle PG (2004) Spinal manipulative therapy for low back pain. Cochrane Database Syst Rev (1):CD000447

Atlas SJ, Volinn E (1997) Classics from the spine literature revisited: a randomized trial of 2 versus 7 days of recommended bed rest for acute low back pain. Spine 22(20):2331–2337

Barr JS (1938) Intervertebral disk lesions as cause of sciatica. Br Med J 2(4067):1247–1251, 1274-1–1274-2

Beurskens AJ, de Vet HC, Köke AJ, Regtop W, van der Heijden GJ, Lindeman E, Knipschild PG (1997) Efficacy of traction for nonspecific low back pain. 12-week and 6-month results of a randomized clinical trial. Spine 22(23):2756–2762

Boden SD, Davis DO, Dina TS, Patronas NJ, Wiesel SW (1990) Abnormal magnetic-resonance scans of the lumbar spine in asymptomatic subjects. A prospective investigation. J Bone Joint Surg Am 72(3):403–408

Borman P, Keskin D, Bodur H (2003) The efficacy of lumbar traction in the management of patients with low back pain. Rheumatol Int 23(2):82–86

Boswell MV, Colson JD, Sehgal N, Dunbar EE, Epter R (2007) A systematic review of therapeutic facet joint interventions in chronic spinal pain. Pain Physician 10(1):229–253

Breckenridge J, Clark JD (2003) Patient characteristics associated with opioid versus nonsteroidal anti-inflammatory drug management of chronic low back pain. J Pain 4(6):344–350

Bronfort G, Haas M, Evans RL, Bouter LM (2004) Efficacy of spinal manipulation and mobilization for low back pain and neck pain: a systematic review and best evidence synthesis. Spine J 4(3): 335–356

Brox JI, Sørensen R, Friis A, Nygaard Ø, Indahl A, Keller A, Ingebrigtsen T, Eriksen HR, Holm I, Koller AK, Riise R, Reikerås O (2003) Randomized clinical trial of lumbar instrumented fusion and cognitive intervention and exercises in patients with chronic low back pain and disc degeneration. Spine 28(17):1913–1921

Brox JI, Reikerås O, Nygaard Ø, Sørensen R, Indahl A, Holm I, Keller A, Ingebrigtsen T, Grundnes O, Lange JE, Friis A (2006) Lumbar instrumented fusion compared with cognitive intervention and exercises in patients with chronic back pain after previous surgery for disc herniation: a prospective randomized controlled study. Pain 122(1–2):145–155

Brox JI, Storheim K, Grotle M, Tveito TH, Indahl A, Eriksen HR (2008) Systematic review of back schools, brief education, and fear-avoidance training for chronic low back pain. Spine J 8(6):948–958

Byröd G, Otani K, Brisby H, Rydevik B, Olmarker K (2000) Methylprednisolone reduces the early vascular permeability increase in spinal nerve roots induced by epidural nucleus pulposus application. J Orthop Res 18(6):983–987

Carette S, Leclaire R, Marcoux S, Morin F, Blaise GA, St-Pierre A, Truchon R, Parent F, Levésque J, Bergeron V, Montminy P, Blanchette C (1997) Epidural corticosteroid injections for sciatica due to herniated nucleus pulposus. N Engl J Med 336(23): 1634–1640

Carey TS, Evans A, Hadler N, Kalsbeek W, McLaughlin C, Fryer J (1995) Care-seeking among individuals with chronic low back pain. Spine 20(3):312–317

Casazza BA, Young JL, Herring SA (1998) The role of exercise in the prevention and management of acute low back pain. Occup Med 13(1):47–60

Chou R, Huffman LH, American Pain Society; American College of Physicians (2007a) Medications for acute and chronic low back pain: a review of the evidence for an American Pain Society/ American College of Physicians clinical practice guideline. Ann Intern Med 147(7):505–514

Chou R, Huffman LH, American Pain Society; American College of Physicians (2007b) Nonpharmacologic therapies for acute and chronic low back pain: a review of the evidence for an American Pain Society/American College of Physicians clinical practice guideline. Ann Intern Med 147(7):492–504

Chou R, Atlas SJ, Stanos SP, Rosenquist RW (2009a) Nonsurgical interventional therapies for low back pain: a review of the evidence for an American Pain Society clinical practice guideline. Spine 34(10):1078–1093

Chou R, Loeser JD, Owens DK, Rosenquist RW, Atlas SJ, Baisden J, Carragee EJ, Grabois M, Murphy DR, Resnick DK, Stanos SP, Shaffer WO, Wall EM, American Pain Society Low Back Pain Guideline Panel (2009b) Interventional therapies, surgery, and interdisciplinary rehabilitation for low back pain: an evidence-based clinical practice guideline from the American Pain Society. Spine 34(10):1066–1077

Cohen JE, Goel V, Frank JW, Bombardier C, Peloso P, Guillemin F (1994) Group education interventions for people with low back pain. An overview of the literature. Spine 19(11):1214–1222

Collacott EA, Zimmerman JT, White DW, Rindone JP (2000) Bipolar permanent magnets for the treatment of chronic low back pain: a pilot study. JAMA 283(10):1322–1325

Deshpande A, Furlan A, Mailis-Gagnon A, Atlas S, Turk D (2007) Opioids for chronic low-back pain. Cochrane Database Syst Rev (3):CD004959

Devor M, Govrin-Lippmann R, Raber P (1985) Corticosteroids suppress ectopic neural discharge originating in experimental neuromas. Pain 22(2):127–137

Deyo RA, Mirza SK, Martin BI (2006) Back pain prevalence and visit rates: estimates from U.S. national surveys, 2002. Spine 31(23):2724–2727

Deyo RA, Mirza SK, Turner JA, Martin BI (2009) Overtreating chronic back pain: time to back off? J Am Board Fam Med 22(1):62–68

Deyo RA, Smith DH, Johnson ES, Donovan M, Tillotson CJ, Yang X, Petrik AF, Dobscha SK (2011) Opioids for back pain patients: primary care prescribing patterns and use of services. J Am Board Fam Med 24(6):717–727

Dreyfuss P, Michaelsen M, Pauza K, McLarty J, Bogduk N (1996) The value of medical history and physical examination in diagnosing sacroiliac joint pain. Spine 21(22):2594–2602

Edlund MJ, Martin BC, Fan MY, Devries A, Braden JB, Sullivan MD (2010) Risks for opioid abuse and dependence among recipients of chronic opioid therapy: results from the TROUP study. Drug Alcohol Depend 112(1–2):90–98

Fishbain DA, Cutler R, Rosomoff HL, Rosomoff RS (1997) Chronic pain-associated depression: antecedent or consequence of chronic pain? A review. Clin J Pain 13(2):116–137

Forssell MZ (1980) The Swedish back school. Physiotherapy 66(4):112–114

Fortin JD, Dwyer AP, West S, Pier J (1994) Sacroiliac joint: pain referral maps upon applying a new injection/arthrography technique. Part I: asymptomatic volunteers. Spine 19(13):1475–1482

Foster L, Clapp L, Erickson M, Jabbari B (2001) Botulinum toxin A and chronic low back pain: a randomized, double-blind study. Neurology 56(10):1290–1293

Furlan AD, van Tulder MW, Cherkin DC, Tsukayama H, Lao L, Koes BW, Berman BM (2005) Acupuncture and dry-needling for low back pain. Cochrane Database Syst Rev (1):CD001351

Harman K, Pivik RT, D'Eon JL, Wilson KG, Swenson JR, Matsunaga L (2002) Sleep in depressed and nondepressed participants with chronic low back pain: electroencephalographic and behaviour findings. Sleep 25(7):775–783

Haroutiunian S, Drennan DA, Lipman AG (2010) Topical NSAID therapy for musculoskeletal pain. Pain Med 11(4):535–549

Hayden JA, van Tulder MW, Malmivaara A, Koes BW (2005) Exercise therapy for treatment of non-specific low back pain. Cochrane Database Syst Rev (3):CD000335

Heymans MW, van Tulder MW, Esmail R, Bombardier C, Koes BW (2005) Back schools for nonspecific low back pain: a systematic review within the framework of the Cochrane Collaboration Back Review Group. Spine 30(19):2153–2163

Indahl A, Velund L, Reikeraas O (1995) Good prognosis for low back pain when left untampered. A randomized clinical trial. Spine 20(4):473–477

Jung AC, Staiger T, Sullivan M (1997) The efficacy of selective serotonin reuptake inhibitors for the management of chronic pain. J Gen Intern Med 12(6):384–389

Karppinen J, Malmivaara A, Kurunlahti M, Kyllönen E, Pienimäki T, Nieminen P, Ohinmaa A, Tervonen O, Vanharanta H (2001) Periradicular infiltration for sciatica: a randomized controlled trial. Spine 26(9):1059–1067

Key JA (1945) Intervertebral disk lesions are the most common cause of low back pain with or without sciatica. Ann Surg 121(4): 534–539

Kochs J (1925) Uber den objektiven tastbefund bei der myalgia. Dtsch Med Wochenschr 15:621

Koes BW, van Tulder MW, van der Windt WM, Bouter LM (1994) The efficacy of back schools: a review of randomized clinical trials. J Clin Epidemiol 47(8):851–862

Koes BW, Assendelft WJ, van der Heijden GJ, Bouter LM (1996) Spinal manipulation for low back pain. An updated systematic review of randomized clinical trials. Spine 21(24):2860–2871; discussion 2872–2873

Kraus H, Fischer AA (1991) Diagnosis and treatment of myofascial pain. Mt Sinai J Med 58(3):235–239

Leclaire R, Fortin L, Lambert R, Bergeron YM, Rossignol M (2001) Radiofrequency facet joint denervation in the treatment of low back pain: a placebo-controlled clinical trial to assess efficacy. Spine 26(13):1411–1416; discussion 1417

Lee HM, Weinstein JN, Meller ST, Hayashi N, Spratt KF, Gebhart GF (1998) The role of steroids and their effects on phospholipase A2. An animal model of radiculopathy. Spine 23(11): 1191–1196

Lethem J, Slade PD, Troup JD, Bentley G (1983) Outline of a Fear-Avoidance Model of exaggerated pain perception–I. Behav Res Ther 21(4):401–408

Lutz GK, Butzlaff M, Schultz-Venrath U (2003) Looking back on back pain: trial and error of diagnoses in the 20th century. Spine 28(16):1899–1905

Madsen MV, Gøtzsche PC, Hróbjartsson A (2009) Acupuncture treatment for pain: systematic review of randomised clinical trials with acupuncture, placebo acupuncture, and no acupuncture groups. BMJ 338:a3115

Maier-Riehle B, Härter M (2001) The effects of back schools – a meta-analysis. Int J Rehabil Res 24(3):199–206

Mäkelä KT, Peltola M, Sund R, Malmivaara A, Häkkinen U, Remes V (2011) Regional and hospital variance in performance of total hip and knee replacements: a national population-based study. Ann Med 43(Suppl 1):S31–S38

Malanga GA, Nadler SF (1999) Nonoperative treatment of low back pain. Mayo Clin Proc 74(11):1135–1148

Martell BA, O'Connor PG, Kerns RD, Becker WC, Morales KH, Kosten TR, Fiellin DA (2007) Systematic review: opioid treatment for chronic back pain: prevalence, efficacy, and association with addiction. Ann Intern Med 146(2):116–127

Martin BI, Deyo RA, Mirza SK, Turner JA, Comstock BA, Hollingworth W, Sullivan SD (2008) Expenditures and health status among adults with back and neck problems. JAMA 299(6):656–664

McGill SM (2010) Core training: evidence translating to better performance and injury prevention. Strength Cond J 32(3):33–46

McQuay HJ, Tramèr M, Nye BA, Carroll D, Wiffen PJ, Moore RA (1996) A systematic review of antidepressants in neuropathic pain. Pain 68(2–3):217–227

Million R, Nilsen KH, Jayson MI, Baker RD (1981) Evaluation of low back pain and assessment of lumbar corsets with and without back supports. Ann Rheum Dis 40(5):449–454

Mirza SK, Deyo RA (2007) Systematic review of randomized trials comparing lumbar fusion surgery to nonoperative care for treatment of chronic back pain. Spine 32(7):816–823

Ng L, Chaudhary N, Sell P (2005) The efficacy of corticosteroids in periradicular infiltration for chronic radicular pain: a randomized, double-blind, controlled trial. Spine 30(8):857–862

Niemistö L, Kalso E, Malmivaara A, Seitsalo S, Hurri H, Cochrane Collaboration Back Review Group (2003) Radiofrequency denervation for neck and back pain: a systematic review within the framework of the cochrane collaboration back review group. Spine 28(16):1877–1888

Oesch P, Kool J, Hagen KB, Bachmann S (2010) Effectiveness of exercise on work disability in patients with non-acute non-specific low back pain: systematic review and meta-analysis of randomised controlled trials. J Rehabil Med 42(3):193–205

Pohjolainen T, Jekunen A, Autio L, Vuorela H (2000) Treatment of acute low back pain with the COX-2-selective anti-inflammatory drug nimesulide: results of a randomized, double-blind comparative trial versus ibuprofen. Spine 25(12):1579–1585

Reyna JR, Leggett SH, Kenney K, Holmes B, Mooney V (1995) The effect of lumbar belts on isolated lumbar muscle. Strength and dynamic capacity. Spine 20(1):68–73

Slipman CW, Bhat AL, Gilchrist RV, Issac Z, Chou L, Lenrow DA (2003) A critical review of the evidence for the use of zygapophysial injections and radiofrequency denervation in the treatment of low back pain. Spine J 3(4):310–316

Staal JB, de Bie RA, de Vet HC, Hildebrandt J, Nelemans P (2009) Injection therapy for subacute and chronic low back pain: an updated Cochrane review. Spine 34(1):49–59

Staiger TO, Gaster B, Sullivan MD, Deyo RA (2003) Systematic review of antidepressants in the treatment of chronic low back pain. Spine (Phila Pa 1976) 28(22):2540–2545

Tveito TH, Hysing M, Eriksen HR (2004) Low back pain interventions at the workplace: a systematic literature review. Occup Med (Lond) 54(1):3–13

UK BEAMT Team (2004) United Kingdom back pain exercise and manipulation (UK BEAM) randomised trial: effectiveness of physical treatments for back pain in primary care. BMJ 329(7479): 1377

van der Heijden GJ, Beurskens AJ, Koes BW, Assendelft WJ, de Vet HC, Bouter LM (1995) The efficacy of traction for back and neck pain: a systematic, blinded review of randomized clinical trial methods. Phys Ther 75(2):93–104 van Middelkoop M, Rubinstein SM, Kuijpers T, Verhagen AP, Ostelo R, Koes BW, Van Tulder M (2011) A systematic review on the effectiveness of physical and rehabilitation interventions for chronic non-specific low back pain. Eur Spine J 20(1):19–39

van Poppel MN, Koes BW, Smid T, Bouter LM (1997) A systematic review of controlled clinical trials on the prevention of back pain in industry. Occup Environ Med 54(12):841–847

van Poppel MN, Koes BW, van der Ploeg T, Smid T, Bouter LM (1998) Lumbar supports and education for the prevention of low back pain in industry: a randomized controlled trial. JAMA 279(22):1789–1794

Van Tulder M, Touray T, Furlan AD, Solway S, Bouter LM, Cochrane Back Review Group (2003) Muscle relaxants for nonspecific low back pain: a systematic review within the framework of the cochrane collaboration. Spine 28(17):1978–1992

Vlaeyen JW, Linton SJ (2000) Fear-avoidance and its consequences in chronic musculoskeletal pain: a state of the art. Pain 85(3): 317–332

Von Korff M, Saunders K (1996) The course of back pain in primary care. Spine 21(24):2833–2837; discussion 2838–2839

Von Korff M, Balderson BH, Saunders K, Miglioretti DL, Lin EH, Berry S, Moore JE, Turner JA (2005) A trial of an activating intervention for chronic back pain in primary care and physical therapy settings. Pain 113(3):323–330

Waddell G, McCulloch JA, Kummel E, Venner RM (1980) Nonorganic physical signs in low-back pain. Spine 5(2):117–125

Waddell G, Newton M, Henderson I, Somerville D, Main CJ (1993) A fear-avoidance beliefs questionnaire (FABQ) and the role of fear-avoidance beliefs in chronic low back pain and disability. Pain 52(2):157–168

Waddell G, Feder G, Lewis M (1997) Systematic reviews of bed rest and advice to stay active for acute low back pain. Br J Gen Pract 47(423):647–652

Walsh NE, Schwartz RK (1990) The influence of prophylactic orthoses on abdominal strength and low back injury in the workplace. Am J Phys Med Rehabil 69(5):245–250

White AP, Arnold PM, Norvell DC, Ecker E, Fehlings M (2011) Pharmacologic management of chronic low back pain: synthesis of the evidence. Spine 36(21 Suppl):S131–S143

Woodhouse ML, McCoy RW, Redondo DR, Shall LM (1995) Effects of back support on intra-abdominal pressure and lumbar kinetics during heavy lifting. Hum Factors 37(3):582–590

Yoon ST (2005) Molecular therapy of the intervertebral disc. Spine J 5(6 Suppl):280S–286S

Zimmerman J, Siguencia J, Tsvang E (1995) Upper gastrointestinal hemorrhage associated with cutaneous application of diclofenac gel. Am J Gastroenterol 90(11):2032–2034

Back Pain and Disc Degeneration: Are They Really Linked?

16

Kjell Olmarker

Contents

K. Olmarker, MD, PhD
Musculoskeletal Research,
Department of Medical Chemistry and Cell biology,
Institute of Biomedicine, Sahlgrenska Academy,
University of Gothenburg, 440, Medicinaregatan 9A,
SE-405 30 Gothenburg, Sweden
e-mail: kjell.olmarker@gu.se

16.1 Introduction and Overview

Back pain or lower back pain (LBP) still remains a controversy, with an apparent lack of understanding of the basic genetic and pathophysiologic mechanisms that predispose patients to this common disabling condition. It has been estimated that LBP affects up to about 80 % of all people during their lifetime (Andersson 1995, 1999). At a given moment, approximately 30 % of the American population suffer from LBP (Frank et al. 1996). LBP thus affects many individuals and is a major societal cost in terms of inability to work, medical treatment, and rehabilitation. In the USA, the total cost was estimated to $50 billion in 1991 (Frymoyer and Cats-Baril 1991) and in Sweden in 1995, with a population of eight million people, to SEK 29.4 billion (approx. US $5 billion) (Nachemson and Jonsson 2000). Low back pain usually has a good prognosis, and most people are able to return to work within a limited period of time, although about 20 % may have recurring problems within 6 months (Cassidy et al. 2005). Also, a considerable number of individuals may suffer from long-lasting low back pain. Because of the lack of knowledge of the underlying causes for back pain and sciatica, it is difficult to define specific treatment modalities.

Based on these facts, numerous studies and theories have been presented regarding a possible cause of LBP. One point that is often overlooked is that LBP is not a specific medical condition with a precise pathogenesis. Instead, it should be looked upon as a mere symptom, like headache of fever, with a variety of potential causes. However, one specific mechanism that has attracted much attention in recent years has been linked to so-called disc degeneration.

Degeneration of the intervertebral as a clinical entity was first described in the 1940s (Epps 1942; Friberg 1948; Friberg and Hirsch 1949; Olsen 1950; Alvik 1950), and at the same time suggestions were made that the intervertebral disc could be a source of back pain (Lindblom 1948). Since then, considerable effort and time has been devoted to establishing specific pathophysiological mechanisms, which could then be used to treat disc degeneration. This has, unfortunately,

I.M. Shapiro, M.V. Risbud (eds.), *The Intervertebral Disc*,
DOI 10.1007/978-3-7091-1535-0_16, © Springer-Verlag Wien 2014

not been entirely successful. The purpose of this chapter is to try to review the rationale and mechanism by which disc degeneration might produce LBP and to briefly discuss treatment strategies that might be used to address this problem.

16.2 Definitions

To form a rational basis for the ensuing discussion, the following definitions will be used:

Pain is derived from the Latin word *poena* meaning "fine" or "penalty." It is defined as "a more or less localized sensation of discomfort, distress, or agony, resulting from the stimulation of specialized nerve endings" (Newman Dorland 2007). In other words, to experience pain, there is a need for transmission of a stimulus from nerve endings or receptors; alternatively, pain is set up by pathophysiologic processes in the axons that are then interpreted as pain stimulus by the central nervous system (neuropathic pain).

Degeneration in turn is derived from the Latin word *degeneratio* which implies "change from a higher form to a lower form; especially change of a tissue to a less functionally active form" (Newman Dorland 2007). This may be interpreted as the result of injury or disease but may also apply to the normal aging process.

16.3 Controversies

The first controversy relates to the disc itself: can the disc per se elicit pain? According to the definition of pain, since nerves must mediate the pain, a tissue producing pain should be innervated. As will be discussed here and in other chapters of the book, the innervation of the intervertebral disc is sparse and normally restricted to the most superficial layers of the annulus fibrosus.

The second controversy concerns what is generally called "disc degeneration" – it begs the question: is it really a pathophysiologic process? Since the intervertebral discs of most individuals exhibit various degrees of "degeneration" and not all experience LBP, it is questioned whether the label "degeneration" is consistent with its pathophysiologic status. It seems even less appropriate to term such changes in the structure of the intervertebral discs as degenerative disc disease, which undoubtedly lends a pathophysiological status to something that might simply reflect normal aging. It must, however, be noted that for 95 % of LBP cases, no specific cause can be found other than exhibiting a radiologic image that suggests rightfully or not that the pain is associated with degenerative disc disease. Probably, with age, the degenerative changes are such that it might possibly be possible to distinguish normal from those associated with pathology. Nevertheless, irrespective of the cause, the term "degeneration" will be used throughout this chapter regarding changes in the intervertebral discs.

16.4 The Basis of Pain: Innervation of the Intervertebral Disc

The innervation of the lumbar intervertebral discs has been studied in detail for many years. The consensus of studies dating back to the early 1930s has been that there are free nerve endings and mechanoreceptors in the superficial layers of the annulus fibrosus and in the posterior longitudinal ligament (Jung and Brunschwig 1932; Roofe 1940; Ehrenhaft 1943; Bogduk et al. 1981; Bogduk 1983; Malinsky 1959; Roberts et al. 1995; Cavanaugh et al. 1997; Palmgren et al. 1999; Fagan et al. 2003) (Fig. 16.1). There are two conjoining nerve plexuses that innervate the anterior and the posterior aspect of the intervertebral disc, respectively, in an overlapping manner (Pedersen et al. 1956; Edgar and Ghadially 1976; Bogduk 1983; Weinstein et al. 1988; Groen et al. 1988). Innervation to the posterior aspect of the disc is mainly provided by the sinuvertebral nerve also known as the nerve of "Luschka"; this nerve penetrates the neuroforamen and supplies the epidural tissues (Luschka 1850). The sinuvertebral nerve was initially thought to innervate only the posterior annulus of the intervertebral disc and the posterior longitudinal ligament, but later studies have demonstrated that there are multiple branches, both ascending and descending, that innervate other structures such as the facet joints (Bogduk and Long 1979; Giles and Taylor 1987; McLain 1993; Masini et al. 2005; Takahashi et al. 2010) and the vertebral end plate (Brown et al. 1997; Fagan et al. 2003; Ohtori et al. 2006; Bailey et al. 2011; Bogduk et al. 1981) and that they overlap within the epidural space (Pedersen et al. 1956; Edgar and Ghadially 1976; Bogduk et al. 1981; Groen et al. 1988). Also, in addition to a pure somatosensory innervation, the intervertebral disc has been found to be innervated by autonomic nerve fibers (Nakamura et al. 1996; Yamada et al. 2001; van Roy et al. 2001; Raoul et al. 2003; Takebayashi et al. 2006; Garcia-Cosamalon et al. 2010).

The overall conflict with the hypothesis that changes in the intervertebral disc would transmit pain to the central nervous system is the observation that the innervation is located only in the superficial layers of the annulus fibrosus (Malinsky 1959; Hirsch et al. 1963; Groen et al. 1988; Ashton et al. 1994; Roberts et al. 1995; Palmgren et al. 1999; Fagan et al. 2003). This is the case in normal nondegenerated discs. On the other hand, degenerated disc specimens exhibit ingrowths of newly sprouted nerves into the deeper portions of the disc. However, this study was performed mainly on the anterior portion of the intervertebral disc, and ingrowths were only demonstrated in the inner part of the annulus fibrosus and, in

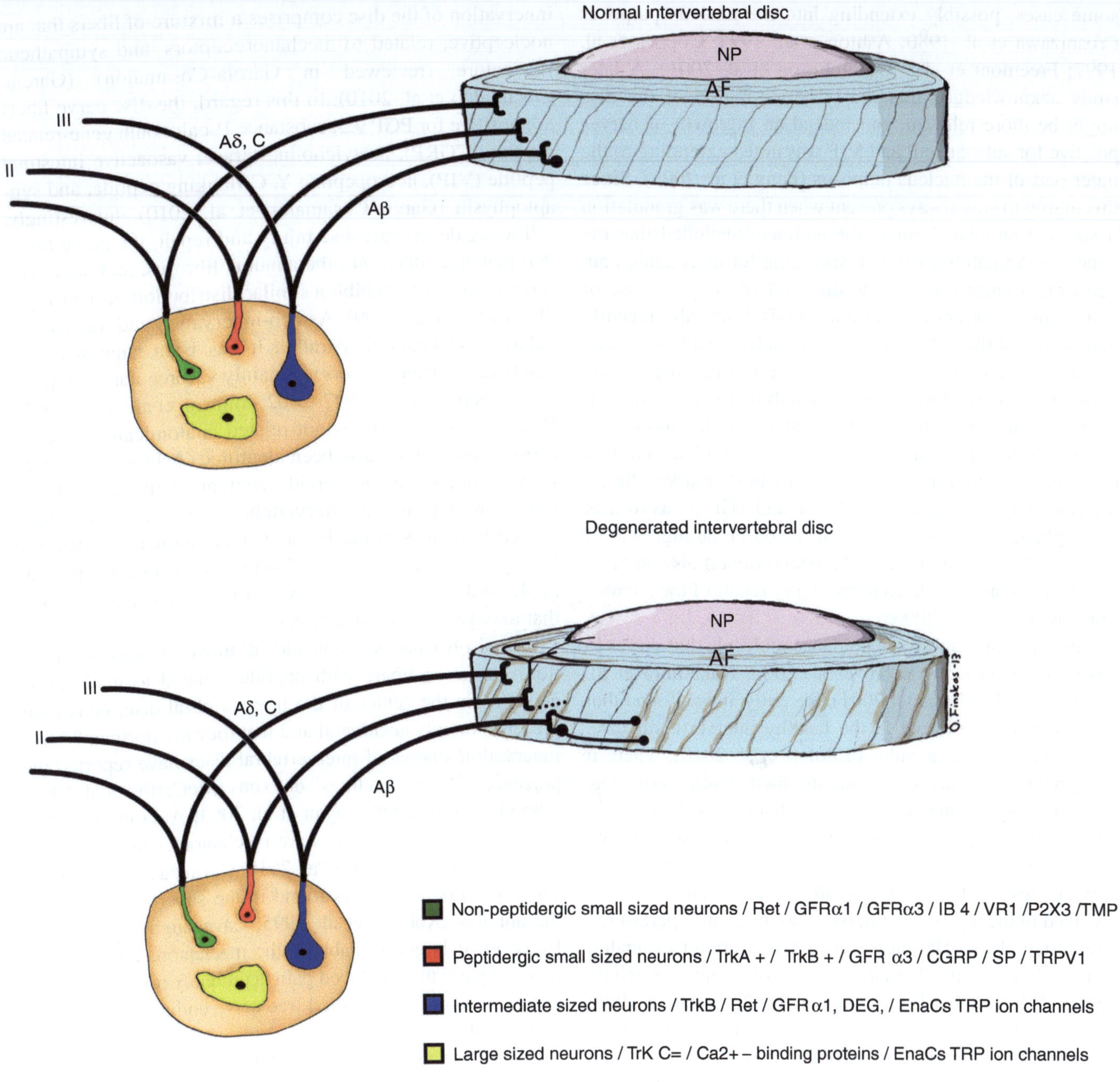

Fig. 16.1 Schematic representation of the innervation of normal (*top*) and degenerated (*bottom*) intervertebral discs (IVDs), as well as the origin of sensory nerve fibers that innervate them. In the normal IVD, innervation is restricted to the outer layers of the annulus fibrosus (*AF*) and consists of small nerve fibers (*red* and *green*) and some large fibers forming mechanoreceptors (*brown*). In the degenerated IVD, nerve fibers are increased in number, and they enter the inner layers of the AF and even the nucleus pulposus (*NP*). Furthermore, in these conditions, the density of mechanoreceptors in the superficial layers of IVDs is increased. Dorsal root ganglions (DRGs) contain different types of sensory neurons that project to the IVD and to the dorsal horn of the spinal cord (DH of SC). Thin myelinated Ad fibers and unmyelinated C fibers arise from small neurons (*red* and *green*), which, in the spinal cord, synapse in laminas I and II and mediate nociception. The myelinated Ab fibers (*brown*) arise from intermediate neurons; at the periphery, they form slowly and rapidly adapting low-threshold mechanoreceptors and synapse in laminas III and IV in the dorsal horn of the spinal cord; they mediate sensations of touch, pressure, and vibration. Most of the sensory nerve fibers innervating the IVD are Ad or C fibers. They originate from small peptidergic neurons expressing TrkA/TrkB (the receptor for nerve growth factor/brain-derived neurotrophic factor, *red*) or non-peptidergic neurons expressing the common signaling receptor for glial cell-derived neurotrophic factor family of neurotrophic factors (Ret) (*red*). Neurons in DRGs can be differentiated based on their pattern of expression of receptors for neurotrophic factors, pattern of expression of different ion channels primarily of the degenerin/epithelial sodium channels (DEG/ENaCs) (ENaCa, ENaCb, and ENaCc), acid-sensing ion channel (ASIC) (ASIC1, ASIC2, and ASIC3) and transient receptor potential (TRP) (TRPA1, TRPC1, TRPC6, and TRPV1–4) families, and peptide content. *CGRP* calcitonin gene-related peptide, *GFRa1 and GFRa3* glial cell line-derived neurotrophic receptor subtypes a1 and a3, *P2X3* ATP-gated ion channel subtype P2X3, *SP* substance P, *TMP* thiamine monophosphatase, *VR1* vanilloid receptor subtype 1 (Modified from Garcia-Cosamalon et al. (2010))

some cases, possibly extending into the nucleus pulposus (Yoshizawa et al. 1980; Ashton et al. 1994; Coppes et al. 1997; Freemont et al. 1997; Johnson et al. 2001). A later study acknowledged that the posterior region of the disc might be more relevant, and indeed an ingrowth of nerves positive for substance P and VIP was noted extending to the outer part of the nucleus pulposus (Peng et al. 2005). Since this ingrowth was always present when there was granulation tissue and annular fissures, the authors concluded that the zone of granulation may be responsible for discogenic pain due to neo-innervation of the disc and possibly a cause of pain from discography (Peng et al. 2005). It was also recently demonstrated that when autologous nucleus pulposus tissue fragments were placed subcutaneously in pigs, there is an ingrowth of newly formed nerves and blood vessels. In contrast, similar ingrowth were not seen when disc tissue was placed in retroperitoneal fat. It was also observed that cytokine inhibitors reduced this ingrowth (Olmarker 2005). It has also been suggested that bFGF and TGF-β1 as well as macrophages and mast cells are involved in the ingrowth of nerves and blood vessels into the intervertebral disc and that this phenomenon is related to the injury repair of the annulus fibrosus (Peng et al. 2006a).

Semaphorin is an axonal guidance molecule that serves to repel axonal growth (Rohm et al. 2000; Nakamura et al. 2000; Liu and Strittmatter 2001). Recently, it was found that this molecule is present in the healthy intervertebral disc, mainly in the outer annulus (Tolofari et al. 2010), where it presumably could prevent axonal ingrowth. Even more interesting is that the same authors found that the levels of semaphorin are lowered in degenerate discs, which would then enhance neo-innervation (Tolofari et al. 2010). Recently, it was suggested that neurotrophins family members were involved in the ingrowth of nerves into the central part of the intervertebral discs (Purmessur et al. 2008; Garcia-Cosamalon et al. 2010). In the human, this family comprises NGF, BDNF, NT-3, and NT-4/5 (Ebendal 1992; Barbacid 1995; Lessmann 1998). The neurotrophins regulate cell proliferation and differentiation via the Trk family of receptor tyrosine kinase and via p75-NTR (Dechant and Barde 1997; Lu et al. 2005; Skaper 2008). Since the neurotrophins seem to be expressed at higher levels in degenerate than in nondegenerate discs, it may be assumed that they may facilitate ingrowth of new nerve fibers into the deeper parts of the intervertebral disc during the degeneration process (Freemont et al. 2002). In summary, based on existing knowledge, there is indeed reason to assume that there is neo-innervation and neovascularization of the annulus fibrosus and nucleus pulposus and that such ingrowth relates to the presence of bioactive substances generated during repair following annular fissures.

Although there may be neo-innervation of injured intervertebral discs, the function and properties of such newly formed nerves are not known (Fig. 16.1). The normal innervation of the disc comprises a mixture of fibers that are nociceptive, related to mechanoreceptors, and sympathetic in nature (reviewed in Garcia-Cosamalón) (Garcia-Cosamalon et al. 2010). In this regard, the disc nerve fibers are positive for PGP 9.5, substance P, calcitonin gene-related peptide (CGRP), acetylcholinesterase, vasoactive intestinal peptide (VIP), neuropeptide Y, C-flanking peptide, and synaptophysin (Garcia-Cosamalon et al. 2010). Interestingly, following degenerate disc injury and repair, the nerve fibers that penetrate deep into the annulus fibrosus, and later even further, appear to exhibit a similar distribution of fiber types (Takahashi et al. 2009). As neo-innervation and the neovascularization occur in parallel, it has been suggested that newly formed nerve fibers are mainly vasoregulatory in function (Freemont et al. 1997, 2002; Johnson et al. 2001, 2007). However, nerve endings not related anatomically to newly formed vessels have also been identified (Ashton et al. 1994). In addition, since the peptide content of the nerve fibers found in degenerate intervertebral discs includes those related to pain transmission and since the nerves related to blood vessels seem to be of sympathetic origin (Yamada et al. 2001), the possibility exists that there are nerve fibers that may be involved in nociception.

Based on what was considered above, it begs the question: are nerve fibers with peptides related to nociception activated in the center of the intervertebral disc, or is their presence merely accidental and that they are dormant? Most innervation studies of intervertebral discs have reported the presence of "nerve endings" or axons (McCarthy et al. 1991; Palmgren et al. 1999; Fagan et al. 2003; Aoki et al. 2004), and the only receptor types are mechanoreceptors (Roberts et al. 1995; Dimitroulias et al. 2010; Cavanaugh et al. 1995). The receptors are always found in the superficial layers of the annulus (Roberts et al. 1995; Cavanaugh et al. 1995). However, it is questionable if the mechanoreceptors could produce pain; thus, induced pain is probably related to direct effects on axons or so-called free nerve endings in the intervertebral disc.

It is known that during degeneration of the nucleus pulposus there are a number of biochemical changes. One such change is the accumulation of metabolites such as lactate and the concomitant pH decrease (Diamant et al. 1968; Nachemson 1969; Buckwalter 1995; Bartels et al. 1998; Keshari et al. 2008; Rajasekaran et al. 2010). Accordingly, pain could be due to chemical excitation of adjacent nerve fibers. Similarly, the increased expression of various bioactive substances, such as members of the neurotrophin family, may activate pain receptors (Freemont et al. 2002; Purmessur et al. 2008; Sugiura et al. 2008; Garcia-Cosamalon et al. 2010; Orita et al. 2011). Biomechanical instability of the motion segment may lead to excess mobility of the degenerated intervertebral disc. Likewise, it has been suggested that such mobility may actively induce signaling in newly formed nerve fibers in the deeper parts of the intervertebral disc, another plausible cause for "disc-triggered" pain (Morgan and King 1957; Kirkaldy-Willis and Farfan 1982; Pope and Panjabi 1985; Bradford 1994; Kim et al. 2005). Finally, injured axons are known to be stimulated by the nerve signals from adjacent axons, so-called cross-excitation (Rasminsky 1987; Lisney and Devor 1987; Devor and Wall 1990; Amir and Devor 1992). Injury can cause a myelin defect due to the loss of its electro-isolating properties: an electrical phenomenon in which nerve impulses in one axons cause an impulse in adjacent axons. Such artificial "ectopic" impulses may be interpreted as pain by the central nervous system, regardless of the axon that originally transmits proprioceptive, temperature, or pressure information (Burchiel 1984; Zimmermann 1984; Devor 1991, 2006; Han et al. 2000; Costigan et al. 2009). Whether this occurs in the intervertebral disc seems unlikely due to its sparse innervation.

In summary, in recent years, knowledge of intervertebral discs innervation has increased tremendously, and the possibility exists that there is "disc-triggered" or "discogenic" pain. However, pain mechanisms still need to be demonstrated convincingly before any conclusions can be drawn as to its clinical relevance.

16.5 Degeneration of the Intervertebral Disc: A Normal Aging Process?

The intervertebral discs are usually referred to as the largest avascular structures of the human body (Holm et al. 1982; Horner and Urban 2001; Roberts 2002; Grunhagen et al. 2011). The nutrition of the cells of the discs, mainly located in the nucleus pulposus, is mainly provided by diffusion from the vertebral end plates. Accordingly, if the nutritional supply becomes insufficient, the nucleus pulposus may undergo changes that may be referred to as age-related or degenerative. This process may be initiated as early as the second decade of life, and its frequency will increase with increasing age (Takatalo et al. 2009; Samartzis et al. 2011). There are reports that 40 % of individuals aged 30 years, 53 in the age group 30–55 years, and 90 % aged 50–55 years exhibit degeneration of one or more discs (Kanayama et al. 2009; Cheung et al. 2009). Degeneration would be expected to lead to changes in the biochemical composition of the disc as well as changes in its mechanical properties. The nucleus pulposus will be more *liquefied,* and there may also be a weakening of the containing structure, the annulus fibrosus. Eventually, the disc will form a more solid and organized structure, which is also usually associated with a reduction of the disc height (Burton et al. 1996; Benneker et al. 2005; Inoue and Espinoza Orias 2011). During the transition from a young healthy disc to the more *solid* state, there is risk of leakage of the liquefied nucleus pulposus with its bioactive components through fissures in the weakened annulus fibrosus into the spinal canal. Similar leakage may also occur on the ventral aspect of the disc and also through the vertebral end plates into the adjacent vertebral bodies (nodes of Schmorl) (Schmorl 1929). What is not known is whether these variants of leakage/herniation produce clinical symptoms (Sward et al. 1990; Takahashi et al. 1995; Zhang et al. 2010). More importantly, the question remains, should these changes in disc structure be considered as normal aging, or should they be described as a degenerative process?

As discussed previously, the term degeneration may be related to the aging process, and hence, the pathophysiological connotation cannot be ignored. Indeed, if the aging processes are shown to induce pain, it might rightfully be termed degeneration. However, signs of spinal pathology, including so-called disc degeneration, are often encountered in asymptomatic individuals (Boden et al. 1990; Jensen et al. 1994; Boos et al. 1995; Stadnik et al. 1998). In this regard, it might be more appropriate to talk about normal and pathological/symptomatic disc aging instead of degeneration. It is thus still not evident how to apply a proper definition to this state. However, according to this author, the term degeneration may be unfortunate and misleading, particularly in persons without any symptoms.

16.6 LBP and Disc Degeneration in Clinical Studies

The literature suggests that there is a strong correlation between degenerative disc changes and LBP (Lindblom 1948; Kelsey and White 1980; Lutz et al. 2003; Chou et al. 2011). However, since no causal link has been confirmed and since a majority of non-symptomatic patients have degenerative disc changes, a causal relationship may be unlikely. This is analogous to the recent discussion on the relationship between Modic-type changes in the vertebrae and LBP. Similar to disc degeneration, there is a correlation between Modic changes and low back clinical pain (Braithwaite et al. 1998; Kjaer et al. 2005; Jensen et al. 2008; Thompson et al. 2009). Again, there is no established causal pathophysiological link. One must therefore consider that there may be a transferred statistical significance, i.e., the Modic changes and low back pain may coexist and have a common pathogenic source but no peer relationship. One such pathogenetic factor might be disc injury. For example, it is known that osteoarthritis in the knee joint may result in changes, fairly similar to the Modic changes, in the femur and that these changes/erosions are considered to be strong indicators of knee cartilage injury (Alexander 1960; Rose and Cockshott 1982; Pattrick et al. 1993). As will be discussed later, disc injury with annular tears and leakage of *liquefied* nucleus pulposus tissue to the superficial and innervated part of the annulus fibrosus could be one cause of low back pain. In this regard, disc injury would be the "common denominator," and an apparent statistical relationship would exist although Modic changes and low back pain merely coexist with no pathophysiologic link. The same phenomenon may be applied to the relationship between disc degeneration and LBP. Since no causal link has been established, there may be another "common denominator" perhaps in this case, secondary to changes in the intervertebral disc.

Box 16.1 Modic Changes

The so-called Modic changes were first described by Michael Modic and collaborators in 1988 (Modic et al. 1998). Magnetic resonance images of vertebral body changes were reviewed of 474 patients. It was found that 4 % of the patients had decreased signal intensity on T1-weighted spin-echo images and increased signal intensity on T2-weighted images, a finding that was given the grade 1. In 16 % of the patients, there was increased signal intensity on T1-weighted images and isointense or slightly increased signal intensity on T2-weighted images, which was graded as 2. A third grade was added later and is defined as bone scar tissue. The authors concluded, "These signal intensity changes appear to reflect a spectrum of vertebral body marrow changes associated with degenerative disk disease." Today it is known that these changes closely correlates to low back pain (Braithwaite et al. 1998; Kjaer et al. 2005; Jensen et al. 2008; Thompson et al. 2009). However, no causal pathophysiological explanation has been found. It is therefore a possibility that there might be a transferred statistical significance, i.e., the Modic changes and low back pain may coexist but have a common pathogenic source and no peer relationship. One such likely source might be disc injury. It is known that there is an increased incidence of Modic changes in patients with disc herniations (Albert and Manniche 2007). If the Modic changes might be responsible for low back pain or not is thus debatable, but it seems plausible that these changes may serve as an indicator of disc injury.

References

Albert HB, Manniche C (2007) Modic changes following lumbar disc herniation. Eur Spine J 16:977–982

Braithwaite I, White J, Saifuddin A et al (1998) Vertebral end-plate (Modic) changes on lumbar spine MRI: correlation with pain reproduction at lumbar discography. Eur Spine J 7:363–368

Jensen TS, Karppinen J, Sorensen JS et al (2008) Vertebral endplate signal changes (Modic change): a systematic literature review of prevalence and association with non-specific low back pain. Eur Spine J 17:1407–1422

Kjaer P, Leboeuf-Yde C, Korsholm L et al (2005) Magnetic resonance imaging and low back pain in adults: a diagnostic imaging study of 40-year-old men and women. Spine (Phila Pa 1976) 30:1173–1180

Modic MT, Steinberg PM, Ross JS et al (1998) Degenerative disk disease: assessment of changes in vertebral body marrow with MR imaging. Radiology 166:193–199

Thompson KJ, Dagher AP, Eckel TS et al (2009) Modic changes on MR images as studied with provocative diskography: clinical relevance – a retrospective study of 2457 disks. Radiology 250:849–855

16.7 Secondary Changes of Disc Degeneration That May Induce Pain

About 80 % of the population worldwide will experience LBP sometime during their lifetime (Andersson 1995, 1999). However, in only a minority of cases, a definitive clinical diagnosis such as vertebral fracture, infection, or tumor will be established (Staiger et al. 1999; Goupille et al. 2000; Della-Giustina and Kilcline 2000; Henschke et al. 2009). The remaining 95 % will therefore be termed idiopathic. Most likely, there may be one or more specific mechanisms that may be hidden within these 95 % that have yet to be discovered. Although events occurring within the disc might theoretically induce LBP (discogenic LBP), the degeneration of the intervertebral disc may also cause secondary changes that could be overlooked.

One such effect is the subsequent reduction of the disc height during the degeneration process. A consequence of this lowered height is that there may be malpositioning of the facet joints (Ghomley 1993; Eisenstein and Parry 1987; Mooney and Robertson 1976). Theoretically such a change could lead to cartilage injury and damage to the capsule facet joint (Fujiwara et al. 2000a, b; Kong et al. 2009). It is known that the facet joints are richly innervated (Bogduk and Long 1979; Bogduk 1983), and attempts have been made to treat facet-joint-related problems with local injections of anesthetics (Carrera 1980; Manchikanti et al. 2007, 2008). However, it is likely that osteoarthritis of these joints and the ensuing production of inflammatory agents that can leak through the injured joint capsule could serve to irritate and stimulate intraspinal nervous structures including the nerve root and nerve endings on the posterior aspect of the intervertebral disc (Hasue 1993; Willburger and Wittenberg 1994; Igarashi et al. 2004).

Another striking feature of the degenerative changes of the intervertebral discs is the formation of annular tears or fissures (Hilton et al. 1980; Videman and Nurminen 2004; Ross et al. 1989; Osti et al. 1992). Such fissures may allow leakage of the degenerated and partly "liquefied" nucleus pulposus (Stadnik et al. 1998; Saifuddin et al. 1999; Derby et al. 2005; Peng et al. 2006b). Biologic product from the degenerative nucleus pulposus could diffuse to the outer annulus fibrosus or even the spinal canal. MRI analysis has shown that a zone of increased inflammatory activity, the high-intensity zone (HIZ), exists in the superficial regions of the annulus (Schellhas et al. 1996; Peng et al. 2006b; Carragee et al. 2000). This zone is associated with LBP although it may also be found in asymptomatic patients (Weishaupt et al. 1998; Stadnik et al. 1998; Carragee et al. 2000; Wang et al. 2008).

It is known that nerve endings and mechanoreceptors exist on the posterior aspect of the annulus fibrosus; while these are normally dormant, they can be activated by inflammatory stimuli (Rang et al. 1991; Dray 1995; Ozaktay et al. 1994; Cavanaugh 1995; Coutaux et al. 2005). It is therefore reasonable to assume that biologically active substances released from the degenerating nucleus pulposus may activate cognate receptors by diffusing into the spinal canal through the annular fissures. One diagnostic approach for assessing symptomatic intervertebral discs is through discography, a procedure in which a fluid is injected under pressure into the center of the disc to provoke pain (Moneta et al. 1994; Schellhas et al. 1996; Carragee 2000; Stout 2010). Possibly, the pain is not related to activation of newly formed nerves within the intervertebral disc, but to a washout of bioactive substances into the spinal canal and the innervated structures including the disc, the longitudinal ligament, and facet-joint capsules.

In a pioneering study, in patients undergoing surgery for disc herniation under local, progressive anesthesia, Kuslich and colleagues stimulated various parts of the spinal complex (Kuslich et al. 1991). They found that stimulation of a nerve root did not generate pain, whereas mechanical stimulation of the nerve root adjacent to the herniated disc produced a radiating pain out into the lower limb, similar to sciatic pain. The most interesting observation, however, was that stimulation of the posterior part of the annulus fibrosus produced pain in the lower back, similar to LBP. The authors concluded that the posterior annulus fibrosus was "the site of back pain" (Kuslich et al. 1991). There is thus compelling evidence that activation of nociceptive nerve endings or receptors in the posterior aspect of the annulus fibrosus (Weber et al. 2006) may produce pain in the lower back; this finding may be due to the release of agents from the nucleus pulposus during discography and also possibly at non-provoked sites (Fig. 16.2).

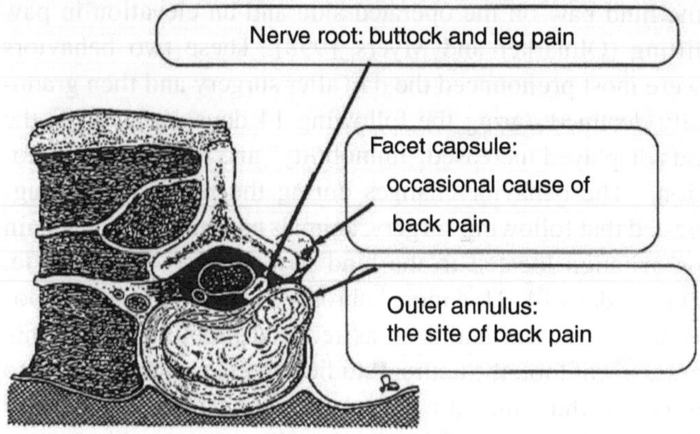

Fig. 16.2 Observations at probing in conscious patients under local anesthesia during laminectomy. Probing of the nerve root adjacent to a disc herniation reproduces buttock and leg pain. Probing of the fact capsule occasionally reproduces back pain, whereas probing of the outer annulus always reproduces back pain and is also concluded to be "the site" of back pain (Republished from Kuslich et al. (1991))

Our group studied whether application of nucleus pulposus samples to the superficial annulus fibrosus might induce LBP in rodents. As discussed in Chap. 18, assessment of LBP in an animal model is a significant challenge. While alterations in specific nerves activity may be assessed by neurophysiologic recordings, pain itself is dependent on its interpretation by the central nervous system. In animals, there is a limitation in available experimental methodologies to assess whether the transmitted signals are perceived as pain. Methods that can be used for assessing pain is through functional MRI (Hsu et al. 1998; Weber et al. 2006; Adamczak et al. 2010) (see Chap. 12); another approach is to study behavioral changes (Kawakami et al. 1994; Abbott et al. 1995; Olmarker and Myers 1998).

In rodents, we have assessed spontaneous behavioral changes following experimental disc herniation (Olmarker et al. 2002). In contrast to most other assessment modalities, spontaneous behavior analysis, which has been used to evaluate psychological parameters (Wuttke and Hoffmeister 1968; Monti and Carlini 1975; Rodriquez-Enchandia et al. 1986; Garcia-Cabrera and Berge 1990), examines an animal's instinctive involuntary activities. Despite the high variation in behavior between animals, changes in spontaneous behavior may reveal discomfort or irritation that is not easily obtained by other behavior modalities. In collaboration with the Department of Physiology, University of Bergen, Norway, spontaneous behavior assessment was adapted to study changes following experimental disc herniation. Procedures used included disc puncture with transfer of the nucleus pulposus tissue to, and a slight mechanical deformation of, the adjacent nerve root (Olmarker and Myers 1998; Olmarker et al. 1998, 2003). The study showed that experimental disc herniation induced an increased rotation of the head towards the hind paw on the operated side and an elevation in paw lifting (Olmarker and Myers 1998). These two behaviors were most pronounced the day after surgery and then gradually declined during the following 14 days. At day 21, the rats displayed increased "immobility" and reduced "locomotion." The behavior changes during the first 14 days suggested that following surgery, animals experienced focal pain or irritation located in the hind paw on the operated side. During days 14–21, a more "chronic" non-focal pain component was present and seen as reduced mobility. Using this assessment tool, the authors studied changes induced by disc puncture, thus simulating a leakage of nucleus pulposus onto the posterior aspect of the annulus fibrosus, but with no contact with the adjacent nerve root. The assumption was that the rats would display reduced motion, analogous to LBP, similar to that reported at 21 days in the radiculopathy model. While the rats did not exhibit reduced mobility, they evidenced increased "grooming" and an uncharacteristic shaking of the head and upper body: both behaviors were displayed significantly more often in disc punctured rats than in rats with non-punctured discs (Olmarker 2008). Increased grooming has been observed in other studies and has been suggested to reflect anxiety, stress, and chronic neuropathic pain (Millan and Emrich 1981; Crawley and Moody 1983; Vos et al. 1994; Deseure and Adriaensen 2002; Eriksson et al. 2005). The observed shaking is commonly seen in psychopharmacological studies and termed wet-dog shakes (WDS): it is a typical sign of withdrawal from opiates, benzodiazepines, and barbiturates (Colasanti and Khazan 1975; Baldino et al. 1979; Horowitz and Allan 1982; Martin et al. 1982). The shakes have also been considered to relate to stress (Treptow et al. 1986; Deschamps and Couture 2005; Brotto et al. 1999) and pain (Papir-Kricheli et al. 1987; Kitamura et al. 2007). It was concluded that rats with punctured discs experienced some kind of discomfort. However, it was not possible to determine if this discomfort was analogous to LBP.

In a follow-up study, we evaluated if the observed behavior changes were induced by disc injury or the presence of nucleus pulposus tissue on the posterior aspect of the annulus fibrosus. It was found that disc puncture and application of nucleus pulposus induced similar behavioral changes. In contrast, the same behavioral changes were not evident following ventral disc puncture and a superficial disc injury without penetration of the annulus fibrosus, with no leakage of nucleus pulposus tissue (Olmarker 2011). It was also observed that inhibition of TNF also markedly reduced the behavioral effects (Nakamae et al. 2011). Interestingly, a recent randomized clinical trial focused on evaluating the effects of epidural TNF inhibition on sciatic pain also revealed that in addition to the inhibitors' beneficial effects on the sciatic pain, it also induced a marked reduction of LBP (Cohen et al. 2009). In summary, there is emerging experimental and clinical evidence that leakage of disc material onto the posterior annulus fibrosus may be an actual cause of LBP possibly mediated through TNF.

Box 16.2 Molecular Events That Are Characteristic of the Aging Process

There is limited information on factors that characterize the normal aging process in the intervertebral disc. However, since the aging disc shares some genetic as well as molecular characteristics of cartilage, changes that are evident in cartilage are listed below:

Mild fibrillation of and softening of the articular surface
Osteophyte formation
Loss of matrix tensile strength and stiffness
Responsiveness to inflammatory stimuli
Changes in metabolism
Accumulation of ROS and glycation products
Changes in IGF, insulin, and growth hormone levels
Progressive chondrocyte senescence
Erosion in of chondrocyte telomere length
Changes in phenotype
Decrease in average size of proteoglycan monomers
Decrease in the aggregation capacity of the proteoglycan monomers
Expression of the senescence-associated enzyme beta-galactosidase
Mitochondrial degeneration

16.8 Therapeutic Strategies: Should the Target Be Nucleus Pulposus Degeneration?

Inevitably, a chapter on disc degeneration and LBP must provide insights into possible therapeutic strategies. Although it is not fully understood if the disc tissue per se can produce clinical pain, the target of much of the work is the degeneration process itself and the disc as a pain generator. Surgically, this has been approached by fusion of the potentially painful disc function unit, a procedure that is frequently performed with varying degrees of success (Gibson and Waddell 2005; Carreon et al. 2008; Glassman et al. 2009). There are also promising attempts to revitalize the disc by injection of stem cells or biological components (Wehling et al. 1997; Nishida et al. 2000; Yoon et al. 2004; Sakai et al. 2003; Brisby et al. 2004; Risbud et al. 2004) (see Chaps. 23 and 24). However, although these procedures might be successful in the future, they do raise a set of new questions. Based on current knowledge, it will be difficult to assess when, how often, and in which discs should such interventions be performed. We know that there are "dangerous years": from the initiation of degeneration/aging, when the disc may leak, herniate, and produce pain, until the end stage when the disc has been transformed to a more solid connective tissue, with less likelihood to produce pain. A provocative but appropriate question would be: would it not be a better strategy to increase the degeneration/aging process so as to shorten the duration of these "dangerous years"? This notion was suggested 50 years ago by Hirsch who recommended that injection of a "chondrolytic enzyme" into the disc would increase the degeneration process and convert the disc to a solid, asymptomatic structure (Hirsch 1959). This original idea was later modified by Smith who indicated that chymopapain would disintegrate the inner structure of the disc and thus be of clinical use for the treatment of sciatica; this procedure was later known as chemonucleolysis (Smith 1964). Bearing this in mind, it might be prudent to consider the apparent risk of delaying the degeneration/aging process of the disc by biological means, in the sense that instead of having mostly "asymptomatic" discs at the age of 60–70, there is the possibility that "symptomatic" discs may be present at much higher ages than would be expected if the disc would be allowed to age normally. The author opines that this potential problem, a reduction in the degeneration process, has not being fully considered and needs to be further explored.

An alternate strategy to that of modifying the degeneration/aging process per se is to control pain pathways. Since the source of the pain has not been identified, this form of "symptomatic" treatment would be analogous to aiming water at flames and not at the source of the fire. In fact, since it is not evident that the disc generates the pain, secondary changes such as loss of disc height might eventually prove to be involved (Twomey and Taylor 1985; Berlemann et al. 1998; Shao et al. 2002). For example, the loss of disc height could influence facet-joint function. Misalignment of the articular surfaces could induce osteoarthritic changes and the release of bioactive molecules. Diffusion of these agents to the intraspinal nervous structures could then induce pain by similar mechanisms to those discussed previously (Hasue 1993; Willburger and Wittenberg 1994; Igarashi et al. 2004).

Another inevitable consequence of degeneration is disarrangement of the fibrils of the annulus fibrosus and leakage of the partly *liquefied* degenerate disc. To the author, this seems to be a very likely scenario and could well be the cause of LBP of "idiopathic origin." Perhaps, in the future, LBP treatment may comprise a dual strategy: epidural administration of agents that inhibit key biological processes and a "sealant" of annular tears, possibly in combination with surgical immobilization of the spinal segment and the preservation of disc height.

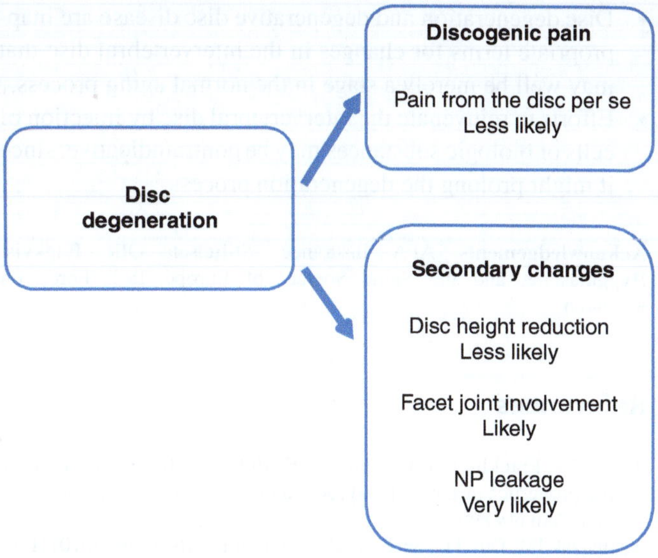

Fig. 16.3 The author's view of pain mechanisms and their likelihood as the result of disc degeneration

16.9 Disc Degeneration and Its Relationship to LBP: Conclusions

Although emerging evidence indicates that degeneration may induce innervation of deeper parts of the intervertebral disc, it seems unlikely that the degenerative process produces pain per se. More likely, it is the result of secondary changes associated with degeneration (Fig. 16.3). As challenging as ever are questions that include whether future treatment strategies should be directed at the degeneration process itself, what is the importance of controlling secondary changes, and should the disc be rejuvenated and when and how should this be accomplished. While this chapter is both speculative and somewhat provocative, it is merely the result of the apparent lack of understanding of the pathophysiologic background of LBP, and it is the hope that this contribution may stimulate continued discussion and research in this complex field both from a basic scientific and a clinical perspective.

16.10 Summary of Critical Concepts Discussed in the Chapter

- The origin of disc pain is still not understood. Pain most likely originates from receptors on nerve fibers on the surface of the posterior aspect of the intervertebral disc.
- Pain activation may be due to leakage of disc-derived biologically active molecules which diffuse through annular tears of the annulus fibrosus.
- The paucity of innervating nerve fibers would indicate that pain is unlikely to originate from the center of the intervertebral disc.

- Disc degeneration and degenerative disc disease are inappropriate terms for changes in the intervertebral disc that may well be merely a stage in the normal aging process.
- Efforts to rejuvenate the intervertebral disc by injection of cells or biologic substances may be contraindicative, since it might prolong the degeneration process.

Acknowledgements AFA Insurance, Stiftelsen Olle Engkvist Byggmästare, and the Spine Society of Europe Task Force on Research

References

Abbott FV, Franklin KB, Westbrook RF (1995) The formalin test: scoring properties of the first and second phases of the pain response in rats. Pain 60(1):91–102

Adamczak JM, Farr TD, Seehafer JU, Kalthoff D, Hoehn M (2010) High field BOLD response to forepaw stimulation in the mouse. Neuroimage 51(2):704–712. doi:10.1016/j.neuroimage.2010.02.083

Alexander C (1960) Erosion of the femoral shaft due to patellofemoral osteoarthritis. Clin Radiol 11:110–113

Alvik I (1950) Degeneration of the lumbar intervertebral disks. Nord Med 44(32):1271–1274

Amir R, Devor M (1992) Axonal cross-excitation in nerve-end neuromas: comparison of A- and C-fibers. J Neurophysiol 68(4):1160–1166

Andersson GBJ (1995) Intervertebral disc herniation: epidemiology and natural history. In: Weinstein JN, Gordon SL (eds) Low back pain. A scientific and clinical overview. American Academy of Orthopaedic Surgeons, Rosemont, pp 7–21

Andersson GB (1999) Epidemiological features of chronic low-back pain. Lancet 354(9178):581–585. doi:10.1016/s0140-6736(99)01312-4

Aoki Y, Ohtori S, Takahashi K, Ino H, Takahashi Y, Chiba T, Moriya H (2004) Innervation of the lumbar intervertebral disc by nerve growth factor-dependent neurons related to inflammatory pain. Spine 29(10):1077–1081

Ashton IK, Roberts S, Jaffray DC, Polak JM, Eisenstein SM (1994) Neuropeptides in the human intervertebral disc. J Orthop Res 12(2):186–192. doi:10.1002/jor.1100120206

Bailey JF, Liebenberg E, Degmetich S, Lotz JC (2011) Innervation patterns of PGP 9.5-positive nerve fibers within the human lumbar vertebra. J Anat 218(3):263–270. doi:10.1111/j.1469-7580.2010.01332.x

Baldino F Jr, Cowan A, Geller EB, Adler MW (1979) Effects of antipsychotic and antianxiety drugs on the morphine abstinence syndrome in rats. J Pharmacol Exp Ther 208(1):63–66

Barbacid M (1995) Structural and functional properties of the TRK family of neurotrophin receptors. Ann N Y Acad Sci 766: 442–458

Bartels EM, Fairbank JC, Winlove CP, Urban JP (1998) Oxygen and lactate concentrations measured in vivo in the intervertebral discs of patients with scoliosis and back pain. Spine (Phila Pa 1976) 23(1): 1–7; discussion 8

Benneker LM, Heini PF, Anderson SE, Alini M, Ito K (2005) Correlation of radiographic and MRI parameters to morphological and biochemical assessment of intervertebral disc degeneration. Eur Spine J 14(1):27–35. doi:10.1007/s00586-004-0759-4

Berlemann U, Gries NC, Moore RJ (1998) The relationship between height, shape and histological changes in early degeneration of the lower lumbar discs. Eur Spine J 7(3):212–217

Boden SD, Davis DO, Dina TS, Patronas NJ, Wiesel SW (1990) Abnormal magnetic-resonance scans of the lumbar spine in asymptomatic subjects. A prospective investigation. J Bone Joint Surg Am 72(3):403–408

Bogduk N (1983) The innervation of the lumbar spine. Spine (Phila Pa 1976) 8(3):286–293

Bogduk N, Long DM (1979) The anatomy of the so-called "articular nerves" and their relationship to facet denervation in the treatment of low-back pain. J Neurosurg 51(2):172–177. doi:10.3171/jns.1979.51.2.0172

Bogduk N, Tynan W, Wilson AS (1981) The nerve supply to the human lumbar intervertebral discs. J Anat 132(Pt 1):39–56

Boos N, Rieder R, Schade V, Spratt KF, Semmer N, Aebi M (1995) 1995 Volvo Award in clinical sciences. The diagnostic accuracy of magnetic resonance imaging, work perception, and psychosocial factors in identifying symptomatic disc herniations. Spine 20(24):2613–2625

Bradford DS (1994) Surgical treatment of low back pain in spine instability. Chir Organi Mov 79(1):63–68

Braithwaite I, White J, Saifuddin A, Renton P, Taylor BA (1998) Vertebral end-plate (Modic) changes on lumbar spine MRI: correlation with pain reproduction at lumbar discography. Eur Spine J 7(5):363–368

Brisby H, Tao H, Ma DD, Diwan AD (2004) Cell therapy for disc degeneration–potentials and pitfalls. Orthop Clin North Am 35(1):85–93. doi:10.1016/s0030-5898(03)00104-4

Brotto LA, Hanson LA, Gorzalka BB (1999) Nefazodone attenuates the stress-induced facilitation of wet dog shaking behaviour but not the facilitation of sexual behaviour in female rats. Eur J Pharmacol 381(2–3):101–104

Brown MF, Hukkanen MV, McCarthy ID, Redfern DR, Batten JJ, Crock HV, Hughes SP, Polak JM (1997) Sensory and sympathetic innervation of the vertebral endplate in patients with degenerative disc disease. J Bone Joint Surg Br 79(1):147–153

Buckwalter JA (1995) Aging and degeneration of the human intervertebral disc. Spine (Phila Pa 1976) 20(11):1307–1314

Burchiel KJ (1984) Spontaneous impulse generation in normal and denervated dorsal root ganglia: sensitivity to alpha-adrenergic stimulation and hypoxia. Exp Neurol 85(2):257–272

Burton AK, Battie MC, Gibbons L, Videman T, Tillotson KM (1996) Lumbar disc degeneration and sagittal flexibility. J Spinal Disord 9(5):418–424

Carragee EJ (2000) Is lumbar discography a determinate of discogenic low back pain: provocative discography reconsidered. Curr Rev Pain 4(4):301–308

Carragee EJ, Paragioudakis SJ, Khurana S (2000) 2000 Volvo Award winner in clinical studies: lumbar high-intensity zone and discography in subjects without low back problems. Spine 25(23):2987–2992

Carreon LY, Glassman SD, Howard J (2008) Fusion and nonsurgical treatment for symptomatic lumbar degenerative disease: a systematic review of Oswestry Disability Index and MOS Short Form-36 outcomes. Spine J 8(5):747–755. doi:10.1016/j.spinee.2007.06.013

Carrera GF (1980) Lumbar facet joint injection in low back pain and sciatica: preliminary results. Radiology 137(3):665–667

Cassidy JD, Cote P, Carroll LJ, Kristman V (2005) Incidence and course of low back pain episodes in the general population. Spine (Phila Pa 1976) 30(24):2817–2823

Cavanaugh JM (1995) Neural mechanisms of lumbar pain. Spine 20(16):1804–1809

Cavanaugh JM, Kallakuri S, Ozaktay AC (1995) Innervation of the rabbit lumbar intervertebral disc and posterior longitudinal ligament. Spine (Phila Pa 1976) 20(19):2080–2085

Cavanaugh JM, Ozaktay AC, Yamashita T, Avramov A, Getchell TV, King AI (1997) Mechanisms of low back pain: a neurophysiologic and neuroanatomic study. Clin Orthop Relat Res 335:166–180

Cheung KM, Karppinen J, Chan D, Ho DW, Song YQ, Sham P, Cheah KS, Leong JC, Luk KD (2009) Prevalence and pattern of lumbar magnetic resonance imaging changes in a population study of one thousand forty-three individuals. Spine (Phila Pa 1976) 34(9): 934–940. doi:10.1097/BRS.0b013e3181a01b3f

Chou D, Samartzis D, Bellabarba C, Patel A, Luk KD, Kisser JM, Skelly AC (2011) Degenerative magnetic resonance imaging changes in patients with chronic low back pain: a systematic review. Spine (Phila Pa 1976) 36(21 Suppl):S43–S53. doi:10.1097/BRS.0b013e31822ef700

Cohen SP, Bogduk N, Dragovich A, Buckenmaier CC 3rd, Griffith S, Kurihara C, Raymond J, Richter PJ, Williams N, Yaksh TL (2009) Randomized, double-blind, placebo-controlled, dose–response, and preclinical safety study of transforaminal epidural etanercept for the treatment of sciatica. Anesthesiology 110(5):1116–1126. doi:10.1097/ALN.0b013e3181a05aa0

Colasanti B, Khazan N (1975) Imipramine-induced changes in the rapid eye movement sleep rebound and wet dog shakes of morphine-abstinent rats. Neuropharmacology 14(5–6):361–367

Coppes MH, Marani E, Thomeer RT, Groen GJ (1997) Innervation of "painful" lumbar discs. Spine 22(20):2342–2349; discussion 2349–2350

Costigan M, Scholz J, Woolf CJ (2009) Neuropathic pain: a maladaptive response of the nervous system to damage. Annu Rev Neurosci 32:1–32. doi:10.1146/annurev.neuro.051508.135531

Coutaux A, Adam F, Willer JC, Le Bars D (2005) Hyperalgesia and allodynia: peripheral mechanisms. Joint Bone Spine 72(5):359–371. doi:10.1016/j.jbspin.2004.01.010

Crawley JN, Moody TW (1983) Anxiolytics block excessive grooming behavior induced by ACTH1-24 and bombesin. Brain Res Bull 10(3):399–401

Dechant G, Barde YA (1997) Signalling through the neurotrophin receptor p75NTR. Curr Opin Neurobiol 7(3):413–418

Della-Giustina D, Kilcline BA (2000) Acute low back pain: a comprehensive review. Compr Ther 26(3):153–159

Derby R, Kim BJ, Lee SH, Chen Y, Seo KS, Aprill C (2005) Comparison of discographic findings in asymptomatic subject discs and the negative discs of chronic LBP patients: can discography distinguish asymptomatic discs among morphologically abnormal discs? Spine J 5(4):389–394

Deschamps K, Couture R (2005) The ventral tegmental area as a putative target for tachykinins in cardiovascular regulation. Br J Pharmacol 145(6):712–727

Deseure KR, Adriaensen HF (2002) Comparison between two types of behavioral variables of non-evoked facial pain after chronic constriction injury to the rat infraorbital nerve. Comp Med 52(1):44–49

Devor M (1991) Chronic pain in the aged: possible relation between neurogenesis, involution and pathophysiology in adult sensory ganglia. J Basic Clin Physiol Pharmacol 2(1–2):1–15

Devor M (2006) Sodium channels and mechanisms of neuropathic pain. J Pain 7(1 Suppl 1):S3–S12. doi:10.1016/j.jpain.2005.09.006

Devor M, Wall PD (1990) Cross-excitation in dorsal root ganglia of nerve-injured and intact rats. J Neurophysiol 64(6):1733–1746

Diamant B, Karlsson J, Nachemson A (1968) Correlation between lactate levels and pH in discs of patients with lumbar rhizopathies. Experientia 24(12):1195–1196

Dimitroulias A, Tsonidis C, Natsis K, Venizelos I, Djau SN, Tsitsopoulos P (2010) An immunohistochemical study of mechanoreceptors in lumbar spine intervertebral discs. J Clin Neurosci 17(6):742–745. doi:10.1016/j.jocn.2009.09.032

Dray A (1995) Inflammatory mediators of pain. Br J Anaesth 75(2):125–131

Ebendal T (1992) Function and evolution in the NGF family and its receptors. J Neurosci Res 32(4):461–470. doi:10.1002/jnr.490320402

Edgar MA, Ghadially JA (1976) Innervation of the lumbar spine. Clin Orthop Relat Res 115:35–41

Ehrenhaft JL (1943) Development of the vertebral column as related to certain congenital and pathological changes. Surg, Gyn Obstr 76:282–292

Eisenstein SM, Parry CR (1987) The lumbar facet arthrosis syndrome. Clinical presentation and articular surface changes. J Bone Joint Surg Br 69(1):3–7

Epps PG (1942) A case of degeneration of the intervertebral disc following lumbar puncture: (section of orthopaedics). Proc R Soc Med 35(3):220–221

Eriksson J, Jablonski A, Persson AK, Hao JX, Kouya PF, Wiesenfeld-Hallin Z, Xu XJ, Fried K (2005) Behavioral changes and trigeminal ganglion sodium channel regulation in an orofacial neuropathic pain model. Pain 119(1–3):82–94

Fagan A, Moore R, Vernon Roberts B, Blumbergs P, Fraser R (2003) ISSLS prize winner: the innervation of the intervertebral disc: a quantitative analysis. Spine (Phila Pa 1976) 28(23):2570–2576. doi:10.1097/01.brs.0000096942.29660.b1

Frank JW, Kerr MS, Brooker AS, DeMaio SE, Maetzel A, Shannon HS, Sullivan TJ, Norman RW, Wells RP (1996) Disability resulting from occupational low back pain. Part I: what do we know about primary prevention? A review of the scientific evidence on prevention before disability begins. Spine (Phila Pa 1976) 21(24):2908–2917

Freemont AJ, Peacock TE, Goupille P, Hoyland JA, O'Brien J, Jayson MI (1997) Nerve ingrowth into diseased intervertebral disc in chronic back pain. Lancet 350(9072):178–181

Freemont AJ, Watkins A, Le Maitre C, Baird P, Jeziorska M, Knight MT, Ross ER, O'Brien JP, Hoyland JA (2002) Nerve growth factor expression and innervation of the painful intervertebral disc. J Pathol 197(3):286–292. doi:10.1002/path.1108

Friberg S (1948) Anatomical studies on lumbar disc degeneration. Acta Orthop Scand 17(3–4):224–230

Friberg S, Hirsch C (1949) Anatomical and clinical studies on lumbar disc degeneration. Acta Orthop Scand 19(2):222–242, illust

Frymoyer JW, Cats-Baril WL (1991) An overview of the incidences and costs of low back pain. Orthop Clin North Am 22(2):263–271

Fujiwara A, Lim TH, An HS, Tanaka N, Jeon CH, Andersson GB, Haughton VM (2000a) The effect of disc degeneration and facet joint osteoarthritis on the segmental flexibility of the lumbar spine. Spine (Phila Pa 1976) 25(23):3036–3044

Fujiwara A, Tamai K, An HS, Kurihashi T, Lim TH, Yoshida H, Saotome K (2000b) The relationship between disc degeneration, facet joint osteoarthritis, and stability of the degenerative lumbar spine. J Spinal Disord 13(5):444–450

Garcia-Cabrera I, Berge OG (1990) Interaction of high pressure and a narcotic dose of ethanol on spontaneous behavior in rats. Pharmacol Biochem Behav 37(3):577–581

Garcia-Cosamalon J, del Valle ME, Calavia MG, Garcia-Suarez O, Lopez-Muniz A, Otero J, Vega JA (2010) Intervertebral disc, sensory nerves and neurotrophins: who is who in discogenic pain? J Anat 217(1):1–15. doi:10.1111/j.1469-7580.2010.01227.x

Ghomley RK (1993) Low back pain with special reference to the articular facets with presentation of an operative procedure. JAMA 101:1773–1777

Gibson JN, Waddell G (2005) Surgery for degenerative lumbar spondylosis. Cochrane Database Syst Rev (4):CD001352. doi:10.1002/14651858.CD001352.pub3

Giles LG, Taylor JR (1987) Innervation of lumbar zygapophyseal joint synovial folds. Acta Orthop Scand 58(1):43–46

Glassman SD, Carreon LY, Djurasovic M, Dimar JR, Johnson JR, Puno RM, Campbell MJ (2009) Lumbar fusion outcomes stratified by specific diagnostic indication. Spine J 9(1):13–21. doi:10.1016/j.spinee.2008.08.011

Goupille P, Avimadje AM, Zerkak D, Valat JP (2000) Clinical elements of the diagnostic guidelines for low back pain. Rev Prat 50(16):1760–1764

Groen GJ, Baljet B, Drukker J (1988) The innervation of the spinal dura mater: anatomy and clinical implications. Acta Neurochir (Wien) 92(1–4):39–46

Grunhagen T, Shirazi-Adl A, Fairbank JC, Urban JP (2011) Intervertebral disk nutrition: a review of factors influencing concentrations of nutrients and metabolites. Orthop Clin North Am 42(4):465–477. doi:10.1016/j.ocl.2011.07.010

Han HC, Lee DH, Chung JM (2000) Characteristics of ectopic discharges in a rat neuropathic pain model. Pain 84(2–3):253–261
Hasue M (1993) Pain and the nerve root. An interdisciplinary approach. Spine (Phila Pa 1976) 18(14):2053–2058
Henschke N, Maher CG, Refshauge KM, Herbert RD, Cumming RG, Bleasel J, York J, Das A, McAuley JH (2009) Prevalence of and screening for serious spinal pathology in patients presenting to primary care settings with acute low back pain. Arthritis Rheum 60(10):3072–3080. doi:10.1002/art.24853
Hilton RC, Ball J, Benn RT (1980) Annular tears in the dorsolumbar spine. Ann Rheum Dis 39(6):533–538
Hirsch C (1959) Studies on the pathology of low back pain. J Bone Joint Surg Br 41-B(2):237–243
Hirsch C, Ingelmark BE, Miller M (1963) The anatomical basis for low back pain. Studies on the presence of sensory nerve endings in ligamentous, capsular and intervertebral disc structures in the human lumbar spine. Acta Orthop Scand 33:1–17
Holm S, Selstam G, Nachemson A (1982) Carbohydrate metabolism and concentration profiles of solutes in the canine lumbar intervertebral disc. Acta Physiol Scand 115(1):147–156
Horner HA, Urban JP (2001) 2001 Volvo Award Winner in Basic Science Studies: effect of nutrient supply on the viability of cells from the nucleus pulposus of the intervertebral disc. Spine (Phila Pa 1976) 26(23):2543–2549
Horowitz GP, Allan AM (1982) Morphine withdrawal in mice selectively bred for differential sensitivity to ethanol. Pharmacol Biochem Behav 16(1):35–39
Hsu EW, Hedlund LW, MacFall JR (1998) Functional MRI of the rat somatosensory cortex: effects of hyperventilation. Magn Reson Med 40(3):421–426
Igarashi A, Kikuchi S, Konno S, Olmarker K (2004) Inflammatory cytokines released from the facet joint tissue in degenerative lumbar spinal disorders. Spine (Phila Pa 1976) 29(19):2091–2095
Inoue N, Espinoza Orias AA (2011) Biomechanics of intervertebral disk degeneration. Orthop Clin North Am 42(4):487–499. doi:10.1016/j.ocl.2011.07.001
Jensen MC, Brant-Zawadzki MN, Obuchowski N, Modic MT, Malkasian D, Ross JS (1994) Magnetic resonance imaging of the lumbar spine in people without back pain. N Engl J Med 331(2):69–73. doi:10.1056/nejm199407143310201
Jensen TS, Karppinen J, Sorensen JS, Niinimaki J, Leboeuf-Yde C (2008) Vertebral endplate signal changes (Modic change): a systematic literature review of prevalence and association with non-specific low back pain. Eur Spine J 17(11):1407–1422. doi:10.1007/s00586-008-0770-2
Johnson WE, Evans H, Menage J, Eisenstein SM, El Haj A, Roberts S (2001) Immunohistochemical detection of Schwann cells in innervated and vascularized human intervertebral discs. Spine (Phila Pa 1976) 26(23):2550–2557
Johnson WE, Patterson AM, Eisenstein SM, Roberts S (2007) The presence of pleiotrophin in the human intervertebral disc is associated with increased vascularization: an immunohistologic study. Spine 32(12):1295–1302
Jung A, Brunschwig A (1932) Rescherches histologique des articulations des corps vertebeaux. La presse Medicale 40:316–317
Kanayama M, Togawa D, Takahashi C, Terai T, Hashimoto T (2009) Cross-sectional magnetic resonance imaging study of lumbar disc degeneration in 200 healthy individuals. J Neurosurg Spine 11(4):501–507. doi:10.3171/2009.5.spine08675
Kawakami M, Weinstein JN, Chatani K, Spratt KF, Meller ST, Gebhart GF (1994) Experimental lumbar radiculopathy. Behavioral and histologic changes in a model of radicular pain after spinal nerve root irritation with chromic gut ligatures in the rat. Spine 19(16): 1795–1802
Kelsey JL, White AA 3rd (1980) Epidemiology and impact of low-back pain. Spine (Phila Pa 1976) 5(2):133–142
Keshari KR, Lotz JC, Link TM, Hu S, Majumdar S, Kurhanewicz J (2008) Lactic acid and proteoglycans as metabolic markers for discogenic back pain. Spine (Phila Pa 1976) 33(3):312–317. doi:10.1097/BRS.0b013e31816201c3
Kim CW, Perry A, Garfin SR (2005) Spinal instability: the orthopedic approach. Semin Musculoskelet Radiol 9(1):77–87. doi:10.1055/s-2005-867098
Kirkaldy-Willis WH, Farfan HF (1982) Instability of the lumbar spine. Clin Orthop Relat Res 165:110–123
Kitamura Y, Kitagawa K, Fujitani Y, Shibata K, Araki H, Sendou T, Gomita Y (2007) The 5-HT(1A) receptor full agonist, 8-OH-DPAT inhibits ACTH-induced 5-HT(2A) receptor hyperfunction in rats: involvement of 5-HT(1A) receptors in the DOI-induced wet-dog shakes in ACTH-treated rats. Biol Pharm Bull 30(1):117–120
Kjaer P, Leboeuf-Yde C, Korsholm L, Sorensen JS, Bendix T (2005) Magnetic resonance imaging and low back pain in adults: a diagnostic imaging study of 40-year-old men and women. Spine (Phila Pa 1976) 30(10):1173–1180
Kong MH, Morishita Y, He W, Miyazaki M, Zhang H, Wu G, Hymanson HJ, Wang JC (2009) Lumbar segmental mobility according to the grade of the disc, the facet joint, the muscle, and the ligament pathology by using kinetic magnetic resonance imaging. Spine (Phila Pa 1976) 34(23):2537–2544. doi:10.1097/BRS.0b013e3181b353ea
Kuslich SD, Ulstrom CL, Michael CJ (1991) The tissue origin of low back pain and sciatica: a report of pain response to tissue stimulation during operations on the lumbar spine using local anesthesia. Orthop Clin North Am 22(2):181–187
Lessmann V (1998) Neurotrophin-dependent modulation of glutamatergic synaptic transmission in the mammalian CNS. Gen Pharmacol 31(5):667–674
Lindblom K (1948) Diagnostic puncture of intervertebral disks in sciatica. Acta Orthop Scand 17(3–4):231–239
Lisney SJ, Devor M (1987) Afterdischarge and interactions among fibers in damaged peripheral nerve in the rat. Brain Res 415(1): 122–136
Liu BP, Strittmatter SM (2001) Semaphorin-mediated axonal guidance via Rho-related G proteins. Curr Opin Cell Biol 13(5):619–626
Lu B, Pang PT, Woo NH (2005) The yin and yang of neurotrophin action. Nat Rev Neurosci 6(8):603–614. doi:10.1038/nrn1726
Luschka H (1850) Die Nerven des menschlichen Wirbelkanales. Laupp und Siebeck, Tübingen
Lutz GK, Butzlaff M, Schultz-Venrath U (2003) Looking back on back pain: trial and error of diagnoses in the 20th century. Spine (Phila Pa 1976) 28(16):1899–1905. doi:10.1097/01.brs.0000083365.41261.cf
Malinsky J (1959) The ontogenetic development of nerve terminations in the intervertebral discs of man. (Histology of intervertebral discs, 11th communication). Acta Anat (Basel) 38:96–113
Manchikanti L, Manchikanti KN, Manchukonda R, Cash KA, Damron KS, Pampati V, McManus CD (2007) Evaluation of lumbar facet joint nerve blocks in the management of chronic low back pain: preliminary report of a randomized, double-blind controlled trial: clinical trial NCT00355914. Pain Physician 10(3):425–440
Manchikanti L, Singh V, Falco FJ, Cash KA, Pampati V (2008) Lumbar facet joint nerve blocks in managing chronic facet joint pain: one-year follow-up of a randomized, double-blind controlled trial: clinical trial NCT00355914. Pain Physician 11(2):121–132
Martin WR, McNicholas LF, Cherian S (1982) Diazepam and pentobarbital dependence in the rat. Life Sci 31(8):721–730
Masini M, Paiva WS, Araujo AS Jr (2005) Anatomical description of the facet joint innervation and its implication in the treatment of recurrent back pain. J Neurosurg Sci 49(4):143–146; discussion 146
McCarthy PW, Carruthers B, Martin D, Petts P (1991) Immunohistochemical demonstration of sensory nerve fibers and endings in lumbar intervertebral discs of the rat. Spine 16(6):653–655

McLain RF (1993) Mechanoreceptor endings in human cervical facet joints. Iowa Orthop J 13:149–154

Millan MJ, Emrich HM (1981) Endorphinergic systems and the response to stress. Psychother Psychosom 36(1):43–56

Moneta GB, Videman T, Kaivanto K, Aprill C, Spivey M, Vanharanta H, Sachs BL, Guyer RD, Hochschuler SH, Raschbaum RF et al (1994) Reported pain during lumbar discography as a function of anular ruptures and disc degeneration. A re-analysis of 833 discograms. Spine (Phila Pa 1976) 19(17):1968–1974

Monti JM, Carlini EA (1975) Spontaneous behavior and sleep-wakefulness cycle in isolated and paired REM sleep deprived-marihuana treated rats. Pharmacol Biochem Behav 3(6):1025–1029

Mooney V, Robertson J (1976) The facet syndrome. Clin Orthop Relat Res 115:149–156

Morgan FP, King T (1957) Primary instability of lumbar vertebrae as a common cause of low back pain. J Bone Joint Surg Br 39-B(1):6–22

Nachemson A (1969) Intradiscal measurements of pH in patients with lumbar rhizopathies. Acta Orthop Scand 40(1):23–42

Nachemson A, Jonsson E (2000) Ont i ryggen, ont i nacken. – En evidensbaserad kunskapssammanställningom orsaker, diagnostik och Behandling. SBU Statens Berednings för medicinsk Utvärdering, Stockholm, Sweden

Nakamae T, Ochi M, Olmarker K (2011) Pharmacological inhibition of tumor necrosis factor may reduce pain behavior changes induced by experimental disc puncture in the rat: an experimental study in rats. Spine 36(15):232–236. doi:10.1097/BRS.0b013e3181d8bef3

Nakamura S, Takahashi K, Takahashi Y, Morinaga T, Shimada Y, Moriya H (1996) Origin of nerves supplying the posterior portion of lumbar intervertebral discs in rats. Spine (Phila Pa 1976) 21(8): 917–924

Nakamura F, Kalb RG, Strittmatter SM (2000) Molecular basis of semaphorin-mediated axon guidance. J Neurobiol 44(2):219–229

Newman Dorland WA (2007) Dorland's illustrated medical dictionary, 31st edn. Saunders/Elsevier, Philadelphia

Nishida K, Gilbertson LG, Robbins PD, Evans CH, Kang JD (2000) Potential applications of gene therapy to the treatment of intervertebral disc disorders. Clin Orthop Relat Res (379 Suppl):S234–S241

Ohtori S, Inoue G, Ito T, Koshi T, Ozawa T, Doya H, Saito T, Moriya H, Takahashi K (2006) Tumor necrosis factor-immunoreactive cells and PGP 9.5-immunoreactive nerve fibers in vertebral endplates of patients with discogenic low back pain and Modic Type 1 or Type 2 changes on MRI. Spine (Phila Pa 1976) 31(9):1026–1031. doi:10.1097/01.brs.0000215027.87102.7c

Olmarker K (2005) Neovascularization and neoinnervation of subcutaneously placed nucleus pulposus and the inhibitory effects of certain drugs. Spine 30(13):1501–1504

Olmarker K (2008) Puncture of a lumbar intervertebral disc induces changes in spontaneous pain behavior: an experimental study in rats. Spine 33(8):850–855

Olmarker K (2011) Puncture of a disc and application of nucleus pulposus induces disc herniation-like changes and osteophytes. An experimental study in rats. Open Orthop J 5:154–159

Olmarker K, Myers RR (1998) Pathogenesis of sciatic pain: role of herniated nucleus pulposus and deformation of spinal nerve root and dorsal root ganglion. Pain 78(2):99–105

Olmarker K, Iwabuchi M, Larsson K, Rydevik B (1998) Walking analysis of rats subjected to experimental disc herniation. Eur Spine J 7(5):394–399

Olmarker K, Storkson R, Berge OG (2002) Pathogenesis of sciatic pain: a study of spontaneous behavior in rats exposed to experimental disc herniation. Spine 27(12):1312–1317

Olmarker K, Nutu M, Storkson R (2003) Changes in spontaneous behavior in rats exposed to experimental disc herniation are blocked by selective TNF-alpha inhibition. Spine 28(15):1635–1641; discussion 1642

Olsen AK (1950) Disc degeneration: a distinct clinical entity. J Nerv Ment Dis 112(3):262–263

Orita S, Eguchi Y, Kamoda H, Arai G, Ishikawa T, Miyagi M, Inoue G, Suzuki M, Toyone T, Aoki Y, Takahashi K, Ohtori S (2011) Brain-derived neurotrophic factor inhibition at the punctured intervertebral disc downregulates the production of calcitonin gene-related peptide in dorsal root ganglia in rats. Spine (Phila Pa 1976) 36(21):1737–1743. doi:10.1097/BRS.0b013e31821d7b9f

Osti OL, Vernon-Roberts B, Moore R, Fraser RD (1992) Annular tears and disc degeneration in the lumbar spine. A post-mortem study of 135 discs. J Bone Joint Surg Br 74(5):678–682

Ozaktay AC, Cavanaugh JM, Blagoev DC, Getchell TV, King AI (1994) Effects of a carrageenan-induced inflammation in rabbit lumbar facet joint capsule and adjacent tissues. Neurosci Res 20(4):355–364

Palmgren T, Gronblad M, Virri J, Kaapa E, Karaharju E (1999) An immunohistochemical study of nerve structures in the anulus fibrosus of human normal lumbar intervertebral discs. Spine 24(20):2075–2079

Papir-Kricheli D, Frey J, Laufer R, Gilon C, Chorev M, Selinger Z, Devor M (1987) Behavioural effects of receptor-specific substance P agonists. Pain 31(2):263–276

Pattrick M, Hamilton E, Wilson R, Austin S, Doherty M (1993) Association of radiographic changes of osteoarthritis, symptoms, and synovial fluid particles in 300 knees. Ann Rheum Dis 52(2):97–103

Pedersen HE, Blunck CF, Gardner E (1956) The anatomy of lumbosacral posterior rami and meningeal branches of spinal nerve (sinu-vertebral nerves); with an experimental study of their functions. J Bone Joint Surg Am 38-A(2):377–391

Peng B, Wu W, Hou S, Li P, Zhang C, Yang Y (2005) The pathogenesis of discogenic low back pain. J Bone Joint Surg Br 87(1):62–67

Peng B, Hao J, Hou S, Wu W, Jiang D, Fu X, Yang Y (2006a) Possible pathogenesis of painful intervertebral disc degeneration. Spine (Phila Pa 1976) 31(5):560–566. doi:10.1097/01.brs.0000201324.45537.46

Peng B, Hou S, Wu W, Zhang C, Yang Y (2006b) The pathogenesis and clinical significance of a high-intensity zone (HIZ) of lumbar intervertebral disc on MR imaging in the patient with discogenic low back pain. Eur Spine J 15(5):583–587

Pope MH, Panjabi M (1985) Biomechanical definitions of spinal instability. Spine (Phila Pa 1976) 10(3):255–256

Purmessur D, Freemont AJ, Hoyland JA (2008) Expression and regulation of neurotrophins in the nondegenerate and degenerate human intervertebral disc. Arthritis Res Ther 10(4):R99. doi:10.1186/ar2487

Rajasekaran S, Vidyadhara S, Subbiah M, Kamath V, Karunanithi R, Shetty AP, Venkateswaran K, Babu M, Meenakshi J (2010) ISSLS prize winner: a study of effects of in vivo mechanical forces on human lumbar discs with scoliotic disc as a biological model: results from serial postcontrast diffusion studies, histopathology and biochemical analysis of twenty-one human lumbar scoliotic discs. Spine (Phila Pa 1976) 35(21):1930–1943. doi:10.1097/BRS.0b013e3181e9a156

Rang HP, Bevan S, Dray A (1991) Chemical activation of nociceptive peripheral neurones. Br Med Bull 47(3):534–548

Raoul S, Faure A, Robert R, Rogez JM, Hamel O, Cuillere P, Le Borgne J (2003) Role of the sinu-vertebral nerve in low back pain and anatomical basis of therapeutic implications. Surg Radiol Anat 24(6):366–371. doi:10.1007/s00276-002-0084-8

Rasminsky M (1987) Spontaneous activity and cross-talk in pathological nerve fibers. Res Publ Assoc Res Nerv Ment Dis 65:39–49

Risbud MV, Shapiro IM, Vaccaro AR, Albert TJ (2004) Stem cell regeneration of the nucleus pulposus. Spine J 4(6 Suppl):348S–353S. doi:10.1016/j.spinee.2004.07.031

Roberts S (2002) Disc morphology in health and disease. Biochem Soc Trans 30(Pt 6):864–869. doi:10.1042/BST0300864

Roberts S, Eisenstein SM, Menage J, Evans EH, Ashton IK (1995) Mechanoreceptors in intervertebral discs. Morphology, distribution, and neuropeptides. Spine (Phila Pa 1976) 20(24):2645–2651
Rodriquez-Enchandia EL, Broitman ST, Foscolo M, Gonzales A (1986) Gamma-vinyl-GABA injection in the locus coeruleus region of the rat. Effect on spontaneous behavior and stress responses. Adv Biochem Psychopharmacol 42:93–102
Rohm B, Ottemeyer A, Lohrum M, Puschel AW (2000) Plexin/neuropilin complexes mediate repulsion by the axonal guidance signal semaphorin 3A. Mech Dev 93(1–2):95–104
Roofe PG (1940) Innervation of annulus fibrosusand posterior longitudinal ligament. Arch Neurol Psychiatry 44:110–113
Rose CP, Cockshott WP (1982) Anterior femoral erosion and patellofemoral osteoarthritis. J Can Assoc Radiol 33(1):32–34
Ross JS, Modic MT, Masaryk TJ (1989) Tears of the anulus fibrosus: assessment with Gd-DTPA-enhanced MR imaging. AJNR Am J Neuroradiol 10(6):1251–1254
Saifuddin A, Mitchell R, Taylor BA (1999) Extradural inflammation associated with annular tears: demonstration with gadolinium-enhanced lumbar spine MRI. Eur Spine J 8(1):34–39
Sakai D, Mochida J, Yamamoto Y, Nomura T, Okuma M, Nishimura K, Nakai T, Ando K, Hotta T (2003) Transplantation of mesenchymal stem cells embedded in Atelocollagen gel to the intervertebral disc: a potential therapeutic model for disc degeneration. Biomaterials 24(20):3531–3541
Samartzis D, Karppinen J, Mok F, Fong DY, Luk KD, Cheung KM (2011) A population-based study of juvenile disc degeneration and its association with overweight and obesity, low back pain, and diminished functional status. J Bone Joint Surg Am 93(7):662–670. doi:10.2106/jbjs.i.01568
Schellhas KP, Pollei SR, Gundry CR, Heithoff KB (1996) Lumbar disc high-intensity zone. Correlation of magnetic resonance imaging and discography. Spine 21(1):79–86
Schmorl G (1929) Über knorpelknoten an der Hinterfläsche der Wirbelbandscheiben. Fortschr Geb Rontgenstr 40:629–634
Shao Z, Rompe G, Schiltenwolf M (2002) Radiographic changes in the lumbar intervertebral discs and lumbar vertebrae with age. Spine (Phila Pa 1976) 27(3):263–268
Skaper SD (2008) The biology of neurotrophins, signalling pathways, and functional peptide mimetics of neurotrophins and their receptors. CNS Neurol Disord Drug Targets 7(1):46–62
Smith L (1964) Enzyme dissolution of the nucleus pulposus in humans. JAMA 187:137–140
Stadnik TW, Lee RR, Coen HL, Neirynck EC, Buisseret TS, Osteaux MJ (1998) Annular tears and disk herniation: prevalence and contrast enhancement on MR images in the absence of low back pain or sciatica. Radiology 206(1):49–55
Staiger TO, Paauw DS, Deyo RA, Jarvik JG (1999) Imaging studies for acute low back pain. When and when not to order them. Postgrad Med 105(4):161–162, 165–166, 171–162
Stout A (2010) Discography. Phys Med Rehabil Clin N Am 21(4):859–867. doi:10.1016/j.pmr.2010.07.002
Sugiura A, Ohtori S, Yamashita M, Inoue G, Yamauchi K, Koshi T, Suzuki M, Norimoto M, Orita S, Eguchi Y, Takahashi Y, Watanabe TS, Ochiai N, Takaso M, Takahashi K (2008) Existence of nerve growth factor receptors, tyrosine kinase a and p75 neurotrophin receptors in intervertebral discs and on dorsal root ganglion neurons innervating intervertebral discs in rats. Spine (Phila Pa 1976) 33(19):2047–2051. doi:10.1097/BRS.0b013e31817f8d58
Sward L, Hellstrom M, Jacobsson B, Peterson L (1990) Back pain and radiologic changes in the thoraco-lumbar spine of athletes. Spine (Phila Pa 1976) 15(2):124–129
Takahashi K, Miyazaki T, Ohnari H, Takino T, Tomita K (1995) Schmorl's nodes and low-back pain. Analysis of magnetic resonance imaging findings in symptomatic and asymptomatic individuals. Eur Spine J 4(1):56–59
Takahashi Y, Ohtori S, Takahashi K (2009) Peripheral nerve pathways of afferent fibers innervating the lumbar spine in rats. J Pain 10(4):416–425. doi:10.1016/j.jpain.2008.10.012
Takahashi Y, Ohtori S, Takahashi K (2010) Dorsoventral organization of sensory nerves in the lumbar spine as indicated by double labeling of dorsal root ganglion neurons. J Orthop Sci 15(4):578–583. doi:10.1007/s00776-010-1482-0
Takatalo J, Karppinen J, Niinimaki J, Taimela S, Nayha S, Jarvelin MR, Kyllonen E, Tervonen O (2009) Prevalence of degenerative imaging findings in lumbar magnetic resonance imaging among young adults. Spine (Phila Pa 1976) 34(16):1716–1721. doi:10.1097/BRS.0b013e3181ac5fec
Takebayashi T, Cavanaugh JM, Kallakuri S, Chen C, Yamashita T (2006) Sympathetic afferent units from lumbar intervertebral discs. J Bone Joint Surg Br 88(4):554–557. doi:10.1302/0301-620X.88B4.17194, 88-B/4/554 [pii]
Thompson KJ, Dagher AP, Eckel TS, Clark M, Reinig JW (2009) Modic changes on MR images as studied with provocative diskography: clinical relevance – a retrospective study of 2457 disks. Radiology 250(3):849–855. doi:10.1148/radiol.2503080474
Tolofari SK, Richardson SM, Freemont AJ, Hoyland JA (2010) Expression of semaphorin 3A and its receptors in the human intervertebral disc: potential role in regulating neural ingrowth in the degenerate intervertebral disc. Arthritis Res Ther 12(1):R1. doi:10.1186/ar2898
Treptow K, Bondarenko NA, Waldmann AW, Oehme P (1986) The effect of substance P on the swimming behavior of rats under stressing and nonstressing conditions. Pharmazie 41(8):578–580
Twomey L, Taylor J (1985) Age changes in lumbar intervertebral discs. Acta Orthop Scand 56(6):496–499
van Roy P, Barbaix E, Clarijs JP, Mense S (2001) Anatomical background of low back pain: variability and degeneration of the lumbar spinal canal and intervertebral disc. Schmerz 15(6):418–424. doi:10.1007/s004820100026
Videman T, Nurminen M (2004) The occurrence of anular tears and their relation to lifetime back pain history: a cadaveric study using barium sulfate discography. Spine 29(23):2668–2676
Vos BP, Strassman AM, Maciewicz RJ (1994) Behavioral evidence of trigeminal neuropathic pain following chronic constriction injury to the rat's infraorbital nerve. J Neurosci 14(5 Pt 1):2708–2723
Wang ZX, Hu YG, Chen XM (2008) Significance of the high-intensity zone located in the posterior annulus fibrosus for diagnosing discogenic low back pain. Zhonghua Yi Xue Za Zhi 88(35):2478–2481
Weber R, Ramos-Cabrer P, Wiedermann D, van Camp N, Hoehn M (2006) A fully noninvasive and robust experimental protocol for longitudinal fMRI studies in the rat. Neuroimage 29(4):1303–1310. doi:10.1016/j.neuroimage.2005.08.028
Wehling P, Schulitz KP, Robbins PD, Evans CH, Reinecke JA (1997) Transfer of genes to chondrocytic cells of the lumbar spine. Proposal for a treatment strategy of spinal disorders by local gene therapy. Spine (Phila Pa 1976) 22(10):1092–1097
Weinstein J, Claverie W, Gibson S (1988) The pain of discography. Spine (Phila Pa 1976) 13(12):1344–1348
Weishaupt D, Zanetti M, Hodler J, Boos N (1998) MR imaging of the lumbar spine: prevalence of intervertebral disk extrusion and sequestration, nerve root compression, end plate abnormalities, and osteoarthritis of the facet joints in asymptomatic volunteers. Radiology 209(3):661–666
Willburger RE, Wittenberg RH (1994) Prostaglandin release from lumbar disc and facet joint tissue. Spine (Phila Pa 1976) 19(18): 2068–2070
Wuttke W, Hoffmeister F (1968) Changes in the spontaneous behavior of cats induced by chlordiazepoxide and chlorpromazine. Naunyn Schmiedebergs Arch Exp Pathol Pharmakol 260(2):221–222
Yamada H, Honda T, Yaginuma H, Kikuchi S, Sugiura Y (2001) Comparison of sensory and sympathetic innervation of the dura

mater and posterior longitudinal ligament in the cervical spine after removal of the stellate ganglion. J Comp Neurol 434(1):86–100

Yoon ST, Park JS, Kim KS, Li J, Attallah-Wasif ES, Hutton WC, Boden SD (2004) ISSLS prize winner: LMP-1 upregulates intervertebral disc cell production of proteoglycans and BMPs in vitro and in vivo. Spine (Phila Pa 1976) 29(23):2603–2611

Yoshizawa H, O'Brien JP, Smith WT, Trumper M (1980) The neuropathology of intervertebral discs removed for low-back pain. J Pathol 132(2):95–104

Zhang N, Li FC, Huang YJ, Teng C, Chen WS (2010) Possible key role of immune system in Schmorl's nodes. Med Hypotheses 74(3):552–554. doi:10.1016/j.mehy.2009.09.044

Zimmermann M (1984) Basic concepts of pain and pain therapy. Arzneimittelforschung 34(9A):1053–1059

Clinical Features and Pathobiology of Chordoma

17

John A. Abraham, Brian Neuman, and Francis J. Hornicek

Contents

J.A. Abraham, MD (✉)
Division of Orthopedic Oncology, Rothman Institute, Philadelphia, PA, USA

Department of Orthopedic Surgery and Radiation Oncology, Thomas Jefferson University, 925 Chestnut Street, Philadelphia, PA 19107, USA
e-mail: john.abraham@rothmaninstitute.com

B. Neuman, MD
Department of Orthopedic Surgery, Thomas Jefferson University, 925 Chestnut Street, Philadelphia, PA 19107, USA
e-mail: bneumy@gmail.com

F.J. Hornicek, MD, PhD
Division of Orthopedic Oncology, Center for Sarcoma and Connective Tissue Oncology, Massachusetts General Hospital Cancer Center, Massachusetts General Hospital, Boston, MA, USA

Department of Orthopedic Surgery, Harvard Medical School, 55 Fruit Street, Boston, MA 02114, USA
e-mail: fhornicek@partners.org

17.1 Introduction and Historical Perspective

Chordoma is the most common primary malignant bone tumor found in the spine and sacrum. While these tumors are relatively slow growing, they do have the potential to recur and metastasize. Chordoma was described histologically long before it was realized that they were probably derived from notochordal precursor cells. Early reports dating back to Virchow in 1857 describe a vacuolated cell type seen in these tumors. These cells were described as physaliferous, from Greek for "having bubbles." It was thought at that early time that they were a cartilaginous tumor, which may have been a result of evaluation of a chondroid variant tumor. By 1923, Burrow and Stewart recognized that chordomas were a "lowly malignant tumor of slow growth, locally invasive and destructive, and only rarely giving rise to metastases." By then, the location at either end of the spine correlated well with contemporary descriptions of the location of vestigial notochordal remnants by Muller. These observations led to the hypothesis that chordomas were not tumors of the intervertebral disc but rather malignant transformation of these notochordal remnants. In 1858, Muller coined the current name by proposing the following hypothesis: "A direct relation of these growths to the chorda dorsalis cannot be overlooked and I consider them to be excessively growing remnants of the chorda. Whosoever likes the name may designate these masses as chordoid tumors, or chordomas." Since these early descriptions, this concept has been supported by significant indirect evidence, although there is a paucity of direct proof.

The early treatment of chordoma focused on surgical removal, but the difficulty in completely resecting these tumors was very quickly recognized. Investigation of the addition of radiation to the treatment regimen with or without surgery was described in the 1970s and continues to be investigated (Pearlman and Friedman 1970; Pearlman et al. 1972). Medical therapies failed to provide any significant benefit, and the search for an effective medical

I.M. Shapiro, M.V. Risbud (eds.), *The Intervertebral Disc*,
DOI 10.1007/978-3-7091-1535-0_17, © Springer-Verlag Wien 2014

agent continues today. This chapter provides a review of the clinical features of chordoma and the current molecular understanding of its pathobiology.

17.2 Epidemiology

Chordoma is the most frequent primary bone tumor found in the spine. Nevertheless, these tumors are rare with the age-adjusted incidence rate of 0.08 per 100,000 (McMaster et al. 2001). Chordomas make up 1–4 % of all primary bone tumors (Healey and Lane 1989; Unni 1996; Papagelopoulos et al. 2004). Approximately 50 % of these tumors are located within the sacrum (Fig. 17.1). The remaining anatomic locations are the skull-base, spheno-occipital region (35 %), and mobile spine (15 %) (Bohlman et al. 1986; Bjornsson et al. 1993; Bergh et al. 2000). The distribution of these tumors within the mobile spine was evaluated by Boriani et al. (2006) in a consecutive series over 50 years. This group demonstrated the highest frequency of involvement in the lumbar spine (57.5 %), followed by the cervical region (29 %), and least frequently in the thoracic spine (13.5 %). Chordomas comprise greater than 50 % of the primary bone tumors found in the sacrum (Boriani et al. 2006). In a recent analysis of 409 patients identified utilizing the California Cancer Registry, the racial distribution was 65 % Caucasian, 23 % Hispanic, 10 % Asian or "other," and 1.7 % African. In this study, in evaluating chordoma-specific survival, there was a significantly decreased risk of death in Hispanics (Lee et al. 2012). In this group, chordomas were also found to be associated with younger age at diagnosis, cranial disease, and a higher rate of surgical intervention, which were all associated with better survival. This observation was surprising as the Hispanic population was associated with low socioeconomic status, and this factor alone should have increased the risk of death. Consistently, studies on gender distribution of chordomas show a 2:1 male predominance (Ashwood et al. 1994; Forsyth et al. 1993). The median age at the time of diagnosis is 58.5 years, while diagnosis is rare in patients younger than 30 years of age (McMaster et al. 2001; Weber and Sim 2002). These tumors are very uncommon in pediatric populations comprising less than 5 % of all chordomas, with the majority of these being skull based (McMaster et al. 2001).

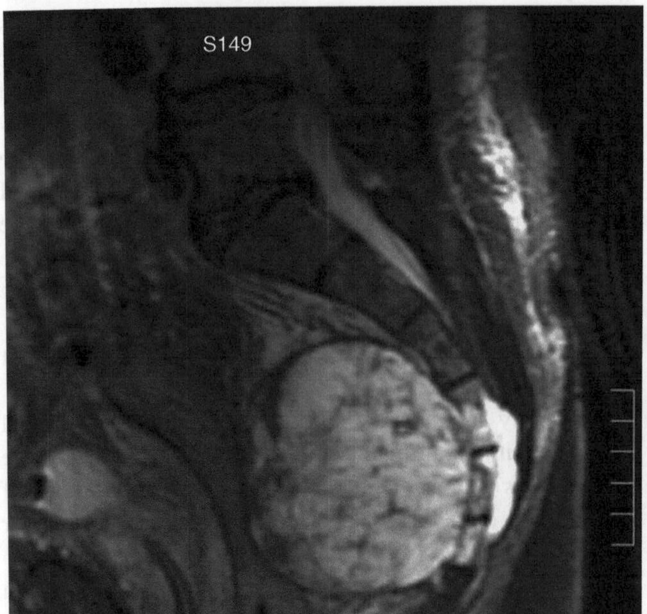

Fig. 17.1 Typical MRI appearance of large sacral chordoma

17.3 Clinical Features

Patients diagnosed with a chordoma most commonly present with pain, regardless of location (Bergh et al. 2000; Boriani et al. 1996, 2006). The second most common presentation is development of neurological symptoms and least commonly a palpable mass (Bergh et al. 2000, Soo 2001). Symptom duration averages 2 years prior to diagnosis, highlighting the slow-growing nature of these tumors (Bergh et al. 2000). If untreated, pain can progress to the point of incapacitation, which in one study was found to be at approximately 50 months from the onset of symptoms (Boriani et al. 2006).

Up to 60 % of the time, chordomas can extend into the spinal canal and in some of these cases can cause significant neurologic symptoms, such as compressive myelopathy or cauda equina (Meyer et al. 1984) (Fig 17.2). Neurological symptoms are most commonly associated with chordomas of

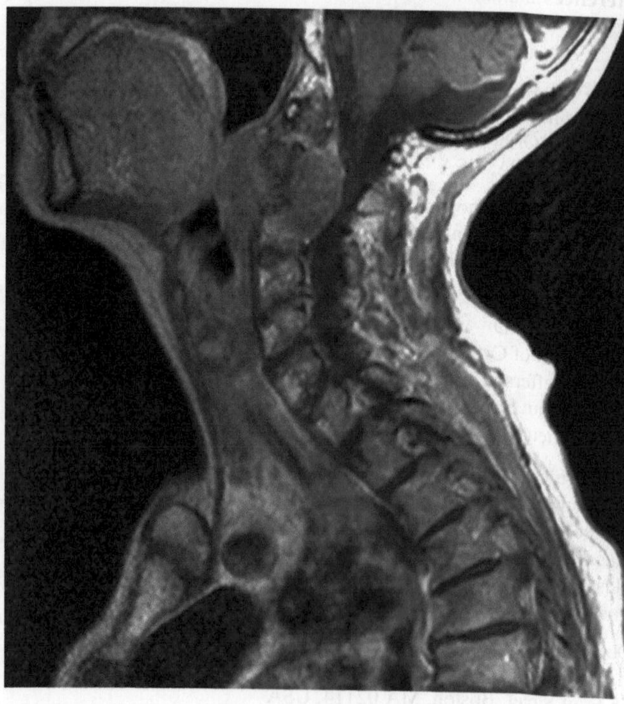

Fig. 17.2 Large cervical spine chordoma at C2 with compression of spinal cord

the mobile spine. The spectrum of neurological symptoms widely ranges depending on the location of the tumor. Severe compression of the spinal cord is a late complication leading to paralysis. Tumors which invade the neural foramina can cause a radicular pattern of symptoms, which includes weakness and sensory deficits in the distribution of a particular nerve root (Sundaresan et al. 1990; Mindell 1981).

Non-neurologic symptoms from chordoma are most commonly due to local effects of the tumor mass. For example, chordomas which develop in the cervical spine may cause throat irritation, dysphagia, esophageal compression, dysphonia, or airway obstruction from compression of critical local structures (Singh et al. 2007; Nicoucar et al. 2008). Horner syndrome has been reported from lower cervical spine chordomas (Leone et al. 2002). Mass effect from of sacral chordomas can cause compression and displacement of the bladder or rectum leading to urinary stress incontinence, constipation, or obstruction. Sacral chordoma of sufficiently large size can be palpated on rectal exam (Fourney and Gokaslan 2003; Atalar et al. 2006).

Box 17.1 The Cauda Equina

Anatomically, the cauda equina, or "horse's tail," is the collection of nerve roots that travels through the spinal canal beyond the termination of the spinal cord. The spinal cord ends at approximately the L1 level in humans, at which point the lumbar (L1–5) and sacral (S1–5) roots have already branched off the spinal cord. However, because these nerve roots exit the spinal canal at successively more inferior levels in the lumbar and sacral bony spine, they travel together for a distance within the spinal canal as a bundle of nerve roots, which is called the cauda equina. Injuries or other conditions which damage the cauda equina cause a specific constellation of symptoms related to dysfunction of these critical nerve roots and is considered a surgical emergency.

Symptoms of cauda equina syndrome from any cause include weakness in the lower extremities, urinary retention due to detrusor muscle weakness, loss of rectal tone due to anal sphincter weakness, and subsequent fecal incontinence. Sexual dysfunction and saddle anesthesia and lower extremity pain may also be present. Lower extremity reflexes are reduced or absent. The causes of cauda equina syndrome are numerous and essentially can be any inciting agent or problem which causes pressure on the cauda equina. Commonly, acutely herniated discs can cause cauda equina syndrome. Other degenerative spinal conditions such as spinal stenosis

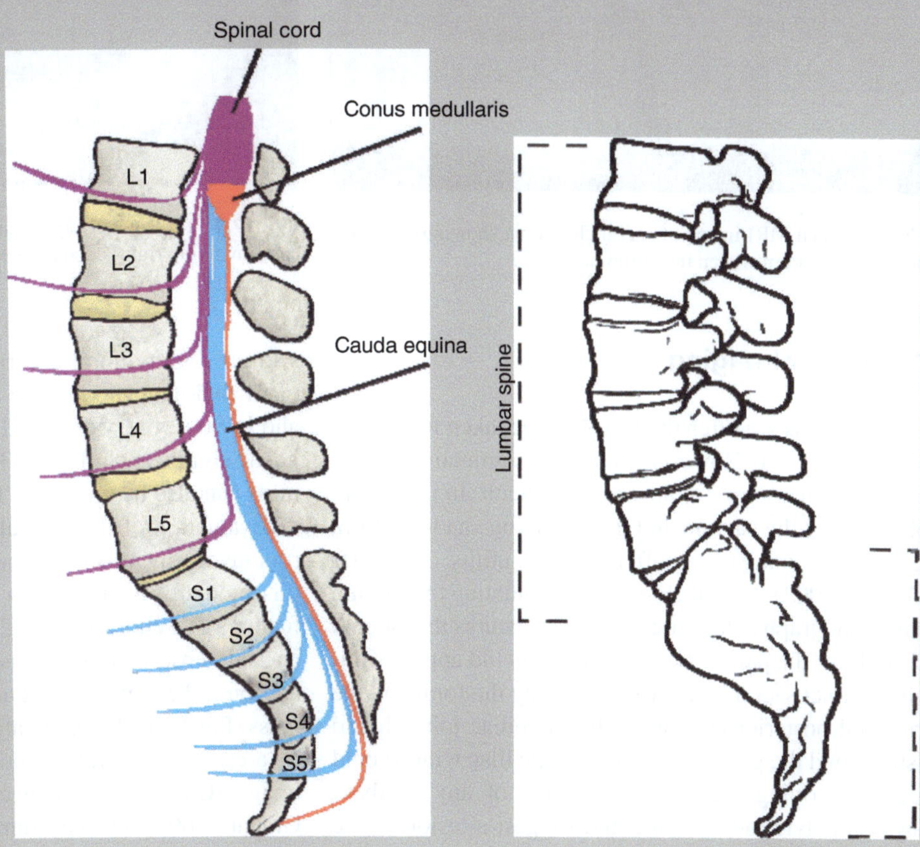

The cauda equina is shown schematically on the *left*, and the osseous anatomy of the lumbar spine and sacrum is shown on the *right*

or spondylolisthesis can contribute as well. Trauma is another common cause, either by direct damage to nerve roots by fracture, dislocation, or penetrating trauma or by hematoma secondary to the initial traumatic injury. Tumors, such as chordoma or more commonly metastatic disease, can also cause a cauda equina syndrome, although in this situation the presenting symptoms are usually more chronic and develop over a longer period of time as the tumor grows.

Treatment of cauda equina syndrome is primarily surgical decompression of the involved nerve roots as well as removal or correction of the inciting mechanical problem. In the case of degenerative and traumatic conditions, every effort is made to preserve the involved nerve roots. In the case of metastatic tumors, intralesional procedures may be performed in conjunction with adjuvant therapies such as radiation. Sacral chordoma requires wide resection, which usually involved resection of some or all of the sacral nerve roots, so the expectation is that the nerve deficits will not recover. It is important to discuss the specific expected deficits with any patient undergoing sacrectomy for chordoma.

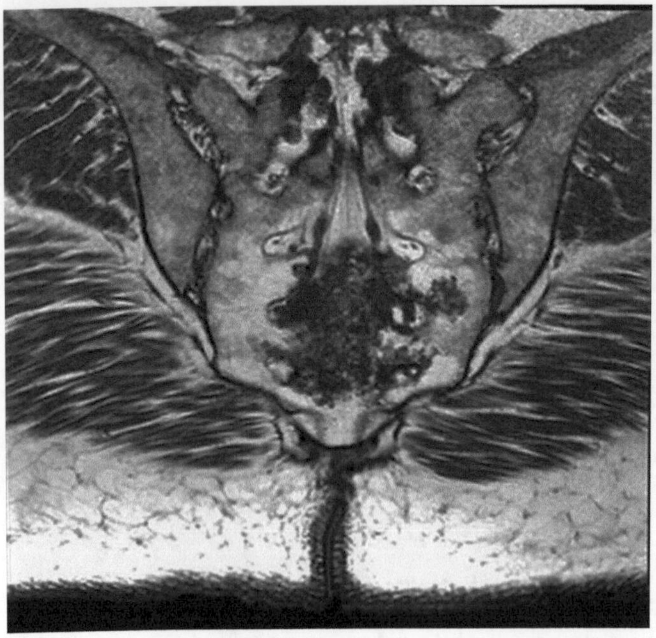

Fig. 17.3 Coronal MRI image of sacral chordoma showing extensive calcifications, sometimes seen in chordoma

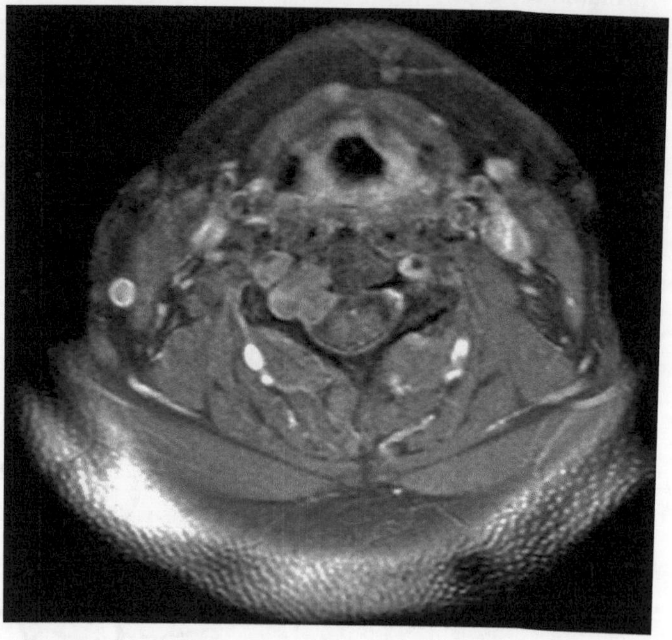

Fig. 17.4 Typical MRI appearance of cervical spine chordoma, in this case involving right-sided pedicle

17.4 Tumor Imaging

Plain radiographs are often the initial image taken for a complaint of back pain. However, detailed examination of the spine with plain imaging alone can be difficult. In particular, the obliquity of the sacrum and the overlying shadows from bowel gas and contents can often limit its utility (Manaster and Graham 2003). Nonetheless, when evaluating the sacrum on plain radiographs, there are particular features that should be scrutinized: the paired sacral foramen should appear similar with distinct sacral boundaries outlining the foramen, the anterior and posterior aspects of the sacroiliac joint should be distinct, and the posterior contour of the iliac wing should be seen underlying the sacral ala. Lack of any of these findings on pelvic radiograph could suggest a lesion of the sacrum. Intratumoral amorphous calcifications are seen on plain radiographs within a chordoma in 50–70 % of cases and in 90 % of cases on CT scan, but have no known prognostic significance (Fig 17.3). An associated large soft tissue mass can also be seen on CT scan or MRI.

Evaluation of the central spinal canal and cord or nerve root involvement is best done with MR imaging, and as such this modality is critical for evaluation of chordomas. MRI features of a chordoma on T1-weighted sequences consist of an isointense or hypointense mass as compared to muscle and on a T2-weighted sequences as a high-signal-intensity mass (Fig 17.4). If calcifications are present, they can appear as areas of low signal intensity on T1- and T2-weighted images. Chordomas enhance with gadolinium (Manaster and Graham 2003). Primary tumors and metastatic lesions both show very high signal intensities on diffusion weighted images, which may help distinguish metastatic nodules from nodules of other unrelated etiologies (Kishimoto et al. 2012). Both MRI and CT scan can show bone destruction and extension of the tumor into the canal (Fig. 17.5). MR imaging can be used to differentiate benign notochordal cell tumors (BNCTs) from chordomas based on the lack of gadolinium uptake, bone sclerosis, and completely intraosseous location seen with BNCTs (Nishiguchi et al. 2011). Chordomas also demonstrate fluorodeoxyglucose avidity on F-18 PET scans (Lin et al. 2006; Miyazaway et al.2008; Park and Kim 2008). Carbon-11-methionine positron emission tomography (MET-PET), used to evaluate the effectiveness of carbon-ion radiotherapy for assessment of rectal cancer and other tumors, has been used to study chordoma treatment. This technology has shown some promise in pre- and posttreatment imaging of chordoma (Zhang et al. 2004).

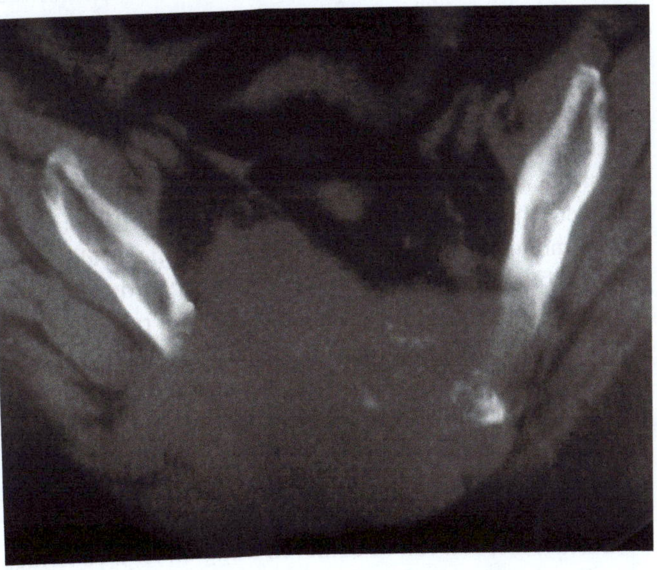

Fig. 17.5 Axial CT scan image showing extensive sacral bone destruction due to chordoma. Note that the tumor is a midline tumor, which can differentiate it from other sacral tumors

17.5 Histopathology and Immunohistochemistry

Virchow's original description of the physaliphorous cell, a vacuolated cell clustered in sheets giving the appearance of "soap bubbles" and demonstrating a lobular pattern of growth, describes the classic histologic features of chordomas (Fig. 17.6). These cells have small round dark staining nuclei with few mitotic figures but demonstrate significant atypia. The sheets of cells are separated by a fibrous septae with areas of calcification or hemorrhage representing necrotic areas (Weber and Sim 2002). These tumors can be separated into three classes: classical or conventional, chondroid, and dedifferentiated (Chugh et al. 2007). The classical form most commonly displays the typical physaliferous features. Chondroid type tumors may exhibit areas of chondrosarcoma-like cartilage as well as features of classic chordoma. Dedifferentiated tumors may have a more highly aggressive sarcomatous histological appearance. Dedifferentiated tumors may display nuclear inclusions, bi- or multinucleation, and sometimes mitotic figures (Crapanzano et al. 2001). Immunohistochemical staining is useful in the evaluation of chordomas. Significant immunoreactivity for S-100, membrane antigen (MUC-1), and cytokeratin is seen in these tumors.

Chondroid tumors are difficult to distinguish from chondrosarcomas, emphasizing the need for specific immunohistochemical markers. Brachyury is a notochordal transcription factor that is expressed in most sporadic chordomas, but not in chondrosarcomas (Vujovic et al. 2006). Interestingly, the

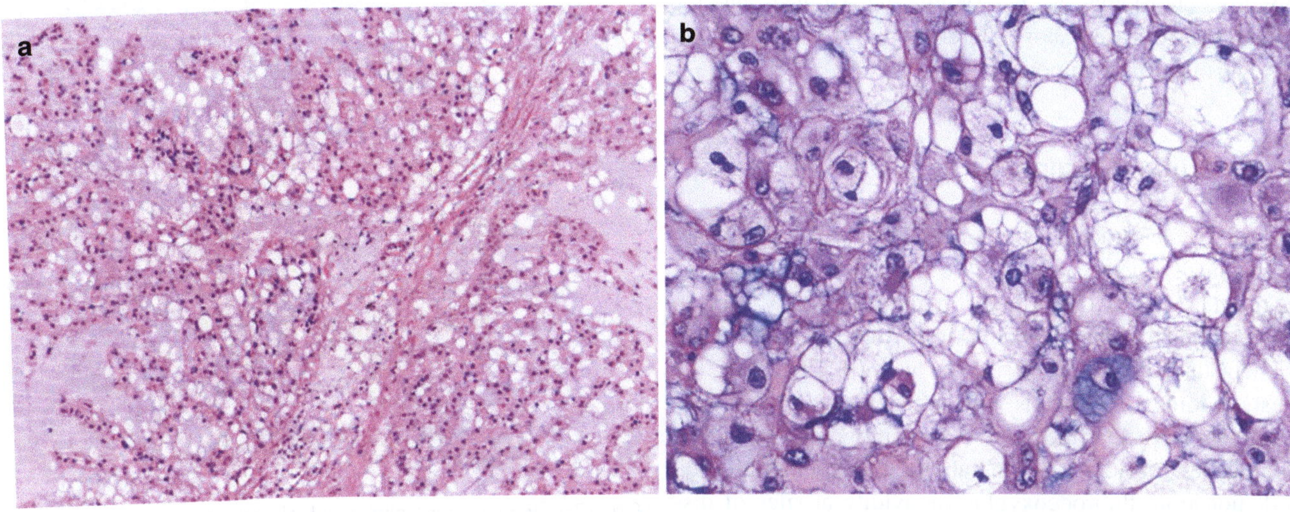

Fig. 17.6 Photomicrograph of chordoma histology demonstrating vacuolated physaliferous cells. (**a**) Low power, 100×; (**b**) high power, 400×

T gene locus containing the brachyury gene has been found to be duplicated in rare familial instances of chordoma, suggesting a critical role in the pathogenesis of this tumor (Yang et al. 2009). The addition of brachyury to the panel of biomarkers used to identify this cell type has improved the sensitivity and specificity for chordoma to 98 and 100 % (Oakley et al. 2008). Other important biomarkers such as ezrin, MMP-9, and COX-2 have also been recently investigated and hold diagnostic promise (Froehlich et al. 2012). The next step in the investigation of these markers is to study their value as potential therapeutic targets.

17.6 Differential Diagnosis

In the differential diagnosis of tumors of the spine, myeloma, plasmacytoma, benign notochordal cell tumor, lymphoma, osteomyelitis, giant cell tumor, and chondrosarcoma need to be considered (Sciubba et al. 2009). Key clinical, radiographic, and histologic findings help distinguish each type of tumor from a chordoma. Plasmacytoma may have a similar radiographic appearance as chordoma. A positive scintigraphy seen with a chordoma may differentiate these tumors (Greenspan et al. 2006). Radiographically, osteomyelitis and lymphoma can be difficult to distinguish from a chordoma; however, their clinical course and laboratory data can usually be used to distinguish these conditions (Sciubba et al. 2009). Benign notochordal cell tumors are usually asymptomatic, may demonstrate a more sclerotic appearance, and have no associated soft tissue mass. Giant cell tumors are benign but locally aggressive tumors that are often seen in the sacrum and can have an appearance similar to that of a chordoma. Chordomas have more of a midline predilection, however, and giant cell tumors often demonstrate a thin rim of peripheral bone encompassing the soft tissue mass which is not typically seen in a chordoma. Chondrosarcoma and chondroid chordomas can have similar appearances, and the biomarkers discussed above therefore play a critical role in distinguishing these tumors.

17.7 Tumor Staging

Staging is the process of defining the local and distant extension of a cancerous disease process. In the case of chordoma, MRI is the primary imaging modality used to evaluate the location and extent of the tumor. The presence of metastatic disease is evaluated using CT scan of the chest, abdomen, and pelvis with intravenous and oral contrast agents. Nuclear medicine bone scintigraphy can show other skeletal lesions. PET metabolic imaging can be used to demonstrate fluorodeoxyglucose avidity at sites of disease, but has some limitations based on lesion size, and is not approved as a first-line modality for this purpose. F-18 PET or MET-PET are potentially promising techniques as described earlier.

17.8 Management

17.8.1 Surgery

The primary treatment of chordoma is wide surgical resection (Fig. 17.7) and the goal of surgery is wide excision with negative margins. This is sometimes an unrealistic goal due to the difficult locations of this tumor, especially clival or skull-base tumors, or high-level sacral tumors. Nonetheless, multiple studies have demonstrated a correlation between recurrence rate and positive margins (Boriani et al. 2006; Bilsky et al. 2004; Fuchs et al. 2005). Boriani et al. (2006) demonstrated that in the absence of negative margins, the recurrence rate was approximately 70 and 100 % following radiation treatment alone, palliative care, or intralesional excision. When wide excision with adequate margins was obtained, there was a recurrence rate of 20 % diagnosed at 56–94 months post surgery. In a group of patients all treated with en bloc excision for sacrococcygeal chordoma, Fuchs et al. (2005) demonstrated an overall survival rate of 74 % at 5 years, 52 % at 10 years, and 47 % at 15 years. Interestingly, the survival rate in this group of patients was significantly higher when negative margins were obtained, and the most significant predictor of survival was a wide margin. The size of the tumor, level of resection, and surgical approach did not significantly impact the survival rate.

Sacral resection can be achieved using either a combined anterior-posterior approach or a posterior-only approach. Generally, for tumors with significant anterior soft tissue

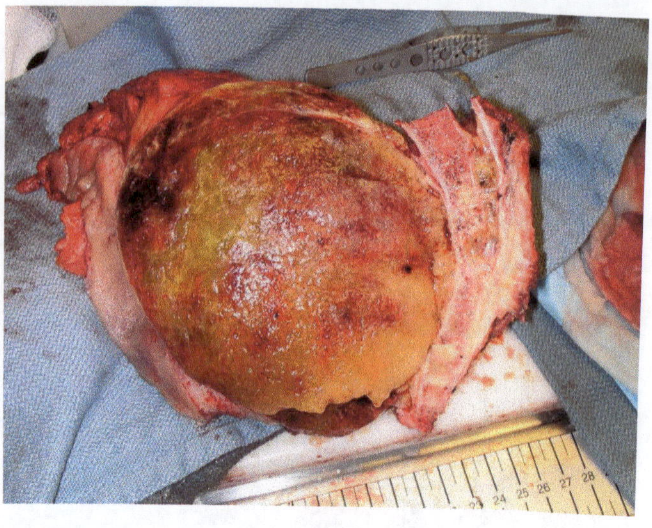

Fig. 17.7 Intraoperative photograph showing sacral chordoma after resection

mass, or high sacral resections, there is a benefit to first performing an anterior dissection prior to resection from a posterior approach. This was best shown by Fuchs et al. (2005) in a series from the Mayo Clinic in which 81 % of patients with combined anterior-posterior approaches had negative margins. Based on these results, it was recommended that a combined dual approach should be used for any patients with tumors above S3.

After chordoma resection, functional deficit is dependent on the extent of the surgery. To maximize survival rates and to prepare patients for postoperative deficits, careful preoperative planning and discussion of possible neurological problems is important. Whether partial or total sacrectomy is performed, usually one or more sacral nerve roots will need to be sacrificed, leading to a motor deficit, sensory impairment, sphincter loss, and/or sexual dysfunction. Fourney et al. (2005) developed a classification system describing the type of sacrectomy based on the level of nerve root sacrificed, as opposed to the site of the osteotomy. The type of resection was defined as low, middle, high sacral amputation, total sacrectomy, or hemicorporectomy. Sacral amputations are considered "low" if at least one S4 nerve root is sacrificed, "middle" if at least one S3 nerve root is sacrificed, and "high" if at least one S2 nerve root is sacrificed. If neither S1 nerve root can be spared, then the required amputation is a total sacrectomy. A hemicorporectomy (translumbar amputation) is performed when the tumor extends to the lumbar spine. Functionally, if both S2 roots can be spared, half of the patients or more will have normal bowel and bladder function. If an S3 root is preserved as well, these odds improve. However, perineal numbness and sexual dysfunction are still commonly observed, the latter more common in the elderly. If one S2 root is sacrificed, typically some amount of voluntary control is compromised. Sacrifice of one S1 or S2 nerve root and all lower roots, as seen in high sacral amputations, commonly leads to urinary or fecal incontinence leading to the possibility for the need of indwelling urinary catheters, intermittent straight catheterization, colostomy, or digital stimulation to defecate (Hulen et al. 2006). Loss of ankle plantar flexion is also seen after the loss of the S1 nerve root.

If resection of the lumbar spine or pelvis is required at the time of sacral amputation, spinopelvic instability must be assessed. If instability is observed, then instrumentation is warranted (Fig. 17.8). In general, about 50 % of the sacroiliac joint can be removed before instability is seen, provided the ligamentous structure of the remainder of the joint is preserved (Gunterberg et al. 1976; Stener and Gunteberg 1978). Chordomas of the mobile spine are also best treated with resection with negative margins. To achieve this goal, a total spondylectomy is the surgery of choice and is generally done through a combined anterior and posterior approach (Boriani et al. 2006).

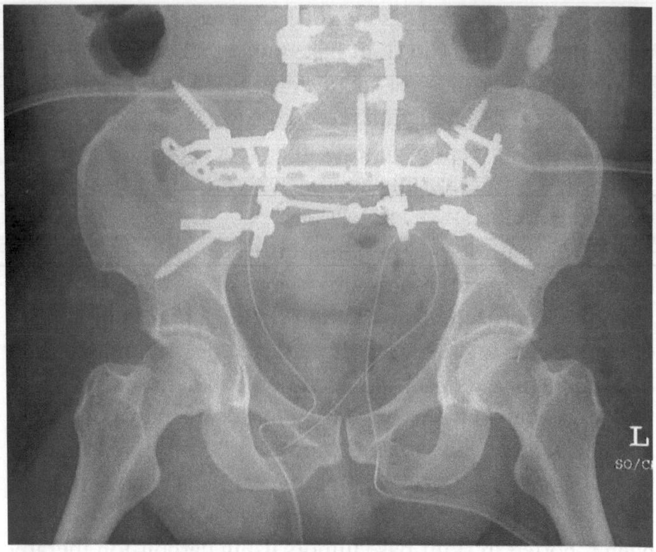

Fig. 17.8 An example of a postoperative reconstruction after resection of entire sacrum

In the skull base, despite multiple surgical approaches, wide resection surgery is rarely possible (Singh et al. 2010; Holzmann et al. 2010). Nonetheless, radiation therapy is effective in managing microscopic or limited gross amounts of residual tumor (Potluri et al. 2011). For this reason the recommended approach in these difficult anatomic areas is aggressive near-total intralesional excision that maximally preserves neurologic function.

17.8.2 Radiation

Radiation therapy has become increasingly important in the management of chordomas. As a result of advances in radiation techniques and modalities, it is now possible to deliver higher doses to the tumor while sparing critical surrounding structures. The limiting factor is the tolerance of the spinal cord, in particular at its upper end, which is lower than the dose needed to effectively treat the tumor. In general, conventional external beam radiation alone, at doses of 40–60 Gy, is suboptimal for treatment of chordoma, resulting in 5-year local control of 10–40 % (Catton et al. 1996; Cummings et al. 1983). Doses of up to 80 Gy have a high rate of associated radiation-induced myelopathy.

Use of high-dose protons and charged particles such as carbon, helium, or neon ions (collectively categorized as hadrons) enables higher doses to be delivered to tumors with limited radiation damage to critical surrounding structures. Indeed, as proton therapy has no measurable exit dose, peripheral structures are spared. Proton beam treatment of chordomas, either alone or in combination with photons, when used in conjunction with primary resection surgery, has proven to be an excellent method for local control

(Hug et al. 1999; Noël et al. 2001; Fuji et al. 2011). This is particularly relevant to skull-base tumors since the tolerance is lower than in the peri-sacral regions. In the sacrum, primary surgery and radiation provide better results when compared with treating chordoma reoccurrence, thereby supporting a role for this approach as an effective first-line treatment option (Park et al. 2006).

Carbon-ion radiotherapy has also been studied in chordoma management. Since carbon ions are heavier than protons, this approach is thought to provide a higher biological effectiveness. Interestingly the effectiveness increases with depth, reaching its peak at the end of the beam's range. This is an extremely attractive property for local control of cancer and as such has led to significant use of carbon-ion therapy in the management of chordoma. 5-year local control rates of 70–88 % and 10-year local control rates of 80–82 % have been reported in skull-base tumors using carbon-ion therapy (Schulz-Ertner et al. 2007; Mizoe et al. 2009; Tsujii and Kamada 2012).

An alternate approach to using hadrons in treatment of chordomas has been the use of highly conformal delivery techniques, such as intensity-modulated radiation therapy (IMRT) or stereotactic radiosurgery (SRS). In a recent study of the North American Gamma Knife Consortium, SRS was found to be an excellent option for small-sized chordomas, especially for young patients, and when combined with surgery, provides an overall 80 % 5-year local control rate (Kano et al. 2011).

17.8.3 Systemic Therapy and Future Directions

Chordomas are generally considered to be insensitive to conventional chemotherapy. Many conventional agents have been tried, with varying levels of response, including anthracycline, cisplatin, alkylating agents, and camptothecin analogues, but no single drug has emerged as a reliable first-line agent. Some small-scale sporadic reports suggest that dedifferentiated chordomas may have an increased sensitivity to aggressive chemotherapy (Fleming et al. 1993), but overall there is no role for chemotherapy in treatment of localized disease. Currently, for metastatic disease, both the timing of initiating treatment and the choice of chemotherapy regimen are generally made on an individualized basis with significant consideration given to limiting the side effect profile.

Based on the observation that chordomas have a high expression of platelet-derived growth factor receptors (PDGFRB and PDGFRA) and KIT receptors (Tamborini et al. 2006), tyrosine kinase inhibitors have been used for the treatment of metastatic chordoma. Imatinib, a tyrosine kinase inhibitor with specificity for PDGFRB and KIT receptors, was initially studied in a small group of chordoma patients with advanced disease (Casali et al. 2005); the promising results of this study led to a larger phase II study with 50 patients (Stacchiotti et al. 2012). This recent study showed only one partial response obtained at 6 months; however, there were 35 patients with stable disease and a 64 % clinical benefit rate, confirming the findings of smaller-scale studies, and certainly warranting further investigation. The EGFR pathway has also been implicated in the pathogenesis of chordoma (Dewaele et al. 2011), leading to study of inhibitors of this pathway, including cetuximab, gefitinib, and erlotinib (Hof et al. 2006; Singhal et al. 2009). A multicenter trial of sunitinib which chordomas, making up 19 % of the study group, demonstrated a 44 % stable disease rate for 16 weeks (George et al. 2009). Current ongoing systemic trials include nilotinib, dasatinib, lapatinib, and everolimus.

Preclinical studies are also accelerating, primarily due to the development of several cell lines which have been characterized, including CH8,GP60, and U-CH-1 (Yang et al. 2010) and more recently CH22 (Liu et al. 2012). The development and characterization of these cell lines may help identify as yet unknown targets and help clarify the role of suspected targets such as brachyury (Hsu et al. 2011), leading to the development of further future clinical trials.

Box 17.2 RTK Inhibition in Chordoma

There is significant interest in the role of receptor tyrosine kinase (RTK) inhibition in the treatment of many sarcomas. Specifically, it has been demonstrated that chordomas express activated platelet-derived growth factor receptors (PDGFRB) (Tamborini et al. 2006). Furthermore, a subset of chordomas are known to express EGFR and c-MET, both of which signal through a tyrosine kinase pathway (Weinberger et al. 2005). mTOR is downstream of the receptor tyrosine kinases and is activated via the MAPK or PI3K/AKT pathways. As the schematic indicates downstream of mTOR, the 40S ribosomal protein S6 kinase ($p70^{s6k}$) and the eukaryotic initiation factor 4E-binding protein-1 (4E-BP1) initiate protein synthesis and promote cell growth and proliferation. eIF4E in an initiation factor that binds to the mRNA cap. When hyperphosphorylated, 4E-BP1 binds to eIF4E repressing its translational initiation.

A recent study investigated the role of RTK inhibition in chordomas (Tamborini et al. 2010). It was noted that activated PDGFR, FLT3, CSF1-R, all components of the PDGFR family, and EGFR family members EGFR, Her2/neu, and HER4 were present in chordoma tissue samples. These findings are in strong support of the concept that the PDGFR and EGFR pathways are activated in chordoma. Another observation was that EGFR and PDGFRB were co-immunoprecipitated, suggesting heterodimer formation. This information could explain why some chordomas are resistant to imatinib treatment. It is possible that a bimodal approach using anti-PDGFR and anti-EGFR agents may be required to fully silence the activation of mTOR in chordomas. Interestingly, in two chordoma patients, there was a clinical response to cetuximab, an anti-EGFR monoclonal antibody (Hof et al. 2006).

With respect to downstream effectors of mTOR, Western blot analysis showed that 14 out of 22 chordomas cases demonstrated eIF4E release from translational repression of 4E-BP1. In 13 of these cases, this was due to hyperphosphorylation of 4E-BP1, and in one case there was an absence of 4E-BP1. At the same time, phospho S6 was only present at low or very low levels in 11 cases; unphosphorylated S6 was found at low levels in 3 cases and not expressed at all in 8 cases. It is unclear if this suggests a tumor suppressor role for S6 or that the majority of downstream effect of mTOR in chordoma is mediated via 4E-BP1/eIF4E, but this discrepancy certainly warrants further study.

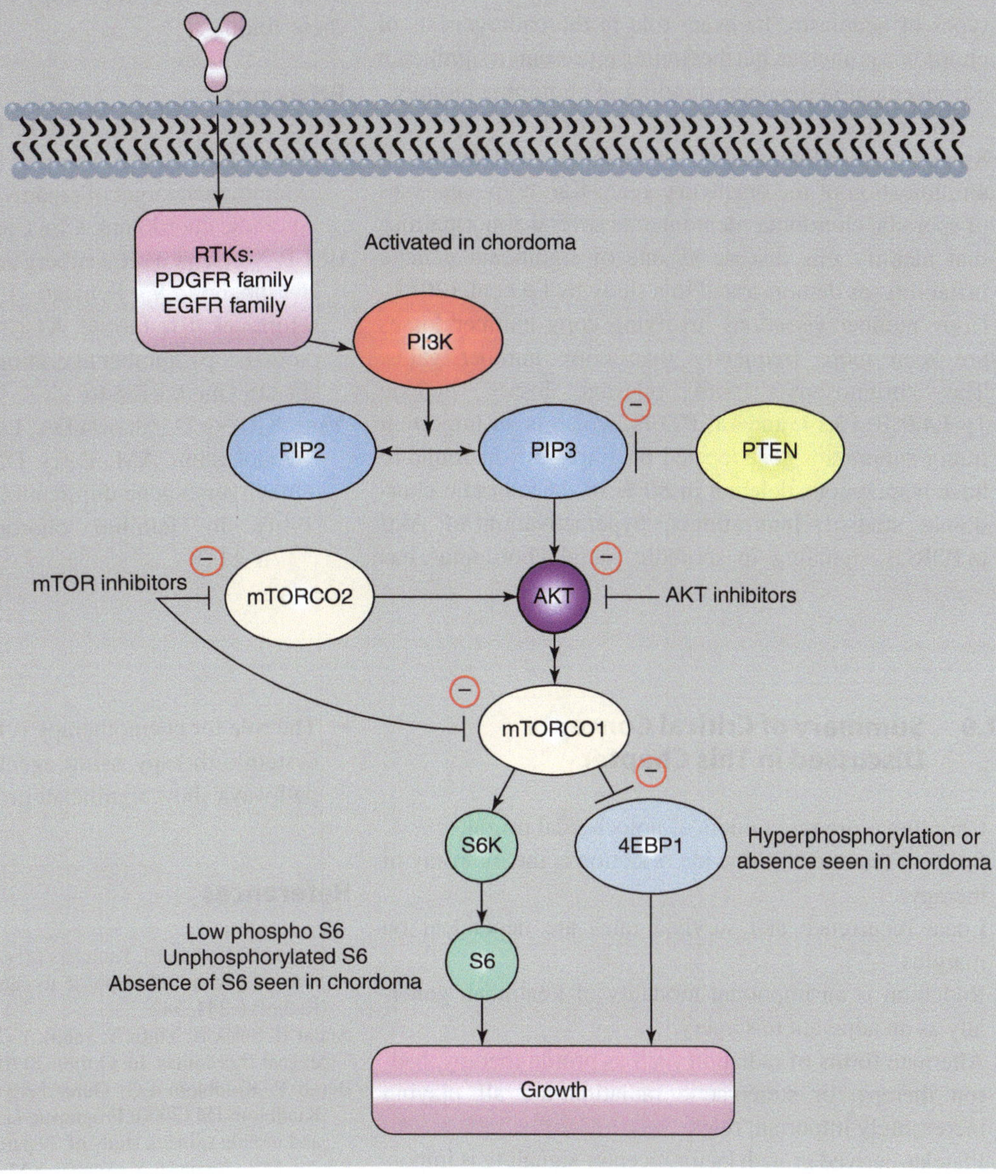

Schematic demonstrating signaling through RTKs via mTOR and critical effectors PTEN, PI3K, and AKT, and downstream effectors S6K and 4EBP1

Box 17.3 Genetics of Chordoma

Molecular studies of tumors from families with familial chordoma syndromes have shed some light on the genetics of chordoma. A recent study by Yang et al. (2009) details the identification of T (brachyury) gene duplication and its role in conferring susceptibility to familial chordoma. These studies were performed using combined genetic linkage and high-resolution array CGH (comparative genomic hybridization) analyses to identify unique duplications of a region on 6q27 in four families with more than three cases or chordoma in each. This locus was found to contain the T (brachyury) gene. Brachyury is a tissue-specific transcription factor expressed in the nucleus of notochord cells. Chordomas express brachyury, but its expression has been studied, and it is not found to be expressed in nonneoplastic tissues and in 42 other types of neoplasm. Its exact role in the pathogenesis of chordoma is unclear, but the finding represents a significant advancement in the understanding of chordoma biology.

The majority of chordomas, however, are sporadic. Sporadic chordomas do not display duplication or amplification of the brachyury gene. Karyotype analyses of sporadic chordomas demonstrate several abnormalities that identify this disease as one of significant genetic instability, as demonstrated in a study by Le et al. (2011). Copy number variations involving copy number losses are seen more frequently than copy number gains. The chromosomes with relevant losses include 1p,3,4,9,10,13,14, and 18. PTEN, which is an important tumor suppressor gene located on 10q23.3, was found to have hemizygous deletion in 80 % of the sporadic chordomas studied. Interestingly, hyperactivation of Akt/mTORC1 signaling in sporadic sacral chordomas has been described and is consistent with loss of PTEN (Han et al. 2009, also see Box 17.2 for a review of RTK signaling in chordoma). CDKN2A is a tumor suppressor gene that inhibits the function of cdk4- and cdk6-cyclin D complexes. These cdk-cyclin complexes regulate the retinoblastoma protein, thereby controlling the G1-S checkpoint of cell cycle progression. This gene was found to be deficient in 80 % of sporadic tumors studied as well.

Although the precise genetic mechanism for the development of chordoma is unclear, these data taken together suggest that T/brachyury is a key figure in the mechanism, at least in the case of familial chordoma. It is possible that T/brachyury is important in sporadic chordoma as well, but if this is the case, then the mechanism must be one other than copy number variation based on these findings.

References

Han S, Polizzano C, Neilsen GP, Hornicek FJ, Rosenberg AE, Ramesh V (2009) Aberrant hyperactivation of akt and Mammalian target of rapamycin complex 1 signaling in sporadic chordomas. Clin Cancer Res 15:1940–1946

Le LP, Nielsen GP, Rosenberg AE, Thomas D, Batten JM, Deshpande V, Schwab J, Duan Z, Xavier RJ, Hornicek FJ, Iafrate AJ (2011) Recurrent chromosomal copy number alterations in sporadic chordomas. PLOS One 6:e18846

Yang XR, Ng D, Alcorta DA, Liebsch NJ, Sheridan E, Li S, Goldstein AM, Parry DM, Kelley MJ (2009) T (brachyury) gene duplication confers major susceptibility to familial chordoma. Nat Genet 41: 1176–1178

17.9 Summary of Critical Concepts Discussed in This Chapter

- Chordomas are rare tumors of notochordal origin.
- Surgical treatment with wide resection is the mainstay of therapy.
- Local recurrence and survival rates are dependent on margins.
- Radiation is an important modality of treatment, generally as an adjuvant to surgery.
- Alternate forms of radiation such as proton therapy, hadron therapy, or stereotactic radiation are all playing increasingly important roles.
- Platelet-derived growth factor receptor signaling is important in the oncogenesis of chordoma.
- The role for chemotherapy is limited but advancements in systemic therapy using agents targeting tyrosine kinase pathways show significant promise.

References

Ashwood N, Hoskin PJ, Saunders MI (1994) Metastatic chordoma: pattern of spread and response to chemotherapy. Clin Oncol (R Coll Radiol) 6:341–342

Atalar H, Selek H, Yildiz Y, Sağlik Y (2006) Management of sacrococcygeal chordomas. Int Orthop 30(6):514–518

Bergh P, Kindblom LG, Gunterberg B, Remotti F, Ryd W, Meis-Kindblom JM (2000) Prognostic factors in chordoma of the sacrum and mobile spine: a study of 39 patients. Cancer 88:2122–2134

Bilsky MH, Yamada Y, Yenice KM, Lovelock M, Hunt M, Gutin PH, Leibel SA (2004) Intensity-modulated stereotactic radiother-

apy of paraspinal tumors: a preliminary report. Neurosurgery 54: 823–830
Bjornsson J, World LE, Ebersold MJ, Laws ER (1993) Chordoma of the mobile spine. A clinicopathological analysis of 40 patients. Cancer 71:735–740
Bohlman HH, Sachs BL, Carter JR, Riley L, Robinson RA (1986) Primary neoplasms of the cervical spine. Diagnosis and treatment of twenty-three patients. J Bone Joint Surg Am 68:483–494
Boriani S, Chevalley F, Weinstein JN, Biagini R, Campanacci L, De Iure F, Piccill P (1996) Chordoma of the spine above the sacrum. Treatment and outcome in 21 cases. Spine 21:1569–1577
Boriani S, Bandiera S, Biagini R, Bacchini P, Boriani L, Cappuccio M, Chevalley F, Gasbarrini A, Picci P, Weinstein JN (2006) Chordoma of the mobile spine: fifty years of experience. Spine 31:493–503
Burrow JF, Stewart MJ (1923) Malignant spheno-occipital chordoma. J Neurol Psychopathol 4(15):205–217
Casali PG, Messina A, Stacchiotti S, Tamborini E, Crippa F, Gronchi A, Orlandi R, Ripamonti C, Spreafico C, Bertieri R, Bertulli R, Colecchia M, Fumagalli E, Greco A, Grosso F, Olmi P, Pierotti MA, Pilotti S (2005) Imatinib mesylate in 18 advanced chordoma patients. J Clin Oncol 23:9012
Catton C, O'Sullivan B, Bell R, Laperriere N, Cummings B, Fornasier V, Wunder J (1996) Chordoma: long-term follow up after radical photon irradiation. Radiother Oncol 41:67–72
Chugh R, Tawbi H, Lucas DR, Biermann JS, Schuetze SM, Baker LH (2007) Chordoma: the nonsarcoma primary bone tumor. Oncologist 12:1344–1350
Crapanzano JP, Ali SZ, Ginsberg MS, Zakowski MF (2001) Chordoma: a cytologic study with histologic and radiologic correlation. Cancer 93:40–51
Cummings BJ, Hodson DI, Bush RS (1983) Chordoma: the results of megavoltage radiation therapy. Int J Radiat Oncol Biol Phys 9: 633–642
Dewaele B, Maggiani F, Floris G, Ampe M, Vanspauwen V, Wozniak A, Debiec-Rychter M, Sciot R (2011) Frequent activation of EGFR in advanced chordomas. Clin Sarcoma Res 1(1):4
Fleming GF, Heimann PS, Stephens JK, Simon MA, Ferguson MK, Benjamin RS, Samuels BL (1993) Dedifferentiated chordoma. Response to aggressive chemotherapy in two cases. Cancer 72(3):714–718
Forsyth PA, Cascino TL, Shaw EG, Scheithauer BW, O'Fallon JR, Dozier JC, Piepgras DG (1993) Intracranial chordomas: a clinicopathological and prognostic study of 51 cases. J Neurosurg 78: 741–747
Fourney DR, Gokaslan ZL (2003) Current management of sacral chordoma. Neurosurg Focus 15:E9
Fourney DR, Rhines LD, Hentschel SJ, Skibber JM, Wolinsky JP, Weber KL, Suki D, Gallia GL, Garonzik I, Gokaslan ZL (2005) En bloc resection of primary sacral tumors: classification of surgical approaches and outcome. J Neurosurg Spine 3:111–122
Froehlich EV, Scheipl S, Lazàry A, Varga PP, Schmid C, Stammberger H, Beham A, Bodo K, Schroettner H, Quehenberger F, Windhager R, Liegl B, Leithner A (2012) Expression of ezrin, MMP-9, and COX-2 in 50 chordoma specimens: a clinical and immunohistochemical analysis. Spine 37(13):E757–E767
Fuchs B, Dickey I, Yaszemski MJ, Inwards CY, Sim FH (2005) Operative management of sacral chordoma. J Bone Joint Surg Am 87:2211–2216
Fuji H, Nakasu Y, Ishida Y, Horiguchi S, Mitsuya K, Kashiwagi H, Murayama S (2011) Feasibility of proton beam therapy for chordoma and chondrosarcoma of the skull base. Skull Base 21(3):201–206
George S, Merriam P, Maki RG, Van den Abbeele AD, Yap JT, Akhurst T, Harmon DC, Bhuchar G, O'Mara MM, D'Adamo DR, Morgan J, Schwartz GK, Wagner AJ, Butrynski JE, Demetri GD, Keohan ML (2009) Multicenter phase II trial of sunitinib in the treatment of nongastrointestinal stromal tumor sarcomas. J Clin Oncol 27(19):3154–3160
Greenspan A, Jundt G, Remagen W (2006) Chordoma, in differential diagnosis in orthopaedic oncology, 2nd edn. Lippincott Williams & Wilkins, Philadelphia, pp 445–446
Gunterberg B, Stener B, Romanus B (1976) Pelvic strength after major amputation of the sacrum. An experimental study. Acta Orthop Scand 47:635–642
Healey JH, Lane JM (1989) Chordoma: a critical review of diagnosis and treatment. Orthop Clin North Am 20:417–426
Hof H, Welzel T, Debus J (2006) Effectiveness of cetuximab/gefitinib in the therapy of a sacral chordoma. Onkologie 29(12):572–574
Holzmann D, Reisch R, Krayenbuhl H, Hug E, Bernays RL (2010) The transnasal transclival approach for clivus chordoma. Minim Invasive Neurosurg 53:211–217
Hsu W, Mohyeldin A, Shah SR, Rhys CM, Johnson LF, Sedora-Roman NI, Kosztowski TA, Awad OA, McCarthy EF, Loeb DM, Wolinsky JP, Gokaslan ZL, Quiñones-Hinojosa A (2011) Generation of chordoma cell line JHC7 and the identification of Brachyury as a novel molecular target. J Neurosurg 115(4):760–769
Hug EB, Loredo LN, Slater JD, DeVries A, Grove RI, Schaefer RA, Rosenberg AE, Slater JM (1999) Proton radiation therapy for chordomas and chondrosarcomas of the skull base. J Neurosurg 91(3): 432–439
Hulen CA, Temple HT, Fox WP, Sama AA, Green BA, Eismont FJ (2006) Oncologic and functional outcome following sacrectomy for sacral chordoma. J Bone Joint Surg Am 88:1532–1539
Kano H, Iqbal FO, Sheehan J, Mathieu D, Seymour ZA, Niranjan A, Flickinger JC, Kondziolka D, Pollock BE, Rosseau G, Sneed PK, McDermott MW, Lunsford LD (2011) Stereotactic radiosurgery for chordoma: a report from the North American Gamma Knife Consortium. Neurosurgery 68(2):379–389
Kishimoto R, Omatsu T, Hasegawa A, Imai R, Kandatsu S, Kamada T (2012) Imaging characteristics of metastatic chordoma. Jpn J Radiol 30(6):509–516
Lee J, Bhatia NN, Hoang BH, Ziogas A, Zell JA (2012) Analysis of prognostic factors for patients with chordoma with use of the California Cancer Registry. J Bone Joint Surg Am 94(4):356–363
Leone A, Cerase A, Tarquini E, Mulè A (2002) Chordoma of the low cervical spine presenting with Horner's syndrome. Eur Radiol 12(Suppl 3):S43–S47
Lin CY, Kao CH, Liang JA, Hsieh TC, Yen KY, Sun SS (2006) Chordoma detected on F-18 FDG PET. Clin Nucl Med 31(8):506–507
Liu X, Nielsen GP, Rosenberg AE, Waterman PR, Yang W, Choy E, Sassi S, Yang S, Harmon DC, Yang C, Schwab JH, Kobayashi E, Mankin HJ, Xavier R, Weissleder R, Duan Z, Hornicek FJ (2012) Establishment and characterization of a novel chordoma cell line: CH22. J Orthop Res. doi:10.1002/jor.22113
Manaster BJ, Graham T (2003) Imaging of sacral tumors. Neurosurg Focus 15(2):E2
McMaster ML, Goldstein AM, Bromley CM, Ishibe N, Parry DM (2001) Chordoma: incidence and survival patterns in the United States, 1973–1995. Cancer Causes Control 12:1–11
Meyer JE, Lepke RA, Lindfors KK, Pagani JJ, Hirschy JC, Hayman LA, Momose KJ, McGinnis B (1984) Chordomas: their CT appearance in the cervical, thoracic and lumbar spine. Radiology 153(3):693–696
Mindell E (1981) Chordoma. J Bone Joint Surg Am 63:501–505
Miyazawa N, Ishigame K, Kato S, Satoh Y, Shinohara T (2008) Thoracic chordoma: review and role of FDG-PET. J Neurosurg Sci 52(4): 117–121
Mizoe JE, Hasegawa A, Takagi R, Bessho H, Onda T, Tsujii H (2009) Carbon ion radiotherapy for skull base chordoma. Skull Base 19(3):219–224
Muller H (1858) Uber das Vorkommen von Resten der Chorda dorsalis bei Menschen nach der Geburt und iiber ihr Verhiiltniss zu den Gallertgeschwiilsten am Clivus. Zeitschr f rat Med ii:202–229

Nicoucar K, Rausch T, Becker M, Dulgucrov P (2008) Cervical chordoma with retropharyngeal extension presenting with impaired voice. Tumori 94:873–876

Nishiguchi T, Mochizuki K, Ohsawa M, Inoue T, Kageyama K, Suzuki A, Takami T, Miki Y (2011) Differentiating benign notochordal cell tumors from chordomas: radiographic features on MRI, CT, and tomography. AJR Am J Roentgenol 196(3): 644–650

Noël G, Habrand JL, Mammar H, Pontvert D, Haie-Méder C, Hasboun D, Moisson P, Ferrand R, Beaudré A, Boisserie G, Gaboriaud G, Mazal A, Kérody K, Schlienger M, Mazeron JJ (2001) Combination of photon and proton radiation therapy for chordomas and chondrosarcomas of the skull base: the centre de Protonthérapie D'Orsay experience. Int J Radiat Oncol Biol Phys 51(2): 392–398

Oakley GJ, Fuhrer K, Seethala RR (2008) Brachyury, SOX-9, and podoplanin, new markers in the skull base chordoma vs chondrosarcoma differential: a tissue microarray-based comparative analysis. Mod Pathol 21:1461–1469

Papagelopoulos PJ, Mavrogenis AF, Currier BL, Katonis P, Galanis EC, Sapkas GS, Korres DS (2004) Primary malignant tumor of the cervical spine. Orthopedics 27:1067–1075

Park SA, Kim HS (2008) F-18 FDG PET/CT evaluation of sacrococcygeal chordoma. Clin Nucl Med 33(12):906–908

Park L, Delaney TF, Liebsch NJ, Hornicek FJ, Goldberg S, Mankin H, Rosenberg AE, Rosenthal DI, Suit HD (2006) Sacral chordomas: impact of high-dose proton/photon-beam radiation therapy combined with or without surgery for primary versus recurrent tumor. Int J Radiat Oncol Biol Phys 65(5):1514–1521

Pearlman AW, Friedman M (1970) Radical radiation therapy of chordoma. Am J Roentgenol Radium Ther Nucl Med 108(2): 332–341

Pearlman AW, Singh RK, Hoppenstein R, Wilder J (1972) Chordoma: combined therapy with radiation and surgery: case report and new operative approach. Bull Hosp Joint Dis 33(1):47–57

Potluri S, Jeffries SJ, Jena R, Harris F, Burton KE, Prevost AT, Burnet NG (2011) Residual postoperative tumor volume predicts outcome after high-dose radiotherapy for chordoma and chondrosarcoma of the skull base and spine. Clin Oncol 32: 199–208

Schulz-Ertner D, Karger CP, Feuerhake A, Nikoghosyan A, Combs SE, Jäkel O, Edler L, Scholz M, Debus J (2007) Effectiveness of carbon ion radiotherapy in the treatment of skull-base chordomas. Int J Radiat Oncol Biol Phys 68(2):449–457

Sciubba D, Cheng JJ, Petteys RJ, Weber KL, Frassica DA, Gokaslan ZL (2009) Chondroma of the sacrum and vertebral bodies. J Am Acad Orthop Surg 17(11):708–717

Singh N, Soo M, De Cruz M, Gomes L, Maclean F, Dandie G (2007) Cervical chordoma presenting as retropharyngeal mass and dysphonia: case report and literature review. Australas Radiol 51(suppl): B183–B188

Singh H, Harrop J, Schiffmacher P, Rosen M, Evans J (2010) Ventral Surgical approaches to craniovertebral junction chordomas. Neurosurgery 66(suppl 3):96–103

Singhal N, Kotasek D, Parnis FX (2009) Response to erlotinib in a patient with treatment refractory chordoma. Anticancer Drugs 20(10):953–955

Soo MY (2001) Chordoma: review of clinicoradiological features and factors affecting survival. Australas Radiol 45:427–434

Stacchiotti S, Longhi A, Ferraresi V, Grignani G, Comandone A, Stupp R, Bertuzzi A, Tamborini E, Pilotti S, Messina A, Spreafico C, Gronchi A, Amore P, Vinaccia V, Casali PG (2012) Phase II study of imatinib in advanced chordoma. J Clin Oncol 30(9): 914–920

Stener B, Gunterberg B (1978) High amputation of the sacrum for extirpation of tumors. Principles and technique. Spine 3:351–366

Sundaresan N, Schmidek HH, Schiller AL, Rosenthal D (1990) Tumors of the spine: diagnosis and clinical management. W.B. Saunders, Philadelphia

Tamborini E, Miselli F, Negri T et al (2006) Molecular and biochemical analyses of platelet-derived growth factor receptor (PDGFR) B, PDGFRA, and KIT receptors in chordomas. Clin Cancer Res 12:6920–6928

Tamborini E, Virdis E, Negri T, Orsenigo M, Brich s, Conca E, Gronchi A, Stacchiotti S, Manenti G, Casali PG, Pierotti MA, Pilotti S (2010) Analysis of receptor tyrosine kinases (RTKs) and downstream pathways in chordomas. Neuro Oncol 12(8):776–789.

Tsujii H, Kamada T (2012) A review of update clinical results of carbon ion radiotherapy. Jpn J Clin Oncol 42(8):670–685

Unni KK (1996) Chordoma. In: Unni KK (ed) Dahlin's bone tumors: general aspects and data on 11,087 cases, 5th edn. Lippincott-Raven, Philadelphia, pp 291–305

Virchow RL (1857) Untersuchungen ueber die Entwicklung des Schaedelgrundes. G Rimer, Berlin

Vujovic S, Henderson S, Presneau N, Odell E, Jacques TS, Tirabosco R, Boshoff C, Flanagan AM (2006) Brachyury, a crucial regulator of notochordal development, is a novel biomarker for chordomas. J Pathol 209:157–165

Weber K, Sim FH (2002) Chordoma. In: Bulstrode C, Buckwalter J, Carr A et al (eds) Oxford textbook of orthopaedics and trauma. Oxford University Press, New York, pp 294–299

Weinberger PM, Yu Z, Kowalski D, Joe J, Manger P, Psyrri A, Sasaki CT (2005) Differential expression of epidermal growth factor receptor, c-Met, and HER2/neu in chordoma compared with 17 other malignancies. Arch Otolaryngol Head Neck Surg 131(8): 707–711.

Yang XR, Ng D, Alcorta DA, Liebsch NJ, Sheridan E, Li S, Goldstein AM, Parry DM, Kelley MJ (2009) T (brachyury) gene duplication confers major susceptibility to familial chordoma. Nat Genet 41(11):1176–1178

Yang C, Hornicek FJ, Wood KB, Schwab JH, Choy E, Iafrate J, Rosenberg A, Nielsen GP, Xavier RJ, Mankin H, Duan Z (2010) Characterization and analysis of human chordoma cell lines. Spine 35(13):1257–1264

Zhang H, Yoshikawa K, Tamura K, Sagou K, Tian M, Suhara T, Kandatsu S, Suzuki K, Tanada S, Tsujii H (2004) Carbon-11-methionine positron emission tomography imaging of chordoma. Skeletal Radiol 33(9):524–530

Part III

Models of Disc Disease and Biological Regeneration

Large Animal Models of Disc Degeneration

18

Shyam A. Patel, Christopher K. Kepler, Thomas P. Schaer, and D. Greg Anderson

Contents

S.A. Patel, BS
Drexel University College of Medicine,
Philadelphia, PA 19107, USA
e-mail: sap.0521@gmail.com

C.K. Kepler, MD
Department of Orthopaedic Surgery,
Thomas Jefferson University, Rothman Institute,
Philadelphia, PA 19107, USA
e-mail: chris.kepler@gmail.com

T.P. Schaer, VMD (✉)
Department of Clinical Studies,
University of Pennsylvania,
School of Veterinary Medicine, New Bolton Center,
Kennett Square, PA 19348, USA
e-mail: tpschaer@vet.upenn.edu

D.G. Anderson, MD
Departments of Orthopaedic Surgery and Neurological Surgery,
Thomas Jefferson University, Rothman Institute,
Philadelphia, PA 19107, USA
e-mail: greg.anderson@rothmanisntitute.com

18.1 Overview

Intervertebral discs are largely of embryonic notochordal origin and impart a unique biomechanical function to the spine of vertebrate animals (Singh et al. 2005). The intervertebral disc is anatomically comprised of two constituents: a proteoglycan-rich nucleus pulposus contained within a collagen 1-rich annulus fibrosus (Singh et al. 2005). Together, these structures effectively dissipate mechanical loads within the spine while allowing controlled motion between adjacent vertebrae. The biologic environment of the disc is uniquely harsh due to the avascular nature of the tissue and the long distance between metabolically active cells and their nutritional source. Tissue degeneration progresses through a well-defined series of changes (Singh et al. 2005) including breakdown of the long-chain proteoglycan constituents of the extracellular matrix, loss of water-binding capacity, decreased cellularity, and annular disorganization/disruption (Lotz 2004).

As discussed in other sections of this book, while degenerative changes within the intervertebral disc are essentially universal, the association between disc degeneration and symptomatic low back pain is unpredictable (Lotz 2004; Alini et al. 2008). Indeed, back pain attributed to disc degeneration is a relatively common phenomenon; however, most individuals have few or no symptoms during the degenerative process. The lack of correlation between degeneration and clinical symptoms has made the study of disc degeneration especially challenging (Lotz 2004). Despite the challenge, the goal of researchers in the field is to identify an effective biologic therapy for painful disc degeneration.

I.M. Shapiro, M.V. Risbud (eds.), *The Intervertebral Disc*,
DOI 10.1007/978-3-7091-1535-0_18, © Springer-Verlag Wien 2014

Human discs are subjected to some unique physical and biomechanical factors that are not easily replicated in animal models. First, humans are bipedal and subject their spines to unique physical forces associated with an upright posture. Second, human discs are significantly larger in size than many common research animals such as rodents and rabbits. This means that the diffusion of nutrients or pharmacologic agents into the central region of the disc is substantially more challenging. In addition, because of the larger size, certain types of physical interventions that would be theoretically possible in humans are difficult to reproduce in small animal models. Third, although the primary symptom attributed to disc degeneration in humans is pain, it is challenging to study pain of spinal origin in animals. Fourth, intervertebral discs from various species differ quite substantially in their cellular makeup. The large physaliferous cells that are felt to be helpful in maintaining the health of the disc are largely absent in adult humans, but remain quite common in some other species. This may affect the response of the disc to various experimental interventions.

Animal research is critical to understanding, developing, and testing biologic interventions for human disc degeneration. Although most of the animal research done to date involves small animals, there are certain limitations in the use of these models mainly due to differences in the relative dimensions of the disc or the cellular makeup of the disc. Thus, large animal disc research is both necessary and important for the development of many disc therapies and is generally required prior to moving a promising therapy into human usage. Large animal models are often specifically required during regulatory approval processes by agencies such as the Food and Drug Administration (FDA), the Central Office for Research Ethics Committees (COREC), the National Institute for Clinical Excellence (NICE), and the Medicines and Healthcare Products Regulatory Agency (MHRA). This chapter will review the status of the large animal models that have been used to study disc degeneration or disc therapeutics.

18.2 History

Historically, large animal veterinary care has played a role in our current understanding of disc pathology and surgical reconstruction. One example is the work of Wagner et al. (1979) who, in 1979, performed cervical fusion using bone from equine cadaver ilia to treat horses with cervical spine disorders. Eleven of the 12 horses achieved a fusion of the operative levels and improved clinically; follow-up necropsies revealed restricted motion at the fusion levels (Wagner et al. 1979). The authors concluded that this technique could be useful in treating dislocations, fractures, and osteolytic processes of the human spine (Wagner et al. 1979). Current prosthetic cages used in spinal fusion can trace their roots to this experiment (Wagner et al. 1979).

18.3 Types of Models Used in Intervertebral Disc Research

Intervertebral disc research involving various regions of the spine has been useful in assessing the physical, histological, and biomechanical characteristics of the disc (Panjabi 1998). In vitro models have also played a substantial role in providing an understanding of the unique cellular biology of the disc. Unfortunately, in vitro models generally lack the complexity of the intact system, which may limit the ability of researchers to draw definitive clinical conclusions from the scientific findings. Additionally, in vitro models generally do not provide an understanding of long-term experimental effects of an intervention.

Advances in computer technology have led to the development of some in silico models. These computer-based simulations are suitable for forming initial hypotheses that may serve as the rationale for further research. Computer simulations also allow the investigator a level of control over experimental variables that is typically not possible with in vitro and in vivo studies. With respect to intervertebral disc research, in silico models have seen limited utilization in the study of mechanical properties of the spine through finite element analysis modeling or the modeling of material properties of the disc (Galbusera et al. 2011).

The testing of novel therapeutics for human applications generally requires the use of in vivo studies. With in vivo research, investigators are able to observe the impact of treatment on a living biologic system (Panjabi 1998). Given the complexity of intervertebral disc tissue and the multifactorial nature of the degenerative process, in vivo research plays a crucial role in the development of human therapeutics (Lotz 2004; Singh et al. 2005). Additionally, before most therapeutics are considered suitable for human use, it is required that they are studied in an animal model with reasonable similarity to the human condition; this often requires the use of a large animal model (Alini et al. 2008).

18.3.1 The Clinical Perspective

From a clinical perspective, the treatment of disc degeneration itself is of limited value as most disc degeneration is not directly responsible for patient symptoms (this concept is discussed in great length in Chap. 16). However, disc degeneration associated with significant pain symptoms is

Box 18.1 Spinal Fusion Basket: Bagby's Basket

Interestingly, the history of spine fusion cages begins with horses. Four decades ago, Dr. George Bagby invented the first cage, also referred to as "Bagby's basket." In collaboration with Dr. Barrie Grant, a veterinarian from Washington State University, the two surgeons explored surgical techniques to treat cervical instability or "wobbler's disease," a neurological condition caused by impingement of the spinal cord in the horse's neck by malformed or degenerated vertebrae. While spinal fusion for human patients has rapidly evolved, cervical interbody fusion using a stainless steel cage remains the only successful surgical intervention to treat this debilitating disease in horses. Digital radiographs[1] (A–D) of a yearling Arabian colt who presented with grade III ataxia in all four limbs. Laboratory findings for EPM (equine protozoal myeloencephalitis) were negative and as was the remainder of cerebral spinal fluid analysis. A myelogram under general anesthesia showed static compression at C6–7 (B, solid arrow) as well as dynamic compression at C3–4 and C4–5 (B, hashed arrow). Ventral stabilization was performed at C6–7 (C&D) 1 month after diagnosis. After surgery, the colt was on stall rest for 1 month, then 1 month of hand-walking, followed by 1 month of round-pen turnout. Exercise level was slowly increased thereafter, the ataxia steadily improved (grade 0.5 in LF/RF/LH and grade 2 RH 9 months after surgery), and now he is showing successfully with full recovery.

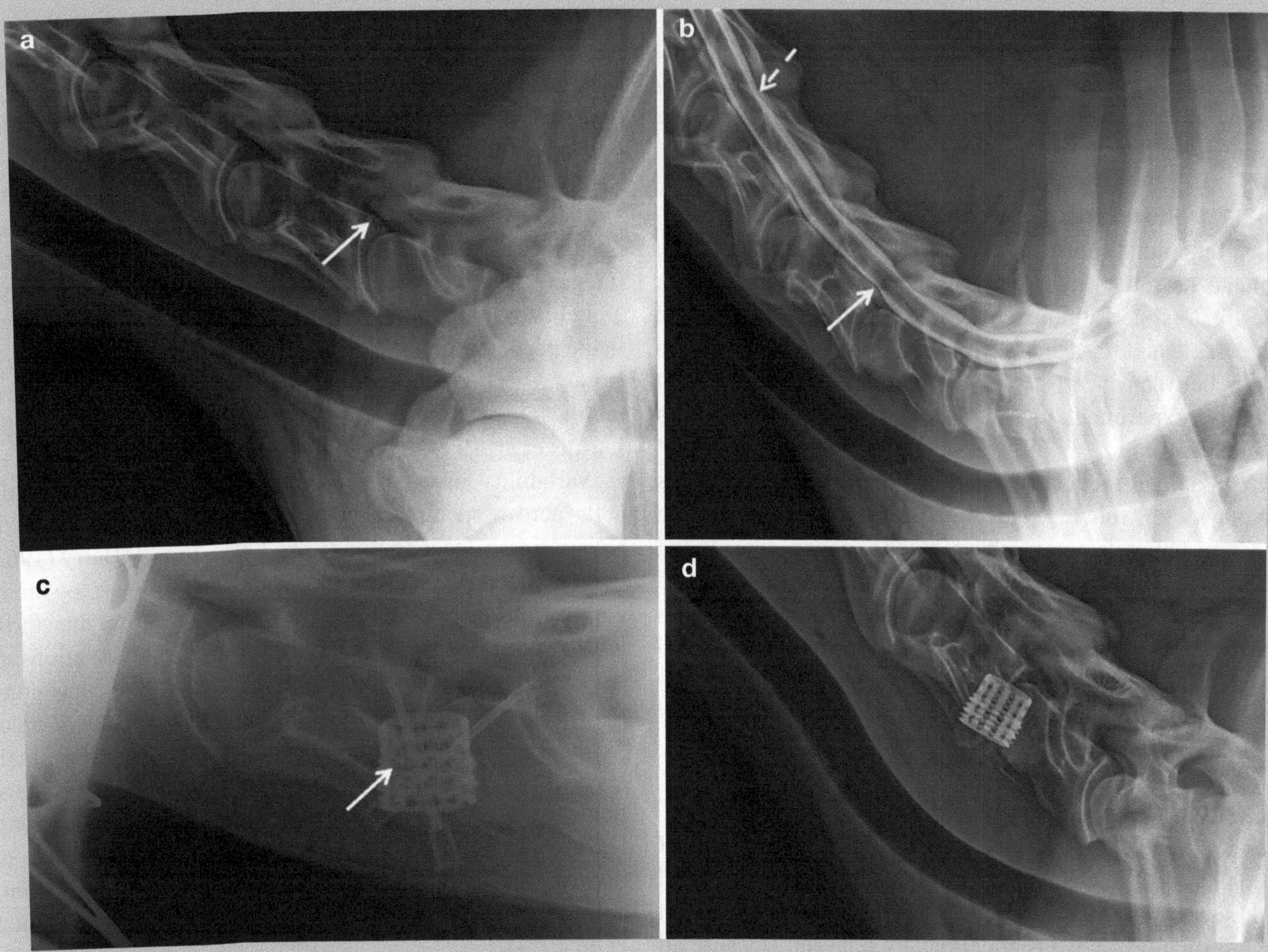

[1]Courtesy of Drs. Reed and Woddie, Rood and Riddle Equine Hospital, Lexington, KY

common, and it is the associated pain and decreased quality of life that are the targets of therapy.

Unfortunately, a reliable means to quantify pain associated with disc degeneration in any animal model has not yet been defined. Therefore, animal research is generally limited to providing a means to study the effects of a potential therapy on the physical, cellular, or chemical milieu of the disc. The hypothesis of this line of research is that an intervention which provides improvement in objective measures of disc health would be likely to provide improvement in the pain associated with the degenerative process in affected human patients. Therefore, although animal testing of potential human therapeutics is important, favorable results still require validation in humans. Thus, animal model testing is just one step in the process of bringing a therapy from the bench top to the clinic (An et al. 2003).

18.3.2 Animal Models in General

As stated, animal models play a vital role in translational research and provide a crucial step in ensuring that a new therapy is valid and safe prior to considering human usage (Smith et al. 2011).

18.3.2.1 Standardization and Reliability

When an animal model is first introduced, it is essential to evaluate its reliability. Using the new model, independent investigators performing similar experiments should find comparable and reproducible results. Significant variation in results between investigators or unpredictable results from repetitive experiments may indicate that the model used is unreliable.

With animal models, standardization of the test animal's age plays a key role in achieving adequate reliability for disc research. Other factors such as breed, gender, size, living conditions, vertebral levels studied, and nutrition could potentially affect the outcome of a study intervention, and so these features should be well controlled in the experimental design. These factors should also be reported by the investigator performing the animal research so that others can replicate the study conditions.

18.3.2.2 Model Fidelity/Validity

Issues of validity and fidelity are important in the design of animal trials. There is little benefit in using an animal model with such substantial differences from human disease that the information gained is not clinically relevant. Because all animal models are significantly different from the human condition, this limitation is one of magnitude. The researcher should seek to use a model that provides the closest possible replication of the human condition, understanding that a perfect match is not possible.

For many studies involving therapeutic interventions, an important factor is identifying a model with similar characteristics in terms of disc size and geometry (Beckstein et al. 2008). Wide variations in disc size across species are obvious, and this can affect the mechanical and biologic properties of the disc (Elliott and Sarver 2004; O'Connell et al. 2007). However, Beckstein et al. (2008) demonstrated that mechanical tissue properties of many species are conserved evolutionarily and that variations with regard to the biomechanical properties of the intervertebral disc are not as drastic as previously thought. Unfortunately, the current literature fails to provide comprehensive comparisons between animal models across a wide range of species. Most comparative studies published to date compare the properties of a specific animal species relative to the human.

18.3.2.3 Complications Associated with Validity/Fidelity

One factor which complicates animal model selection is related to intervertebral disc development. The nucleus pulposus is embryologically derived from notochordal cells. In humans, notochordal cells which are common at birth become rare following the first decade of life (Urban et al. 2000). Notochordal cells are believed to produce greater amounts of proteoglycan than other disc cells and contribute positively to the maintenance of disc extracellular matrix integrity (Palmer and Lotz 2004; Aguiar et al. 1999; Kalichman and Hunter 2008). In addition to wide variation in the persistence of these cells on a species-by-species basis, exposure to high biomechanical loads on the spine may hasten the disappearance of notochordal cells (Lotz et al. 1998; Iatridis et al. 1999; Palmer and Lotz 2004).

Variability in the presence and number of notochordal cells across species is important given their potential in resisting disc degeneration (Lotz 2004). In fact, Berry (1961) demonstrated that a breed of pin-tailed mice with low notochordal mitotic rates develops degeneration earlier than those with a more rapid rate of cell replication. This relationship between notochordal cells and disc degenerations may complicate the validity of many current animal models (Omlor et al. 2009) as certain species, particularly small animals (Higuchi et al. 1982) and dogs (Aguiar et al. 1999), have notochordal cells present throughout most of their lives. Differences in the number or qualitative characteristics of notochordal cells across species may manifest itself clinically as variation in the onset of disc degeneration (Hunter et al. 2004).

Animal models may also differ in the mechanism leading to the onset of the degradative process in the disc. Generally speaking, the etiology of disc degeneration in an animal model can be divided into spontaneous and experimentally induced degeneration (Lotz 2004) with the latter being further subdivided into models which are induced by either mechanical or structural alterations (Lotz 2004). Mechanical perturbations involve changes in the distribution or magnitude of loads placed on a disc, whereas structural perturbations involve chemical or physical injury to the disc itself (Lotz 2004). In contrast, human intervertebral disc degeneration usually occurs spontaneously (Lotz 2004) or possibly in response to a poorly defined mechanism of injury. Although spontaneous disc degeneration is present in many animal species, well-characterized models of spontaneous degeneration generally have involved smaller animals such as the Mediterranean sand rat (Silberberg 1988) and genetically altered mice (Lotz 2004). The value of the sand rat in disc research is discussed in considerable detail in Chap. 20. One counterexample, however, is chondrodystrophic dogs which have an abnormality in chondrocyte proliferation and maturation that also impacts the cells of the nucleus pulposus. With chondrodystrophy, there is accelerated disc degeneration, making these dogs a potential preclinical model for the human condition.

18.4 Large Animal Models

Sheep, goats, pigs, mini pigs, runt cows, nonhuman primates, dogs, chickens, kangaroos, and ostriches are all large animal species that have been used or discussed for disc research. However, the most commonly used species to date have been the pig, sheep, goat, and dog (Wilke et al. 1997a, b).

One concern regarding the use of the most commonly used large animal models relates to their quadruped nature (Wilke et al. 1997a, b). Unlike quadrupeds, humans are bipedal, using unique motions and body positions during ambulation and rest (Zhang et al. 2011a, b). This biomechanical limitation must be acknowledged when considering quadrupedal animals for research. Although some animals use bipedal ambulation (e.g., kangaroo, ostrich) and some could be considered partial bipeds (nonhuman primates), none provide an accurate replication of human gait including the upright torso position, sagittal balance of the spine, and the almost horizontally positioned discs during ambulation. Tissue processing of large animal spine specimen can be a challenge at times. To process isolated motion segments containing various devices often requires resorting to un-decalcified histology using plastic embedding. Careful tissue processing starting with adequate tissue fixation yields good-quality histological sections at an average thickness of 8 μm. Figures 18.1, 18.2, and 18.3 represent key features from ovine lumbar intervertebral discs with various degrees of degeneration. While there is little evidence of intervertebral disc degeneration days following the surgical intervention (chemonucleolysis using chondroitinase ABC), at 6 and 18 months, the degenerative process is well advanced. Specimens were stained using a Sirius red/Alcian Blue stain developed in our laboratory as a method for morphologic identification of collagen and proteoglycans in sections of non-decalcified disc specimens embedded in methyl methacrylate and sectioned on a rotary microtome at 4–8 μm.

18.4.1 Porcine

Multiple studies of the intervertebral disc have relied on porcine models. A number of lines of evidence suggest that the porcine model is a reasonably good model of the human disc. At the gene expression level, changes associated with aging in swine are similar to those observed in humans (Cho et al. 2011). Substantial morphologic similarities have been observed in the porcine disc post-nucleotomy and the human degenerative disc. Omlor et al. (2009) found significant decreases in disc height, MRI signal intensity, and notochordal cell number in the porcine disc after nucleotomy (Omlor et al. 2009). Kaapa et al. (1994b, c) studied the effect of pig disc injury on collagen content and metabolism and found dramatic alterations in collagen levels and collagen biosynthesis along with decreased intradiscal water content. Holm et al. (2007) used a structural porcine disc injury model, in which intradiscal pressure was used to assess degeneration. Using two separate injuries (one to the annulus and the other to the endplate), intradiscal pressure was measured while applying biomechanical loads (Holm et al. 2007). The authors found that the ratio of injured to adjacent disc pressure was highest in the annulus injury model, signifying that the endplate injury was a more severe type of injury. Although this type of injury may lead to morphologic and biochemical changes which replicate human disc degeneration, the traumatic effects of the disc injury may also introduce unintended effects that limit the interpretation of this type of research.

Other studies have used pigs to assess the therapeutic value of various interventions or to examine specific changes associated with degeneration. Buser et al. (2011) evaluated the use of fibrin sealant after nucleotomy to determine if intradiscal injection of the sealant had a therapeutic effect on the degenerating intervertebral disc. With injection of the sealant, the authors observed an inhibition of fibrosis and improvements in proteoglycan levels (Buser et al. 2011). Similarly, Chiang et al. (2011) demonstrated that sealing of annular defects via the modified purse-string suture reduced degenerative changes in the disc following the injury.

Kaapa et al. studied porcine disc innervation and the effects of degeneration on nerve topography. The authors characterized nerve density, finding that in common with humans, the outer annulus contained most of the nerve

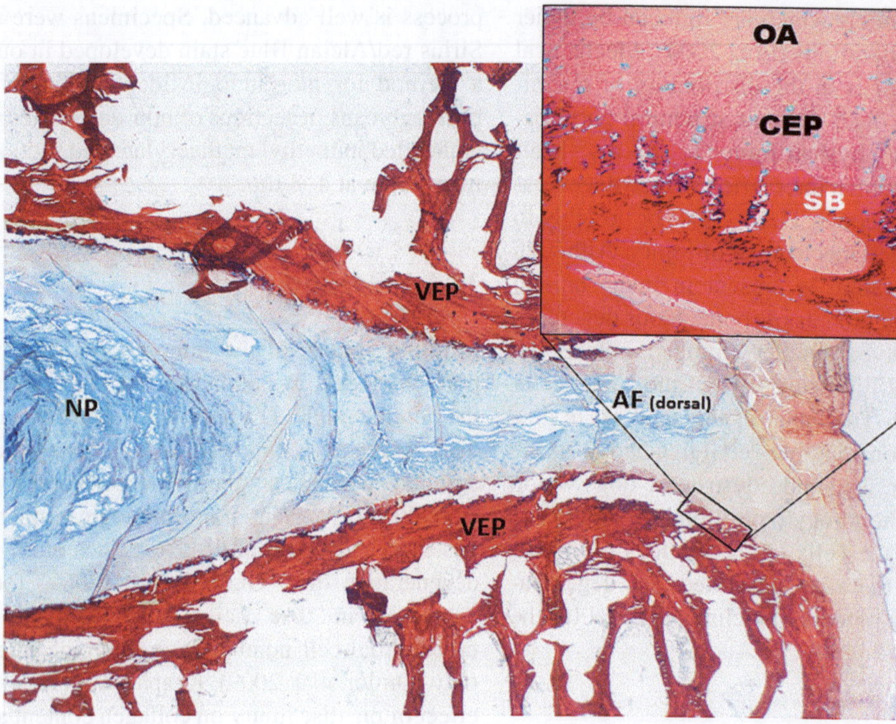

Fig. 18.1 Sections of two ovine vertebral bodies (L4–L5) and intervertebral disc. Low-power (orig mag ×1) view of a section stained with Picrosirius Red/Alcian Blue demonstrates normal intervertebral disc morphology consisting of vertebral endplates (*VEP*, annulus fibrosus *AF*, and nucleus pulposus *NP*). The cartilaginous disc stains an intense blue. Note the high content of collagen (*red*) in cortical and trabecular bone and the distinctly heterogeneous staining of collagen (*red*) and proteoglycan (*blue*) in the disc. Insert: high-power view of Picrosirius Red/Alcian Blue stained section (×40). Proteoglycan-positive chondrocytes and surrounding matrix stain *blue*. Residual collagen stains *red* (*SB* subchondral bone, *CEP* cartilaginous endplate, *OA* outer annulus); unstained areas (picric acid) appear *yellow*

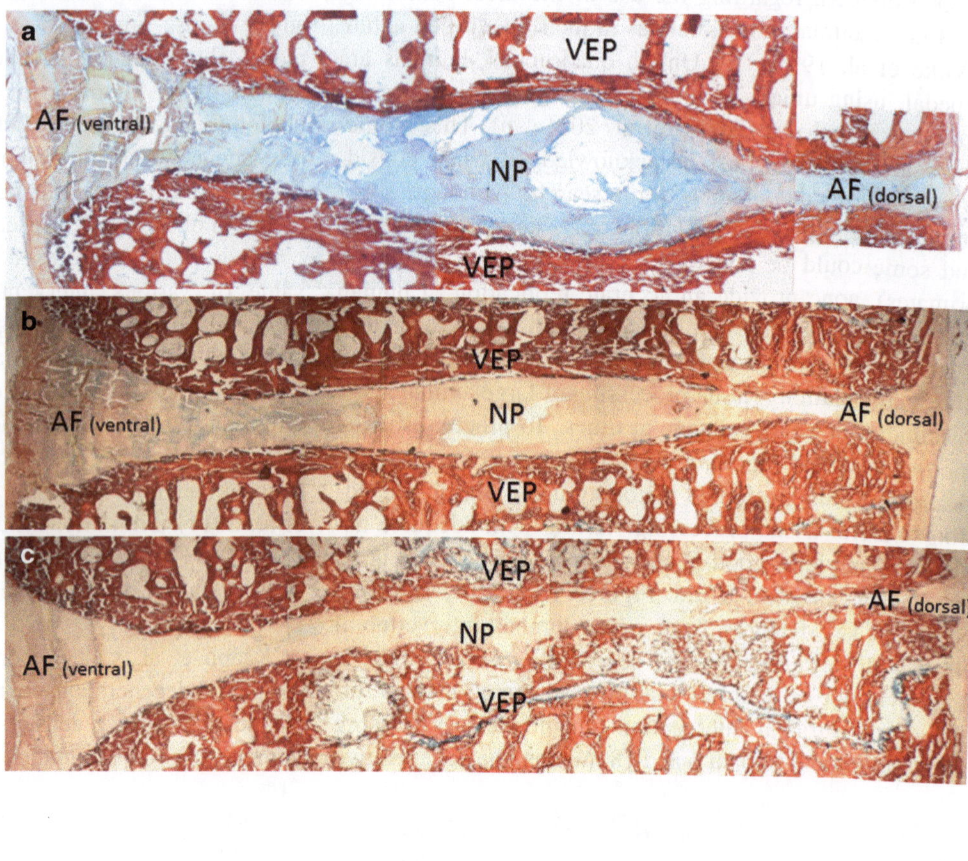

Fig. 18.2 Plastic embedded sagittal sections of ovine lumbar motion segments (L4–5) stained with Picrosirius Red/Alcian Blue at day 0 (**a**), 6 months (**b**), and 18 months (**c**) postoperative. Choosing a left lateral percutaneous approach through a 19-g docking needle, sheep were injected with 300 μl of chondroitinase ABC via the dorsolateral corner into the center of L4–5 discs using a 22-g spinal needle. Figure (a–c) demonstrates progressive loss of overall disc height associated with decreased proteoglycan content in the nucleus pulposus (*NP*) and loss of vertebral endplate integrity with established subchondral bone thickening (**b, c**). *VEP* vertebral endplate. Sections were photographed at 4×

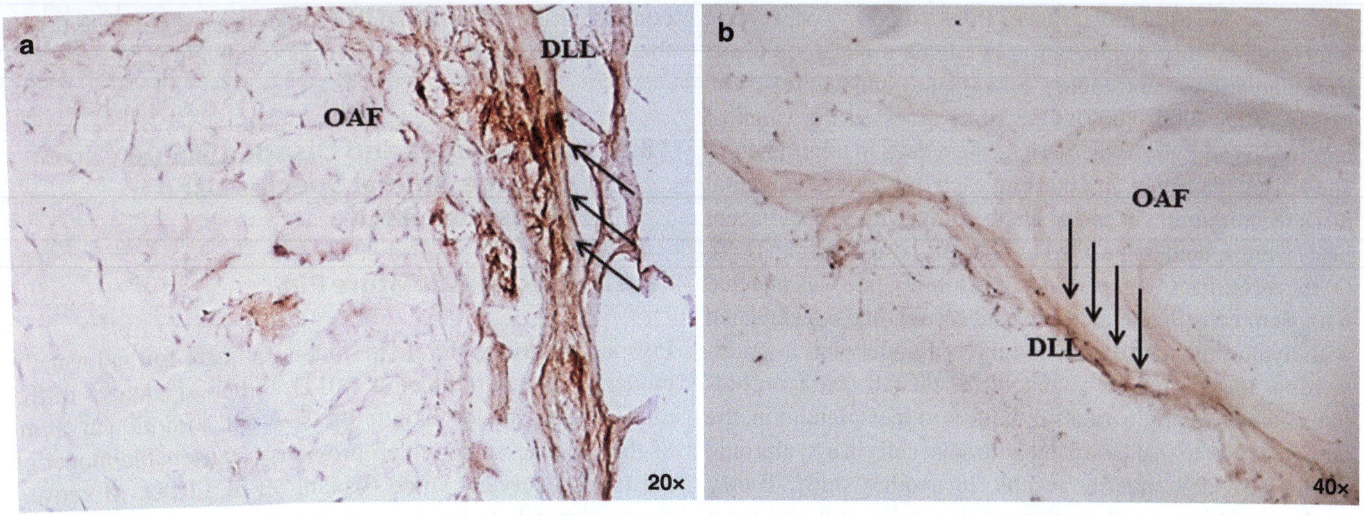

Fig. 18.3 Intervertebral disc degeneration (IVDD) per se is not a basis for clinical intervention: identification of specific features underlying discogenic pain is of the utmost importance to advance the current level of care and identify novel therapeutic targets. One critical deficiency in large animal models (sheep, goat, and cattle) is the lack of perceptible pain during surgically induced IVDD. Symptoms derived from degenerating discs may be classified into two types: (1) radicular pain secondary to stenosis and nerve-root or cord irritation and (2) discogenic pain due to internal disc disruption. These syndromes may have distinct etiologic bases. Certain dog breeds that exhibit an insidious onset of IVDD may provide clues to the pathophysiology of discogenic pain. A preclinical model correlating the clinical course of IVDD as it is seen in the humans would greatly enhance the predictability of clinical outcome when evaluating novel therapeutic concepts. Figure (**a**) and (**b**) demonstrates sparse positive immunoreactivity (*arrows*) to CGRP and SP confined to the dorsal longitudinal ligament (*DLL*) and outermost annulus fibrosus (*OAF*) in the lumbar disc of dogs without clinical history of back problems. These findings support current knowledge of neuroanatomic similarities between the healthy human and canine intervertebral discs

endings (Kaapa et al. 1994a). Interestingly, this study found that disc injury had no effect on nerve topography (Kaapa et al. 1994c).

18.4.2 Ovine

The ovine model has also been used widely as a model for disc research. Melrose et al. (2012) used annular incisions to create mechanical destabilization and degeneration in sheep. Three months after surgery, MRI examination demonstrated a reduction in disc height. Biomechanical testing to assess range of motion and to measure the neutral zone was performed along with histopathological examination. Measurement of aggrecan breakdown along with the expression of proteoglycan and collagen indicated that there were progressive degradative changes. In an earlier study, 8 months after annular injury of the lumbar discs of sheep, Melrose et al. (1992) found that while proteoglycan and collagen levels had decreased, the amount of non-collagenous protein had increased. The changes were primarily found in the nucleus pulposus and not the annulus fibrosus (Melrose et al. 1992). A subsequent study by the same investigators revealed increased expression of decorin and biglycan after annular damage. These proteins exhibit adverse effects on cell proliferation in vitro and may further suppress the limited ability of the disc to heal after injury (Melrose et al. 1997). A later study by Melrose et al. (2002) suggested that the ovine annular lesion model can be extended to study neural and vascular ingrowth during the degradative process, a phenomenon hypothesized to play a role in the pain experienced by some human patients.

18.4.3 Canine

The canine model has also been popular in disc research. Various insults have been applied to canine discs in order to induce disc degeneration. Hutton et al. (2004) hypothesized that disc degeneration could be produced in canine models by limiting nutritional flow through application of bone cement to the endplates; however, 70 weeks postsurgery, no changes were observed (Hutton et al. 2004). In other studies, canine lumbar discs were subjected to compressive forces using springs (Hutton et al. 1998, 2000). Despite application of springs over an entire year, the authors reported that there were no gross discal changes. They did, however, find differences in proteoglycan and collagen content between the control and experimental groups. A study by Hasegawa et al. (1995) demonstrated that fatigue loading was more detrimental to vertebral bodies adjacent to nucleotomized discs when compared to controls. Cyclic compression loading of nucleotomized discs resulted in an increase in microcrack density on the adjacent vertebral bodies suggesting a possible microtrauma mechanism for progressive disc degeneration (Hasegawa et al. 1995).

Several investigations have tried to slow or reverse intervertebral disc degeneration in canine models via direct transplantation of autologous cells (Ganey and Meisel 2002; Ganey et al. 2003, 2009). One study assessed the value of autologous adipose tissue-derived stem cells in treating damaged discs (Ganey et al. 2009). In each dog, three sequential discs were injured via partial nucleotomy, while two adjacent discs were spared and served as controls (Ganey et al. 2009). Of the three discs with partial nucleotomies, one was injected with stem cells in a hyaluronic acid carrier, one was injected with hyaluronic acid alone, and the last underwent no intervention. Based on assessments of the overall disc morphology and matrix production subsequent to transplantation, the authors reported that treatment with stem cells in a hyaluronic carrier provided superior results. In another study, Ganey et al. (2003) harvested autologous disc cells, cultured them ex vivo, and returned them to the original canine disc via a percutaneous method. Not only did the transplanted cells successfully reintegrate into the disc, they also produced extracellular matrix. With respect to disc water content, follow-up MRI was consistent with disc regeneration. Similarly, Hiyama et al. (2008) were also able to show signs of regeneration in a canine post-nucleotomy model through the injection of autologous disc cells expanded in culture.

In contrast to the canine disc injury models, chondrodystrophic breeds have the potential to serve as a model for spontaneous disc degeneration. The genetic defect which influences disc cell proliferation and maturation leads to an increased pace of disc degeneration. These dogs experience the early disappearance of notochordal cells, and there is replacement of the nucleus pulposus with fibrocartilage (Melrose et al. 1996). Thus, they provide a unique model to study a spontaneous degenerative process within the disc of a larger animal model. Additionally, investigations into disc innervations have thus far revealed the sparse presence of nociceptive fibers (Fig. 18.3). Whether there is indeed an increase of nociception during disc injury or degenerative processes in this species is subject of ongoing investigations.

18.4.4 Caprine

Attempts have also been made to induce disc disease in caprine models. Hoogendoorn et al. (2008) successfully injected chondroitinase ABC directly into goat discs. A subsequent study by Zhang et al. (2011a, b) demonstrated that a 4.5-mm drill bit inserted 15 mm into the disc resulted in significantly greater histological changes consistent with disc degeneration compared to disc injuries using a scalpel blade. This group also studied the effects of injecting caprine bone marrow stromal cells into degenerating discs and reported this intervention increased the proteoglycan content. It should be noted that the degree of degeneration in these studies prior to injection was relatively mild.

18.5 Advantages and Disadvantages of Large Animal Species Used in Disc Research

18.5.1 Porcine/Miniature Pig

Pigs are relatively simple to obtain and care for and usually moderate in cost (Cho et al. 2011). Other advantages of the mini-porcine model include the size and lordotic curvature of the cervical spine which provides a reasonable model of the human cervical spine (Chiang et al. 2011). Moreover, biomechanical studies have shown that porcine and human spines are similar with respect to spinal flexibility and disc dimensions (Lundin et al. 2000; Park et al. 2005). Although pigs are quadrupeds, biomechanical evidence suggests that the forces acting on their spines are primarily along the long axis, similar to humans (Alini et al. 2008).

Pig spines are most similar to human spines between the T6 and T10 vertebral levels making these levels ideal for modeling thoracic conditions (Sheng et al. 2010). Moreover, pig discs are relatively large, facilitating surgical interventions (Omlor et al. 2009). From a biochemical perspective, the extracellular matrix composition and chondroitin sulfate to keratan sulfate ratios in humans and pig discs are similar (Kaapa et al. 1994b). Pigs, like dogs, retain notochordal cells through adult life which may make the pig disc more resistant to degeneration and afford them greater regenerative potential compared to humans (Omlor et al. 2009).

The primary disadvantage of using full-sized porcine models is the rapid growth rate of most breeds; because of the subsequent weight gain, they are costly for long-term studies and also difficult to use for surgical interventions (Sheng et al. 2010). To overcome this limitation, some workers have turned to the mini pig model. Yoon et al. (2008) were able to induce slow progressive disc degeneration, confirmed by histopathology and MRI imaging, in miniature pigs after annular injury.

Another shortcoming of the pig (as with most large animal models) is that young animals generally do not experience spontaneous degeneration. Therefore, the degenerative process must be induced by annular or endplate injury (Yoon et al. 2008; Omlor et al. 2009).

18.5.2 Ovine

Sheep are also relatively easy to obtain and moderate in cost. In contrast to dogs and pigs, sheep are similar to humans with regard to the absence of notochordal cells in adulthood (Osti et al. 1990; Melrose et al. 1992; Alini et al. 2008). They also exhibit similarities in water content, collagen content, and fiber orientation angles (Reid et al. 2002). Despite the similarity in cellular composition, sheep have relatively smaller spines and substantial anatomic incongruences when compared to humans. Upon comparing the anatomic dimensions of sheep and human discs, Wilke et al. (1997a, b) found that the greatest similarities were in the thoracic and lumbar regions; however, there were disparities in all regions in terms of disc height: disc height in humans is greatest in the lumbar region, while sheep have greater disc heights in the cervical region. In addition, there are fundamental anatomic differences including variations of the atlas and axis vertebrae, pedicles, and posterior vertebral body heights (Wilke et al. 1997a, b). The range of motion between vertebral regions (e.g., cervical, thoracic, lumbar) is similar to the human (Wilke et al. 1997a, b). Kandziora et al. (2001) evaluated 20 human and Merino sheep spines and concluded that despite significant differences in anatomy, the two were similar enough to use for in vivo modeling of human diseases, specifically endorsing the C3–4 motion segment as a reliable model of human cervical motion.

18.5.3 Canine

Although dogs are abundant and relatively inexpensive to maintain, their use for research in many communities provokes ethical scrutiny. Moreover, due to the unique relationship between humans and dogs, attitudes regarding the use of canine models in research vary (Zhang et al. 2011a, b). In some cases, social norms complicate the use of dogs in biomedical research, and ethical scrutiny has led to an increased regulatory burden when performing canine research (Zhang et al. 2011).

Nonetheless, because dog intervertebral discs have been observed to have certain favorable similarities to humans, the canine model has been used extensively (Nguyen et al. 1989). The major differences between the dog and human spine have been described by Nguyen et al. (1989) and include their smaller size and dissimilar disc shape (Nguyen et al. 1989; Zhang et al. 2011a, b).

In terms of motion, lateral bending and axial rotation are coupled differently in humans and dogs at the C4–5 vertebral levels. The dog cervical spine appears to have more coupled motion with regard to lateral bending and axial rotation compared to human spinal motion segments (Hofstetter et al. 2009). However, compressive and torsional stiffness along with the relative contribution of the posterior elements, discs, and ligament is similar between dog and human (Zimmerman et al. 1992).

As previously mentioned, non-chondrodystrophic canine breeds have persistent notochordal cells which may be protective against degenerative changes and promote regeneration following mild injuries. Chondrodystrophic breeds experience spontaneous degeneration, although the genetic basis for the degenerative process is quite different from that of normal human discs (Sakai et al. 2009).

18.5.4 Caprine

Goats are robust animals that are relatively easy to obtain and moderate in cost. One advantage of the caprine model is that the disc height, size, and shape of certain breeds are similar to those of humans (Zhang et al. 2011a, b). The C3–4 intervertebral disc in goats is particularly useful for modeling the C5–6 disc in humans (Hu et al. 2006). Grossly, goat spines have similar geometric, anatomic, and loading characteristics, while the nucleus pulposus displays comparable mechanical properties (Zhang et al. 2011a, b).

The weight range of goats is similar to humans, they tolerate surgery and anesthesia well, and they do not gain enough weight to interfere with surgical manipulation (Zhang et al. 2011a, b). Due to the shape of the goat torso, which is much thinner side to side than the anterior-posterior dimension, a lateral approach to the lumbar spine is relatively easy and can be performed using a minimally invasive approach (Zhang et al. 2011a, b). A disadvantage of the goat model is that it has not been used as widely in disc research as some other large animal models.

18.5.5 Nonhuman Primates

From an evolutionary perspective, nonhuman primates have the greatest genetic similarity to humans and theoretically should have the most conserved disc biology. Not surprisingly, the baboon and human cervical spines are very similar in terms of geometry and anatomic shape (Sheng et al. 2010).

However, the lumbar region of the spine does exhibit notable differences that relate to upright posture and ambulation in the human. Nonhuman primates do not require the lordotic posture of humans in the lumbar region. Additionally, human lumbar discs (especially in the lower two lumbar segments) are wedge shaped with greater anterior disc height. This allows for a greater range of extension and reduced flexion (Farfan 1978).

In spite of the genetic similarities, the principal barriers to the use of nonhuman primates for disc research are the substantially greater cost of acquiring and maintaining these relatively rare and highly social animals and the ethical scrutiny that must be met before utilizing these intelligent animals for biomedical research.

18.6 Guide to Selecting the Most Useful Animal Model

The selection of an animal model should be guided by the unique research objectives of the specific study. No single animal model identically reproduces all of the clinically relevant variables associated with the human disc (Alini et al. 2008); however, different animal models share with humans' specific anatomic and biologic characteristics which may be relevant to a particular investigation. If the topic of interest is focused on an area in which a particular large animal model shares favorable anatomic, biomechanical, or biochemical features with the human, the choice is fairly straightforward (Alini et al. 2008).

Assessing disc torsional biomechanics and collagen content across an assortment of species, Showalter et al. (2012) provided loose guidelines as to which species are the most favorable for modeling of human disc degeneration. With respect to torsional mechanics, they found that 9 out of 11 species were similar to humans; however, sheep and pig discs exhibited a significantly higher torsional stiffness. Calf, pig, baboon, goat, sheep, lumbar discs, and cow caudal discs are the most preferable species for studies investigating torsional forces on the spine. With regard to collagen content, although the authors noted differences between species with regard to specific disc regions, in general, they concluded there was relatively little variation across species. Unfortunately, few other similar cross-species studies have been performed to date.

Cost-effectiveness is an important factor in choosing an animal species for investigational studies. Larger, more intelligent animals are expensive to acquire and maintain. Typically, such animals require specialized housing and may need trained handlers. Furthermore, some animals take longer to manifest degenerative changes after an experimental intervention, which can contribute to both study cost and length (Singh et al. 2005).

The methods used to evaluate experimental results may also play a role in model selection. Histological examination, mechanical testing, and gene expression analysis all provide different levels of information regarding the extent of disc degeneration and the success of potential therapeutic interventions (Chan et al. 2011). In vivo postoperative monitoring is critical and helps reduce animal numbers. Methodologies may include digital radiography, computed tomography, or magnetic resonance imaging. Digital radiography can be a cost-effective tool to monitor, i.e., disc space as a function of efficacy testing of an experimental intervention. Collapsing disc space is one radiographic hallmark of disc degeneration. Subjective radiographic assessments require perfect lateral projections and are imprecise at best. A robust method to assess radiographic findings can be a powerful tool to corroborate findings from preclinical animal trials (Fig. 18.4). Careful pre-experimental planning is required to ensure that the minimal numbers of animals used for the study are adequate to address the research question and avoid performing an underpowered study. Gene expression studies generally require DNA sequence information which is more readily available in certain animal species. Studies in which the research objectives can be completed using advanced imaging, without animal sacrifice, may allow animals to be used for additional research so long as it does not confound the results of the first set of experiments (Chan et al. 2011).

When selecting an animal model for a specific purpose, such as medical device development, anatomic dimensions may be of particular importance. For example, in order to test a novel posterior instrumentation system, the investigator may want to use an animal model with more humanlike pedicle morphology and vertebral body size. For testing interbody cages or an intervertebral disc prosthesis, disc and vertebral body dimensions must to be taken into account (McLain et al. 2002).

For studies of spinal motion, it is important that the model is biomechanically similar to humans. As an example, Schmidt et al. (2005) found that the porcine model was biomechanically similar to humans in flexion/extension, but markedly different for lateral bending and axial rotation. Thus, the porcine model would be best suited for the study of flexion/extension and not for lateral bending and rotation.

Finally, when working with large animal models, safety is always a concern. The most obvious cause for concern is the potential for injury (bites, kicks); however, there are other less obvious hazards (Langley 1999). These include, but are not limited to, needle puncture and scalpel cuts, allergies related to dander or hair, and fall-related injuries on floors slippery from animal urine, food, or feces (Langley 1999). Zoonotic diseases are also a potential concern (Weigler et al. 2005). Appropriate protocols and training should be set in place and communicated to all staff working with animals to insure that precautions are taken to reduce the risk of injury or disease exposure (Weigler et al. 2005).

18.7 Summary of Critical Concepts Discussed in the Chapter

Many small animal models are useful for studies involving intervertebral disc disease; however, large animal models are required for certain types of research and for regulatory agency approval of certain medical devices.

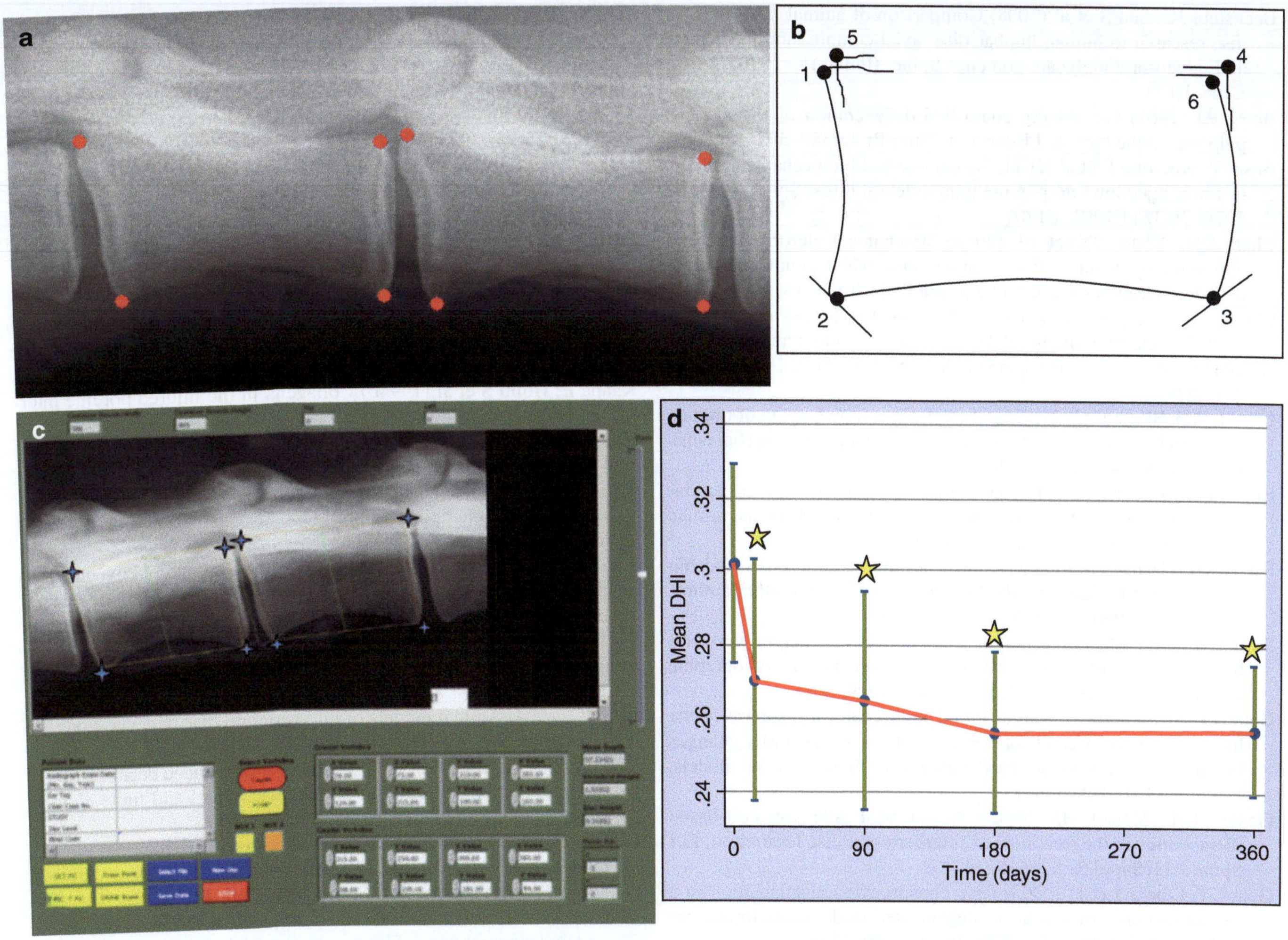

Fig. 18.4 To evaluate disc height changes over time, a robust methodology adapted from Frobin et al. (1997) was developed and validated in a cohort of sheep enrolled in an IVDD study involving chemonucleolysis with chondroitinase ABC at L4–5. Digital radiographs in the lateral projection of the lumbar spine were obtained at 0, 2, 12, 26, and 52 weeks (**a**). Radiographs were imported into LabVIEW (**c**) where disc height changes were measured using specific anatomic landmarks (**b**) and the disc height index (*DHI*) calculated by blinded observers. The DHI for normal discs was consistent and reliable for multiple observers. The disc collapsed after C-ABC injection by 12 % after 12 weeks postoperative and maximally by 16 % at 6 months before stabilizing (**d**). DHI at all time points following C-ABC injection were lower than at time zero ($p<0.01$). This imaging analysis allows for effective in vivo monitoring during preclinical intervertebral disc research trials

- Large animal models can be used for studying disc biology, biomechanics, regeneration strategies, and medical device development.
- Validation of each animal model is necessary. Significant differences exist between species with regard to the presence of notochordal cells, the biologic predilection towards disc degeneration, and the anatomic and physiologic features of the intervertebral disc. Thus, selection of the best animal model for a particular investigation will depend on the goals of the study.
- Large animal model potentially useful for the study of degenerative disc disease includes sheep, goat, pig/miniature pigs, runt cow, nonhuman primates, dog, chicken, kangaroo, and ostrich.
- For a specific study, the research objectives, ethical considerations, budget, and availability of the model should be considered when choosing the preferred animal model.

References

Aguiar DJ, Johnson SL et al (1999) Notochordal cells interact with nucleus pulposus cells: regulation of proteoglycan synthesis. Exp Cell Res 246(1):129–137

Alini M, Eisenstein SM et al (2008) Are animal models useful for studying human disc disorders/degeneration? Eur Spine J 17(1):2–19

An H, Boden SD et al (2003) Summary statement: emerging techniques for treatment of degenerative lumbar disc disease. Spine (Phila Pa 1976) 28(15 Suppl):S24–S25

Beckstein JC, Sen S et al (2008) Comparison of animal discs used in disc research to human lumbar disc: axial compression mechanics and glycosaminoglycan content. Spine (Phila Pa 1976) 33(6): E166–E173

Berry RJ (1961) Genetically controlled degeneration of the nucleus pulposus in the mouse. J Bone Joint Surg Br 43:387–393

Buser Z, Kuelling F et al (2011) Biological and biomechanical effects of fibrin injection into porcine intervertebral discs. Spine (Phila Pa 1976) 36(18):E1201–E1209

Chan DD, Khan SN et al (2011) Mechanical deformation and glycosaminoglycan content changes in a rabbit annular puncture disc degeneration model. Spine (Phila Pa 1976) 36(18):1438–1445

Chiang CJ, Cheng CK et al (2011) The effect of a new anular repair after discectomy in intervertebral disc degeneration: an experimental study using a porcine spine model. Spine (Phila Pa 1976) 36(10): 761–769

Cho H, Park SH et al (2011) Snapshot of degenerative aging of porcine intervertebral disc: a model to unravel the molecular mechanisms. Exp Mol Med 43(6):334–340

Elliott DM, Sarver JJ (2004) Young investigator award winner: validation of the mouse and rat disc as mechanical models of the human lumbar disc. Spine (Phila Pa 1976) 29(7):713–722

Farfan HF (1978) The biomechanical advantage of lordosis and hip extension for upright activity. Man as compared with other anthropoids. Spine (Phila Pa 1976) 3(4):336–342

Frobin W et al (1997) Precision measurement of disc height, vertebral height and sagittal plane displacement from lateral radiographic views of the lumbar spine. Clin Biomech 12:S1–S63

Galbusera F, Schmidt H et al (2011) The mechanical response of the lumbar spine to different combinations of disc degenerative changes investigated using randomized poroelastic finite element models. Eur Spine J 20(4):563–571

Ganey TM, Meisel HJ (2002) A potential role for cell-based therapeutics in the treatment of intervertebral disc herniation. Eur Spine J 11(Suppl 2):S206–S214

Ganey T, Libera J et al (2003) Disc chondrocyte transplantation in a canine model: a treatment for degenerated or damaged intervertebral disc. Spine (Phila Pa 1976) 28(23):2609–2620

Ganey T, Hutton WC et al (2009) Intervertebral disc repair using adipose tissue-derived stem and regenerative cells: experiments in a canine model. Spine (Phila Pa 1976) 34(21):2297–2304

Hasegawa K, Turner CH et al (1995) Effect of disc lesion on microdamage accumulation in lumbar vertebrae under cyclic compression loading. Clin Orthop Relat Res 311:190–198

Higuchi M, Kaneda K et al (1982) Age-related changes in the nucleus pulposus of intervertebral disc in mice. An electronmicroscopic study. Nihon Seikeigeka Gakkai Zasshi 56(4):321–329

Hiyama A, Mochida J et al (2008) Transplantation of mesenchymal stem cells in a canine disc degeneration model. J Orthop Res 26(5): 589–600

Hofstetter M, Gedet P et al (2009) Biomechanical analysis of the three-dimensional motion pattern of the canine cervical spine segment C4-C5. Vet Surg 38(1):49–58

Holm S, Ekstrom L et al (2007) Intradiscal pressure in the degenerated porcine intervertebral disc. Vet Comp Orthop Traumatol 20(1): 29–33

Hoogendoorn RJ, Helder MN et al (2008) Reproducible long-term disc degeneration in a large animal model. Spine (Phila Pa 1976) 33(9): 949–954

Hu N, Cunningham BW et al (2006) Porous coated motion cervical disc replacement: a biomechanical, histomorphometric, and biologic wear analysis in a caprine model. Spine (Phila Pa 1976) 31(15): 1666–1673

Hunter CJ, Matyas JR et al (2004) Cytomorphology of notochordal and chondrocytic cells from the nucleus pulposus: a species comparison. J Anat 205(5):357–362

Hutton WC, Toribatake Y et al (1998) The effect of compressive force applied to the intervertebral disc in vivo. A study of proteoglycans and collagen. Spine (Phila Pa 1976) 23(23):2524–2537

Hutton WC, Ganey TM et al (2000) Does long-term compressive loading on the intervertebral disc cause degeneration? Spine (Phila Pa 1976) 25(23):2993–3004

Hutton WC, Murakami H et al (2004) The effect of blocking a nutritional pathway to the intervertebral disc in the dog model. J Spinal Disord Tech 17(1):53–63

Iatridis JC, Mente PL et al (1999) Compression-induced changes in intervertebral disc properties in a rat tail model. Spine (Phila Pa 1976) 24(10):996–1002

Kaapa E, Gronblad M et al (1994a) Neural elements in the normal and experimentally injured porcine intervertebral disk. Eur Spine J 3(3): 137–142

Kaapa E, Holm S et al (1994b) Collagens in the injured porcine intervertebral disc. J Orthop Res 12(1):93–102

Kaapa E, Holm S et al (1994c) Proteoglycan chemistry in experimentally injured porcine intervertebral disk. J Spinal Disord 7(4):296–306

Kalichman L, Hunter DJ (2008) Diagnosis and conservative management of degenerative lumbar spondylolisthesis. Eur Spine J 17(3):327–335

Kandziora F, Pflugmacher R et al (2001) Comparison between sheep and human cervical spines: an anatomic, radiographic, bone mineral density, and biomechanical study. Spine (Phila Pa 1976) 26(9): 1028–1037

Langley R (1999) Physical hazards of animal handlers. Occup Med 14(2):181–194

Lotz JC (2004) Animal models of intervertebral disc degeneration: lessons learned. Spine (Phila Pa 1976) 29(23):2742–2750

Lotz JC, Colliou OK et al (1998) Compression-induced degeneration of the intervertebral disc: an in vivo mouse model and finite-element study. Spine (Phila Pa 1976) 23(23):2493–2506

Lundin O, Ekstrom L et al (2000) Exposure of the porcine spine to mechanical compression: differences in injury pattern between adolescents and adults. Eur Spine J 9(6):466–471

McLain RF, Yerby SA et al (2002) Comparative morphometry of L4 vertebrae: comparison of large animal models for the human lumbar spine. Spine (Phila Pa 1976) 27(8):E200–E206

Melrose J, Ghosh P et al (1992) A longitudinal study of the matrix changes induced in the intervertebral disc by surgical damage to the annulus fibrosus. J Orthop Res 10(5):665–676

Melrose J, Taylor TK et al (1996) Variation in intervertebral disc serine proteinase inhibitory proteins with ageing in a chondrodystrophoid (beagle) and a non-chondrodystrophoid (greyhound) canine breed. Gerontology 42(6):322–329

Melrose J, Ghosh P et al (1997) Elevated synthesis of biglycan and decorin in an ovine annular lesion model of experimental disc degeneration. Eur Spine J 6(6):376–384

Melrose J, Roberts S et al (2002) Increased nerve and blood vessel ingrowth associated with proteoglycan depletion in an ovine anular lesion model of experimental disc degeneration. Spine (Phila Pa 1976) 27(12):1278–1285

Melrose J, Shu C et al (2012) Mechanical destabilization induced by controlled annular incision of the intervertebral disc dysregulates metalloproteinase expression and induces disc degeneration. Spine (Phila Pa 1976) 37(1):18–25

Nguyen CM, Haughton VM et al (1989) A model for studying intervertebral disc degeneration with magnetic resonance and a nucleotome. Invest Radiol 24(5):407–409

O'Connell GD, Vresilovic EJ et al (2007) Comparison of animals used in disc research to human lumbar disc geometry. Spine (Phila Pa 1976) 32(3):328–333

Omlor GW, Nerlich AG et al (2009) A new porcine in vivo animal model of disc degeneration: response of anulus fibrosus cells, chondrocyte-like nucleus pulposus cells, and notochordal nucleus pulposus cells to partial nucleotomy. Spine (Phila Pa 1976) 34(25): 2730–2739

Osti OL, Vernon-Roberts B et al (1990) 1990 Volvo Award in experimental studies. Anulus tears and intervertebral disc degeneration. An experimental study using an animal model. Spine (Phila Pa 1976) 15(8):762–767

Palmer EI, Lotz JC (2004) The compressive creep properties of normal and degenerated murine intervertebral discs. J Orthop Res 22(1): 164–169

Panjabi MM (1998) Cervical spine models for biomechanical research. Spine (Phila Pa 1976) 23(24):2684–2700

Park C, Kim YJ et al (2005) An in vitro animal study of the biomechanical responses of anulus fibrosus with aging. Spine (Phila Pa 1976) 30(10):E259–E265

Reid JE, Meakin JR et al (2002) Sheep lumbar intervertebral discs as models for human discs. Clin Biomech (Bristol, Avon) 17(4): 312–314

Sakai D, Nakai T et al (2009) Differential phenotype of intervertebral disc cells: microarray and immunohistochemical analysis of canine nucleus pulposus and anulus fibrosus. Spine (Phila Pa 1976) 34(14): 1448–1456

Schmidt R, Richter M et al (2005) Limitations of the cervical porcine spine in evaluating spinal implants in comparison with human cervical spinal segments: a biomechanical in vitro comparison of porcine and human cervical spine specimens with different instrumentation techniques. Spine (Phila Pa 1976) 30(11): 1275–1282

Sheng SR, Wang XY et al (2010) Anatomy of large animal spines and its comparison to the human spine: a systematic review. Eur Spine J 19(1):46–56

Showalter BL, Beckstein JC et al (2012) Comparison of animal discs used in disc research to human lumbar disc: torsion mechanics and collagen content. Spine (Phila Pa 1976) 37(15):E900–E907

Silberberg R (1988) Histologic and morphometric observations on vertebral bone of aging sand rats. Spine (Phila Pa 1976) 13(2): 202–208

Singh K, Masuda K et al (2005) Animal models for human disc degeneration. Spine J 5(6 Suppl):267S–279S

Smith LJ, Nerurkar NL et al (2011) Degeneration and regeneration of the intervertebral disc: lessons from development. Dis Model Mech 4(1):31–41

Urban JP, Roberts S et al (2000) The nucleus of the intervertebral disc from development to degeneration. Am Zool 40:53–61

Wagner PC, Bagby GW et al (1979) Surgical stabilization of the equine cervical spine. Vet Surg 8(1):7–12

Weigler BJ, Di Giacomo RF et al (2005) A national survey of laboratory animal workers concerning occupational risks for zoonotic diseases. Comp Med 55(2):183–191

Wilke HJ, Kettler A et al (1997a) Are sheep spines a valid biomechanical model for human spines? Spine (Phila Pa 1976) 22(20): 2365–2374

Wilke HJ, Kettler A et al (1997b) Anatomy of the sheep spine and its comparison to the human spine. Anat Rec 247(4):542–555

Yoon SH, Miyazaki M et al (2008) A porcine model of intervertebral disc degeneration induced by annular injury characterized with magnetic resonance imaging and histopathological findings. Laboratory investigation. J Neurosurg Spine 8(5):450–457

Zhang Y, Drapeau S et al (2011a) Histological features of the degenerating intervertebral disc in a goat disc-injury model. Spine (Phila Pa 1976) 36(19):1519–1527

Zhang Y, Drapeau S et al (2011b) Transplantation of goat bone marrow stromal cells to the degenerating intervertebral disc in a goat disc injury model. Spine (Phila Pa 1976) 36(5):372–377

Zimmerman MC, Vuono-Hawkins M et al (1992) The mechanical properties of the canine lumbar disc and motion segment. Spine (Phila Pa 1976) 17(2):213–220

pulposus cells in partial meniscectomy. Spine (Phila Pa 1976) 34(5): 423–429

Intervertebral Disc Herniation: Pathophysiology and Emerging Therapies

19

Beth A. Winkelstein, Kyle D. Allen, and Lori A. Setton

Contents

B.A. Winkelstein, PhD
Departments of Bioengineering and Neurosurgery,
University of Pennsylvania,
Philadelphia, PA, USA
e-mail: winkelst@seas.upenn.edu

K.D. Allen, PhD
J. Crayton Pruitt Family Department of Biomedical Engineering,
University of Florida, Gainesville, FL, USA
e-mail: kyle.allen@bme.ufl.edu

L.A. Setton, PhD (✉)
Departments of Biomedical Engineering and Orthopaedic Surgery,
Duke University, 136 Hudson Hall, 90281,
Durham, NC 27708, USA
e-mail: setton@duke.edu

I.M. Shapiro, M.V. Risbud (eds.), *The Intervertebral Disc*,
DOI 10.1007/978-3-7091-1535-0_19, © Springer-Verlag Wien 2014

19.1 Introduction

Approximately 2.6 % of the US population visits a physician for treatment of spinal disorders annually (Fraser 2009) with costs of $7.1 billion from lost work days alone (Ricci et al. 2006). "Herniation" of the intervertebral disc is one of the several spinal disorders that contribute to this very high incidence, with potential to cause significant pain, neurological deficit, and functional disability in affected individuals. Herniation presents as a protrusion or extrusion of discal tissue into the epidural cavity, resulting in nerve root impingement and disc tissue exposure (Fig. 19.1). Both mechanical compression and tissue exposure contribute to pain and disability associated with intervertebral disc herniation (Goupille et al. 1998; Mixter et al. 1934; Olmarker and Rydevik 1991). In areas innervated by the affected nerves, it is commonly seen as low back pain, radiating leg pain (i.e., radiculopathy or sciatica), muscle weakness, gait abnormality, muscle atrophy, asymmetric reflexes, or loss of function (Atlas et al. 2005; Frymoyer 1988; Hart et al. 1995). The incidence of sciatica related to intervertebral disc herniation peaks between the fourth and fifth decades of life and is most frequently associated with herniations between the L3 and S1 vertebral levels (Atlas et al. 2005; Awad and Moskovich 2006). The severity of herniation symptoms in the cervical or lumbar regions has been shown to relate to the size or nature of the herniated fragment, whether it is simply protruding into the neural cavity, extruded, or completely sequestered from the parent structure.

Intervertebral disc herniation may also occur in association with disc degeneration, wherein degenerated nucleus pulposus fragments migrate into previously established defects in the anulus fibrosus (Moore et al. 1996). A desiccated and fibrous nucleus pulposus is associated with loss of disc height and an increased axial disc bulge with compressive loading (Adams and Roughley 2006); the altered tissue can generate untoward stresses upon the anulus fibrosus leading to tissue fragment extrusion. Thus, while intervertebral disc degeneration is positively associated with disc herniation,

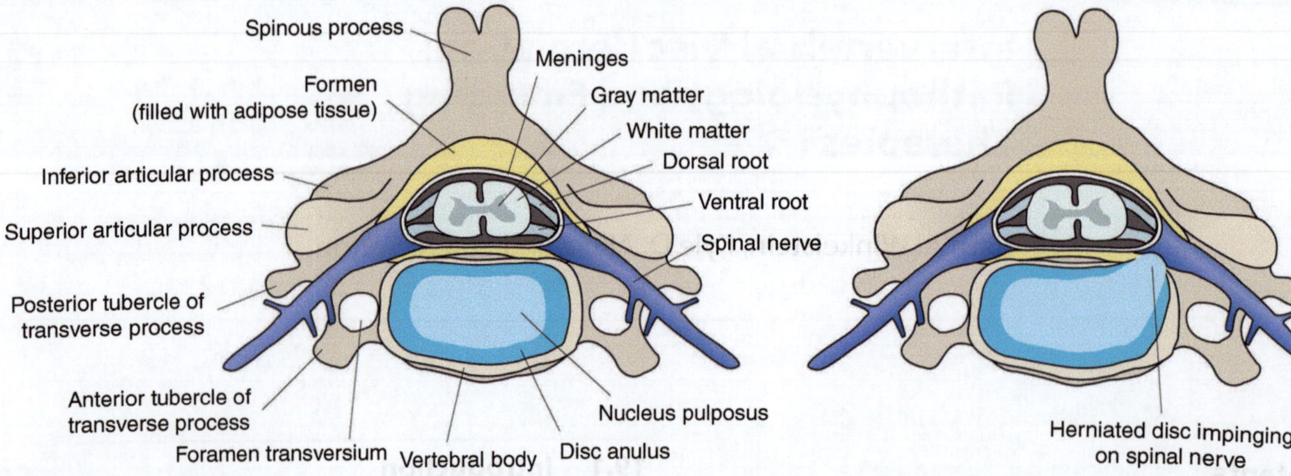

Fig. 19.1 Schema showing a cross section of the intervertebral disc and anatomy of the spinal cord and posterior vertebral processes. (*Left*) Normal anatomy showing labels identifying the intervertebral disc anulus fibrous and nucleus pulposus, as well as the nerve roots which come together as spinal nerves as they exit through the intervertebral foramen. (*Right*) Schema of anatomic changes typical of a posterolateral intervertebral disc herniation, suggesting nerve root impingement (Used under CCL3.0, http://en.wikipedia.org/wiki/File:Cervical_vertebra_english.png)

it can be difficult to identify the specific contributions of biomechanical, environmental, or genetic factors. Once the tissue is protruded or herniated, there is evidence for increased angiogenesis, macrophage infiltration, and proteinase production in the tissue fragment that can contribute to its resorption over a period of months to years (Komori et al. 1996).

The factors listed above are also believed to play important roles in the etiology and pathophysiology of intervertebral disc herniation (Adams and Roughley 2006; Battie and Videman 2006). Mechanical loading of the lumbar spine in work-related loading conditions may be sufficient to cause disc herniation. Epidemiological studies further suggest a role for mechanical factors and nutrient transport in intervertebral disc herniation with higher incidences of herniation and sciatica associated with obesity, smoking, and heavy physical work (this topic is discussed in considerable detail in Chap. 9) (Battie et al. 2009; Bostman 1993; Heliovaara 1987a, b; Heliovaara et al. 1987a, b). Genetic predisposition to lumbar radiculopathy may also exist, with data suggesting that disc herniation may be associated with genetic mutations in the α2 and α3 chains of collagen IX or the regulatory cytokines interleukin-1β (IL-1β) and interleukin-6 (IL-6) (see Chap. 11).

For intervertebral disc herniation, the first treatment of choice is conservative, unless motor weakness or loss of function is a significant concern. Lifestyle modifications, in particular exercise and physical therapy, can provide symptomatic relief and reduce the need for operative treatment, although they are not generally considered to be disease-modifying therapies (Weinstein et al. 2006a, b). In addition, conventional pharmacological interventions are widely prescribed for sciatica including orally administered anti-inflammatory and opioid analgesics. While more invasive, epidural administration of anesthetics, such as bupivacaine, and/or corticosteroids, like methylprednisolone or triamcinolone, shows some efficacy in providing symptom relief, although again without evidence of disease modification (Buenaventura et al. 2009; Staal et al. 2008).

While nonsurgical care is the first treatment option (see Chap. 15), surgical intervertebral disc excision is the most frequently performed musculoskeletal procedure in the USA, affecting 0.3 % of the population with hospitalization costs of $9.5 billion (Fraser 2009; Ricci et al. 2006). The surgical approach for painful disc herniation is simply to remove the inflammatory material and to unload and decompress the adjacent neural structures (Loupasis et al. 1999). While frequently successful in providing relief, compression-relieving discectomy may not prevent recurrence of pain, prompting the need for additional surgeries, or in 20–60 % of patients, there may be repeat herniations (Weinstein et al. 2006a, b).

19.2 Pathophysiology and Pain of Intervertebral Disc Herniation

Both chemical and mechanical factors are widely believed to contribute to radicular pain subsequent to intervertebral disc herniation (Olmarker 2001). The herniated fragment may impinge upon the exiting spinal nerve and contribute to nerve root compression with many associated deleterious effects. The root consists of both anterior and posterior rootlets exiting from the spinal nerve that combine to form the dorsal and ventral nerve roots containing sensory and efferent fibers, respectively (Fig. 19.2). The roots come together in the region

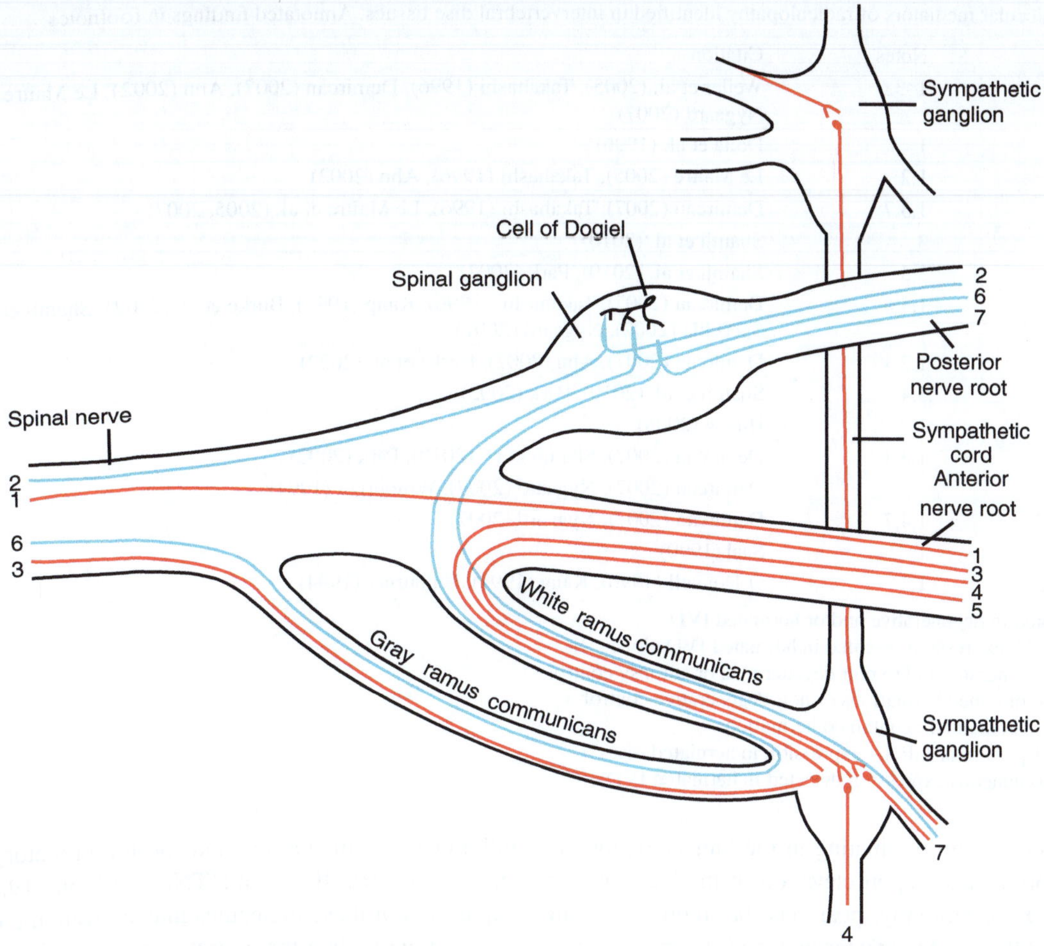

Fig. 19.2 Scheme showing structure of a typical spinal nerve and spinal ganglion. *1* Somatic efferent, *2* somatic afferent, *3, 4, 5* sympathetic efferent, *6, 7* sympathetic afferent (Figure 799 from Gray's Anatomy (Used under CCL3.0, http://en.wikipedia.org/wiki/File:Gray799.svg))

of the neural foramen and continue more distally into the periphery of the spinal nerve to innervate the structures outside of the spinal column. Unlike nerves, the nerve roots are not enclosed by a thick epineural sheath, and so they lack the mechanical resilience of their peripheral counterparts; hence, their structural anatomy places them at particular risk for injurious mechanical loading under intervertebral disc herniation. In addition, the cell bodies of peripheral nerves are housed in the dorsal root ganglion (DRG) and can respond to even slight compression with sustained neuronal activity and pain (Hanai et al. 1996; Hu and Xing 1998; Van Zundert et al. 2006). Intraoperative studies in patients with disc herniation and associated root impingement demonstrate decreases in the amplitude of compound muscle action potentials following electrical stimulation to the affected nerve root (Morishita et al. 2006; Takamori et al. 2011). This work provides direct support for the clinical observation that functional impairment is associated with disc herniation. Reproduction of pain generating straight-leg raises in patients undergoing surgery showed that the amplitude of the evoked action potentials decreased 41 % at as early as 1 min following positioning and decreased by 63 % after 3 min (Takamori et al. 2011). The change in evoked action potential continued to develop through the period of nerve root impingement, demonstrating that time-dependent electrophysiologic responses occur in the nerve root with compression. These changes in neuronal signaling probably contribute to radiculopathy symptoms. Together, the magnitude, duration, and rate of compression of the nerve root modulate both the extent of the local tissue damage and the degree and duration of the pain symptoms (Kobayashi et al. 2005b; Olmarker et al. 1989; Rothman et al. 2010; Rydevik et al. 1991; Winkelstein et al. 2002).

As indicated above, intervertebral disc herniation can contribute to a type of neuropathic pain that has, as its most common characteristic symptom, radicular pain or radiculopathy. Self-reported pain and disability scales, such as the visual analogue scale (VAS) or Oswestry Disability Index, are often used to provide measures of pain or functional loss associated with disc herniation. Clinically, the straight-leg raise test (or SLR) is considered the most sensitive approach for quantifying the

Table 19.1 Molecular mediators of radiculopathy identified in intervertebral disc tissues. Annotated findings in footnotes

Mediator	Notes	Citation
TNF-α	1–3,6	Weiler et al. (2005), Takahashi (1996), Demircan (2007), Ahn (2002), Le Maitre et al. (2007), Nygaard (2007)
ICAM-1	1	Doita et al. (1996)
Interleukin-1α	1,2	Le Maitre (2005), Takahashi (1996), Ahn (2002)
Interleukin-1β	1,3,7	Demircan (2007), Takahashi (1996), Le Maitre et al. (2005, 2007)
Interleukin-17	3	Shamji et al. (2010)
Interleukin-4	3,5	Shamji et al. (2010), Park (2002)
Interleukin-6	1,3,6	Demircan (2007), Takahashi (1996), Kang (1997), Burke et al. (2002), Shamji et al. (2010), Specchia (2002), Nygaard (2007)
Interleukin-8	1,2,4	Demircan (2007), Ahn (2002), Burke et al. (2002)
Interleukin-12	3,4	Shamji et al. (2010), Park (2002)
Interleukin-20	1	Huang (2008)
Interferon-γ	1,3,4	Demircan (2007), Shamji et al. (2010), Park (2002)
Leukotriene-B4		Demircan (2007), Nygaard (2007), Willburger (1994)
Thromboxane-B2	1,4,7	Demircan (2007), Nygaard (2007)
Phospholipase A	1	Saal (1990)
Prostaglandin E2	1,3	O'Donnell (1996), Kang (1997), Wilburger (1994)

1. Expression noted in degenerative and/or herniated IVD
2. Protein or mRNA expression revealed in herniated IVD alone
3. Herniated or degenerated IVD > non-degenerative or autopsy control
4. Uncontained > contained herniations or non-degenerative control
5. Expression in uncontained < contained herniations
6. No evidence of protein or mRNA expression in herniated discs
7. Little or no spontaneous expression detected in herniated IVD

degree of radicular pain originating in the lumbar region, as pain is more pronounced upon elevation of the leg (van der Windt et al. 2010). Similarly, positions that reproduce pain such as forward flexion, hyperextension, and slump are sometimes used to corroborate findings of radicular pain, although imaging is commonly needed to confirm the pain source is related to intervertebral disc herniation. In patients, physical tests of muscle weakness, impaired reflexes, and sensory deficits or hypersensitivity may also be used to detect impairment associated with radiculopathy. These diagnostic and quantitative assessments are relevant to animal models as no diagnostic biomarkers that span human to animal models have yet been developed for intervertebral disc herniation radiculopathy (Brisby et al. 2002; Gajendran et al. 2011; Tokunaga et al. 2010). Tests of hypersensitivity to non-noxious (allodynia) and noxious stimuli (hyperalgesia) serve as surrogate measures of sensory changes with disc herniation and can serve as indicators of neuropathic pain in both human subjects and animals. A heightened response to a light brush of the skin would be considered a sign of mechanical allodynia, while a heightened response to pinch would be considered a sign of mechanical hyperalgesia. Patients presenting with herniation may experience either or both mechanical or/and thermal allodynia, and these serve as important metrics of pain-related behaviors in animal models of intervertebral disc herniation.

Separate from nerve root compression, a herniated disc fragment may evoke an inflammatory and immune response near an affected root (Olmarker and Larsson 1998). Indeed, the herniated tissue fragment is a known generator of many inflammatory mediators and proinflammatory cytokines, such as IL-1α, IL-6, and TNF-α (Table 19.1). Elevated expression of these molecules may activate the immune system and upregulate the expression of proteinases important for fragment resorption; nerve root compression alone may also upregulate the expression of many of these same inflammatory mediators (Kobayashi et al. 2005b). Many mediators are known generators of pain, such that they have become therapeutic targets for new and emerging studies (reviewed at the end of this chapter).

19.3 Animal Models of Intervertebral Disc Herniation

To advance therapeutic options that can change disc herniation outcomes, it is of critical importance to understand the molecular mechanisms that regulate pain, muscle changes, and dysfunction. Animal models of herniation have been extensively studied for this purpose. These models fall into two categories: (1) models designed to mimic direct nerve root compression in a well-controlled manner using plungers, constriction, or graded compression (Hou et al. 2003; Kallakuri et al. 2005; Kawakami et al. 2003; Onda et al. 2005; Sekiguchi et al. 2009); (2) models designed to mimic chemical injury that can elicit an inflammatory response through the use of chemical irritants (Colburn et al. 1999; Hashizume et al. 2000a; Hubbard and Winkelstein 2005; Kajander et al. 1996; Kawakami et al. 1994a, b; Maves et al.

1993; Olmarker et al. 1993; Winkelstein and DeLeo 2004); or (3) direct application of nucleus pulposus tissue to the nerve root (Allen et al. 2011; Brisby et al. 2000; Cuellar et al. 2005; Kawakami et al. 1999; McCarron et al. 1987; Olmarker et al. 1997; Olmarker and Myers 1998; Otani et al. 1997; Sekiguchi et al. 2008; Shamji et al. 2009). All of these animal models mimic key features of painful radiculopathy such as limb allodynia or hyperalgesia. The most commonly reported measure of limb hypersensitivity in preclinical models of intervertebral disc herniation is mechanical allodynia, detected using von Frey microfilaments applied to the plantar region of an animal's paw (Fig. 19.5) (Colburn et al. 1999; Kallakuri et al. 2005; Kobayashi et al. 2005b; Shamji et al. 2009; Rothman et al. 2010; van der Windt et al. 2010). By measuring the frequency or response of withdrawal from a given filament, the sensitivity of a limb to non-noxious mechanical stimuli can be assessed. Mechanical hyperalgesia is also a measure of limb sensitivity and can be determined by recording the time spent grooming following a pinprick or assessing the mechanical pinch force required to initiate an animal response (Randall–Selitto device). These measures have some gross relationships to pain and serve as surrogate measures of underlying neuropathology with intervertebral disc herniation.

Pain or dysesthesia can also elicit changes in grooming, locomotion, or sensorimotor skills in animal models. Pain in disc herniation models has been identified by recording key features of animal behavior over a period of time, such as the frequency of head turns toward a respective limb, leg lifts, duration of spontaneous grooming activity on a given limb, and "wet-dog shakes" (see Chap. 16) (Nakamae et al. 2011; Nilsson et al. 2011; Olmarker 2008; Olmarker et al. 2002, 2003). Alternatively, quantitative measures of gait have been used to identify compensations and disabilities resulting from intervertebral disc herniation (Allen et al. 2011; Shamji et al. 2009), made easier by the recent introduction of digitized gait apparata including the CatWalk™, Treadscan™, and Digigait™ systems (Beare et al. 2009; Berryman et al. 2009; Gensel et al. 2006; Piesla et al. 2009; Vrinten and Hamers 2003). Tracking of spatial and temporal gait parameters, such as the geometric position of the limb and paw ground contact times, can be used to obtain measures such as stride length, step width, toe-out angle, stance times, gait symmetry (a measure of limping), and running velocity (Fig. 19.3). Dynamic data describe forces and moments that occur during a gait cycle and include measures such as ground reaction forces and moments (Crawley 2007; Whishaw and Kolb 2005). These parameters are standard analytical tools in the study of musculoskeletal injury and pathology and are more recently being used to objectively quantify pain-related behaviors and functional losses in animal models of disc herniation. The major models used to study mechanisms that contribute to symptoms of intervertebral disc herniation are reviewed here, followed by an overview of developments in the area of emerging nonsurgical therapies.

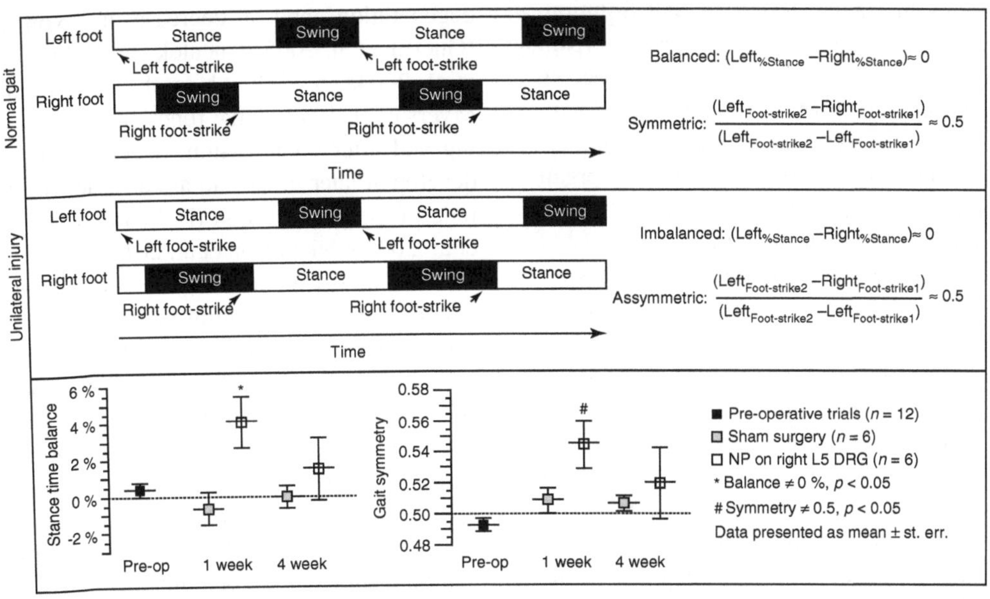

Fig. 19.3 Definitions of temporal parameters obtained from quantitative gait analysis. Rats freely ambulate across a clear gait chamber while digital video is acquired for determination of geometric positions of both hindpaws during each gait cycle. As shown, parameters of stance time, gait symmetry, as well as self-selected velocity, stance width, stride length, and more can be measured. (*Top*) Schema of a normal gait sequence wherein stance times are similar on the left and right hind limbs and a right foot-strike event occurs at the midpoint between two left foot-strike events. (*Middle*) For unilateral right limb injury, increased time is spent on the left limb and decreased time is spent on the right limb, as seen relative shifts in stance times. Also, the foot-strike sequence becomes syncopated in time, with the right limb foot strike occurring past the midway point of two left limb foot strikes. (*Bottom*) Data for stance time imbalance and gait symmetry of rats in a nucleus pulposus injury model of radiculopathy as compared to sham controls (Plotted from Hwang et al. (2012), used under CCL3.0)

Box 19.1 DRG and Neuronal Cell Culture

Intervertebral disc herniation can initiate cellular-level changes in the neurons and afferents in the dorsal root ganglion (DRG). Because many of these neuronal changes can contribute to central sensitization that induces sustained nociceptive responses in the spinal cord as well as pain, DRG culture studies are a useful proxy for investigating the pathophysiology of disc herniation. In particular, cell culture systems have the potential to recapitulate the cellular environment of primary afferents of the DRG via chemical and/or mechanical stimuli. In some cases, multi-compartment in vitro systems enable more complicated systems approaches to modeling synaptic connections, and integration of multi-electrode arrays in these setups also enables neuron-level assessments of function. In addition, culture preparations have been used to evaluate neuronal responses to challenges such as cytokines and other inflammatory mediators known to be involved in disc-mediated pain.

A variety of specialized techniques have been developed to isolate, maintain, and manipulate isolated neurons and intact DRGs from rodents. Briefly, immediately following perfusion with Krebs–Ringer bicarbonate buffer, laminectomies and facetectomies are performed to expose the DRG which is removed and immediately placed in Krebs buffer on ice. For isolation of intact neurons, the DRG is digested in collagenase under sterile conditions in Hank's Balanced Salt Solution, trypsinized, and dissociated by trituration. After trypsin inactivation, cells are resuspended in Dulbecco's Modified Eagle Medium (DMEM) supplemented with fetal bovine serum, growth factors, and antibiotics. Intact rodent DRGs may also be incubated with organ culture medium (DMEM and serum that is supplemented with glucose and nerve growth factor). Isolated neurons can be cultured on a variety of different substrates and exhibit varied responses depending on the substrate stiffness. Typically, cells are plated with culture media on glass-bottom dishes coated with poly-D-lysine in borate buffer and laminin in borate buffer. It is possible to phenotype DRG cultures to identify afferent populations using immunohistochemistry techniques to identify A fibers (by positive NF200 labeling), C fibers (negative for NF200 labeling), and also peptidergic (substance P positive) and non-peptidergic fibers (IB4 positive).

Although these culture techniques have been widespread in the neuroscience community for quite some time, they are becoming more common for understanding disc-mediated pain since they can provide a cellular-level characterization of neuronal responses to relevant stimuli related to disc herniation. They enable dose–response studies and real-time functional assays, as well as provide an exciting platform for screening potential therapeutics.

19.3.1 Mechanical Factors in Intervertebral Disc Herniation

Nerve root compression in association with disc herniation can result from acute insult to the axonal, connective, and vascular tissues of the nerve root and initiate a cascade of related and integrated neuronal, inflammatory, and degenerative changes (Kobayashi et al. 2004b; Rydevik et al. 1984, 1994; Winkelstein et al. 2002). From this perspective, mechanical injury and inflammatory injury are not unique, nor unlinked, events. Nerve root compression following acute mechanical loading can induce long-term nerve root pathophysiology, such as edema, inflammation, and thickening of connective tissues (Beck et al. 2010; Jancalek and Dubovy 2007; Kobayashi et al. 2004b; Mosconi and Kruger 1996), as well as the development of evoked pain via modified communication with the spinal cord. Following mechanical trauma and compression, injured axons exhibit axonal swelling, loss of cytoskeleton proteins, separation and disorganization of the myelin sheath, loss of axonal transport, Wallerian degeneration, and a decrease in axon packing density (Guertin et al. 2005; Jancalek and Dubovy 2007; Kobayashi et al. 2004a, b, 2005a, b, c, d; Mosconi and Kruger 1996; Myers et al. 1993). Like functional changes in neurons during and after compression, degenerative changes in axons develop at later times and are also dependent on the magnitude of the compression (Hubbard et al. 2008b; Kobayashi et al. 2005b; Nicholson et al. 2011).

Cells that respond to injury include microglia (resident macrophages in the central nervous system) and astrocytes. These cells have many roles in both the peripheral and central nervous systems, including the maintenance of homeostasis at neuronal synapses. Both types of glial cells respond to injury by changing their morphology, proliferating, upregulating cell surface markers, and releasing several inflammatory mediators (Cao and Zhang 2008; DeLeo et al. 2004; Saab et al. 2008; Suter et al. 2007). A peripheral stimulus by some neurotransmitters/neuromodulators (e.g., excitatory amino acids, substance P, ATP) (Cao and Zhang 2008; Marriott 2004) can activate early release of proinflammatory cytokines as well as nitric oxide, prostaglandins, and nerve growth factor (DeLeo et al. 2004; Inoue 2006). These mediators, in turn, induce an exaggerated release of neurotransmitters

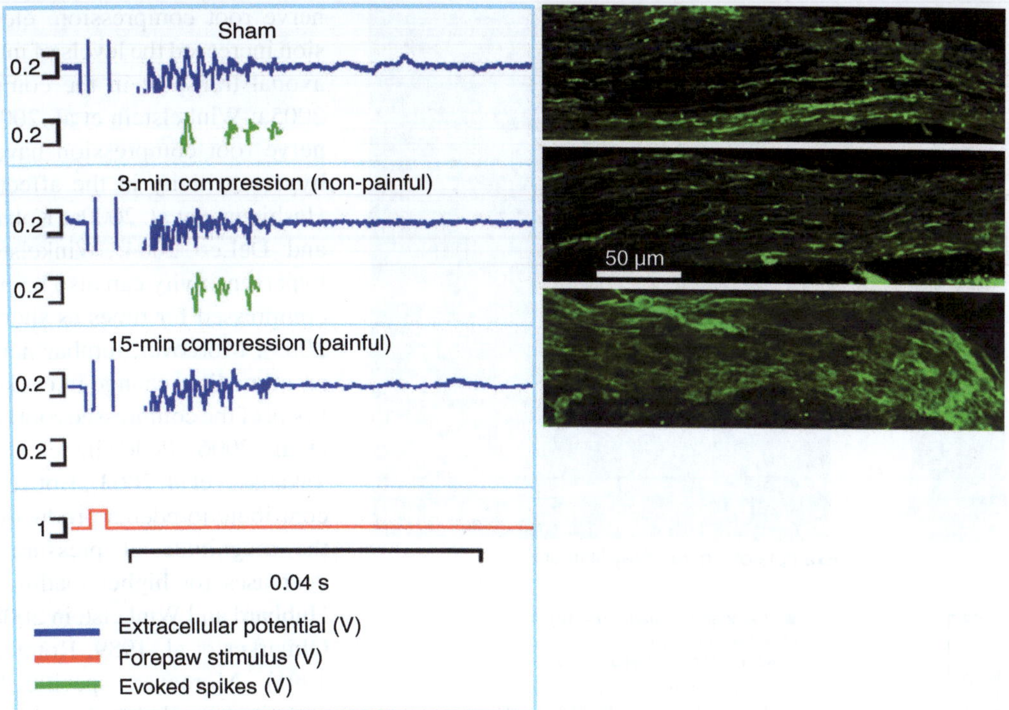

Fig. 19.4 Both the spinal extracellular potential (*blue trace*) and number of spikes evoked by electrical stimulus (*green traces*) generated following a nerve root compression are modified by the duration of the applied compression. The longer duration (15 min) compression that produces pain symptoms also causes an abolishment of evoked responses and decrease in EC response. In addition, that loading scenario also produces axonal swelling in the unmyelinated nerve fibers of the root that is absent in the 3-min (non-painful) compression

from presynaptic neurons, sensitize the postsynaptic membrane, activate neighboring astrocytes, and enhance microglial activity (DeLeo et al. 2004; Inoue 2006). This positive feedback sustains the release of pain mediators, facilitating the development of neuronal hypersensitivity and can lead to the persistent pain that is often associated with a herniated disc or inflamed nerve root. Following such neural insults, spinal glial cells become activated and modulate other immunologic changes via cytokine and growth factor production, leading to persistent pain (DeLeo and Yezierski 2001; Hashizume et al. 2000a; Obata et al. 2004; Winkelstein et al. 2001a). In particular, greater nerve root compression leads to increased activation of spinal astrocytes that is apparent as early as 1 day and is sustained in parallel with persistent symptoms of mechanical allodynia (Rothman and Winkelstein 2007). These observations suggest that spinal astrocytes may directly respond to the changes in the dorsal horn that are induced by damaged primary afferents (Hogan 2007; Sapunar et al. 2005) (Fig. 19.4).

Severe axonal injury can also induce Wallerian degeneration of the axonal process distal to the cell body (Stoll and Jander 1999; Stoll and Muller 1999). For the central axons of primary afferents, which make up the dorsal nerve root, Wallerian degeneration can occur proximal to the site of injury (Hubbard and Winkelstein 2008; Kobayashi et al. 2008). Axonal degeneration, marked by neurofilament degradation and loss of axonal integrity, is evident as early as 15 min after trauma, but is more commonly present at time points in the order of weeks (Kobayashi et al. 2008; Ramer et al. 2004). The extent of degeneration is modulated by the mechanics of the insult and is associated with persistent pain and hypersensitivity after a compression to the nerve root (Dyck et al. 1990; Hubbard et al. 2008a, b; Kobayashi et al. 2008; Nicholson et al. 2011) (Fig. 19.5). Disruption to the axonal structure has been found to be more pronounced for greater loads applied for longer durations (Dyck et al. 1990; Hubbard et al. 2008a; Kobayashi et al. 2005a, 2008; Nicholson et al. 2011). Further, the extent of damage and Wallerian degeneration of the axons in the compressed nerve root is directly related to the development of persistent hypersensitivity (Hubbard et al. 2008a, b; Hubbard and Winkelstein 2008).

The severity of nerve root injury and the intensity of pain after nerve root injury inflammation strongly relate to neuropeptide depletion in the DRG and spinal cord together with axonal degeneration (Hubbard et al. 2008a, b; Rothman et al. 2005). For example, persistent allodynia, due to higher magnitudes of dorsal nerve root compression, is associated with greater sensitivity at 1 week or later (Hubbard et al. 2008a, b). This is accompanied by a corresponding depletion of the nociceptive neuropeptide, substance P, in the DRG that similarly varies with the magnitude of the initiating compressive load (Hubbard et al. 2008b; Kobayashi et al. 2005b). Spinal expression of another potent neuropeptide for regulating pain, calcitonin gene-related peptide (CGRP), also decreases with increased painful loading to the nerve root (Hubbard et al. 2008a, b). Together with the

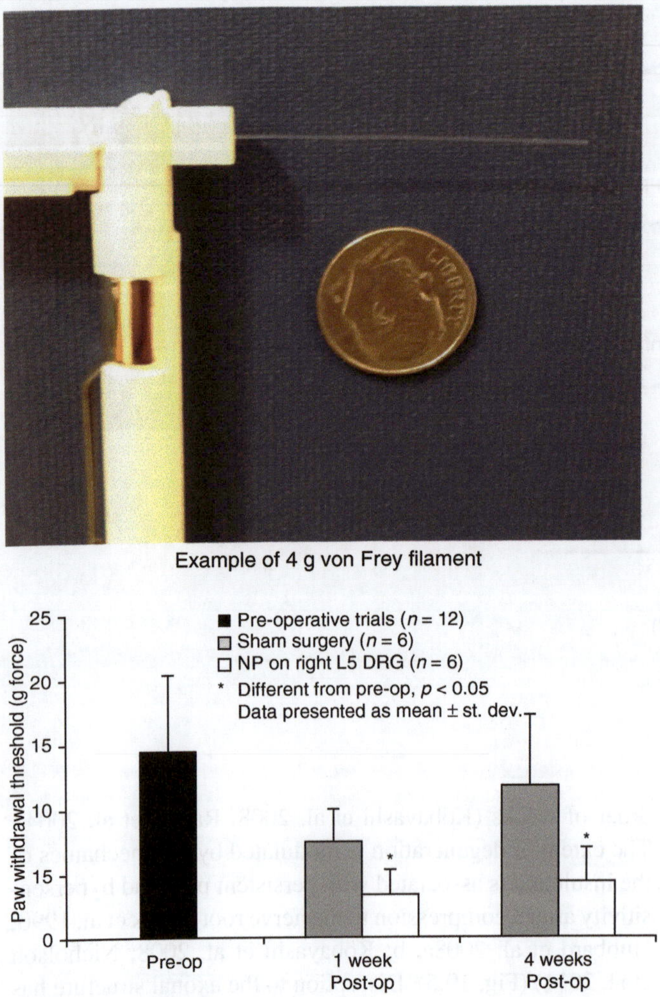

Fig. 19.5 Apparata and typical results for measuring mechanical allodynia in a rodent model of radiculopathy. (*Left*) von Frey filaments are logarithmically graded (e.g., 4g as shown) by buckling load upon compressive application. (*Right*) When filaments of varying strengths are applied to the hindpaw of a rat following placement of nucleus pulposus tissue upon the lumbar dorsal root ganglion (*DRG*), paw withdrawal is recorded over multiple trials and filaments. Data for paw withdrawal threshold of rats in an NP injury model of radiculopathy as compared to sham controls. Data show that nucleus pulposus placement upon a naïve DRG induces a paw withdrawal at lower filament strength, indicative of a persistent sensitivity to non-noxious stimuli (mechanical allodynia) (Plotted from Hwang et al. (2012), used under CCL3.0)

effects of neural trauma described above, these mechanically deleterious events can dramatically contribute to reduced transport of neuropeptides and neurotrophic factors from neurons, where these factors are synthesized, to their release from the presynaptic terminals in the spinal cord.

In animal models, the magnitude, duration, and rate of the nerve root compression have been shown to modulate the extent of the local tissue damage to the root and the degree and duration of the pain-related behaviors (Kobayashi et al. 2005a; Olmarker et al. 1989; Rothman et al. 2010; Rydevik et al. 1991; Winkelstein et al. 2002). In rodent models of nerve root compression, elevated magnitudes of compression increased the levels of mechanical allodynia and reduced axonal transport in the compressed root (Kobayashi et al. 2005a; Winkelstein et al. 2002). Although animal models of nerve root compression have shown sustained mechanical hypersensitivity in the affected limb (Colburn et al. 1999; Hashizume et al. 2000a; Kobayashi et al. 2005a; Winkelstein and DeLeo 2004; Winkelstein et al. 2002), mechanical hypersensitivity can also be produced when the nerve root is compressed for times as short as 2 s (Sekiguchi et al. 2003, 2009). Moreover, lumbar nerve root compression produces an immediate change in evoked signal conduction along the fibers of the compressed root (Fumihiko et al. 1996; Morishita et al. 2006; Pedowitz et al. 1992; Rydevik et al. 1991; Takahashi et al. 2003). Both compression rate and magnitude contribute to edema production in the nerve root, such that the magnitude of pressure required to produce edema decreases for higher loading rates (Hubbard et al. 2008b; Hubbard and Winkelstein 2008; Nicholson et al. 2011, 2012; Olmarker et al. 1989; Rothman et al. 2010; Rydevik et al. 1991). Moreover, specific loading parameters, such as magnitude and duration, likely play a role in modulating electrophysiologic responses. Animal models of nerve root compression in the cauda equina demonstrate that evoked neuronal signaling is altered during and after compression (Fumihiko et al. 1996; Garfin et al. 1990; Pedowitz et al. 1992; Rydevik et al. 1991) and decreases in the amplitude of electrically evoked compound nerve action potentials due to cauda equina compression may persist after removal of the compressive force (Pedowitz et al. 1992; Rydevik et al. 1991). These changes are corroborated by measurements in human subjects with intervertebral disc herniation that similarly show changes in evoked nerve action potentials upon straight-leg raise.

The results of studies of mechanically compressed nerve roots together with the widespread molecular changes can be integrated into a generalized schema. As early as 1 h following even a transient nerve root compression that is sufficient to produce persistent behavioral sensitivity, inflammatory cytokines, IL-6 and TNF-α, and mRNA expression levels are elevated in the ipsilateral DRG and also in the spinal cord (Rothman et al. 2009b). Within 1 day of that event, behavioral sensitivity develops along with hallmarks of spinal inflammation, including activation and proliferation of microglia (Rothman et al. 2009a). By 7 days after injury, axons of the injured nerve root show signs of degeneration, and the spinal inflammation becomes even more pronounced, and both astrocytes and microglia become activated (Hubbard and Winkelstein 2005, 2008). These changes together with the decrease in neuropeptides in the spinal cord at this same time point (Hubbard et al. 2008b) may lead to alterations in neuronal signaling in the spinal cord following a painful injury.

19.3.2 Role of Chemical and Inflammatory Mediators in Disc Herniation

As mentioned above, contributing to a cascade of chemical injuries at the affected nerve are elevated levels of inflammatory mediators, infiltration of macrophages, and activation of glial cells. To further examine these effects, animal models have been developed that mimic features of both inflammation and immune system function in intervertebral disc herniation. Both behavioral hypersensitivity and widespread immune responses are produced when chromic gut suture pieces are placed in contact with the nerve root without any mechanical perturbation (Colburn et al. 1999; Hashizume et al. 2000a; Hou et al. 2003; Hubbard and Winkelstein 2005; Kajander et al. 1996; Kawakami et al. 1994a, b; Maves et al. 1993; Murata et al. 2004a, b; Olmarker et al. 1993; Rothman and Winkelstein 2007; Rutkowski et al. 2002; Winkelstein and DeLeo 2004). Gut suture ligation simultaneously compresses the nerve root by ligation, while the chromic salts and pyrogallol in the suture serve as irritants (Colburn et al. 1999; Hashizume et al. 2000a; Kajander et al. 1996; Kawakami et al. 1994a, b; Maves et al. 1993; Robinson and Meert 2005; Winkelstein and DeLeo 2004; Xu et al. 1996). A consistent response to the chromic gut suture by the nerve root damage is the induction of thermal hyperalgesia (decreased latency to withdraw from thermal stimuli) that is transient and dose dependent; this form of hyperalgesia is not consistently present in intervertebral disc herniation models that mimic the compressive stimuli alone (Maves et al. 1993; Yamamoto and Nozaki-Taguchi 1995). The mechanisms governing the neuronal responses to chromic gut salts appear to be related to early immune activation characterized by Schwann cell proliferation, macrophage infiltration, and microglial activation. Along with these changes are molecular events including a depleted neuropeptide expression and an early expression of cell adhesion molecules such as ICAM-1 and PECAM. These adhesion molecules would serve to promote recruitment of circulating monocytes to the injured nerve root (Chang and Winkelstein 2011; Hashizume et al. 2000a; Rothman et al. 2010; Rutkowski et al. 2002; Xu et al. 1996; Yamamoto and Nozaki-Taguchi 1995). These studies indicate that, despite similarities in sensitivity to chromic gut suture and mechanical compression, differences in the pattern of hypersensitivity and molecular changes may reflect only limited injury etiologies. Nonetheless, use of chromic gut sutures as a chemical injury model for nerve root damage is popular for evaluating treatments that can interfere in the perception of disc herniation-related pain.

Soft tissues of the disc are believed to be immune privileged, in that the internal structures of the intervertebral disc do not come into contact with the systemic circulation under normal conditions and express the Fas ligand that can promote an autoimmune response. With degeneration and damage, the internal structures of the intervertebral disc can come in contact with adjacent tissues, producing an immune response that is the subject of extensive investigation. Intervertebral disc tissues contain high levels of CD68+ immunoreactive macrophages, as well as lesser quantities of T and B lymphocytes (Doita et al. 1996;

Box 19.2 Historical Information on Sciatica

What we currently understand as "sciatica" was originally considered an "evil display of demon magic" by the earliest civilizations to provide written record (Sigerist 1934). The Greeks of fifth century BC provide documentation of early attempts at treating the sudden shots of pain that were common to the spine–hip–joint complex. In Hippocratic times, corrective traction was often undertaken, with more conservative treatment that included massage, heat, dietary alterations, bed rest, and music "to pipe away pain." A particular Roman physician of the fourth century AD, Caelius Aurelianus, is noted for providing some attempt at explaining the etiopathogenesis and anatomic origins of sciatica (Drabkin ed 1950). Caelius Aurelianus believed that a sciatic attack could be caused by a sudden jerk or movement during exercise, lifting a heavy object, a sudden shock, or fall and that this presentation was most common for middle-aged persons. Surprisingly, these early Roman observations are all consistent with our present-day understanding. Further, Caelius Aurelianus believed that sciatica could be caused by a "deep-seated congelation," referring to a cutting off of squeezing of nervous tissue. In the day of Caelius Aurelianus, patients afflicted with sciatica may have been treated with a mixture of "sweet marjoram, rosemary leaf, wine, and olive oil," as well as bed rest, massage, heat, and passive range-of-motion exercises. If met with failure, a Roman may have undergone treatment with leeches, hot coals, skin hooks, and bloodletting.

References

Aurelianus, Caelius. Edited by Israel E. Drabkin, New ed., based on the first printed editions, of Caelii Aureliani Methodici Siccensis celerum vel acutarum passionum and Caelii Aureliani Methodici Siccensis tardarum passionum, Chicago : University of Chicago Press 1950.

Sigerist HE. A history of medicine (German). Oxford U.P, 1951.

Source: Adapted from Karampelas et al. Neurosurgery Focus V16: pp. 1–4, 2004

Box 19.3 Glossary of Terms

Schober index Schober index measures a patient's ability to flex the lumbar region of his or her back. In a normal standing posture, a mark is made 5 cm above and 10 cm below the iliac spine. The patient then bends to full flexion, and the distance between the two marks is measured. A distance above 20 cm in flexion is considered normal, where distances below 20 cm during flexion suggest a limited range of motion.

Oswestry Disability Index The Oswestry Disability Index is a validated questionnaire commonly used to evaluate the principal conditions associated with spinal disorders. The Oswestry Disability Index evaluates self-reports of pain intensity, emotional well-being, and ability to perform common tasks.

Visual analogue scale (VAS) Visual analogue scales are commonly used in questionnaires and surveys as ranking statistics, where subjective semiquantitative ranks are used to assess a patient's relative improvement or decline.

Radiculopathy A medical condition where one or more nerves do not function properly resulting in radicular pain, numbness, and weakness and dysfunction.

Sciatica A sharp pain sensation or series of painful sensations affecting the back, hip, or leg. Sciatica can result from compression or inflammation of the spinal nerve root in the lower back and is often described as "shooting pain" down the leg.

N-Methyl-D-aspartic acid (NMDA) receptor NMDA receptors are ionotropic glutamate receptors that help to control synaptic plasticity and regulate nociception. NMDA receptors have been identified as key regulators of peripheral and central sensitization in lumbar radiculopathy.

Allodynia Allodynia is the sensation of pain from stimuli that would not typically cause pain. Mechanical allodynia, a heightened sensitivity to light touch, and cold allodynia, a heightened sensitivity to cold, have been observed in several models of lumbar radiculopathy.

Hyperalgesia Hyperalgesia is a prolonged or exaggerated pain response to stimuli that typically would cause pain. Thermal hyperalgesia, a heightened sensitivity to heat, and mechanical hyperalgesia, a heightened sensitivity to a pinch or pinprick, have been observed in several models of lumbar radiculopathy.

Dysesthesia Dysesthesia is a sensation described as unpleasant or abnormal, but not considered painful. Dysesthesia is among the symptoms reported from neuropathies and is often associated with descriptions of limb weakness and numbness.

Ground reaction force Ground reaction forces occur as a limb contacts the ground during motion and are typically described by three ground reaction force components. Vertical ground reaction forces help to support body weight during motion. Braking and propulsive ground reaction forces occur in the direction of travel and help to propel the body forward during locomotion. Mediolateral ground reaction forces are directed toward an animal's or person's midline and help to stabilize and balance the body during locomotion.

Wet-dog shake A characteristic shaking motion resembling a wet dog shaking out its coat. The frequency of wet-dog shake motions increases in rat models of lumbar radiculopathy.

Freemont et al. 2002; Gronblad et al. 1994; Roberts et al. 2006; Shamji et al. 2010). In addition, the disc tissues secrete numerous proinflammatory cytokines and inflammatory mediators, such as interleukin-1α (IL-1α), interleukin-6 (IL-6), interleukin-17 (IL-17), and tumor necrosis factor-α (TNF-α); these cytokines may be produced by primary disc cells or by infiltrating monocytes (Bachmeier et al. 2009; Burke et al. 2002; Le Maitre et al. 2007; Murata et al. 2004a; Saal 1995; Shamji et al. 2010; Weiler et al. 2005, 2011) (Table 19.1). Numerous studies have documented the molecular effects of the herniated discal tissues (Mulleman et al. 2006a, b). Models used for these studies have included harvest of tail nucleus pulposus tissue for placement at a lumbar nerve root or cauda equina (Allen et al. 2011; Aoki et al. 2002; Brisby et al. 2000; Cuellar et al. 2005; Kawakami et al. 1999; Shamji et al. 2009; Skouen et al. 1999; Yabuki et al. 1998) or lumbar disc puncture to promote nucleus pulposus herniation (Olmarker et al. 1998; Olmarker and Myers 1998; Otani et al. 1997). Physiological changes noted in these models include reduced nerve conduction velocities, lowered endoneurial pressure for dorsal horn or sensory neurons, and elevated nitric oxide synthase activity in spinal nerve roots at 1–4 weeks following exposure to discal tissues. In addition, there is increased expression of neurotrophins, IL-1β, TNF-α, phospholipase-1, and/or nitric oxide synthase in the applied nucleus pulposus tissues or in cell bodies and intercellular domains around the DRG (Kallakuri et al. 2005; Kawakami et al. 1999; Murata et al. 2004a; Onda et al. 2002). Disc-associated cytokines (IL-1β, TNF-α, IFN-γ) applied directly to nerve roots, as opposed to cytokines secreted by nucleus fragments, have also been shown to induce electrophysiological changes, consistent with a heightened sensitivity (Ozaktay et al. 2002; 2006). It is likely that these cytokines bind to receptors for TNF-α and IL-1β on the sensory neurons (Binshtok et al. 2008; Verri et al. 2006). While these findings clearly indicate a role for inflammation and inflammatory mediators in regulating neuronal sensitivity in intervertebral disc herniation, it must be noted that many changes in the nucleus pulposus-induced or chemical injury models of radiculopathy overlap with those reported for direct compression neuropathy.

As with direct nerve root compression or chromic gut suture exposure, application of nucleus pulposus tissue to a naïve nerve root induces limb hypersensitivity that is largely characterized by a mechanical allodynia (Hou et al. 2003; Mulleman et al. 2006a, b) (Fig. 19.5). Many studies of nucleus pulposus-induced radiculopathy following disc puncture to induce nucleus herniation or placement of nucleus pulposus tissue upon the nerve root report evidence of allodynia as early as 2 days that may persist out to 3 weeks (Kawakami et al. 1999; Obata et al. 2002). Early studies also report functional changes following nucleus pulposus-induced radiculopathy, including altered footprints and visual evidence of limping, paw lift, or rotation of the head (Olmarker et al. 1998, 2002). With the use of quantitative gait analysis, our laboratories have further demonstrated gait asymmetries between ipsi- and contralateral hind limbs out to 3 or 4 weeks postoperatively, indicative of limping (Shamji et al. 2009) (Fig 19.3). Static and dynamic gait analyses indicate that animals with radiculopathy bear less weight on their affected hindpaw in both stance and during locomotion (Allen et al. 2012).

The findings discussed above suggest that radiculopathy induced by DRG exposure to nucleus pulposus tissue, as a model of intervertebral disc herniation, can repeatedly mimic key characteristics of prolonged pain sensitivity in the human patient (Allen et al. 2011; Shamji et al. 2009). The finding of persistence of sensitivity supports the notion that the molecular responses of an inflamed disc may influence sensory changes during intervertebral disc herniation. The persistent sensitivity changes, extending beyond fragment removal or resorption, imply that the widespread responses imitated in the CNS and even systemically are not ameliorated. Once initiated, the neuroimmune cascade involves activation of many nonneuronal cells in the peripheral tissues (DeLeo and Yezierski 2001; Julius and Basbaum 2001; Moalem and Tracey 2006). These resident cells, including mast and Schwann cells, release mediators such as histamine, prostaglandins, cytokines, and chemokines that also lead to the recruitment of other infiltrating immune cells (e.g., neutrophils, macrophages, lymphocytes) (DeLeo and Yezierski 2001; Moalem and Tracey 2006; Verri et al. 2006). Proinflammatory cytokines also trigger the release of many other inflammatory mediators that can sensitize nociceptors, further maintaining neuronal excitability and sensitization and leading to dysfunction and pain (Moalem and Tracey 2006; Verri et al. 2006). Nonetheless, the persistence of pain observed in some human subjects following intervertebral disc herniation that may continue for months and even years has not been replicated in these animal models, where mechanical allodynia or thermal hyperalgesia can recover to control or preoperative values at later times after surgery. Additional studies of CNS sensitization in human and animal models of disc herniation are needed to better understand the role of these important pathway changes in the pathogenesis of disc pain.

Taken together, with knowledge gained from direct nerve root compression studies, it becomes clear that many of the sensitization and functional changes associated with disc herniation may reflect contributions from both compressive trauma as well as inflammatory agents in the disc. While somewhat intuitive, the more severe nerve root injuries (with greater degrees of tissue impingement) produce more pain-associated behavioral sensitivity than those injuries with less tissue compression (Hubbard et al. 2008b; Hubbard and Winkelstein 2005; Winkelstein et al. 2001b, 2002). This graded relationship has been shown to hold true regardless of the absence or presence of molecular challenges (Winkelstein and DeLeo 2004). Indeed, evidence that the duration of the mechanical trauma modulates several different pain pathways strongly supports the concept that a more permanent mechanical insult would produce a similar or even more robust deleterious clinical effect. Based on these understandings, clinical interventions, and specifically nonsurgical therapies, are focused on alleviating the persistent sensitivity that is associated with a transient or more chronic compressive trauma to the nerve root and the associated inflammatory events. This topic is briefly covered in the next section on emerging pharmacological approaches to treat intervertebral disc herniation-associated radiculopathy.

19.4 Emerging Therapies for Intervertebral Disc-Associated Radiculopathy

As mentioned in Sect. 19.1, in the absence of motor weakness or related loss of function, conservative care is the preferred treatment for a patient presenting with pain and symptoms of radiculopathy secondary to an intervertebral disc herniation. Conservative care most frequently involves lifestyle modifications as well as orally administered nonsteroidals or opioid analgesics. Commonly prescribed selective or nonselective nonsteroidal drugs include ibuprofen, indomethacin, diclofenac, piroxicam, diflunisal, and celecoxib, few of which have demonstrated significant effects on radicular pain associated with disc herniation (Chou and Huffman 2007) (also see Chap. 15). In animal models, indomethacin, ibuprofen, diclofenac, and celecoxib have been shown to reverse allodynia following peripheral or nerve root compression and may work by lowering prostaglandins and inhibiting the resulting decreases in nerve conduction velocity and decreased intraneural blood flow (see Table 19.2). Epidural administration of anesthetics such as bupivacaine and/or corticosteroids, including methylprednisolone, is also widely used for treatment of symptoms with

Table 19.2 Summary of compounds under investigation for treatment of IVD herniation-associated radiculopathy

Agent	Route	Model description	Reference	Observations
Anti-inflammatories				
Indomethacin	Oral	Canine lumbar nerve injury	Arai et al. (2004)	Reversed changes in intraneural blood flow and nerve conduction
Ketoprofen	Systemic (i.m.)	Porcine nerve root constriction or NP tissue placement	Cornefjord et al. (2001)	Partly reversed decreased nerve conduction velocity in constriction but not NP exposure
Diclofenac	Systemic (i.m.)	Porcine nerve root constriction or NP tissue placement	Cornefjord et al. (2001)	Partly reversed decreased nerve conduction velocity
Ibuprofen	Oral	Rat sciatic nerve compression injury	Schafers et al. (2004)	Reduced mechanical allodynia at short times after injury, reduced PGE2 levels in nerve and DRG
COX-2 inhibitor celecoxib	Oral	Rat sciatic nerve compression injury	Schafers et al. (2004)	Reduced mechanical allodynia at short times after injury, reduced PGE2 levels in nerve
NO synthase inhibitor (L-NAME)	Intrathecal	Rat lumbar DRG compression injury	Ding et al. (2010)	Some reversal of thermal hyperalgesia, decreased nitrite in DRG
Prostaglandin E2 receptor antagonist (EP1-RA)	Oral	Rat exposure of lumbar DRG to NP	Sekiguchi et al. (2011)	Reduced mechanical allodynia, attenuated increased activating transcription factor-3 (ATF3) immunoreactive positive cells induced by NP
Thromboxane A2 synthetase inhibitor	Epidural	Rat exposure of lumbar DRG to NP	Kawakami et al. (2001)	Reduced mechanical allodynia
Leukotriene B4 receptor antagonist (LTB4 receptor antagonist)	Epidural	Rat exposure of lumbar DRG to NP	Kawakami et al. (2001)	Reduced mechanical allodynia
COX-2 antibody	Intrathecal	Rat exposure of lumbar DRG to NP	Ohtori et al. (2004)	Reduced mechanical allodynia
Neuronal receptor modifiers				
NMDA receptor antagonist, MK-801	Intraspinal or systemic (i.p.)	Rat spinal nerve or sciatic nerve constriction injury	Chaplan et al. (1997), Uceyler et al. (2008)	Reversed molecular changes in CNS, partly reversed motor changes
Gabapentin	Systemic i.p. or local (perineural) delivery	Rat sciatic nerve or lumbar nerve root constriction injury	Abe et al. (2002), Zanella et al. (2008)	Some reversal of mechanical allodynia
Sarpogrelate hydrochloride (5-HT2A receptor antagonist: 5-HTRA)	Systemic	Canine or rat DRG exposure to NP	Sekiguchi et al. (2008), Hashizume et al. (2007)	Decreased blood vessel diameter and increased blood flow in nerve roots inflamed by NP application, partly reversed mechanical allodynia
Cell cycle modifiers				
Minocycline	Systemic i.v. and prophylactic delivery	Rat cervical nerve root compression and chromic gut exposure	Rothman et al. (2009b)	Some reversal of mechanical allodynia, no changes in spinal microglial proliferation
Methotrexate	Intrathecal or local	Rat lumbar DRG constriction with chromic gut	Hashizume et al. (2000b)	Reduced allodynia, no changes in spinal glial activation
Pathway inhibitors				
Ruthenium red (TRPV4 antagonist) or TRPV4 antisense oligonucleotide (TRPV4 AS)	Intrathecal	Rat lumbar DRG compression injury	Ding et al. (2010)	Some reversal of thermal hyperalgesia, decreased nitrite in DRG
Soluble guanylate cyclase inhibitor (1H-[1,2,4]-oxadiazolo[4,3-a] quinoxalin-1-one, ODQ)	Intrathecal or perineural	Rat lumbar DRG compression injury, rat lumbar nerve root compression via steel rod	Song et al. (2006), Ding et al. (2010)	Some reversal of thermal hyperalgesia
8-(4-chlorophenylthio)-guanosine 3′,5′-cyclic monophosphorothioate	Intrathecal	Rat lumbar DRG compression injury	Ding et al. (2010)	Some reversal of thermal hyperalgesia

(continued)

Table 19.2 (continued)

Agent	Route	Model description	Reference	Observations
PKA antagonist (SQ22536)	Perineural	Rat lumbar nerve root compression via steel rod	Song et al. (2006)	Some reversal of thermal hyperalgesia
NF-kappa B decoy-FITC	Intrathecal	Rat L5 DRG compression and NP placement	Suzuki et al. (2009)	Reversed molecular changes in DRG, partly reversed mechanical allodynia, and thermal hyperalgesia
PKG inhibitor Rp-isomer sodium salt (Rp-8-pCPT-cGMPS)	Intrathecal	Rat lumbar nerve root compression via steel rod, rat lumbar DRG compression injury	Song et al. (2006), Ding et al. (2010)	Some reversal of thermal hyperalgesia
Protease or cytokine inhibitors				
Hydroxamic acid-based metalloproteinase inhibitor, TAPI	Epineural	Rat sciatic nerve constriction injury	Sommer et al. (1997)	Reduced thermal hyperalgesia and mechanical allodynia, reduced TNF immunoreactivity in epineurium
sTNFRI	Intrathecal or systemic	Lumbar or cervical nerve root compression with, or without chromic gut exposure	Winkelstein et al. (2001a), Rothman et al. (2009b, 2010)	Some reversal of mechanical allodynia, reduced spinal astrocytic reactivity
sTNFRII	Systemic i.p. or local (perineural)	Rat constriction nerve injury or ligation, rat DRG exposure to NP	Schafers et al. (2003), Allen et al. (2011), Zanella et al. (2008)	Some reversal of allodynia, restored normal gait
IL-1Ra	Intrathecal or systemic	Lumbar or cervical nerve root compression with or without chromic gut exposure	Winkelstein et al. (2001b), Rothman et al. (2009b, 2010)	Some reversal of allodynia, and reduced spinal astrocytic reactivity
Salmon fibrin and thrombin	Perineural	Rat cervical nerve root compression	Weisshaar et al. (2011)	Partly reversed mechanical allodynia and reduced macrophage recruitment

radiculopathy, and they appear to have some efficacy as measured with both objective (e.g., straight-leg raising test) and self-reported outcomes (e.g., VAS) (Buenaventura et al. 2009; Staal et al. 2008). Methylprednisolone and other corticosteroids may work by inhibiting the increase in endoneurial vascular permeability and the decrease in nerve conduction velocity that follows injury to the nerve root upon exposure to nucleus pulposus tissue or chemical injury (Byrod et al. 2000; Olmarker et al. 1994). Regardless of the mechanism, use of these NSAIDs and corticosteroids is generally considered safe and a first line of treatment for patients presenting with pain from intervertebral disc herniation.

The current standard of care does not address the underlying pathology of intervertebral disc herniation, which clearly involves inflammatory, proteolytic, and immune-mediated pathways. As new knowledge from animal models is gained, an understanding of the role of inflammatory mediators in mediating responses to nerve root injury has emerged; the focus here is on cytokines that regulate immune system involvement, such as TNF-α, or those that mediate pain sensitivity such as α2 adrenergic receptor and serotonin receptor antagonists. Pharmacological approaches that target perception of pain and restoration of functional losses with radiculopathy, as well as those that influence disease pathways, have great potential to reduce the duration of symptoms and disability associated with disc herniation and may even play a role in reducing the need for surgical intervention. Here, we will briefly review ongoing investigations to pharmacologically treat radiculopathy associated with disc herniation and to identify those with the most promising therapeutic potential.

19.4.1 Cytokine Antagonism

Given the documented increase of TNF-α and IL-1β expression in degenerated and herniated discal tissues, as well as clear evidence of a role for the cytokine TNF-α in reproducing many symptoms of radiculopathy in animal models (Allen et al. 2011; Olmarker 2001; Onda et al. 2002; Rothman and Winkelstein 2010; Winkelstein et al. 2001a), cytokine antagonism has received considerable attention. In our prior studies, we have demonstrated an ability for IL-1β antagonists (IL-1Ra or Kineret™) to partially reverse mechanical allodynia and spinal astrocytic reactivity following nerve root compression (Rothman and Winkelstein 2010; Winkelstein et al. 2001a, Table 2). The finding that TNF antagonists (blocking antibodies) influence peripheral nerve injury (DeLeo et al. 2000; Lindenlaub et al. 2000; Sommer et al. 2001) and attenuate allodynia in constriction injury models, and that overexpression of TNF could elevate allodynia in the same model, has evoked considerable interest in this class of compounds. Application of exogenous TNF-α to lumbar nerve roots in the rat reproduces many of the neurophysiology changes described earlier for compression-induced nerve root injury, including decreased nerve conduction velocity, glial activation, and inflammatory changes in the ganglion (Aoki et al. 2002; Igarashi et al. 2000;

Onda et al. 2002; Ozaktay et al. 2002). Furthermore, systemic treatment with the TNF-blocking antibody, Remicade® (infliximab, intravenous or intraperitoneal), reduced pain-related movements in rats, as well as the expression of key neurotrophins in the DRG and spinal cord (Murata et al. 2004b; Olmarker et al. 2003; Olmarker and Rydevik 2001; Onda et al. 2004; Sasaki et al. 2007). In other animal studies, including our own, local delivery of a soluble TNF receptor type II analogue (etanercept or Enbrel®) has been shown to restore normal gait patterns and reverse the heightened allodynia response to nucleus pulposus placement upon the DRG as a model of intervertebral disc herniation (Allen et al. 2011; Cuellar et al. 2004). These results add strength to the notion that TNF inhibition can attenuate or reverse changes in animal locomotion, nerve electrophysiology, and pathology due to nucleus pulposus exposure in the short term (<7 days). For these reasons, the hypothesis has evolved that, in response to disc herniation, TNF-α serves as the critical cytokine mediating nerve sensitivity and inflammation. This plausible mechanism is supported by the elevated tissue levels of TNF-α in the degenerative disc as well the increased number of activated macrophages and lymphocytes in herniated tissue fragments that secrete the cytokine. Thus, it is plausible that TNF-α contributes, at least in part, to the perception of pain and promotes neuroinflammation following disc herniation. For this reason, to date, clinical studies that target symptoms of disc herniation-associated radiculopathy have focused largely on TNF antagonists.

In a first study of TNF inhibitors to antagonize pain associated with intervertebral disc herniation, patients with a history of herniation-associated sciatica (average duration of symptoms = 7 weeks) were given a single intravenous infusion of infliximab ($n = 10$, 3 mg/kg, Karppinen et al. 2003) or treated with periradicular saline as a "historical control" ($n = 62$). Outcomes of visual analogue scale (VAS), straight-leg raising test, low back pain severity, and Oswestry Disability Index were measured at baseline and out to 3 months after treatment. All outcomes outperformed the saline control, with the exception of a decrease in leg pain reported at 1 h after the infusion, and sustained out to 3 months (88 and 51 % change from baseline, infliximab vs. saline). Similar changes supportive of infliximab treatment were noted in low back pain severity, straight-leg raising test results, the Schöber index, and the Oswestry index. No patients required surgery and none experienced adverse effects of infliximab, while motor and sensory loss resolved in patients within 1–3 months. A later study evaluated the efficacy of subcutaneous injections of etanercept (25 mg every 3 days, 3 injections) in ten patients with acute severe sciatica (mean symptom duration of 2–7 weeks (Genevay et al. 2004)). Visual analogue scales (VAS) for leg and back pain, as well as Oswestry Disability Index and modified Roland–Morris Disability Questionnaire, were obtained after 10 days and 6 weeks. A good clinical response was observed in nine or ten patients at 6 weeks after treatment, although no control group was cited in this study. Over the years, multiple clinicians have individually described case reports of their experiences with delivery of infliximab or etanercept for the treatment of disc herniation-related radiculopathy that was otherwise nonresponsive to treatment (Atcheson and Dymeck 2004; Tobinick and Britschgi-Davoodifar 2003). Decreases in pain scores and improved disability indices are generally reported, leading to the emergence of TNF inhibitors as available strategies for clinical treatment of pain associated with intervertebral disc herniation.

The first randomized controlled trial of TNF antagonism for radiculopathy (termed FIRST II, Finnish Infliximab Related Study) (Korhonen et al. 2006; Korhonen et al. 2005) was reported in 2006. Patients ($n = 40$ with symptomatic disc herniation on MRI, leg pain <12 weeks. ≤60° on the straight-leg raising test) were treated with a single intravenous infusion of infliximab (5 mg/kg) and compared against a placebo. Straight-leg raise, motor and sensory defects, leg and back pain (VAS), Oswestry disability, quality of life (RAND-36), and more parameters were compared between the treatment and placebo groups out to 1 year following treatment. Results were not supportive of infliximab therapy, however, with 67 and 63 % of all patients reporting no pain in the infliximab and placebo groups, respectively. Similar values were observed between treatment groups for other outcomes, although a subgroup of patients in the infliximab group appeared to especially benefit from the infliximab treatment (an L4–L5 or L3–L4 herniation with a Modic change at the symptomatic level). The authors concluded that further study of this subgroup of patients may yield insights about the potential for TNF antagonists to modify clinical outcomes for intervertebral disc herniation.

A recent study of epidural etanercept for radiculopathy (Cohen et al. 2009) provided a more promising result. Patients with unresolved symptoms ($n = 12$, >2 months in duration) received 2 injections of etanercept (2, 4, or 6 mg). A majority of patients noted complete resolution of pain by 3 months after treatment with etanercept; this was much higher than the 17 % for the epidural saline control group. While a small study, it nonetheless illustrates the potential for local administration of TNF antagonists to modify radicular pain associated with disc herniation.

19.4.2 Neuronal Receptor Blockers

Another set of targets proposed for the treatment of intervertebral disc herniation-associated pain centers around blocking receptors involved in neuronal activation. Compounds shown in Table 19.2 generally act by competitively binding to receptors that control neuronal excitation and downstream effectors. When delivered systemically, their activity is not localized to the affected nerve and can involve the CNS and other sites. In preclinical models, an NMDA receptor antagonist, administered systemically following sciatic nerve ligation, reversed mRNA changes induced by peripheral nerve constriction (Uceyler et al. 2008). When administered locally, this NMDA receptor antagonist was also capable of partly reversing motor deficits and allodynia following lumbar spinal nerve ligation (Chaplan et al. 1997). In animal models, the GABA analogue, gabapentin, whether delivered locally or systemically also caused a similar reversal of allodynia (Abe et al. 2002; Zanella et al. 2008). Indeed, orally prescribed gabapentin has been shown to relieve symptoms associated with radiculopathy from lumbar disc herniation when measured by the VAS or self-reported disability indices; on the other hand, systemic delivery is associated with frequent and adverse side effects (Kasimcan and Kaptan 2010; Yildirim et al. 2009). Nevertheless, this class of receptor blockers appears to be of use for the treatment of radiculopathy and superior to nonsteroidal anti-inflammatory drugs, especially when delivered locally.

The serotonin receptor, 5-HT(2A), blocker, sarpogrelate hydrochloride, has been used for both animal model and clinical studies for the treatment of sciatica. In a rat model, 5-HT(2A) receptor blockers were shown to decrease blood flow to a nerve inflamed by placement of nucleus pulposus tissue upon the nerve root and to reverse allodynia (Hashizume et al. 2007; Sekiguchi et al. 2008). In patients, high doses (300 mg) of sarpogrelate hydrochloride given orally led to significant improvements in VAS scales of sciatic pain in a majority of patients, with few patients (<20 %) needing to go on to surgery (Kanayama et al. 2003). Patients with an "uncontained disc herniation," or one that is extruded or sequestered from the parent disc, responded more favorably to the 5-HT(2A) blocker treatment with few side effects, suggesting this approach may be useful for alleviating symptoms associated with intervertebral disc herniation.

19.4.3 Cell Cycle Modifiers

A number of therapeutic approaches have been proposed to target the microglia that are believed to be activated early in the inflammation cascade that follows compression or chemical injury to the nerve root. The neuroprotective antibiotic minocycline, as well as the antimetabolite methotrexate, attenuates allodynia induced by DRG constriction injury, yet does not appear to act through attenuation of glial activation following injury (Table 19.2).

19.4.4 Pathway Inhibitors

New developing therapies that target the NF-κB or protein kinase pathways have been proposed (Table 19.2). Results of animal studies show that pathway inhibitors are able to partly reverse thermal hyperalgesia induced by DRG compression or nucleus pulposus placement. Importantly, inhibition of NF-κB, a key mediator of TNF-α signaling, appears to also reverse changes in the mRNA profile downstream of DRG compression. As for cell cycle modifiers, additional studies are required to promote the concept that any specific inhibitor can influence neuroinflammation linked to intervertebral disc herniation.

19.5 Final Comments

This review focuses on pathological events associated with disc herniation, in particular the grade of nerve root compression and the exposure and presence of nucleus pulposus tissue. The impact of herniation can thus be viewed as not one disorder, but perhaps two or three distinct conditions that can benefit from distinctly different therapeutic approaches. A contained or protruding herniation that is linked to prolonged nerve root compression may be associated with electrophysiological changes that can benefit from early intervention including the use of agents to attenuate glial activation and mediate pain sensitivity (e.g., neuronal receptor modifiers). An uncontained or extruded disc herniation that has components of both nerve root compression and tissue-mediated inflammation may be better addressed with a combined anti-inflammatory approach including the use of cytokine antagonists and protein kinase or NF-κB inhibitors. In all cases, it appears that systemic delivery of these agents will be associated with lower efficacy and higher risk of side effects than local drug delivery; this view is supported by the increased interest in epidural administration of immunosuppressants like the TNF antagonists and advancement of novel, depot-based delivery systems (Hubbard et al. 2009; Shamji et al. 2008; Zanella et al. 2008). Of course, surgery for disc fragment removal remains an option for patients that are nonresponsive to pharmacologic and alternate approaches. However, it is becoming clear that residual and persistent hypersensitivity from long-term nerve root compression can be a deleterious event and a constant source of intense pain. Thus, demand will continue for strategies that attenuate the neuropathy associated with intervertebral disc herniation, shorten the symptom period, and promote functional recovery.

19.6 Summary of Critical Concepts Discussed in the Chapter

Fragments of intervertebral disc that "herniate" into the extra-discal space and impinge upon, or contact, the spinal nerve roots can cause significant pain, neurological deficits, and functional disability in a large number of affected individuals.

- Nerve root impingement due to a herniated disc can result in nerve root pathophysiology, including edema, inflammation, disorganization of the myelin sheath, decreased axonal packing, Wallerian degeneration of the peripheral axons, and loss of axonal transport and decreased amplitudes of evoked action potentials.
- Nerve root changes are associated with developing hypersensitivity to non-noxious (allodynia) and noxious stimuli (hyperalgesia) that serve as useful indicators of neuropathic pain in both human subjects and animals.
- The magnitude, duration, and rate of compression of the nerve root promote local nerve root damage and the degree and duration of the pain symptoms.
- Herniated intervertebral disc exhibits increased angiogenesis, macrophage and lymphocyte infiltration, and proinflammatory cytokine and proteinase activity that can contribute to sustained painful symptoms over a period of months to years.
- Herniated disc fragments may activate the immune system when in contact with the systemic circulation, glial cells of the affected nerves, and the central nervous system (microglia and astrocytes). The activated microglia will release increased levels of neurotransmitters from presynaptic neurons, sensitize the postsynaptic membrane, activate neighboring astrocytes, and enhance microglial activity. Hence, the initiation of nerve root damage by a herniated disc can drive a positive feedback loop that can promote a sustained painful neuropathy.
- While surgical removal of the herniated disc fragment can alleviate many of the pathological symptoms, pharmacological interventions and lifestyle modifications are the first line of treatment for pain from disc herniation.
- The use of NSAIDs and corticosteroids with herniation-associated radiculopathy is safe, but provides no means to modify pathology or outcomes. Emerging pharmacological therapies provide some promise here and are focused on antagonizing the many proinflammatory cytokines implicated in radiculopathy, most notably tumor necrosis factor (TNF-α).
- Pharmacologic interventions that show promise in the treatment of herniation-associated radiculopathy include the class of competitive inhibitors of neuronal receptors (e.g., serotonin receptor antagonists), inhibitors of glial proliferation (e.g., minocycline) or metabolism (e.g., methotrexate), and inhibitors of the cellular inflammatory pathways (e.g., NF-κB or PKC inhibitors).
- Additional work is needed to reveal the role of central nervous system sensitization and remodeling in response to disc herniation and to better understand its role in the persistent neuropathy.

In summary, there is a growing demand for strategies that attenuate neuropathy associated with intervertebral disc herniation and shorten the duration of pain and functional recovery.

Acknowledgments This work was supported by grants from the NIH R00AR057426 (KDA), R01AR047442 (LAS), P01AR050245 (LAS), DOD (BAW), and the Catherine Sharpe Foundation (BAW).

References

Abe M, Kurihara T, Han W, Shinomiya K, Tanabe T (2002) Changes in expression of voltage-dependent ion channel subunits in dorsal root ganglia of rats with radicular injury and pain. Spine (Phila Pa 1976) 27:1517–1524; discussion 1525

Adams MA, Roughley PJ (2006) What is intervertebral disc degeneration, and what causes it? Spine (Phila Pa 1976) 31:2151–2161

Ahn SH, Cho YW, Ahn MW, Jang SH, Sohn YK, Kim HS (2002) mRNA expression of cytokines and chemokines in herniated lumbar intervertebral discs. Spine 27(9):911–917

Allen KD, Shamji MF, Mata BA, Gabr MA, Sinclair SM, Schmitt DO, Richardson WJ, Setton LA (2011) Kinematic and dynamic gait compensations in a rat model of lumbar radiculopathy and the effects of tumor necrosis factor-alpha antagonism. Arthritis Res Ther 13:R137

Allen KD, Mata BA, Gabr MA, Huebner JL, Adams SB Jr, Kraus VB, Schmitt DO, Setton LA (2012) Kinematic and dynamic gait compensations resulting from knee instability in a rat model of osteoarthritis. Arthritis Res Ther 14:R78

Aoki K, Rydevik B, Kikuchi S, Olmarker K (2002) Local application of disc-related cytokines on spinal nerve roots. Spine 27: 1614–1617

Arai I, Mao GP, Otani K, Konno S, Kikuchi S, Olmarker K (2004) Indomethacin blocks the nucleus pulposus-induced effects on nerve root function. An experimental study in dogs with assessment of nerve conduction and blood flow following experimental disc herniation. Eur Spine J 13(8):691–694

Atcheson SG, Dymeck T (2004) Rapid resolution of chronic sciatica with intravenous infliximab after failed epidural steroid injections. Spine 29:E248–E250

Atlas SJ, Keller RB, Wu YA, Deyo RA, Singer DE (2005) Long-term outcomes of surgical and nonsurgical management of lumbar spinal stenosis: 8 to 10 year results from the maine lumbar spine study. Spine (Phila Pa 1976) 30:936–943

Awad JN, Moskovich R (2006) Lumbar disc herniations: surgical versus nonsurgical treatment. Clin Orthop Relat Res 443:183–197

Bachmeier BE, Nerlich A, Mittermaier N, Weiler C, Lumenta C, Wuertz K, Boos N (2009) Matrix metalloproteinase expression levels suggest distinct enzyme roles during lumbar disc herniation and degeneration. Eur Spine J 18:1573–1586

Battie MC, Videman T (2006) Lumbar disc degeneration: epidemiology and genetics. J Bone Joint Surg Am 88(Suppl 2):3–9

Battie MC, Videman T, Kaprio J, Gibbons LE, Gill K, Manninen H, Saarela J, Peltonen L (2009) The twin spine study: contributions to a changing view of disc degeneration. Spine J 9:47–59

Beare JE, Morehouse JR, DeVries WH, Enzmann GU, Burke DA, Magnuson DS, Whittemore SR (2009) Gait analysis in normal and spinal contused mice using the treadscan system. J Neurotrauma 26:2045–2056

Beck KD, Nguyen HX, Galvan MD, Salazar DL, Woodruff TM, Anderson AJ (2010) Quantitative analysis of cellular inflammation after traumatic spinal cord injury: evidence for a multiphasic inflammatory response in the acute to chronic environment. Brain 133:433–447

Berryman ER, Harris RL, Moalli M, Bagi CM (2009) Digigait quantitation of gait dynamics in rat rheumatoid arthritis model. J Musculoskelet Neuronal Interact 9:89–98

Binshtok AM, Wang H, Zimmermann K, Amaya F, Vardeh D, Shi L, Brenner GJ, Ji RR, Bean BP, Woolf CJ, Samad TA (2008) Nociceptors are interleukin-1beta sensors. J Neurosci 28: 14062–14073

Bostman OM (1993) Body mass index and height in patients requiring surgery for lumbar intervertebral disc herniation. Spine (Phila Pa 1976) 18:851–854

Brisby H, Byrod G, Olmarker K, Miller VM, Aoki Y, Rydevik B (2000) Nitric oxide as a mediator of nucleus pulposus-induced effects on spinal nerve roots. J Orthop Res 18:815–820

Brisby H, Olmarker K, Larsson K, Nutu M, Rydevik B (2002) Proinflammatory cytokines in cerebrospinal fluid and serum in patients with disc herniation and sciatica. Eur Spine J 11:62–66

Buenaventura RM, Datta S, Abdi S, Smith HS (2009) Systematic review of therapeutic lumbar transforaminal epidural steroid injections. Pain Physician 12:233–251

Burke JG, Watson RW, McCormack D, Dowling FE, Walsh MG, Fitzpatrick JM (2002) Intervertebral discs which cause low back pain secrete high levels of proinflammatory mediators. J Bone Joint Surg Br 84:196–201

Byrod G, Otani K, Brisby H, Rydevik B, Olmarker K (2000) Methylprednisolone reduces the early vascular permeability increase in spinal nerve roots induced by epidural nucleus pulposus application. J Orthop Res 18:983–987

Cao H, Zhang YQ (2008) Spinal glial activation contributes to pathological pain states. Neurosci Biobehav Rev 32:972–983

Chang YW, Winkelstein BA (2011) Schwann cell proliferation and macrophage infiltration are evident at day 14 after painful cervical nerve root compression in the rat. J Neurotrauma 28:2429–2438

Chaplan SR, Malmberg AB, Yaksh TL (1997) Efficacy of spinal NMDA receptor antagonism in formalin hyperalgesia and nerve injury evoked allodynia in the rat. J Pharmacol Exp Ther 280:829–838

Chou R, Huffman LH (2007) Medications for acute and chronic low back pain: a review of the evidence for an American Pain Society/ American College of Physicians clinical practice guideline. Ann Intern Med 147:505–514

Cohen SP, Bogduk N, Dragovich A, Buckenmaier CC 3rd, Griffith S, Kurihara C, Raymond J, Richter PJ, Williams N, Yaksh TL (2009) Randomized, double-blind, placebo-controlled, dose–response, and preclinical safety study of transforaminal epidural etanercept for the treatment of sciatica. Anesthesiology 110:1116–1126

Colburn RW, Rickman AJ, DeLeo JA (1999) The effect of site and type of nerve injury on spinal glial activation and neuropathic pain behavior. Exp Neurol 157:289–304

Cornefjord M, Olmarker K, Otani K, Rydevik B (2001) Effects of diclofenac and ketoprofen on nerve conduction velocity in experimental nerve root compression. Spine (Phila Pa 1976) 26(20):2193–2197

Crawley JN (2007) What's wrong with my mouse? Behavioral phenotyping of transgenic and knockout mice. Wiley-Interscience, Hoboken

Cuellar JM, Montesano PX, Carstens E (2004) Role of TNF-alpha in sensitization of nociceptive dorsal horn neurons induced by application of nucleus pulposus to L5 dorsal root ganglion in rats. Pain 110:578–587

Cuellar JM, Montesano PX, Antognini JF, Carstens E (2005) Application of nucleus pulposus to L5 dorsal root ganglion in rats enhances nociceptive dorsal horn neuronal windup. J Neurophysiol 94:35–48

DeLeo JA, Yezierski RP (2001) The role of neuroinflammation and neuroimmune activation in persistent pain. Pain 90:1–6

DeLeo JA, Rutkowski MD, Stalder AK, Campbell IL (2000) Transgenic expression of TNF by astrocytes increases mechanical allodynia in a mouse neuropathy model. Neuroreport 11:599–602

DeLeo JA, Tanga FY, Tawfik VL (2004) Neuroimmune activation and neuroinflammation in chronic pain and opioid tolerance/hyperalgesia. Neuroscientist 10:40–52

Demircan MN, Asir A, Cetinkal A, Gedik N, Kutlay AM, Colak A et al. (2007) Is there any relationship between proinflammatory mediator levels in disc material and myelopathy with cervical disc herniation and spondylosis? A non-randomized, prospective clinical study. Eur Spine J 16(7):983–986

Ding XL, Wang YH, Ning LP, Zhang Y, Ge HY, Jiang H, Wang R, Yue SW (2010) Involvement of TRPV4-NO-cGMP-PKG pathways in the development of thermal hyperalgesia following chronic compression of the dorsal root ganglion in rats. Behav Brain Res 208(1):194–201

Doita M, Kanatani T, Harada T, Mizuno K (1996) Immunohistologic study of the ruptured intervertebral disc of the lumbar spine. Spine 21:235–241

Dyck PJ, Lais AC, Giannini C, Engelstad JK (1990) Structural alterations of nerve during cuff compression. Proc Natl Acad Sci U S A 87:9828–9832

Fraser I (2009) Statistics on hospital-based care in the United States. Agency for Healthcare Research and Quality, Rockville

Freemont AJ, Watkins A, Le Maitre C, Jeziorska M, Hoyland JA (2002) Current understanding of cellular and molecular events in intervertebral disc degeneration: implications for therapy. J Pathol 196:374–379

Frymoyer JW (1988) Back pain and sciatica. N Engl J Med 318:291–300

Fumihiko H, Nobuo M, Nobuo H (1996) Changes in responses of wide dynamic range neurons in the spinal dorsal horn after dorsal root or dorsal root ganglion compression. Spine (Phila Pa 1976) 21:1408–1414

Gajendran VK, Reuter MW, Golish SR, Hanna LS, Scuderi GJ (2011) Is the fibronectin-aggrecan complex present in cervical disk disease? PM R 3:1030–1034

Garfin SR, Cohen MS, Massie JB, Abitbol JJ, Swenson MR, Myers RR, Rydevik BL (1990) Nerve-roots of the cauda equina. The effect of hypotension and acute graded compression on function. J Bone Joint Surg Am 72:1185–1192

Genevay S, Stingelin S, Gabay C (2004) Efficacy of etanercept in the treatment of acute, severe sciatica: a pilot study. Ann Rheum Dis 63:1120–1123

Gensel JC, Tovar CA, Hamers FP, Deibert RJ, Beattie MS, Bresnahan JC (2006) Behavioral and histological characterization of unilateral cervical spinal cord contusion injury in rats. J Neurotrauma 23:36–54

Goupille P, Jayson MI, Valat JP, Freemont AJ (1998) The role of inflammation in disk herniation-associated radiculopathy. Semin Arthritis Rheum 28:60–71

Gronblad M, Virri J, Tolonen J, Seitsalo S, Kaapa E, Kankare J, Myllynen P, Karaharju EO (1994) A controlled immunohistochemical study of inflammatory cells in disc herniation tissue. Spine (Phila Pa 1976) 19:2744–2751

Guertin AD, Zhang DP, Mak KS, Alberta JA, Kim HA (2005) Microanatomy of axon/glial signaling during Wallerian degeneration. J Neurosci 25:3478–3487

Hanai F, Matsui N, Hongo N (1996) Changes in responses of wide dynamic range neurons in the spinal dorsal horn after dorsal root or dorsal root ganglion compression. Spine 21:1408–1414; discussion 1414–1415

Hart LG, Deyo RA, Cherkin DC (1995) Physician office visits for low back pain. Frequency, clinical evaluation, and treatment patterns from a US national survey. Spine (Phila Pa 1976) 20: 11–19

Hashizume H, DeLeo JA, Colburn RW, Weinstein JN (2000a) Spinal glial activation and cytokine expression after lumbar root injury in the rat. Spine (Phila Pa 1976) 25:1206–1217

Hashizume H, Rutkowski MD, Weinstein JN, DeLeo JA (2000b) Central administration of methotrexate reduces mechanical allodynia in an animal model of radiculopathy/sciatica. Pain 87(2):159–169

Hashizume H, Kawakami M, Yoshida M, Okada M, Enyo Y, Inomata Y (2007) Sarpogrelate hydrochloride, a 5-HT2a receptor antagonist, attenuates neurogenic pain induced by nucleus pulposus in rats. Spine (Phila Pa 1976) 32:315–320

Heliovaara M (1987a) Body height, obesity, and risk of herniated lumbar intervertebral disc. Spine (Phila Pa 1976) 12:469–472

Heliovaara M (1987b) Occupation and risk of herniated lumbar intervertebral disc or sciatica leading to hospitalization. J Chronic Dis 40:259–264

Heliovaara M, Impivaara O, Sievers K, Melkas T, Knekt P, Korpi J, Aromaa A (1987a) Lumbar disc syndrome in Finland. J Epidemiol Community Health 41:251–258

Heliovaara M, Knekt P, Aromaa A (1987b) Incidence and risk factors of herniated lumbar intervertebral disc or sciatica leading to hospitalization. J Chronic Dis 40:251–258

Hogan QH (2007) Role of decreased sensory neuron membrane calcium currents in the genesis of neuropathic pain. Croat Med J 48:9–21

Hou SX, Tang JG, Chen HS, Chen J (2003) Chronic inflammation and compression of the dorsal root contribute to sciatica induced by the intervertebral disc herniation in rats. Pain 105:255–264

Hu SJ, Xing JL (1998) An experimental model for chronic compression of dorsal root ganglion produced by intervertebral foramen stenosis in the rat. Pain 77:15–23

Huang KY, Lin RM, Chen WY, Lee CL, Yan JJ, Chang MS (2008) IL-20 may contribute to the pathogenesis of human intervertebral disc herniation. Spine 33(19):2034–2040

Hubbard RD, Winkelstein BA (2005) Transient cervical nerve root compression in the rat induces bilateral forepaw allodynia and spinal glial activation: mechanical factors in painful neck injuries. Spine (Phila Pa 1976) 30:1924–1932

Hubbard RD, Winkelstein BA (2008) Dorsal root compression produces myelinated axonal degeneration near the biomechanical thresholds for mechanical behavioral hypersensitivity. Exp Neurol 212:482–489

Hubbard RD, Chen Z, Winkelstein BA (2008a) Transient cervical nerve root compression modulates pain: load thresholds for allodynia and sustained changes in spinal neuropeptide expression. J Biomech 41:677–685

Hubbard RD, Quinn KP, Martinez JJ, Winkelstein BA (2008b) The role of graded nerve root compression on axonal damage, neuropeptide changes, and pain-related behaviors. Stapp Car Crash J 52:33–58

Hubbard RD, Martinez JJ, Burdick JA, Winkelstein BA (2009) Controlled release of GDNF reduces nerve root-mediated behavioral hypersensitivity. J Orthop Res 27:120–127

Hwang PY, Allen KD, Shamji MF, Jing L, Mata BA, Gabr MA, Huebner JL, Kraus VB, Richardson WJ, Setton LA (2012) Changes in midbrain pain receptor expression, gait and behavioral sensitivity in a rat model of radiculopathy. Open Orthop J 6:383–391. PubMed Central PMCID: PMC3434701

Igarashi T, Kikuchi S, Shubayev V, Myers RR (2000) 2000 Volvo Award winner in Basic Science Studies: exogenous tumor necrosis factor-alpha mimics nucleus pulposus-induced neuropathology. Molecular, histologic, and behavioral comparisons in rats. Spine 25:2975–2980

Inoue K (2006) The function of microglia through purinergic receptors: neuropathic pain and cytokine release. Pharmacol Ther 109: 210–226

Jancalck R, Dubovy P (2007) An experimental animal model of spinal root compression syndrome: an analysis of morphological changes of myelinated axons during compression radiculopathy and after decompression. Exp Brain Res 179:111–119

Julius D, Basbaum AI (2001) Molecular mechanisms of nociception. Nature 413:203–210

Kajander KC, Pollock CH, Berg H (1996) Evaluation of hindpaw position in rats during chronic constriction injury (CCI) produced with different suture materials. Somatosens Mot Res 13:95–101

Kallakuri S, Takebayashi T, Ozaktay AC, Chen C, Yang S, Wooley PH, Cavanaugh JM (2005) The effects of epidural application of allografted nucleus pulposus in rats on cytokine expression, limb withdrawal and nerve root discharge. Eur Spine J 14:956–964

Kanayama M, Hashimoto T, Shigenobu K, Yamane S (2003) Efficacy of serotonin receptor blocker for symptomatic lumbar disc herniation. Clin Orthop Relat Res (411):159–165

Kang JD, Stefanovic-Racic M, McIntyre LA, Georgescu HI, Evans CH (1997) Toward a biochemical understanding of human intervertebral disc degeneration and herniation. Contributions of nitric oxide, interleukins, prostaglandin E2, and matrix metalloproteinases. Spine 22(10):1065–1073

Karppinen J, Korhonen T, Malmivaara A, Paimela L, Kyllonen E, Lindgren KA, Rantanen P, Tervonen O, Niinimaki J, Seitsalo S, Hurri H (2003) Tumor necrosis factor-alpha monoclonal antibody, infliximab, used to manage severe sciatica. Spine 28:750–753; discussion 753–754

Kasimcan O, Kaptan H (2010) Efficacy of gabapentin for radiculopathy caused by lumbar spinal stenosis and lumbar disk hernia. Neurol Med Chir (Tokyo) 50:1070–1073

Kawakami M, Weinstein JN, Chatani K, Spratt KF, Meller ST, Gebhart GF (1994a) Experimental lumbar radiculopathy. Behavioral and histologic changes in a model of radicular pain after spinal nerve root irritation with chromic gut ligatures in the rat. Spine (Phila Pa 1976) 19:1795–1802

Kawakami M, Weinstein JN, Spratt KF, Chatani K, Traub RJ, Meller ST, Gebhart GF (1994b) Experimental lumbar radiculopathy. Immunohistochemical and quantitative demonstrations of pain induced by lumbar nerve root irritation of the rat. Spine (Phila Pa 1976) 19:1780–1794

Kawakami M, Matsumoto T, Kuribayashi K, Tamaki T (1999) mRNA expression of interleukins, phospholipase A2, and nitric oxide synthase in the nerve root and dorsal root ganglion induced by autologous nucleus pulposus in the rat. J Orthop Res 17:941–946

Kawakami M, Matsumoto T, Tamaki T (2001) Roles of thromboxane A2 and leukotriene B4 in radicular pain induced by herniated nucleus pulposus. J Orthop Res 19(3):472–477

Kawakami M, Hashizume H, Nishi H, Matsumoto T, Tamaki T, Kuribayashi K (2003) Comparison of neuropathic pain induced by the application of normal and mechanically compressed nucleus pulposus to lumbar nerve roots in the rat. J Orthop Res 21:535–539

Kobayashi S, Yoshizawa H, Yamada S (2004a) Pathology of lumbar nerve root compression. Part 1: intraradicular inflammatory changes induced by mechanical compression. J Orthop Res 22:170–179

Kobayashi S, Yoshizawa H, Yamada S (2004b) Pathology of lumbar nerve root compression. Part 2: morphological and immunohistochemical changes of dorsal root ganglion. J Orthop Res 22:180–188

Kobayashi S, Baba H, Uchida K, Kokubo Y, Kubota C, Yamada S, Suzuki Y, Yoshizawa H (2005a) Effect of mechanical compression on the lumbar nerve root: localization and changes of intraradicular inflammatory cytokines, nitric oxide, and cyclooxygenase. Spine 30:1699–1705

Kobayashi S, Kokubo Y, Uchida K, Yayama T, Takeno K, Negoro K, Nakajima H, Baba H, Yoshizawa H (2005b) Effect of lumbar nerve root compression on primary sensory neurons and their central branches: changes in the nociceptive neuropeptides substance P and somatostatin. Spine (Phila Pa 1976) 30:276–282

Kobayashi S, Meir A, Baba H, Uchida K, Hayakawa K (2005c) Imaging of intraneural edema by using gadolinium-enhanced MR imaging: experimental compression injury. AJNR Am J Neuroradiol 26:973–980

Kobayashi S, Sasaki S, Shimada S, Kaneyasu M, Mizukami Y, Kitade I, Ogawa M, Kawahara H, Baba H, Yoshizawa H (2005d) Changes of calcitonin gene-related peptide in primary sensory neurons and their central branch after nerve root compression of the dog. Arch Phys Med Rehabil 86:527–533

Kobayashi S, Uchida K, Kokubo Y, Takeno K, Yayama T, Miyazaki T, Nakajima H, Nomura E, Mwaka E, Baba H (2008) Synapse involvement of the dorsal horn in experimental lumbar nerve root compression: a light and electron microscopic study. Spine (Phila Pa 1976) 33:716–723

Komori H, Shinomiya K, Nakai O, Yamaura I, Takeda S, Furuya K (1996) The natural history of herniated nucleus pulposus with radiculopathy. Spine (Phila Pa 1976) 21:225–229

Korhonen T, Karppinen J, Paimela L, Malmivaara A, Lindgren KA, Jarvinen S, Niinimaki J, Veeger N, Seitsalo S, Hurri H (2005) The treatment of disc herniation-induced sciatica with infliximab: results of a randomized, controlled, 3-month follow-up study. Spine 30:2724–2728

Korhonen T, Karppinen J, Paimela L, Malmivaara A, Lindgren KA, Bowman C, Hammond A, Kirkham B, Jarvinen S, Niinimaki J, Veeger N, Haapea M, Torkki M, Tervonen O, Seitsalo S, Hurri H (2006) The treatment of disc-herniation-induced sciatica with infliximab: one-year follow-up results of first ii, a randomized controlled trial. Spine 31:2759–2766

Le Maitre CL, Freemont AJ, Hoyland JA (2005) The role of interleukin-1 in the pathogenesis of human intervertebral disc degeneration. Arthritis Res Ther 7(4):R732–R745

Le Maitre CL, Hoyland JA, Freemont AJ (2007) Catabolic cytokine expression in degenerate and herniated human intervertebral discs: IL-1beta and TNFalpha expression profile. Arthritis Res Ther 9:R77

Lindenlaub T, Teuteberg P, Hartung T, Sommer C (2000) Effects of neutralizing antibodies to TNF-alpha on pain-related behavior and nerve regeneration in mice with chronic constriction injury. Brain Res 866:15–22

Loupasis GA, Stamos K, Katonis PG, Sapkas G, Korres DS, Hartofilakidis G (1999) Seven- to 20-year outcome of lumbar discectomy. Spine (Phila Pa 1976) 24:2313–2317

Marriott I (2004) The role of tachykinins in central nervous system inflammatory responses. Front Biosci 9:2153–2165

Maves TJ, Pechman PS, Gebhart GF, Meller ST (1993) Possible chemical contribution from chromic gut sutures produces disorders of pain sensation like those seen in man. Pain 54:57–69

McCarron RF, Wimpee MW, Hudkins PG, Laros GS (1987) The inflammatory effect of nucleus pulposus. A possible element in the pathogenesis of low-back pain. Spine (Phila Pa 1976) 12: 760–764

Mixter CG, Blumgart HL, Berlin DD (1934) Total ablation of the thyroid for angina pectoris and congestive heart failure: results of eighteen months' experience. Ann Surg 100:570–577

Moalem G, Tracey DJ (2006) Immune and inflammatory mechanisms in neuropathic pain. Brain Res Rev 51:240–264

Moore RJ, Vernon-Roberts B, Fraser RD, Osti OL, Schembri M (1996) The origin and fate of herniated lumbar intervertebral disc tissue. Spine 21:2149–2155

Morishita Y, Hida S, Naito M, Arimizu J, Matsushima U, Nakamura A (2006) Measurement of the local pressure of the intervertebral foramen and the electrophysiologic values of the spinal nerve roots in the vertebral foramen. Spine (Phila Pa 1976) 31:3076–3080

Mosconi T, Kruger L (1996) Fixed-diameter polyethylene cuffs applied to the rat sciatic nerve induce a painful neuropathy: ultrastructural morphometric analysis of axonal alterations. Pain 64:37–57

Mulleman D, Mammou S, Griffoul I, Watier H, Goupille P (2006a) Pathophysiology of disk-related low back pain and sciatica. II. Evidence supporting treatment with TNF-alpha antagonists. Joint Bone Spine 73:270–277

Mulleman D, Mammou S, Griffoul I, Watier H, Goupille P (2006b) Pathophysiology of disk-related sciatica. I – Evidence supporting a chemical component. Joint Bone Spine 73:151–158

Murata Y, Onda A, Rydevik B, Takahashi K, Olmarker K (2004a) Distribution and appearance of tumor necrosis factor-alpha in the dorsal root ganglion exposed to experimental disc herniation in rats. Spine (Phila Pa 1976) 29:2235–2241

Murata Y, Onda A, Rydevik B, Takahashi K, Olmarker K (2004b) Selective inhibition of tumor necrosis factor-alpha prevents nucleus pulposus-induced histologic changes in the dorsal root ganglion. Spine 29:2477–2484

Myers RR, Yamamoto T, Yaksh TL, Powell HC (1993) The role of focal nerve ischemia and wallerian degeneration in peripheral nerve injury producing hyperesthesia. Anesthesiology 78: 308–316

Nakamae T, Ochi M, Olmarker K (2011) Pharmacological inhibition of tumor necrosis factor may reduce pain behavior changes induced by experimental disc puncture in the rat: an experimental study in rats. Spine (Phila Pa 1976) 36:E232–E236

Nicholson KJ, Quindlen JC, Winkelstein BA (2011) Development of a duration threshold for modulating evoked neuronal responses after nerve root compression injury. Stapp Car Crash J 55:1–24

Nicholson KJ, Guarino BB, Winkelstein BA (2012) Transient nerve root compression load and duration differentially mediate behavioral sensitivity and associated spinal astrocyte activation and mGLuR5 expression. Neuroscience 209:187–195

Nilsson E, Nakamae T, Olmarker K (2011) Pain behavior changes following disc puncture relate to nucleus pulposus rather than to the disc injury per se: an experimental study in rats. Open Orthop J 5:72–77

Nygaard OP, Mellgren SI, Osterud B (1997) The inflammatory properties of contained and noncontained lumbar disc herniation. Spine 22(21):2484–2488

Obata K, Tsujino H, Yamanaka H, Yi D, Fukuoka T, Hashimoto N, Yonenobu K, Yoshikawa H, Noguchi K (2002) Expression of neurotrophic factors in the dorsal root ganglion in a rat model of lumbar disc herniation. Pain 99:121–132

Obata K, Yamanaka H, Dai Y, Mizushima T, Fukuoka T, Tokunaga A, Noguchi K (2004) Activation of extracellular signal-regulated protein kinase in the dorsal root ganglion following inflammation near the nerve cell body. Neuroscience 126:1011–1021

O'Donnell JL, O'Donnell AL (1996) Prostaglandin E2 content in herniated lumbar disc disease. Spine 21(14):1653–1655; discussion 1655–1656

Ohtori S, Takahashi K, Aoki Y, Doya H, Ozawa T, Saito T, Moriya H (2004) Spinal neural cyclooxygenase-2 mediates pain caused in a rat model of lumbar disk herniation. J Pain 5(7):385–391

Olmarker K (2001) Radicular pain – recent pathophysiologic concepts and therapeutic implications. Schmerz 15:425–429

Olmarker K (2008) Puncture of a lumbar intervertebral disc induces changes in spontaneous pain behavior: an experimental study in rats. Spine 33:850–855

Olmarker K, Larsson K (1998) Tumor necrosis factor alpha and nucleus-pulposus-induced nerve root injury. Spine (Phila Pa 1976) 23:2538–2544

Olmarker K, Myers R (1998) Pathogenesis of sciatic pain: role of herniated nucleus pulposus and deformation of spinal nerve root and dorsal root ganglion. Pain 78:99–105

Olmarker K, Rydevik B (1991) Pathophysiology of sciatica. Orthop Clin North Am 22:223–234

Olmarker K, Rydevik B (2001) Selective inhibition of tumor necrosis factor-alpha prevents nucleus pulposus-induced thrombus formation, intraneural edema, and reduction of nerve conduction velocity: possible implications for future pharmacologic treatment strategies of sciatica. Spine 26:863–869

Olmarker K, Rydevik B, Holm S (1989) Edema formation in spinal nerve roots induced by experimental, graded compression. An experimental study on the pig cauda equina with special reference to differences in effects between rapid and slow onset of compression. Spine (Phila Pa 1976) 14:569–573

Olmarker K, Rydevik B, Nordborg C (1993) Autologous nucleus pulposus induces neurophysiologic and histologic changes in porcine cauda equina nerve roots. Spine (Phila Pa 1976) 18:1425–1432

Olmarker K, Byrod G, Cornefjord M, Nordborg C, Rydevik B (1994) Effects of methylprednisolone on nucleus pulposus-induced nerve root injury. Spine (Phila Pa 1976) 19:1803–1808

Olmarker K, Brisby H, Yabuki S, Nordborg C, Rydevik B (1997) The effects of normal, frozen, and hyaluronidase-digested nucleus pulposus on nerve root structure and function. Spine 22:471–475; discussion 476

Olmarker K, Iwabuchi M, Larsson K, Rydevik B (1998) Walking analysis of rats subjected to experimental disc herniation. Eur Spine J 7:394–399

Olmarker K, Storkson R, Berge OG (2002) Pathogenesis of sciatic pain: a study of spontaneous behavior in rats exposed to experimental disc herniation. Spine 27:1312–1317

Olmarker K, Nutu M, Storkson R (2003) Changes in spontaneous behavior in rats exposed to experimental disc herniation are blocked by selective TNF-alpha inhibition. Spine 28:1635–1641; discussion 1642

Onda A, Hamba M, Yabuki S, Kikuchi S (2002) Exogenous tumor necrosis factor-alpha induces abnormal discharges in rat dorsal horn neurons. Spine (Phila Pa 1976) 27:1618–1624; discussion 1624

Onda A, Murata Y, Rydevik B, Larsson K, Kikuchi S, Olmarker K (2004) Infliximab attenuates immunoreactivity of brain-derived neurotrophic factor in a rat model of herniated nucleus pulposus. Spine 29:1857–1861

Onda A, Murata Y, Rydevik B, Larsson K, Kikuchi S, Olmarker K (2005) Nerve growth factor content in dorsal root ganglion as related to changes in pain behavior in a rat model of experimental lumbar disc herniation. Spine (Phila Pa 1976) 30:188–193

Otani K, Arai I, Mao GP, Konno S, Olmarker K, Kikuchi S (1997) Experimental disc herniation: evaluation of the natural course. Spine (Phila Pa 1976) 22:2894–2899

Ozaktay AC, Cavanaugh JM, Asik I, DeLeo JA, Weinstein JN (2002) Dorsal root sensitivity to interleukin-1 beta, interleukin-6 and tumor necrosis factor in rats. Eur Spine J 11:467–475

Ozaktay AC, Kallakuri S, Takebayashi T, Cavanaugh JM, Asik I, DeLeo JA, Weinstein JN (2006) Effects of interleukin-1 beta, interleukin-6, and tumor necrosis factor on sensitivity of dorsal root ganglion and peripheral receptive fields in rats. Eur Spine J 15:1529–1537

Park JB, Chang H, Kim YS (2002) The pattern of interleukin-12 and T-helper types 1 and 2 cytokine expression in herniated lumbar disc tissue. Spine (Phila Pa 1976) 27(19):2125–2128

Pedowitz RA, Garfin SR, Massie JB, Hargens AR, Swenson MR, Myers RR, Rydevik BL (1992) Effects of magnitude and duration of compression on spinal nerve root conduction. Spine (Phila Pa 1976) 17:194–199

Piesla MJ, Leventhal L, Strassle BW, Harrison JE, Cummons TA, Lu P, Whiteside GT (2009) Abnormal gait, due to inflammation but not nerve injury, reflects enhanced nociception in preclinical pain models. Brain Res 1295:89–98

Ramer LM, Richter MW, Roskams AJ, Tetzlaff W, Ramer MS (2004) Peripherally-derived olfactory ensheathing cells do not promote primary afferent regeneration following dorsal root injury. Glia 47:189–206

Ricci JA, Stewart WF, Chee E, Leotta C, Foley K, Hochberg MC (2006) Back pain exacerbations and lost productive time costs in United States workers. Spine (Phila Pa 1976) 31:3052–3060

Roberts S, Evans H, Trivedi J, Menage J (2006) Histology and pathology of the human intervertebral disc. J Bone Joint Surg Am 88(Suppl 2):10–14

Robinson I, Meert TF (2005) Stability of neuropathic pain symptoms in partial sciatic nerve ligation in rats is affected by suture material. Neurosci Lett 373:125–129

Rothman SM, Winkelstein BA (2007) Chemical and mechanical nerve root insults induce differential behavioral sensitivity and glial activation that are enhanced in combination. Brain Res 1181:30–43

Rothman SM, Winkelstein BA (2010) Cytokine antagonism reduces pain and modulates spinal astrocytic reactivity after cervical nerve root compression. Ann Biomed Eng 38(8):2563–2576

Rothman SM, Kreider RA, Winkelstein BA (2005) Spinal neuropeptide responses in persistent and transient pain following cervical nerve root injury. Spine (Phila Pa 1976) 30:2491–2496

Rothman SM, Guarino BB, Winkelstein BA (2009a) Spinal microglial proliferation is evident in a rat model of painful disc herniation both in the presence of behavioral hypersensitivity and following minocycline treatment sufficient to attenuate allodynia. J Neurosci Res 87:2709–2717

Rothman SM, Huang Z, Lee KE, Weisshaar CL, Winkelstein BA (2009b) Cytokine mRNA expression in painful radiculopathy. J Pain 10(1):90–99

Rothman SM, Nicholson KJ, Winkelstein BA (2010) Time-dependent mechanics and measures of glial activation and behavioral sensitivity in a rodent model of radiculopathy. J Neurotrauma 27: 803–814

Rutkowski MD, Winkelstein BA, Hickey WF, Pahl JL, DeLeo JA (2002) Lumbar nerve root injury induces central nervous system neuroimmune activation and neuroinflammation in the rat: relationship to painful radiculopathy. Spine (Phila Pa 1976) 27:1604–1613

Rydevik B (1994) Sciatica and herniated disk. Current aspects of pathophysiology and pain mechanisms. Nord Med 109:74–76, 80

Rydevik B, Brown MD, Lundborg G (1984) Pathoanatomy and pathophysiology of nerve root compression. Spine (Phila Pa 1976) 9:7–15

Rydevik BL, Pedowitz RA, Hargens AR, Swenson MR, Myers RR, Garfin SR (1991) Effects of acute, graded compression on spinal nerve root function and structure. An experimental study of the pig cauda equina. Spine (Phila Pa 1976) 16:487–493

Saab CY, Waxman SG, Hains BC (2008) Alarm or curse? The pain of neuroinflammation. Brain Res Rev 58:226–235

Saal JS (1995) The role of inflammation in lumbar pain. Spine (Phila Pa 1976) 20:1821–1827

Saal JS, Franson RC, Dobrow R, Saal JA (1990) High levels of inflammatory phospholipase A2 activity in lumbar disc herniations. Spine 15:674–678

Sapunar D, Ljubkovic M, Lirk P, McCallum JB, Hogan QH (2005) Distinct membrane effects of spinal nerve ligation on injured and adjacent dorsal root ganglion neurons in rats. Anesthesiology 103:360–376

Sasaki N, Kikuchi S, Konno S, Sekiguchi M, Watanabe K (2007) Anti-TNF-alpha antibody reduces pain-behavioral changes induced by epidural application of nucleus pulposus in a rat model depending on the timing of administration. Spine (Phila Pa 1976) 32: 413–416

Schafers M, Svensson CI, Sommer C, Sorkin LS (2003) Tumor necrosis factor-alpha induces mechanical allodynia after spinal nerve ligation by activation of p38 MAPK in primary sensory neurons. J Neurosci 23(7):2517–2521

Schafers M, Marziniak M, Sorkin LS, Yaksh TL, Sommer C (2004) Cyclooxygenase inhibition in nerve-injury- and TNF-induced hyperalgesia in the rat. Exp Neurol 185(1):160–168

Sekiguchi Y, Kikuchi S, Myers RR, Campana WM (2003) ISSLS prize winner: erythropoietin inhibits spinal neuronal apoptosis and pain following nerve root crush. Spine (Phila Pa 1976) 28:2577–2584

Sekiguchi M, Otoshi K, Kikuchi S, Konno S (2011) Analgesic effects of prostaglandin E2 receptor subtype EP1 receptor antagonist: experimental study of application of nucleus pulposus. Spine 36(22):1829–1834
Sekiguchi M, Konno S, Kikuchi S (2008) The effects of a 5-HT2A receptor antagonist on blood flow in lumbar disc herniation: application of nucleus pulposus in a canine model. Eur Spine J 17:307–313
Sekiguchi M, Sekiguchi Y, Konno S, Kobayashi H, Homma Y, Kikuchi S (2009) Comparison of neuropathic pain and neuronal apoptosis following nerve root or spinal nerve compression. Eur Spine J 18:1978–1985
Shamji MF, Whitlatch L, Friedman AH, Richardson WJ, Chilkoti A, Setton LA (2008) An injectable and in situ-gelling biopolymer for sustained drug release following perineural administration. Spine (Phila Pa 1976) 33:748–754
Shamji MF, Allen KD, So S, Jing L, Adams SB Jr, Schuh R, Huebner J, Kraus VB, Friedman AH, Setton LA, Richardson WJ (2009) Gait abnormalities and inflammatory cytokines in an autologous nucleus pulposus model of radiculopathy. Spine (Phila Pa 1976) 34:648–654
Shamji MF, Setton LA, Jarvis W, So S, Chen J, Jing L, Bullock R, Isaacs RE, Brown C, Richardson WJ (2010) Proinflammatory cytokine expression profile in degenerated and herniated human intervertebral disc tissues. Arthritis Rheum 62:1974–1982
Skouen J, Brisby H, Otani K, Olmarker K, Rosengren L, Rydevik B (1999) Protein markers in cerebrospinal fluid in experimental nerve root injury. A study of slow-onset chronic compression effects or the biochemical effects of nucleus pulposus on sacral nerve roots. Spine 24:2195–2200
Sommer C, Schmidt C, George A, Toyka KV (1997) A metalloprotease-inhibitor reduces pain associated behavior in mice with experimental neuropathy. Neurosci Lett 237(1):45–48
Sommer C, Schafers M, Marziniak M, Toyka KV (2001) Etanercept reduced hyperalgesia in experimental painful neuropathy. J Peripher Nerv Syst 6:67–72
Song XJ, Wang ZB, Gan Q, Walters ET (2006) cAMP and cGMP contribute to sensory neuron hyperexcitability and hyperalgesia in rats with dorsal root ganglia compression. J Neurophysiol 95(1):479–492
Specchia N, Pagnotta A, Toesca A, Greco F (2002) Cytokines and growth factors in the protruded intervertebral disc of the lumbar spine. Eur Spine J 11:145–151
Staal JB, de Bie R, de Vet HC, Hildebrandt J, Nelemans P (2008) Injection therapy for subacute and chronic low-back pain. Cochrane Database Syst Rev (3):CD001824
Stoll G, Jander S (1999) The role of microglia and macrophages in the pathophysiology of the CNS. Prog Neurobiol 58:233–247
Stoll G, Muller HW (1999) Nerve injury, axonal degeneration and neural regeneration: basic insights. Brain Pathol 9:313–325
Suter MR, Wen YR, Decosterd I, Ji RR (2007) Do glial cells control pain? Neuron Glia Biol 3:255–268
Suzuki M, Inoue G, Gemba T, Watanabe T, Ito T, Koshi T, Yamauchi K, Yamashita M, Orita S, Eguchi Y, Ochiai N, Kishida S, Takaso M, Aoki Y, Takahashi K, Ohtori S (2009) Nuclear factor-kappa B decoy suppresses nerve injury and improves mechanical allodynia and thermal hyperalgesia in a rat lumbar disc herniation model. Eur Spine J 18(7):1001–1007
Takahashi H, Suguro T, Okazima Y, Motegi M, Okada Y, Kakiuchi T (1996) Inflammatory cytokines in the herniated disc of the lumbar spine. Spine (Phila Pa 1976) 21(2):218–224
Takahashi N, Yabuki S, Aoki Y, Kikuchi S (2003) Pathomechanisms of nerve root injury caused by disc herniation: an experimental study of mechanical compression and chemical irritation. Spine (Phila Pa 1976) 28:435–441
Takamori Y, Arimizu J, Izaki T, Naito M, Kobayashi T (2011) Combined measurement of nerve root blood flow and electrophysiological values: intraoperative straight-leg-raising test for lumbar disc herniation. Spine (Phila Pa 1976) 36:57–62
Tobinick EL, Britschgi-Davoodifar S (2003) Perispinal TNF-alpha inhibition for discogenic pain. Swiss Med Wkly 133:170–177
Tokunaga S, Yamanokuchi K, Yabuki A, Fujiki M, Misumi K (2010) Cartilage oligomeric matrix protein in canine spinal cord appears in the cerebrospinal fluid associated with intervertebral disc herniation. Spine (Phila Pa 1976) 35:4–9
Uceyler N, Tscharke A, Sommer C (2008) Early cytokine gene expression in mouse CNS after peripheral nerve lesion. Neurosci Lett 436(2):259–264
van der Windt DAWM, Simons E, Riphagen II, Ammendolia C, Verhagen AP, Laslett M, Devillé W, Deyo RA, Bouter LM, de Vet HCW, Aertgeerts B (2010) Physical examination for lumbar radiculopathy due to disc herniation in patients with low-back pain. Cochrane Database Syst Rev (2):CD007431
Van Zundert J, Harney D, Joosten EA, Durieux ME, Patijn J, Prins MH, Van Kleef M (2006) The role of the dorsal root ganglion in cervical radicular pain: diagnosis, pathophysiology, and rationale for treatment. Reg Anesth Pain Med 31:152–167
Verri WA Jr, Cunha TM, Parada CA, Poole S, Cunha FQ, Ferreira SH (2006) Hypernociceptive role of cytokines and chemokines: targets for analgesic drug development? Pharmacol Ther 112:116–138
Vrinten DH, Hamers FF (2003) 'Catwalk' automated quantitative gait analysis as a novel method to assess mechanical allodynia in the rat; a comparison with von Frey testing. Pain 102:203–209
Weiler C, Nerlich AG, Bachmeier BE, Boos N (2005) Expression and distribution of tumor necrosis factor alpha in human lumbar intervertebral discs: a study in surgical specimen and autopsy controls. Spine (Phila Pa 1976) 30:44–53; discussion 54
Weiler C, Lopez-Ramos M, Mayer HM, Korge A, Siepe CJ, Wuertz K, Weiler V, Boos N, Nerlich AG (2011) Histological analysis of surgical lumbar intervertebral disc tissue provides evidence for an association between disc degeneration and increased body mass index. BMC Res Notes 4:497
Weinstein JN, Lurie JD, Tosteson TD, Skinner JS, Hanscom B, Tosteson AN, Herkowitz H, Fischgrund J, Cammisa FP, Albert T, Deyo RA (2006a) Surgical vs nonoperative treatment for lumbar disk herniation: the spine patient outcomes research trial (sport) observational cohort. JAMA 296:2451–2459
Weinstein JN, Tosteson TD, Lurie JD, Tosteson AN, Hanscom B, Skinner JS, Abdu WA, Hilibrand AS, Boden SD, Deyo RA (2006b) Surgical vs nonoperative treatment for lumbar disk herniation: the spine patient outcomes research trial (sport): a randomized trial. JAMA 296:2441–2450
Weisshaar CL, Winer JP, Guarino BB, Janmey PA, Winkelstein BA (2011) The potential for salmon fibrin and thrombin to mitigate pain subsequent to cervical nerve root injury. Biomaterials 32(36):9738–9746
Whishaw IQ, Kolb B (2005) The behavior of the laboratory rat: a handbook with tests. Oxford University Press, Oxford/New York
Willburger RE, Wittenberg RH (1994) Prostaglandin release from lumbar disc and facet joint tissue. Spine (Phila Pa 1976) 19(18): 2068–2070
Winkelstein BA, DeLeo JA (2004) Mechanical thresholds for initiation and persistence of pain following nerve root injury: mechanical and chemical contributions at injury. J Biomech Eng 126: 258–263
Winkelstein BA, Rutkowski MD, Sweitzer SM, Pahl JL, DeLeo JA (2001a) Nerve injury proximal or distal to the DRG induces similar spinal glial activation and selective cytokine expression but differential behavioral responses to pharmacologic treatment. J Comp Neurol 439(2):127–139
Winkelstein BA, Rutkowski MD, Weinstein JN, DeLeo JA (2001b) Quantification of neural tissue injury in a rat radiculopathy model: comparison of local deformation, behavioral outcomes, and spinal cytokine mRNA for two surgeons. J Neurosci Methods 111: 49–57

Winkelstein BA, Weinstein JN, DeLeo JA (2002) The role of mechanical deformation in lumbar radiculopathy: an in vivo model. Spine (Phila Pa 1976) 27:27–33

Xu J, Pollock CH, Kajander KC (1996) Chromic gut suture reduces calcitonin-gene-related peptide and substance P levels in the spinal cord following chronic constriction injury in the rat. Pain 64:503–509

Yabuki S, Kawaguchi Y, Nordborg C, Kikuchi S, Rydevik B, Olmarker K (1998) Effects of lidocaine on nucleus pulposus-induced nerve root injury: a neurophysiologic and histologic study of the pig cauda equina. Spine 23:2383–2389

Yamamoto T, Nozaki-Taguchi N (1995) Role of cholecystokinin-B receptor in the maintenance of thermal hyperalgesia induced by unilateral constriction injury to the sciatic nerve in the rat. Neurosci Lett 202:89–92

Yildirim K, Deniz O, Gureser G, Karatay S, Ugur M, Erdal A, Senel K (2009) Gabapentin monotherapy in patients with chronic radiculopathy: the efficacy and impact on life quality. J Back Musculoskelet Rehabil 22:17–20

Zanella JM, Burright EN, Hildebrand K, Hobot C, Cox M, Christoferson L, McKay WF (2008) Effect of etanercept, a tumor necrosis factor-alpha inhibitor, on neuropathic pain in the rat chronic constriction injury model. Spine (Phila Pa 1976) 33(3):227–234

The Sand Rat (*Psammomys obesus obesus*) Model of Spontaneous, Age-Related Intervertebral Disc Degeneration

20

Helen E. Gruber and Edward N. Hanley Jr.

Contents

H.E. Gruber, PhD (✉)
Department of Orthopaedic Surgery, Cannon Research Center, Room 304, Carolinas Medical Center, 32861, Charlotte, NC 28232, USA
e-mail: helen.gruber@carolinashealthcare.org

E.N. Hanley Jr., MD
Department of Orthopaedic Surgery, Carolinas Medical Center, 1025 Morehead Medical Drive, Suite 300, Charlotte, NC, USA
e-mail: edward.hanley@carolinashealthcare.org

20.1 Introduction

20.1.1 Need for a Reliable, Economical Small Animal Model for Degenerative Disc Research

With its associated low back pain, disc degeneration is a major health-care concern causing disability. It plays a major role in the US medical, social, and economic structure. Low back pain is devastating and influences the quality of life for millions. The lifetime prevalence of low back pain approximates 80 % with an estimated direct cost burden of $86 billion per year. Patients with back pain incur higher health-care costs and utilization and greater work loss than do patients without back pain. These health-care statistics point to the need for appropriate animal models for translational research efforts directed towards a greater understanding of disc degeneration and models to test potential new therapies.

In November 1995, an NIH workshop was held on "New Horizons in Low Back Pain." The publication which grew from this workshop emphasized the importance of this costly health-care problem and recommended areas of future research, including the importance of animal models for the study of disc degeneration. In his review of animal models, Krag commented that "…the usefulness of a particular model derives not from the extent to which it mimics reality (because that cannot be known in advance), but rather from the extent to which it facilitates the formulation and subsequent testing of hypotheses that lead to an improved understanding of that reality" (Krag 1996).

In the search for a reliable and economical species, the authors reviewed the value of possible animal models that can be utilized for studies of disc degeneration. From those discussions, the laboratory has chosen to utilize the sand rat (*Psammomys obesus obesus*). This desert mammal, indigenous to land bounded by the eastern Mediterranean, is the only small animal model with spontaneous, age-related disc degeneration.

I.M. Shapiro, M.V. Risbud (eds.), *The Intervertebral Disc*,
DOI 10.1007/978-3-7091-1535-0_20, © Springer-Verlag Wien 2014

20.1.2 Animal Models Using the Stab Technique to Induce Degeneration Are Not Optimum

The goal of this chapter is to review past literature and summarize recent findings using the sand rat model. There are a number of reasons why this is an extremely important and valuable model for disc degeneration. First, as noted above, these animals undergo spontaneous, age-related disc degeneration. Degeneration in the commonly employed rabbit models must be induced by a scalpel blade stab. Sobajima et al. (2005) have noted that the classic stab model causes immediate herniation of the nucleus pulposus, and thus it cannot mimic slower changes in the nucleus or annulus associated with onset and progression of degenerative disc disease. It is also not appropriate as a model to test therapies which focus upon the early stages of degeneration. Second, as the sand rat is a small rodent, its use avoids the high costs of larger animal models such as the canine or even the rabbit. Finally, modern custom diets, such as that used in the authors' laboratory, can be designed with low-calorie formulations (see below), thus avoiding the onset of nutrition-related type 2 diabetes associated with ad lib feeding of high-caloric diets as evidenced in the diabetes-prone strain of the sand rat.

20.2 Review of the Early Literature on Disc Degeneration in the Sand Rat

The sand rat (*Psammomys obesus*) is a very attractive model which avoids problems linked with chemonucleolysis or surgical injury. In the older literature, spine studies on the sand rat were primarily derived from one research group, their subsequent collaborators (Adler et al. 1983; Moskowitz et al. 1990; Silberberg et al. 1979, 1989; Silberberg 1988a, b; Silberberg and Adler 1983; Ziran et al. 1994; Ziv et al. 1992), and notations in later reviews (Krag 1996; Matsuzaki and Wakabayashi 1999). Published studies focused primarily on histologic and radiologic changes in animals aged 2, 3, 6, and 18–30 months of age and documented the presence of granular debris in the nucleus, small annular tears, herniations into and through cartilage end plates, and ligament calcification.

20.3 Newer Findings on Sand Rat Disc Degeneration

20.3.1 Morphologic Changes with Aging

Midsagittal histologic studies have documented the features of disc degeneration in older animals which include irregular disc margins, disc space narrowing, wedging, and end plate calcification (Gruber et al. 2005). Morphologic changes beginning in younger animals have received less attention, however. As previously recognized with radiologic analyses, lower lumbar vertebrae show the earliest signs of degeneration (Gruber et al. 2002a). Figure 20.1 illustrates the striking morphologic changes in the nucleus pulposus with aging. At age 3 weeks (Fig. 20.1a), the notochordal syncytium makes up the nucleus pulposus. Notochordal cells can still be prominent up to 2–3 months of age in upper lumbar discs. Notochordal cells are shown in high magnification in Fig. 20.1b. In lower discs at 3 months, notochordal cells begin to undergo fragmentation and cell death (Fig. 20.1c); by 11.7 months the demarcation between annulus and nucleus becomes less distinct, and it appears that annulus cells begin to occupy the proteoglycan-rich nucleus pulposus (Fig. 20.1d, e). By 17 months, the nucleus shows marked degenerative changes. Nuclear material can be found projecting into regions of herniation in the dorsal margin of the disc by 18–36 months of age (Fig. 20.1g). Often, these nucleus matrix sites become sequestered (Fig. 20.1h) and can be quite large (Fig. 20.1i) extending dramatically towards the spinal cord (Fig. 20.1j).

Analyses of live and dead cells in the aging sand rat have also been carried out using fluorescent markers (Gruber et al. 2008a). This work utilized animals aged 2–6, 13–19, and 26–38 months of age. The percentages of dead cells for the entire annulus were 46.1, 48.1, and 76.8 %, respectively, for the three age groups studied. The percentage of dead cells correlated significantly with end plate bone mineral density ($p<0.02$). (Bone mineral density studies are discussed in greater detail below.) This study also confirmed the progressive death of notochordal cells in the nucleus during aging as previously noted in morphologic studies.

Sand rat disc tissue has also been extremely valuable when used in parallel with human disc tissue for specialized studies and for immunohistochemical investigations. Like human disc tissue (Gruber and Hanley 1998), sand rat discs

Fig. 20.1 Representative light microscopic images of the aging sand rat lumbar disc: (**a**) Lumbar disc at 3 weeks of age: image shows nucleus pulposus filled with notochordal cells, annulus, and end plates (scale = 200 μm). (**b**) Higher-resolution view of the syncytial network of the notochord (scale = 20 μm). (**c**) The nucleus pulposus in a 3-month-old animal. Note that the notochordal cells have begun to fragment (scale = 50 μm). (**d**) Annulus-nucleus transition zone lacks clear definition in this specimen from an 11.7-month-old animal (scale = 50 μm). (**e, f**) Images of the nucleus from an 11.7-month-old (e) and 17-month-old (f) animals show progressive degeneration of matrix and cells (scale on $E=50$ μm and on $F=200$ μm). (**g–j**) Low magnification images of lumbar discs showing herniations in the dorsal portions of lumbar discs. Note the greatly narrowed nucleus regions. (**g**) 18-month-old animal (scale = 200 μm). (**h**) 28-month-old animal with regions of sequestered nucleus pulposus matrix isolated in the herniation region (scale = 200 μm). (**i**) 30-month-old animal. (scale = 500 μm). (**j**) 36-month-old animal (scale = 500 μm) (*SP* spinal cord, Masson-trichrome staining)

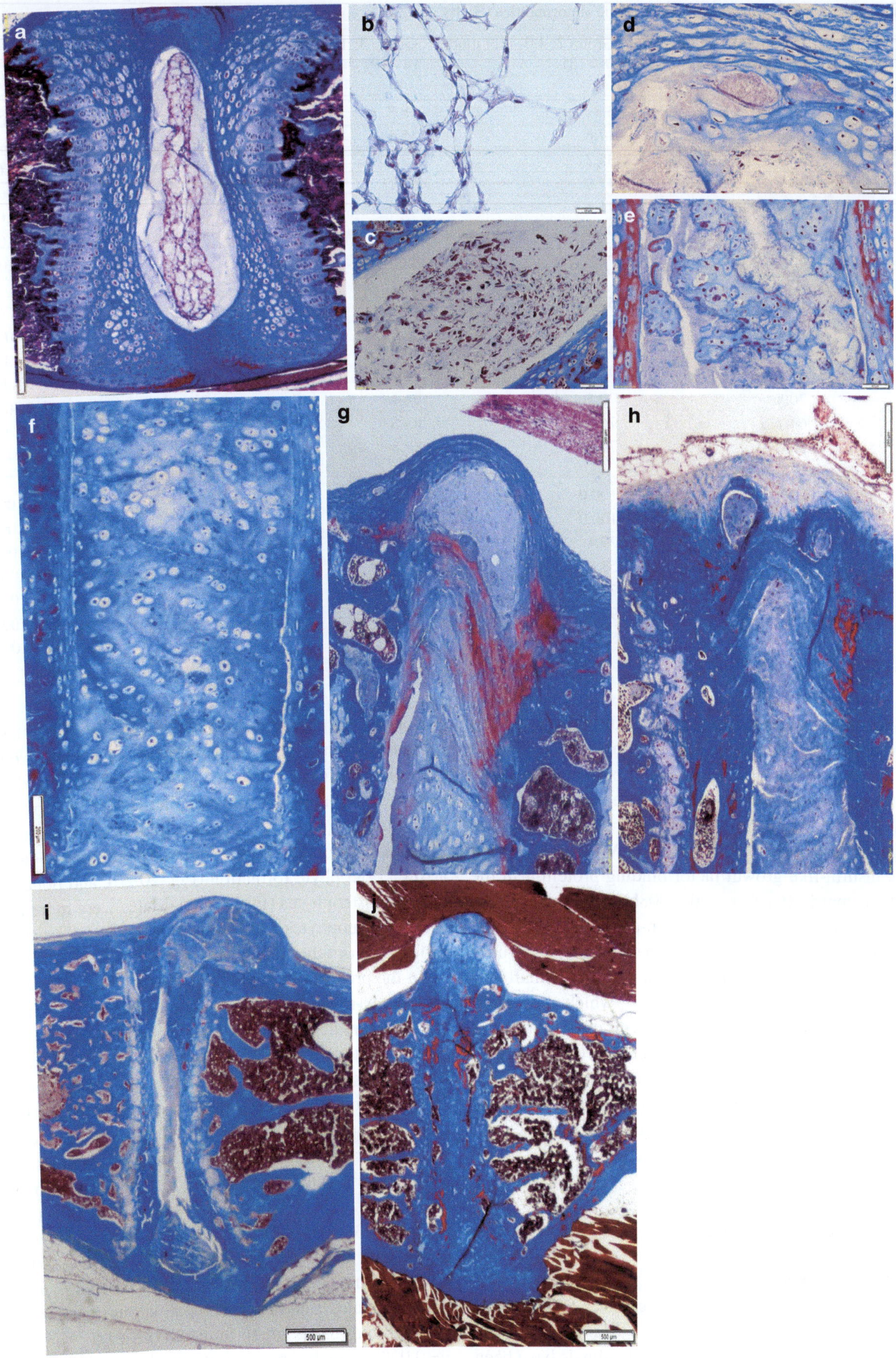
a
b
c
d
e
f
g
h
i
j
500 µm
500 µm

Table 20.1 Analysis of the incidence of radiologic abnormalities (%) by age group

	Group 1: 1–3.9 months (*n*=36)	Group 2: 4.0–11.9 months (*n*=18)	Group 3: 12–23.9 months (*n*=19)	Group 4: 24–46 months (*n*=26)	*P* value[a]
Narrowing					
L_{1-2}	4.0	5.8	38.8	34.6	0.01
L_{2-3}	29.4	17.6	55.5	42.3	NS (0.08)
L_{3-4}	29.4	35.2	55.5	88.4	<0.001
L_{4-5}	35.2	47.0	61.1	88.4	0.0005
L_{5-6}	38.2	41.1	66.6	96.1	<0.001
L_{6-7}	50.0	94.1	88.8	100.0	<0.001
L_{7-S}	44.1	82.3	88.8	100.0	<0.001
Wedging					
L_{1-2}	11.7	5.8	33.3	26.9	NS (0.08)
L_{2-3}	14.7	29.4	55.5	46.1	0.01
L_{3-4}	29.4	41.1	50.0	65.3	0.04
L_{4-5}	55.8	70.5	72.2	88.4	NS (0.056)
L_{5-6}	70.5	70.5	94.4	100.0	0.005
L_{6-7}	64.7	76.4	83.3	92.3	NS (0.075)
L_{7-S}	82.3	70.5	88.8	100.0	0.04
End plate calcification					
L_{1-2}	2.9	100.0	44.4	100.0	<0.001
L_{2-3}	2.9	100.0	61.1	96.1	<0.001
L_{3-4}	2.9	29.4	83.3	96.1	<0.001
L_{4-5}	8.8	58.8	88.8	100.0	<0.001
L_{5-6}	26.4	70.5	100.0	100.0	<0.001
L_{6-7}	47.0	94.1	100.0	100.0	<0.001
L_{7-S}	47.0	82.3	100.0	100.0	<0.001

[a]Analysis by chi-square

show the presence of programmed cell death (apoptosis) and cell senescence (Gruber et al. 2007b). Immunolocalization studies in the sand rat disc have shown patterns similar to those present in human discs for the presence of thrombospondin (Gruber et al. 2006b), myocilin (Gruber et al. 2006a), and pregnancy-associated plasma protein-A (PAPP-A) which unmasks insulin-like growth factor binding protein-4 in the extracellular matrix (Gruber et al. 2008b). The sand rat disc shows a pattern of localization of brain-derived neurotrophic factor (BDNF) similar to that seen in the human disc (Gruber et al. 2008c). Asporin, a member of the family of small leucine-rich proteoglycan (SLRP) family which has been reported to have a genetic association with osteoarthritis, is present in both the human and sand rat disc (Gruber et al. 2009b). Periostin, a matricellular protein in the fasciclin family expressed in tissues subjected to constant mechanical stress, has also been shown to be present within both the sand rat and human disc (Gruber et al. 2011a).

20.3.2 Radiology and Micro-CT

20.3.2.1 Lumbar Spine

The sand rat spine contains seven lumbar discs (Table 20.1). Radiologic characterizations of degenerating discs in both cross-sectional and prospective groups of animals have been performed (Gruber et al. 2002a, 2007a) (Table 20.1). Cross-sectional studies showed significant age-related changes comprising irregular disc margins, disc wedging, disc narrowing, end plate and ligament calcification, and osteophyte formation. Figure 20.2 illustrates radiologic changes at 12, 29, and 30 months of age, including wedging (Fig. 20.2a, arrow), osteophyte formation (Fig. 20.2b), and bone bridges between osteophytes (Fig, 20.2c). Males were more likely to develop osteophytes than were females. There was no gender difference for other radiographic features.

In the prospective study, 22 sand rats were followed with monthly X-rays from age 2 to 12 months; 11 were males and 11 were females (Gruber et al. 2002a). Statistical analysis showed that wedging, narrowing, end plate calcification, and irregular disc margins were all significantly more common at 12 months of age than at 2 months of age ($p=0.0001$). Tests for differences in radiologic disc features related to gender were performed at 2, 3, 6, and 12 months. Males showed a statistically greater incidence (%) of wedging at 6 months (6.4 ± 1.6 vs. 4.8 ± 1.1, $p=0.024$) and at 12 months (7.8 ± 0.6 vs. 6.3 ± 1.3, $p=0.004$) than females. Narrowing was more frequent in males at age 2 months (1.5 ± 1.6 vs. 0.3 ± 0.5, $p=0.028$) and age 6 months (5.8 ± 1.8 vs. 4.1 ± 1.6, $p=0.025$) than in females. End plate calcification was more common in 2-month-old males than females (1.8 ± 1.5 vs. 1.2 ± 1.7, $p=0.028$). Females, however, showed a greater incidence of

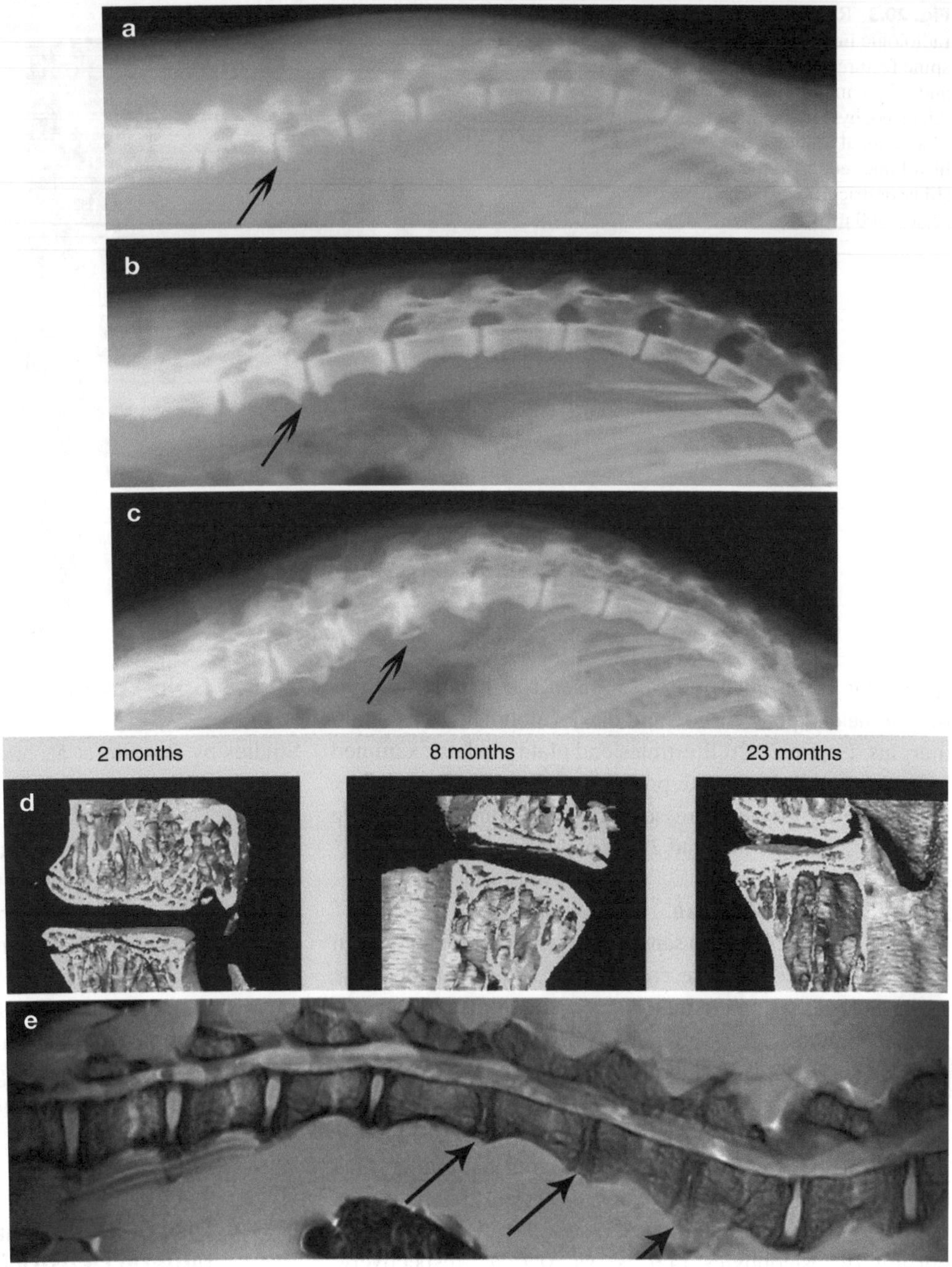

Fig. 20.2 (**a–c**) Representative radiographic images of the lumbar spine showing wedging (*arrow*, **a**), osteophyte formation (*arrow*, **b**), and bony bridging across osteophytes (*arrow*, **c**). (**a**) 12-month-old animal; (**b**) 29-month-old animal; (**c**) 30-month-old animal. (**d**) Micro-CT models with cuts revealing interior features of the end plate in 2-, 8-, and 23-month-old animals. Note the progressive loss of porosity in end plates. (**e**) High-resolution spin-lock (T_{1r}) image of the lumbar spine representative of degenerative changes in older animals. *Arrows mark* disc space narrowing and loss of proteoglycan content (Image courtesy of Dr. Ravinder Regatte, Depts. of Orthopaedic Surgery and Radiology, New York University School of Medicine)

end plate calcification at 6 months of age than did males (5.5 ± 1.2 vs. 3.9 ± 0.2, $p = 0.009$). No gender differences were found for irregular disc margin incidence at 2, 3, 6, or 12 months of age.

Lumbar spine radiographs showing degenerative features in the sand rat have been utilized for development of an automated computer-assisted procedure that analyzed digitized X-rays (Wilson et al. 2003). Techniques were developed to automate the quantitative processing of vertebral radiographic images that may be applicable to modeling of human disc degeneration. Microcomputerized tomography (CT) has been applied to the development of three-dimensional (3D) models of vertebral bone and the disc space (Gruber et al. 2005).

In humans, and in the sand rat, advanced disc degenerative changes and end plate calcification (sclerosis) have been documented. Most notably, Modic et al. have contributed the major study of end plates in degenerating human discs (Modic et al. 1988). As noted above, a positive correlation was observed between the percentages of dead cells in the aging sand rat disc and end plate bone mineral density.

Micro-CT model formulation provided an additional novel, nondestructive technique to assess the end plate-disc interface and the vascular canal network within the end plate of the sand rat spine (Gruber et al. 2005). This technique revealed a solid bony surface to the end plate that was not penetrated by vasculature. Models constructed from

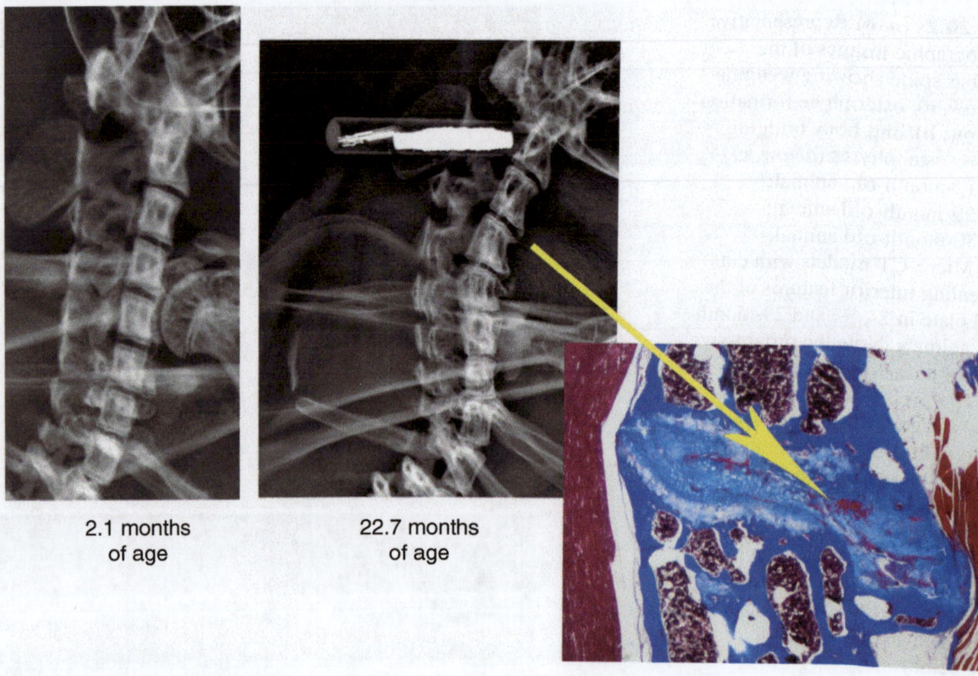

Fig. 20.3 Representative radiologic images of cervical spine features in a 2-month-old and a 22.7-month-old sand rat. An osteophyte marked in the older animal is shown in histologic section in the insert (Masson-trichrome stain; image scale = 500 μm)

specimens from older animals showed roughening and pitting of the end plate surface and the development of irregular margins. Figure 20.2d illustrates end plate models examined in sagittal section to make porosity of the end plate visible. Note the progressive decrease in canals within the end plate from age 2 months to 6 and 23 months of age.

20.3.2.2 Cervical Spine

Data are now available on sand rat cervical disc degeneration (Gruber et al. 2011b). Recent findings show that the same major features seen in human disc degeneration and sand rat lumbar spine disc degeneration are also present in the aging sand rat cervical discs. Scoring of digital X-rays of cervical and lumbar sites in the same animals showed that in younger animals, cervical discs exhibited a significantly greater proportion of irregular margins compared to lumbar sites (96.5 % vs. 86.2 %, respectively, $p = 0.001$). In older animals, cervical discs also showed a significantly greater proportion of osteophytes (4.9 % vs. 0.7 %, respectively, $p < 0.0001$) compared to lumbar sites. Since animal models for cervical disc degeneration are rare, the sand rat fills an important need and provides spontaneous, age-related degeneration in both lumbar and cervical spines. Figure 20.3 illustrates cervical radiologic features in a 2.1-month-old animal and compares that with degenerative changes present in a 22.7-month-old animal. In the older animal, the inset highlights the histologic features of the osteophyte marked in the digital radiograph.

20.3.3 Spin-Lock (T_{1r}) Imaging

Studies by Regatte et al. have utilized spin-lock (T_{1r}) imaging to study the sand rat model of disc degeneration (Regatte et al. 2004; also see Chap. 12). High-spatial-resolution images documented disc changes in both sagittal and cross-sectional planes of the disc. Figure 20.2e illustrates a sagittal plane image that shows prominent disc space narrowing (arrows) in a 4–5-month-old animal. These investigators also quantified spatial variation in the T_{1r} relaxation times in annulus and nucleus regions. These values were in the range of 100–120 ms and 50–60 ms, respectively, at 500 Hz. Proteoglycan imaging was excellent based on exchange of protons on glycosaminoglycans with bulk water.

20.3.4 Disc Cell Death and End Plate Bone Mineral Density (BMD)

As noted above, the degenerating disc exhibits increasing end plate calcification. The bone mineral density (BMD) of cranial and caudal end plates of the sand rat lumbar vertebrae was significantly greater in older animals (Table 20.2), and caudal end plates usually had significantly greater BMD values than did cranial plates (Gruber et al. 2008a). These same specimens were used to obtain viability assays for live/dead cells within the annulus. The percentage of dead

Table 20.2 Analysis of the averaged end plate BMD (g/cm²) per level in the age groups

Level	Group 1: 1–3.9 months ($n=36$)	Group 2: 4.0–11.9 months ($n=18$)	Group 3: 12–23.9 months ($n=19$)	Group 4: 24–46 months ($n=26$)	P value[a]
L_{1-2}	0.064±0.013	0.102±0.016	0.113±0.014	0.128±0.022	<0.001
L_{2-3}	0.068±0.015	0.101±0.020	0.118±0.016	0.134±0.023	<0.001
L_{3-4}	0.084±0.016	0.120±0.019	0.133±0.019	0.153±0.028	<0.001
L_{4-5}	0.094±0.018	0.138±0.022	0.146±0.023	0.177±0.027	<0.001
L_{5-6}	0.100±0.018	0.145±0.026	0.159±0.026	0.197±0.031	<0.001
L_{6-7}	0.108±0.019	0.157±0.028	0.167±0.032	0.204±0.036	<0.001
L_{7-S}	0.121±0.024	0.180±0.029	0.199±0.033	0.214±0.030	<0.001

[a]Data are expressed as mean±SD. Analysis by ANOVA for each disc site for the four groups. Note: P values were <0.001 for each disc site when analyses were also run on either cranial or caudal BMD data separately. ANOVA analysis for all sites comparing the four age groups was also performed. With this analysis, Group 1 was differed significantly from Groups 2, 3, and 4, and Group 3 vs. 4 was also significant ($p=0.05$)

cells in the annulus correlated in a significant, positive manner with end plate BMD ($p=0.02$, $r=0.347$). Vertebral end plate sclerosis and disc cell viability are probably associated because diffusion of nutrients through the end plate and disc margin provides the only source of nutrition for the adult avascular disc. It is believed that end plate calcification, followed by its replacement by bone, impedes nutrient flow into the disc (Bernick et al. 1991; Bernick and Caillet 1982). In these experiments the sand rat model provided excellent information directly relevant to human disc degeneration.

20.3.5 Vascular Supply to the Disc

In order to more carefully and accurately study the relationship between vascular supply through the end plate and disc degeneration, studies have been performed using a fluorescent vascular tracer in vivo with subsequent visualization of the tracer with UV microscopy (Gruber et al. 2005). No penetration of the vascular tracer was seen into the disc; this was verified by immunocytochemical staining for blood vessels. Only small vasculature features were identified on the dorsal and ventral margins of the annulus.

20.4 Spine Fusion Model

The potential for long-term adjacent segment degeneration at a fused clinical site remains a complex topic of great interest. An economical small animal model for lumbar fusion would be a useful research tool in investigations of lumbar fusion and degenerative changes in adjacent discs or facet joints caused by mechanical loading after fusion. A recent study has shown the relevance of the sand rat model for this need (Gruber et al. 2009a). A small segment of the outer annulus of lumbar discs was surgically removed, the animals allowed to recover, and then allowed to age 1–26 months postsurgery. Analysis of adjacent segment changes was not able to identify significant differences in cranial vs. caudal disc changes based on age at surgery or time of harvest postsurgery.

20.5 Autologous Disc Cell Implantation and Annulus Fibrosus Cell Culture

With other researchers, the Gruber/Hanley laboratory shares a great enthusiasm for the potential of biologic therapies for disc degeneration, especially cell-based therapies (see Chaps. 6, 23, and 27 and An et al. 2003; Anderson et al. 2005; Fassett et al. 2009; Ganey and Meisel 2002; Gruber and Hanley 2003; Phillips et al. 2003). The sand rat has been shown to be an excellent model for proof-of-concept studies for cell-based autologous disc cell therapy (Gruber et al. 2002b). For this purpose, cells were harvested from a healthy disc, expanded in culture, and implanted into a degenerating disc in the older donor animal. Immunohistochemical identification of the implanted cells showed that they integrated well into the normal matrix at time points up to 8 months post-engraftment. Although this work was technically challenging, the sand rat proved to be a valuable model for these autologous disc cell studies.

Sand rat annulus cells have been cultured in both monolayer and in three-dimensional agarose culture (see Box 20.1). Annulus cells also attached well and proliferated within collagen three-dimensional sponges and after 10 days of culture produced extracellular matrix containing collagen I and II, keratin sulfate, and chondroitin sulfate (Gruber et al. 2002b).

Box 20.1 Culture of Cells from the Sand Rat Annulus

The sand rat has been utilized to demonstrate the feasibility of cell-based autologous disc cell therapy (Gruber et al. 2002b). Figure (a) presents a view of a surgical field during opening of a lumbar disc for gentle curetting and sterile removal of annulus fragments for culture. Annulus fragments are then minced and cultured in 35 % Dulbecco's Modified Eagle's Medium, 35 % Ham's/F-12 nutrient mixture, and 30 % fetal bovine serum. Fragments are anchored in 24-well tissue culture plates using sterile SpectraMesh (104 μm mesh opening, Spectrum Laboratories Inc.) trimmed to fit the well. Cells are fed every 48 h and cultured until confluent (~6–8 weeks of culture). Next, cells can be labeled for immunohistochemical identification postimplantation (with carboxyfluorescein diacetate succinimidyl ester (CFSE) or 5-bromo-2′-deoxyuridine (BrdU)), rinsed, trypsinized, and carefully placed within a 2-mm^3-3D carrier (Gelfoam, Pfizer) for implantation in the donor animal. On average, 10,000–21,000 cells can be loaded into Gelfoam for implantation. In monolayer, sand rat annulus cells are spindle-shaped (illustration B) but assume a rounded morphology when cultured in 3D in agarose (illustration C). In agarose culture, cells proliferate more slowly than in monolayer; over 10 days of culture in agarose, ~40 % of seeded cells form multicellular colonies. It is important to note that in our experience cultures derived from younger animals (aged 2–3.9 months) yielded disc tissue with successful long-term annulus cultures 60 % of the time. Old animals, aged 8–10 months, yielded successful long-term cultures ~20 % of the time (Figs. b and c, original magnification ×200)

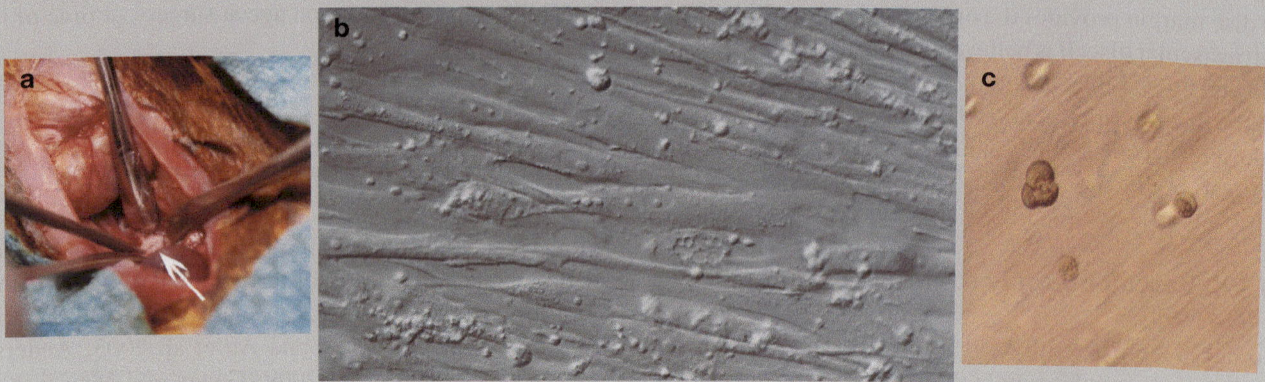

Box 20.2 Advantages and Disadvantages of the Sand Model for Disc Research

Advantages of the sand rat model:

- Only natural model with spontaneous, age-related disc degeneration.
- Economically advantageous small animal model that is available commercially via Harlan Laboratories, Inc.
  - Note that Harlan requires investigators to sign an agreement that purchased animals and their descendants be used solely for research purposes at that institution and not be further distributed to any third party or utilized for development of breeding colonies outside that institution.
- Radiologic and histologic changes mimic those in the aging/degenerating human lumbar and cervical spines (see below).
- Radiologic and histologic changes are reliable and well characterized in cross-sectional and prospective analyses.
- Small size advantageous for viewing the entire lumbar or cervical spine in a single radiologic or histologic field.

Shortcomings of the sand rat model:

- A nontraditional species with few colonies now in research use.
- More costly than other rodent models (such as rats and mice).
- Colony requires specialized low-caloric diet.
- Colony requires separate housing with controlled access.
- Small litter sizes (commonly four pups/litter).
- Genome not fully sequenced.
- Small animal size may make disc surgical procedures challenging.

Parallels with human lumbar and cervical disc degeneration:

- Age-related disc degeneration.
- Degeneration of both cervical and lumbar levels.
- Exhibits radiologic features present in the degenerating human lumbar and cervical spine, including:
  - Disc space narrowing, wedging, end plate calcification, and irregular disc margins.
- Exhibits histologic disc features present in the degenerating human lumbar and cervical spine, including:
  - Development of disc cell death, disc cell senescence, and disc cell apoptosis.
  - Dehydration/loss of recognizable nucleus pulposus in lower lumbar sites with progressive degeneration.
- MRI examination shows loss of hydration features present in the degenerating human lumbar and cervical spine.

20.6 Utility and Challenges of the Sand Rat Model

In addition to studies of age-induced spontaneous disc degeneration in the sand rat, this animal model is valuable for other types of research. Many laboratories utilize the sand rat specified as diabetes prone in nutritionally induced type 2 diabetes research [see (Collier et al. 2002) for a review] and for research on cataract formation (Chenault et al. 2002; Pollack et al. 1999).

20.6.1 A Nontraditional Species

Also called the fat or obese sand rat, desert sand rat, or the diurnal sand rat, the common nomenclature is misleading because these animals are of the genus *Psammomys*, a ratlike gerbil with a heavy body type and a fully haired and tufted tail, small ears, and short hindfoot (Harrison 1964). Figure 20.4a illustrates an adult female and offspring. The sand rat is found in Algeria, Libya, Egypt, Sudan, Israel, and Saudi Arabia (Strasser 1968).

Sand rats generally have a pleasant disposition and the animal caretakers enjoy working with these animals. Animals in the facility are individually housed with the exception of old mated pairs and same-sex littermates which have been housed together since weaning. All adult animals should have implantable micro identification chips to assure correct individual animal identification.

20.6.1.1 Need for Separate Housing with Restricted Access

There is the need to maintain restricted personnel access to nontraditional species such as the sand rat. A dedicated housing room should be maintained and special animal handling procedures employed. Animal caretakers usually work in this room as their final daily task and may wear protective disposable lab coats and booties.

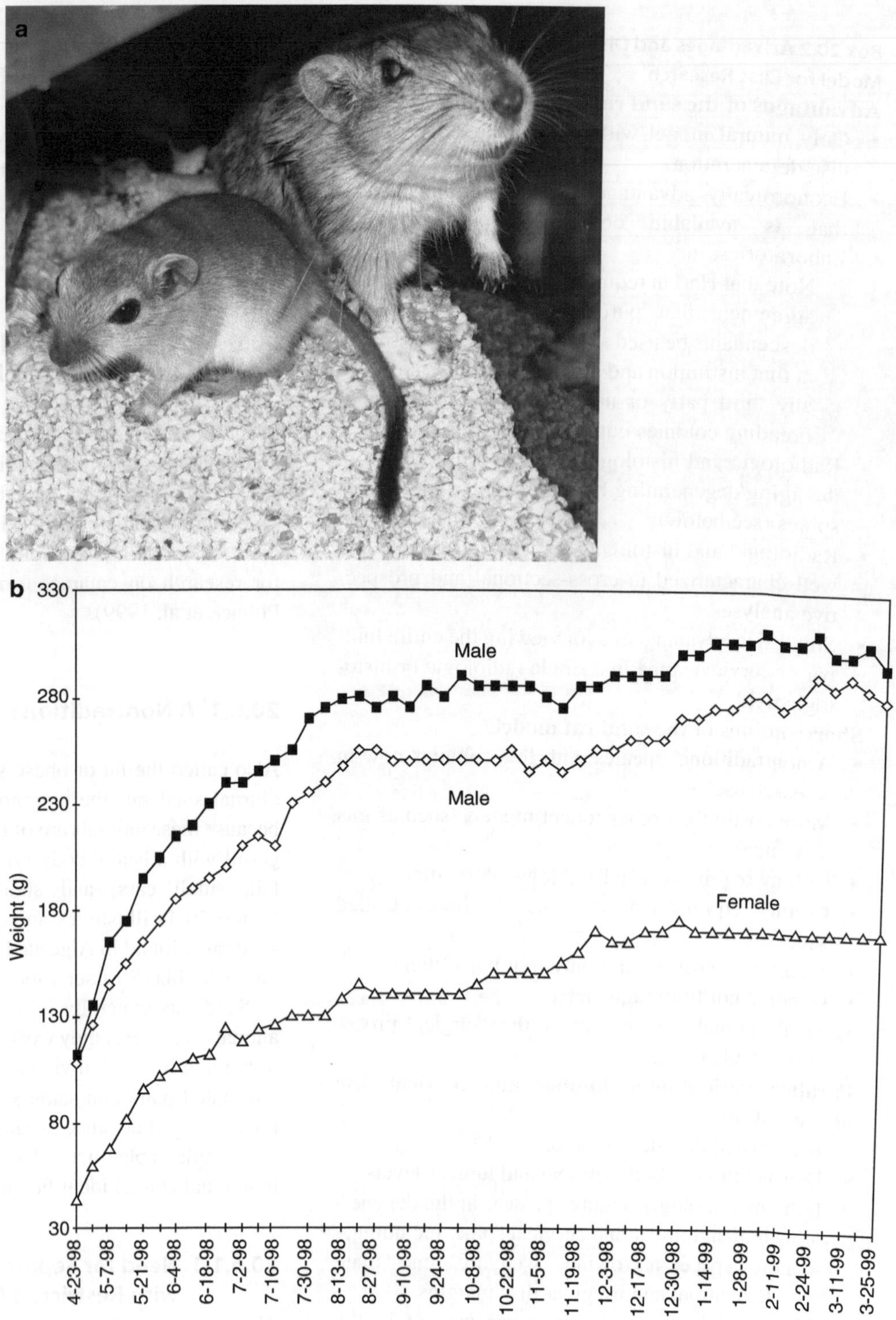

Fig. 20.4 (**a**) Dam (*right*) and offspring (*left*). Note the small ears and furred tail, with slight tufting at the tip. (**b**) Representative normal body weights for male and female animals

Table 20.3 Age and body weight demographics

Group	Mean age ± SD (*n*) in months	Mean body weight ± SD (*n*) in grams	Gender distribution[a]
Group 1: 1–3.9 months	2.13 ± 0.50 (36)	137.86 ± 23.41 (36)	15 F, 21 M
Group 2: 4.0–11.9 months	6.92 ± 1.57 (18)	189.72 ± 30.22 (18)	5 F, 13 M
Group 3: 12–23.9 months	16.05 ± 4.06 (19)	212.37 ± 53.76 (19)	9 F, 10 M
Group 4: 24–46 months	33.54 ± 5.01 (26)	175.04 ± 33.74 (26)	20 F, 6 M

[a]*F* female, *M* male. Chi-square analysis showed a significant difference in gender distribution between groups, $p = 0.0069$

20.6.1.2 Colony Monitoring Challenges

Sentinel animals occasionally housed within the sand rat colony have never shown positive disease serology, but the value of available non-sand-rat-specific serology tests continues to be an issue of discussion. Due to lack of specificity, such monitoring may not be accurate.

20.6.1.3 Breeding

In captivity, the sand rat breeds best in the springtime, possibly related to airborne pollen which reaches the colony. Animals are fed ad lib only when they are paired for breeding or when the dam has pups in the cage. Animals can be considered sexually mature by 12 weeks of age. When first paired, males and females should be checked for compatibility. Several articles in the older literature have addressed the topic of sand rat breeding (Adler et al. 1976; Frenkel et al. 1972; Strasser 1968).

20.6.1.4 Litter Size

Litter sizes are small; rarely are there six pups/litter, and four pups/litter is more common. It is advisable to always have pairs set up for mating within the colony.

20.6.1.5 Low-Calorie Diet Essential

All animals should be fed the Purina special formulated sand rat diet (Purina custom sand rat diet #5L09 with 2.42 kcal/g metabolizable energy). 100–120 g (50–60 g/sand rat) is placed in cages twice a week. This low-caloric diet serves to minimize development of diabetes (El Aoufi et al. 2007), and adults, breeders, and young animals do well on it due to their ability to ferment materials in their hind gut for nutrition.

20.6.2 Other Topics Related to Animal Husbandry

20.6.2.1 Body Weight Is the Best Health Indicator

Experience has shown that body weight is the best index of sand rat health (Fig. 20.4b, Table 20.3). For adult breeders, if 20 % of initial body weight is lost, this may be seen as a criterion for euthanization. Body weight should be monitored weekly and water consumption and body fur evaluated (animals which are not thriving look "scruffy" in appearance).

20.6.2.2 Teeth Need to Be Clipped Periodically

If animals are losing weight, they should be promptly examined for possible overgrowth of incisors which might be interfering with chewing. If malocclusion is noted, teeth are trimmed and weight monitored for a return to normal. The state of other dental issues in older sand rats have been reported in the literature (Ulmansky et al. 1984).

20.6.2.3 Blood Testing

Since the sand rat has a fully haired tail, blood sampling is accomplished via orbital eye sinus puncture or via the saphenous vein.

20.7 Importance of Animal Models Such as the Sand Rat for Disc Research

The discovery and maintenance of relevant animal models for human disease should remain a high priority among researchers. Although the creation of animal models through genetic engineering continues to be highly important (Schulhof 2000), support and maintenance of naturally occurring animal models needs to be encouraged. Animal models which closely resemble the progression of human diseases, such as the sand rat model of spontaneous, age-related disc degeneration, are an especially important tool in orthopedic research. In addition, as seen in the use of autologous disc cell therapy in the sand rat model, they can bridge the gap between in vitro studies and initial human clinical trials (An and Friedman 1999; Gruber et al. 2002b).

As utilization of the sand rat model increases, knowledge will be gained of its molecular biology. This will be aided by ongoing research into genome sequencing that is being developed for diabetes research at various centers (IREN cDNA libraries of insulin-producing cells 2011).

20.8 Summary of Critical Concepts Discussed in the Chapter

- The sand rat (*Psammomys obesus*) exhibits age-related spontaneous degeneration of the intervertebral disc. As such it is a very important, economical model which avoids the use of chemonucleolysis or surgical injury to induce disc degeneration.
- Radiologic cross-sectional and prospective studies have characterized disc changes with aging in the sand rat. These changes mimic human disc degeneration, including disc wedging, disc space narrowing, end plate calcification, and osteophyte formation.
- Micro-CT models and spin-lock (T_{1r}) imaging studies provided additional confirmation of the presence of wedging, disc space narrowing, end plate calcification, and osteophyte formation.

- Micro-CT models also provide an excellent experimental approach for the analysis of end plate porosity and vascular canals.
- Because of the importance of cell-based therapies for disc degeneration, the sand rat has been used to demonstrate the practicality of autologous disc cell transplantation.
- Morphologic studies of the aging sand rat disc show strong parallels with the aging human disc, including the presence of programmed cell death and cell senescence, the formation of concentric layers of extracellular matrix around disc cells, and cell clustering. Asporin, pregnancy-associated plasma protein-A, and brain-derived neurotrophic factor are present in both human and sand rat discs.
- Highlights on animal husbandry issues with the nontraditional species are provided.

Acknowledgments The authors wish to thank the Brooks Back Pain Research Endowment for support. We thank Michelle V. Chenault, Ph.D., for her assistance in providing animals for the early establishment of our colony, and Brian Gordon, D.V.M., Kim Mihalko, D.V.M., and Dr. Chenault for assistance with animal husbandry. Thanks are also due to Cliff Williams, Karen D. Fay, and Juanita C. Jolly for colony maintenance and to Jane A. Ingram and Natalia Zinchenko for assistance with morphology and radiology studies. We also thank our previous coauthors on past sand rat publications for their many contributions.

References

Adler JH, Roderig C, Gutman Z (1976) Breeding sand rats (Psammomys obesus) with a diabetic predisposition for laboratory investigation. Refuah Vet 33:1–8

Adler JH, Schoenbaum M, Silberberg R (1983) Early onset of disk degeneration and spondylosis in sand rats (Psammomys obesus). Vet Pathol 20:13–22

An YH, Friedman RJ (1999) Animal selections in orthopaedic research. In: An YH, Friedman RJ (eds) Animal models in orthopaedic research, 1st edn. CRC Press LLC, Boca Raton, pp 39–57

An HS, Thonar EJ, Masuda K (2003) Biological repair of intervertebral disc. Spine 28:S86–S92

Anderson DG, Yoon T, Shen F, Kang J, Phillips F, An H (2005) Summary statement: biologic repair or regeneration of the intervertebral disc. Spine J 5:304s

Bernick S, Caillet R (1982) Vertebral end-plate changes with aging of human vertebrae. Spine 7:97–102

Bernick S, Walker JM, Paule WJ (1991) Age changes to the anulus fibrosus in human intervertebral discs. Spine 16:520–524

Chenault VM, Ediger MN, Ansari RR (2002) In vivo assessment of diabetic lenses using dynamic light scattering. Diabetes Technol Ther 4:651–659

Collier G, Walder K, De Silva A, Tenne-Brown J, Sanigorski A, Segal D, Kantham L, Augert G (2002) New approaches to gene discovery with animal models of obesity and diabetes. Ann N Y Acad Sci 967:403–413

El Aoufi S, Gendre P, Sennoune SR, Rigoard P, Maxixent JM, Griene L (2007) A high calorie diet induces type 2 diabetes in the desert sand rat (*Psammomys obesus*). Cell Mol Biol 53:943–953

Fassett DR, Kurk MF, Vaccaro AR (2009) Biologic solutions for degenerative disk disease. J Spinal Disord Tech 22:297–308

Frenkel G, Shaham Y, Kraicer PF (1972) Establishment of conditions for colony-breeding of the sand-rat Psammomys obesus. Lab Anl Sci 22:40–47

Ganey TM, Meisel HJ (2002) A potential role for cell-based therapeutics in the treatment of intervertebral disc herniation. Eur Spine J 11(suppl 2):S206–S214

Gruber HE, Hanley EN Jr (1998) Analysis of aging and degeneration of the human intervertebral disc – comparison of surgical specimens with normal controls. Spine 23:751–757

Gruber HE, Hanley EN Jr (2003) Biologic strategies for the therapy of intervertebral disc degeneration. Expert Opin Biol Ther 3:1209–1214

Gruber HE, Johnson T, Norton HJ, Hanley EN Jr (2002a) The sand rat model for disc degeneration: radiologic characterization of age-related changes. Cross-sectional and prospective analyses. Spine 27:230–234

Gruber HE, Johnson TL, Leslie K, Ingram JA, Martin D, Hoelscher G, Banks D, Phieffer L, Coldham G, Hanley EN Jr (2002b) Autologous intervertebral disc cell implantation: a model using *Psammomys obesus*, the sand rat. Spine 27:1626–1633

Gruber HE, Ashraf N, Kilburn J, Williams C, Norton HJ, Gordon BE, Hanley EN (2005) Vertebral endplate architecture and vascularization: application of micro-computerized tomography, a vascular tracer, and immunocytochemistry in analyses of disc degeneration in the aging sand rat. Spine 30:2593–2600

Gruber HE, Ingram JA, Hanley EN Jr (2006a) Cellular immunohistochemical localization of the matricellular protein myocilin in the intervertebral disc. Biotech Histochem 81:119–124

Gruber HE, Ingram JA, Hanley EN Jr (2006b) Immunolocalization of thrombospondin in the human and sand rat intervertebral disc. Spine 31:2556–2561

Gruber HE, Gordon B, Williams C, Norton HJ, Hanley EN (2007a) Vertebral endplate and disc changes in the aging sand rat lumbar spine: cross-sectional analyses of a large male and female population. Spine 32:2529–2536

Gruber HE, Ingram JA, Hoelscher G, Norton HJ, Hanley EN (2007b) Senescence in cells of the aging and degenerating intervertebral disc: immunolocalization of senescence associated-ß-galactosidase in human and sand rat discs. Spine 32:321–327

Gruber HE, Gordon B, Norton HJ, Kilburn J, Williams C, Zinchenko N, Heath J, Ingram J, Hanley EN Jr (2008a) Analysis of cell death and vertebral endplate bone mineral density in the annulus of the aging sand rat. Spine J 8:475–481

Gruber HE, Hoelscher GL, Ingram JA, Hanley EN (2008b) Immunolocalization and biochemical evidence of pregnancy-associated plasma protein-A (PAPP-A) in the intervertebral disc. Spine 33:E447–E454

Gruber HE, Ingram JA, Hoelscher G, Zinchenko N, Norton HJ, Hanley EN Jr (2008c) Brain-derived neurotrophic factor and its receptor in the human and the sand rat intervertebral disc. Biomed Cent Arthritis Res Ther 10:R82

Gruber HE, Gordon B, Williams C, Ingram JA, Norton HJ, Hanley EN Jr (2009a) A new small animal model for the study of spine fusion in the sand rat: pilot studies. Lab Anim 43:272–277

Gruber HE, Ingram JA, Hoelscher GL, Zinchenko N, Hanley EN Jr, Sun Y (2009b) Asporin, a susceptibility gene in osteoarthritis, is expressed at higher levels in the more degenerated human intervertebral disc. Arthritis Res Ther 11:R47

Gruber HE, Norris RA, Kern MJ, Hoelscher GL, Ingram JA, Zinchenko N, Hanley EN Jr (2011a) Periostin is expressed by cells of the human and sand rat intervertebral discs. Biotech Histochem 86:199–206

Gruber HE, Phillips R, Zinchenko N, Ingram JA, Norton HJ, Hanley EN (2011b) Spontaneous, age-related cervical spine degeneration in the sand rat: a new research application for this animal model. Cervical Spine Research Society, Scottsdale

Harrison DL (1964) The mammals of Arabia, 1st edn. Stechert-Hafner Service Agency, New York, pp 597–602

IREN cDNA libraries of insulin-producing cells (2011) Sand rat islet cDNA library. http://www99.mh-hannover.de/institute/clinbiochemistry/iren/libraries.htm.

Krag M (1996) In: Weinstein JN, Gordon SL (eds) Low back pain: a scientific and clinical overview, 1st edn. American Academy of Orthopaedic Surgeons, Rosemont, pp 479–492

Matsuzaki H, Wakabayashi K (1999) In: An YH, Friedman RJ (eds) Animal models in orthopaedic research, 1st edn. CRC Press, Boca Raton, pp 539–547

Modic MT, Steinberg PM, Ross JS, Masaryk TJ, Carter JR (1988) Degenerative disk disease: assessment of changes in vertebral body marrow with MR imaging. Radiology 166:193–199

Moskowitz RW, Ziv I, Denko CW, Boja B, Jones PK, Adler JH (1990) Spondylosis in sand rats: a model of intervertebral disc degeneration and hyperostosis. J Orthop Res 8:401–411

Phillips FM, An H, Kang JD, Boden SD, Weinstein J (2003) Biologic treatment for intervertebral disc degeneration – summary statement. Spine 28:S99

Pollack A, Oren P, Stark AH, Eisner Z, Nyska A, Madar Z (1999) Cataract development in sand and galactosemic rats fed a natural tomato extract. J Agric Food Chem 47:5122–5126

Regatte RR, Akella SVS, Dodge GR, Reddy R (2004) Spin-lock (T_{1r}) MRI of the sand rat: A new approach to study this model of disc degeneration. 5th Combined Meeting of the Orthopaedic Research Societies of Canada, USA, Japan and Europe, podium presentation No. 048

Schulhof J (2000) Restocking the ark: supporting the discovery, creation, and maintenance of new animal models. Lab Anim 29:25–29

Silberberg R (1988a) Histologic and morphometric observations on vertebral bone of aging sand rats. Spine 13:202–208

Silberberg R (1988b) The vertebral column of diabetic sand rats (Psammomys obesus). Expt Cell Biol 56:217–220

Silberberg R, Adler JH (1983) Comparison of truncal and caudal lesions in the vertebral column of the sand rat (Psammomys obesus). Isr J Med Sci 19:1064–1071

Silberberg R, Aufdermaur M, Adler JH (1979) Degeneration of the intervertebral disks and spondylosis in aging sand rats. Arch Pathol Lab Med 103:231–235

Silberberg R, Meier-Ruge W, Odermatt B (1989) Age-related changes in fibronectin in annulus fibrosus of the sand rat (Psammomys obesus). Expl Cell Biol 57:233–237

Sobajima S, Kompel JF, Kim JS, Wallach CJ, Robertson DD, Vogt MT, Kang JD, Gilbertson LG (2005) A slowly progressive and reproducible animal model of intervertebral disc degeneration characterized by MRI, x-ray, and histology. Spine 30:15–24

Strasser H (1968) A breeding program for spontaneously diabetic experimental animals: *psammomys obesus* (sand rat) and *acomys cahirinus* (spiny mouse). Lab Anim Care 18:328–338

Ulmansky M, Ungar H, Adler JH (1984) Dental abnormalities in aging sand rats (*Psammomys obesus*). J Oral Pathol 13:366–372

Wilson C, Brown D, Najarian K, Hanley EN Jr, Gruber HE (2003) Computer aided vertebral visualization and analysis: a methodology using the sand rat, a small animal model of disc degeneration. BMC Musculoskelet Disord 4:4

Ziran BH, Pineda S, Pokharna H, Esteki A, Mansour JM, Moskowitz RW (1994) Biomechanical, radiologic, and histopathologic correlations in the pathogenesis of experimental intervertebral disc disease. Spine 19:2159–2163

Ziv I, Moskowitz RW, Kraise I, Adler JH, Maroudas A (1992) Physicochemical properties of the aging and diabetic sand rat intervertebral disc. J Orthop Res 10:205–210

[illegible] (2000) Extending the [illegible] supporting the discovery, development and management of new animal models. Lab Anim 29:23–26

Use of Knockout and Transgenic Mouse Models in Disc Research

21

Laura Mangiavini, Rita Gerard-O'Riley, and Ernestina Schipani

Contents

L. Mangiavini, MD • R. Gerard-O'Riley, BS
E. Schipani, MD, PhD (✉)
Department of Medicine,
Cancer Center, Indiana University, 980 W. Walnut Street, R3 C102, Indianapolis, IN 46202, USA

Department of Anatomy and Cell Biology,
Cancer Center, Indiana University,
980 W. Walnut Street, R3 C102, Indianapolis, IN 46202, USA
e-mail: laumangi@iu.edu; rloriley@iu.edu; eschipan@iu.edu

21.1 Introduction

21.1.1 Brief Anatomical Description of the Intervertebral Disc and Its Embryonic Origin

The intervertebral disc is a fibrocartilaginous structure that is located between two vertebral bodies; it transmits loads through the spine and allows bending, flexion, and torsion of the column. The intervertebral disc consists of an outer ring of fibrous cartilage called the annulus fibrosus and an inner gelatinous structure, the nucleus pulposus. The nucleus pulposus is a gelatinous structure mainly formed by sparse chondrocyte-like cells embedded in a highly hydrated aggrecan-containing gel (Raj 2008). For more details of the structure of the disc, see Chaps. 4 and 5. The annulus fibrosus is composed of an outer layer of collagen I and an inner region containing collagen II. The collagen fibers are arranged in parallel lamellae, and elastin fibers are interposed between the lamellae.

The annulus fibrosus and the nucleus pulposus follow different developmental pathways. The annulus fibrosus is derived from the condensation of sclerotome cells. Signals from the notochord induce migration, condensation, and differentiation of sclerotome cells into the annulus fibrosus and vertebrae (Risbud et al. 2010). Still uncertain is the origin of the nucleus pulposus, although recent experimental evidence showed that the nucleus pulposus cells in mice derive from the notochord (Choi et al. 2008); notochordal cells probably undergo hypertrophy to form the nucleus pulposus (Aszódi et al. 1998; Hunter et al. 2004; Sakai et al. 2009). However, the mechanism by which notochordal cells differentiate into nuclei pulposi is not completely understood.

The notochord thus appears to have a double function: directly forming the nucleus pulposus and indirectly controlling the formation of vertebral bodies and the annulus fibrosus. The development of the disc is described in detail in Chap. 3.

I.M. Shapiro, M.V. Risbud (eds.), *The Intervertebral Disc*,
DOI 10.1007/978-3-7091-1535-0_21, © Springer-Verlag Wien 2014

21.1.2 Genetic Factors Involved in Disc Degeneration in Humans

Aging leads to numerous changes in the structure of the intervertebral disc such as shape, vascular supply, and matrix composition including proteoglycan accumulation and water content. With degeneration and age, the extracellular matrix of the nucleus pulposus is progressively reduced. It is likely that the decreased aggrecan content in the aging nucleus pulposus impairs its hydration status resulting in unequal distribution of compressive forces on the spine and, eventually, to disc herniation. For detailed analysis of this topic, see Chaps. 2, 7 and 19.

Degenerative disc disease (DDD) and disc herniation are the most common cause of low back pain in modern society (Frymoyer 1988; Frymoyer and Cats-Baril 1991; Wisneski et al. 1992; Anderson and Weinstein 1996; Komori et al. 1996). Curiously, however, their precise etiology is still largely unknown (Sambrook et al. 1999; Ala-Kokko 2002; Battie et al. 2004). Familial studies have established that disc herniation is influenced, not surprisingly, by genetic and familial factors (Varlotta et al. 1991; Battie et al. 1995; Matsui et al. 1997; Zhang et al. 2008). In the last decade, degenerative disc disease in humans has been associated with different mutations in genes encoding matrix proteins such as collagen I (Pluijm et al. 2004; Tilkeridis et al. 2005), collagen IX (Annunen et al. 1999; Paassilta et al. 2001), and aggrecan (Kawaguchi et al. 1999; Roughley et al. 2006). Moreover, the three master transcription factors of chondrogenesis, Sox5, Sox6, and Sox9; cytokines such as interleukin-1 (Solovieva et al. 2004) and interleukin-6 (Noponen-Hietala et al. 2005); and, lastly, the vitamin D receptor (Videman et al. 2001) have been also involved in the pathogenesis of DDD. The role of each of these genes is described in detail in Chap. 10.

21.2 Animal Models

21.2.1 General Considerations

In recent years, different animal models have been characterized in order to reach a better understanding of the development and function of the intervertebral disc in humans. Generally speaking, a series of variables need to be considered when choosing an adequate animal model to study the nucleus pulposus, such as availability, size, and cost, but knowledge of the similarities and differences in biomechanical and biochemical properties between the model and the human discs is of utmost importance. Larger animals are good models as they recapitulate the human disc with respect to biomechanics, geometry, and structure. However, large animals require long time frames in order to analyze the different developmental stages and/or to generate disc degeneration. Moreover, husbandry and housing are often cost-prohibitive (Singh et al. 2005). For further discussion of the pros and cons of large animal models, see Chap. 18.

On the other hand, smaller animals like rats and mice are less expensive and easy to handle. Moreover, intervertebral disc development and subsequent degeneration occur in a shorter time period, making the use of these models more cost-effective. In addition, a variety of markers and probes are available for murine tissues. Lastly, mouse models are ideal for studies of the intervertebral disc because they can be genetically manipulated. Taken altogether, genetically engineered mice provide an important new tool to test hypotheses related to disc function, degeneration mechanisms, and nonsurgical treatments for disc degeneration. Of course there are limitations for their use: first, anatomical differences exist between humans and mice; second, because of costs, young mice are often analyzed and they may not faithfully reproduce adult human conditions (Alini et al. 2008). In this chapter, mouse models that have promoted a critical new understanding of the human intervertebral disc will be reviewed.

21.2.2 Genetically Modified Mice

Genetically manipulated mice have contributed enormously to identification of genes controlling intervertebral disc development and to the elucidation of their mechanisms of action (Table 21.1).

A genetically modified mouse is a mouse whose genome has been altered through the use of genetic engineering techniques. Different genetic techniques are available to examine the effects of mutant gene products and their roles in the intervertebral disc. In the next section, we will briefly discuss some of them.

21.2.2.1 Transgenic and Global Knockout Approaches

There are two basic genetic technical approaches to produce either transgenic mice or gene-targeted mutant mice, respectively. In the transgenic approach, new genetic information is inserted into the mouse genome via injection of a full-length coding sequence (cDNA) of the gene of interest cloned downstream of a specific promoter sequence into the pronuclei of fertilized mouse oocytes, with subsequent random integration of this cDNA sequence into the host genome. A major limitation of the transgenic approach is that overexpression models often produce nonphysiological levels of the protein of interest, and this can confound interpretation of the physiological role of the gene. Also, the site of transgene integration can have consequences on tissue specificity and levels of expression of the transgene. Moreover, even

Table 21.1 Knockout and transgenic mouse models in the intervertebral disc

Gene of interest	Knockout	Annulus fibrosus	Nucleus pulposus	References
GDF-5	Universal	Abnormal	Abnormal	Li et al. (2004)
Col2a1	Universal	Abnormal	Normal	Sahlman et al. (2001)
Col1a1	Universal	Abnormal	Normal	Sarver and Elliott (2004)
Col9a1	Universal	Abnormal	Normal	Boyd et al. (2008) Allen et al. (2009)
Biglycan	Universal	Abnormal	Abnormal	Furukawa et al. (2009)
Danforth's short tail (Sd)	Universal	Abnormal	Absent	Lane and Birkenmeiser (1993), Alfred et al. (1997)
Sickle tail (Skt)	Universal	Abnormal	Abnormal	Semba et al. (2006)
Sox5 and Sox6	Universal	Deficiency of the inner annulus	Absent	Smits and Lefebvre (2003)
Pax-1	Universal	Abnormal	Abnormal	Wallin et al. (1994)
Pax-9	Universal	Abnormal	Abnormal	Peters et al. (1998)
Has2	Conditional Knockout in cartilage	Abnormal	Abnormal	Roughley et al. (2011)
c-Jun	Conditional Knockout in axial skeleton, sclerotome, notochord	Normal	Abnormal	Behrens et al. (2003)
Ext1	Conditional Knockout in the developing joints	Abnormal	Abnormal	Mundy et al. (2011)
Smoothened	Conditional Knockout in the notochord	Normal	Abnormal	Choi and Harfe (2011)
Tgfbr2	Conditional Knockout in growth plate chondrocytes and inner annulus fibrosus cells in the postnatal stage	Deficiency of the inner annulus	Normal	Jin et al. (2011)
Wnt/β-catenin	Conditional Knockout in axial skeleton	Abnormal	Abnormality due to degeneration of the growth plate	Kondo et al. (2011)

well-characterized promoters can be expressed at low levels in nontarget tissues, so rigorous analysis should include examination of expression of the transgene in a large range of tissues.

The second approach, homologous recombination, involves modifying a specific gene in embryonic stem cells with a DNA construct containing DNA sequences homologous to the target gene. Embryonic stem cells carrying the recombined genomic DNA are selected and are then injected into mouse blastocysts. As a result, mutant genes with either loss-of-function or gain-of-function mutations can be generated (Fig. 21.1).

If the mutated gene is a null allele, a global knockout for that targeted gene is then generated. Global knockouts provide direct insight into the physiological role of the ablated gene product. Moreover, novel actions of the targeted genes can emerge because, unlike transgenic models, global knockout models are not limited to a particular tissue or system. A disadvantage of the global knockout approach is that deletion of genes that are essential for early development may result in early lethality. On the other hand, because of functional redundancy, many knockout strains do not exhibit an obvious phenotype. In this case, creation of double or even triple knockouts may be necessary. Another consideration is that global knockouts usually contain a modified allele in which the selectable cassette used to screen the ES colonies is often retained in the locus of interest. In this case, this could have effects on neighboring genes.

If the mutated gene carries loss-of-function or gain-of-function mutations, a global knock-in for that targeted gene is then generated.

Instead of using a "targeted" strategy, global knockouts can be generated using a high-throughput mutagenesis strategy. One of the most widely used strategies involves the production of random insertional mutations in ES cells using vectors that contain a promoterless reporter gene.

21.2.2.2 Tissue-Specific Knockout Models

Conventional gene targeting generates a modified allele in all cells of the mouse from fertilization on; therefore, it is an extremely useful tool for investigating gene function during development and adulthood. However, if the inactivation of the target gene results in early embryonic lethality, the functions of the gene in specific tissues cannot be studied. Further, universal gene targeting can make it difficult to distinguish direct effects of ablating a gene in a particular tissue from the

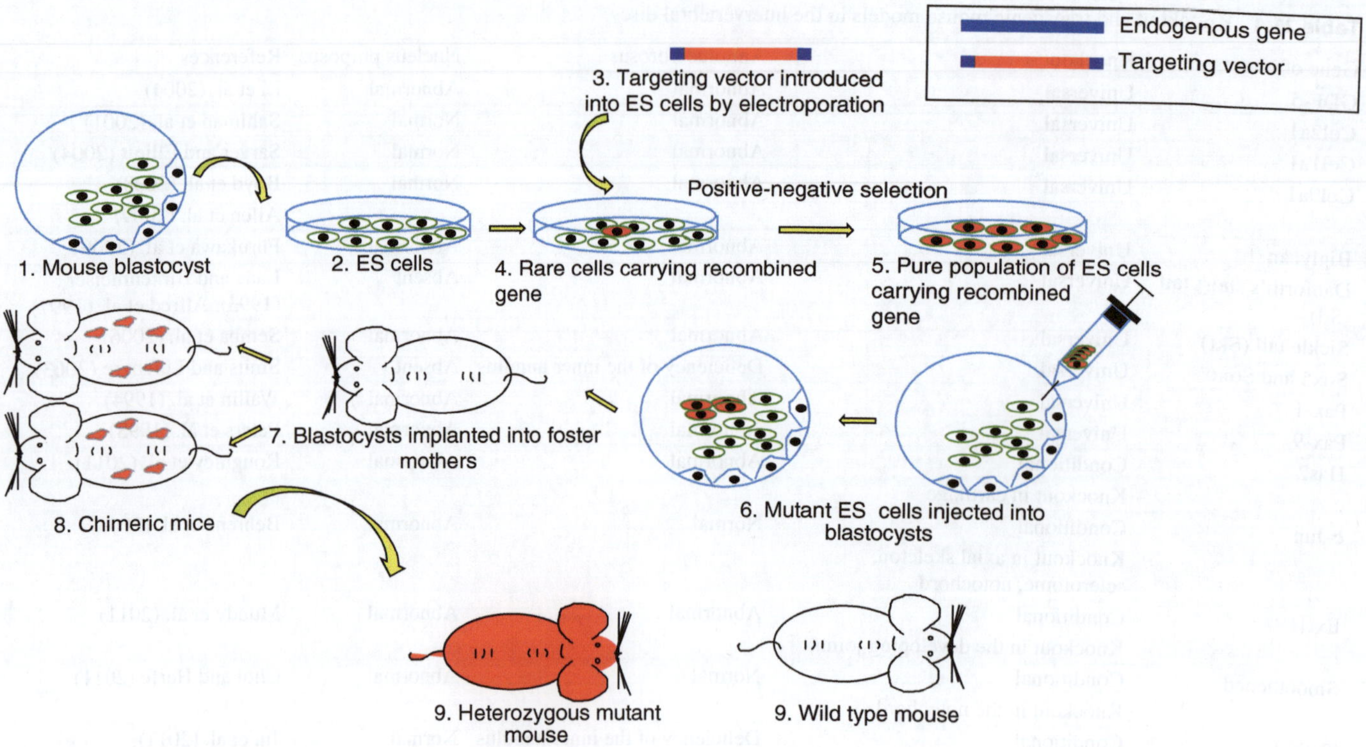

Fig. 21.1 Schematic representation of gene targeting in mice. Embryonic stem cells (ES) are collected from mouse blastocysts (*1*). ES are cultivated in vitro (*2*) and a targeting vector is introduced by electroporation. The targeting vector contains fragments of DNA that are homologous to the endogenous gene (*3*). Homologous recombination occurs between the targeting vector and the endogenous gene (*4*). ES carrying the recombined gene are selected (*5*). The targeted ES are injected into blastocysts (*6*). The blastocysts are implanted into foster mothers (*7*) and they give birth to chimeric mice (*8*). The breeding between chimeric mice produces mice heterozygous for the targeted gene and wild-type mice (*9*)

more indirect effects of ablating the gene in all tissues. The Cre recombinase-loxP (Cre-loxP) system was developed to overcome these limitations and to inactivate genes in a conditional manner in the living mouse as well (Orban et al. 1992; Sauer 1998). "Conditional" gene targeting refers to a gene modification in the mouse that is restricted either to certain cell types (tissue specific), to a specific developmental stage (temporally specific), or to both (Lewandoski 2001).

The regional and temporal specificity provided by conditional gene targeting allows a better analysis of the gene function in different ways. The tissue specificity allows the study of a gene in a particular cell lineage without being influenced by gene loss in adjacent tissues, as the rest of the embryo is genetically wild type. Moreover, the temporal specificity does not permit the organism to adapt to the genetic change, as the wild-type gene product was previously present. Therefore, compensatory responses, which can alter interpretation of conventional germ line mutations, are mitigated, providing a more precise link between genotype and phenotype. Lastly, if null mutations lead to a severe or lethal phenotype during embryonic development, conditional gene targeting can also be used to investigate gene function at late embryonic stages or in adulthood.

To date, the Cre-loxP system is the best-characterized system for conditional gene inactivation in mice (Wilson and Kola 2001; Le and Sauer 2001). The Cre-loxP system is comprised of two elements: the Cre recombinase enzyme and a small stretch of DNA recognized by the recombinase (loxP site) (Stark et al. 1992; Van Duyne 2001). The Cre recombinase is produced by the bacteriophage P1 and is a member of the integrase superfamily of site-specific recombinases that cleave DNA at a distinct target sequence and ligate it to the cleaved DNA of a second identical site to generate a contiguous strand. The loxP site consists of 34 base pairs, a size that is unlikely to occur randomly in even the largest vertebrate genome and yet small enough to be effectively neutral toward gene expression when positioned in chromosomal DNA for genetic manipulations. The orientation of these target sites relative to each other on a segment of DNA directs the type of modification catalyzed by the recombinase; more specifically, in order to achieve excision of the intervening DNA, the two loxP sites must be oriented in the same direction.

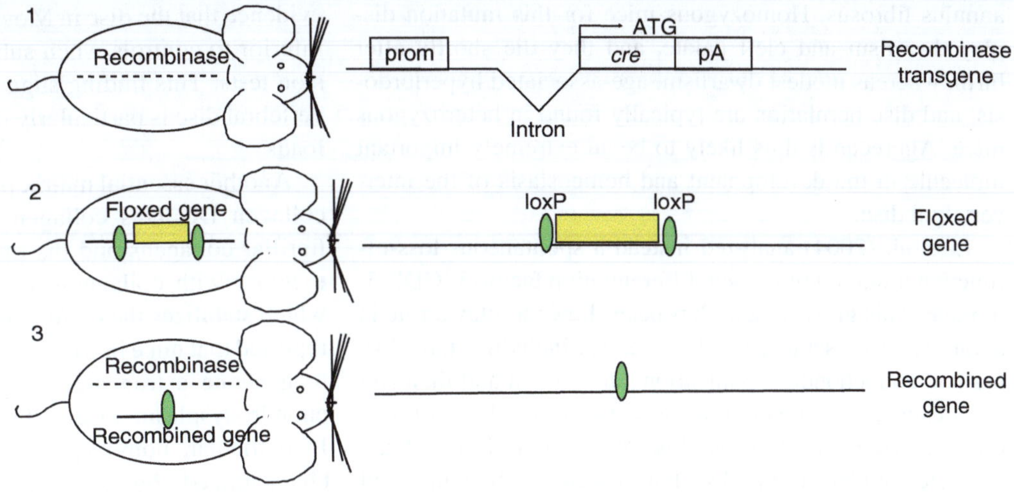

Fig. 21.2 Cre-loxP strategy. Two separate mouse strains are typically generated and intercrossed for a conditional gene targeting experiment. One mouse strain expresses the Cre recombinase in selected tissues (*1*); the mate carries a gene segment flanked (floxed) by the loxP sites (*2*). In offspring (*3*), cells expressing the recombinase delete the target gene segment

Two separate mouse strains are typically generated and intercrossed for a conditional gene targeting experiment. One mouse strain expresses the Cre recombinase in selected tissues, depending on which promoter has been selected to drive recombinase expression; the mate carries a gene segment flanked (floxed) by the loxP sites (Fig. 21.2). The location of the loxP sites must be appropriately chosen so that the function of the gene is not affected and that deletion of the floxed gene segment will lead to inhibition of transcription and/or translation of the gene of interest or to the synthesis of a nonfunctional protein. In offspring, cells expressing the recombinase delete the target gene segment, while the target gene remains functional in cells of all other tissues where Cre is not expressed (Schipani 2002).

The ability to achieve site-specific recombination has revolutionized genetic analysis of skeletal cell function; it is important to bear in mind that it may be difficult to find a promoter that drives Cre expression with sufficient activity to result in complete excision of the target gene.

21.2.3 Studies of Disc Development and Function Using Genetically Modified Mice

21.2.3.1 Spontaneous Gene Mutations Causing Impaired Disc Function and/or Structure

Numerous animal models with spontaneous disc degeneration have been described. In these animals, the mutation is not artificially induced as the animals develop the pathological condition naturally.

The *sand rat* and the *pintail mouse* are the first spontaneous models that have been reported (Singh et al. 2005). As was discussed in Chap. 20, in the *sand rat* (*Psammomys obesus*), cysts and tears in the annulus fibrosus and even herniation of the nucleus pulposus are evident. These conditions resemble the pathological aspects of the degenerate human intervertebral discs. This phenotype may be related to aging but is mainly attributed to an altered metabolism. In fact, diabetic *sand rats* show a decrease in disc hydration, which leads to less advantageous biomechanical properties and eventually to degeneration of the disc (Silberberg et al. 1979; Ziv et al. 1992).

Another spontaneous disc degeneration mouse model is the *pintail mouse* (*Anas acuta*). The nuclei pulposi in the subcervical region have a low mucopolysaccharide content as in the degenerate human discs. This phenotype is stronger in homozygotes. This mouse model was the first evidence that deterioration of the human disc could indeed have a genetic correlate (Berry 1961).

Transcription factors of the Pax family play a major role in intervertebral disc development. Pax-1 is a transcription factor critically involved in various aspects of mammalian organogenesis (Chalepakis et al. 1992). It is expressed in the sclerotome and is implicated in the formation of ventral vertebral structures. Pax-1 is a critical modulator of the cross-talk between notochord and sclerotome in early development (Wallin et al. 1994). For further information on this gene, please see Chap. 3.

Mice carrying a naturally occurring mutation of the Pax-1 gene demonstrate impaired development of both the vertebral bodies and intervertebral discs (Wallin et al. 1994). In particular, both vertebral bodies and intervertebral discs may be either absent or severely deformed. The defects are especially evident in the lumbar region and in the tail. The malformations appear at an early embryonic stage and they affect both the sclerotome and the notochord. However, this phenotype most likely involves additional genes, as a targeted null mutation of Pax-1 causes a less severe phenotype (see below).

Watanabe et al. (1997) and, later, Wai et al. (1998) reported that the "cmd" (cartilage matrix deficiency) mouse carries an autosomal recessive mutation in the gene encoding aggrecan, which is expressed in both the nucleus pulposus and the annulus fibrosus. Homozygous mice for this mutation display dwarfism and cleft palate, and they die shortly after birth, whereas modest dwarfism, age-associated hyperlordosis, and disc herniation are typically found in heterozygous mice. Aggrecan is thus likely to be an extremely important molecule in the development and homeostasis of the intervertebral disc.

Li et al. (2004) analyzed instead a spontaneous loss-of-function mutation of growth differentiation factor-5 (GDF-5) in mice. This growth factor has been shown to play a role in a variety of musculoskeletal processes, including joint formation, endochondral ossification, and tendon and ligament maintenance and repair (Francis-West et al. 1999). Mutant mice carrying a spontaneous loss of function of GDF-5 are characterized by short limbs, abnormalities of the joints, and a reduction in the number of phalanges in the second through fifth digits (Merino et al. 1999). More importantly, these mice demonstrate abnormalities of both the annulus fibrosus and the nucleus pulposus, resembling changes seen in some animal models of disc degeneration. In particular, young adult mice displayed decreased water content of the nucleus pulposus as indicated by MRI analysis. Moreover, the mutant nucleus pulposus is smaller and the glycosaminoglycan content of the disc is diminished, although the amount of total collagen is not altered. In addition, the annulus fibrosus in these mutant mice is characterized by loss of the lamellar organization. All of these abnormalities can be corrected by treatment with recombinant GDF-5. Consistent with these data, conditional knockout (see subsequent paragraph) of GDF-5 further highlighted the importance of this growth factor in the biology of the nucleus pulposus.

21.2.3.2 Global Knockout of Genes Encoding Extracellular Matrix Proteins

Sahlman et al. (2001) reported that mice heterozygous for a Col2a1 null allele develop abnormalities in the vertebral bodies and in the disc. In particular, their vertebral end plates undergo premature ossification, which is associated with a mild grade of degeneration of the disc and with a significantly reduced ability to run, likely secondary to the discomfort caused by the anatomical abnormalities. Of note, collagen II is poorly expressed in the nucleus pulposus, though it is a classical marker of the fibrocartilage that forms the annulus fibrosus. Mice homozygous for a null mutation of Col2a1 show abnormalities in both vertebral bodies and intervertebral discs: the vertebral bodies enlarge gradually and they never initiate endochondral ossification; moreover, the notochord persists, leading to a failure in the development of the intervertebral disc (Aszódi et al. 1998).

Along these lines, Sarver and Elliott (2004) created a transgenic mouse with reduced collagen I expression (Mov13 strain). Collagen I is particularly abundant in the matrix of the outer annulus fibrosus. Mechanical testing provided evidence that the disc in Mov13 mutant mice is mechanically inferior to controls when subjected to compression and torsion tests. This finding suggests that collagen I in the intervertebral disc is particularly important in absorbing torsional loads.

Another essential matrix protein of the annulus fibrosus is collagen IX. This collagen acts as a bridge between the fibrillar collagens and the other components of the matrix; together with collagens II and XI, it forms a heterofibril, which stabilizes the cartilaginous tissue. Nakata et al. (1993) reported that mice in which a gene construct has been inserted to generate a truncated $\alpha 1$ chain of collagen IX develop chondrodysplasia, osteoarthritis, and corneal abnormalities. In particular, homozygous mice exhibit spine deformities characterized by shortening of the vertebrae, matrix disorganization within the annulus fibrosus, and end-plate irregularities (Kimura et al. 1996).

More recently, another study demonstrated that mice homozygous for a loss-of-function mutation of the Col9a1 gene have early-onset osteoarthritis around 6 months of age, secondary to degeneration both in the annulus fibrosus and in the end plate. Interestingly, in this mouse model, the changes in the intervertebral disc are already clearly detectable at 3 months of age and thus precede the degeneration of the vertebral end plate. Notably, disc degeneration occurs in the annulus fibrosus and it is mainly characterized by tears of this structure, whereas the nucleus pulposus is virtually unaffected (Boyd et al. 2008; Allen et al. 2009).

Furukawa et al. (2009) analyzed the function of another component of the extracellular matrix in the intervertebral disc by knocking out biglycan, which is a member of the family of small leucine repeat proteoglycans (SLRPs); SLRPs bind to TGF-βs, collagens, and other matrix proteins. In humans, biglycan is mostly expressed in the outer layer of the annulus fibrosus, while its concentration is very low in the nucleus pulposus. Advancing age leads to an increase in biglycan content in the early stages of degeneration and then, eventually, to a progressive decrease (Cs-Szabo et al. 2002). Previous studies showed that biglycan-deficient mice developed premature osteoarthritis (Ameye et al. 2002). In this study, the authors provide evidence that the absence of biglycan leads to an early degeneration of the intervertebral disc. Using morphometrical and histological analyses, the authors reported that the size of the nucleus pulposus decreases with age in the mutant mice and that, notably, at 6 months of age, mice display an abnormal proliferation of chondrocyte-like cells within the nucleus pulposus. Later, both the nucleus pulposus and the annulus fibrosus in biglycan-deficient mice are characterized by tears associated with "mucous degeneration" of the nucleus. Therefore, biglycan is likely to be an important factor in the maintenance of the intervertebral disc. There are different mechanisms to explain why loss of biglycan accelerates disc degeneration: its loss might cause instability of the extracellular matrix, or it might increase the mechanical stress on the intervertebral disc. The absence of biglycan may also inhibit TGF-β signaling, and this could suppress the damage repair response in the extracellular matrix.

21.2.3.3 Global Knockouts of Genes Affecting Disc Development

In recent years, numerous mouse mutants with abnormalities of the intervertebral disc have been generated by deleting genes of interest by homologous recombination. This knockout strategy has allowed researchers to define the role of different genes in disc development.

For instance, transcription factors important in chondrogenesis have also been shown to play a critical role in disc development and homeostasis. In particular, Smits and Lefebvre (2003) have provided evidence that Sox5 and Sox6 are expressed not only in the chondrocyte precursors that form the vertebral bodies and the annulus fibrosus but also in the notochord and are critically important for disc development. *Sox5* and *Sox6* encode two identical transcription factors (L-Sox5 and Sox6); moreover, *Sox5* also encodes a short protein (Sox5) that lacks the N-terminal of L-Sox5. L-Sox5 and Sox6 are co-expressed in all cartilages and in a few other tissues. In vitro data have shown that these two transcription factors cooperate with Sox9 in the activation of the collagen II gene (Lefebvre et al. 1998). Moreover, Sox5 and Sox6 have redundant roles in chondrogenesis, and knockout mice for these two transcription factors are characterized by a severe chondrodysplasia (Smits et al. 2001). In a more recent work, Smits and Lefebvre analyzed the spine phenotype of mice lacking *Sox5*, *Sox6*, or both through RNA in situ hybridization, cell proliferation, and death assays. First, they showed that *Sox5*$^{-/-}$/*Sox6*$^{-/-}$ mice lack the nucleus pulposus and that the annulus fibrosus has a deficient extracellular matrix. At earlier developmental ages, mutant embryos display an abnormal development of the notochord secondary to massive cell death. Analysis of the possible different genotypes led to the conclusion that *Sox5* and *Sox6* have redundant functions in notochord development, though *Sox6* could be slightly more important.

Taken together, these findings demonstrate that Sox5 and Sox6 are not necessary in early notochord formation but in the survival of notochordal cells. Moreover, these data are consistent with the notion that the nucleus pulposus is derived from the notochord (Choi et al. 2008).

Homozygous Pax-1$^{-/-}$ mice display abnormalities in the shape of the vertebrae, and the intervertebral discs are replaced by a ventral cartilaginous rodlike structure (Wilm et al. 1998). In contrast to Pax-1 mutants, Pax-9$^{-/-}$ mutant mice do not exhibit morphological abnormalities of the axial skeleton (Peters et al. 1998). However, double mutants lacking both Pax-1 and Pax-9 have a more severe phenotype in both vertebral bodies and intervertebral discs when compared to single Pax-1 null mice (Peters et al. 1999). This study indicates that Pax-1 can completely compensate for the absence of Pax-9 during early development of vertebral bodies and intervertebral discs, whereas Pax-9 has a redundant role in the formation of these structures.

Gene-trap mutagenesis in mice has revealed a critical role for genes located on chromosome 2 in development and homeostasis of the nucleus pulposus. In particular, the so-called Danforth's short tail (*Sd*) mouse shows a complete absence of the nucleus along with severe abnormalities of the notochord and vertebral bodies as early as E9.5 that lead to the characteristic short tail (Lane and Birkenmeiser 1993; Alfred et al. 1997). In another mouse model (the enhancer trap line *Etl4*^{lacZ}, located also on chromosome 2), a reporter (lacZ) is inserted near the *Sd* locus, and the resulting phenotype is characterized by kinks in the caudal region of the tail (Zachgo et al. 1998). Interestingly, loss-of-function mutations in the Sickle tail (*Skt*) gene, which is located on chromosome 2 near the *Sd* locus, also lead to severe abnormalities of the notochord and of the nucleus pulposus, resulting in a kinky-tail phenotype in adults (Semba et al. 2006). The nucleus pulposus in homozygous mice is degenerated at its periphery, and also the annulus fibrosus shows some abnormalities such as thin fibrous layers and lack of adhesion to the vertebral bodies: this phenotype is particularly pronounced in the tail, although some degree of abnormality is also present in other regions of the spine. Mutant mice carrying both mutations, *Sd and Skt*, display a phenotype that appears to be the cumulative result of phenotypic abnormalities due to the individual mutations. However, the detailed

Box 21.1 Procedures to Phenotype a Mutant Mouse Disc

1. Genomic PCR analysis to confirm the genotype
2. Macroscopic evaluation of the spine
3. Whole mount Alizarin Red S/Alcian Blue stain to visualize cartilage and ossified skeletal elements
4. Harris hematoxylin and eosin stain to analyze the morphology of the cells
5. Alcian Blue stain to identify the presence of glycosaminoglycans
6. PAS stain to identify the presence of glycogen
7. BrdU immunohistochemistry to quantify cell proliferation
8. Tunel assay to examine cell death
9. Immunohistochemistry to detect the presence of specific proteins
10. In situ hybridization to detect the presence of specific mRNAs
11. Use of reporter mice
12. Biomechanical tests (tension, compression, torsion)

functional and genetic relations between the two loci are still largely unknown. Generally speaking, *Sd* controls an early stage of mesoderm development and thus affects both sclerotome and notochord, while *Skt* is important at a later stage and is essentially involved in the growth and hypertrophy of cells of the nucleus pulposus.

21.2.3.4 Tissue-Specific Knockouts of Genes Encoding Extracellular Matrix Proteins

Conditional knockouts of matrix proteins, signaling molecules, or transcription factors have identified essential players in the biology of the intervertebral disc. Roughley et al. (2011) conditionally knocked out hyaluronan synthase-2 (Has2) in cartilage by using Col2-Cre transgenic mice. Has2 is responsible for most of the hyaluronan production in the body and its universal knockout is embryonic lethal. In the intervertebral disc, hyaluronan forms the core of the proteoglycan aggregates that are responsible for the osmotic properties that allow the disc to resist compression. The knockout of Has2 specifically in cartilage confers a phenotype characterized by a shortening in the spine, long bones, ribs, and snout. Notably, disappearance of the notochord appears to be delayed.

Mundy et al. (2011) have analyzed the role of heparan sulfate proteoglycans (HSPGs) in the development of intervertebral discs. HPSGs modulate numerous developmental processes, and they regulate cell-matrix interactions. Mundy et al. conditionally knocked out Ext1, which is responsible for heparan sulfate synthesis, in developing fibrous/synovial joints by using GDF5-Cre transgenic mice. Of note, by using ROSA26 reporter mice, the authors provided evidence that expression of the Cre was restricted to the annulus fibrosus and did not involve the nucleus pulposus. The mutant mice die from respiratory failure at birth, and they demonstrate severe abnormalities of the intervertebral discs; some discs are missing and the adjacent vertebrae are fused, while the remaining discs contain a hypocellular annulus fibrosus. These abnormalities could be due, at least in part, to a failure of annulus fibrosus progenitor cells to migrate or to proliferate. In conclusion, these data indicate that Ext1 and, consequently, heparan sulfate proteoglycans are necessary for the formation of the annulus fibrosus.

21.2.3.5 Tissue-Specific Knockouts of Genes Affecting Disc Development

The conditional knockout of a variety of genes has revealed an important function for many of these genes in notochord and/or nucleus pulposus development.

β-catenin-dependent Wnt signaling is one of the central regulators of endochondral bone development (Tamamura et al. 2005; Enomoto-Iwamoto et al. 2002); but little is known about the function of this pathway in intervertebral disc development. A series of conditional in vivo gain-of-function and loss-of-function mutations of β-catenin achieved using transgenic mice in which Cre recombinase was driven by fragment of Col11a1 or Col2a1 promoters have provided unequivocal evidence that Wnt/β-catenin signaling supports organization of the annulus fibrosus and that this signaling pathway is critical for maintenance of intervertebral disc structures during development (Kondo et al. 2011).

TGF-β signaling has also been involved in disc formation during embryonic development (Battie et al. 2004). Mice in which Tgfb receptor 2 (Tgfbr2) had been conditionally knocked out in the axial skeleton using a fragment of the Col2a1 promoter displayed abnormal intervertebral discs. Along these lines, postnatal deletion of Tgfbr2, achieved using Col2a1-CreERT2 transgenic mice, led to severe abnormalities of both the vertebral end plate and the inner annulus fibrosus, whereas the nucleus pulposus was virtually intact (Jin et al. 2011). These findings are consistent with the higher content of collagen II, and thus likely of Cre recombinase activity, in the vertebral bodies and in the annulus fibrosus in comparison with the nucleus pulposus. Of course, they do not exclude the possibility that Tgfbr2 could also play an important role in homeostasis of the nucleus upon expression of Cre recombinase specifically in the nucleus pulposus itself.

Behrens et al. conditionally deleted the transcription factor c-Jun in the notochord, sclerotome, and cartilage using a Cre recombinase driven by a fragment of the collagen II promoter (Col2a1; $Jun^{\Delta/\Delta}$). In this way, they provided clear evidence that this transcription factor has an essential role in the development of the intervertebral disc. The Col2a1; $Jun^{\Delta/\Delta}$ mice exhibited a scoliotic vertebral column and abnormal morphogenesis of the ribs. Interestingly, the overall length and morphology of bones in the limbs appear normal in the adult mice. Moreover, the absence of c-Jun does not severely affect chondrogenesis, and the skeletal defects are mainly limited to the developing spine. Consistent with the high levels of expression of c-Jun in the notochord, the mutant mice displayed a dramatic reduction in the size of the nucleus pulposus, but not of the annulus fibrosus. Notably, the reduced size of the nucleus pulposus is likely the result of increased cell death (Behrens et al. 2003).

Sonic Hedgehog (Shh) is expressed in the notochord, in the floorplate, and in the posterior margins of the limb buds (Chiang et al. 1996). Embryos (E9.5) homozygous for a Shh null allele do not form both the vertebral column and the nucleus pulposus, whereas differentiation of the annulus fibrosus is unaffected. Notably, their notochord progressively degenerates as demonstrated by the loss of expression of Brachyury. Two elegant lineage studies achieved by knocking in the cDNA encoding Cre recombinase into the Shh locus (Choi et al. 2008; Maier et al. 2011) have provided the first genetic evidence that nucleus pulposus cells are derived from the notochord. Moreover, deletion of Smoothened, receptor for Shh, achieved using a conditional knockout in which Cre recombinase expression is driven by Shh promoter (Choi and Harfe 2011), has shown that Hedgehog signaling is indeed required for notochord sheath formation and for development of the nucleus pulposus. Interestingly, induction of Cre recombinase at a later stage of development when the notochord sheath had already formed using a tamoxifen-inducible Cre allele (ShhcreERT2) did not affect differentiation of the nucleus pulposus. Taken together, these data strongly support the notion that the notochord gives origin to the nucleus pulposus and indicate that hedgehog signaling, though not required for differentiation of the notochord into nucleus pulposus cells, is essential for subsequent development of the notochord. In this regard, a transgenic mouse in which Cre recombinase is expressed under the control of the Foxa2 promoter (Uetzmann et al. 2008; Park et al. 2008) has been recently generated. Foxa2-Cre recombination activity can be detected in the endoderm but also in the node, floorplate, and notochord. Therefore, in the future, this particular mouse line could be an extremely useful tool for notochord-specific knockouts.

21.3 Summary of Critical Concepts Discussed in the Chapter

- Spontaneous mutation models have enhanced the understanding of the role of genes in disc function.
- Global gene targeting has significantly expanded our knowledge of the molecular mechanisms that regulate disc development, homeostasis, and degeneration.
- Conditional gene targeting has overcome the limitations of universal gene targeting, allowing the analysis of the genes of interest at different embryological stages and in different tissues, without affecting mouse viability. This technique has also led to the discovery of the embryological origin of the nucleus pulposus.
- Future research related to the intervertebral disc will involve a considerable extension of the use of tissue-specific and temporally inducible knockout models, further expanding our knowledge of the development of these important tissues and providing direction in the search for therapies.

Acknowledgements This work was supported by the NIH RO1 AR04819 grant (to E.S.).

References

Ala-Kokko L (2002) Genetic risk factors for lumbar disc disease. Ann Med 34:42–47

Alfred JB, Rance K, Taylor BA, Phillips SJ, Abbott CM et al (1997) Mapping in the region of Danforth's short tail and the localization of tail length modifiers. Genome Res 7:108–117

Alini M, Eisenstein SM, Ito K, Little C, Kettler AA, Masuda K, Melrose J, Ralphs J, Stokes I, Wilke HJ (2008) Are animal models useful for studying human disc disorders/degeneration? Eur Spine J 17(1):2–19

Allen KD, Griffin TM, Rodriguiz RM, Wetsel WC, Kraus VB, Huebner JL, Boyd LM, Setton LA (2009) Decreased physical function and increased pain sensitivity in mice deficient for type IX collagen. Arthritis Rheum 60(9):2684–2693

Ameye L, Aria D, Jepsen K et al (2002) Abnormal collagen fibrils in tendons of biglycan/fibromodulin- deficient mice lead to gait impairment, ectopic ossification, and osteoarthritis. FASEB J 16:673–680

Anderson GBJ, Weinstein JN (1996) Disc herniation. Spine 21:1S

Annunen S, Paassilta P, Lohiniva J, Perälä M, Pihlajamaa T, Karppinen J, Tervonen O, Kröger H, Lähde S, Vanharanta H, Ryhänen L, Göring HH, Ott J, Prockop DJ, Ala-Kokko L (1999) An allele of COL9A2 associated with intervertebral disc disease. Science 285:409–412

Aszódi A, Chan D, Hunziker E, Bateman JF, Fässler R (1998) Collagen II is essential for the removal of the notochord and the formation of intervertebral discs. J Cell Biol 143(5):1399–1412

Battie MC, Videman T, Gibbon LE, Fisher LD, Manninen H, Gill K (1995) Determinants of lumbar disc degeneration: a study relating lifetime exposures and magnetic resonance imaging findings in identical twins. Spine 20:2601–2612

Battie MC, Videman T, Parent E (2004) Lumbar disc degeneration: epidemiology and genetic influences. Spine 29:2679–2690

Behrens A, Haigh J, Mechta-Grigoriou F, Nagy A, Yaniv M, Wagner EF (2003) Impaired intervertebral disc formation in the absence of Jun. Development 130(1):103–109

Berry R (1961) Genetically controlled degeneration of the nucleus pulposus in the mouse. J Bone Joint Surg 43B:387–393

Boyd LM, Richardson WJ, Allen KD, Flahiff C, Jing L, Li Y, Chen J, Setton LA (2008) Early-onset degeneration of the intervertebral disc and vertebral end plate in mice deficient in type IX collagen. Arthritis Rheum 58(1):164–171

Chalepakis G, Tremblay P, Gruss P (1992) Pax genes, mutants and molecular function. J Cell Sci 16(Suppl):61–67

Chiang C, Litingtung Y, Lee E, Young KE, Corden JL, Westphal H, Beachy PA (1996) Cyclopia and defective axial patterning in mice lacking sonic hedgehog gene function. Nature 383(6599): 407–413

Choi KS, Harfe BD (2011) Hedgehog signaling is required for formation of the notochord sheath and patterning of nuclei pulposi within the intervertebral discs. Proc Natl Acad Sci U S A 108(23):9484–9489

Choi KS, Cohn MJ, Harfe BD (2008) Identification of nucleus pulposus precursor cells and notochordal remnants in the mouse: implications for disk degeneration and chordoma formation. Dev Dyn 237(12):3953–3958

Cs-Szabo G, Ragasa-San Juan D, Turumella V, Masuda K, Thonar EJ, An HS (2002) Changes in mRNA and protein levels of proteoglycans of the annulus fibrosus and nucleus pulposus during intervertebral disc degeneration. Spine (Phila Pa 1976) 27(20): 2212–2219

Enomoto-Iwamoto M, Kitagaki J, Koyama E et al (2002) The Wnt antagonist Frzb-1 regulates chondrocyte maturation and long bone development during limb skeletogenesis. Dev Biol 251:142–156

Francis-West PH, Abdelfattah A, Chen P et al (1999) Mechanisms of GDF-5 action during skeletal development. Development 126:1305–1315

Frymoyer JW (1988) Back pain and sciatica. N Engl J Med 318:291–300

Frymoyer JW, Cats-Baril WL (1991) An overview of the incidence and costs of low back pain. Orthop Clin North Am 22:263–271
Furukawa T, Ito K, Nuka S, Hashimoto J, Takei H, Takahara M, Ogino T, Young MF, Shinomura T (2009) Absence of biglycan accelerates the degenerative process in mouse intervertebral disc. Spine (Phila Pa 1976) 34(25):E911–E917
Hunter CJ, Matyas JR, Duncan NA (2004) Cytomorphology of notochordal and chondrocytic cells from the nucleus pulposus: a species comparison. J Anat 205:357–362
Jin H, Shen J, Wang B, Wang M, Shu B, Chen D (2011) TGF-β signaling plays an essential role in the growth and maintenance of intervertebral disc tissue. FEBS Lett 585(8):1209–1215
Kawaguchi Y, Osada R, Kanamori M, Ishihara H, Ohmori K, Matsui H et al (1999) Association between an aggrecan gene polymorphism and lumbar disc degeneration. Spine 24:2456–2460
Kimura T, Nakata K, Tsumaki N, Miyamoto S, Matsui Y, Ebara S, Ochi T (1996) Progressive degeneration of articular cartilage and intervertebral discs. An experimental study in transgenic mice bearing a type IX collagen mutation. Int Orthop 20(3):177–181
Komori H et al (1996) The natural history of herniated nucleus pulposus with radiculopathy. Spine 21:225–229
Kondo N, Yuasa T, Shimono K, Tung W, Okabe T, Yasuhara R, Pacifici M, Zhang Y, Iwamoto M, Enomoto-Iwamoto M (2011) Intervertebral disc development is regulated by Wnt/β-catenin signaling. Spine (Phila Pa 1976) 36(8):E513–E518
Lane PW, Birkenmeiser CS (1993) Urogenital syndrome (us): a developmental mutation on chromosome 2 of the mouse. Mamm Genome 4:481–484
Le Y, Sauer B (2001) Conditional gene knockout using Cre recombinase. Mol Biotechnol 17(3):269–275
Lefebvre V, Li P, de Crombrugghe B (1998) A new long form of Sox5 (L-Sox5), Sox6 and Sox9 are co-expressed in chondrogenesis and cooperatively activate the type II collagen gene. EMBO J 17:5718–5733
Lewandoski M (2001) Conditional control of gene expression in the mouse. Nat Rev Genet 2(10):743–755. Review
Li X, Leo BM, Beck G et al (2004) Collagen and proteoglycan abnormalities in the GDF-5- deficient mice and molecular changes when treating disk cells with recombinant growth factor. Spine (Phila Pa 1976) 29(20):2229–2234
Maier JA, Harfe BD (2011) Nuclei pulposi formation from the embryonic notochord occurs normally in GDF5-deficient mice. Spine (Phila Pa 1976) 36(24):E1555–E1561
Matsui H, Maeda A, Tsuji H, Naruse Y (1997) Risk indicators of low back pain among workers in Japan. Association of familial and physical factors with low back pain. Spine 22:1242–1247
Merino R, Macias D, Ga√±an Y, Economides AN, Wang X, Wu Q, Stahl N, Sampath KT, Varona P, Hurle JM (1999) Expression and function of Gdf-5 during digit skeletogenesis in the embryonic chick leg bud. Dev Biol 206(1):33–45
Mundy C, Yasuda T, Kinumatsu T, Yamaguchi Y, Iwamoto M, Enomoto-Iwamoto M, Koyama E, Pacifici M (2011) Synovial joint formation requires local Ext1 expression and heparan sulfate production in developing mouse embryo limbs and spine. Dev Biol 351(1):70–81
Nakata K, Ono K, Miyazaki J, Olsen BR, Muragaki Y, Adachi E, Yamamura K, Kimura T (1993) Osteoarthritis associated with mild chondrodysplasia in transgenic mice expressing alpha 1(IX) collagen chains with a central deletion. Proc Natl Acad Sci U S A 90(7):2870–2874
Noponen-Hietala N, Virtanen I, Karttunen R, Schwenke S, Jakkula E, Li H et al (2005) Genetic variations in IL6 associated with intervertebral disc disease characterized by sciatica. Pain 114:186–194
Orban PC, Chui D, Marth JD (1992) Tissue- and site-specific DNA recombination in transgenic mice. Proc Natl Acad Sci U S A 89(15):6861–6865
Paassilta P, Lohiniva J, Goring HH, Perala M, Raina SS, Karppinen J et al (2001) Identification of a novel common risk factor for lumbar disc disease. JAMA 285:1843–1849
Park EJ, Sun X, Nichol P, Saijoh Y, Martin JF, Moon AM (2008) System for tamoxifen-inducible expression of cre-recombinase from the Foxa2 locus in mice. Dev Dyn 237(2):447–453
Peters H, Neubüser A, Kratochwil K, Balling R (1998) Pax9- deficient mice lack pharyngeal pouch derivatives and teeth and exhibit craniofacial and limb abnormalities. Genes Dev 12:2735–2747
Peters H, Wilm B, Sakai N, Imai K, Maas R, Balling R (1999) Pax1 and Pax9 synergistically regulate vertebral column development. Development 126(23):5399–5408
Pluijm SM, van Essen HW, Bravenboer N, Uitterlinden AG, Smit JH, Pols HA, Lips P (2004) Collagen type I alpha1 Sp1 polymorphism, osteoporosis, and intervertebral disc degeneration in older men and women. Ann Rheum Dis 63:71–77
Raj PP (2008) Intervertebral disc: anatomy-physiology-pathophysiology-treatment. Pain Pract 8(1):18–44. Review
Risbud MV, Schaer TP, Shapiro IM (2010) Toward an understanding of the role of notochordal cells in the adult intervertebral disc: from discord to accord. Dev Dyn 239(8):2141–2148. Review
Roughley P, Martens D, Rantakokko J, Alini M, Mwale F, Antoniou J (2006) The involvement of aggrecan polymorphism in degeneration of human intervertebral disc and articular cartilage. Eur Cell Mater 11:1–7; discussion 7. Review
Roughley PJ, Lamplugh L, Lee ER, Matsumoto K, Yamaguchi Y (2011) The role of hyaluronan produced by Has2 gene expression in development of the spine. Spine (Phila Pa 1976) 36(14):E914–E920
Sahlman J, Inkinen R, Hirvonen T, Lammi MJ, Lammi PE, Nieminen J et al (2001) Premature vertebral endplate ossification and mild disc degeneration in mice after inactivation of one allele belonging to the Col2a1 gene for type II collagen. Spine 26:2558–2565
Sakai D, Nakai T, Mochida J, Alini M, Grad S (2009) Differential phenotype of intervertebral disc cells: microarray and immunohistochemical analysis of canine nucleus pulposus and annulus fibrosus. Spine (Phila Pa 1976) 34(14):1448–1456
Sambrook PN, MacGregor AJ, Spector TD (1999) Genetic influences on cervical and lumbar disc degeneration: a magnetic resonance imaging study in twins. Arthritis Rheum 42:366–372
Sarver JJ, Elliott DM (2004) Altered disc mechanics in mice genetically engineered for reduced type I collagen. Spine 29:1094–1098
Sauer B (1998) Inducible gene targeting in mice using the Cre/lox system. Methods 14(4):381–392. Review
Schipani E (2002) Conditional gene inactivation using cre recombinase. Calcif Tissue Int 71(2):100–102. Epub 2002 Jul 24. Review
Semba K, Araki K, Li Z, Matsumoto K, Suzuki M, Nakagata N, Takagi K, Takeya M, Yoshinobu K, Araki M, Imai K, Abe K, Yamamura K (2006) A novel murine gene, Sickle tail, linked to the Danforth's short tail locus, is required for normal development of the intervertebral disc. Genetics 172(1):445–456
Silberberg R, Aufdermaur M, Adler JH (1979) Degeneration of the intervertebral disks and spondylosis in aging sand rats. Arch Pathol Lab Med 103(5):231–235
Singh K, Masuda K, An HS (2005) Animal models for human disc degeneration. Spine J 5(6 Suppl):267S–279S. Review
Smits P, Lefebvre V (2003) Sox5 and Sox6 are required for notochord extracellular matrix sheath formation, notochord cell survival and development of the nucleus pulposus of intervertebral discs. Development 130(6):1135–1148
Smits P, Li P, Mandel J, Zhang Z, Deng JM, Behringer RR, de Crombrugghe B, Lefebvre V (2001) The transcription factors L-Sox5 and Sox6 are essential for cartilage formation. Dev Cell 1(2):277–290
Solovieva S, Leino-Arjas SK, Ala-Kokko L, Luomo K, Raininko R, Saarela J et al (2004) Interleukin 1 polymorphisms and intervertebral disc degeneration. Epidemiology 15:626–633

Stark WM, Boocock MR, Sherratt DJ (1992) Catalysis by site-specific recombinases. Trends Genet 8(12):432–439. Review

Tamamura Y, Otani T, Kanatani N, Koyama E, Kitagaki J, Komori T, Yamada Y, Costantini F, Wakisaka S, Pacifici M, Iwamoto M, Enomoto-Iwamoto M (2005) Developmental regulation of Wnt/β-catenin signals is required for growth plate assembly, cartilage integrity, and endochondral ossification. J Biol Chem. 280(19): 19185–19195

Tilkeridis C, Bei T, Garantziotis S, Stratakis C (2005) Association of a COL1A1 polymorphism with lumbar disc disease in young military recruits. J Med Genet 42:e44

Uetzmann L, Burtscher I, Lickert H (2008) A mouse line expressing Foxa2-driven Cre recombinase in node, notochord, floorplate, and endoderm. Genesis 46(10):515–522

Van Duyne GD (2001) A structural view of cre-loxp site-specific recombination. Annu Rev Biophys Biomol Struct 30:87–104. Review

Varlotta GP, Brown MD, Kelsey JL, Golden AL (1991) Familial predisposition for herniation of a lumbar disc in patients who are less than twenty-one years old. J Bone Joint Surg Am 73:124–128

Videman T, Gibbons LE, Battie MC, Maravilla K, Vanninen E, Leppavuori J et al (2001) The relative roles of intragenic polymorphisms of the vitamin D receptor gene in lumbar spine degeneration and bone density. Spine 26:A1–A6

Wai AW, Ng LJ, Watanabe H, Yamada Y, Tam PP, Cheah KS (1998) Disrupted expression of matrix genes in the growth plate of the mouse cartilage matrix deficiency (cmd) mutant. Dev Genet 22(4): 349–358

Wallin J, Wilting J, Koseki H, Fritsch R, Christ B, Balling R (1994) The role of Pax-1 in axial skeleton development. Development 120(5):1109–1121

Watanabe H, Nakata K, Kimata K, Nakanishi I, Yamada Y (1997) Dwarfism and age-associated spinal degeneration of heterozygote cmd mice defective in aggrecan. Proc Natl Acad Sci U S A 94(13): 6943–6947

Wilm B, Dahl E, Peters H, Balling R, Imai K (1998) Targeted disruption of Pax1 defines its null phenotype and proves haploinsufficiency. Proc Natl Acad Sci U S A 95(15):8692–8697

Wilson TJ, Kola I (2001) The LoxP/CRE system and genome modification. Methods Mol Biol 158:83–94. Review

Wisneski RJ, Garfin SR, Rothman RH (1992) Lumbar disc disease. In: Rothman RH, Simeone FA (eds) The spine, 3rd edn. W.B. Saunders Co, Philadelphia, p 671

Zachgo J, Korn R, Gossler A (1998) Genetic interactions suggest that Danforth's short tail (Sd) is a gain-of-function mutation. Dev Genet 23(1):86–96

Zhang Y, Sun Z, Liu J, Guo X (2008) Advances in susceptibility genetics of intervertebral degenerative disc disease. Int J Biol Sci 4(5):283–290

Ziv I, Moskowitz RW, Kraise I, Adler JH, Maroudas A (1992) Physicochemical properties of the aging and diabetic sand rat intervertebral disc. J Orthop Res 10:205–210

22 Intervertebral Disc Culture Models and Their Applications to Study Pathogenesis and Repair

Svenja Illien-Jünger, Benjamin A. Walter, Jillian E. Mayer, Andrew C. Hecht, and James C. Iatridis

Contents

22.1 Introduction

The intervertebral disc is the largest avascular and aneural structure in the human body (Holm et al. 1981) and composed of a number of interacting and interdependent tissues. While there are numerous clinical studies of the human disc, there remains a great deal to learn concerning its basic biology, alterations during disease, and treatment strategies. One important approach to studying the pathophysiology and the repair of the degenerative disc is through the use of animal models that approximate its unique anatomy and physiology. Although many relevant animal systems are available, because of the relatively small size of the disc, differences in cell and tissue function, and confounding biologic factors that include nutrient transport and metabolic activity, it is difficult to generate models that are comparable to the human. Simulating the disc niche is one of the greatest challenges in intervertebral disc degeneration research and a major obstacle in preventing the direct translation of findings relevant to cell culture and small animal model studies to the human condition. This chapter describes historical advancements in techniques used for intervertebral disc organ culture models and their applications to study disc physiology, pathogenesis of disease, and repair.

S. Illien-Jünger, PhD • B.A. Walter, MS
A.C. Hecht, MD • J.C. Iatridis, PhD (✉) • J.E. Mayer, BS
Leni and Peter W. May Department of Orthopaedics,
Icahn School of Medicine at Mount Sinai,
1 Gustave Levy Place, 1188, New York, NY 10029-6574, USA
e-mail: svenja.illien-juenger@mssm.edu; benjamin.walter@mssm.edu; andrew.hecht@mountsinai.org; james.iatridis@mssm.edu; jillian.mayer@mssm.edu

I.M. Shapiro, M.V. Risbud (eds.), *The Intervertebral Disc*,
DOI 10.1007/978-3-7091-1535-0_22, © Springer-Verlag Wien 2014

22.1.1 Animal, Cell, and Organ Culture Models

The current understanding of the biology of the intervertebral disc and its associated diseases has been established through studies using human cadaveric tissue, surgical samples, and animal models. While animal models are essential for hypothesis testing and therapeutic screening, as will be discussed later, they can differ both structurally and cellularly from the human disc. Small and large animal in vivo models are ideal for investigating interactions between the intervertebral disc and surrounding spinal tissues as well as developmental studies of systemic inflammation, healing, or pain. However, in vivo conditions cannot be precisely controlled as in vitro models. Live animal testing is costly from both economic and ethical perspectives, and for large animal models, the capacity for high-throughput or long-term in vivo studies is limited. Despite these drawbacks, large animal models are most appropriate for evaluating late-stage therapeutic interventions and treatment strategies.

Studies of surgical and cadaveric tissue are of great relevance to the human condition. Human cadaveric tissue is required for spine biomechanical testing and for studies of surgical repair but is limited in terms of measurements of biologic change in response to interventions. Biochemical and histological analyses facilitate investigations of cellularity, inflammation, matrix composition, and other biological, structural, and mechanical questions even on postmortem tissue. When cadaveric human tissue is obtained within approximately 24 h of death, intervertebral disc cells can also be harvested for long-term cell and organ culture experiments. Human surgical samples are the most clinically relevant, yet the quantity (i.e., for multiple dependent variable measurements) is often limited. Surgical tissue quality can also be highly variable preventing clear distinction between nucleus pulposus, annulus fibrosus, and herniation tissue. Furthermore, surgical samples, almost by definition, exclude healthy tissues.

Intervertebral disc cell culture experiments are used for therapeutic screening and also for hypothesis testing. Most cell culture techniques extract and then harvest cells from the native matrix, thereby altering the important interactions between matrix and cells. Both matrix constituents and novel biomaterials provide high-quality 3D cell culture environments, but these model systems all differ from the native tissue niche.

Organ culture is a variant of more traditional cell culture systems where instead of extracting and culturing the tissue cellular components, the entire intervertebral disc is collected and maintained in culture. Ex vivo organ culture also allows more precise control over mechanical and chemical boundary conditions of the disc compared with in vivo models. A key strength of organ culture techniques is that native cellular matrix connectivity and other niche characteristics are retained, which is important because cellular behavior is greatly influenced by the surrounding environment (Risbud et al. 2003).

22.1.2 The Intervertebral Disc Niche

The intervertebral niche is formed by the intimate connection between cells and their surroundings, and in the mature human adult, this niche is strongly influenced by the nutritional environment, the presence of cytokines, and the composition of the extracellular matrix. The specific structure and niche environment undergoes age-dependent adaptive changes that can lead to the accumulation of toxic metabolites. Nutrients and metabolites are transported into the nucleus pulposus by fluid exchange mediated by the diffusion of molecules through the cartilaginous endplates or outer annulus fibrosus. As a result, oxygen tension and glucose concentrations within the central region of the disc are generally low; the acidic by-products of anaerobic metabolism and the slow transport of waste products out of the disc induce a decrease in environmental pH, typically composed of lactic acid (Urban et al. 2004). It is assumed that the low concentrations of required nutrients and metabolites and the relatively high concentration of waste products provide a physicochemical environment that is supportive of a small cell number (4,000–9,000 cells) and slow metabolic rate (Bibby et al. 2005; Maroudas et al. 1975).

22.2 Objectives

Based on its anatomy and physiology, there are many unique challenges for simulating and studying the mechanism by which the intervertebral disc functions in health and disease. While all model systems have limitations, retaining mechanical, chemical, and biological characteristics that are similar to, or mimic, the human disc is a priority; this chapter focuses on specific techniques and advantages of organ culture models. The purpose of this chapter, therefore, is to provide an overview of intervertebral disc organ culture systems, the historical aspects of method development, technical considerations required for successful implementation of organ culture, its importance as an experimental model for the study of intervertebral disc pathology, and finally as a screening tool for implementation of therapeutic repair.

Box 22.1 Intervertebral Disc Organ Culture System Development

A historical survey of published papers, found using online search engines, demonstrates that there has been a substantial increase in the number of papers published on intervertebral disc organ culture systems. Notably, approximately 10 years ago, there were less than two papers on the topic published per year, and in 2011 there were seven papers published in the first 10 months of the year (Table 22.1). Similar trends were found in the Transactions of the Orthopaedic Research Society. Why are so many research groups adopting these novel techniques? There are at least four answers to this question:

Technical advance. Since the first disc organ culture paper was published in 1979 (Oegema et al. 1979), several dissection procedures, bioreactor systems, and cell culture technologies have been developed. It was necessary to overcome two major technical obstacles. The first involved tissue processing procedures that allow transport of nutrients into and waste products out of the intervertebral disc. The second involved the development of improved dissection procedures and bioreactors to inhibit axial swelling and apply physiological loading. Comprehensive techniques for organ culture are described in Sect. 22.3.5.

Need for human-relevant models of intervertebral discs. The discs of most animal models have nutrient transport mechanisms, micro-architecture, and cell metabolic rates that are different from the mature human intervertebral disc. Rodents have small intervertebral discs with a more gelatinous nucleus pulposus structure, a predominantly notochordal cell composition, and higher cell metabolism rates than the mature human intervertebral disc. In contrast, the intervertebral discs of some large animals are closer in structure, size, and cellularity to the mature human discs. The expenses and ethical costs of large animal in vivo testing make large animal organ culture models an attractive option. Comparison with other animal models can be found in Sect. 22.3.1.

Need to quickly test novel hypotheses and screen therapeutic strategies. The high degree of control over mechanical and chemical boundary conditions of organ culture models is an advantage over in vivo systems. The elaborate 3D cellular niche of intervertebral disc cells can be maintained in organ culture and provide major advantages when compared with more traditional cell culture systems especially with respect to testing novel scientific hypotheses and screening of therapeutics. Organ culture models that describe pathophysiology of degeneration and intervertebral disc repair are described in Sects. 23.5 and 23.6.

Because human intervertebral discs can be maintained in culture. There are many practical and ethical constraints on human subject testing. The capacity to maintain viable human intervertebral discs in organ culture provides a new and important preclinical tool that offers promise for screening therapeutic agents in a way that complements live animal testing. The use of human discs in organ culture is described in Sect. 23.7.

Table 22.1 Publication history of intervertebral disc organ culture systems

Date range	www.pubmed.gov	www.ors.org
2011	7	5
2006–2010	26	11
2001–2005	7	3
1996–2000	8	0
1991–1995	6	na
>1990	4	na

Survey of the number of intervertebral disc organ culture papers published over the last two decades based on electronic searches of Medline (www.pubmed.gov; keywords "intervertebral organ culture"; date 9/27/2011) and of the Transactions of the Orthopaedic Research Society Meeting (www.ors.org, keywords "intervertebral organ culture"; date 9/27/2011); note that electronic search spans 1999–2011. The table demonstrates the recent growth in the number of papers on the topic of organ culture

22.3 Organ Culture Model Development

Organ culture models have been developed over the last few decades using animal discs of various sizes in either simple or complex bioreactor systems to provide controlled in vitro conditions that simulate the in vivo situation. The earliest organ culture systems faced many challenges in establishing effective and relevant culture conditions that were adequate to maintain tissue integrity and intervertebral disc cell viability and metabolism. The most modern systems are computer controlled and capable of maintaining multiple intervertebral discs from large animals with loading in multiple degrees of freedom. The following sections provide an overview of the historical progression and diversity of organ culture models that have been developed.

22.3.1 Choice of Animal Models

When compared to the human, small animal models (including mice, rats, and rabbits) have enhanced nutrient and waste transport characteristics. Small animal models also have higher matrix water content, greater distinction between annulus fibrosus and nucleus pulposus, and a larger number of notochordal cells that persist to older ages; the latter cells exhibit an elevated metabolic activity when compared with chondrocytic nucleus pulposus cells (Aguiar et al. 1999; Oegema et al. 2000). Indeed, the notochordal population in human intervertebral discs is greatly reduced if not entirely absent by puberty (Hunter et al. 2004). Sakai et al. (2009) found considerable interspecies differences when comparing gene expression levels of notochordal and non-notochordal animal discs with cells of human intervertebral discs. The high metabolic rate, relatively rapid aging process, and low cost of small animal models are all very attractive research features. However, these advantages ignore major differences between animal and human disc cells. From this perspective, therapeutic interventions that may be successful in small animal models may not succeed in large animal models or humans. Depending on the biologic or biomechanical question, small animal models can also be of limited value as they lack sufficient tissue for multiple measurements.

The intervertebral discs of large animal models are of comparable size to the human, and nutrient transport, disc structure, cellularity, and metabolic rates are similar. Nutritional and transport limitations in the large human intervertebral discs have long been considered a key factor in slowing successful repair (Kandel et al. 2008) and in contributing to the uniquely challenging disc cell niche. These large diffusion distances that human disc cells experience are likely to become a critical issue as research becomes more clinically translatable. Recently developed bioreactor systems are designed to handle the size and loading requirements of bovine and ovine intervertebral coccygeal discs which are among the most commonly used tissue sources.

There are differences in the types of loading that intervertebral discs of quadrupeds experience when compared to bipeds. This difference reflects the orientation of the spine with respect to gravity and biomechanical differences between anatomic regions (tails vs. spines). Surprisingly, since the dominant loading forces on the spine of all animals are associated with muscle action along the axis of the spine, these biomechanical differences are often smaller than one might expect and are most relevant when considering instrumentation design. Even loading on the tail is dominated by axial musculature, so that loading differences between ovine, bovine, rodent, and other coccygeal intervertebral discs models are typically no more significant than the biological differences between species. These biomechanical similarities are highlighted by the findings that the effective axial stress (axial force normalized by cross-sectional area) required to restrain swelling of tail intervertebral discs (0.1–0.3 MPa) is similar to the in vivo intradiscal pressure measured in human lumbar discs in the prone position (0.1–0.3 MPa; see also Sect. 22.3.4). The range of motion and peak stresses do vary across intervertebral discs levels and species (Alini et al. 2008; Demers et al. 2004; MacLean et al. 2005; Oshima et al. 1993; Wilke et al. 1999). These differences are paramount when considering final geometry and material choices for instrumentation and implants at final stages of product development.

Most commonly, the intervertebral discs of large animals are smaller in size than human lumbar discs. However, human intervertebral discs have a greater disc height (height = 11.3 ± 0.3 mm) and they are elliptical in cross section (medial-lateral diameter = 55.9 ± 9.4 mm and anterior-posterior diameter = 37.2 ± 4.7 mm). Bovine caudal discs are smaller than human lumbar discs (bovine disc height = 6.90 ± 0.35 mm) and circular in cross section (diameter = 28.9 ± 2.0 mm). The normalized transport distance or aspect ratios (disc height normalized to lateral diameter) are similar for human (0.202) and bovine (0.239; O'Connell et al. 2007). A comparison of intervertebral disc dimensions and differences in tissue composition of commonly used animal models is shown in Fig. 22.1. The most obvious difference between the discs is the size: bovine coccygeal discs have diameter of ~22 mm (30 % smaller than human discs), followed by lumbar porcine (~18 mm), coccygeal ovine (~15 mm), rat (~4 mm), and mice (~2 mm). The coccygeal discs of bovine and ovine are approximately round in the transverse plane compared to the human and porcine which are kidney bean shaped and typically approximate to an ellipse. Similar to the healthy human nucleus pulposus, the nucleus of bovine and ovine coccygeal intervertebral discs appears white and fibrous, whereas the gelatinous nucleus of the porcine and rodent lumbar discs clearly differs in composition. Several authors have provided a more comprehensive comparison of bovine coccygeal intervertebral discs with the human (Demers et al. 2004; Oshima et al. 1993). Furthermore, most smaller species retain notochordal cells throughout aging, while bovine and ovine species do not (Hunter et al. 2004).

Taken together, coccygeal intervertebral discs from bovine and ovine are of large size with similar aspect ratios, transport distances, and composition as human discs and are becoming accepted tissues for large animal organ culture systems.

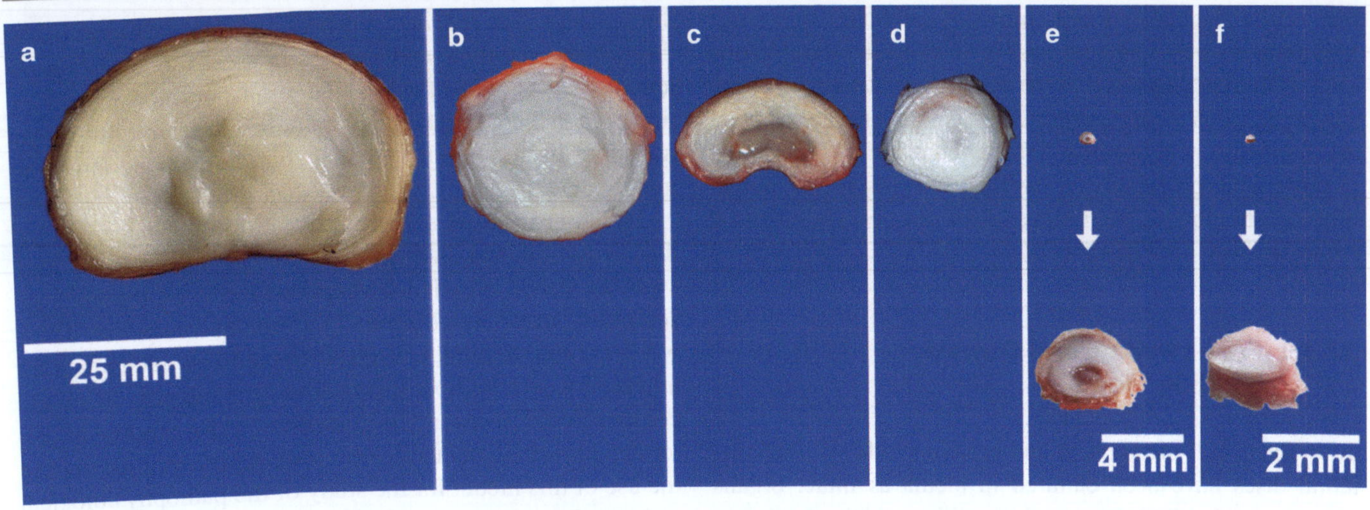

Fig. 22.1 Disc species comparison. Transverse sections from **(a)**, human (lumbar); **(b)**, bovine (coccygeal); **(c)**, porcine (lumbar); **(d)**, ovine (coccygeal); **(e)**, rat (lumbar); and **(f)**, mouse (lumbar) intervertebral discs

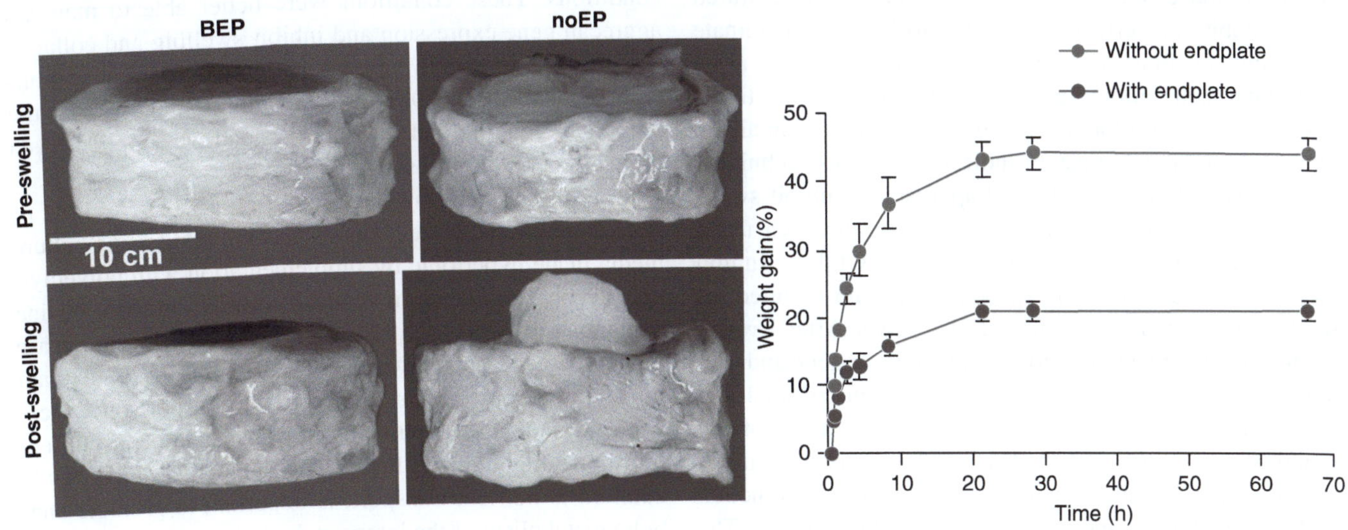

Fig. 22.2 Free swelling of disc explants. *Left*: comparison of swelling capacity and deformation of intervertebral discs with and without bone endplates. *Right*: change in wet weight of intervertebral discs without endplates and cartilage endplate cultures after 66 h ($n=4$, error bars indicate standard deviation; modified from Gawri et al. 2011)

22.3.2 Intervertebral Disc Swelling

A significant challenge for intervertebral disc research, regardless of species, is to maintain the original tissue structure. When muscular loading is removed and intervertebral discs are isolated, the tissue exhibits a propensity to swell in standard culture media as a result of development of large osmotic gradients (Urban and Maroudas 1981). Notably, if the disc is isolated without the superior and inferior endplates, its weight increases drastically compared to discs with bone-covered endplates. This rapid increase in wet weight of intervertebral discs without endplates is apparent within the first 1.5 h (% increase of initial wet weight for discs after 10, 20, and 90 min was 10, 16, and 22 % for intervertebral discs without endplates, while the change was 2, 4, and 5 % for discs with bone-covered endplates (Fig. 22.2)). After 15 h, the weight of discs without endplates increased around 22 % compared to 10 % when cultured with bone-covered endplates. A similar finding was observed by Gawri et al. (2011) who compared swelling of intervertebral discs with cartilage endplates vs. discs without endplates; after 66 h in culture, the observed increase in wet weight was 21 % in the cartilage endplate group, compared with 44 % for the discs without endplates (Gawri et al. 2011). When disc tissue was isolated as fragments, the wet weight was elevated to an even greater extent (Urban and Maroudas 1981). In response to swelling, disc cells increase expression of catabolic and proinflammatory genes and can undergo cell death (Haschtmann et al. 2008a). Conversely, as the disc dehydrates in air, exposure to aqueous media is required to maintain tissue structure and biomechanical integrity (Pflaster et al. 1997). To counter or prevent this propensity for swelling and preserve the physiological structure of the intervertebral disc, ex vivo, several strategies have been developed.

22.3.3 Free-Swelling and Osmotic Loading Models

To evaluate cell metabolism and protein synthesis, intervertebral discs have been cultured in media as intact organs (Oegema et al. 1979). Despite the swelling which can disrupt structure and promote loss of glycosaminoglycans (GAGs) and structural proteins, cells in the disc remain metabolically active (Chiba et al. 1998). Chiba and coworkers cultured whole rabbit intervertebral disc for up to 1 month in alginate to inhibit swelling using techniques adapted from more traditional cell culture protocols. In this system, tissue integrity and biosynthetic activities were maintained. However, other investigators indicated that this technique, and its general nonphysiological approach to inhibit swelling, required further optimization. A new approach using hyperosmotic media (supplemented with TGFβ) to inhibit swelling was described by Risbud et al. who cultured rat lumbar intervertebral discs for 1 and 3 weeks. After 1 week, no differences in cell viability, morphology, or gene and protein expression profiles were found between cultured and control discs, whereas after 3 weeks in culture, a loss of cell function was observed (Risbud et al. 2003). This was a novel approach for investigating the nucleus pulposus function under physiological and pathophysiological conditions. The model also demonstrated that even if swelling of the intervertebral disc could be prevented, cell viability could not be maintained, suggesting that inhibition of swelling was not sufficient to maintain physiological levels of nucleus pulposus cell viability and function in long-term culture.

To prevent swelling of the intervertebral disc in small animals, a further refinement of this technique involved retention of the surrounding tissues. Lim et al. (2006) cultured rat motion segments (the disc with the adjacent vertebrae) for 4 weeks under free-swelling conditions; they reported that after 14 days, nucleus pulposus and annulus fibrosus cell viability (~95 %) was maintained; after 21 days, only 25 % of the cells were viable and viability decreased even further after 28 days (9 %). Thus, the authors demonstrated that rigid fixation of the disc through the vertebral bodies inhibited tissue swelling in media. However, similar to the study by Risbud and coworkers, the loss of cell viability was problematic at longer time intervals. Together, these studies support the concept that reduced nutrient and metabolite transport through the vertebrae and annulus in these models is a problem. It is also notable that endplate transport may be a limitation even in these small animal models which have diffusional transport distances much smaller than human and large animal models.

Haschtmann et al. (2006a) cultured rabbit intervertebral discs with retained endplates in standard media under free-swelling conditions. It was hypothesized that the endplate served to "naturally constrain" the nucleus pulposus. These workers observed that cell viability could be maintained for at least 4 weeks without losing structural integrity or matrix composition. However, "degenerative" gene expression pattern and lowered metabolic rate were reported, thus limiting the use of this model for the study of the pathophysiological and long-term changes in the disc (Haschtmann et al. 2006a). In a subsequent study, rabbit intervertebral discs were cultured with endplates with diurnal changes in hyperosmotic conditions. These conditions were better able to maintain aggrecan gene expression and inhibit swelling and collagen I expression than conventional static osmolarity conditions (Haschtmann et al. 2006b). This finding suggests that the amount of loading and the way the load was applied has a large effect on disc biosynthetic activity.

In a further study by Van Dijk et al. (2011), swelling of nucleus pulposus tissue explants was inhibited using culture media made hypertonic by supplementation with polyethylene glycol. Tissue integrity and cell viability of these bovine explants was maintained for 21 days. However, the decrease in matrix gene expression observed in this tissue explant model (a best case scenario for nutrient transport since there were no endplates or annulus fibrosus to impede nutrient transport) highlighted that biomechanical stimulation, in addition to nutrient transport, is important to promote anabolic metabolism of the intervertebral disc.

22.3.4 Static and Diurnal Compression Loading Models

Oshima et al. (1993) evaluated the axial load required to prevent swelling. These workers estimated that the intervertebral disc experiences an effective mechanical stress of ~0.3 MPa in vivo. In a short 12-h study, both tissue hydration and matrix synthesis were affected by varying the static axial loading. In vivo levels were maintained when the effective stress ranged between 0.13 and 0.26 MPa (Ohshima et al. 1995). This early work established what is now considered to be appropriate baseline loads for large animal disc organ culture and showed the feasibility of this model for studies of the mechanobiology of the intervertebral disc (Fig. 22.3a). Baseline axial compression levels of similar values ~0.15 MPa were also found to retain in vivo disc height in rat

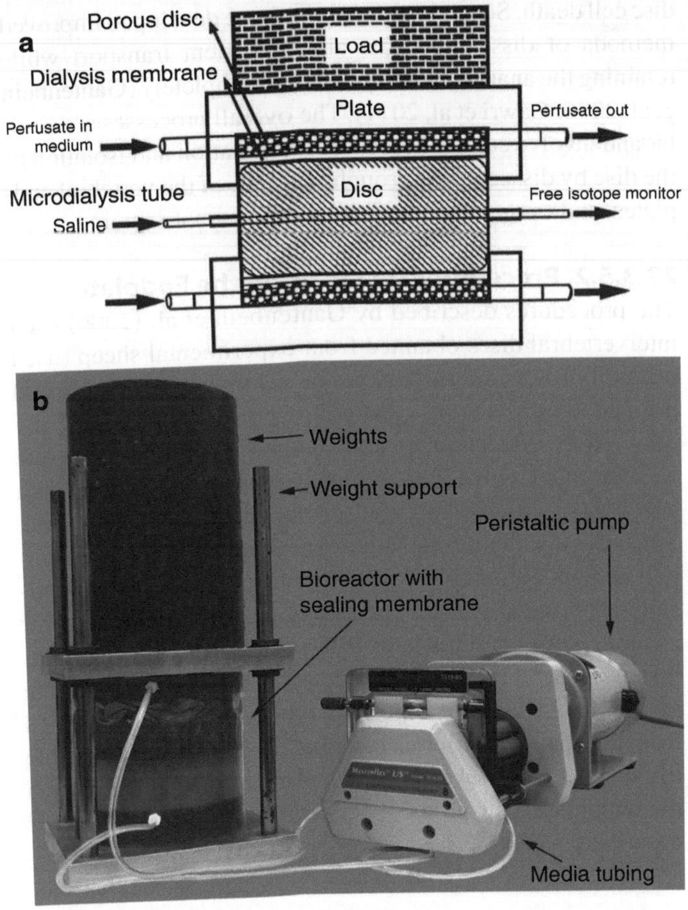

Fig. 22.3 Static and diurnal organ culture models. (**a**) Schematic representation of the first axial compression bioreactor for large animal organ culture designed by Ohshima et al. (1995). (**b**) Load frame to allow diurnal loading on the Ohshima-style static bioreactor

caudal discs (MacLean et al. 2005). From these and other studies, it was concluded that for a number of animal species and vertebrae levels, to prevent disc swelling, an effective compressive stress of ~0.1–0.2 MPa is a reasonable baseline loading condition.

Lee et al. (2006) created a bioreactor system for longer-term culture using the same static compression loading design of Ohshima and coworkers. This system successfully maintained cell viability for up to 7 days; although the GAG synthesis rates dropped by 70–80 % after only 2 days of culture, the cells remained sensitive to mechanical stimulation. Lee and coworkers concluded that this drop in GAG synthesis was the result of static loading, since in vivo experiments demonstrated decreased cell metabolism with loading and enhanced biosynthesis under dynamic compression loading (Maclean et al. 2004; MacLean et al. 2003). Lee and coworkers also evaluated the possibility of culturing intervertebral discs with intact endplates, which by anchoring the annulus fibrosus fibers and retaining nucleus pulposus, pressurization would maintain the biomechanical integrity of the disc. However, culturing discs with endplates drastically reduced cell viability within 1 week, especially in the nucleus. The reduced viability was hypothesized to be associated with formation of blood clots in the vertebral endplates that inhibited nutrient transport. A further validation of bovine organ culture explants without endplates was performed by Korecki et al. (2007; Fig. 22.3b) who found that static as well as diurnal loading conditions maintained GAG content and had similar cell metabolism rates.

22.3.5 Improved Dissection Procedures for Disc Organ Culture

As nucleus pulposus viability in organ culture requires the retention of the endplate cartilage, it was necessary to improve current methods for isolating these regions of the intervertebral disc. Gantenbein et al. (2006) obtained intervertebral discs from sheep that had been treated with a systemic anticoagulant before death. The endplates were cleaned thoroughly with a debridement tool to ensure vasculature channel competence and facilitate nutrient transport. Intervertebral discs with endplates were cultured either under static (0.2 MPa/24 h) or diurnal loading (0.2 MPa/6 h and 0.8 MPa/16 h) for 4 days in media supplemented with 50 mol/l of dextran conjugated with a fluorescent label. They demonstrated that when discs are loaded diurnally, the fluorophores diffused to a greater extent through the annulus fibrosus and endplate towards the disc center than when loaded statically. This was the first study to demonstrate a technique in which (1) large animal intervertebral discs could be cultured with endplates under diurnal loading conditions and (2) cell viability and GAG synthesis could be maintained for 7 days. However, gene expression data indicated possible catabolic changes in cell activity, which was likely associated with a lack of cyclic loading stimulus.

Free-swelling studies by Gawri et al. (2011) on human intervertebral discs and Jim et al. (2011) on bovine discs evaluated if the cartilaginous endplates promoted tissue structure and cell viability and metabolism. In both studies, the vertebral endplates were prepared by removing bone with a high-speed drill until only the cartilage endplates remained. Disc explants with cartilage endplates in free-swelling conditions were cultured for up to 4 months in medium containing high or low glucose levels with high or low concentrations of fetal bovine serum (FBS) (high glucose = 4.5 g/l; low glucose = 1 g/l; high FBS = 5 %; low FBS = 1 %). Importantly, cell viability of these free-swelling explants with cartilage endplates was very high (>95 %) for up to 4 months for all nutritional culture conditions, indicating that adequate waste and nutrition exchange was taking place. However, after

4 weeks in culture, the increase in disc height was about 21 %, and matrix degradation was observed to have increased, independent of the various culture conditions. Similar to other studies, they reported high cell viability but GAG loss in free-swelling culture conditions, suggesting that physiological axial loading may be necessary to regulate cellular metabolism and retain GAG content.

22.3.5.1 Dissection Procedures That Retain Structural Integrity of the Explants

The method of removing and preparing discs from the surrounding tissues is an intricate multistep process. The procedure utilizes bovine caudal intervertebral discs; these discs are freely available and similar to the human lumbar disc (Sect. 22.3.1). It can be adapted for use with other animals, other spine levels, and human specimens. As demonstrated by Lee et al. (2006), without thorough cleaning of blood clots within the endplates, there is inhibition of nutrient and waste transport and nucleus pulposus cell death. In contrast to the earlier techniques that serve to completely dissect the disc from the vertebrae using a straight edge razor or cutting tool to insure straight, parallel cuts (Korecki et al. 2007), the current procedure maintains the cartilaginous and/or vertebral endplates as part of the disc organ system. This technique creates a more anatomically complete structure; it inhibits aberrant swelling, maintains collagen connectivity, and reduces disc cell death. Several investigators have developed improved methods of dissections that allow nutrient transport while retaining the anatomic structure more completely (Gantenbein et al. 2006; Gawri et al. 2011). The overall processes are similar and involve coarse dissection, sterilization and isolation of the disc by dissection, thorough cleaning of the vertebral endplates, and eventual placement in a bioreactor system.

22.3.5.2 Procedures for Cleaning the Endplate

The procedures described by Gantenbein et al. (2006) used intervertebral discs obtained from experimental sheep (used primarily for an alternate experiment) that were heparinized prior to death, making cleaning of the endplates relatively easy. After dissection, residual blood within the endplate was aspirated with a Pasteur pipette and using a syringe with an 18-gauge needle and a jet of phosphate-buffered saline. Since the availability of large experimental animals is limited and obtaining only the tail can be costly both economically and ethically, it was necessary to develop methods for cleaning vertebral endplates that were effective for animals that were not heparinized prior to death, thus creating the possibility of using bovine tails which are easily obtained from the abattoir. Different cleaning procedures are available to clean the vertebral capillaries and enable diffusion through the endplates. Our protocol for removal of clotted blood is described in Box 22.2.

Box 22.2 Refined Dissection Procedures for Isolation of Disc Explants with Vertebral Endplates

- The whole tail should be disinfected before dissection. To access the discs, soft tissue should be removed from the caudal spine.
- For better accessibility, the spinous and transverse processes of the vertebrae can be removed. In our laboratory, we use a simple histological saw. After removal of surrounding tissue, muscles, nerves, and blood vessels should be removed carefully to avoid cutting into the disc.
- To make exact cutting possible, the vertebrae should be rough-cut approximately in half to facilitate the successive precision cutting.
- A high precision histological band saw (e.g., Exakt Apparatebau, GmbH, Norderstedt, Germany) should be used to make two parallel transverse cuts through the vertebral endplate just proximal and distal to the cartilage (1–2 mm adjacent to the disc; Fig. 22.4a).
- After dissection, residual tissue (Fig. 22.4b), cutting debris, and blood clots need to be removed. A commercially available wound debridement irrigation system (Inter Pulse® handpiece set; Stryker, Kalamazoo, MI, USA), commonly used in many surgical procedures, can be used (Fig. 22.4c).

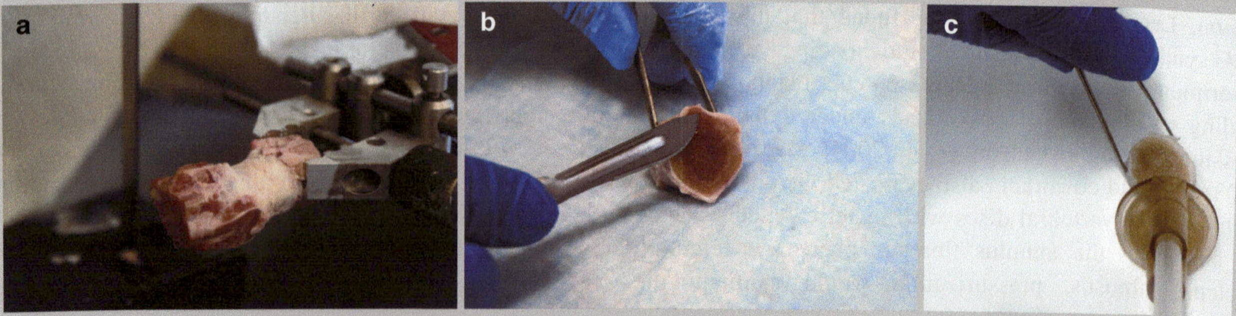

Fig. 22.4 Dissection procedure for cultures with vertebral endplates. (**a**) Isolation of the intervertebral discs from vertebrae; (**b**) growth plate removal; (**c**) intervertebral discs bone-covered endplate cleaning

An alternate procedure used for organ culture loading involves removal of vertebral endplates and retention of just the cartilaginous portion of the plate. Instead of cleaning the residual ossified vertebral tissue, the discs are further processed by surgically ablating the vertebral bone with a surgical round-end bit attached to a high-speed drill, until the cartilage surface is exposed (Gawri et al. 2011; Jim et al. 2011). Intervertebral discs with cartilage endplates and no calcified bone can be maintained in culture or loaded into a bioreactor (Haglund et al. 2011). It is notable that for the dissections that retain the cartilage endplates, the loading surfaces are not straight and parallel, so loading platens that accommodate the unique curvature and size of the cartilaginous EPs are required (Haglund et al. 2011) and as such are a challenge for precise loading.

22.4 Dynamic Compression Loading Models

The addition to dynamic compression loading to intervertebral disc cultures with retained bone-covered endplates provided another significant technical advance in organ culture techniques (Jünger et al. 2009). This method comprised a pneumatically actuated bioreactor loading system capable of loading and culturing whole intervertebral discs with bone endplates and able to simultaneously apply compression loads to 4 individually controlled discs. Physiological loading was simulated with a rest phase at force equivalent of 0.2 MPa for 8 h (representing sleep), an active phase of 0.6 MPa for the remaining 16 h (to simulate time awake), and 2 simulated bouts of exercise lasting 4 h at 0.2 Hz and ±0.2 MPa (i.e., spanning from 0.4 to 1.0 MPa during the active phase). These simulated physiological loading cycles proved beneficial to ovine disc explant cultures as there were no changes in metabolic activity observed after 3 weeks of culture (Jünger et al. 2009). The design specifications of the chambers and pneumatic actuator were optimized for culturing relatively small discs with a diameter of ~15 mm (Fig. 22.5a).

Haglund et al. (2011) developed an organ culture loading device for culturing intervertebral discs with cartilage endplates (based on the dissection technique described by Gawri et al. (2011)) for 4 weeks. During the first week, the discs were cultured without external load, followed by 2-day static load (0.1 MPa) and 19 days with a dynamic loading regimen consisting of 0.1 MPa static loading with 2 periods of sinusoidal dynamic loading between 0.1 and 0.3 MPa load at 0.1 Hz for 2 h separated by a 6-h 0.1 MPa static load period (Haglund et al. 2011). In this model, cell viability was maintained for up to 4 weeks, and Western blot analysis revealed that the dynamic loading regimen preserved intact aggrecan and prevented the increase in degraded aggrecan that was observed under free-swelling culture conditions. The culture chambers were designed to accommodate discs between 20 and 60 mm, making them sufficient in size for bovine and human intervertebral discs (Fig. 22.5b, Haglund et al. 2011). Another multi-chamber organ culture device is being developed by our group that is capable of dynamically loading bovine coccygeal or human lumbar discs in organ culture in axial compression under relatively high loading conditions. The device is designed to fit in an incubator; it is hydraulically actuated, controlled via proportional solenoids, and capable of applying high forces required for large human lumbar intervertebral discs (up to ~5.5 kN; ~2 MPa; Fig. 22.5c). An additional device under development allows loading both in axial compression and in torsion so that the explants can be loaded in multiple degrees of freedom simultaneously (Fig. 22.5d; Walser et al. 2012).

Overall, organ culture has evolved from the first studies, where intervertebral discs were simply placed in culture media and allowed to free swell, to the current elegant computer-controlled systems capable of loading several disc organs simultaneously, in multiple degrees of freedom. The major advances involved controlling swelling, retaining endplates to allow nutrient transport, and applying physiological loads. The next sections describe the usage of these models for degenerative and regenerative studies.

Organ culture permits the investigation of concurrent changes in both structure and cellular responses in a specific and controlled environment. As these models are well controlled, they can be used to determine how multiple factors individually and together contribute to changes in the intervertebral disc biology and degeneration. These organ culture models have been used to address the following scientific questions:

1. What factor(s) causes and/or contributes to pathogenesis of disc degeneration?
2. What potential therapeutic approaches can be used to prevent and/or slow the degeneration process?
3. Can human intervertebral discs be maintained in culture? Research on human tissues addresses issues most directly relevant to health.

22.5 Insights into Mechanism of Degeneration Using Disc Organ Culture

Intervertebral disc degeneration has been defined as "an aberrant, cell-mediated response to progressive structural failure" (Adams and Roughley 2006) with multiple factors thought to be involved in its initiation and progression. The role of these factors is reviewed in other chapters of this book. The majority of current degeneration models are induced using mechanical, structural, nutritional, or inflammatory challenges. This work is providing an improved understanding of individual and interacting factors that cause or lead to degenerative disc disease.

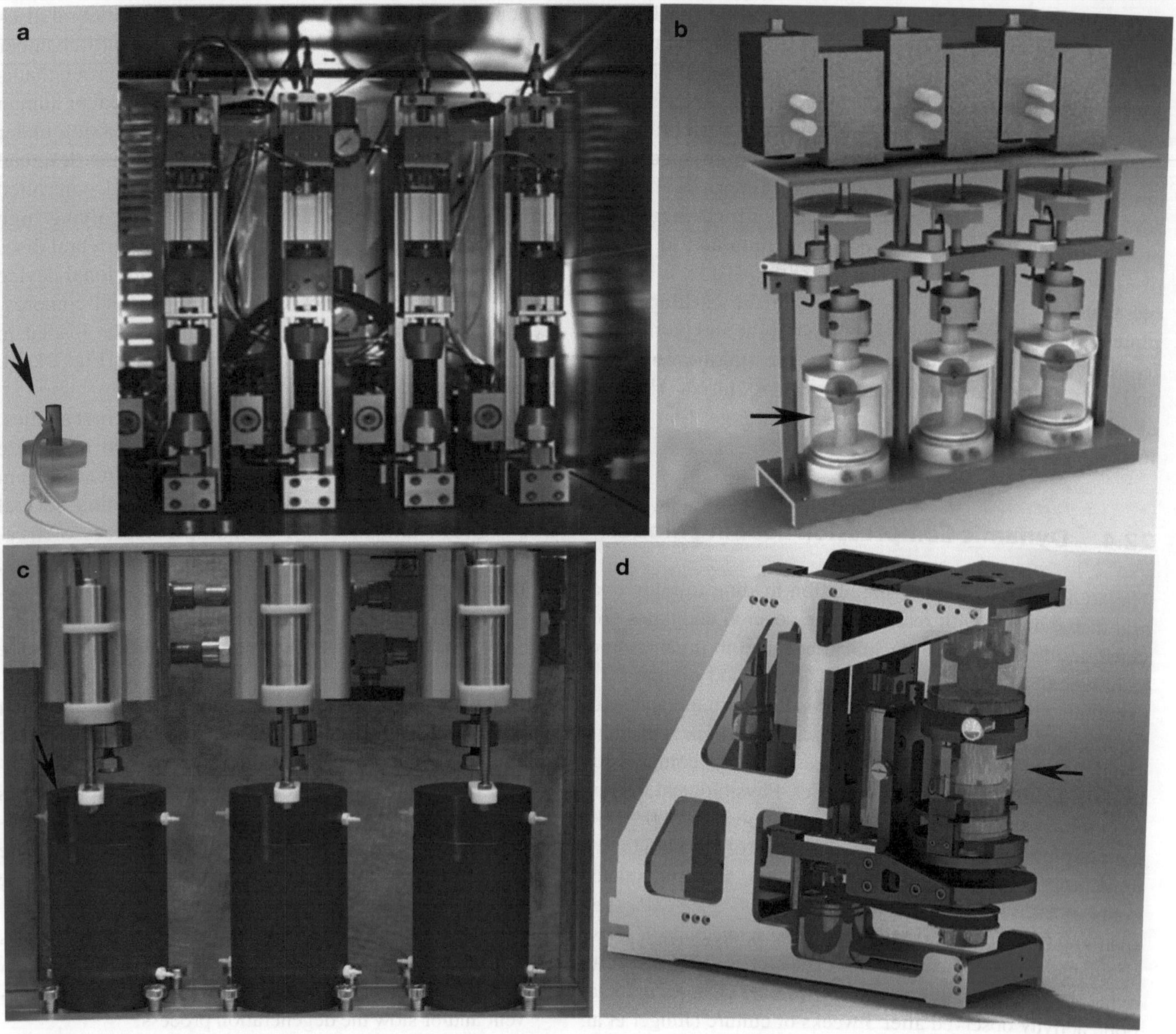

Fig. 22.5 Computer-controlled organ culture loading devices. (**a**) Pneumatically actuated multi-chamber system for axially loading intervertebral discs of medium size (up to 15 mm in diameter) (system described in Jünger et al. 2009). (**b**) Pneumatically actuated multi-chamber system for axially loading of bovine or human discs (Figure modified from Haglund et al. 2011). (**c**) Hydraulically actuated multi-chamber system for applying high magnitudes of axial loading on bovine or human intervertebral discs (Ben Walter and James Iatridis). (**d**) Pneumatically actuated device for axial and torsional loading on bovine discs (With kind permission of Benjamin Gantenbein-Ritter; system described in Walser et al. 2012). All of these loading devices incorporate mechanical parts including a displacement sensor, a load sensor, and a pneumatic or hydraulic actuator

22.5.1 Altered Media Conditions

When compared with in vivo studies that are directed at assessing nutrient transport and uptake by the tissues of the disc, organ culture models provide a much simpler approach to elucidating the importance of this confounding factor. The relevance of nutrient transport as a predisposing factor was demonstrated using nucleus pulposus cell culture (Bibby et al. 2005; Horner and Urban 2001). However, some in vivo models have failed to show that limited nutrition induces degeneration (Hutton et al. 2004; Krebs et al. 2007), possibly due to the lack of precise control over chemical or nutritional boundary conditions. A whole-organ culture study in which there was excellent control over nutrient levels was able to address this controversy (Jünger et al. 2009). Jünger et al. (2009) cultured intervertebral discs under limiting glucose conditions and found that low glucose concentrations (2 g/l vs. 4.5 g/l in normal media) reduced the viability of ovine caudal discs by 40–50 %. However, they also noted that the remaining viable cells exhibited no changes in cellular metabolism, suggesting that limited nutrition alone was not sufficient to initiate a degenerative cascade.

Pro-inflammatory cytokines, specifically tumor necrosis factor-α (TNFα) and interleukin-1-β (IL-1β), are associated with increased degeneration (Le Maitre et al. 2005). Since both cytokines are known to induce catabolic shifts in gene expression and influence the activation of proteases (Hoyland et al. 2008; Seguin et al. 2005), these pro-inflammatory cytokines have served as an attractive target for studies of the degenerative process. Bovine discs that were treated with media containing 200 ng/ml of TNFα for 7 days experienced dramatic losses of aggrecan and altered gene expression that continued following cytokine removal (Walter et al. 2012). Thus, from a mechanistic viewpoint, the effects of injury may be directly linked to upregulation of this and other cytokines.

22.5.2 Mechanical and Nutritional Challenges

Mechanical loading is known to alter metabolic activity and matrix integrity (Iatridis et al. 2006; Walsh et al. 2000), and hence a threshold of "healthy" loading has been described in which immobilization (or underloading) and overloading can both lead to deleterious or degenerative changes (Stokes and Iatridis 2004). Immobilization reduces anabolic metabolism, and overloading can induce micro-injuries (or even larger injuries) which can accumulate and contribute to the degenerative process.

Korecki et al. (2008) found that when bovine intervertebral discs (without endplates) were loaded in compression at 1 Hz, even up to 2.5 MPa, there were no detrimental effects on cellular metabolism or disc structure and there was a dose-dependent increase in sulfate incorporation and collagen I and II gene expression in the annulus fibrosus (Korecki et al. 2008). This finding indicated that moderate dynamic compression increases disc cell metabolism and can thus be considered as healthy loading conditions. These observations were consistent with mechanobiology studies using in vivo rat tail models that showed that only small amounts of damage accumulated when loading was applied at excessive magnitudes and duty cycles in dynamic compression (Maclean et al. 2004; Wuertz et al. 2009). Taken together, these investigations support the concept that endplates are the point of greatest weakness under axial compression in the motion segment, as was demonstrated previously with in vitro biomechanical testing (Adams et al. 2000).

To evaluate how biomechanical loading interacts with reduced nutrition, Illien-Jünger et al. (2010) examined the effects of high-frequency loading at 10 Hz (extreme high-frequency dynamic axial compression) and 0.2 Hz (considered a beneficial moderate dynamic compression) on intervertebral disc explants. These explants were also cultured in media with sufficient (4.5 g/l) or limited (2 g/l) glucose concentrations (to simulate reduced nutrition resulting from endplate sclerosis and calcification). Both high-frequency loading and limited glucose nutrition resulted in increased cell death, and the combination of high frequency and limited nutrition caused an additive increase in cell death and increased MMP13 gene expression. These findings suggested that high-frequency loading may increase cell metabolism without sufficient time to allow transport of nutrients to the disc cells. As a result, there would be an accumulation of acidic metabolites within the explants, and the reduced pH of the microenvironment would accelerate cell death. This phenomenon was further enhanced when disc explants were loaded under nutrient-depleted conditions. The shift in mRNA expression suggested that if cultured for longer durations, more substantial structural changes would be evident (Illien-Jünger et al. 2010).

The response of intervertebral disc explants to short-term repetitive cyclic torsion was evaluated using bovine caudal tissue in organ culture. It was found that small angles (±2°) of torsion increased nucleus pulposus cell viability, whereas apoptosis was observed at larger torsion angles (±5°) (Chan et al. 2011). These results are consistent with the in vivo rat tail studies of Barbir et al. (2011) who found that high magnitudes of cyclic torsion increased pro-inflammatory cytokine production. While these tail model studies applied torsional magnitudes well above the physiological range for human lumbar discs of ±2° (Adams and Hutton 1981), it is also known that tail discs have a larger physiological range of motion than those in the lumbar spine (Elliott and Sarver 2004). In contrast, low and moderate dynamic axial compression loading modes such as torsion, that produce high fiber strains with minimal pressurization, have the capacity to increase cell death, promote the expression of pro-inflammatory cytokines, and enhance catabolism, without provoking an anabolic response.

Noteworthy, complex loading involves multiple loading modes, for example, compression with bending. When complex loading is excessive, e.g., hyperflexion, it can cause herniation in the motion segment (Adams and Hutton 1982). In the bovine intervertebral disc, complex loading of 0.2 MPa compression at an applied wedge angle of 15° was shown to induce a rapid increase in apoptosis, a raised level of catabolic and pro-inflammatory gene expression, and disruption of the annulus fibrosus (Walter et al. 2011). Although vertebral endplates were absent in this model making it a hyperphysiological simulation, the results indicated that annulus fibrosus structural disruption can rapidly induce apoptosis and inflammation and promote a strong catabolic response (Fig. 22.6a).

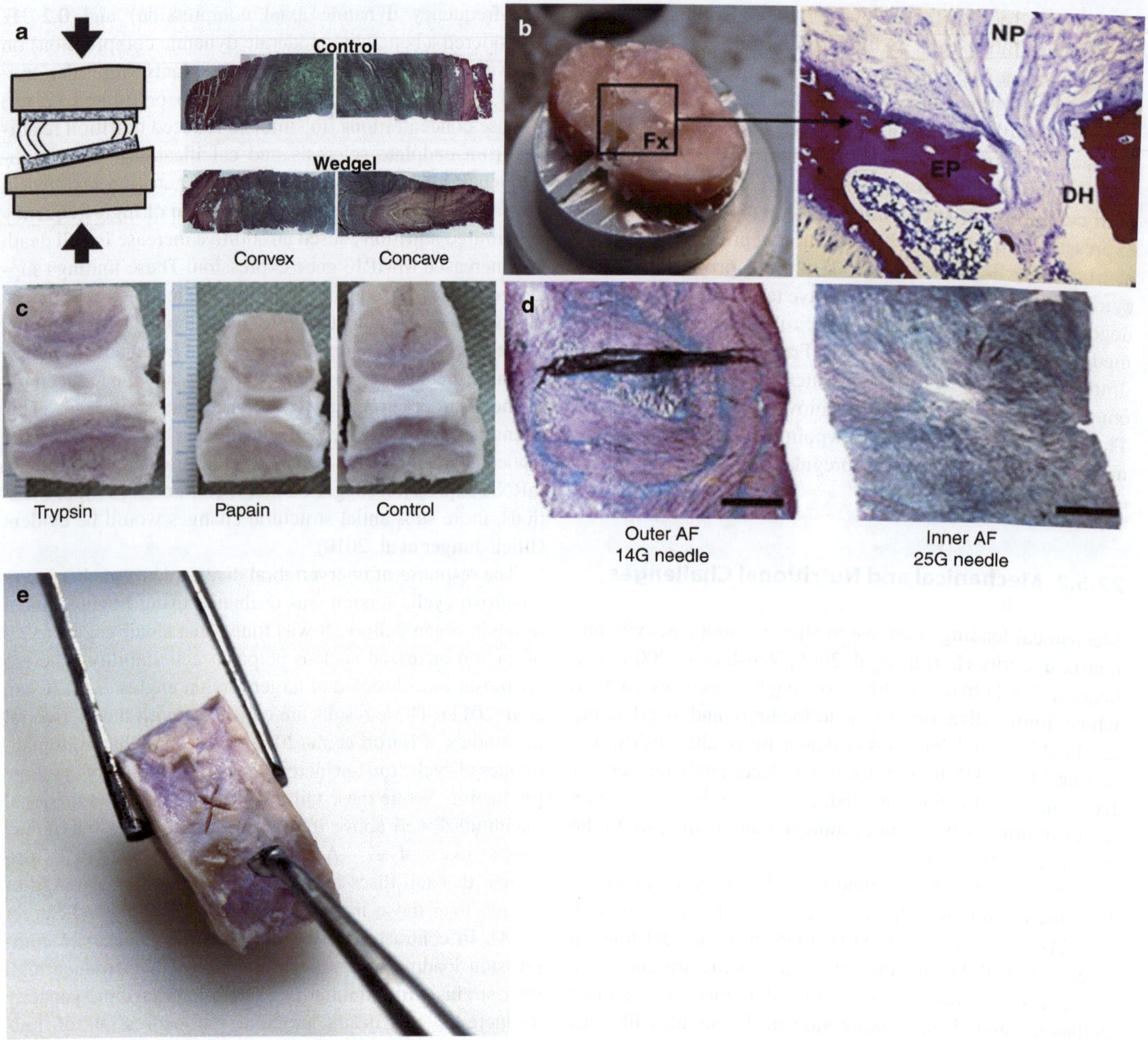

Fig. 22.6 Intervertebral discs organ culture injury models. (**a**) Complex loading of 0.2 MPa axial compression applied at a wedged angle of 15° (Figure modified from Walter et al. 2011); (**b**) vertebral endplates fracture (Haschtmann et al. 2008a, b); (**c**) enzyme digestion to induce degenerative changes (Roberts et al. 2008); (**d**) needle injury simulation in organ culture (Figure modified from Korecki et al. 2008); (**e**) surgical micro-discectomy simulation (Illien-Jünger et al. 2012a)

22.5.3 Surgical and Chemical Challenges

Endplate fractures after spinal trauma can induce rapid degenerative changes in the intervertebral disc. To investigate posttraumatic degenerative changes, Haschtmann et al. (2008b) developed an endplate trauma model based on their established rabbit organ culture system. Endplate burst fractures (Fig. 22.6b) were induced in the disc with a custom-made fracture device and cultured for 9 days. Within the first 3 days, the injuries resulted in immediate cell damage (necrosis) and apoptosis. Continued expression of pro-apoptotic proteins FasL and TNFα was observed in the nucleus pulposus, cytokines that might be expected to cause apoptosis. As cell death is an early response of disc degeneration, this system could represent a reproducible model for investigating degenerative processes after trauma.

Since one sign of degeneration is loss of pressurization of the nucleus pulposus and overall decrease in structural integrity, some studies have directly altered the disc structure by treatment with proteases such as trypsin and papain.

Bovine intervertebral discs that were injected with trypsin were found to have a reduced swelling pressure in the nucleus and a corresponding loss of intact GAGs (Fig. 22.6c; Jim et al. 2011; Roberts et al. 2008). Trypsin had no significant effect on cell viability, but significantly altered the disc structure (Jim et al. 2011); however, the effect on cellular phenotype remains uninvestigated. These models have the advantage of quickly creating a structurally degenerate disc and suggest that they could be used to evaluate or screen therapeutic agents. However, this technique does not reflect the "typical" pathophysiological history of disc degeneration.

Needle puncture is a mild surgical intervention that is important therapeutically and in the context of disc degeneration warrants investigation (Fig. 22.6d). Needle injection simulates discography, a common diagnostic procedure used to inform surgical treatments for low back pain. Needle injection through the annulus fibrosus is also known to induce degenerative changes in several animal models (Masuda et al. 2005). It was shown that bovine caudal discs that were punctured with a needle prior to culturing experienced a rapid change in mechanical function, assessed via measurement of the dynamic modulus, and there was localized cell death at the injection site (Korecki et al. 2008). This finding suggested that the degenerative changes observed in vivo can be associated with compromised mechanical behavior and that following large or small injuries, it is critical that function is restored to the intervertebral disc.

Micro-discectomies can provide back and leg pain relief by removing herniated fragments of tissue that impact nerve roots in the spinal canal of back pain patients. While micro-discectomy surgery can provide immediate benefits, the treated disc continues to degenerate. Post-discectomy disc degeneration often occurs rapidly and leads to significant back pain and occasionally to re-herniation. So as to develop repair strategies, we are currently investigating the direct response of the cells remaining after discectomy using a bovine organ culture system (Fig. 22.6e; Illien-Jünger et al. 2012a).

Several organ culture models have been used to study the pathology of intervertebral disc degeneration. The systems permit analysis of multiple causes of degeneration, including intrinsic factors like altered nutrition and inflammation and extrinsic initiators represented by different loading patterns. Based on these models, novel regeneration therapies are being developed, as described in the next section.

22.6 Mechanisms of Repair and Organ Culture Models of Disc Regeneration

Disc organ culture models have been used to assess the feasibility of potential therapeutic treatments, with the aim of maintaining the extracellular matrix and/or promoting its nutritional status. To investigate the utility of drugs, mouse disc models can be a useful and relatively simple means to assess the effects of an intervention. In contrast, for studies of growth factor therapy, screening can be performed in a small animal model, but the potential clinical efficacy may require additional testing using a large animal. A critical scientific question has focused on long-term evaluation of biosynthesis rates, cell survival, and mechanobiology. For this purpose, rigorous dissection and loading techniques are required that enhance transport as well as simulated physiological loading.

22.6.1 Screening of Potential Therapeutic Agents

The activities of cells of the intervertebral disc are regulated by the interplay of cytokines, proteolytic enzymes, enzyme inhibitors, and growth factors (Masuda and An 2004) (see also Chaps. 8 and 25). Recent in vitro and in vivo studies have generated methods to upregulate the synthesis of the major structural proteins like aggrecan or to downregulate catabolic proteins that are induced by pro-inflammatory cytokines, such as interleukin-1 (IL-1) or tumor necrosis factor-α (TNFα) (Masuda and An 2004; Seguin et al. 2005). Some studies have investigated these effects in vitro using organ culture. In 2006, Risbud et al. cultured rat lumbar intervertebral discs with endplates for 1 week in media supplemented with TGFβ-1 or TGFβ-3. They found that by elevating the levels of activated ERK1/2, which in turn promoted the expression of receptors for TGFβ-1 and TGFβ-1I, TGFβ-3 maintained the in vivo phenotype and biological properties of the disc tissues.

Using mouse functional spine units, Wang et al. (2011) studied the effect of an anesthetic commonly used for the management of back pain. Discs of functional spinal units were treated with the anesthetic for up to 4 weeks in organ culture. Compared to the control group, there was dramatic decrease in cell viability and matrix protein synthesis, demonstrating that the anesthetic, at clinical relevant doses, is toxic to tissues of the intervertebral disc.

22.7 Stem Cells in the Intervertebral Disc

Adult mesenchymal stem cells (MSCs) are a promising cell source for tissue repair and regeneration therapies. While these cells are found in various tissues including skeletal muscle, periosteum, and synovium, the most well-studied sources of MSCs are from bone marrow and adipose. One practical advantage of using MSCs is that they proliferate rapidly, while retaining their multi-lineage potential to commit to a number of phenotypes including bone, cartilage, muscle, ligament, tendon, adipose, and stromal tissues (Pittenger et al. 1999). In vitro and in vivo studies have indicated the potential of MSCs to differentiate towards a phenotype similar to nucleus pulposus cells (Risbud et al. 2004; Steck et al. 2005). In addition, MSCs are known to have immunosuppressive properties and are regarded as nonimmunogenic, rendering them particularly attractive for tissue engineering and cell and gene therapies (Di Nicola et al. 2002). This general topic is discussed further in Chaps. 23 and 24.

22.7.1 Fate of Injected Stem Cells

In 2009, Le Maitre et al. presented a model in which labeled human MSCs were injected into healthy bovine nucleus pulposus explants and cultured for up to 4 weeks. MSCs were identified in all tissue samples, and viability was maintained throughout the whole culture period. Immunohistochemical staining for Sox-9, aggrecan, and collagen II revealed a spontaneous expression of nucleus pulposus markers, whereas no collagen I or X or alizarin red staining was detected at any time point. The authors concluded that cellular hypertrophy and calcification were not induced, i.e., the MSCs differentiated into nucleus pulposus cells rather than annulus fibrosus cells or hypertrophic chondrocytes (Le Maitre et al. 2009). Disc organ culture is therefore a promising tool for future studies to evaluate the fate of injected cells. The technology would help define optimal conditions for cell survival and phenotypic maintenance following injection. For further information on the use of MSC and stem cells in repair of the discal tissue, see Chaps. 23 and 24.

22.7.2 Homing of MSCs

Besides their potential to differentiate into a nucleus pulposus-like phenotype, MSCs also have the ability to engraft into different tissues after site-directed and systematic administration, in particular after injury or disease. The direct migration into areas of tissue damage was demonstrated in bone defects (Kitaori et al. 2009), myocardial infarction (Barbash et al. 2003; Kawada et al. 2004), ischemic cerebral injury (Ji et al. 2004), nephropathy (Hauger et al. 2006), pulmonary fibrosis, and wound healing (Mackenzie and Flake 2001). It has been suggested that trophic factors and cytokines released from those tissues are involved in this migration process. Several studies have reported the functional expression of various chemokine receptors on MSCs (Honczarenko et al. 2006; Nasef et al. 2007), and inflammatory cytokines have been shown to trigger MSC chemotactic migration through extracellular matrix structures (Ries et al. 2007). Recently, it was demonstrated that migration of MSCs into injured discs in organ culture was significantly higher than migration into healthy tissue (Illien-Jünger et al. 2012b). In this model, disc degeneration was induced using needle puncture injury combined with 10 Hz high-frequency dynamic compression. Bovine intervertebral disc was pre-cultured either under simulated physiological or degenerating conditions. At 8–12 days, fluorescently labeled MSCs were added to the culture, and discs were further cultured under static conditions. After 14 days, migration of MSCs into the discs was visualized using fluorescent microscopy (Illien-Jünger et al. 2012b). The results of this study confirm that organ culture is a useful paradigm in which to investigate MSC homing and migration into the disc as well as offering a promising tool for potential regenerative treatments.

22.8 Biomaterials for Intervertebral Disc Repair

Several types of biomaterials and gels have been developed to support the regeneration of the herniated or degenerated intervertebral disc (Grad et al. 2010). The ideal biomaterial should resemble the composition of the native disc in that it should provide a 3D matrix to retain cells or drugs and partially replace the loss of disc tissue, while also providing mechanical support.

The screening of biomaterials in organ culture provides a strategy that complements in vivo implantation studies in animal models. Recent in vitro and in vivo studies have shown that hydrogels consisting of collagen and hyaluronan, a composition similar to the native components of the nucleus pulposus extracellular matrix, are suitable biomaterial substitutes (Collin et al. 2011; Sakai et al. 2006). Peroglio et al. (2011) designed an injectable thermoreversible hyaluronan-based hydrogel (HA-pNIPAM) as a nucleus pulposus cell carrier. In the first step they compared bovine nucleus pulposus cells seeded in HA-pNIPAM and pNIPAM alone. They showed that cell morphology and the GAG synthesis rate were similar in both hydrogels. Gene expression analyses revealed that after expansion, the hydrogels induced a redifferentiation towards the nucleus pulposus phenotype. Compared to alginate beads, HA-pNIPAM promoted hyaluronan synthase 1 gene expression. In a bovine disc culture, they showed that when cells were suspended in the thermoreversible hydrogel, they could be injected through a 22-G needle with cell viability above 80 % after 1 week in culture. The authors concluded that HA-pNIPAM is a suitable, injectable carrier that is capable of maintaining the nucleus pulposus phenotype and promoting disc matrix generation (Peroglio et al. 2011).

22.9 Human Organ Culture Models

Human intervertebral disc organ culture models remain at an early stage of development. As with all research involving human tissue, sample procurement and usage must follow federal guidelines including removal of any identifying information and receive the approval of relevant ethical committees. Whole intervertebral discs with endplates are currently obtained from cadavers following autopsy or from organ donors usually 12–30 h postmortem. Due to the avascular nature of the tissues, cadaveric discs remain viable for 30 h postmortem with cell viability >90 %.

After obtaining specimens, it is important to assess the degenerative grade of the tissue. This can be achieved using X-ray and MRI analysis and graded using the modified Thompson and Pfirrmann classification (Pfirrmann et al. 2001; Thompson et al. 1990). While it is not known whether all grades can be used, the clinical relevance of culturing an end-stage degenerated disc is arguable. Nevertheless, depending on the question being assessed, the development of criteria for including human discs in culturing experiments is helpful and requires degenerative grade assessment. Thorough cleaning of the bone endplate is absolutely necessary to enhance transport of nutrients and waste products.

Organ donor intervertebral disc explants with cartilage endplates have been cultured in free-swelling conditions, for up to 4 months with high cell viability (Gawri et al. 2011). This method has been further improved for culturing human discs with cartilage endplates under diurnal (0.1 MPa/0.3 MPa) and sinusoidal (0.2 Hz) loads (Fig. 22.5b; Haglund et al. 2011). A high-speed grinding drill is used to completely remove vertebral endplates and isolate whole discs with cartilage endplates. In this case, bioreactors must be of sufficient size to accommodate human lumbar intervertebral discs. These discs have an average diameter of approx. 34–35 mm in length and 41–47 mm in width (L1–L5; Panjabi et al. 1992). In turn, the bioreactors must accommodate a large volume of media and to simulate daily loading to be able to withstand forces of 1,500 N (Adams and Hutton 1983). For dynamic compression, computer-controlled loading devices have been developed as shown in Fig. 22.5. The bioreactor chambers are composed of a bottom chamber and a top loading piston with sintered porous loading platens on both ends. Tubing underneath/above the lower/upper platen provides equal distribution of media through and around the disc (Fig. 22.3).

22.10 Limitations of Organ Culture Models

Whole disc organ culture models have become an essential tool that is available to address important intervertebral disc research questions. Some intrinsic drawbacks of these model systems impact the types of questions that can be addressed. The largest limitations relate to questions of age and pain.

22.10.1 Age Changes and Use of Human Tissues

The structure and composition of the human intervertebral disc changes with age, with older discs typically showing more signs of degeneration. When large animal discs are used to model the human, as they are obtained from abattoirs, they are typically younger and healthier than the clinically relevant human intervertebral disc. Not surprisingly, the healthy human disc is structurally similar to the bovine and ovine (Fig. 22.1), but compared to the animal spine, the moderately degenerate human discs display a more fibrous nucleus pulposus, the tissue appears brownish in color, and the demarcation between the nucleus and the annulus is less distinct (Fig. 22.7). With progressing degeneration, the nucleus pulposus becomes more fibrous and it is hardly distinguishable from the annulus; in some severely degenerated discs, there is also vascular ingrowth (Fig. 22.7c). In the light of these pathological differences, it is difficult to extrapolate information generated from discs of young healthy animals to answer questions concerning severely degenerate human discs.

Large animal organ culture models of disc degeneration differ substantially from the human. The intervertebral specimens are from the young, meaning that they did not develop, grow, remodel, accumulate injury, undergo endplate calcification, and respond to pro-inflammatory cytokines. In other words, animal intervertebral discs are generally "healthier," and most suitable for studies aimed at understanding the biology of the young and healthy human intervertebral tissues (up to ~40 years of age), but are probably not reliable models for aging studies (Demers et al. 2004). This topic is considered in detail in Chap. 18.

Accordingly, because of their high reproducibility, uniformity, and availability, animal disc models have considerable advantages when used for screening therapeutic agents or addressing mechanistic questions regarding degenerative changes and responsiveness to injurious and environmental conditions. Human discs are the gold standard when investigating aging and degeneration changes. However, inconsistencies between human disc specimens are high, and the limited number of available discs exacerbates this variability. Nevertheless, human rather than animal organ culture models are most valuable for evaluating disc treatment options.

22.10.2 Measurements of Predictors of Painful Conditions

Low back pain is often associated with disc degeneration (Biering-Sorensen et al. 1985) (see also Chaps. 16 and 19). It is difficult, if not impossible, to directly measure pain in a whole-organ culture model due to its subjective nature. However, while direct clinical measures of pain cannot be

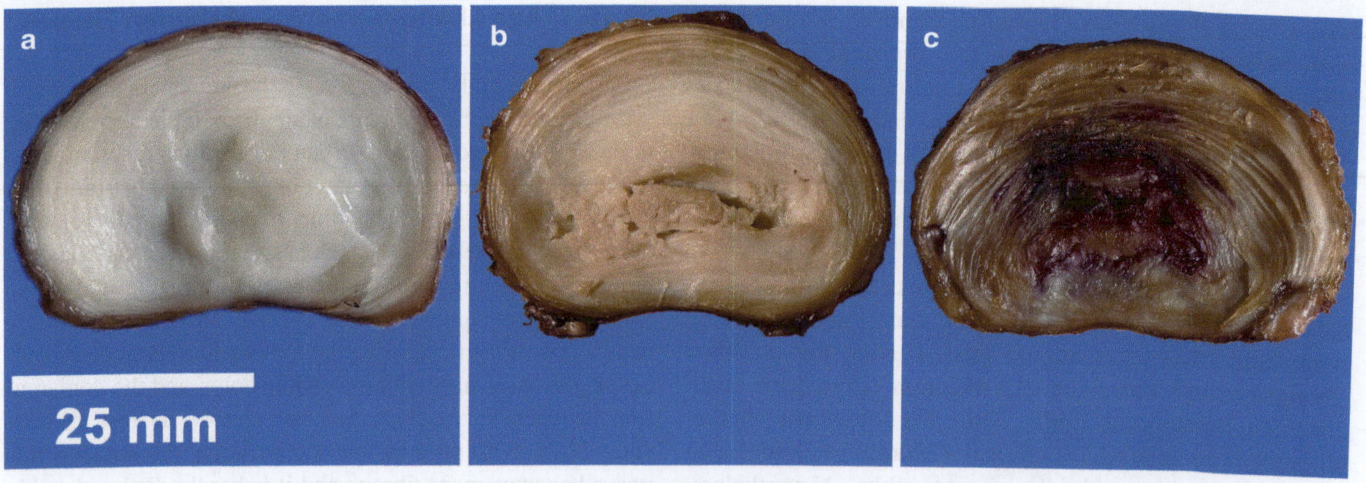

Fig. 22.7 Human healthy and degenerate intervertebral discs. (**a**) Healthy intervertebral discs (grade I); (**b**) moderate degeneration (grade III); (**c**) severe degeneration (grade IV). Grading is based on the Thompson degeneration scale

assessed in vitro, it is possible to measure the secretion or expression of selected neurotrophic agents and growth factors (Jung et al. 2011; Purmessur et al. 2008). Assessing these factors may indicate potential induction or relief of pain; however, the actual pain cannot be measured. Interestingly, most patients who have degenerative discs are asymptomatic. What makes the degenerative disc painful in one patient and asymptomatic in another remains unknown. Differentiating the normal aging process from pathologic disc degeneration also remains a very challenging if not impossible endeavor at this time. Further details on neurogenic pain are discussed in Chap. 16.

22.11 Conclusions

Disc degeneration is a widely investigated disorder strongly associated with low back pain. The highly structured extracellular matrix and harsh physicochemical microenvironment of human intervertebral tissues create a unique niche with low cellularity and metabolic activity. This niche is not well simulated with current cell culture techniques or small animal models. The development of organ culture models has the capacity to better simulate the important 3D connectivity and other niche characteristics found in the human disc with precise control over the mechanical and chemical boundary conditions. Intervertebral disc organ culture techniques have advanced from simple free-swelling tissue models to computer-controlled and elegantly designed multiaxis and multi-chamber systems with the capacity to maintain disc structure, control nutritional factors, and simulate physiological or damaging loads. Successful organ culture experiments can now be designed to focus on critical scientific questions, having developed procedures that inhibit the high swelling propensity of the matrix and enable nutrient transport. The high repeatability, uniformity, similar aspect ratios, and metabolic rates of bovine or ovine caudal discs make them valuable tissues for disc organ culture to be used for screening therapeutic agents that are in development and for answering mechanistic questions concerning the pathogenesis of degenerative events and progress in response to physicochemical challenges. These models represent the initial battleground for exploring therapies that will inhibit catabolic and promote anabolic processes in the disc. Experimental variation in human discs is high, and specimen procurement is challenging so that human organ cultures are best suited for evaluating refined treatment options.

While animal organ culture models are valuable tools for the evaluation of therapeutic interventions, almost all models require degeneration to be induced before a repair strategy can be implemented. The use of human intervertebral discs provides a model with naturally occurring degeneration and can therefore serve as a useful tool in validating therapeutic interventions for repair of early- to moderate-stage disc degeneration. Due to slow disc cell metabolism, long-term cultures will be needed to measure a significant change in disc matrix composition during repair. Thus, organ cultures provide an important link between conventional in vitro and in vivo technologies and offer a means of significantly reducing the use of animal models.

22.12 Summary of Critical Concepts Discussed in the Chapter

- The native cellular niche of disc cells can be maintained in organ culture providing an important advantage over the more traditional 2D and 3D cell culture studies.

- Intervertebral disc organ cultures allow precise control over mechanical and chemical boundary conditions, facilitating more targeted mechanistic hypothesis testing compared with in vivo models.
- Intervertebral disc culture under free-swelling conditions results in GAG loss, a decrease in anabolic activity, and an increase in the expression of catabolic genes. Retention of the endplate in culture maintains collagen connectivity, reduces disc cell death near the cut edge of the disc, and inhibits swelling.
- Axial loading is required to fully inhibit swelling, preserve the complex extracellular environment of the intervertebral disc, and simulate diurnal loading and daily activities that are necessary to maintain physiological biosynthesis rates of disc cells.
- Development of animal models enhances the study of agents that promote degeneration and promote tissue regeneration models in a defined and reproducible manner with minimal donor variability.
- Human discs can be maintained in organ culture and provide an important preclinical technique for screening therapies in a way that complements and minimizes in vivo animal testing.

Acknowledgments The research reported in this chapter was supported by the National Institute of Arthritis and Musculoskeletal and Skin Diseases of the National Institutes of Health under Award Numbers R01AR057397 and R01AR051146. The authors would like to thank Marianna Peroglio, Benjamin Gantenbein-Ritter, and Jochen Walser.

References

Adams MA, Hutton WC (1981) The relevance of torsion to the mechanical derangement of the lumbar spine. Spine (Phila Pa 1976) 6(3):241–248

Adams MA, Hutton WC (1982) Prolapsed intervertebral disc. A hyperflexion injury 1981 Volvo Award in basic science. Spine (Phila Pa 1976) 7(3):184–191

Adams MA, Hutton WC (1983) The effect of fatigue on the lumbar intervertebral disc. J Bone Joint Surg Br 65(2):199–203

Adams MA, Roughley PJ (2006) What is intervertebral disc degeneration, and what causes it? Spine (Phila Pa 1976) 31(18):2151–2161

Adams MA, Freeman BJ, Morrison HP, Nelson IW, Dolan P (2000) Mechanical initiation of intervertebral disc degeneration. Spine (Phila Pa 1976) 25(13):1625–1636

Aguiar DJ, Johnson SL, Oegema TR (1999) Notochordal cells interact with nucleus pulposus cells: regulation of proteoglycan synthesis. Exp Cell Res 246(1):129–137

Alini M, Eisenstein SM, Ito K, Little C, Kettler AA, Masuda K, Melrose J, Ralphs J, Stokes I, Wilke HJ (2008) Are animal models useful for studying human disc disorders/degeneration? Eur Spine J 17(1):2–19

Barbash IM, Chouraqui P, Baron J, Feinberg MS, Etzion S, Tessone A, Miller L, Guetta E, Zipori D, Kedes LH, Kloner RA, Leor J (2003) Systemic delivery of bone marrow-derived mesenchymal stem cells to the infarcted myocardium: feasibility, cell migration, and body distribution. Circulation 108(7):863–868

Barbir A, Godburn KE, Michalek AJ, Lai A, Monsey RD, Iatridis JC (2011) Effects of torsion on intervertebral disc gene expression and biomechanics, using a rat tail model. Spine (Phila Pa 1976) 36(8):607–614

Bibby SR, Jones DA, Ripley RM, Urban JP (2005) Metabolism of the intervertebral disc: effects of low levels of oxygen, glucose, and pH on rates of energy metabolism of bovine nucleus pulposus cells. Spine (Phila Pa 1976) 30(5):487–496

Biering-Sorensen F, Hansen FR, Schroll M, Runeborg O (1985) The relation of spinal x-ray to low-back pain and physical activity among 60-year-old men and women. Spine (Phila Pa 1976) 10(5):445–451

Chan SC, Ferguson SJ, Wuertz K, Gantenbein-Ritter B (2011) Biological response of the intervertebral disc to repetitive short term cyclic torsion. Spine (Phila Pa 1976) 36:2021–2030

Chiba K, Andersson GB, Masuda K, Momohara S, Williams JM, Thonar EJ (1998) A new culture system to study the metabolism of the intervertebral disc in vitro. Spine (Phila Pa 1976) 23(17):1821–1827; discussion 28

Collin EC, Grad S, Zeugolis DI, Vinatier CS, Clouet JR, Guicheux JJ, Weiss P, Alini M, Pandit AS (2011) An injectable vehicle for nucleus pulposus cell-based therapy. Biomaterials 32(11):2862–2870

Demers CN, Antoniou J, Mwale F (2004) Value and limitations of using the bovine tail as a model for the human lumbar spine. Spine (Phila Pa 1976) 29(24):2793–2799

Di Nicola M, Carlo-Stella C, Magni M, Milanesi M, Longoni PD, Matteucci P, Grisanti S, Gianni AM (2002) Human bone marrow stromal cells suppress T-lymphocyte proliferation induced by cellular or nonspecific mitogenic stimuli. Blood 99(10): 3838–3843

Elliott DM, Sarver JJ (2004) Young investigator award winner: validation of the mouse and rat disc as mechanical models of the human lumbar disc. Spine (Phila Pa 1976) 29(7):713–722

Gantenbein B, Grunhagen T, Lee CR, van Donkelaar CC, Alini M, Ito K (2006) An in vitro organ culturing system for intervertebral disc explants with vertebral endplates: a feasibility study with ovine caudal discs. Spine (Phila Pa 1976) 31(23):2665–2673

Gawri R, Mwale F, Ouellet J, Roughley P, Steffen T, Antoniou J, Haglund L (2011) Development of an organ culture system for long term survival of the intact human intervertebral disc. Spine (Phila Pa 1976) 36:1835–1842

Grad S, Mauro A, Eglin D, Sakai D, Mochida J, Mahor S, Collin E, Dash B, Pandit A (2010) Cells and biomaterials for intervertebral disc regeneration. In: Athanasiou KA (ed) Cell therapy for nucleus pulposus regeneration. Morgan & Claypool, Davis, pp 1–39

Haglund L, Moir J, Beckman L, Mulligan KR, Jim B, Ouellet JA, Roughley P, Steffen T (2011) Development of a bioreactor for axially loaded intervertebral disc organ culture. Tissue Eng Part C Methods 17:1011–1019

Haschtmann D, Stoyanov JV, Ettinger L, Nolte LP, Ferguson SJ (2006a) Establishment of a novel intervertebral disc/endplate culture model: analysis of an ex vivo in vitro whole-organ rabbit culture system. Spine (Phila Pa 1976) 31(25):2918–2925

Haschtmann D, Stoyanov JV, Ferguson SJ (2006b) Influence of diurnal hyperosmotic loading on the metabolism and matrix gene expression of a whole-organ intervertebral disc model. J Orthop Res 24(10):1957–1966

Haschtmann D, Ferguson SJ, Stoyanov JV (2008a) Apoptosis and gene expression of collagenases but not gelatinases in rabbit disc fragment cultures. J Neurosurg Spine 8(6):552–560

Haschtmann D, Stoyanov JV, Gedet P, Ferguson SJ (2008b) Vertebral endplate trauma induces disc cell apoptosis and promotes organ degeneration in vitro. Eur Spine J 17(2):289–299

Hauger O, Frost EE, van Heeswijk R, Deminiere C, Xue R, Delmas Y, Combe C, Moonen CT, Grenier N, Bulte JW (2006) MR evaluation of the glomerular homing of magnetically labeled mesenchymal stem cells in a rat model of nephropathy. Radiology 238(1): 200–210

Holm S, Maroudas A, Urban JP, Selstam G, Nachemson A (1981) Nutrition of the intervertebral disc: solute transport and metabolism. Connect Tissue Res 8(2):101–119

Honczarenko M, Le Y, Swierkowski M, Ghiran I, Glodek AM, Silberstein LE (2006) Human bone marrow stromal cells express a distinct set of biologically functional chemokine receptors. Stem Cells 24(4):1030–1041

Horner HA, Urban JP (2001) 2001 Volvo Award Winner in Basic Science Studies: effect of nutrient supply on the viability of cells from the nucleus pulposus of the intervertebral disc. Spine (Phila Pa 1976) 26(23):2543–2549

Hoyland JA, Le Maitre C, Freemont AJ (2008) Investigation of the role of IL-1 and TNF in matrix degradation in the intervertebral disc. Rheumatology (Oxford) 47(6):809–814

Hunter CJ, Matyas JR, Duncan NA (2004) Cytomorphology of notochordal and chondrocytic cells from the nucleus pulposus: a species comparison. J Anat 205(5):357–362

Hutton WC, Murakami H, Li J, Elmer WA, Yoon ST, Minamide A, Akamaru T, Tomita K (2004) The effect of blocking a nutritional pathway to the intervertebral disc in the dog model. J Spinal Disord Tech. 17(1):53–63

Iatridis JC, MacLean JJ, Roughley PJ, Alini M (2006) Effects of mechanical loading on intervertebral disc metabolism in vivo. J Bone Joint Surg Am 88(Suppl 2):41–46

Illien-Jünger S, Gantenbein-Ritter B, Grad S, Lezuo P, Ferguson SJ, Alini M, Ito K (2010) The combined effects of limited nutrition and high-frequency loading on intervertebral discs with endplates. Spine (Phila Pa 1976) 35(19):1744–1752

Illien-Jünger SM, Mayer JE, Walter BA, Qureshi S, Hecht AC, Iatridis JC (2012a) Intervertebral disc whole organ culture model to investigate the effect of TGFβ3 after discectomy. Trans Orthop Res Soc 12: Abstract 1192

Illien-Jünger S, Pattappa G, Peroglio M, Benneker LM, Stoddart MJ, Sakai D, Mochida J, Grad S, Alini M (2012b) Homing of mesenchymal stem cells in induced degenerative intervertebral discs in a whole organ culture system. Spine (Phila Pa 1976) 15;37(22): 1865–1873

Ji JF, He BP, Dheen ST, Tay SS (2004) Interactions of chemokines and chemokine receptors mediate the migration of mesenchymal stem cells to the impaired site in the brain after hypoglossal nerve injury. Stem Cells 22(3):415–427

Jim B, Steffen T, Moir J, Roughley P, Haglund L (2011) Development of an intact intervertebral disc organ culture system in which degeneration can be induced as a prelude to studying repair potential. Eur Spine J 20(8):1244–1254

Jung WW, Kim HS, Shon JR, Lee M, Lee SH, Sul D, Na HS, Kim JH, Kim BJ (2011) Intervertebral disc degeneration-induced expression of pain-related molecules: glial cell-derived neurotropic factor as a key factor. J Neurosurg Anesthesiol 23:329–334

Jünger S, Gantenbein-Ritter B, Lezuo P, Alini M, Ferguson SJ, Ito K (2009) Effect of limited nutrition on in situ intervertebral disc cells under simulated-physiological loading. Spine (Phila Pa 1976) 34(12):1264–1271

Kandel R, Roberts S, Urban JP (2008) Tissue engineering and the intervertebral disc: the challenges. Eur Spine J 17(Suppl 4):480–491

Kawada H, Fujita J, Kinjo K, Matsuzaki Y, Tsuma M, Miyatake H, Muguruma Y, Tsuboi K, Itabashi Y, Ikeda Y, Ogawa S, Okano H, Hotta T, Ando K, Fukuda K (2004) Nonhematopoietic mesenchymal stem cells can be mobilized and differentiate into cardiomyocytes after myocardial infarction. Blood 104(12): 3581–3587

Kitaori T, Ito H, Schwarz EM, Tsutsumi R, Yoshitomi H, Oishi S, Nakano M, Fujii N, Nagasawa T, Nakamura T (2009) Stromal cell-derived factor 1/CXCR4 signaling is critical for the recruitment of mesenchymal stem cells to the fracture site during skeletal repair in a mouse model. Arthritis Rheum 60(3):813–823

Korecki CL, MacLean JJ, Iatridis JC (2007) Characterization of an in vitro intervertebral disc organ culture system. Eur Spine J 16(7):1029–1037

Korecki CL, MacLean JJ, Iatridis JC (2008) Dynamic compression effects on intervertebral disc mechanics and biology. Spine (Phila Pa 1976) 33(13):1403–1409

Krebs J, Aebli N, Goss BG, Wilson K, Williams R, Ferguson SJ (2007) Cardiovascular changes after pulmonary cement embolism: an experimental study in sheep. AJNR Am J Neuroradiol. 28(6):1046–1050

Le Maitre CL, Freemont AJ, Hoyland JA (2005) The role of interleukin-1 in the pathogenesis of human intervertebral disc degeneration. Arthritis Res Ther 7(4):R732–R745

Le Maitre CL, Baird P, Freemont AJ, Hoyland JA (2009) An in vitro study investigating the survival and phenotype of mesenchymal stem cells following injection into nucleus pulposus tissue. Arthritis Res Ther 11(1):R20

Lee CR, Iatridis JC, Poveda L, Alini M (2006) In vitro organ culture of the bovine intervertebral disc: effects of vertebral endplate and potential for mechanobiology studies. Spine (Phila Pa 1976) 31(5):515–522

Lim TH, Ramakrishnan PS, Kurriger GL, Martin JA, Stevens JW, Kim J, Mendoza SA (2006) Rat spinal motion segment in organ culture: a cell viability study. Spine (Phila Pa 1976) 31(12):1291–1297

Mackenzie TC, Flake AW (2001) Human mesenchymal stem cells persist, demonstrate site-specific multipotential differentiation, and are present in sites of wound healing and tissue regeneration after transplantation into fetal sheep. Blood Cells Mol Dis 27(3):601–604

MacLean JJ, Lee CR, Grad S, Ito K, Alini M, Iatridis JC (2003) Effects of immobilization and dynamic compression on intervertebral disc cell gene expression in vivo. Spine (Phila Pa 1976) 28(10):973–981

Maclean JJ, Lee CR, Alini M, Iatridis JC (2004) Anabolic and catabolic mRNA levels of the intervertebral disc vary with the magnitude and frequency of in vivo dynamic compression. J Orthop Res 22(6):1193–1200

MacLean JJ, Lee CR, Alini M, Iatridis JC (2005) The effects of short-term load duration on anabolic and catabolic gene expression in the rat tail intervertebral disc. J Orthop Res 23(5):1120–1127

Maroudas A, Stockwell RA, Nachemson A, Urban J (1975) Factors involved in the nutrition of the human lumbar intervertebral disc: cellularity and diffusion of glucose in vitro. J Anat 120(Pt 1):113–130

Masuda K, An HS (2004) Growth factors and the intervertebral disc. Spine J 4(6 Suppl):330S–340S

Masuda K, Aota Y, Muehleman C, Imai Y, Okuma M, Thonar EJ, Andersson GB, An HS (2005) A novel rabbit model of mild, reproducible disc degeneration by an annulus needle puncture: correlation between the degree of disc injury and radiological and histological appearances of disc degeneration. Spine (Phila Pa 1976) 30(1):5–14

Nasef A, Chapel A, Mazurier C, Bouchet S, Lopez M, Mathieu N, Sensebe L, Zhang Y, Gorin NC, Thierry D, Fouillard L (2007) Identification of IL-10 and TGF-beta transcripts involved in the inhibition of T-lymphocyte proliferation during cell contact with human mesenchymal stem cells. Gene Expr 13(4–5):217–226

O'Connell GD, Vresilovic EJ, Elliott DM (2007) Comparison of animals used in disc research to human lumbar disc geometry. Spine (Phila Pa 1976) 32(3):328–333

Oegema TR Jr, Bradford DS, Cooper KM (1979) Aggregated proteoglycan synthesis in organ cultures of human nucleus pulposus. J Biol Chem 254(21):10579–10581

Oegema TR Jr, Johnson SL, Aguiar DJ, Ogilvie JW (2000) Fibronectin and its fragments increase with degeneration in the human intervertebral disc. Spine (Phila Pa 1976) 25(21):2742–2747

Ohshima H, Urban JP, Bergel DH (1995) Effect of static load on matrix synthesis rates in the intervertebral disc measured in vitro by a new perfusion technique. J Orthop Res 13(1):22–29

Oshima H, Ishihara H, Urban JP, Tsuji H (1993) The use of coccygeal discs to study intervertebral disc metabolism. J Orthop Res 11(3): 332–338

Panjabi MM, Goel V, Oxland T, Takata K, Duranceau J, Krag M, Price M (1992) Human lumbar vertebrae. Quantitative three-dimensional anatomy. Spine (Phila Pa 1976) 17(3):299–306

Peroglio M, Grad S, Mortisen D, Sprecher CM, Illien-Jünger S, Alini M, Eglin D (2011) Injectable thermoreversible hyaluronan-based hydrogels for nucleus pulposus cell encapsulation. Eur Spine J 21:S839–S849

Pfirrmann CW, Metzdorf A, Zanetti M, Hodler J, Boos N (2001) Magnetic resonance classification of lumbar intervertebral disc degeneration. Spine (Phila Pa 1976) 26(17):1873–1878

Pflaster DS, Krag MH, Johnson CC, Haugh LD, Pope MH (1997) Effect of test environment on intervertebral disc hydration. Spine (Phila Pa 1976) 22(2):133–139

Pittenger MF, Mackay AM, Beck SC, Jaiswal RK, Douglas R, Mosca JD, Moorman MA, Simonetti DW, Craig S, Marshak DR (1999) Multilineage potential of adult human mesenchymal stem cells. Science 284(5411):143–147

Purmessur D, Freemont AJ, Hoyland JA (2008) Expression and regulation of neurotrophins in the nondegenerate and degenerate human intervertebral disc. Arthritis Res Ther 10(4):R99

Purmessur D, Walter BA, Roughley PJ, Laudier DM, Hecht AC, Iatridis J (2013) A role for TNFα in intervertebral disc degeneration: a non-recoverable catabolic shift. Biochem Biophys Res Commun 433(1): 151–156

Ries C, Egea V, Karow M, Kolb H, Jochum M, Neth P (2007) MMP-2, MT1-MMP, and TIMP-2 are essential for the invasive capacity of human mesenchymal stem cells: differential regulation by inflammatory cytokines. Blood 109(9):4055–4063

Risbud MV, Izzo MW, Adams CS, Arnold WW, Hillibrand AS, Vresilovic EJ, Vaccaro AR, Albert TJ, Shapiro IM (2003) An organ culture system for the study of the nucleus pulposus: description of the system and evaluation of the cells. Spine (Phila Pa 1976) 28(24):2652–2658; discussion 58–59

Risbud MV, Albert TJ, Guttapalli A, Vresilovic EJ, Hillibrand AS, Vaccaro AR, Shapiro IM (2004) Differentiation of mesenchymal stem cells towards a nucleus pulposus-like phenotype in vitro: implications for cell-based transplantation therapy. Spine (Phila Pa 1976) 29(23):2627–2632

Risbud MV, Di Martino A, Guttapalli A, Seghatoleslami R, Denaro V, Vaccaro AR, Albert TJ, Shapiro IM (2006) Toward an optimum system for intervertebral disc organ culture: TGF-beta 3 enhances nucleus pulposus and annulus fibrosus survival and function through modulation of TGF-beta-R expression and ERK signaling. Spine (Phila Pa 1976) 31(8):884–890

Roberts S, Menage J, Sivan S, Urban JP (2008) Bovine explant model of degeneration of the intervertebral disc. BMC Musculoskelet Disord 9:24

Sakai D, Mochida J, Iwashina T, Watanabe T, Suyama K, Ando K, Hotta T (2006) Atelocollagen for culture of human nucleus pulposus cells forming nucleus pulposus-like tissue in vitro: influence on the proliferation and proteoglycan production of HNPSV-1 cells. Biomaterials 27(3):346–353

Sakai D, Nakai T, Mochida J, Alini M, Grad S (2009) Differential phenotype of intervertebral disc cells: microarray and immunohistochemical analysis of canine nucleus pulposus and annulus fibrosus. Spine (Phila Pa 1976) 34(14):1448–1456

Seguin CA, Pilliar RM, Roughley PJ, Kandel RA (2005) Tumor necrosis factor-alpha modulates matrix production and catabolism in nucleus pulposus tissue. Spine (Phila Pa 1976) 30(17): 1940–1948

Steck E, Bertram H, Abel R, Chen B, Winter A, Richter W (2005) Induction of intervertebral disc-like cells from adult mesenchymal stem cells. Stem Cells 23(3):403–411

Stokes IA, Iatridis JC (2004) Mechanical conditions that accelerate intervertebral disc degeneration: overload versus immobilization. Spine (Phila Pa 1976) 29(23):2724–2732

Thompson JP, Pearce RH, Schechter MT, Adams ME, Tsang IK, Bishop PB (1990) Preliminary evaluation of a scheme for grading the gross morphology of the human intervertebral disc. Spine (Phila Pa 1976) 15(5):411–415

Urban JP, Maroudas A (1981) Swelling of the intervertebral disc in vitro. Connect Tissue Res 9(1):1–10

Urban JP, Smith S, Fairbank JC (2004) Nutrition of the intervertebral disc. Spine (Phila Pa 1976) 29(23):2700–2709

van Dijk B, Potier E, Ito K (2011) Culturing bovine nucleus pulposus explants by balancing medium osmolarity. Tissue Eng Part C Methods 17:1089–1096

Walser J, Ferguson SJ, Gantenbein-Ritter B (2012) Design of a mechanical loading device to culture intact bovine caudal motional segments of the Spine under twisting motion. In: Davies J (ed) Replacing animal models: a practical guide to creating and using biomimetic alternatives. John Wiley & Co., Chichester

Walsh WR, Harrison J, Loefler A, Martin T, Van Sickle D, Brown MK, Sonnabend DH (2000) Mechanical and histologic evaluation of Collagraft in an ovine lumbar fusion model. Clin Orthop Relat Res 375:258–266

Walter BA, Korecki CL, Purmessur D, Roughley PJ, Michalek AJ, Iatridis JC (2011) Complex loading affects intervertebral disc mechanics and biology. Osteoarthritis Cartilage 19(8): 1011–1018

Wang D, Vo NV, Sowa GA, Hartman RA, Ngo K, Choe SR, Witt WT, Dong Q, Lee JY, Niedernhofer LJ, Kang JD (2011) Bupivacaine decreases cell viability and matrix protein synthesis in an intervertebral disc organ model system. Spine J 11(2):139–146

Wilke HJ, Neef P, Caimi M, Hoogland T, Claes LE (1999) New in vivo measurements of pressures in the intervertebral disc in daily life. Spine (Phila Pa 1976) 24(8):755–762

Wuertz K, Godburn K, MacLean JJ, Barbir A, Donnelly JS, Roughley PJ, Alini M, Iatridis JC (2009) In vivo remodeling of intervertebral discs in response to short- and long-term dynamic compression. J Orthop Res 27(9):1235–1242

Sato M, Kikuchi M, Ishihara M, Ishihara M, Asazuma T, Kikuchi T, Masuoka K, Hattori H, Fujikawa K (2003) Tissue engineering of the intervertebral disc with cultured annulus fibrosus cells using atelocollagen honeycomb-shaped scaffold with a membrane seal (ACHMS scaffold). [illegible] nucleus pulposus cells forming nuclei pulposus-like tissue in vitro: influence on the proliferation and proteoglycan production. HNPSV-1 cell. Biomaterials 2(3):346–351

Use of Stem Cells for Regeneration of the Intervertebral Disc

23

Daisuke Sakai and Joji Mochida

Contents

D. Sakai, MD, PhD (✉) • J. Mochida, MD, PhD
Department of Orthopaedic Surgery, Surgical Science, Research Center for Regenerative Medicine, Tokai University School of Medicine, Shimokasuya 143, Isehara, Kanagawa 259-1193, Japan
e-mail: daisakai@is.icc.u-tokai.ac.jp; jomo@is.icc.u-tokai.ac.jp

I.M. Shapiro, M.V. Risbud (eds.), *The Intervertebral Disc*, DOI 10.1007/978-3-7091-1535-0_23, © Springer-Verlag Wien 2014

23.1 Evolution of Stem Cell Biology in Musculoskeletal Tissues

The ability of a tissue to respond to stress or injury requires the involvement and functions of stem cells resident in tissue-specific microenvironmental niches. Aging has been shown to result in a decrease in stem cell number as well as loss of ability to maintain tissue homeostasis and regenerate lost tissue function. Therefore, it is of critical importance to identify stem/progenitor cell populations in different tissues, determine how these cells function in tissue homeostasis, and ascertain their potential utility in tissue engineering.

Classically, stem cells of the musculoskeletal region were defined as undifferentiated cells, found in small numbers in the periosteum or the bone marrow (Caplan 1991; Deans and Moseley 2000). Subsequently, these small populations of cells have been found in other stem cell pools, such as the adipose tissues, synovial tissues, perivascular regions in the surrounding tissue environment, and even in the matrix component of tissues (Bianco et al. 2001; Crisan et al. 2008). They were designated "mesenchymal stem cells" because from a developmental perspective, they were thought to be mesenchymal in origin. These cells can undergo sustained proliferation in vitro and potentially give rise to multiple mesenchymal cell lineages, including osteocytes, chondrocytes, and adipocytes. Since then, many researchers have reported studies of mesenchymal stem cells using different methods of isolation and expansion. With the increasing difficulties encountered in comparing and contrasting study outcomes, these cells are now preferentially called "multipotent mesenchymal stromal cells" (multipotent MSCs). The Tissue Stem Cell Committee of the International Society for Cellular Therapy has proposed minimal criteria to define human MSC (Dominici et al. 2006). First, MSC must be adherent to plastic when maintained under standard culture conditions. Second, MSC must express the surface molecules CD105, CD73, and CD90, and not express CD45, CD34, CD14, CD11b, CD79α, CD19, or HLA-DR. Third, MSC must differentiate into osteoblasts, adipocytes, or chondroblasts in vitro. Despite these

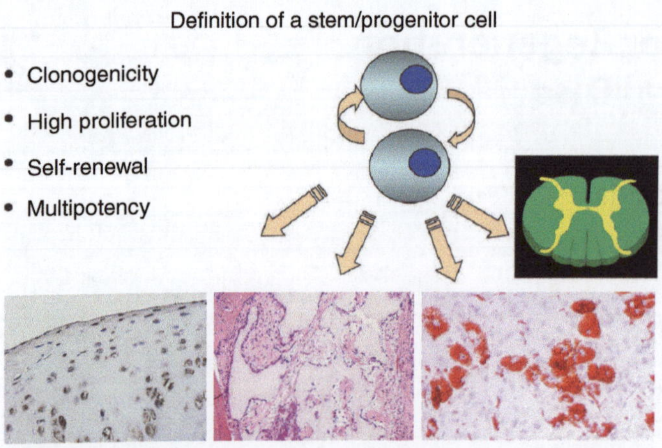

Fig. 23.1 Definition of a stem/progenitor cell. Criteria of stem/progenitor cell include clonogenicity, high proliferative capacity, self-renewal capability (from a single cell to reconstitute a tissue in which the cell was derived), and multipotency

minimal criteria to identify MSC, it is difficult to define MSC other than by the operational definition of self-renewal and differentiation potential in vitro. Therefore, our knowledge of MSC is based solely on the characterization of cultured cells. We still lack any knowledge of their in vivo characteristics, such as their development, exact tissue localization, and physiological roles.

Despite these difficulties, the considerable therapeutic potential of human MSC has generated marked and increasing interest within a wide variety of biomedical disciplines, including studies of the intervertebral disc. Published studies involving MSC have increased markedly in this field and may in the long run provide new and useful information on disc biology, the pathogenesis of intervertebral disc degeneration, and possibly offer new therapeutic strategies (Sakai 2011). However, as with any area of study, researchers must share similar definitions, terminologies, and methods to ensure that their findings can be compared. It is important for scientists to know the essential features of a stem cell: its capacity for self-renewal and the ability of a single cell to regenerate all the cell types and matrices of the lineage from which the cell was derived (Fig. 23.1) (Blanpain et al. 2004). Accordingly, the experimental design and the types of stem cells used in investigational studies and translational cell therapies involving the intervertebral disc must be selected with care.

23.2 Evidence of a Stem Cell System in the Intervertebral Disc

As mentioned above, investigation of the tissue-specific stem cell niche is a key factor in understanding the degenerative processes and tissue regeneration. Although research into the stem cell system in the intervertebral disc is still in its infancy, recent studies have shown evidence of a potential stem cell niche in the intervertebral disc region. Henriksson et al. (2009) attempted to detect cell proliferation zones and label-retaining cells with in vivo 5-bromo-2′-deoxyuridine (BrdU) labeling in rabbit discs. They also investigated the localization of progenitor cell markers (Notch1, Delta4, Jagged1, C-KIT, KI67, and Stro-1) with immunohistochemistry in the degenerated intervertebral discs of rabbits, rats, mini pigs, and humans. Although slow, ongoing proliferation was detectable in both the nucleus pulposus and annulus fibrosus regions. They also found a high number of BrdU-positive cells at the annulus fibrosus borders with the ligament zone and the perichondrium region at early time points, whereas only a few label-retaining cells were observed at later time points, identifying a stem cell niche-like pattern. This may support the findings of Melrose et al. (2007), who demonstrated spatial annular remodeling in experimentally injured ovine discs.

The recruitment of cells from the surrounding environment is another phenomenon often seen in the regenerative process. Using the BrdU in vivo labeling technique described above, Henriksson et al. (2011) observed BrdU-labeled cells in the intervertebral disc niche, adjacent to the epiphyseal plate at early time points, but at later time points, these cells were mainly in the outer region of the annulus fibrosus, suggesting possible migratory pathway. Tzaan and Chen (2011) have extended this concept by enhancing bone marrow cell migration to the disc by stimulation with granulocyte colony-stimulating factor. However, their results only demonstrated increased bone marrow cells in the endplate. Cell migration processes are thus underdefined and require substantial investigation.

There is increasing evidence that stem/progenitor cells are present in the intervertebral disc. Risbud et al. (2007) reported that cells isolated from degenerative human disc tissues expressed CD105, CD166, CD63, CD49a, CD90, CD73, p75 low-affinity nerve growth factor receptor, and CD133/1, proteins that are characteristic of MSC and represent the differentiation capacity of these cells toward osteogenesis, adipogenesis, and chondrogenesis. Feng et al. (2010) have demonstrated that the human degenerative annulus contains cells that express the MSC markers CD29, CD49e, CD51, CD73, CD90, CD105, CD166, CD184, and Stro-1 and two neuronal stem cell markers, nestin and neuron-specific enolase. In an in vitro assay, they differentiated annulus fibrosus-derived cells into adipocytes, osteoblasts, chondrocytes, neurons, and endothelial cells. Blanco et al. (2010) investigated MSC markers in nucleus pulposus cells isolated from degenerated discs and compared their differentiation capacities with those of bone marrow-derived MSC from the same patient. They found that nucleus pulposus-derived MSC fulfilled almost all the morphological, immunophenotypical, and differentiation criteria for MSC

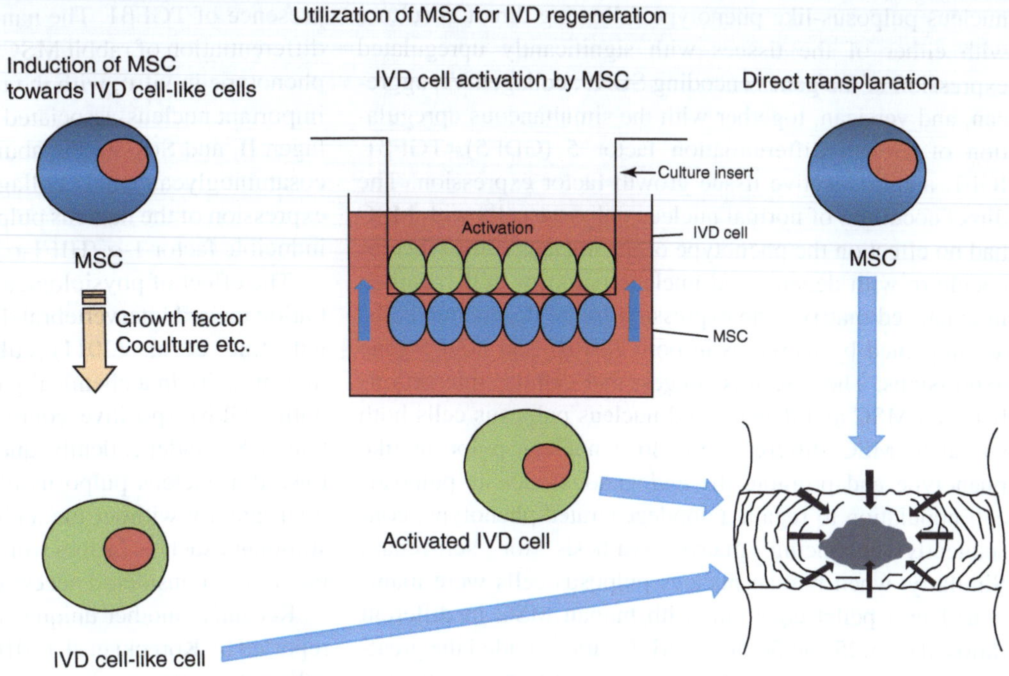

Fig. 23.2 Utilization of multipotent mesenchymal stromal cells for disc regeneration. Mesenchymal stem cells (*MSCs*) can be directly induced to differentiate toward an intervertebral disc cell (*IVD*) using growth factor and coculture techniques (*left*). In addition, activation can be achieved using coculture systems in which there is direct cell–cell contact (*middle*). Alternatively, MSC can be directly transplanted into the disc and commitment enhanced by the local conditions and the presence of resident host cells (*right*)

described by the International Society of Cell Therapy, except that nucleus-derived MSCs were unable to differentiate into adipocytes. Likewise, Liu et al. (2011) investigated the characteristics of MSC derived from degenerated human disc cartilage endplates and reported that the morphology, proliferation rate, cell cycle, immunophenotype, and expression of stem cell genes were similar to those isolated from the bone marrow. These research findings suggest that the stimulation of endogenous stem cell populations may be an effective strategy for treating intervertebral disc degeneration or to provide cells for the allogeneic transplantation of somatic-tissue-specific stem cells.

23.3 Commitment of Stem Cells Toward an Intervertebral Disclike Cell

In contrast to the small steps yet taken in investigating the endogenous stem cell system in the intervertebral disc, a number of studies have reported the utilization of MSC in new, targeted therapeutic strategies (Fig. 23.2). MSC utilization can be subdivided into three main types of studies. The first approach utilizes the multipotent differentiation capacity of MSC to induce stem cells to commit toward an intervertebral disclike cell. A considerable number of studies in the literature describe this strategy (Risbud et al. 2004; Li et al. 2005; Steck et al. 2005; Richardson et al. 2006; Sobajima et al. 2008; Vadalà et al. 2008; Wuertz et al. 2008; Chen et al. 2009; Kim et al. 2009; Le Maitre et al. 2009; Wei et al. 2009a; Korecki et al. 2010; Strassburg et al. 2010; Bertolo et al. 2012; Choi et al. 2011; Feng et al. 2011a; Luo et al. 2011; Purmessur et al. 2011; Ruan et al. 2012; Stoyanov et al. 2011). Various methods to induce MSC differentiation have been evaluated such as stimulation with growth factors under specific culture conditions, coculture with terminally differentiated intervertebral disc cells, or seeding cells onto a microenvironment-mimicking scaffold. Steck et al. (2005) compared the molecular phenotypes of human disc cells and articular chondrocytes to determine whether MSC can differentiate toward both cell types after transforming growth factor-β (TGFβ)-mediated induction in vitro. Their results demonstrated that the gene expression profile adopted by MSC resembled that of native disc tissue more closely than that of native joint cartilage. As well as TGFβ3, insulin-like growth factor 1 (IGF1), fibroblast growth factor 2, and platelet-derived growth factor BB have been shown to induce MSC differentiation toward nucleus pulposus-like cells (Ehlicke et al. 2010). Richardson et al. (2006) assessed the value of a coculture system with or without cell–cell contact to induce MSC differentiation toward a nucleus pulposus-like phenotype. Real-time quantitative polymerase chain reaction (RT-PCR) demonstrated a significant increase in the expression of nucleus pulposus marker genes in stem cells when the cells were cocultured with contact for 7 days, and this change was regulated by the cell ratio. However, no significant changes in marker gene expression was observed when the cells were cultured with either the nucleus pulposus cells or stem cells without contact, indicating a requirement for cell–cell contact in this induction process.

In a follow-up study, Strassburg et al. (2010) used human nucleus pulposus cells from degenerate and nondegenerate intervertebral discs to show that MSC differentiated into a nucleus pulposus-like phenotype following direct coculture with either of the tissues with significantly upregulated expression of the genes encoding SOX9, collagen VI, aggrecan, and versican, together with the simultaneous upregulation of growth differentiation factor 5 (GDF5), TGFβ1, IGF1, and connective tissue growth factor expression. The direct coculture of normal nucleus pulposus cells with MSC had no effect on the phenotype of the nucleus cells, whereas coculture with degenerated nucleus pulposus cells resulted in enhanced matrix gene expression in the degenerate cells, accompanied by increases in both *TGFB1* and *GDF5* gene expressions. These results suggest that cellular interactions between MSC and degenerated nucleus pulposus cells both stimulate MSC differentiation to a nucleus pulposus-like phenotype and promote the endogenous nucleus pulposus cell population to regain a nondegenerated phenotype, consequently enhancing matrix synthesis for self-repair. Similarly, when human nucleus pulposus cells were maintained in a pellet coculture with human MSC in different ratios, the 75:25 and 50:50 NP:MSC ratios yielded the greatest increases in extracellular matrix (ECM) production (Sobajima et al. 2008). Vadalà et al. (2008) also reported a reduction in the expression of collagen I and an increase in the expression of collagen II and aggrecan in MSCs after coculture with nucleus pulposus cells in alginate hydrogels, which allowed short-distance paracrine cell interactions. Stoyanov et al. (2011) have shown the important role of hypoxia, together with the addition of GDF5, in enhancing the expression of nucleus pulposus markers in a bone marrow-derived MSC coculture.

MSCs from sources other than the bone marrow have also been examined. Lu et al. (2007) studied the interactions between human nucleus pulposus cells and adipose-tissue-derived stem cells in Transwell coculture, using both monolayer and micromass configurations. A similar coculture study was performed by Chen et al. (2009) utilizing synovium-derived MSC. Vadalà et al. (2008) investigated muscle-derived MSC, and Ruan et al. (2012) assessed whether Wharton's jelly cells could be induced to differentiate toward nucleus pulposus-like cells in similar coculture studies.

The effects of scaffold properties on the differentiation of MSC toward intervertebral disc cells have also been investigated. Bertolo et al. (2012) evaluated four types of matrices as scaffolds, approved as medical devices for other applications: two made of equine or porcine collagen, one of gelatin, and one of chitosan. They showed that although the collagen scaffolds induced better chondrogenic differentiation than the other scaffolds, the phenotype of the MSC was not fully equivalent to that of nucleus pulposus cells. Feng et al. (2011a) investigated the use of three-dimensional (3D) nanofibrous poly(L-lactide) scaffolds seeded with rabbit MSCs which were induced to differentiate along the nucleus pulposus pathway in a hypoxic chamber (2 % O_2) in the presence of TGFβ1. The nanofibrous scaffold supported the differentiation of rabbit MSC toward a nucleus pulposus-like phenotype in vitro, with the upregulated expression of a few important nucleus-associated genes (encoding aggrecan, collagen II, and Sox-9), the abundant deposition of ECM (glycosaminoglycan and collagen II), and the continuous expression of the nucleus pulposus-specific marker, hypoxia-inducible factor 1-α (HIF1-α).

The effect of physiological stimulation on MSC differentiation toward intervertebral disclike cells has also been studied. Luo et al. (2011) cultured MSC under simulated microgravity in a chemically defined medium supplemented with TGFβ1 (positive control group). The results showed that MSC independently and spontaneously differentiated toward a nucleus pulposus-like phenotype under simulated microgravity without the addition of any external bioactive stimulant, such as factors from the TGFβ family, which were previously considered necessary.

Recently, another unique approach to inducing MSC was reported by Korecki et al. (2010). Because notochord-derived cells play a major role in nucleus development, they tested whether the culture medium from porcine notochordal cells could direct the differentiation of MSCs. Human MSC pellets were cultured first in serum-free medium for 4 days and then in notochordal cell-conditioned medium for 7 days. It was found that there was glycosaminoglycan accumulation and increased gene expression toward a nucleus pulposus-like phenotype, together suggesting that there was differentiation toward that of the intervertebral disc phenotype.

The results of these studies suggest that MSC from any source can be forced to express some of the molecular markers of intervertebral disc cells in vitro and many external stimuli can accelerate differentiation. However, at the end of the day, they do not develop beyond nucleus pulposus-like cells because the default differentiation pathway is determined by the localization of the MSC. The most important factor in studying the induction of MSC toward intervertebral disclike cells is to demonstrate their functional capacity in vivo.

23.4 Stem Cell Promotion of Disc Cell Differentiation

Another approach to the utilization of stem cells is to exploit their capacity to nourish other cells. Stem cells can act as feeder cells to stimulate target cells directly through cell–cell contact or indirectly through the secretion of various factors. In a rabbit disc cell culture, Yamamoto et al. (2004) showed that direct cell–cell contact between nucleus pulposus cells and MSC occurred across a membrane with 0.45 mm pores, which allowed only the cell processes to adhere to each other, without any more extensive contact between the cultured cells. Compared with the culture systems with no cell–cell contact, a coculture system that allowed intercellular adhesion between nucleus pulposus cells and MSC yielded a marked increase in target cell proliferation, DNA synthesis, and proteoglycan synthesis. This is possibly attributable to the increased secretion of cytokines found in the culture system.

An interesting study by He and Pei (2012) tested the effects of the ECM deposited by synovium-derived MSC on the rejuvenation of nucleus pulposus cells. The nucleus pulposus cells that were expanded on ECM grew much faster, were smaller, and had a more fibroblastic shape than those expanded in plastic flasks. ECM-treated nucleus pulposus cells acquired enhanced CD90 expression and higher mRNA levels of collagen I, collagen II, and collagen X and aggrecan as well as a robust redifferentiation capacity for up to six passages. The authors concluded that the ECM provides a tissue-specific microenvironment for the rejuvenation of nucleus pulposus cells with a higher proliferation rate and greater redifferentiation capacity. These characteristics may improve any future autologous disc cell-based minimally invasive therapeutic approach to the physiological reconstruction of a biologically functional disc in the clinical setting.

Another use of MSC is in the delivery of bioactive factors to resident disc cells. Meyerrose et al. (2010) suggested the use of MSC for the sustained in vivo production of supraphysiological levels of cytokines to support co-transplanted stem cells and resident cells in intervertebral disc therapies.

23.5 Stem Cell Transplantation for Intervertebral Disc Tissue Engineering and Regeneration

The final approach to MSC utilization in intervertebral disc tissue engineering and regeneration involves the construction of a disclike tissue in vitro and its transplantation or the direct delivery of stem cells into the intervertebral disc. Gaetani et al. (2008), Nesti et al. (2008), Driscoll et al. (2011), and See et al. (2011) have all attempted to construct this type of tissue in vitro. To improve the quality of in vitro-reconstructed tissue, Gaetani et al. (2008) constructed a nucleus pulposus-like tissue using a 3D culture of nucleus cells and adipose-derived MSC. To develop a biphasic construct, Nesti et al. (2008) seeded MSC onto a hyaluronic acid–nanofibrous scaffold that consisted of an electrospun, biodegradable nanofibrous scaffold enveloping a hyaluronic acid hydrogel center. The seeded MSCs were induced to undergo chondrogenesis in vitro in the presence of TGFβ for up to 28 days. The cartilaginous hyaluronic acid–nanofibrous scaffold construct resembled a native disc architecturally, with an outer annulus fibrosus-like region and an inner nucleus-like region. Histological and biochemical analyses, immunohistochemistry, and gene expression profiling revealed the time-dependent development of the chondrocytic phenotype of the seeded cells. The cells also maintained the microarchitecture of the native disc. An electrospun nanofibrous scaffold has also been used to examine the native biomechanics of the annulus fibrosus (Driscoll et al. 2011). Previous studies have shown that the tensile and shear properties of the native tissue are dependent on the fiber angle and the sample aspect ratio, respectively, so the effects of changing the fiber angle and the sample aspect ratio on the shear properties of aligned electrospun poly(ε-caprolactone) scaffolds were evaluated. How ECM deposition by the resident MSC modulates the measured shear response was also determined. This team showed that the fiber orientation and sample aspect ratio significantly influenced the response of scaffolds in shear; indeed, the shear properties of both cellular and cell-seeded formulations can match or even exceed the native tissue.

A different approach to tissue engineering the annulus fibrosus was reported by See et al. (2011). They constructed cell sheets from bone marrow MSC and incorporated them onto silk scaffolds to simulate the native lamellae of the annulus fibrosus. They then wrapped the construct around silicone nucleus pulposus, mimicking an intervertebral disc construct, and used a bioreactor to provide compressive mechanical stimulation to the silicone disc. Under static conditions, the MSC sheets remained viable, with no significant change in cell numbers for 4 weeks. A histological analysis showed that the MSC sheets adhered well to the silk scaffolds and glycosaminoglycans were detected within the ECM. The ratio of collagen I to collagen II within the ECM of the MSC sheets also decreased significantly over the period of culture. These results suggest that extensive remodeling of the ECM occurred within the simulated disclike assembly and that this assembly is suitable for the regeneration of the inner annulus fibrosus.

Finally, there have been several attempts to supplement viable cells in the disc by direct stem cell transplantation. The thought behind this concept is the finding that degeneration is initiated by reductions in the numbers, viability, and functions of disc cells, especially those of the nucleus pulposus. Basic in vitro studies have shown that disc cells have a low proliferative capacity and that most cells in the adult human disc are in a senescent state. These facts have led researchers to focus on the idea of transplanting stem cells, which may show transplanted site-dependent differentiation and function to produce a functional ECM.

Sakai et al. (2003) reported the first MSC transplantation study in a rabbit model of disc degeneration. In follow-up studies (Sakai et al. 2005, 2006), they showed that transplanted MSCs survive, proliferate, and differentiate into cells expressing chondroitin sulfate; keratan sulfate; collagen I, collagen II, and collagen IV; HIF1-α and HIF1-β; HIF2-α

Table 23.1 Summary of in vivo animal experimental studies on stem cell transplantation therapy for intervertebral disc degeneration

Stem cell type	Mode	Animal model	Author	Year
Bone marrow MSCs	(Autologous MSCs expanded)	Rabbit (nucleus aspiration)	Sakai et al.	2003, 2005, 2006
Bone marrow MSCs	(MSCs expanded)	Rat (no injury)	Crevensten et al.	2004
Bone marrow MSCs	(Allogeneic MSCs expanded)	Rabbit no injury	Zhang et al.	2005
Bone marrow MSCs	(Allogeneic MSCs expanded)	Rabbit (nucleus puncture)	Leung et al.	2006
Bone marrow MSCs	(Autologous MSCs expanded)	Canine (nucleotomy)	Hiyama et al.	2008
Adipose MSCs	(Autologous MSCs expanded)	Goat (ABC chondroitinase)	Hoogendoorn et al.	2008
Adipose MSCs	(Autologous MSCs expanded)	Canine (nucleotomy)	Ganey et al.	2009
Bone marrow human MSCs	(Xenogeneic MSC expanded)	Rat (no injury)	Wei et al.	2009a and 2009b
Bone marrow human MSCs	(Xenogeneic MSC expanded)	Porcine(nucleus aspiration)	Henriksson et al.	2009
Synovial MSCs	(Allogeneic MSCs expanded)	Rabbit (nucleus puncture)	Miyamoto et al.	2010
Bone marrow MSCs	(Autologous MSCs expanded)	Rabbit (nucleus aspiration)	Yang et al.	2010
Bone marrow human MSCs	(Xenogeneic MSC expanded)	Rat (nucleotomy)	Allon et al.	2010
Bone marrow MSC + autologous NP cells	(Autologous MSCs expanded)	Rabbit (nucleus aspiration)	Feng et al.	2010
Bone marrow MSCs	(Autologous MSCs expanded)	Mini pig (annulus incision)	Bendtsen et al.	2011
Adipose human MSCs	(Xenogeneic MSCs expanded)	Rabbit (nucleus puncture)	Chun et al.	2012

and HIF2-β; glucose transporter type 1 (GLUT1) and GLUT3; and matrix metalloproteinase 2 (MMP2), proteins that characterize the native nucleus pulposus cells. They also used RT-PCR to quantify the expression of the genes encoding aggrecan, versican, collagen I and II, interleukin 1β (IL1β), IL6, tumor necrosis factor-α, MMP9, and MMP13, thus demonstrating the increased expression of nucleus pulposus cell markers and the downregulated expression of inflammatory genes. Magnetic resonance imaging (MRI) and radiography confirmed the regenerative effects of the procedure, showing that MSC transplanted into degenerating discs in vivo can survive, proliferate, and differentiate into cells that express the phenotype of nucleus pulposus cells, with suppressed inflammatory gene expression. Since then, numerous similar studies have used different animal models and cell carriers and MSC from various sources (Table 23.1) (Crevensten et al. 2004; Zhang et al. 2005; Hiyama et al. 2008; Hoogendoorn et al. 2008; Ganey et al. 2009; Wei et al. 2009a).

Crevensten et al. (2004) used a 15 % hyaluronan gel as the carrier and injected fluorescently labeled MSC into rat coccygeal discs. Although the number of MSCs retained decreased significantly during the first 2 weeks after injection, the initial cell number was restored after 4 weeks, and cell viability and disc height were maintained. These results indicate that the injected cells had started to proliferate within the rat disc. Zhang et al. (2005) implanted allogeneic MSC containing the marker gene *lacZ* from young rabbits into rabbit intervertebral discs to determine the potential of this cell-based approach. As the transplanted allogeneic MSC survived and increased the proteoglycan content within the disc, it lent strong support to the notion that these cells could be used as a potential treatment for intervertebral disc degeneration. Along the same lines, Hiyama et al. (2008) injected one million autologous MSCs into lumbar discs 4 weeks after nucleus pulposus aspiration in mature beagle dogs (a chondrodystrophoid breed), and the animals were followed for another 8 weeks. Radiological, histological, biochemical, immunohistochemical, and gene expression analyses demonstrated the clear regenerative effects of the transplanted cells. Importantly, MSC found in the nucleus 8 weeks after transplantation expressed Fas-ligand protein, which has not been detected in MSCs before transplantation. Fas-ligand, which is present in tissues with isolated immune privilege, including the nucleus pulposus, plays an important role in nucleus maintenance. The expression of Fas-ligand indicates that MSC transplantation may also contribute to the preservation of the immune privilege of the disc environment. In a follow-up study using the same model, Serigano et al. (2010) investigated the effects of the numbers of MSC transplanted. To determine the optimal number of MSCs for transplantation, 10^5, 10^6, and 10^7 MSCs were transplanted, and their survival and apoptosis after transplantation were compared, together with their regenerative effects, which were assessed with histology, radiography, and MRI images. The transplantation of 10^6 MSCs, rather than 10^5 or 10^7 cells, best maintained the structure of the intervertebral disc and optimally inhibited degeneration. This study demonstrates that the number of cells transplanted affects the regenerative capacity of MSC transplants in animal models of disc degeneration and addresses the importance of cell number in the clinical application of MSC transplantation.

Leung et al. (2006) investigated the allogeneic transplantation of MSC and reported many advantages of such transplantations in treating disc disease. They reasoned that if the nucleus pulposus is an immunoprivileged environment, then by presenting fewer antigens, MSC should escape alloantigen recognition. Wei et al. (2009b) have also reported the xenogeneic transplantation of bone marrow-derived MSC in rats, and Henriksson et al. (2009) transplanted human bone marrow MSC into a porcine model of disc degeneration, producing a regenerative effect.

Various stem cells have already been tested as cell sources. Hoogendoorn et al. (2008) reported that adipose-derived MSC may be beneficial in cell-based therapies for intervertebral disc disease because they are isolated more easily than are bone marrow MSC. Ganey et al. (2009) studied the efficacy of autologous adipose-tissue-derived stem cells in promoting disc regeneration in a canine model of disc injury and found enhanced disc matrix production and improved overall disc morphology. A recent study by Chun et al. (2012) in a rabbit trauma model has also shown that the transplantation of adipose-derived MSC increased ECM secretion, with little ossification of the damaged cartilage in the nucleus pulposus compared with degenerated control discs. MSC purified from the synovial tissue of knee joints demonstrated superior proliferative ability and greater chondrogenic differentiation capacity than those of bone marrow MSC. Miyamoto et al. (2010) transplanted allogeneic synovial MSC into rabbits and found that synovial MSC injected into the nucleus pulposus space promoted the synthesis of collagen II in the remaining nucleus pulposus cells and inhibited the expressions of degradative enzymes and inflammatory cytokines. This allowed the structure of the intervertebral disc to be maintained.

Although evidence of the regenerative effects of MSC transplantation has accrued, whether MSCs perform better than transplanted nucleus pulposus cells is as yet unknown. Feng et al. (2011b) compared the regenerative effects of nucleus pulposus cell and MSC transplantation in a rabbit model. No significant differences in gene expression were observed between the groups transplanted with nucleus cells or MSCs, supporting the role of MSC as a useful cell therapy substitute for nucleus pulposus cells for intervertebral disc degeneration. Furthermore, recent studies have explored various modifications to this method to enhance its effect. In vitro studies have shown that the coculture of nucleus pulposus cells and MSC promotes ECM production. The use of bilaminar coculture pellets (BCPs) of MSC and nucleus pulposus cells has also been explored by Allon et al. (2010). BCPs, in which MSCs are enclosed in a shell of nucleus pulposus cells, were transplanted into denucleated rat-tail discs with a fibrin-sealant carrier. Cell retention was higher in the BCP-treated group than in the control group. The disc height and disc grade increased over time only in the BCP-treated group. Only after transplantation with BCPs was proteoglycan staining evident in the nuclear space after 35 days. This approach has been combined with growth factor therapy (Yang et al. 2010). MSC transplanted with pure fibrinous gelatin-TGFβ1 resulted in less degeneration and a reduction in apoptotic cells in rabbits.

The modalities used to evaluate disc degeneration have advanced markedly with the evolution of MRI technology. Bendtsen et al. (2011) investigated the regenerative effects of MSC transplantation with or without hydrogel in mini pigs, using dynamic contrast-enhanced MRI to focus on endplate function. They showed that MSC transplantation partly regenerated the degenerative disc and maintained the perfusion and permeability characteristics of the vertebral endplate and subchondral bone.

With increasing evidence of the efficacy of MSC transplantation therapy in promoting intervertebral disc regeneration, three reports of stem cell transplantation in humans have been published. Haufe and Mork (2006) injected hematopoietic stem cells from the bone marrow into ten patients with discogenic back pain, diagnosed with provocative discogram. There was no improvement in any patient after 1 year. This study cautions that the appropriate selection of patients, cells, and methods must be made with care before the clinical application of this technique. Yoshikawa et al. (2010) transplanted autologous bone marrow MSC into discs showing the vacuum phenomenon and instability in two patients undergoing decompression surgery for spinal stenosis. The MSCs were cultured in medium containing autologous serum. During surgery, the stenosed spinal canal was fenestrated, and pieces of collagen sponge containing autologous MSCs were then grafted percutaneously onto the degenerated disc. Two years after surgery, radiography and computed tomography showed improvements in the vacuum phenomenon in both patients. T2-weighted MRI showed high signal intensity in the intervertebral discs treated with cell grafts, indicating a high moisture content, and dynamic radiography showed less lumbar disc instability. Orozco et al. (2011) also transplanted autologous bone marrow MSC into ten patients with chronic back pain, diagnosed with lumbar disc degeneration with an intact annulus fibrosus. The feasibility and safety of the treatment were confirmed and strong indications of its clinical efficacy identified. The patients displayed rapid improvement in their pain and disability (to 85 % of maximum in 3 months), which approached 71 % of optimal efficacy, comparing favorably with the results for other procedures, such as spinal fusion and total disc replacement. MRI evaluations 1 year after transplantation showed that although the disc height was not restored, the water content was significantly elevated. They concluded that MSC therapy might be a valid alternative treatment for chronic back pain caused by degenerative disc disease. Its advantages over the current gold standard treatments include that it is a simpler and more conservative intervention, without surgery, it preserves the normal biomechanics of the intervertebral disc, and it offers the same or better pain relief.

23.6 Perspectives on the Role of Stem Cell Biology in the Treatment of Intervertebral Disc Disease

Recent advances in stem cell biology offer a number of enticing possible avenues for intervertebral disc research, with therapeutic potential. Undoubtedly, studies of the applications of stem cell biology will increase; however, as already discussed, it is important that investigators share a common stem cell terminology. There is an increasing interest in this field and evidence of endogenous stem/progenitor cells within the intervertebral disc. Identification of these stem/progenitor cells in their niche and the fates of these cells should provide insight into the key elements in the pathogenesis of disc degeneration and the endogenous repair system of the intervertebral disc. This insight is required for potential therapeutic interventions. For instance, molecules that enhance the recruitment and function of disc stem/progenitor cells may enhance the longevity of the tissue itself. This area of research is still underdefined and awaits rigorous investigation. Supporting this insight, an epoch making finding that nucleus pulposus progenitor cell exhaustion relates to aging and degeneration has been recently reported (Sakai et al. 2012). In this study, the authors sorted human and mouse nucleus pulposus cells using various surface markers and then scored their ability to form colonies. They identified nucleus pulposus progenitor cells that formed spheroid colonies in Tie2$^+$ and disialoganglioside GD2$^+$ population. These spheroid colonies demonstrated superior aggrecan and collagen II production capability compared to other colonies (Fig. 23.3). Clonal analyses of Tie2$^+$GD2$^+$ human nucleus pulposus cell demonstrated that these cells are highly proliferative and clonally capable of differentiation into multiple mesenchymal and nucleus pulposus lineages. Moreover, this multipotent ability is sustained through long-term engraftment and was demonstrated to include the ability for self-renewal. Analyses in clinically obtained tissue provided new concept in the underdefined pathology of disc degeneration by showing a gradual exhaustion of Tie2$^+$ cells in the disc correlating with aging and degeneration in humans. Moreover, they defined the importance of Tie2/angiopoietin-1 niche (Fig. 23.4) in maintenance of Tie2$^+$ nucleus pulposus progenitor cells, which may lead to new treatment targets. To induce MSC to differentiate into intervertebral disc cells, an obstacle that must be overcome is that induced MSCs never proceed beyond intervertebral disclike cells. This problem is exacerbated by the lack of a specific marker or assays that defines a cell as an intervertebral disc cell. Fundamental studies that can define a cell as a disc cell that can function in vitro will be most useful in this field. The use of MSC as an activation tool for drug delivery systems may still offer a novel strategy for tissue repair. In the developmental and maturation stages of the disc, the mesenchymal cells surrounding the nucleus pulposus are

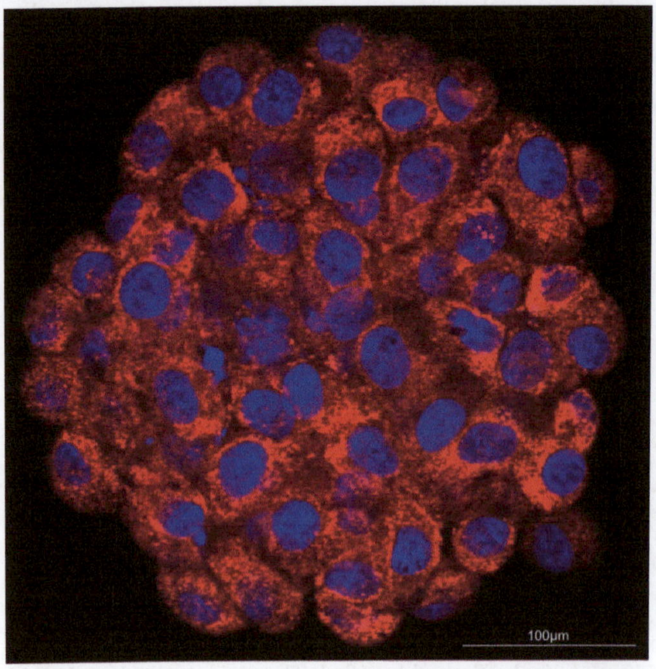

Fig. 23.3 Spheroid colony derived from nucleus pulposus progenitor cells. These cells express abundant aggrecan (*red*), the major extracellular matrix component of the nucleus pulposus (*blue* indicates nuclear staining with diamidino-2-phenylindole) (Reproduced from Sakai et al. 2012)

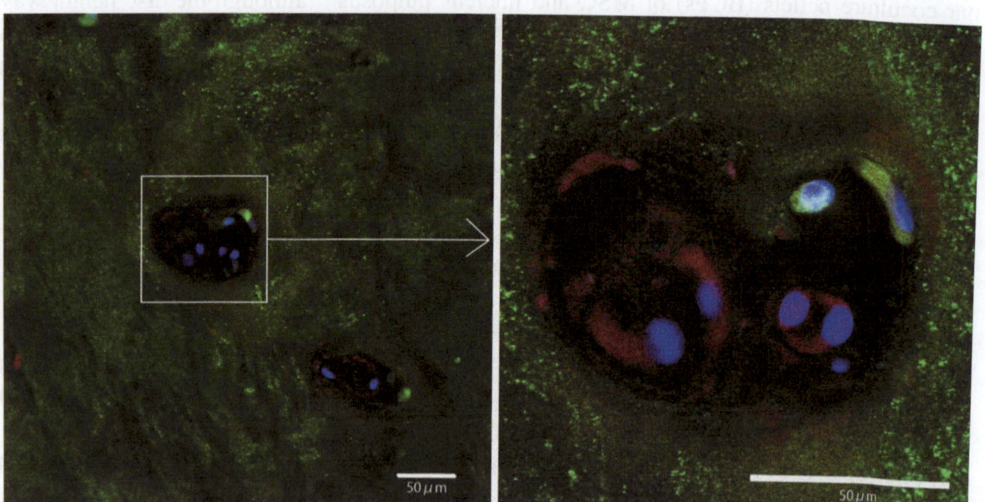

Fig. 23.4 Tie2/angiopoietin-1 signaling maintains progenitor cells in the nucleus pulposus of the intervertebral disc. Both Tie2 (*red*) and Ang-1 (*green*) are expressed in cluster of cells found in the nucleus pulposus (*blue* indicates nuclear staining with diamidino-2-phenylindole) (Reproduced from Sakai et al. 2012)

thought to be influenced by notochord-derived cells. Knowledge of the interactions between the components that participate in disc development will certainly provide new information on tissue regeneration and tissue engineering. Finally, more clinical trials of actual MSC transplantation for intervertebral disc repair will also undoubtedly be reported in the future, using various techniques and stem cells from various sources. However, caution is strongly warranted. For example, using a rabbit model, Vadalà et al. (2012) reported that cell leakage after MSC injection into the intervertebral disc can cause osteophyte formation. They suggest that cell carriers or annulus-sealing techniques should be assessed or perhaps postsurgical rehabilitation protocols investigated, to minimize leakage. Unintended differentiation and tumorigenesis are also potential risks usually faced in stem cell therapies. Although many animal studies and preliminary human trials have supported the promising future of stem cell therapy for disc disease, careful application of cells and techniques, with the selection of the appropriate types of patients in a strictly controlled manner, are key elements in ensuring the success of these therapies.

23.7 Summary of Critical Concepts Discussed in the Chapter

- While definition of stem cells in the mesenchymal tissues has changed with time, there is still a lack of knowledge of their in vivo characteristics, and therefore, selection of stem cells for regeneration of the intervertebral disc needs to be carefully evaluated.
- It is important that investigators share a common stem cell terminology in designing experiments to evaluate the use of stem cells for intervertebral disc research.
- Laboratory investigations have revealed that a stem cell system is present in the intervertebral disc and that its exhaustion may be related to aging and degeneration.
- Stem cells can be induced to express some of the characteristics of intervertebral disc cells.
- Stem cells are capable of stimulating intervertebral disc cell metabolism.
- Stem cells can facilitate intervertebral disc tissue engineering and repair.
- Investigation of intervertebral disc stem/progenitor cells in their niche and the fates of these cells should provide insight into key events in the pathogenesis of disc degeneration and the endogenous repair system. This information should be of great use in the design of new biological therapies.

Acknowledgments The authors are grateful to the staff of the Education and Research Support Center, Tokai University. This work was supported in part by a Grant-in-Aid for Scientific Research from the Ministry of Education, Culture, Sports, Science and Technology of Japan and a grant from AOSpine International and AO Foundation to D.S.

References

Allon AA, Aurouer N, Yoo BB, Liebenberg EC, Buser Z, Lotz JC (2010) Structured coculture of stem cells and disc cells prevent disc degeneration in a rat model. Spine J 10:1089–1097

Bendtsen M, Bünger CE, Zou X, Foldager C, Jørgensen HS (2011) Autologous stem cell therapy maintains vertebral blood flow and contrast diffusion through the endplate in experimental intervertebral disc degeneration. Spine (Phila Pa 1976) 36:E373–E379

Bertolo A, Mehr M, Aebli N, Baur M, Ferguson SJ, Stoyanov JV (2012) Influence of different commercial scaffolds on the in vitro differentiation of human mesenchymal stem cells to nucleus pulposus-like cells. Eur Spine J 21:S826–S838

Bianco P, Riminucci M, Gronthos S, Robey PG (2001) Bone marrow stromal stem cells: nature, biology, and potential applications. Stem Cells 19:180–192

Blanco JF, Graciani IF, Sanchez-Guijo FM, Muntion S, Hernandez-Campo P, Santamaria C, Carrancio S, Barbado MV, Cruz G, Gutierrez-Cosio S, Herrero C, San Miguel JF, Brinon JG, del Canizo MC (2010) Isolation and characterization of mesenchymal stromal cells from human degenerated nucleus pulposus: comparison with bone marrow mesenchymal stromal cells from the same subjects. Spine (Phila Pa 1976) 35:2259–2265

Blanpain C, Lowry WE, Geoghegan A, Polak L, Fuchs E (2004) Self-renewal, multipotency, and the existence of two cell populations within an epithelial stem cell niche. Cell 118:635–648

Caplan AI (1991) Mesenchymal stem cells. J Orthop Res 9:641–650

Chen WH, Liu HY, Lo WC, Wu SC, Chi CH, Chang HY, Hsiao SH, Wu CH, Chiu WT, Chen BJ, Deng WP (2009) Intervertebral disc regeneration in an ex vivo culture system using mesenchymal stem cells and platelet-rich plasma. Biomaterials 30:5523–5533

Choi EH, Park H, Park KS, Park KS, Kim BS, Han IB, Shin DA, Lee SH (2011) Effect of nucleus pulposus cells having different phenotypes on chondrogenic differentiation of adipose-derived stromal cells in a coculture system using porous membranes. Tissue Eng Part A 17:2445–2451

Chun HJ, Kim YS, Kim BK, Kim EH, Kim JH, Do BR, Hwang SJ, Hwang JY, Lee YK (2012) Transplantation of human adipose-derived stem cells in a rabbit model of traumatic degeneration of lumbar discs. World Neurosurg 78:364–371

Crevensten G, Walsh AJ, Ananthakrishnan D, Page P, Wahba GM, Lotz JC, Berven S (2004) Intervertebral disc cell therapy for regeneration: mesenchymal stem cell implantation in rat intervertebral discs. Ann Biomed Eng 32:430–434

Crisan M, Yap S, Casteilla L, Chen CW, Corselli M, Park TS, Andriolo G, Sun B, Zheng B, Zhang L, Norotte C, Teng PN, Traas J, Schugar R, Deasy BM, Badylak S, Buhring HJ, Giacobino JP, Lazzari L, Huard J, Péault B (2008) A perivascular origin for mesenchymal stem cells in multiple human organs. Cell Stem Cell 3:301–313

Deans RJ, Moseley AB (2000) Mesenchymal stem cells: biology and potential clinical uses. Exp Hematol 2:875–884

Dominici M, Le Blanc K, Mueller I, Slaper-Cortenbach I, Marini F, Krause D, Deans R, Keating A, Prockop DJ, Horwitz E (2006) Minimal criteria for defining multipotent mesenchymal stromal cells. The International Society for Cellular Therapy position statement. Cytotherapy 8:315–317

Driscoll TP, Nerurkar NL, Jacobs NT, Elliott DM, Mauck RL (2011) Fiber angle and aspect ratio influence the shear mechanics of oriented electrospun nanofibrous scaffolds. J Mech Behav Biomed Mater 4:1627–1636

Ehlicke F, Freimark D, Heil B, Dorresteijn A, Czermak P (2010) Intervertebral disc regeneration: influence of growth factors on differentiation of human mesenchymal stem cells (hMSC). Int J Artif Organs 33:244–252

Feng G, Yang X, Shang H, Marks IW, Shen FH, Katz A, Arlet V, Laurencin CT, Li X (2010) Multipotential differentiation of human annulus fibrosus cells: an in vitro study. J Bone Joint Surg Am 92:675–685

Feng G, Jin X, Hu J, Ma H, Gupte MJ, Liu H, Ma PX (2011a) Effects of hypoxias and scaffold architecture on rabbit mesenchymal stem cell differentiation toward a nucleus pulposus-like phenotype. Biomaterials 32:8182–8189

Feng G, Zhao X, Liu H, Zhang H, Chen X, Shi R, Liu X, Zhao X, Zhang W, Wang B (2011b) Transplantation of mesenchymal stem cells and nucleus pulposus cells in a degenerative disc model in rabbits: a comparison of 2 cell types as potential candidates for disc regeneration. J Neurosurg Spine 14:322–329

Gaetani P, Torre ML, Klinger M, Faustini M, Crovato F, Bucco M, Marazzi M, Chlapanidas T, Levi D, Tancioni F, Vigo D, Rodriguez y Baena R (2008) Adipose-derived stem cell therapy for intervertebral disc regeneration: an in vitro reconstructed tissue in alginate capsules. Tissue Eng Part A 14:1415–1423

Ganey T, Hutton WC, Moseley T, Hedrick M, Meisel HJ (2009) Intervertebral disc repair using adipose tissue-derived stem and regenerative cells: experiments in a canine model. Spine (Phila Pa 1976) 34:2297–2304

Haufe SM, Mork AR (2006) Intradiscal injection of hematopoietic stem cells in an attempt to rejuvenate the intervertebral discs. Stem Cells Dev 15:136–137

He F, Pei M (2012) Rejuvenation of nucleus pulposus cells using extracellular matrix deposited by synovium-derived stem cells. Spine (Phila Pa 1976) 37:459–469

Henriksson H, Thornemo M, Karlsson C, Hagg O, Junevik K, Lindahl A, Brisby H (2009) Identification of cell proliferation zones, progenitor cells and a potential stem cell niche in the intervertebral disc region: a study in four species. Spine (Phila Pa 1976) 34:2278–2287

Henriksson HB, Svala E, Skioldebrand E, Lindahl A, Brisby H (2011) Support of concept that migrating progenitor cells from stem cell niches contribute to normal regeneration of the adult mammal intervertebral disc: a descriptive study in the New Zealand white rabbit. Spine (Phila Pa 1976) 37:722–732

Hiyama A, Mochida J, Iwashina T, Omi H, Watanabe T, Serigano K, Tamura F, Sakai D (2008) Transplantation of mesenchymal stem cells in a canine disc degeneration model. J Orthop Res 26:589–600

Hoogendoorn RJ, Lu ZF, Kroeze RJ, Bank RA, Wuisman PI, Helder MN (2008) Adipose stem cells for intervertebral disc regeneration: current status and concepts for the future. J Cell Mol Med 12:2205–2216

Kim DH, Kim SH, Heo SJ, Shin JW, Lee SW, Park SA, Shin JW (2009) Enhanced differentiation of mesenchymal stem cells into NP-like cells via 3D co-culturing with mechanical stimulation. J Biosci Bioeng 108:63–67

Korecki CL, Taboas JM, Tuan RS, Iatridis JC (2010) Notochordal cell conditioned medium stimulates mesenchymal stem cell differentiation toward a young nucleus pulposus phenotype. Stem Cell Res Ther 1:18

Le Maitre CL, Baird P, Freemont AJ, Hoyland JA (2009) An in vitro study investigating the survival and phenotype of mesenchymal stem cells following injection into nucleus pulposus tissue. Arthritis Res Ther 11:R20

Leung VY, Chan D, Cheung KM (2006) Regeneration of intervertebral disc by mesenchymal stem cells: potentials, limitations, and future direction. Eur Spine J 15(Suppl 3):S406–S413

Li X, Lee JP, Balian G, Greg AD (2005) Modulation of chondrocytic properties of fat-derived mesenchymal cells in co-cultures with nucleus pulposus. Connect Tissue Res 46:75–82

Liu LT, Huang B, Li CQ, Zhuang Y, Wang J, Zhou Y (2011) Characteristics of stem cells derived from the degenerated human intervertebral disc cartilage endplate. PLoS One 6:e26285

Lu ZF, Zandieh Doulabi B, Wuisman PI, Bank RA, Helder MN (2007) Differentiation of adipose stem cells by nucleus pulposus cells: configuration effect. Biochem Biophys Res Commun 359:991–996

Luo W, Xiong W, Qiu M, Lv Y, Li Y, Li F (2011) Differentiation of mesenchymal stem cells toward a nucleus pulposus-like phenotype utilizing simulated microgravity in vitro. J Huazhong Univ Sci Technolog Med Sci 31:199–203

Melrose J, Smith SM, Fuller ES, Young AA, Roughley PJ, Dart A, Little CB (2007) Biglycan and fibromodulin fragmentation correlates with temporal and spatial annular remodelling in experimentally injured ovine intervertebral discs. Eur Spine J 16:2193–2205

Meyerrose T, Olson S, Pontow S, Kalomoiris S, Jung Y, Annett G, Bauer G, Nolta JA (2010) Mesenchymal stem cells for the sustained in vivo delivery of bioactive factors. Adv Drug Deliv Rev 62:1167–1174

Miyamoto T, Muneta T, Tabuchi T, Matsumoto K, Saito H, Tsuji K, Sekiya I (2010) Intradiscal transplantation of synovial mesenchymal stem cells prevents intervertebral disc degeneration through suppression of matrix metalloproteinase-related genes in nucleus pulposus cells in rabbits. Arthritis Res Ther 12:R206

Nesti LJ, Li WJ, Shanti RM, Jiang YJ, Jackson W, Freedman BA, Kuklo TR, Giuliani JR, Tuan RS (2008) Intervertebral disc tissue engineering using a novel hyaluronic acid-nanofibrous scaffold (HANFS) amalgam. Tissue Eng Part A 14:1527–1537

Orozco L, Soler R, Morera C, Alberca M, Sánchez A, García-Sancho J (2011) Intervertebral disc repair by autologous mesenchymal bone marrow cells: a pilot study. Transplantation 92:822–828

Purmessur D, Schek RM, Abbott RD, Ballif BA, Godburn KE, Iatridis JC (2011) Notochordal conditioned media from tissue increases proteoglycan accumulation and promotes a healthy nucleus pulposus phenotype in human mesenchymal stem cells. Arthritis Res Ther 13:R81

Richardson SM, Walker RV, Parker S, Rhodes NP, Hunt JA, Freemont AJ, Hoyland JA (2006) Intervertebral disc cell-mediated mesenchymal stem cell differentiation. Stem Cells 24:707–716

Risbud MV, Albert TJ, Guttapalli A, Vresilovic EJ, Hillibrand AS, Vaccaro AR, Shapiro IM (2004) Differentiation of mesenchymal stem cells towards a nucleus pulposus-like phenotype in vitro: implications for cell-based transplantation therapy. Spine (Phila Pa 1976) 29:2627–2632

Risbud MV, Guttapalli A, Tsai TT, Lee JY, Danielson KG, Vaccaro AR, Albert TJ, Gazit Z, Gazit D, Shapiro IM (2007) Evidence for skeletal progenitor cells in the degenerate human intervertebral disc. Spine (Phila Pa 1976) 32:2537–2544

Ruan D, Zhang Y, Wang D, Zhang C, Wu J, Wang C, Shi Z, Xin H, Xu C, Li H, He Q (2012) Differentiation of human Wharton's jelly cells toward nucleus pulposus-like cells after coculture with nucleus pulposus cells in vitro. Tissue Eng Part A 18:167–175

Sakai D (2011) Stem cell regeneration of the intervertebral disk. Orthop Clin North Am 42:555–562, viii–ix. Review

Sakai D, Mochida J, Yamamoto Y, Nomura T, Okuma M, Nishimura K, Nakai T, Ando K, Hotta T (2003) Transplantation of mesenchymal stem cells embedded in Atelocollagen gel to the intervertebral disc: a potential therapeutic model for disc degeneration. Biomaterials 24:3531–3541

Sakai D, Mochida J, Iwashina T, Watanabe T, Nakai T, Ando K, Hotta T (2005) Differentiation of mesenchymal stem cells transplanted to a rabbit degenerative disc model: potential and limitations for stem cell therapy in disc regeneration. Spine (Phila Pa 1976) 30:2379–2387

Sakai D, Mochida J, Iwashina T, Hiyama A, Omi H, Imai M, Nakai T, Ando K, Hotta T (2006) Regenerative effects of transplanting mesenchymal stem cells embedded in atelocollagen to the degenerated intervertebral disc. Biomaterials 27:335–345

Sakai D, Nakamura Y, Nakai T, Mishima T, Kato S, Grad S, Alini M, Risbud M, Chan D, Cheah K, Yamamura K, Masuda K, Okano H, Ando K, Mochida J (2012) Exhaustion of nucleus pulposus progenitor cells with ageing and degeneration of the intervertebral disc. Nat Commun 3:1264

See EY, Toh SL, Goh JC (2011) Simulated intervertebral disc-like assembly using bone marrow-derived mesenchymal stem cell sheets and silk scaffolds for annulus fibrosus regeneration. J Tissue Eng Regen Med. doi:10.1002/term.457

Serigano K, Sakai D, Hiyama A, Tamura F, Tanaka M, Mochida J (2010) Effect of cell number on mesenchymal stem cell transplantation in a canine disc degeneration model. J Orthop Res 28:1267–1275

Sobajima S, Vadalà G, Shimer A, Kim JS, Gilbertson LG, Kang JD (2008) Feasibility of a stem cell therapy for intervertebral disc degeneration. Spine J 8:888–896

Steck E, Bertram H, Abel R, Chen B, Winter A, Richter W (2005) Induction of intervertebral disc-like cells from adult mesenchymal stem cells. Stem Cells 23:403–411

Stoyanov JV, Gantenbein-Ritter B, Bertolo A, Aebli N, Baur M, Alini M, Grad S (2011) Role of hypoxia and growth and differentiation factor-5 on differentiation of human mesenchymal stem cells toward intervertebral nucleus pulposus-like cells. Eur Cell Mater 21:533–547

Strassburg S, Richardson SM, Freemont AJ, Hoyland JA (2010) Co-culture induces mesenchymal stem cell differentiation and modulation of the degenerate human nucleus pulposus cell phenotype. Regen Med 5:701–711

Tzaan WC, Chen HC (2011) Investigating the possibility of intervertebral disc regeneration induced by granulocyte colony stimulating factor-stimulated stem cells in rats. Adv Orthop 2011:602089. Epub 2010 Nov 21

Vadalà G, Studer RK, Sowa G, Spiezia F, Iucu C, Denaro V, Gilbertson LG, Kang JD (2008) Coculture of bone marrow mesenchymal stem cells and nucleus pulposus cells modulate gene expression profile without cell fusion. Spine (Phila Pa 1976) 33:870–876

Vadalà G, Sowa G, Hubert M, Gilbertson LG, Denaro V, Kang JD (2012) Mesenchymal stem cells injection in degenerated intervertebral disc: cell leakage may induce osteophyte formation. J Tissue Eng Regen Med 6:348–355. doi:10.1002/term.433

Wei A, Chung SA, Tao H, Brisby H, Lin Z, Shen B, Ma DD, Diwan AD (2009a) Differentiation of rodent bone marrow mesenchymal stem cells into intervertebral disc-like cells following coculture with rat disc tissue. Tissue Eng Part A 15:2581–2595

Wei A, Tao H, Chung SA, Brisby H, Ma DD, Diwan AD (2009b) The fate of transplanted xenogeneic bone marrow-derived stem cells in rat intervertebral discs. J Orthop Res 27:374–379

Wuertz K, Godburn K, Neidlinger-Wilke C, Urban J, Iatridis JC (2008) Behavior of mesenchymal stem cells in the chemical microenvironment of the intervertebral disc. Spine (Phila Pa 1976) 33:1843–1849

Yamamoto Y, Mochida J, Sakai D, Nakai T, Nishimura K, Kawada H, Hotta T (2004) Upregulation of the viability of nucleus pulposus cells by bone marrow-derived stromal cells: significance of direct cell-to-cell contact in coculture system. Spine (Phila Pa 1976) 29:1508–1514

Yang H, Wu J, Liu J, Ebraheim M, Castillo S, Liu X, Tang T, Ebraheim NA (2010) Transplanted mesenchymal stem cells with pure fibrinous gelatin–transforming growth factor-β1 decrease rabbit intervertebral disc degeneration. Spine J 10:802–810

Yoshikawa T, Ueda Y, Miyazaki K, Koizumi M, Takakura Y (2010) Disc regeneration therapy using marrow mesenchymal cell transplantation: a report of two case studies. Spine (Phila Pa 1976) 35:E475–E480

Zhang YG, Guo X, Xu P, Kang LL, Li J (2005) Bone mesenchymal stem cells transplanted into rabbit intervertebral discs can increase proteoglycans. Clin Orthop Relat Res 430:219–226

Gene Therapy Approaches for Disc Regeneration

24

Zulma Gazit, Nadav Kimelman-Bleich, Olga Mizrahi, and Dan Gazit

Contents

Z. Gazit (✉) • D. Gazit
Skeletal Biotechnology Laboratory,
Hadassah Faculty of Dental Medicine, Hebrew University,
12272, Ein Kerem, Jerusalem 91120, Israel
e-mail: zulma.gazit@csmc.edu; dan.gazit@csmc.edu

Department of Surgery,
Regenerative Medicine Institute, Cedars-Sinai Medical Center,
8700 Beverly Blvd AHSP-8108, Los Angeles, CA 90048, USA

N. Kimelman-Bleich • O. Mizrahi
Skeletal Biotechnology Laboratory,
Hadassah Faculty of Dental Medicine, Hebrew University,
12272, Ein Kerem, Jerusalem 91120, Israel
e-mail: nadav.kimelman@gmail.com; golzand@gmail.com

24.1 Introduction: Use of Gene Therapy for the Treatment of Disease

One of the first articles describing the use of gene therapy was published in *Science* in 1972. In that paper, Friedmann and Roblin described how they induced mammalian cells to express bacterial and viral DNA, demonstrating the possibility that this method could later be used to promote therapies for treatment of human genetic diseases (Friedmann and Roblin 1972). Today, scientists are exploring the therapeutic use of gene therapy for the treatment of numerous pathological conditions including Parkinson disease (Yasuda et al. 2011), glioma (Lee et al. 2011), X-linked severe combined immunodeficiency (SCID-X) (Huston et al. 2011), diabetes (Rowzee et al. 2011), bone fractures (Sheyn et al. 2008; Kimelman-Bleich et al. 2011), and heart failure (Muona et al. 2012; Pleger et al. 2011). During the last two decades, efforts have been made to enhance the safety and efficiency of gene therapy. Despite numerous advances, the immune response, which led to the death of a patient in one clinical trial (Somia and Verma 2000), and insertional mutagenesis, which

I.M. Shapiro, M.V. Risbud (eds.), *The Intervertebral Disc*,
DOI 10.1007/978-3-7091-1535-0_24, © Springer-Verlag Wien 2014

triggered the development of leukemia in several patients (Hacein-Bey-Abina et al. 2003; Cavazzana-Calvo et al. 2004), continue to pose a major barrier to the clinical use of gene therapy. Fortunately, improvements are constantly being made in protocols as well as in the safety features of some vectors, such as exogenous control of gene expression or the use of nonviral gene delivery methods (Herzog et al. 2010). Hundreds of clinical trials involving gene delivery are currently being conducted in the USA for the treatment of various diseases, ranging from cystic fibrosis to HIV (Flotte 2007).

Although most developments in gene therapy have as their aim treatment of systemic diseases and disorders, a few focus on tissue regeneration (Edelstein et al. 2007). In orthopedics, gene therapy is studied for its usefulness in bone-tissue engineering (Bueno and Glowacki 2009), because even transient expression of the *bone morphogenetic protein* (*BMP*)*-2*, *BMP-6*, or BMP-*9* gene is sufficient to promote bone generation. Gene therapy is also being explored for its value in creating cartilage (Menendez et al. 2011) and tendon (Xia et al. 2010), although success has been limited when direct gene delivery approaches are used.

Viral vectors, primarily adenovirus and retrovirus, are the main vectors used in clinical trials involving gene therapy (Edelstein et al. 2007). However, to avoid the safety issues associated with viral vectors (discussed earlier), there is increasing reliance on nonviral techniques (Edelstein et al. 2007). Nonviral vectors are easy to prepare and scale up for production (Schmidt-Wolf and Schmidt-Wolf 2003; Aslan et al. 2006). They also exhibit a high potential for orthopedic applications, since bone formation requires short-term expression of osteogenic genes (Noel et al. 2004). Gene therapy can be performed either directly, by injection of a gene-carrying vector into the target area, or ex vivo, by inserting the gene into harvested cells and then implanting the modified cells into the desired tissue (Wehling 2001). Current studies are underway to explore various gene delivery techniques.

One of the first studies in which gene therapy was used for the treatment of intervertebral disc degeneration was published in 1997 (Wehling et al. 1997). End plate chondrocytes were isolated and induced to express an anti-inflammatory gene using a retrovirus. This was a feasibility study demonstrating that gene therapy can be applied to intervertebral disc cells. Since then, many studies have been conducted to locate target genes, improve gene delivery mechanisms, and provide preliminary proof of the therapeutic potential of gene therapy in the organ. However, until now no clinical trial involving gene therapy for disc disease or disorder has been listed in the clinical trial database of the NIH (www.clinicaltrails.gov).

Currently, three groups of genes are being used in studies that explore intervertebral disc gene therapy. First, reporter genes (Wehling et al. 1997), such as *green fluorescence protein* (*GFP*) and *luciferase*, are used for proof-of-concept studies to demonstrate the feasibility of gene delivery and to further understand how gene insertion influences the cell's phenotype. Second, anti-inflammatory or "anti-degeneration" genes, such as *interleukin-1* (*IL-1*), *tissue inhibitors of metalloproteinases-1* (*TIMP-1*), and *Fas ligand* (*FasL*) (Wallach et al. 2003b; Le Maitre et al. 2007; Seki et al. 2009; Suzuki et al. 2009), are used to stop the degeneration process or to minimize it. Third, anabolic genes, such as *growth and differentiation factor-5* (*GDF-5*), *BMPs*, *transforming growth factor-beta* (*TGF-β*), and *Sox-9*, are used not only to mitigate the degenerative process but also to promote tissue regeneration (Nishida et al. 1999; Lee et al. 2001; Paul et al. 2003; Cui et al. 2008; Reddi and Reddi 2009; Wang et al. 2011). In this chapter, insight is provided into the current status of intervertebral disc gene therapy. Also discussed are future directions and current hurdles that need to be surmounted to promote gene therapy as a therapeutic option for intervertebral disc degeneration.

24.2 Importance of Reporter Genes for Studies of Gene Delivery

24.2.1 In Vitro Approaches Using Animal Cells

Several studies have been conducted to deliver reporter genes into disc cells that have been isolated from animal tissues. The goal of these experiments is usually to evaluate the feasibility and limitations of gene delivery into disc-derived cells, specifically annulus fibrosus, nucleus pulposus, and end plate chondrocytes. Early attempts at delivery of reporter genes to intervertebral disc cells used a retroviral vector with a bacterial *LacZ* gene which was transfected into bovine end plate cells (Wehling et al. 1997) and delivery of the same gene into rabbit nucleus pulposus cells using adenovector (Nishida et al. 1998). While only 1 % of the end plate cells were successfully transduced, the use of adenovector yielded much higher levels of *LacZ* expression (detected by X-gal staining) after in vivo infection (Wehling et al. 1997; Nishida et al. 1998). In another study, the effect of different doses of baculovirus encoding the *GFP* reporter gene in rabbit nucleus pulposus cells was evaluated. A direct correlation between *GFP* expression and the multiplicity of infection (MOI) of the vector was noted up to a maximum of 87 % expressing cells at an MOI of 200, with gene expression observable up to 21 days after infection (Liu et al. 2006). RNA interference (RNAi), first described at 1998 (Fire et al. 1998), was also evaluated as a gene therapy tool, aimed at silencing specific genes involved in the disc degeneration process. Kakutani and colleagues used small interfering RNA (siRNA, 21 nt in length) to assess the use of this strategy in nucleus pulposus cells that had been isolated from rats and humans (Kakutani et al. 2006). These researchers showed that after a single transfection, siRNA could prevent *luciferase* and *GFP* expression for 2 weeks. Moreover, no differences were found between rat and human nucleus pulposus cells (Kakutani et al. 2006). Based on these studies, it is concluded that siRNA may represent a therapeutic strategy which could stop or slow disc degeneration.

24.2.2 Use of Reporter Genes for Assessment of Gene Delivery: In Vitro Studies Using Human Cells

Following studies performed on animal cells, researchers turned their attention to the delivery of reporter genes to human intervertebral disc cells. Moon and colleagues were among the first to analyze the value of adenovectors for gene delivery into human disc cells (nucleus pulposus and annulus fibrosus cells) isolated from healthy and degenerate discs. They reported that in vitro, an adenovector harboring the *LacZ* or *luciferase* reporter genes was able to transduce 100 % of cultured cells, regardless of the disc's degenerative state or the anatomical location of the transfected intervertebral disc cells (Moon et al. 2000). As it became clear that human disc cells could be genetically engineered, efforts were made to use more complex expression strategies, such as exogenous regulation of gene expression. Vadala and colleagues reported that a Tet-Off system, in which gene expression is shut down by tetracycline could be used to control *GFP* expression in human nucleus pulposus cells (Vadala et al. 2007). Lipid-based nonviral gene delivery systems were also used to deliver plasmid DNA encoding the *GFP* reporter into human nucleus pulposus cells, with high efficiency (Morrey et al. 2008).

24.2.3 Use of Reporter Genes for Assessment of Gene Delivery: In Vivo Studies Using Animal Models

Nishida and colleagues reported the first successful in vivo gene delivery into an intervertebral disc in 1998 (Wallach et al. 2003a, b). After in vitro delivery of the *LacZ* reporter gene into rabbit nucleus pulposus cells using an adenovector, the same virus was injected into the intervertebral discs; gene delivery was analyzed up to 3 months postinjection. Gene expression was evident, and no pathological changes were noted in the injected discs (Nishida et al. 1998). Moreover, in a follow-up study, protein expression was detected up to 1 year after gene delivery. The fact that no pathological changes were noted was encouraging (Wallach et al. 2003a, b). Another paper described the use of the *luciferase* reporter gene in noninvasive monitoring of gene expression following both ex vivo (cell mediated) and in vivo (adenovector injection) gene delivery into rat discs (Leo et al. 2004). The authors compared direct injection of the viral vector with the use of three different cell types as gene vehicles: (1) disc cells, a mix of nucleus pulposus and annulus fibrosus cells; (2) adipose-derived rat mesenchymal stem cells (ASCs); and (3) bone marrow-derived rat mesenchymal stem cells (MSCs). Of the three groups of cells, the most potent gene expressers were the genetically induced disc cells (Leo et al. 2004). This was the first report of bioluminescence imaging performed in the intervertebral disc, and it demonstrated the feasibility of noninvasive imaging of gene expression in this tissue. The use of *GFP*-encoding baculovirus as a gene delivery vehicle was also tested in vivo. *GFP* expression in the intervertebral disc was noted as long as 13 days after gene delivery (Liu et al. 2006). Following these feasibility studies, the effect of dosing and vector choice on the safety aspects of gene delivery into the disc was evaluated. When different doses of both adenovector and adeno-associated viral (AAV) vector encoding either *GFP* or *LacZ* were injected into rabbit intervertebral discs, no clinical, biochemical, or histological pathological deficits were noted. However, this was not the case when *BMP-2* or *TGF-β* was delivered (Levicoff et al. 2008). One take home message from these studies is that a range of markers need to be evaluated to assess the safety of gene delivery systems.

Box 24.1 Bioluminescence: BLI

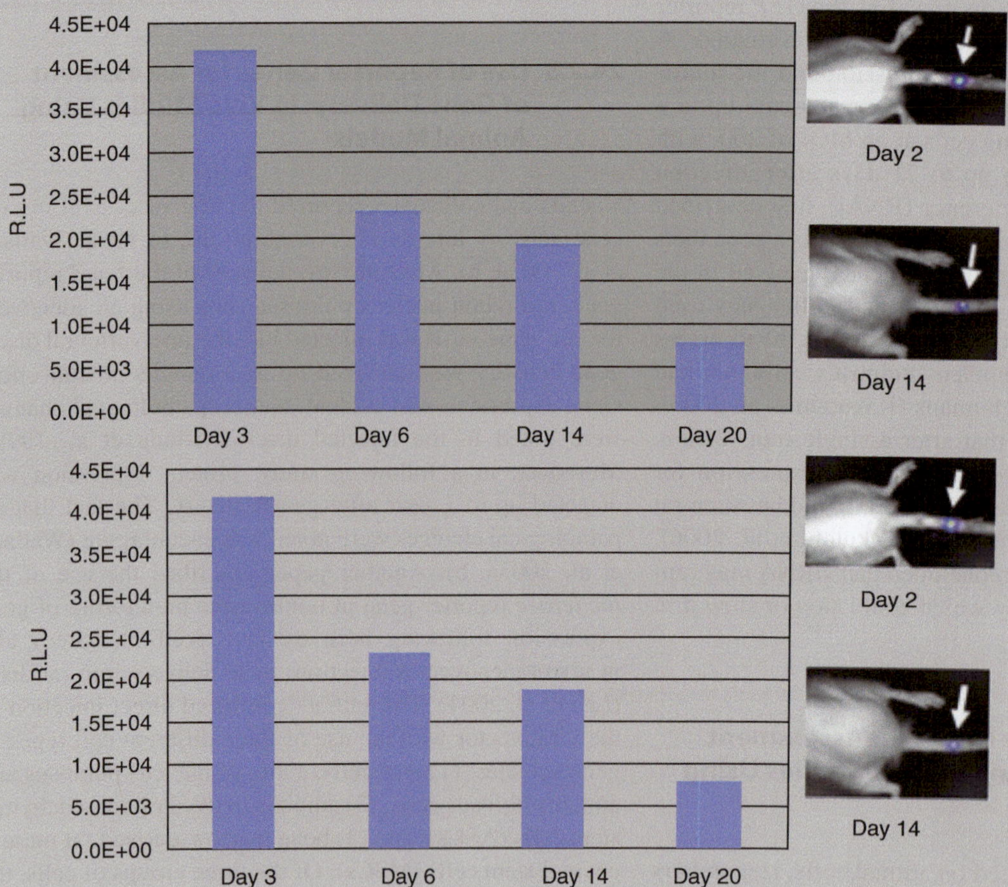

Survival of *luciferase*-expressing stem cells following implantation into the intervertebral disc region. Stem cells expressing the *luciferase* gene were implanted in a caudal disc space in the rat. At each time point listed, luciferin was injected into the implantation site. Images and quantified data were generated using the BLI system. *Arrows* indicate *luciferase*-expressing cells in the disc region. *RLU* relative luminescence unit

Bioluminescence imaging can be used to monitor cell survival over time both in vitro and in vivo. To apply this method, *luciferase*-expressing cells are required. Following gene delivery and cell culture or implantation, the *luciferase* substrate luciferin is added to cells in culture or injected into the implantation area in the animal. In vitro and in vivo imaging is performed using a cooled charge-coupled device (CCCD), which can detect light (photons) emitted from tissue following luciferin degradation by *luciferase* (Sheyn et al. 2011).

Reference

Sheyn D, Kallai I et al (2011) Gene-modified adult stem cells regenerate vertebral bone defect in a rat model. Mol Pharm 8:1592–1601

Following the use of viral vectors, there was an assessment of nonviral vectors for gene therapy. When *GFP*- and *luciferase*-encoding plasmid DNAs were delivered into rat discs via sonoporation (an ultrasound technique that enhances gene delivery), prolonged expression of the reporter genes was noted. Expression of *GFP* was evident after 7 days, and *luciferase* activity was recorded up to 24 weeks following gene delivery (Nishida et al. 2006). This finding – remarkable because nonviral gene delivery is usually transient – was probably due to low cellular metabolic activity and proliferation in the disc. It also demonstrated the advantage of using nonviral gene delivery techniques in this organ.

Exogenously controlled gene delivery was assessed not only in vitro (Vadala et al. 2007) but also in vivo (Sowa et al. 2011). A novel ligand-based system for gene expression control (RheoSwitch) was successfully used in a rabbit model. *GFP* expression was controlled both in vitro and in vivo, demonstrating this system's potential and enhanced safety features (Sowa et al. 2011).

Finally, ex vivo gene delivery of reporter genes was used to assess gene delivery into discs in a preclinical large-animal model. Omlor and colleagues used a retroviral vector to generate stable *luciferase*-expressing porcine MSCs. These cells were subsequently implanted into the intervertebral discs of Gottingen minipigs. The animals were sacrificed on the same day or 3 days later, and a *luciferase* assay was performed to assess gene activity. Activity on Day 3 postimplantation was reduced to 7 % of initial values, indicating massive cell loss following implantation (Omlor et al. 2010).

Recently, siRNA was also used in vivo in a rat model to analyze the feasibility of this gene-silencing tool in the intervertebral disc. The siRNA downregulated the activity of the *luciferase* reporter gene up to 24 weeks following transfection performed using the ultrasound technique. At that time, gene activity remained at 80 % of control values (Suzuki et al. 2009). These findings indicate that siRNA can be used in the disc with high efficiency.

24.3 Delivery and Activity of Anti-inflammatory/Anti-degeneration Genes

As discussed in other chapters of the book, during disc degeneration there is a progressive loss of water, proteoglycans, and collagen II from the matrix of the nucleus pulposus. Although the events that lead to these degenerative changes have not been clearly defined, there is overwhelming evidence to indicate that inflammatory mediators are elevated during degeneration. Kang et al. (1997) showed that cells obtained from normal, nondegenerate human discs and cultured for 72 h with interleukin (IL)-1β were biologically responsive and increased their production of matrix metalloproteinases, nitric oxide, IL-6, and prostaglandin E2. The effect was significantly higher in normal, nondegenerate discs, in which spontaneous synthesis of these mediators is low. These agents are inhibitors of proteoglycan synthesis, but IL-1 is likely to have a direct effect on proteoglycan breakdown through activation of members of the metalloproteinase (MMP) family of enzymes.

Aside from the interleukins, Seguin et al. (2005) studied the in vitro effect of TNF-α on nucleus pulposus tissue from bovine caudal spines. These studies reported decreased proteoglycan and collagen gene expression and protein synthesis and activation of aggrecanase-mediated proteoglycan degradation, involving MMPs, and ADAMTS. Since MMP activity is normally inhibited within the matrix by tissue inhibitors of MMPs (TIMPs) (Nagase and Woessner 1999), it is reasonable that members of this family were used to explore whether candidate genes would stop or slow the disc degradation process.

24.3.1 Anti-inflammatory/Anti-degeneration Gene Delivery into Animal and Human Cells: In Vitro and In Vivo Studies

In 2003, Wallach et al. (2003b) isolated cells from degenerate intervertebral disc obtained from patients undergoing elective surgical procedures and infected the cells with an adenoviral-tissue inhibitor of metalloproteinase-1 (Adeno-TIMP-1) construct. Gene delivery of TIMP-1 increased proteoglycan synthesis in a dose–response manner. Disc cells treated with Adeno-TIMP-1 demonstrated an optimal response at an MOI of 100; cell pellets treated with Adeno-TIMP-1 at 100 MOI were consistently larger than controls and pellets treated with other virus concentrations. Successful delivery of the anticatabolic gene *TIMP-1* resulted in increased levels of proteoglycan in three-dimensional cultures of degenerate disc cells. It is likely that TIMP-1 had no direct effect on proteoglycan synthesis, but rather inhibited proteoglycan degradation, thus promoting its accumulation in the culture. In addition, these results may reflect a secondary effect, that is, inhibition of aggrecanase-1 (ADAMTS-4), which is also inhibited by the TIMP family, as reported elsewhere (Hashimoto et al. 2001).

In a more recent study, Liu et al. (2010) investigated the effect of combined *connective tissue growth factor* (*CTGF*) and *TIMP-1* expression mediated by AAV. These researchers isolated rhesus monkey lumbar disc nucleus pulposus cells; cultured and transduced the cells with rAAV2-CTGF-IRES-TIMP-1 (a vector that elicits both *CTGF* and *TIMP-1* expression), rAAV2-CTGF, or rAAV2-TIMP-1 at an MOI of 10^6; and then measured the expression of collagen II and proteoglycan using reverse transcription polymerase chain reaction (RT-PCR) analysis and Western blotting. By comparing transduced with nontransduced cells, these researchers showed that *CTGF* induced the synthesis of collagen II and proteoglycan, whereas *TIMP-1* enhanced expression of proteoglycan, but had no effect on collagen. Expression of both genes in the lumbar disc nucleus pulposus cells significantly increased the synthesis of proteoglycan and collagen II. In this particular case, single gene transduction of *CTGF* or *TIMP-1* increased proteoglycan synthesis (Lee et al. 2001). Overexpression of *CTGF* caused an increase in collagen II protein synthesis. Combined transduction of both *CTGF* and *TIMP-1* significantly promoted the expression of proteoglycan and collagen II to levels greater than that achieved using each of the individual genes. This finding is of considerable importance as it supports the concept that one approach to preventing degradation is by promoting inhibition of catabolic processes. It thus serves as a promising avenue of research for the treatment of degenerative disc disease via gene therapy.

IL-1 is an inflammatory mediator implicated in the degeneration of intervertebral discs, especially the nucleus pulposus matrix (Elfervig et al. 2001; Shen et al. 2003;

Jimbo et al. 2005; Le Maitre et al. 2005). In 2006, Le Maitre et al. targeted the IL-1 receptor using an *IL-1 receptor antagonist (IL-1Ra)* gene that was transferred ex vivo to the intervertebral disc. Normal and degenerate human disc cells, growing in a monolayer or in alginate beads, were infected with an adenoviral vector carrying the *IL-1Ra* gene (Adeno-IL-1Ra). Protein production was measured, and the ability of the infected cells to inhibit the effects of IL-1 was assessed. In addition, normal and degenerate intervertebral disc cells infected with Adeno-IL-1Ra were injected into degenerate disc tissue explants, and IL-1Ra production in these discs was evaluated. Nucleus pulposus cells and annulus fibrosus cells infected with Adeno-IL-1Ra produced elevated levels of IL-1Ra for prolonged time periods, and the infected cells were unaffected by IL-1. IL-1Ra protein expression was increased and maintained for 2 weeks when infected cells were injected into disc explants. In a further study by the same group (Le Maitre et al. 2007), Adeno-IL-1Ra was introduced into degenerate disc explants directly or via genetically engineered nucleus pulposus cells. This resulted in cessation of degenerate intervertebral disc matrix, degradation; in situ zymographic and immunohistochemical investigations showed that there was downregulation of MMP-1, MMP-3, MMP-7, and MMP-13 expression as well as ADAMTS4 expression. Single injections of disc cells engineered to overexpress IL-1Ra significantly inhibited degradation enzyme expression for 2 weeks. These studies indicated that since IL-1 is a key cytokine that promotes matrix degradation, direct delivery of IL-1Ra or direct delivery by gene therapy provides a powerful new way to prevent or inhibit disc matrix degradation.

In 2005 Glasson and colleagues reported on the prevention of cartilage degradation in a murine model of osteoarthritis by deletion of the *ADAMTS5* "a disintegrin and metalloproteinase with thrombospondin motifs" gene (Glasson et al. 2005). To pursue the goal of looking for additional candidate genes that would stop or slow the disc degeneration process, the effect of ADAMTS5 was investigated by Seki using siRNA oligonucleotide in a rabbit annulus needle-puncture model (Seki et al. 2009). The efficiency of the siRNA constructs was first evaluated by growing rabbit NP cells in culture and transfecting them with the siRNA oligonucleotide specific to *ADAMTS5*. Compared with control, the *ADAMTS5* siRNA-transfected cells displayed an approximately 75 % decrease in levels of *ADAMTS5* mRNA. For the in vivo portion of the study, the nucleus pulposus was punctured, and 7 days later the *ADAMTS5* siRNA oligonucleotide was injected into the rabbit nucleus. The early timing of the injection was to ascertain the impact of *ADAMTS5* siRNA during the acute phase of disc degeneration. Eight weeks after the siRNA oligonucleotide injection, the rabbit spines were examined ex vivo by using MRI. The T2 signal intensity was stronger in *ADAMTS5* siRNA-injected nucleus pulposi than in the control siRNA-injected nucleus. Histological studies supported the MRI results, showing partial maintenance of nucleus pulposus tissues in the *ADAMTS5* siRNA-injected group, compared with the control group.

24.3.2 Fas-Fas Ligand (L) and the Intervertebral Disc as an Immune-Privileged Tissue

Since the concept of immune privilege is of high relevance in the biology of the intervertebral disc, the concept is discussed further in the accompanying box. Early in 1995, Griffith et al. (1995) published a paper showing that Fas-FasL interactions appear to be an important mechanism for the maintenance of immune privilege. That publication had as its focus the compartmentalization of tissues of the eye. In a related publication, Takada and his group reported that FasL exists in the intervertebral disc and confers immune privilege (Takada et al. 2002). In their study, Takada et al. (2002) used immunohistochemical and RT-PCR analysis to ascertain if FasL was present in human and rat disc specimens. They reported that nucleus pulposus cells of human and rat origin exhibited intense positive reactions for FasL. Outer annulus fibrosus cells and notochordal cells exhibited weak immunostaining. The results of RT-PCR confirmed the existence of FasL in the rat disc cells, but analysis was not performed on human tissues.

Results of investigations reported by Han et al. (2009) showed that FasL-induced apoptosis of rat nucleus pulposus cells was sharply reduced by Fas siRNA, suggesting that it is feasible to suppress nucleus cell death using an RNAi approach. The authors recognized that this was successful in short-term in vitro assays, but for research purposes and especially as a therapeutic strategy a much longer period of inhibition may be required. Because nucleus pulposus cells reportedly express FasL constitutively and since *FasL* is recognized as a marker gene, a study led by Suzuki et al. (2009) investigated the applicability of RNAi technology to downregulate the expression of this endogenous gene in rat intervertebral discs in vivo. As mentioned earlier in this chapter, the Suzuki group previously used RNAi in cultured nucleus pulposus cells in vitro, targeting two exogenous reporter luciferase plasmids, *firefly* and *Renilla* (Kakutani et al. 2006). For the endogenous *FasL* gene study, siRNAs that target rat *FasL* was injected into coccygeal intervertebral discs. After the injection, therapeutic ultrasound was applied to the skin surface covering the injected discs. There was significant inhibition (53 %) of endogenous *FasL* gene expression compared with the control group, which was transfected with nonspecific siRNA, at both 4 and 20 weeks posttransfection. One important conclusion from this study is that there is long-term downregulation, which is mediated by siRNA for the endogenous gene *Fas* in discs in vivo. Besides the techniques used for Fas-FasL genetic manipulation, it is important to take into consideration the actual debate on the paradoxical role of FasL. Reports have indicated that FasL is involved in the formation of the intervertebral disc and its immune privilege, and also that the expression of FasL is decreased in degenerate discs, but does not vary with age (Kaneyama et al. 2008). On the other hand, FasL has also been found to have a close relationship with disc cell apoptosis and is seen as another factor involved in disc degeneration (Han et al. 2009).

Box 24.2 Immune Privilege

Immune privilege (IP) is the ability of certain organs to suppress the immune response to foreign bodies or organisms within their specific boundaries. IP was first described by Sir Peter Medawar in 1948, based on the prolonged survival of an allogenic tissue graft that had been placed in the anterior chamber of the eye (Hori et al. 2010). Additional sites of IP include the brain, pregnant uterus, and testis. Recent studies have led to the identification of more tissues with IP-like characteristics (i.e., tissues that adopt IP mechanisms and hence avoid a destructive immune response) such as the gut, skin, and lung (Arck et al. 2008). The oral mucosa displays a similar tolerance: it rarely exhibits acute inflammatory or allergic reactions to high levels of bacterial colonization or frequent contacts with allergens (Novak et al. 2008). Although IP was first thought to be a passive process, it soon became evident that many active immunoregulatory processes take place in maintenance of IP (Hong and Van Kaer 1999; Arck et al. 2008; Novak et al. 2008; Hori et al. 2010). This phenomenon is believed to be an evolutionary protective mechanism designed to prevent a destructive inflammatory immune response in critical parts of the body (Hong and Van Kaer 1999; Arck et al. 2008). The potential clinical use of IP is clear. From allogenic cornea replacement (Hori et al. 2010) to implantation of xenogenic pancreatic islets performed in both rodents and large-animal models (Gores et al. 2003), the possibility of exploiting sites of IP to avoid the immune response to implanted tissue is attractive. In addition, the inherent IP properties of stem cells overcome the host immune rejection response, as in the case of ex vivo expanded hematopoietic stem cells, which when used in allogenic transplantation in a mouse model surmounts the major histocompatibility complex barrier (Zheng et al. 2011). Translated to humans, this strategy can significantly enhance the availability of implanted tissues and organs as well as promote novel therapies.

References

Arck PC, Gilhar A et al (2008) The alchemy of immune privilege explored from a neuroimmunological perspective. Curr Opin Pharmacol 8:480–489

Gores PF, Hayes DH et al (2003) Long-term survival of intratesticular porcine islets in nonimmunosuppressed beagles Transplantation 75:613–618

Hong, SL, Van Kaer L (1999) Immune privilege: keeping an eye on natural killer T cells. J Exp Med 190:1197–1200

Hori J, Vega JL et al (2010) Review of ocular immune privilege in the year 2010: modifying the immune privilege of the eye. Ocul Immunol Inflamm 18:325–333

Novak N, Haberstok J et al (2008) The immune privilege of the oral mucosa. Trends Mol Med 14:191–198

Zheng J, Umikawa M et al (2011) Ex vivo expanded hematopoietic stem cells overcome the MHC barrier in allogeneic transplantation. Cell Stem Cell 9:119–130

24.4 Gene Targeting of Growth and Transcription Factors

To maintain the health and integrity of the intervertebral disc, both in the nucleus pulposus and annulus fibrosus, there should be a balance among systems that regulate the synthesis, breakdown, and accumulation of macromolecules in the matrix. When reviewing work published to date on the gene therapy approach to treat disc degeneration, four main intracellular regulators were found: BMPs and TGF-β as morphogens and LMP-1 and Sox-9. Growth factors are polypeptides that bind to cell membranes and regulate matrix production and regeneration of various cell types in paracrine and autocrine pathways (Masuda and An 2004) (see also Chap. 25). In normal conditions, intervertebral disc cells express and secrete anabolic growth factors to maintain the balance between normal matrix synthesis and degradation. Included in this group of molecules is insulin-like growth factor (IGF), transforming growth factor-beta (TGF-β), and members of the BMP family (Thompson et al. 1991; Osada et al. 1996; Cui et al. 2008). Another group of targets includes transcriptional factors that are "master regulators" of the chondrogenic and osteogenic phenotype. Sox-9 is one such factor that has received study for cartilage and intervertebral disc basic and preclinical research; retroviral expression of Sox-9 can also efficiently induce ASCs differentiation into chondrocyte-like cells. Thus, Sox-9 is a candidate gene for use as a possible therapeutic tool for the treatment of degenerative disc diseases (Yang et al. 2011). LIM mineralization protein-1 (LMP-1) is another regulatory protein that positively regulates BMP secretion (Boden et al. 1998). The activities of both anabolic growth factors and selected transcription factors have been used to promote regeneration through augmentation of matrix production thereby impacting disc height and function (Zhang et al. 2006).

24.4.1 In Vitro Gene Delivery of Growth and Transcription Factors

Most experiments conducted in this field are still performed in vitro. Research is focused on finding the set of genes and cells that will elicit the most promising results (Zhang et al. 2006; Bron et al. 2009; Zhang et al. 2009). Most experiments are conducted in 3D cultures known to support chondrogenesis and nucleus pulposus-like differentiation (Risbud et al. 2004). Another established method for in vitro differentiation is a whole-disc culture model, which mimics the in vivo environment (Zhang et al. 2008).

Originally identified by their ability to induce the formation of bone and cartilage, BMPs are regarded today as key signaling proteins responsible for organization of tissue architecture throughout the entire body. Today, 20 proteins are known to be associated with this group. The Food and Drug Administration has recently allowed the initiation of Investigational New Drug clinical trials on osteogenic protein-1 and growth differentiation factor-5 in the United States (Reddi and Reddi 2009; Zhang et al. 2011). Zhang and colleagues compared the effects of overexpression of recombinant adenoviral vectors expressing various BMPs (BMP-2, BMP-3, BMP-4, BMP-5, BMP-7, BMP-8, BMP-10, BMP-11, BMP-12, BMP-13, BMP-14, and BMP-15) on extracellular matrix accumulation by bovine intervertebral disc cells. Of the 12 vectors evaluated by these researchers, BMP-2 and BMP-7 (also known as OP-1) were best at stimulating proteoglycan accumulation in nucleus pulposus cells, whereas BMP-4 and BMP-14 (also known as GDF-5) optimally stimulated collagen production (Zhang et al. 2006, 2009). Similar results were seen using the AAV-BMP-7 vector in canine nucleus pulposus cells (Wang et al. 2011). In another study, researchers injected knee chondrocytes transduced with Adeno-BMP-7 or Adeno-BMP-10 into whole intervertebral disc explants cultured in vitro. Discs treated with chondrocytes expressing BMP-7 demonstrated a 50 % increase in proteoglycan within the nucleus pulposus, whereas discs treated with chondrocytes expressing BMP-10 evidenced no increase in proteoglycan accumulation (Zhang et al. 2008).

GDF-5 (BMP-14) is known for its participation in joint formation and endochondral ossification (Cui et al. 2008). It is also known that a deficiency in GDF-5 leads to abnormalities in intervertebral disc structure (Li et al. 2004). Studies have shown that overexpression of GDF-5 in disc cells using viral (adenoviral vector) and nonviral (nucleofection) methods augments expression of proteoglycan proteins and collagen (Cui et al. 2008; Feng et al. 2009). LMP-1 is an

Box 24.3 Viral Vector Used to Monitor Bone Formation

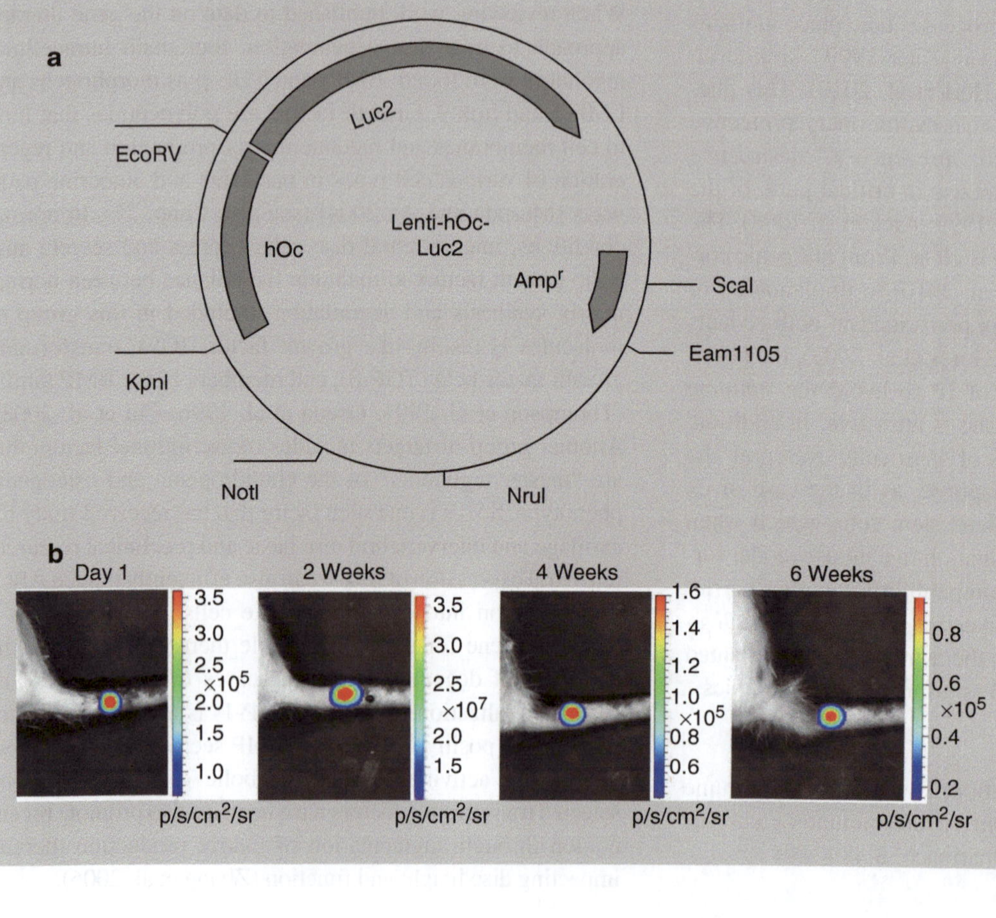

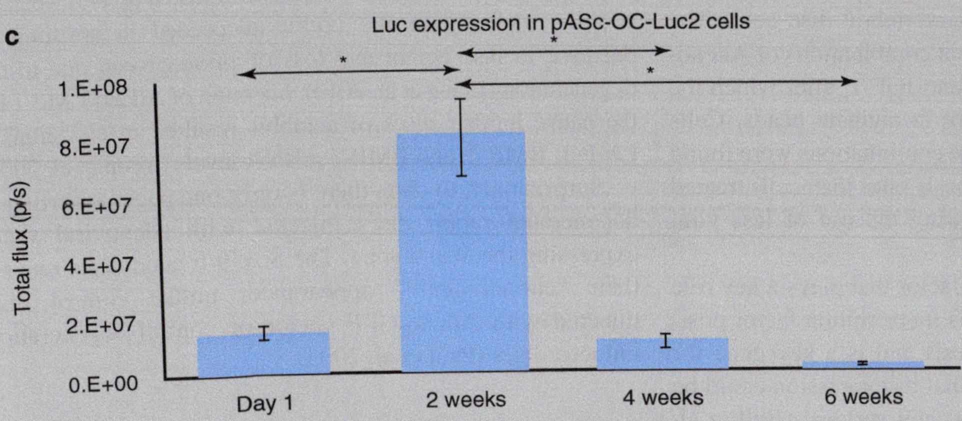

Vector used to monitor bone formation when applied in vertebral bone defect regeneration. (**a**) *Osteocalcin*-driven *luciferase* construct. To monitor bone formation noninvasively in real time, the *osteocalcin* promoter was cloned into the commercial reporter Luc2 vector (pGL.4, Promega). The *luciferase* gene was expressed as new bone formed. (**b**, **c**) Stem cells expressing the *osteocalcin*-driven *luciferase* gene were implanted in a bone defect created in a rat caudal vertebra. At each time point displayed, luciferin was injected in situ. Images and quantified data were generated using the BLI system. (Figures **b** and **c** are reprinted (adapted) with permission from Sheyn et al. (2011). Copyright (2011) American Chemical Society

Osteocalcin is one of the pivotal genes expressed during new bone formation in rodents. In transgenic mice, when the *osteocalcin* promoter is used to control expression of the reporter gene *luciferase*, bone formation (or osteogenic activity) can be monitored using the BLI system (Iris et al. 2003; Kimelman-Bleich et al. 2009). The activity of implanted cells can also be monitored using the *osteocalcin*-driven *luciferase* gene (Sheyn et al. 2011).

References

Iris B, Zilberman Y et al (2003) Molecular imaging of the skeleton: quantitative real-time bioluminescence monitoring gene expression in bone repair and development. J Bone Miner Res 18:570–578

Kimelman-Bleich N, Pelled G et al (2009) The use of a synthetic oxygen carrier-enriched hydrogel to enhance mesenchymal stem cell-based bone formation in vivo. Biomaterials 30:4639–4648

Sheyn D, Kallai I et al (2011) Gene-modified adult stem cells regenerate vertebral bone defect in a rat model. Mol Pharm 8:1592–1601

intracellular regulatory molecule known to induce secretion of multiple BMPs from leukocytes and osteoblasts (Boden et al. 1998). Boden and colleagues used this activity to increase proteoglycan production by intervertebral disc cells (Yoon et al. 2004; Kuh et al. 2008). They have shown that transduction of rat disc cells in a 3D culture or in a monolayer with Adeno-LMP1 results in significant increases in proteoglycan and aggrecan mRNA levels as well as elevations in BMP-2 and BMP-7 mRNA levels.

A nonviral gene delivery system is a promising alternative that avoids the risks of insertional mutagenesis of retroviruses, immunogenicity of adenoviruses, and acquisition of replication competence (Nishida et al. 2000). Using a gene gun, Matsumoto et al. demonstrated successful transfection of bovine intervertebral disc cells with BMP-7, which led to a higher proteoglycan content (Matsumoto et al. 2001).

In common with the BMPs discussed above, TGF-β is a secreted signaling protein that regulates many aspects of development and tissue homeostasis, including growth, patterning, and cellular differentiation. Three isoforms of TGF-β (1, 2, and 3) act through the same heteromeric receptor complex (Baffi et al. 2004). TGF-β signaling plays a key role in the development and maintenance of cartilage and, in particular, the intervertebral disc (Nishida et al. 1999). Lee and colleagues examined the effect of TGF-β on human disc cells in vitro. Disc cells were transfected with an adenovector expressing TGF-β, after which the cells were grown in 3D pellets. In response to this treatment, the cells increased synthesis of proteoglycan and collagen II (Lee et al. 2001).

Although positive results have been achieved with gene therapy, mainly when using adenoviral vectors, transfer of a single gene using high doses of viral vector can produce hazardous systemic effects, in particular cytotoxicity, and an immune response (Lohr et al. 2001). It is likely that these effects can be mitigated by administration of several vectors so as to decrease the level of a single vector and possibly augment the regenerative potential. Moon and colleagues tested this concept in human intervertebral disc cells. The cells were transduced with different combinations of Adeno-TGF-β1, Adeno-BMP-2, and Adeno-IGF-1, after which the cells were placed in a 3D culture in alginate beads. Cells treated with double and triple gene combinations were found to have higher proteoglycan synthesis rates than cells treated with a single vector, hence allowing the use of less viral vector (Moon et al. 2008).

Sox-9 is another transcription factor that plays a key role in the differentiation process. This transcription factor positively controls collagen II synthesis and is a key gene for chondrogenesis, thus suggesting that its expression could be used to promote nucleus pulposus cell survival (Bell et al. 1997; Paul et al. 2003; Yang et al. 2011). After infection with Adeno-Sox-9 vector, cells from a chondroblast line, human disc cells derived from degenerated discs, and bovine nucleus pulposus-derived cells demonstrated elevated collagen II mRNA expression and raised protein levels (Paul et al. 2003; Zhang et al. 2006). In another study, rat ASCs were infected with a retro-Sox-9 vector based on the murine leukemia virus. In a 3D culture system, supplemented with TGF-β, these genetically modified cells demonstrated increased levels of Sox-9 and collagen II. These researchers also cocultured these genetically modified ASCs with nucleus pulposus cells. The coculturing technique has been shown to enhance differentiation toward a nucleus pulposus-like fate since the ASC secrete growth factors into the culture medium. When this was performed, a marked increase in proteoglycan and collagen II production by the nucleus pulposus cells was noted (Yang et al. 2011).

24.4.2 In Vivo Gene Delivery of Growth and Transcription Factors: Animal Models

There are few published studies dealing with gene therapy for intervertebral disc regeneration in vivo. The experiments described in this section are all focused on early stages of development and were performed to evaluate the feasibility and safety of using gene therapy as a tool for disc regeneration. The model used for these studies is based on intradiscal injection of a therapeutic vector into the degenerated intervertebral disc and takes advantage of the avascularity and immune privilege of the disc (Nishida et al. 2008).

Nishida and colleagues evaluated injections of Adeno-TGF-β into rabbit IVDs. The discs were harvested 1 week after virus injection and were subjected to histological analysis and biochemical assays. The injected discs showed extensive increases in TGF-β expression and production, as well as in proteoglycan synthesis (Nishida et al. 1999). In a similar study, Adeno-GDF-5 or Adeno-Luc vector was injected directly into mouse lumbar degenerated intervertebral discs. Gene expression of the delivered vector lasted up to 6 weeks. In addition, delivery of the vector succeeded in arresting the decrease in disc height and loss of proteoglycan due to disc degeneration (Liang et al. 2010). Injection of Adeno-LMP-1 into the native lumbar discs of a rabbit resulted in elevations of LMP-1, BMP-2, and BMP-7 mRNA levels (Yoon et al. 2004).

Surprisingly, to date, there is only one paper reporting on degenerated rabbit discs injected with adenoviral vector expressing the *Sox-9* gene. The Sox-9-treated discs retained their "chondrogenic" appearance, unlike control discs injected with Adeno-GFP vector or control degeneration-induced discs (Paul et al. 2003).

24.5 Use of Gene Therapy for Intervertebral Disc Repair: Theoretical and Practical Consideration

Concomitant with increased human life expectancy, disc degeneration and associated spinal disorders are a major health concern. Due to the limited regenerative capacity of the disc tissues, it is almost impossible to reverse or even stop the process of degeneration, a topic extensively discussed in this book. Thus, there is increasing interest in developing new biological approaches to regenerating the degenerating disc. In this chapter, we have reviewed how this can be achieved through genetic modification of intradiscal gene expression via gene therapy. Other therapeutic approaches to disc regeneration include injection of growth factors, with or without a carrier, and use of mature cells, progenitor cells, and stem cells, with or without scaffolding, topics addressed in other chapters of this book.

Accordingly, we have reviewed studies of intervertebral disc gene therapy performed in the last decade, summarized in Table 24.1. The vast majority of the investigations performed in vitro use reporter genes as proof of concept. Several studies were conducted to deliver reporter genes into disc cells isolated from animal tissues. Those experiments addressed the feasibility and limitations of gene delivery into intervertebral disc-derived cells. *LacZ* and *GFP* genes were used in various animal and human cells and were delivered via viral and nonviral methods. Small iRNA technology was also used in vitro in rat and human nucleus pulposus cells to downregulate *luciferase* activity. Following studies performed on animal cells, the delivery of reporter genes to human disc cells was also pursued. Adenovector harboring the *LacZ* or *luciferase* reporter genes transduced 100 % of cultured human intervertebral disc cells, healthy or degenerate. Another in vitro study demonstrated that it is possible to exert exogenous control over gene activity using human cells in vitro. To date, both viral and nonviral vectors have been used to deliver reporter genes into intervertebral discs in vivo. When different doses of both adenovector and AAV encoding

Table 24.1 Summary table of genes, vehicles, experimental models, and main results obtained in the last decade

Gene	Vector	Experimental system	Findings	Author (year)
ADAMTS5	siRNA, specific for ADAMTS5 (a) Transfection in vitro	(a) In vitro, rabbit NP cells both in monolayer and alginate bead cultures	(a) *ADAMTS5* gene suppression was 70 % compared with the control upon IL-1 stimulation	Seki et al. (2009)
	(b) Injection, in vivo	(b) In vivo by using the rabbit annular needle-puncture model and intradiscal injection	(b) The injection of anti-*ADAMTS5* oligonucleotide in vivo resulted in improved MRI scores	
BMP-2	Adenovirus	Efficiency of different BMPs in bovine NP cells in culture	Most effective in stimulating proteoglycan accumulation	Zhang et al. (2006)
		Cells from human degenerated disc cultured in monolayer	Cells treated with Ad-BMP-2 demonstrated a progressive increase in proteoglycan synthesis with increasing viral concentrations	Wallach et al. (2003a)
BMP-7 (OP-1)	Adenovirus	Efficiency of different BMPs in bovine NP cells in culture	Best at stimulating proteoglycan synthesis	Zhang et al. (2006), Zhang et al. (2009)
	Adeno-associated virus (AAV)	Canine NP cells growing in culture	Promoted proteoglycan and collage-II production	Wang et al. (2011)
	Gene gun	Bovine IVD cells cultured in monolayer	High proteoglycan synthesis in IVD cells	Matsumoto et al. (2001)
BMP-14 (GDF-5)	Nucleofection	Mouse disc cells cultured in monolayer	Elevated collagen type II and aggrecan genes expression	Cui et al. (2008)
	Adenovirus	Efficiency of different BMPs in bovine NP cells in culture	Best in stimulating collagen production	Zhang et al. (2006)
		Rabbit knee chondrocytes injected in disc explants	50 % increase in proteoglycan within the NP	Zhang et al. (2008)
		Intradiscal injection to degenerated mouse IVD	Successful arrest of the typical decrease in disc height and proteoglycan content	Liang et al. (2010)
CTGF	AAV	Rhesus monkey lumbar IVD NP cells in monolayer	CTGF promoted the synthesis of collagen type II and proteoglycan	Liu et al. (2010)
FasL	siRNA specific for FasL, delivered by ultrasound	siRNA delivered in vivo into coccygeal IVD of Sprague–Dawley rats	The siRNA transfection inhibited endogenous FasL expression by 53 % compared with the control	Suzuki et al. (2009)
IL-1Ra	Adenovirus	(a) Normal and degenerate human IVD cells growing in monolayer or alginate cultures	(a) Cells infected with Ad-IL-1Ra produced elevated levels of IL-1Ra for prolonged time periods, and the infected cells were resistant to IL-1	LeMaitre et al. (2007)
		(b) Normal and degenerate IVD cells infected with Ad-IL-1Ra were injected into degenerate disc tissue explants	(b) IL-1Ra protein expression was increased which was maintained for 2 weeks	
LMP-1	Adenovirus	Rat IVD cells cultured in vitro in 3D and monolayer	Significant increase in proteoglycan and BMP-2 and BMP-7 mRNA levels	Yoon et al. (2004), Kuh et al. (2008)
		Injection into native rabbit lumbar discs	Elevation of LMP-1, BMP-2, and BMP-7 mRNA levels	Yoon et al. (2004)

(continued)

Table 24.1 (continued)

Gene	Vector	Experimental system	Findings	Author (year)
Sox-9	Adenovirus	Chondroblastic cell line and human degenerated disc cells and bovine NP cells	Increased level of RNA and protein of collagen type II	Paul et al. (2003), Zhang et al. (2006)
	Retro (murine leukemia) virus	Rat ASCs cultured in 3D	Increase levels of collagen type II and Sox-9	Yang et al. (2011)
		Coculture of the transfected cells with NP cells	Increased collagen type II and proteoglycan production	
TGF-ß	Adenovirus	Human IVD cells cultured in 3D pellets	Increased synthesis of proteoglycan and collagen II	Lee et al. (2001)
		Human IVD cells treated with different combinations of TGF- ß, BMP-2, and IGF and grown in 3D alginate culture	Cells treated with triple and double combinations showed higher proteoglycan content	Moon et al. (2008)
		Chondroblastic cell line and human degenerated disc cells and bovine NP cells	Increased level of RNA and protein of collagen type II	Paul et al. (2003), Zhang et al. (2006)
		Intradiscal injection to rabbit IVD	Increase in TGF-β expression and production and in proteoglycan synthesis 1 week after injection	Nishida et al. (1999)
		Intradiscal injection into degenerated rabbit IVDs	The injected discs retained their chondrogenic appearance	Paul et al. (2003)
TIMP-1	Adenovirus	Degenerated human IVD cells cultured in 3D pellet	Increased measured proteoglycan in cultured degenerated disc cells	Wallach et al. (2003b)
	AAV	Rhesus monkey lumbar IVD NP cells in culture	Enhancing effect on the expression of proteoglycan but no effect on collagen type II	Liu et al. (2010)

NP nucleus pulposus, *AF* annulus fibrosus, *IVD* intervertebral disc either *GFP* or *LacZ* were injected into rabbit discs, no clinical, biochemical, or histological deficits were noted. However, this was not the case when *BMP-2* or *TGF-β* was delivered (Levicoff et al. 2008). It is therefore probable that the safety of gene delivery cannot be assessed using only reporter genes. Cell- or stem cell-mediated gene therapy is another tactic of choice and is viewed as a "more physiological" approach to regulating gene expression. *Luciferase*-expressing porcine MSCs were implanted into a minipig disc, but massive cell loss followed implantation. siRNA against the exogenous *Luciferase* gene was used in a rat model in vivo. Because the *luciferase* gene was silenced for 24 weeks, the siRNA activity was active for a considerable time period (Suzuki et al. 2009).

Despite these positive results, transitions into preclinical and clinical studies require further safety and dose–response studies designed to mimic conditions anticipated in human disease. There is always concern that the proximity of the disc to the spinal canal may result in exposure of cord cells to the viral vector and/or therapeutic cDNA/protein (Wallach et al. 2006). Thus, we find it relevant at this point to consider the safety aspect of gene therapy as a therapeutic approach to overcome disease. Overall, safety studies that mimic possible hazardous situations, such as injection of a wrong dose of vector, have produced contradictory results. The groups of Wallach and Levicoff mimicked injections of an incorrect dosage to assess safety concerns and possible complications involving viral vectors carrying BMPs; the results of the two investigations were contradictory (Wallach et al. 2006; Levicoff et al. 2008). Levicoff and colleagues reported that up to 80 % of rabbits injected with adeno-based vector developed significant morbidity, whereas rabbits injected with AAV, a less immunogenic vector, displayed no clinical signs of morbidity. In another study, only rabbits that received a high dose of Adeno-TGF-β exhibited signs of paralysis; rabbits injected with Adeno-BMP-2 did not. However, both studies concluded that with appropriate dosing, the therapeutic benefits of gene therapy may compensate for its risks.

Intradiscal injections of therapeutic vectors carrying anabolic genes/transcription factors provide a possible approach to treating or preventing disc degeneration. Moreover, the authors opine that injections of cells genetically manipulated to express the genes discussed earlier (as shown in models mentioned in the in vitro section) provide an attractive approach to enhancing the abilities of cells and therapeutic genes to repair the degenerate intervertebral disc.

Undoubtedly, there are many obstacles to be overcome and issues to be resolved concerning the timing and the control of therapeutic gene delivery before this type of remediation can be clinically relevant. As with all innovative therapeutic approaches, preclinical research, translational research, and clinical trials will be needed to assess safety before focusing on clinical efficacy. Given what we have learned to date, we postulate that in the future a good treatment strategy may improve vectors – viral- or nonviral-encoding multiple genes. Perhaps a combination of anti-inflammatory and anabolic genes, which in different combinations and stoichiometry, will regenerate the extracellular matrix or, if prevention should prove feasible, will mitigate the altered homeostasis brought about by the degeneration process in the intervertebral disc.

24.6 Summary of Critical Concepts Discussed in the Chapter

- Almost all of the gene therapy studies in the last decade were performed in vitro, using reporter genes, *LacZ* and *GFP*, in various animal and human cells, delivered via viral and nonviral methods, as a proof of concept.
- In specific cases, gene delivery of TIMP-1 increased proteoglycan synthesis at each concentration assessed.
- Adenoviral vector carrying the *IL-1Ra* gene can be transferred to nucleus pulposus cells and annulus fibrosus cells; of IL-1Ra levels were elevated for prolonged time periods and the infected cells were unaffected by the IL-1
- Fas siRNA mediated a long-term downregulation of the endogenous gene *FasL*, showing that RNAi can be used to suppress apoptosis in cultured rat nucleus pulposus cells and in discs in vivo.
- ADAMTS5 siRNA restrained intervertebral disc degeneration in a rabbit model.
- Plasmids containing *BMP-*, *LMP-1-*, *TGF-β-*, and *Sox-9-* encoding genes can be used to transfect nucleus pulposus cells. Adenoviral vectors bearing the *BMP-2* or *BMP-7* (OP-1) genes were found to be most potent in stimulating proteoglycan synthesis, whereas *BMP-4* and *BMP-14* (*GDF-5*) genes showed more affinity and potency in stimulating collagen production.
- Degenerated rabbit intervertebral discs served as a relevant model of disease for studies utilizing adenoviral vector expressing Sox-9. The architecture and histology of the nucleus pulposus were preserved over a 5-week study period.
- Doses of both adenovector and AAV encoding either *GFP* or *LacZ* injected into rabbit intervertebral discs elicited no detrimental clinical, biochemical, or histological changes. Nevertheless, safety studies that mimic possible hazardous situations, such as injection of a wrong dose of vector, have produced contradictory results.

Acknowledgments The authors wish to thank the NIH and NIAMS for ongoing support through grant RO3AR057143 and the Israel Science Foundation (ISF) grants and the Levi Eshkol Scholarship for PhD Students, the Ministry of Science, Culture and Sport of the State of Israel.

References

Aslan H, Zilberman Y, Arbeli V, Sheyn D, Matan Y, Liebergal M, Li J, Helm GA, Gazit D, Gazit Z (2006) Nucleofection-based ex vivo nonviral gene delivery to human stem cells as a platform for tissue regeneration. Tissue Eng 12(4):877–889

Baffi MO, Slattery E, Sohn P, Moses HL, Chytil A, Serra R (2004) Conditional deletion of the TGF-beta type II receptor in Col2a expressing cells results in defects in the axial skeleton without alterations in chondrocyte differentiation or embryonic development of long bones. Dev Biol 276(1):124–142

Bell DM, Leung KK, Wheatley SC, Ng LJ, Zhou S, Ling KW, Sham MH, Koopman P, Tam PP, Cheah KS (1997) SOX9 directly regulates the type-II collagen gene. Nat Genet 16(2):174–178

Boden SD, Liu Y, Hair GA, Helms JA, Hu D, Racine M, Nanes MS, Titus L (1998) LMP-1, a LIM-domain protein, mediates BMP-6 effects on bone formation. Endocrinology 139(12):5125–5134

Bron JL, Helder MN, Meisel HJ, Van Royen BJ, Smit TH (2009) Repair, regenerative and supportive therapies of the annulus fibrosus: achievements and challenges. Eur Spine J 18(3):301–313

Bueno EM, Glowacki J (2009) Cell-free and cell-based approaches for bone regeneration. Nat Rev Rheumatol 5(12):685–697

Cavazzana-Calvo M, Thrasher A, Mavilio F (2004) The future of gene therapy. Nature 427(6977):779–781

Cui M, Wan Y, Anderson DG, Shen FH, Leo BM, Laurencin CT, Balian G, Li X (2008) Mouse growth and differentiation factor-5 protein and DNA therapy potentiates intervertebral disc cell aggregation and chondrogenic gene expression. Spine J 8(2):287–295

Edelstein ML, Abedi MR, Wixon J (2007) Gene therapy clinical trials worldwide to 2007–an update. J Gene Med 9(10):833–842

Elfervig MK, Minchew JT, Francke E, Tsuzaki M, Banes AJ (2001) IL-1beta sensitizes intervertebral disc annulus cells to fluid-induced shear stress. J Cell Biochem 82(2):290–298

Feng G, Wan Y, Shen FH, Li X (2009) Nucleus pulposus explant culture model. J Orthop Res 27(6):814–819

Fire A, Xu S, Montgomery MK, Kostas SA, Driver SE, Mello CC (1998) Potent and specific genetic interference by double-stranded RNA in Caenorhabditis elegans. Nature 391(6669):806–811

Flotte TR (2007) Gene therapy: the first two decades and the current state-of-the-art. J Cell Physiol 213(2):301–305

Friedmann T, Roblin R (1972) Gene therapy for human genetic disease? Science 175(25):949–955

Glasson SS, Askew R, Sheppard B, Carito B, Blanchet T, Ma HL, Flannery CR, Peluso D, Kanki K, Yang Z, Majumdar MK, Morris EA (2005) Deletion of active ADAMTS5 prevents cartilage degradation in a murine model of osteoarthritis. Nature 434(7033): 644–648

Griffith TS, Brunner T, Fletcher SM, Green DR, Ferguson TA (1995) Fas ligand-induced apoptosis as a mechanism of immune privilege. Science 270(5239):1189–1192

Hacein-Bey-Abina S, Von Kalle C, Schmidt M, McCormack MP, Wulffraat N, Leboulch P, Lim A, Osborne CS, Pawliuk R, Morillon E, Sorensen R, Forster A, Fraser P, Cohen JI, de Saint BG, Alexander I, Wintergerst U, Frebourg T, Aurias A, Stoppa-Lyonnet D, Romana S, Radford-Weiss I, Gross F, Valensi F, Delabesse E, Macintyre E, Sigaux F, Soulier J, Leiva LE, Wissler M, Prinz C, Rabbitts TH, Le Deist F, Fischer A, Cavazzana-Calvo M (2003) LMO2-associated clonal T cell proliferation in two patients after gene therapy for SCID-X1. Science 302(5644):415–419

Han D, Ding Y, Liu SL, Wang G, Si IC, Wang X, Cui L, Huang D (2009) Double role of Fas ligand in the apoptosis of intervertebral disc cells in vitro. Acta Biochim Biophys Sin (Shanghai) 41(11):938–947

Hashimoto G, Aoki T, Nakamura H, Tanzawa K, Okada Y (2001) Inhibition of ADAMTS4 (aggrecanase-1) by tissue inhibitors of metalloproteinases (TIMP-1, 2, 3 and 4). FEBS Lett 494(3): 192–195

Herzog RW, Cao O, Srivastava A (2010) Two decades of clinical gene therapy–success is finally mounting. Discov Med 9(45):105–111

Huston MW, van Til NP, Visser TP, Arshad S, Brugman MH, Cattoglio C, Nowrouzi A, Li Y, Schambach A, Schmidt M, Baum C, von Kalle C, Mavilio F, Zhang F, Blundell MP, Thrasher AJ, Verstegen MM, Wagemaker G (2011) Correction of murine SCID-X1 by lentiviral gene therapy using a codon-optimized IL2RG gene and minimal pretransplant conditioning. Mol Ther 19:1867–1877

Jimbo K, Park JS, Yokosuka K, Sato K, Nagata K (2005) Positive feedback loop of interleukin-1beta upregulating production of inflammatory mediators in human intervertebral disc cells in vitro. J Neurosurg Spine 2(5):589–595

Kakutani K, Nishida K, Uno K, Takada T, Shimomura T, Maeno K, Kurosaka M, Doita M (2006) Prolonged down regulation of specific gene expression in nucleus pulposus cell mediated by RNA interference in vitro. J Orthop Res 24(6):1271–1278

Kaneyama S, Nishida K, Takada T, Suzuki T, Shimomura T, Maeno K, Kurosaka M, Doita M (2008) Fas ligand expression on human nucleus pulposus cells decreases with disc degeneration processes. J Orthop Sci 13(2):130–135

Kang JD, Stefanovic-Racic M, McIntyre LA, Georgescu HI, Evans CH (1997) Toward a biochemical understanding of human intervertebral disc degeneration and herniation. Contributions of nitric oxide, interleukins, prostaglandin E2, and matrix metalloproteinases. Spine (Phila Pa 1976) 22(10):1065–1073

Kimelman-Bleich N, Pelled G, Zilberman Y, Kallai I, Mizrahi O, Tawackoli W, Gazit Z, Gazit D (2011) Targeted gene-and-host progenitor cell therapy for nonunion bone fracture repair. Mol Ther 19(1):53–59

Kuh SU, Zhu Y, Li J, Tsai KJ, Fei Q, Hutton WC, Yoon ST (2008) The AdLMP-1 transfection in two different cells; AF cells, chondrocytes as potential cell therapy candidates for disc degeneration. Acta Neurochir (Wien) 150(8):803–810

Le Maitre CL, Freemont AJ, Hoyland JA (2005) The role of interleukin-1 in the pathogenesis of human intervertebral disc degeneration. Arthritis Res Ther 7(4):R732–R745

Le Maitre CL, Hoyland JA, Freemont AJ (2007) Interleukin-1 receptor antagonist delivered directly and by gene therapy inhibits matrix degradation in the intact degenerate human intervertebral disc: an in situ zymographic and gene therapy study. Arthritis Res Ther 9(4):R83

Lee JY, Hall R, Pelinkovic D, Cassinelli E, Usas A, Gilbertson L, Huard J, Kang J (2001) New use of a three-dimensional pellet culture system for human intervertebral disc cells: initial characterization and potential use for tissue engineering. Spine (Phila Pa 1976) 26(21):2316–2322

Lee EX, Lam DH, Wu C, Yang J, Ng WH, Wang S (2011) Glioma gene therapy using induced pluripotent stem cell-derived neural stem cells. Mol Pharm 8:1515–1524

Leo BM, Li X, Balian G, Anderson DG (2004) In vivo bioluminescent imaging of virus-mediated gene transfer and transduced cell transplantation in the intervertebral disc. Spine (Phila Pa 1976) 29(8):838–844

Levicoff EA, Kim JS, Sobajima S, Wallach CJ, Larson JW 3rd, Robbins PD, Xiao X, Juan L, Vadala G, Gilbertson LG, Kang JD (2008) Safety assessment of intradiscal gene therapy II: effect of dosing and vector choice. Spine (Phila Pa 1976) 33(14):1509–1516; discussion 1517

Li X, Leo BM, Beck G, Balian G, Anderson GD (2004) Collagen and proteoglycan abnormalities in the GDF-5-deficient mice and molecular changes when treating disk cells with recombinant growth factor. Spine (Phila Pa 1976) 29(20):2229–2234

Liang H, Ma SY, Feng G, Shen FH, Joshua Li X (2010) Therapeutic effects of adenovirus-mediated growth and differentiation factor-5 in a mice disc degeneration model induced by annulus needle puncture. Spine J 10(1):32–41

Liu X, Li K, Song J, Liang C, Wang X, Chen X (2006) Efficient and stable gene expression in rabbit intervertebral disc cells transduced with a recombinant baculovirus vector. Spine (Phila Pa 1976) 31(7):732–735

Liu Y, Kong J, Chen BH, Hu YG (2010) Combined expression of CTGF and tissue inhibitor of metalloprotease-1 promotes synthesis of proteoglycan and collagen type II in rhesus monkey lumbar intervertebral disc cells in vitro. Chin Med J (Engl) 123(15):2082–2087

Lohr F, Huang Q, Hu K, Dewhirst MW, Li CY (2001) Systemic vector leakage and transgene expression by intratumorally injected recombinant adenovirus vectors. Clin Cancer Res 7(11):3625–3628

Masuda K, An HS (2004) Growth factors and the intervertebral disc. Spine J 4(6 Suppl):330S–340S

Matsumoto T, Masuda K, Chen S, An H, Andersson G, Aota Y, Horvath E, Thonar E (2001) Transfer of osteogenic protein-1 gene by gene gun system promotes matrix synthesis in bovine intervertebral disc and articular cartilage cells. Trans Orthop Res Soc 26:30

Menendez MI, Clark DJ, Carlton M, Flanigan DC, Jia G, Sammet S, Weisbrode SE, Knopp MV, Bertone AL (2011) Direct delayed human adenoviral BMP-2 or BMP-6 gene therapy for bone and cartilage regeneration in a pony osteochondral model. Osteoarthritis Cartilage 19(8):1066–1075

Moon SH, Gilbertson LG, Nishida K, Knaub M, Muzzonigro T, Robbins PD, Evans CH, Kang JD (2000) Human intervertebral disc cells are genetically modifiable by adenovirus-mediated gene transfer: implications for the clinical management of intervertebral disc disorders. Spine (Phila Pa 1976) 25(20):2573–2579

Moon SH, Nishida K, Gilbertson LG, Lee HM, Kim H, Hall RA, Robbins PD, Kang JD (2008) Biologic response of human intervertebral disc cells to gene therapy cocktail. Spine (Phila Pa 1976) 33(17):1850–1855

Morrey ME, Anderson PA, Chambers G, Paul R (2008) Optimizing nonviral-mediated transfection of human intervertebral disc chondrocytes. Spine J 8(5):796–803

Muona K, Makinen K, Hedman M, Manninen H, Yla-Herttuala S (2012) 10-year safety follow-up in patients with local VEGF gene transfer to ischemic lower limb. Gene Ther 19:392–395

Nagase H, Woessner JF Jr (1999) Matrix metalloproteinases. J Biol Chem 274(31):21491–21494

Nishida K, Kang JD, Suh JK, Robbins PD, Evans CH, Gilbertson LG (1998) Adenovirus-mediated gene transfer to nucleus pulposus cells. Implications for the treatment of intervertebral disc degeneration. Spine (Phila Pa 1976) 23(22):2437–2442; discussion 2443

Nishida K, Kang JD, Gilbertson LG, Moon SH, Suh JK, Vogt MT, Robbins PD, Evans CH (1999) Modulation of the biologic activity of the rabbit intervertebral disc by gene therapy: an in vivo study of adenovirus-mediated transfer of the human transforming growth factor beta 1 encoding gene. Spine (Phila Pa 1976) 24(23): 2419–2425

Nishida K, Gilbertson LG, Robbins PD, Evans CH Kang JD (2000) Potential applications of gene therapy to the treatment of intervertebral disc disorders. Clin Orthop Relat Res (379 Suppl): S234–S241

Nishida K, Doita M, Takada T, Kakutani K, Miyamoto H, Shimomura T, Maeno K, Kurosaka M (2006) Sustained transgene expression in intervertebral disc cells in vivo mediated by microbubble-enhanced ultrasound gene therapy. Spine (Phila Pa 1976) 31(13): 1415–1419

Nishida K, Suzuki T, Kakutani K, Yurube T, Maeno K, Kurosaka M, Doita M (2008) Gene therapy approach for disc degeneration and associated spinal disorders. Eur Spine J 17(Suppl 4):459–466

Noel D, Gazit D, Bouquet C, Apparailly F, Bony C, Plence P, Millet V, Turgeman G, Perricaudet M, Sany J, Jorgensen C (2004) Short-term BMP-2 expression is sufficient for in vivo osteochondral differentiation of mesenchymal stem cells. Stem Cells 22(1):74–85

Omlor GW, Bertram H, Kleinschmidt K, Fischer J, Brohm K, Guehring T, Anton M, Richter W (2010) Methods to monitor distribution and metabolic activity of mesenchymal stem cells following in vivo injection into nucleotomized porcine intervertebral discs. Eur Spine J 19(4):601–612

Osada R, Ohshima H, Ishihara H, Yudoh K, Sakai K, Matsui H, Tsuji H (1996) Autocrine/paracrine mechanism of insulin-like growth factor-1 secretion, and the effect of insulin-like growth factor-1 on proteoglycan synthesis in bovine intervertebral discs. J Orthop Res 14(5):690–699

Paul R, Haydon RC, Cheng H, Ishikawa A, Nenadovich N, Jiang W, Zhou L, Breyer B, Feng T, Gupta P, He TC, Phillips FM (2003) Potential use of Sox9 gene therapy for intervertebral degenerative disc disease. Spine (Phila Pa 1976) 28(8):755–763

Pleger ST, Shan C, Ksienzyk J, Bekeredjian R, Boekstegers P, Hinkel R, Schinkel S, Leuchs B, Ludwig J, Qiu G, Weber C, Raake P, Koch WJ, Katus HA, Muller OJ, Most P (2011) Cardiac AAV9-S100A1 gene therapy rescues post-ischemic heart failure in a preclinical large animal model. Sci Transl Med 3(92):92ra64

Reddi AH, Reddi A (2009) Bone morphogenetic proteins (BMPs): from morphogens to metabologens. Cytokine Growth Factor Rev 20(5–6):341–342

Risbud MV, Albert TJ, Guttapalli A, Vresilovic EJ, Hillibrand AS, Vaccaro AR, Shapiro IM (2004) Differentiation of mesenchymal stem cells towards a nucleus pulposus-like phenotype in vitro: implications for cell-based transplantation therapy. Spine (Phila Pa 1976) 29(23):2627–2632

Rowzee AM, Cawley NX, Chiorini JA, Di Pasquale G (2011) Glucagon-like Peptide-1 gene therapy. Exp Diabetes Res 2011:601047

Schmidt-Wolf GD, Schmidt-Wolf IG (2003) Non-viral and hybrid vectors in human gene therapy: an update. Trends Mol Med 9(2): 67–72

Seguin CA, Pilliar RM, Roughley PJ, Kandel RA (2005) Tumor necrosis factor-alpha modulates matrix production and catabolism in nucleus pulposus tissue. Spine (Phila Pa 1976) 30(17): 1940–1948

Seki S, Asanuma-Abe Y, Masuda K, Kawaguchi Y, Asanuma K, Muehleman C, Iwai A, Kimura T (2009) Effect of small interference RNA (siRNA) for ADAMTS5 on intervertebral disc degeneration in the rabbit anular needle-puncture model. Arthritis Res Ther 11(6):R166

Shen B, Melrose J, Ghosh P, Taylor F (2003) Induction of matrix metalloproteinase-2 and –3 activity in ovine nucleus pulposus cells grown in three-dimensional agarose gel culture by interleukin-1beta: a potential pathway of disc degeneration. Eur Spine J 12(1):66–75

Sheyn D, Kimelman-Bleich N, Pelled G, Zilberman Y, Gazit D, Gazit Z (2008) Ultrasound-based nonviral gene delivery induces bone formation in vivo. Gene Ther 15(4):257–266

Somia N, Verma IM (2000) Gene therapy: trials and tribulations. Nat Rev Genet 1(2):91–99

Sowa G, Westrick E, Pacek C, Coelho P, Patel D, Vadala G, Georgescu H, Vo N, Studer R, Kang J (2011) In vitro and in vivo testing of a novel regulatory system for gene therapy for intervertebral disc degeneration. Spine (Phila Pa 1976) 36(10):E623–E628

Suzuki T, Nishida K, Kakutani K, Maeno K, Yurube T, Takada T, Kurosaka M, Doita M (2009) Sustained long-term RNA interference in nucleus pulposus cells in vivo mediated by unmodified small interfering RNA. Eur Spine J 18(2):263–270

Takada T, Nishida K, Doita M, Kurosaka M (2002) Fas ligand exists on intervertebral disc cells: a potential molecular mechanism for immune privilege of the disc. Spine (Phila Pa 1976) 27(14): 1526–1530

Thompson JP, Oegema TR Jr, Bradford DS (1991) Stimulation of mature canine intervertebral disc by growth factors. Spine (Phila Pa 1976) 16(3):253–260

Vadala G, Sowa GA, Smith L, Hubert MG, Levicoff EA, Denaro V, Gilbertson LG, Kang JD (2007) Regulation of transgene expression using an inducible system for improved safety of intervertebral disc gene therapy. Spine (Phila Pa 1976) 32(13):1381–1387

Wallach CJ, Gilbertson LG, Kang JD (2003a) Gene therapy applications for intervertebral disc degeneration. Spine (Phila Pa 1976) 28(15 Suppl):S93–S98

Wallach CJ, Sobajima S, Watanabe Y, Kim JS, Georgescu HI, Robbins P, Gilbertson LG, Kang JD (2003b) Gene transfer of the catabolic inhibitor TIMP-1 increases measured proteoglycans in cells from degenerated human intervertebral discs. Spine (Phila Pa 1976) 28(20):2331–2337

Wallach CJ, Kim JS, Sobajima S, Lattermann C, Oxner WM, McFadden K, Robbins PD, Gilbertson LG, Kang JD (2006) Safety assessment of intradiscal gene transfer: a pilot study. Spine J 6(2):107–112

Wang C, Ruan DK, Zhang C, Wang DL, Xin H, Zhang Y (2011) Effects of adeno-associated virus-2-mediated human BMP-7 gene transfection on the phenotype of nucleus pulposus cells. J Orthop Res 29(6):838–845

Wehling P (2001) Transfer of genes to intervertebral disc cells: proposal for a treatment strategy of spinal disorders by local gene therapy. Joint Bone Spine 68(6):554–556

Wehling P, Schulitz KP, Robbins PD, Evans CH, Reinecke JA (1997) Transfer of genes to chondrocytic cells of the lumbar spine. Proposal for a treatment strategy of spinal disorders by local gene therapy. Spine (Phila Pa 1976) 22(10):1092–1097

Xia C, Ding C, Yang X, Sun K, Tian S (2010) Effects of antisense transforming growth factor-beta1 gene transfer on the biological activities of tendon sheath fibroblasts. Orthopedics 33(8)

Yang Z, Huang CY, Candiotti KA, Zeng X, Yuan T, Li J, Yu H, Abdi S (2011) Sox-9 facilitates differentiation of adipose tissue-derived stem cells into a chondrocyte-like phenotype in vitro. J Orthop Res 29(8):1291–1297

Yasuda T, Hayakawa H, Nihira T, Ren YR, Nakata Y, Nagai M, Hattori N, Miyake K, Takada M, Shimada T, Mizuno Y, Mochizuki H (2011) Parkin-mediated protection of dopaminergic neurons in a chronic MPTP-minipump mouse model of Parkinson disease. J Neuropathol Exp Neurol 70:686–697

Yoon ST, Park JS, Kim KS, Li J, Attallah-Wasif ES, Hutton WC, Boden SD (2004) ISSLS prize winner: LMP-1 upregulates intervertebral disc cell production of proteoglycans and BMPs in vitro and in vivo. Spine (Phila Pa 1976) 29(23):2603–2611

Zhang Y, An HS, Thonar EJ, Chubinskaya S, He TC, Phillips FM (2006) Comparative effects of bone morphogenetic proteins and sox9 overexpression on extracellular matrix metabolism of bovine nucleus pulposus cells. Spine (Phila Pa 1976) 31(19): 2173–2179

Zhang Y, Phillips FM, Thonar EJ, Oegema T, An HS, Roman-Blas JA, He TC, Anderson DG (2008) Cell therapy using articular chondrocytes overexpressing BMP-7 or BMP-10 in a rabbit disc organ culture model. Spine (Phila Pa 1976) 33(8):831–838

Zhang Y, Markova D, Im HJ, Hu W, Thonar EJ, He TC, An HS, Phillips FM, Anderson DG (2009) Primary bovine intervertebral disc cells transduced with adenovirus overexpressing 12 BMPs and Sox9 maintain appropriate phenotype. Am J Phys Med Rehabil 88(6): 455–463

Zhang Y, Chee A, Thonar EJ, An HS (2011) Intervertebral disk repair by protein, gene, or cell injection: a framework for rehabilitation-focused biologics in the spine. PM R 3(6 Suppl):S88–S94

Enhancing Disc Repair by Growth Factors and Other Modalities

25

Won C. Bae and Koichi Masuda

Contents

W.C. Bae, PhD
Department of Radiology,
University of California, San Diego,
408 Dickinson Street, San Diego, CA 92103-8226, USA
e-mail: wbae@ucsd.edu

K. Masuda, MD (✉)
Department of Orthopaedic Surgery,
University of California, San Diego,
9500 Gilman Dr. MC0863, La Jolla, CA 92093-0863, USA
e-mail: koichimasuda@ucsd.edu

I.M. Shapiro, M.V. Risbud (eds.), *The Intervertebral Disc*,
DOI 10.1007/978-3-7091-1535-0_25, © Springer-Verlag Wien 2014

25.1 Disc Degeneration: Imbalance of Anabolic and Catabolic Activities

Recent studies have found an association between disc degeneration and genes related to the extracellular matrices of the disc, such as those encoding collagen I (Tilkeridis et al. 2005), collagen IX (Annunen et al. 1999; Solovieva et al. 2006), aggrecan (Kawaguchi et al. 1999), matrix metalloprotease-2 (MMP-2) (Dong et al. 2007), MMP-3 (Takahashi et al. 2001), interleukin-1β (IL-1β) (Solovieva et al. 2004), IL-6 (Noponen-Hietala et al. 2005), vitamin D receptor (Videman et al. 1998), asporin (Song et al. 2008), and cartilage intermediate layer protein (CILP) (Seki et al. 2005; Virtanen et al. 2007). These observations suggest that proteins in the extracellular matrix (ECM) or cytokines that may degrade the matrix may play a role in disc degeneration.

Homeostasis of the extracellular matrix of the nucleus pulposus and annulus fibrosus is conserved by the activities of the resident disc cells that maintain a balance between anabolism and catabolism. In the young human nucleus pulposus, there exists a large population of notochordal cells (Trout et al. 1982), which by maturity is replaced by or differentiates into a population of chondrocyte-like cells. Both cell types synthesize proteoglycans (Kim et al. 2009) which constitute the bulk of the nucleus pulposus tissue (Aguiar et al. 1999). In common with articular cartilage, proteoglycans interact extracellularly with hyaluronan to form aggregates that become entangled in a fibrillar network composed primarily of collagen II (Scott and Haigh 1986). Together, the large hydrophilic proteoglycan aggregates and the collagen network provide the intrinsic mechanical properties of the nucleus pulposus. The annulus fibrosus contains a relatively homogeneous population of cells that synthesize a matrix richer in collagen and poorer in proteoglycans than the nucleus pulposus; as a result. The annulus fibrosus is a dense lamellar tissue that contains fibrillar layers rich in collagen I and in the deeper regions collagen II (Schollmeier et al. 2000). For a detailed discussion of collagen and proteoglycans of the disc, see Chaps. 4 and 5.

Molecules that regulate the anabolic state of the intervertebral disc include polypeptide growth factors, such as insulin-like growth factor (IGF-1), transforming growth factor-β (TGF-β), and the bone morphogenetic proteins (BMPs) (Thompson et al. 1991; Osada et al. 1996). Catabolic regulators include cytokines, such as IL-1 (Ahn et al. 2002a; Takahashi et al. 1996a) and tumor necrosis factor-α (TNF-α) (Ahn et al. 2002a; Miyamoto et al. 2000; Takahashi et al. 1996a), which influence the synthesis of matrix-degrading enzymes. Alterations in both anabolic and catabolic processes are thought to play key roles in the onset and progression of disc degeneration (Masuda and An 2006).

While the upregulation of anabolic genes and regulators has been studied (Gokorsch et al. 2005; Desmoulin et al. 2011), a far greater number of investigations have focused on biochemical changes of the intervertebral disc under pathologic conditions. These conditions include intervertebral disc degeneration (Patel et al. 2007), injury (e.g., puncture or stab wounds) (Anderson et al. 2002; Sobajima et al. 2005), and abnormal mechanical loading (Yurube et al. 2010; Iatridis et al. 2011). In these conditions, the cells of the disc express and synthesize cytokines that can tilt the balance towards catabolism. Increases in IL-1 mRNA and protein levels and its major regulator, TNF-α, have been observed in degenerated or herniated discal tissues in culture (Ahn et al. 2002b; Burke et al. 2003; Kang et al. 1996; Weiler et al. 2005; Igarashi et al. 2000; Olmarker and Larsson 1998; Le Maitre et al. 2005, 2007a). The catabolic processes induced by cytokines, such as IL-1, may be mediated by a number of enzymes, including collagenase (Sakuma et al. 2002), cycloxygenase-2 (COX-2) (Kang et al. 1997), prostaglandin E2 (PGE2) (Takahashi et al. 1996a; Rannou et al. 2000), MMP-1 (Jimbo et al. 2005), MMP-3, (Jimbo et al. 2005), MMP-13 (Miyamoto et al. 2005; Le Maitre et al. 2004), and the aggrecanases, such as a disintegrin and metalloproteinase with thrombospondin motifs-4 (ADAMTS-4) (Patel et al. 2007). It is also interesting to note that in articular cartilage, low concentrations of IL-1, in addition to inducing tissue degradation, can also inhibit the synthesis of proteoglycans, mainly aggrecan (Arner and Pratta 1989; Benton and Tyler 1988; Dingle et al. 1991).

25.2 Biologic Treatments of Degenerative Disc Diseases

There are several strategies being pursued for biologic repair or regeneration of the disc. A widely used strategy, and also the focus of this chapter, is to directly inject therapeutic agents into the intervertebral disc. The agents used include those aimed at stimulating the anabolism of the host disc, providing an environment conducive for biologic repair, and those that inhibit or compete with catabolic regulators and enzymes that may exist in degenerated disc tissues. Anabolic agents include growth factors [e.g., osteogenic protein-1 (OP-1; otherwise known as BMP-7), other BMPs, and TGF-β], materials containing multiple growth factors (e.g., platelet-rich plasma), and cells transfected with therapeutic genes (e.g., TGF-β). Gel-based biomaterials can provide several benefits conducive to biologic repair: Gels that have similar mechanical properties to the nucleus pulposus tissue can provide immediate load support and may promote hydration. Moreover, they can be mixed or cross-linked with growth factors to provide long-lasting anabolic effects compared to the growth factors alone. Inhibitory agents include those that inhibit expression of catabolic genes [e.g., small interference RNA (siRNA) for ADAMTS-5], antagonists for IL-1 receptors, and TNF-α (i.e., soluble TNF receptor type II). Tables 25.1 and 25.2 summarize some of the therapeutic agents that have been studied in vitro and in vivo, respectively.

Table 25.1 The in vitro effects of injectable therapeutic agents

Agent	Target	Effect	Reference
TGF-β	Mature canine IVD	PG synthesis increased up to 5X; higher in NP than AF	Thompson et al. (1991)
IGF-1	Mature canine IVD	PG synthesis marginally increased in NP	Thompson et al. (1991)
TGF-β	Human annulus cells, 3D culture	Cell proliferation and PG synthesis increased; reduced apoptosis with serum depletion	Gruber et al. (1997)
IGF-1	Young and old bovine NP cells	Cell proliferation and matrix synthesis stimulated; more IGF-1 receptors	Osada et al. (1996)
OP-1	Young rabbit NP and AF cells; alginate beads	Increased PG and collagen production and content	Masuda et al. (2003)
BMP-2	Rat IVD cells monolayer	Increased cell number, GAG, expression for collagen, aggrecan at higher doses	Yoon et al. (2003)
OP-1	Human NP and AF cells, alginate beads	Maintained cell density, increased PG synthesis and accumulation	Imai et al. (2007a)
OP-1	Rabbit IVD cells; alginate beads: IL-1α preexposure	IL-1 decreased PG and collagen; reversed and exceeded with OP-1	Takegami et al. (2002)

Table 25.1 (continued)

Agent	Target	Effect	Reference
OP-1	Rabbit IVD cells; alginate bead: C-ABC preexposure	OP-1 upregulated PG synthesis. Greater effect on C-ABC preexposure than control	Takegami et al. (2005)
BMP-2	Human IVD cells	Increased PG synthesis, expression of aggrecan, collagen types I and II; no bone formation	Kim et al. (2003)
rhBMP-2 and BMP-12	Human IVD cells in monolayer	PG, collagen synthesis increased in NP cells; minimal effect on AF cells	Gilbertson et al. (2008)
GDF-5	Bovine IVD cells; alginate bead	Increased DNA and PG content; at higher dose, PG and collagen synthesis increased	Chujo et al. (2006)
PRP	Porcine IVD cells; alginate bead	Mild increase in cell proliferation; marked increase in PG and collagen synthesis and PG accumulation	Akeda et al. (2006)
TGF-β1 and PRP	Human NP cells	NP cell proliferation and aggregation; increase in mRNA of SOX-9, collagen type II, aggrecan	Chen et al. (2006)
Ad-TIMP-1, Ad-BMP-2	IVD cells from human degenerated IVD	2,000 pg/ml production of TIMP w/100 MOI at day 4. PG synthesis increased with both Ad-TIMP-1 and Ad-BMP-2	Wallach et al. (2003)
Dexamethasone	Human disc herniation tissue explants	Decreased MMP-1 and MMP-3 levels	Genevay et al. (2009)
IL-1ra	Human disc herniation tissue explants	Decreased MMP-3 levels	Genevay et al. (2009)
IL-1ra	Human normal and degenerated disc tissues in situ with IL-1 treatment	IL-1ra reduced cytokine levels (MMP-3, MMP-7, MMP-13) and matrix degradation in all tissue types	Le Maitre et al. (2007b)
IL-1ra/ELP	Human IVD cells (grades 2–3); alginate beads: IL-1ra pre-Tx then IL-1β insult	Reduced ADAMTS-4, MMP-3 transcription	Shamji et al. (2007)
p38 MAPK inhibitor (SB 202190)	Rabbit NP cells pretreated with IL-1	Decreased message for collagen, aggrecan, IGF-1. Increased message for iNOS, COX-2, MMP-3, IL-6	Studer et al. (2008)
TNF inhibitor mAb	Human IVD herniation tissue explants	Decreased MMP-3 levels	Genevay et al. (2009)
PDGF, bFGF, IGF-I	Human NP and AF cells	Increased DNA synthesis via ERK and Akt pathways	Pratsinis et al. (2012)
TGFb3 + Dex, notochordal conditioned media	Degenerated human NP cells	Stimulated NP cell proliferation and decreased ADAMTS-5, MMP-1 expression	Abbott et al. (2012)
Lactoferricin	Bovine NP cells	Increased PG accumulation and expression of SOX-9, aggrecan, TIMP-family genes. Decreased expression of MMPs and ADAMTSs in dose-dependent manner	Kim et al. (2012)
IGF-1, BMP-7, IGF-1 + BMP-7	Bovine NP cells	Synergistically increased anabolic gene expression, PG synthesis, and PG accumulation	Kim et al. (2010)

TGF-β transforming growth factor-β, *IVD* intervertebral disc, *PG* proteoglycan, *NP* nucleus pulposus, *AF* annulus fibrosus, *IGF-1* insulin-like growth factor-1, *3D* three dimensional, *OP-1* osteogenic protein-1, *BMP-2* bone morphogenetic protein-2, *GAG* glycosaminoglycan, *IL-1* interleukin-1, *C-ABC* chondroitinase ABC, *rh* recombinant human, *GDF-5* growth and differentiation factor-5, *SOX-9* sex determining region Y-box 9 gene, *PRP* platelet-rich plasma, *Ad-TIMP-1* adenoviral vector delivering cDNA of tissue inhibitor of matrix metalloproteinases-1, *Ad-BMP-2* adenoviral vector delivering cDNA of BMP-2, *MOI* multiplicity of infection, *MMP* matrix metalloproteinase, *IL-1ra* IL-1 receptor antagonist, *ELP* elastin-like polypeptide, *Tx* treatment, *ADAMTS a disintegrin and metalloproteinase with thrombospondin motifs*, *MAPK* mitogen-activated protein kinase, *iNOS* inducible nitric oxide synthase, *COX-2* cyclooxygenase-2, *TNF* tumor necrosis factor, *mAb* monoclonal antibody, *PDGF* platelet-derived growth factor, *bFGF* basic fibroblast growth factor, *ERK* extracellular signal-regulated kinases, *Akt* protein kinases, *Dex* dexamethasone

Table 25.2 The in vivo effects of intradiscal injection treatments

Agent	Species	Site	Model	Effect	Reference
IGF-1	Rat	Tail	Static compression	Clustering of inner annulus cells after single injection	Walsh et al. (2004)
GDF-5	Rat	Tail	Static compression	Clustering of cells, increase in disc height (single injection)	Walsh et al. (2004)
TFG-β	Rat	Tail	Static compression	Proliferation of cells (multiple injections)	Walsh et al. (2004)
bFGF	Rat	Tail	Static compression	No response	Walsh et al. (2004)
OP-1	Rabbit	Lumbar	None (normal)	Increased disc height and PG content in NP	An et al. (2005)

(continued)

Table 25.2 (continued)

Agent	Species	Site	Model	Effect	Reference
OP-1	Rabbit	Lumbar	C-ABC: co-injection	Increased disc height and PG content in NP	Imai et al. (2003)
OP-1	Rabbit	Lumbar	Needle puncture: Tx 4 weeks later	Increased disc height and PG content in NP and AF, improvement of MRI and histology grades	Masuda et al. (2006)
OP-1	Rabbit	Lumbar	Needle puncture	Increased disc height and viscoelastic properties	Miyamoto et al. (2006b)
OP-1	Rabbit	Lumbar	C-ABC: Tx 4 weeks later	Increased disc height, PG content in NP and AF	Imai et al. (2007b)
GDF-5	Rabbit	Lumbar	Needle puncture: Tx 4 weeks later	Increased disc height, improvement of MRI and histology grades	Chujo et al. (2006)
GDF-5	Rabbit	Lumbar	Thrombin degraded: Tx 4 weeks later	Increased disc height, improved T1rho and T2 values. Decreased ADAMTS-4 and ADAMTS-5 and COX-2 expression	Bae et al. (2009)
BMP-2	Rabbit	Lumbar	Annular stab (5×7 mm)	More degeneration, vascularity, and fibroblast	Huang et al. (2007)
PRP	Rabbit	Lumbar	Nucleotomy, immediate Tx	PRP+GHM group had less degeneration and increased PG; PRP+PBS group showed no differences	Nagae et al. (2007)
PRP	Rabbit	Lumbar	Nucleotomy, immediate Tx	PRP+GHM had greater disc height, water content, mRNA for PG core protein, and collagen type II; fewer apoptotic cells in NP	Sawamura et al. (2009)
BMP-17	Sheep	Lumbar	Annular stab (3×6 mm), immediate Tx	BMP-17 maintained disc height, MRI and histology scores, NP cell density; increased PG and collagen synthesis	Wei et al. (2009)
ADAMTS-5 siRNA	Rabbit	Lumbar	Needle puncture: Tx 4 weeks later	Improved MRI and histology scores	Seki et al. (2009)
8K-NBD peptide (NF-κB inhibitor)	Mouse	Lumbar	Progeroid Ercc1 p65 KO	Restored total NP GAG and PG synthesis	Nasto et al. (2012)
allograft MSC or JC in fibrin	Minipig	Lumbar	1 cm incision and nucleotomy; evaluate at 3, 6, 12 months	JC Tx: high GAG content at 12 months, rich in collagen type II	Acosta et al. (2011)
Link N protein	Rabbit	Lumbar	Needle puncture: Tx 4 weeks later	Increased aggrecan gene expression and decreased proteinase gene expression	Mwale et al. (2011)

IGF-1 insulin-like growth factor-1, *GDF-5* growth differentiation factor-5, *TGF-β* transforming growth factor-β, *bFGF* basic fibroblast growth factor, *OP-1* osteogenic protein-1, *PG* proteoglycan, *NP* nucleus pulposus, *C-ABC* chondroitinase ABC, *Tx* treatment, *AF* annulus fibrosus, *MRI* magnetic resonance imaging, *ADAMTS a disintegrin and metalloproteinase with thrombospondin motifs*, *COX* cyclooxygenase, *BMP* bone morpho genetic protein, *PRP* platelet-rich plasma, *GHM* gelatin hydrogel microspheres, *PBS* phosphate-buffered saline, *siRNA* small interference RNA (siRNA), *8K-NBD* Nemo-binding domain, *NF-κB* nuclear factor kappa-light-chain-enhancer of activated B cells, *Ercc1* excision repair cross-complementing rodent repair deficiency, complementation group 1, *KO* knock out, *MSC* mesenchymal stem cell, *JC* juvenile chondrocytes, *GAG* glycosaminoglycan, *Link N* amino terminal peptide of link protein (DHLSDNYTLDHDRAIH)

25.3 Model Systems and Outcome Measures to Evaluate Treatment Efficacy

For evaluation of the efficacy of various biologic treatments, a number of in vitro and in vivo model systems are routinely used. Isolated nucleus pulposus and annulus fibrosus cells from intervertebral discs are seeded in monolayer and treated with specific cytokines (e.g., IL-1, TNF-α) to model degenerative conditions. Cells from discs with varying degrees of degeneration are also used. In these systems, the efficacy of therapeutic agents can be determined at several levels. In cells, a decrease in the gene expression of catabolic enzymes, such as aggrecanases and proteinases, as well as vascular factors and pain-related factors may be assessed using PCR techniques. Anabolic genes of interest may include those molecules comprising the extracellular matrix, such as collagen and aggrecan, and anabolic regulators, such as TGF-β, IGF-1, and growth and differentiation factor-5 (GDF-5). At the protein level, the synthesis of collagen and proteoglycans can be assessed, using radiolabeled ^{3}H and ^{35}S, respectively, by determining their incorporation from the media into the cells. Other factors can be assessed by enzyme-linked immunosorbent assay (ELISA) or multiplex cytokine assay.

Pellets of cells surrounded by three-dimensional extracellular matrices, recovered after alginate culture (Masuda et al. 2000), for example, have also been used. The presence of the extracellular matrix better mimics the microenvironment of disc cells. In addition to treatments using a monolayer system, pellet cultures may be treated with agents to alter or deplete specific matrix components (e.g., using chondroitinase ABC to deplete proteoglycans); this is not feasible using monolayer culture. For outcome measurements, the biochemical content of the matrix can be determined. For example, the dimethylmethylene blue (DMMB) assay can be used to assess the proteoglycan content, while western blot and PCR can be used to assess protein and gene expression levels.

25.4 Effect of Growth Factors on Intervertebral Disc Cells and Tissues

A variety of anabolic growth factors and cytokines alter intervertebral disc homeostasis and stimulate extracellular matrix synthesis (Masuda et al. 2004). OP-1 (Masuda et al. 2003), a member of the BMP family and TGF-β superfamily (Fig. 25.1), upregulates proteoglycan metabolism in intervertebral disc cells. OP-1 strongly stimulated the production and formation of extracellular matrix by rabbit disc cells (Masuda et al. 2003); similar effects have been noted using human intervertebral disc cells (Imai et al. 2007a). OP-1 also replenished proteoglycans and collagens after depletion of the matrix following exposure of intervertebral disc pellets to IL-1 (Takegami et al. 2002) or chondroitinase ABC (C-ABC) (Takegami et al. 2005). The efficacy of OP-1 injection has also been evaluated in a number of in vivo animal models. In adolescent rabbits, an injection of recombinant human OP-1 (rhOP-1), but not the lactose vehicle, reversed the reduction in disc height and improved the magnetic resonance imaging (MRI) grade caused by a needle puncture of the annulus fibrosus (Masuda et al. 2006). In another rabbit study (Miyamoto et al. 2006b), OP-1 restored dynamic viscoelastic biomechanical properties, in

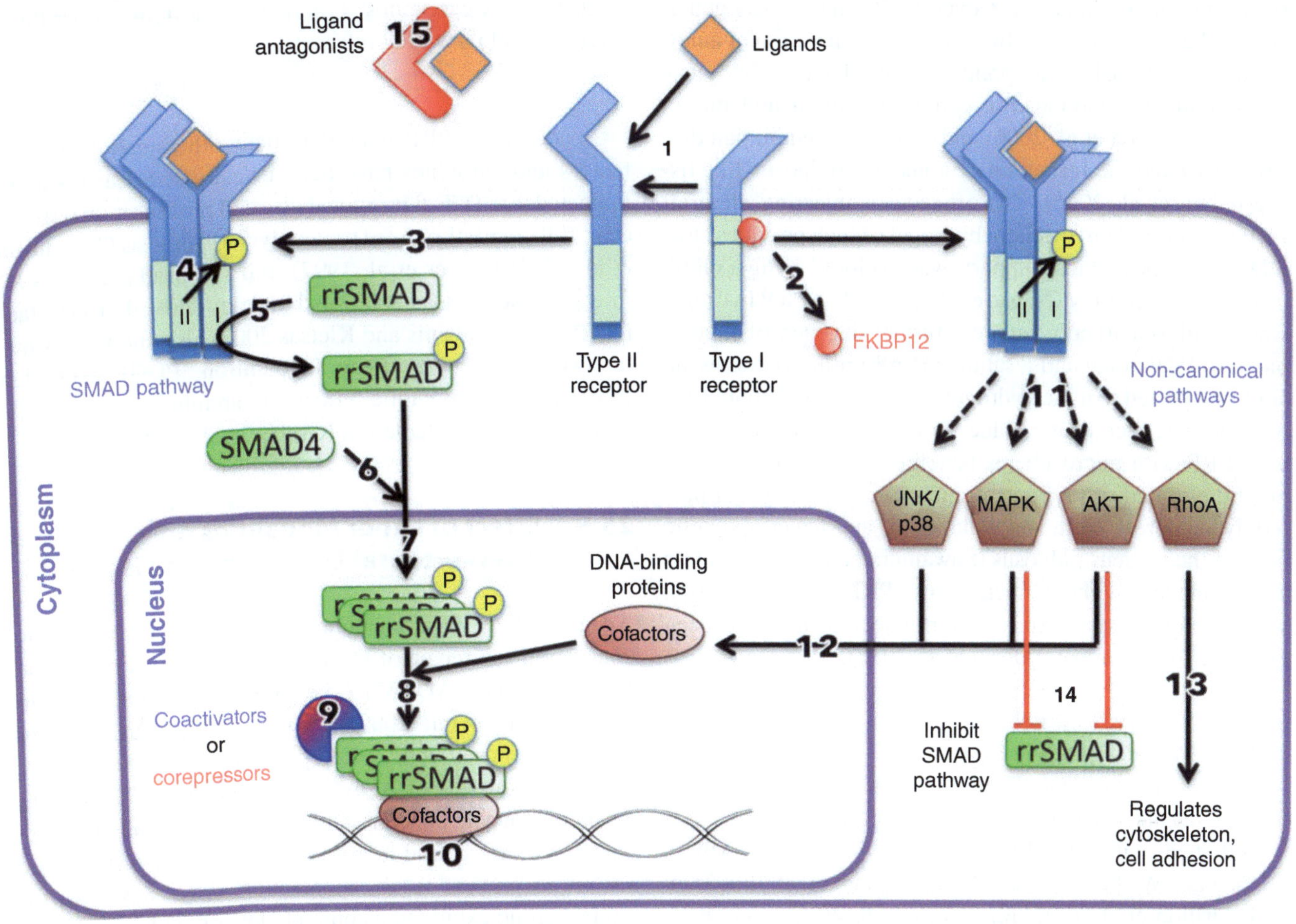

Fig. 25.1 TGF-β signaling pathways. Ligand binds with types I and II receptors (*1*), which releases FKBP12 (*2*) from the GS domain of the type I receptor and forms a ligand-receptor complex (*3*). The type I receptor is phosphorylated by type II receptor (*4*). The activated type I receptors phosphorylate receptor-regulated SMADs (*rrSMAD*) (*5*), which associate with SMAD4 (*6*) and move into the nucleus (*7*). The SMAD complex associates with DNA-binding cofactors (*8*) along with coactivators or corepressors (*9*) to activate or repress transcription of genes (*10*). The activated ligand-receptor complex can begin other non-canonical pathways (*11*), which can affect cofactors (*12*), regulate cytoskeletal organization and cell adhesion (*13*), or inhibit the SMAD pathway (*14*). In addition, ligand antagonists can sequester ligands extracellularly (*15*)

needle-punctured intervertebral discs (Miyamoto et al. 2006b). It was also effective in restoring discs that have been chemically degraded with C-ABC, which has been considered as an alternative to chymopapain for chemonucleolysis (Eurell et al. 1990; Fry et al. 1991; Henderson et al. 1991; Kato et al. 1992; Ando et al. 1995; Sugimura et al. 1996; Takahashi et al. 1996b; Yamada et al. 2001), in animal models of disc degeneration such as the rat tail (Norcross et al. 2003; Hoogendoorn et al. 2007, 2008; Boxberger et al. 2008) and goat (Hoogendoorn et al. 2007, 2008). When OP-1 or vehicle was injected into rabbit discs degraded with C-ABC for 4 weeks, the disc height was initially decreased (~34 %), then recovered, and gradually approached the level of the control (Imai et al. 2007b).

A number of autologous agents have been shown to be clinically useful. For example, platelet-rich plasma (PRP) contains high levels of multiple growth factors and as such it has been used in disc repair in animal studies and in a clinical study ongoing in Japan. Moreover, PRP can be easily generated in the operating room by centrifugal separation of autologous blood using a point-of-care device. In vitro, PRP-stimulated porcine disc cell proliferation and matrix synthesis (Akeda et al. 2006) and using isolated human disc cells provoked the formation of a nucleus pulposus-like tissue (Chen et al. 2006). The efficacy of injecting allograft PRP with or without a gelatin hydrogel (which provides slow release and mechanical support) was explored using a rabbit model of nucleotomy (Nagae et al. 2007). The PRP hydrogel was found to markedly suppress further degeneration, compared to PRP alone and a saline control group. A follow-up study suggested that the hydrogel microspheres without PRP did not have therapeutic value. In contrast, animals treated with PRP with microspheres benefited from increased disc height, elevated water content, increased expression of proteoglycan core protein and collagen II, and fewer apoptotic cells in the nucleus pulposus (Sawamura et al. 2009). In less severe models without nucleotomy, PRP (after activation with autologous serum and calcium) injection alone has been effective for disc repair (Obata et al. 2012).

Box 25.1 Platelet-Rich Plasma

Platelet-rich plasma (PRP) injection is increasingly used as an off-label procedure before resorting to orthopedic surgery. PRP contains a mixture of growth factors (Weibrich et al. 2002; Okuda et al. 2003; Dugrillon et al. 2002; Mazzocca et al. 2012) such as transforming growth factor (TGF)-β1 and TGF-β2, vascular endothelial growth factor (VEGF), platelet-derived growth factor (PDGF), and insulin-like growth factor (IGF), which are naturally released from platelets after being activated by calcium or thrombin (Tozum and Demiralp 2003; Arpornmaeklong et al. 2004). Among these growth factors, TGF-β1 exists in the highest concentration (Weibrich et al. 2002) and may be the core ingredient and the indicator for applying PRP. These growth factors appear to play an important role in wound healing and are assumed to facilitate hard and soft tissue regeneration.

The efficacy of PRP injection for disc regeneration is still being investigated; however, promising results such as upregulation of proteoglycan anabolism and restoration of disc height have been seen in a number of in vitro studies on disc cell (Akeda et al. 2006; Chen et al. 2006), on explants (Chen et al. 2009), as well as in animal models (Nagae et al. 2007; Chen et al. 2009; Obata et al. 2012). PRP is often used in conjunction with biomaterials such as gelatin (Nagae et al. 2007) and mesenchymal stem cells (Chen et al. 2006, 2009). PRP has been used without activation (Nagae et al. 2007); however, most commercial systems (Castillo et al. 2011) use PRP releasate.

In addition to PRP and OP-1, many other anabolic growth factors and cytokines have been investigated. Early studies indicated that TGF-β promoted disc cell proliferation (Gruber et al. 1997) and stimulated proteoglycan synthesis (Thompson et al. 1991; Gruber et al. 1997). IGF-1 (Osada et al. 1996; Pratsinis and Kletsas 2007) and platelet-derived growth factor (PDGF) (Pratsinis and Kletsas 2007) also showed a similar cell-proliferative effect. In addition, PDGF exerted a protective, antiapoptotic effect on annulus fibrosus cells induced by serum depletion (Gruber et al. 2000).

25.5 Effect of Other Modalities on Intervertebral Disc Cells and Tissues

Agents other than anabolic growth factors are being considered for repair of the degenerate intervertebral disc. In a recent study, ADAMTS-5 expression was silenced using siRNA (Seki et al. 2009). In vitro studies, using rabbit nucleus pulposus cells, were performed to determine the extent of reduction of ADAMTS-5 expression. Then, using an annular needle puncture rabbit model, MRI and histological analysis were used to assess the efficacy of ADAMTS-5 siRNA to prevent tissue degradation. After 8 weeks, the control group exhibited a complete loss of nucleus pulposus tissue, while the ADAMTS-silenced animals maintained disc structure (Seki et al. 2009).

IL-1 receptor antagonist (IL-1ra) is another inhibitory agent that has been studied. When applied in vitro to degenerated (Le Maitre et al. 2007b) and herniated (Genevay et al. 2009) human disc tissues, IL-1ra reduced the expression of MMP-3 (Le Maitre et al. 2007b;

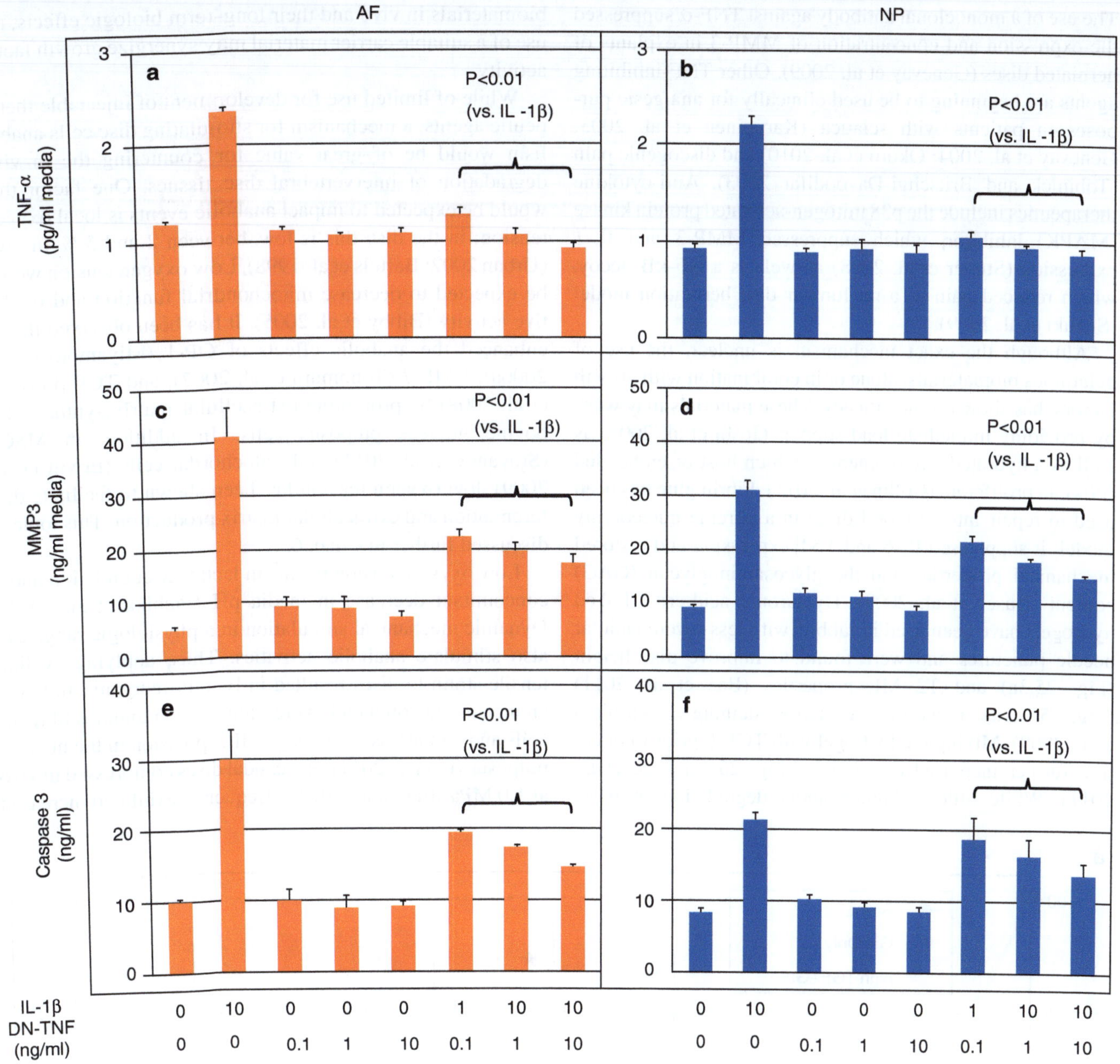

Fig. 25.2 Dominant-negative tumor necrosis factor (*DN-TNF*) effectively antagonizes interleukin-1β (*IL-1β*)-induced catabolic changes in human intervertebral disc cells. Human nucleus pulposus (*NP*) and annulus fibrosis (*AF*) cells were isolated from cadaveric intervertebral disc (*IVD*) tissues (average of ~60 years old) and cultured in alginate beads for 7 days. Cells were serum starved for 1 day and treated for 2 days in media containing a combination of IL-1β and DN-TNF. Levels of TNF-α, matrix metalloproteinase-3 (*MMP-3*), and caspase 3 released into the media were measured. DN-TNF treatment suppressed release of (**a**, **b**) TNF-α, (**c**, **d**) MMP-3, and (**e**, **f**) caspase 3 by both AF and NP cells, suggesting DN-TNF may be effective in suppressing catabolic cytokines, matrix-degrading enzymes, and cell apoptosis (Modified from Pichika et al. (2011))

Genevay et al. 2009). In addition, following pretreatment of degenerated human nucleus pulposus cells with IL-1ra and subsequent treatment with IL-1, there was reduced expression of ADAMTS-4 and MMP-3 (Shamji et al. 2007).

Yet another target for inhibition is TNF-α. In human disc cells, the use of soluble TNF receptors along with IL-1ra significantly upregulated proteoglycan synthesis (Kakutani et al. 2008), while co-treatment with TNF-α suppressed nitric oxide and IL-6 production (Sinclair et al. 2011). Although dominant-negative TNF (DN-TNF) does not activate TNF receptors, it effectively competes with soluble TNF. When applied to human intervertebral disc cells challenged with IL-1β (Pichika et al. 2011), DN-TNF effectively reduced the concentration of TNF-α (Fig. 25.2a, b), levels of MMP-3 in the media (Fig. 25.2c, d), the expression of intracellular caspase 3 (Fig. 25.2e, f), and the production of PGE2.

The use of a monoclonal antibody against TNF-α suppressed the expression and concentration of MMP-3 in explants of herniated discs (Genevay et al. 2009). Other TNF-inhibiting agents are beginning to be used clinically for analgesic purposes in patients with sciatica (Karppinen et al. 2003; Genevay et al. 2004; Okoro et al. 2010) and discogenic pain (Tobinick and Britschgi-Davoodifar 2003). Anti-cytokine therapeutics include the p38 mitogen-activated protein kinase (MAPK) inhibitor, which suppressed MMP-3 and IL-1 expression (Studer et al. 2008) as well as a NF-κB decoy, which reduced pain in a rat lumbar disc herniation model (Suzuki et al. 2009).

Although the exact mechanism is unclear, the use of gelatinous biomaterials, alone or in combination with growth factors, has shown some efficacy. These materials may work by providing immediate load support (Joshi et al. 2005) as well as a hydrated environment in which host or embedded cells can proliferate (Collin et al. 2011). Fibrin glue has been used to repair intervertebral discs in a porcine nucleotomy model: it suppressed IL-6 and TNF expression and restored mechanical properties and the glycosaminoglycan (GAG) content (Buser et al. 2009). Hyaluronic acid-cross-linked hydrogels have been used in rabbits with less severe annular needle punctures and were found to improve disc height (Fig. 25.3a) and T2 MR properties (Bae et al. 2011) (Fig. 25.3a–d), as well as safranin O staining (Nakashima et al. 2009). Mixing the hydrogel with TGF-β prior to injection further increased disc height (Fig. 25.3a) (Bae et al. 2011). While little is known about degradation of these biomaterials in vivo and their long-term biologic effects, the use of a suitable carrier material may synergize growth factor activity.

While of limited use for development of injectable therapeutic agents, a mechanism for stimulating disc cells anabolism would be of great value for countering the in vivo degradation of intervertebral disc tissues. One factor that would be expected to impact anabolic events is local oxygen tension; in the disc this is low, between 2 and 5 % in vivo (Urban 2002; Bartels et al. 1998). Low oxygen tension would be expected to decrease mitochondrial function and oxidative activity (Bibby et al. 2005). It has been observed that it enhanced the anabolic effects of OP-1 (Miyamoto et al. 2006a), BMP-7 (Tonomura et al. 2007), and TGF-β3 (Abe et al. 2008) by promoting extracellular matrix synthesis by bovine nucleus pulposus cells. In addition, in MSCs (Stoyanov et al. 2011) and notochordal cells (Erwin et al. 2009), low oxygen tension has been shown to facilitate differentiation and extracellular matrix production. This topic is discussed further in Chap. 6.

Low oxygen tension results in lactate accumulation and a concomitant decrease in media pH (Pichika et al. 2012). Dynamic mechanical stimulation in a physiologic range can also stimulate anabolic activities. Thus, applying cycling tensile strain to discs resulted in F-actin reorganization and an increase in collagen I expression in outer annulus fibrosus cells and an increase of collagen II expression in the nucleus pulposus (Li et al. 2011). Rat caudal discs compressed in vivo at 1.0 MPa stress and 0.01 Hz frequency exhibited increased

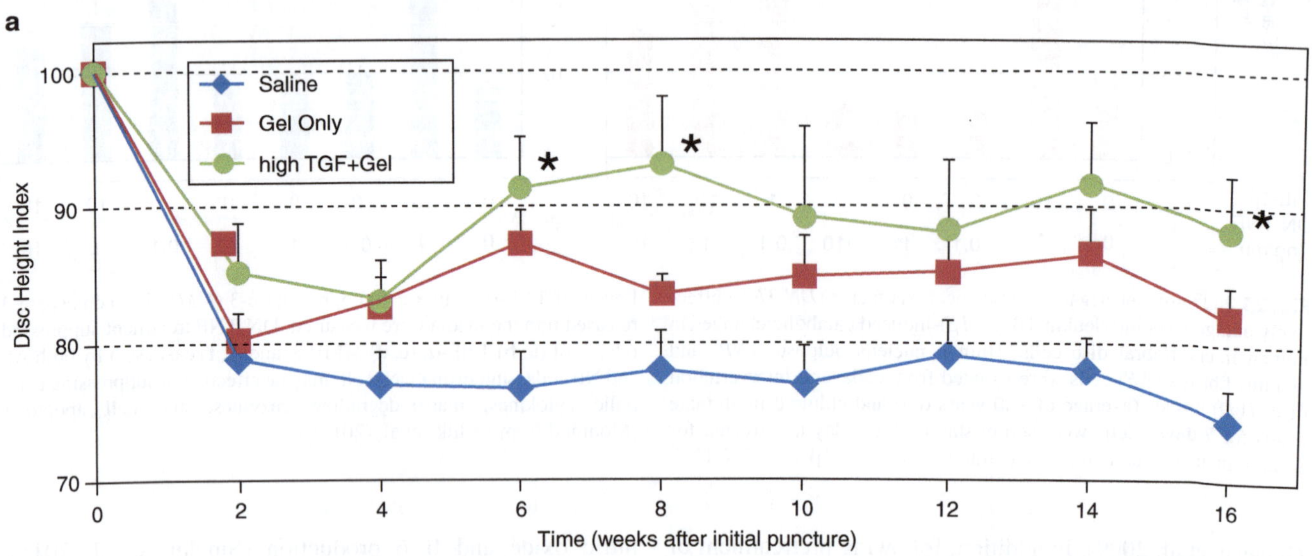

Fig. 25.3 Treatment of intervertebral disc degeneration using injectable hydrogel. Adult (~9 months old) rabbits received annular puncture. After 4 weeks, animals were divided into three groups and received an injection of either saline, hyaluronic acid-based hydrogel, or transforming growth factor β3 (TGFβ3) mixed with the hydrogel. Lateral plane radiographs were taken biweekly. At week 16, animals were sacrificed and MRI was performed to determine T2 relaxation properties of the discs. (**a**) Disc height index was higher for hydrogel samples than saline samples, consistent with (**b**) MRI showing larger nucleus pulposus (NP) morphology for the hydrogel samples. (**c**) T2 property of the NP also showed a trend of being higher for the hydrogel group, while (**d**) that of the AF did not show much variation. The addition of TGFβ3 increased disc height even more (a) but had no effect on the T2 property. *ROI* region of interest (Reproduced from Bae et al. (2011), abstract)

Fig. 25.3 (continued)

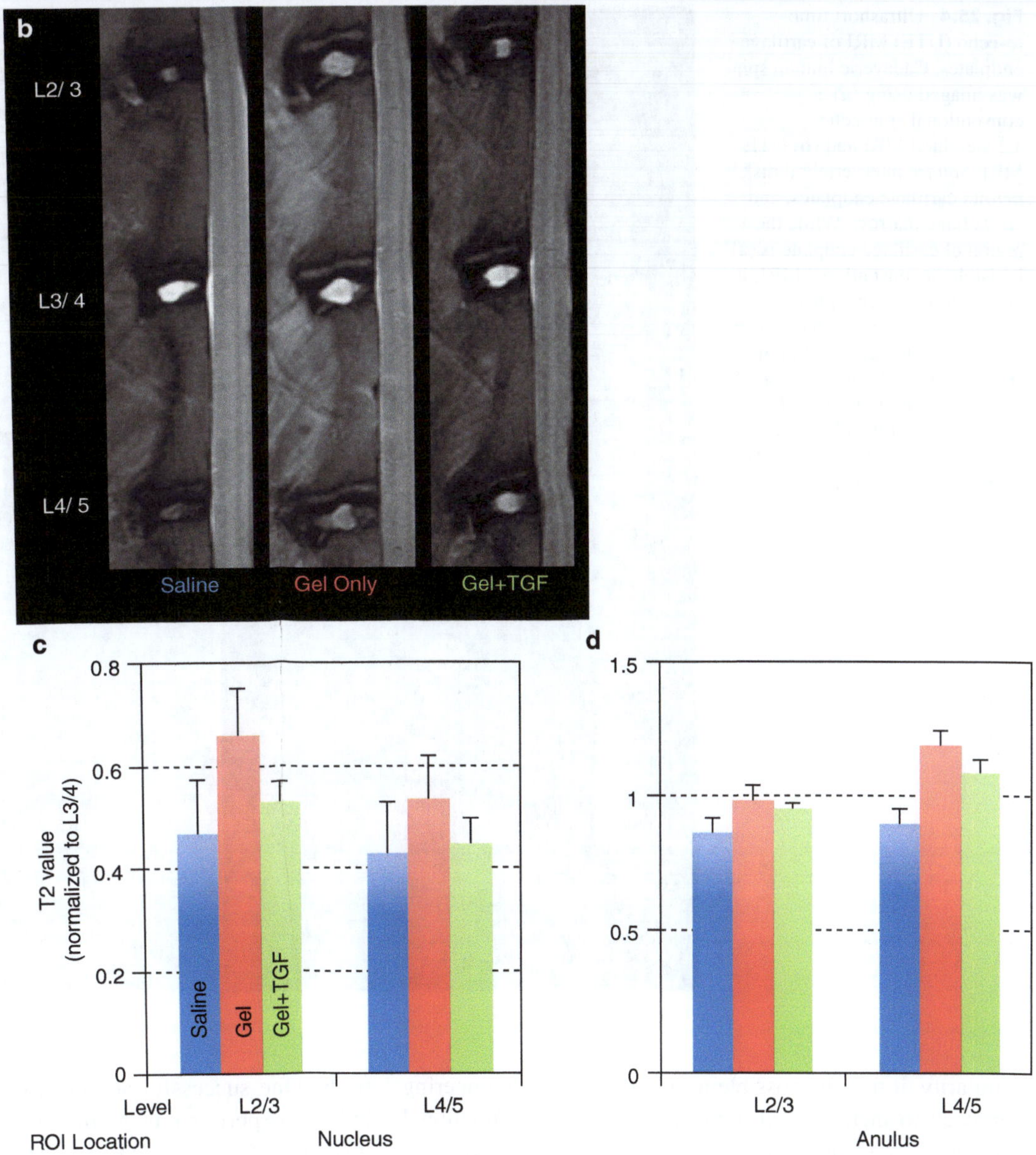

expression of anabolic genes (Maclean et al. 2004). For tissue-engineering applications, these techniques may be combined with growth factors and scaffold or gel biomaterials to help optimize the function of disc tissues (this topic is discussed in detail in Chap. 26).

25.6 Limitations of Injection Therapy

While the effects of growth factors on disc cells and tissues have been widely studied, questions still remain regarding their long-term effects. A major factor influencing efficiency is the residence time of an injected protein/compound in the disc, which for most agents has not been established. For OP-1, while some studies have suggested a short half-life (~minutes) (Larson et al. 2006), others, using radiolabeling, have noted times longer than 1 month (Pierce et al. 2006). This is consistent with a study suggesting that OP-1 binds to collagen molecules (Reddi 2000); a physical interaction between the proteins would slow degradation and thereby explain the long residence time. There are other confounding factors, such as physical characteristics of the intervertebral disc tissue, the nature of the carrier or vehicle, as well as the injection location and technique. In addition, the duration and time course of the anabolic effect resulting from a single exposure to a growth factor remain to be established.

Many injectable therapies have inherent limitations that are dependent on the stage of disc degeneration. Growth factor injection requires the presence of viable and functional cells in the intervertebral disc. In end-stage disc degeneration, very little tissue and cells remain (Gruber and Hanley 1998). Even if viable cells are present in the degenerate discs, they may exhibit a poor response to the growth factor (Le Maitre et al. 2008). For intervertebral disc with very low

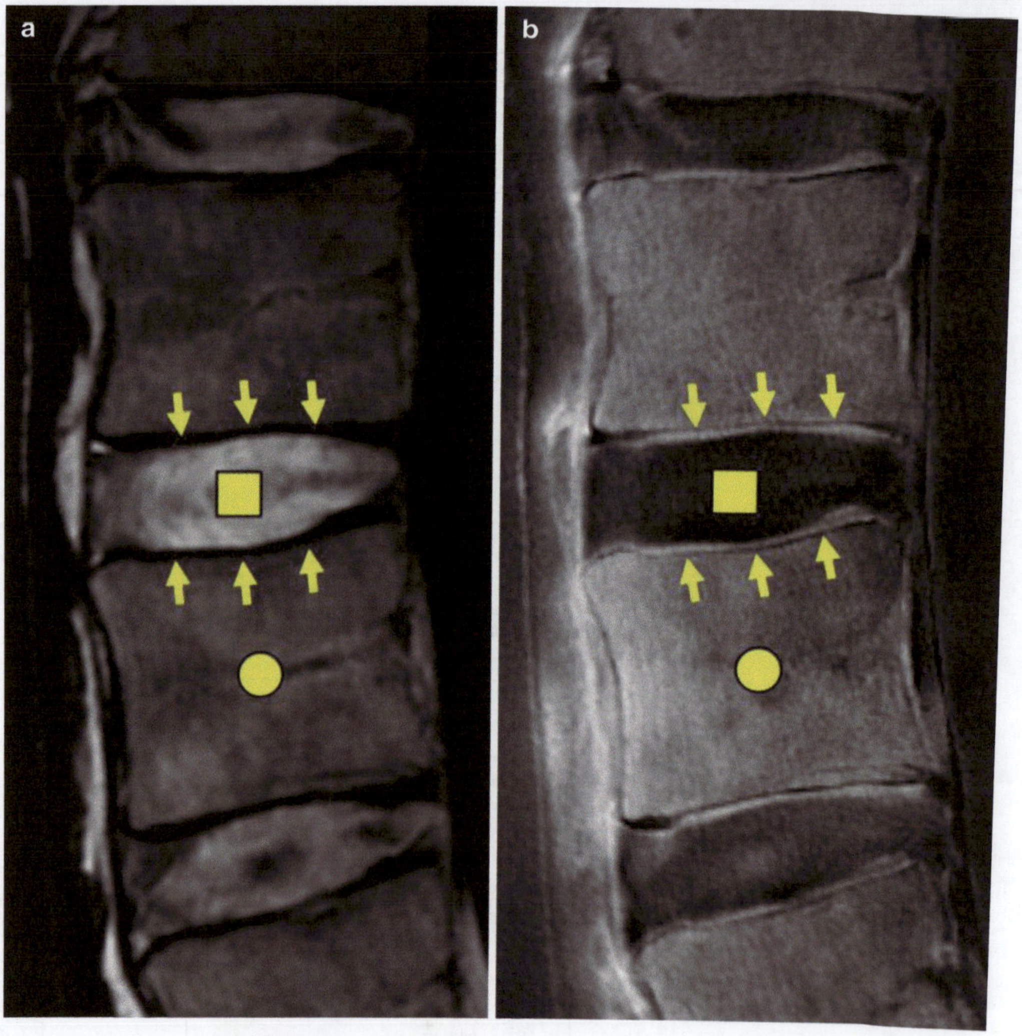

Fig. 25.4 Ultrashort time-to-echo (UTE) MRI of cartilage endplates. Cadaveric human spine was imaged using (**a**) a conventional spin-echo T2-weighted MRI and (**b**) UTE MRI. *Square* intervertebral disk, *arrows* cartilage endplates, and *circle* bone marrow. While the region of cartilage endplate is (a) invisible in conventional MRI, it is shown with high signal intensity and contrast in (b) UTE MRI. Novel imaging techniques such as UTE MRI may be useful for evaluation of nutritional environment of the disks, as well as selection of suitable subjects for receiving biological therapeutics

cellularity, it may be possible to utilize a tissue-engineering approach to increase cell number. For example, functional cells recovered from herniated tissues could be used or even MSCs derived from bone marrow or other tissue sites (Nishimura and Mochida 1998; Okuma et al. 2000; Anderson et al. 2005; Gruber et al. 2002; Ganey et al. 2003).

Another consideration is that the level of nutrients in the disc may be low (Urban et al. 2004) due to vertebral endplate sclerosis or cartilage endplate calcification (Bae et al. 2010). This region can be visualized using novel imaging techniques such as ultrashort time-to-echo MRI (Fig. 25.4) (Bae et al. 2010, 2012). The perfusion of solutes from the vertebral body into intervertebral disc has been assessed indirectly using contrast-enhanced MRI in human subjects (Rajasekaran et al. 2004, 2008). It remains to be determined if these techniques provide information on the time course of subsequent disc degeneration.

Lastly, assessment of pain reduction is difficult when using a preclinical animal model; this is of critical importance, as pain is the primary outcome measure for clinical trials. One successful attempt to address this issue was an indirect experiment using the rat tail compression model. In this study, OP-1 was injected into the disc, which was then transplanted into the dorsal root ganglion in the same rat (Kawakami et al. 2005). It was noted that the animal exhibited less allodynia after OP-1 injection. Other approaches include behavioral (Olmarker 2008) or gait analysis (Shamji et al. 2009). Results of these studies provide preliminary evidence that an injection therapy is effective in reducing pain. Moreover, they permit pain generation to be related to changes in the biochemical profile of disc tissues following treatment.

25.7 Conclusion

This chapter outlined approaches using injectable therapeutics to enhance biologic repair or regeneration of the intervertebral disc and described methods available to evaluate the efficacy of the treatment. Using intervertebral disc cells in vitro and discs in animal models in vivo, there is abundant evidence supporting the use and efficacy of treatment using growth factors and agents that exert anti-catabolic activity. In current preclinical animal studies, outcomes focus mainly on structural modification, and little is known about pain reduction. More behavioral studies, animal models of pain, and other novel methods such as functional MRI may be needed to better understand this important issue. In addition, further studies on large animals with intervertebral disc biology similar to humans are desired. Ultimately, using agents discussed earlier, intradiscal injections offer great potential for treatment of patients with chronic discogenic low back pain. Results of clinical trials currently underway will provide important initial safety and efficacy information.

25.8 Summary of Critical Concepts Discussed in the Chapter

- Intervertebral disc degeneration involves an imbalance between the anabolic and catabolic activities of disc cells and a decrease in the number of functional cells.
- Therapeutic agents that can alter the activities of the intervertebral disc cells by direct injections are being actively pursued.
- Therapeutic agents include anabolic growth factors, biostimulatory biomaterials, and agents antagonistic to matrix-degrading enzymes and cytokines, some of which are currently under clinical trials.
- The efficacy of candidate agents is initially evaluated in vitro using various cell and explant culture models and in vivo using preclinical animal models.
- There is a need for continued development of model systems and evaluation techniques to assess the efficacy and safety aspects of injected agents, as well as an understanding of the pathogenesis and progression of degenerative disc disease.

Acknowledgements This work was supported in part by NIH P01AR48152 and K01AR059764.

Disclosures Koichi Masuda, M.D.: Research/Institutional Support: Medtronic, Nippon Zoki, Nuvasive, Biotime

References

Abbott RD, Purmessur D, Monsey RD, Iatridis JC (2012) Regenerative potential of TGFbeta3 + Dex and notochordal cell conditioned media on degenerated human intervertebral disc cells. J Orthop Res 30(3):482–488. doi:10.1002/jor.21534

Abe Y, Asanuma K, Tonomura H, Kimura T, An H, Masuda K (2008) Transforming growth factor-ß3 and low oxygen tension stimulate synthesis of proteoglycan and collagen by bovine intervertebral disc cells in alginate beads. In: 54th annual meeting of Orthopedic Research Society, San Francisco, p 1413

Acosta FL Jr, Metz L, Adkisson HD, Liu J, Carruthers-Liebenberg E, Milliman C, Maloney M, Lotz JC (2011) Porcine intervertebral disc repair using allogeneic juvenile articular chondrocytes or mesenchymal stem cells. Tissue Eng Part A 17(23–24):3045–3055. doi:10.1089/ten.tea.2011.0229

Aguiar DJ, Johnson SL, Oegema TR (1999) Notochordal cells interact with nucleus pulposus cells: regulation of proteoglycan synthesis. Exp Cell Res 246(1):129–137

Ahn S-H, Teng P-N, Niyibizi C, Gilbertson L, Kang J (2002a) The effects of BMP-12 and BMP-2 on proteoglycan and collagen synthesis in nucleus pulposus cells from human degenerated discs. In: The International Society for the Study of the Lumbar Spine, 29th Annual Meeting Proceeding, Cleveland, 14–18 May 2002, p 49

Ahn SH, Cho YW, Ahn MW, Jang SH, Sohn YK, Kim HS (2002b) MRNA expression of cytokines and chemokines in herniated lumbar intervertebral discs. Spine 27(9):911–917

Akeda K, An HS, Pichika R, Attawia M, Thonar EJ, Lenz ME, Uchida A, Masuda K (2006) Platelet-rich plasma (PRP) stimulates the extracellular matrix metabolism of porcine nucleus pulposus and anulus fibrosus cells cultured in alginate beads. Spine 31(9):959–966

An HS, Takegami K, Kamada H, Nguyen CM, Thonar EJ, Singh K, Andersson GB, Masuda K (2005) Intradiscal administration of osteogenic protein-1 increases intervertebral disc height and proteoglycan content in the nucleus pulposus in normal adolescent rabbits. Spine 30(1):25–31

Anderson DG, Izzo MW, Hall DJ, Vaccaro AR, Hilibrand A, Arnold W, Tuan RS, Albert TJ (2002) Comparative gene expression profiling of normal and degenerative discs: analysis of a rabbit annular laceration model. Spine 27(12):1291–1296

Anderson DG, Albert TJ, Fraser JK, Risbud M, Wuisman P, Meisel HJ, Tannoury C, Shapiro I, Vaccaro AR (2005) Cellular therapy for disc degeneration. Spine 30(17 Suppl):S14–S19

Ando T, Kato F, Mimatsu K, Iwata H (1995) Effects of chondroitinase ABC on degenerative intervertebral discs. Clin Orthop 318:214–221

Annunen S, Paassilta P, Lohiniva J, Perala M, Pihlajamaa T, Karppinen J, Tervonen O, Kroger H, Lahde S, Vanharanta H, Ryhanen L, Goring HH, Ott J, Prockop DJ, Ala-Kokko L (1999) An allele of COL9A2 associated with intervertebral disc disease. Science 285(5426):409–412

Arner EC, Pratta MA (1989) Independent effects of interleukin-1 on proteoglycan breakdown, proteoglycan synthesis, and prostaglandin E2 release from cartilage in organ culture. Arthritis Rheum 32: 288–297

Arpornmaeklong P, Kochel M, Depprich R, Kubler NR, Wurzler KK (2004) Influence of platelet-rich plasma (PRP) on osteogenic differentiation of rat bone marrow stromal cells. An in vitro study. Int J Oral Maxillofac Surg 33(1):60–70. doi:10.1054/ijom.2003.0492

Bae WC, Yoshikawa T, Kakutani K, Hammed A, Znamirowski R, Chung CB, Bydder GM, Masuda K (2009) Effect of rhGDF-5 on the thrombin model of rabbit intervertebral disc degeneration; T2 Quantification Using 3T MRI. Orthop Res Soc Trans:2129

Bae WC, Du J, Bydder GM, Chung CB (2010) Conventional and ultrashort time-to-echo magnetic resonance imaging of articular cartilage, meniscus, and intervertebral disk. Top Magn Reson Imaging 21(5):275–289. doi:10.1097/RMR.0b013e31823ccebc

Bae WC, Yoshikawa T, Yamaguchi T, Hemmad AR, Rana S, Inoue N, Bydder GM, Masuda K (2011) Repair of intervertebral disc degeneration using injectable hydrogel: imaging assessments. Trans Orthop Res Soc 36:362

Bae WC, Statum S, Zhang Z, Yamaguchi T, Wolfson T, Gamst AC, Du J, Bydder GM, Masuda K, Chung CB (2012) Morphology of the cartilaginous endplates in human intervertebral disks with ultrashort echo time MR imaging. Radiology. doi:10.1148/radiol.12121181

Bartels EM, Fairbank JC, Winlove CP, Urban JP (1998) Oxygen and lactate concentrations measured in vivo in the intervertebral discs of patients with scoliosis and back pain. Spine 23(1):1–7

Benton HP, Tyler JA (1988) Inhibition of cartilage proteoglycan synthesis by interleukin I. Biochem Biophys Res Commun 154(1): 421–428

Bibby SR, Jones DA, Ripley RM, Urban JP (2005) Metabolism of the intervertebral disc: effects of low levels of oxygen, glucose, and pH on rates of energy metabolism of bovine nucleus pulposus cells. Spine 30(5):487–496

Boxberger JI, Auerbach JD, Sen S, Elliott DM (2008) An in vivo model of reduced nucleus pulposus glycosaminoglycan content in the rat lumbar intervertebral disc. Spine 33(2):146–154. doi:10.1097/BRS.0b013e31816054f8, 00007632-200801150-00005 [pii]

Burke JG, Watson RW, Conhyea D, McCormack D, Dowling FE, Walsh MG, Fitzpatrick JM (2003) Human nucleus pulposus can respond to a pro-inflammatory stimulus. Spine 28(24):2685–2693

Buser Z, Kuelling F, Jane L, Liebenberg E, Tang J, Thorne K, Coughlin D, Lotz J (2009) Fibrin injection stimulates early disc healing in the porcine model. Spine J 9(10 Suppl):105S. doi:10.1016/j.spinee.2009.08.241

Castillo TN, Pouliot MA, Kim HJ, Dragoo JL (2011) Comparison of growth factor and platelet concentration from commercial platelet-rich plasma separation systems. Am J Sports Med 39(2):266–271. doi:10.1177/0363546510387517

Chen WH, Lo WC, Lee JJ, Su CH, Lin CT, Liu HY, Lin TW, Lin WC, Huang TY, Deng WP (2006) Tissue-engineered intervertebral disc and chondrogenesis using human nucleus pulposus regulated through TGF-beta1 in platelet-rich plasma. J Cell Physiol 209(3):744–754. doi:10.1002/jcp.20765

Chen WH, Liu HY, Lo WC, Wu SC, Chi CH, Chang HY, Hsiao SH, Wu CH, Chiu WT, Chen BJ, Deng WP (2009) Intervertebral disc regeneration in an ex vivo culture system using mesenchymal stem cells and platelet-rich plasma. Biomaterials 30(29):5523–5533. doi:10.1016/j.biomaterials.2009.07.019

Chujo T, An HS, Akeda K, Miyamoto K, Muehleman C, Attawia M, Andersson G, Masuda K (2006) Effects of growth differentiation factor-5 on the intervertebral disc–in vitro bovine study and in vivo rabbit disc degeneration model study. Spine 31(25):2909–2917

Collin EC, Grad S, Zeugolis DI, Vinatier CS, Clouet JR, Guicheux JJ, Weiss P, Alini M, Pandit AS (2011) An injectable vehicle for nucleus pulposus cell-based therapy. Biomaterials 32(11):2862–2870. doi:10.1016/j.biomaterials.2011.01.018

Desmoulin GT, Hewitt CR, Hunter CJ (2011) Disc strain and resulting positive mRNA expression from application of a noninvasive treatment. Spine 36(14):E921–E928. doi:10.1097/BRS.0b013e3181fd78b3

Dingle JT, Horner A, Shield M (1991) The sensitivity of synthesis of human cartilage matrix to inhibition by IL-1 suggests a mechanism for the development of osteoarthritis. Cell Biochem Funct 9(2):99–102

Dong DM, Yao M, Liu B, Sun CY, Jiang YQ, Wang YS (2007) Association between the -1306C/T polymorphism of matrix metalloproteinase-2 gene and lumbar disc disease in Chinese young adults. Eur Spine J 16(11):1958–1961. doi:10.1007/s00586-007-0454-3

Dugrillon A, Eichler H, Kern S, Kluter H (2002) Autologous concentrated platelet-rich plasma (cPRP) for local application in bone regeneration. Int J Oral Maxillofac Surg 31(6):615–619

Erwin WM, Las Heras F, Islam D, Fehlings MG, Inman RD (2009) The regenerative capacity of the notochordal cell: tissue constructs generated in vitro under hypoxic conditions. J Neurosurg Spine 10(6):513–521. doi:10.3171/2009.2.SPINE08578

Eurell JA, Brown MD, Ramos M (1990) The effects of chondroitinase ABC on the rabbit intervertebral disc. A roentgenographic and histologic study. Clin Orthop 256:238–243

Fry TR, Eurell JC, Johnson AL, Brown MD, Losonsky JM, Schaeffer DJ (1991) Radiographic and histologic effects of chondroitinase ABC on normal canine lumbar intervertebral disc. Spine 16(7):816–819

Ganey T, Libera J, Moos V, Alasevic O, Fritsch KG, Meisel HJ, Hutton WC (2003) Disc chondrocyte transplantation in a canine model: a treatment for degenerated or damaged intervertebral disc. Spine 28(23):2609–2620

Genevay S, Stingelin S, Gabay C (2004) Efficacy of etanercept in the treatment of acute, severe sciatica: a pilot study. Ann Rheum Dis 63(9):1120–1123

Genevay S, Finckh A, Mezin F, Tessitore E, Guerne PA (2009) Influence of cytokine inhibitors on concentration and activity of MMP-1 and MMP-3 in disc herniation. Arthritis Res Ther 11(6):R169. doi:10.1186/ar2858

Gilbertson L, Ahn SH, Teng PN, Studer RK, Niyibizi C, Kang JD (2008) The effects of recombinant human bone morphogenetic protein-2, recombinant human bone morphogenetic protein-12, and adenoviral bone morphogenetic protein-12 on matrix synthesis in human annulus fibrosis and nucleus pulposus cells. Spine J 8(3):449–456. doi:10.1016/j.spinee.2006.11.006, S1529-9430(06)01068-0 [pii]

Gokorsch S, Weber C, Wedler T, Czermak P (2005) A stimulation unit for the application of mechanical strain on tissue engineered anulus fibrosus cells: a new system to induce extracellular matrix synthesis by anulus fibrosus cells dependent on cyclic mechanical strain. Int J Artif Organs 28(12):1242–1250

Gruber HE, Hanley EN Jr (1998) Analysis of aging and degeneration of the human intervertebral disc. Comparison of surgical specimens with normal controls. Spine 23(7):751–757

Gruber HE, Fisher EC Jr, Desai B, Stasky AA, Hoelscher G, Hanley EN Jr (1997) Human intervertebral disc cells from the annulus: three-dimensional culture in agarose or alginate and responsiveness to TGF-beta1. Exp Cell Res 235(1):13–21

Gruber HE, Norton HJ, Hanley EN Jr (2000) Anti-apoptotic effects of IGF-1 and PDGF on human intervertebral disc cells in vitro. Spine 25(17):2153–2157

Gruber HE, Johnson TL, Leslie K, Ingram JA, Martin D, Hoelscher G, Banks D, Phieffer L, Coldham G, Hanley EN Jr (2002) Autologous intervertebral disc cell implantation: a model using Psammomys obesus, the sand rat. Spine 27(15):1626–1633

Henderson N, Stanescu V, Cauchoix J (1991) Nucleolysis of the rabbit intervertebral disc using chondroitinase ABC. Spine 16(2):203–208

Hoogendoorn RJ, Wuisman PI, Smit TH, Everts VE, Helder MN (2007) Experimental intervertebral disc degeneration induced by chondroitinase ABC in the goat. Spine 32(17):1816–1825. doi:10.1097/BRS.0b013e31811ebac5, 00007632-200708010-00004 [pii]

Hoogendoorn RJ, Helder MN, Kroeze RJ, Bank RA, Smit TH, Wuisman PI (2008) Reproducible long-term disc degeneration in a large animal model. Spine 33(9):949–954. doi:10.1097/BRS.0b013e31816c90f0, 00007632-200804200-00004 [pii]

Huang KY, Yan JJ, Hsieh CC, Chang MS, Lin RM (2007) The in vivo biological effects of intradiscal recombinant human bone morphogenetic protein-2 on the injured intervertebral disc: an animal experiment. Spine 32(11):1174–1180

Iatridis JC, Godburn K, Wuertz K, Alini M, Roughley PJ (2011) Region-dependent aggrecan degradation patterns in the rat intervertebral disc are affected by mechanical loading in vivo. Spine 36(3):203–209. doi:10.1097/BRS.0b013e3181cec247

Igarashi T, Kikuchi S, Shubayev V, Myers RR (2000) 2000 Volvo Award winner in basic science studies: exogenous tumor necrosis factor-alpha mimics nucleus pulposus-induced neuropathology. Molecular, histologic, and behavioral comparisons in rats. Spine 25(23):2975–2980

Imai Y, An H, Thonar E, Muehleman C, Okuma M, Matsumoto T, Andersson G, Masuda K (2003) Co-injected recombinant human osteogenic protein-1 minimizes chondroitinase ABC-induced intervertebral disc degeneration: an in vivo study using a rabbit model. Trans Orthop Res Soc:1143

Imai Y, Miyamoto K, An HS, Thonar EJ, Andersson GB, Masuda K (2007a) Recombinant human osteogenic protein-1 upregulates proteoglycan metabolism of human anulus fibrosus and nucleus pulposus cells. Spine 32(12):1303–1309; discussion 1310

Imai Y, Okuma M, An H, Nakagawa K, Yamada M, Thonar E, Muehleman C, Masuda K (2007b) Restoration of disc height loss by recombinant human osteogenic protein-1 injection into intervertebral discs undergoing degeneration induced by an intradiscal injection of chondroitinase ABC. Spine 32(11):1197–1205

Jimbo K, Park JS, Yokosuka K, Sato K, Nagata K (2005) Positive feedback loop of interleukin-1beta upregulating production of inflammatory mediators in human intervertebral disc cells in vitro. J Neurosurg Spine 2(5):589–595

Joshi A, Mehta S, Vresilovic E, Karduna A, Marcolongo M (2005) Nucleus implant parameters significantly change the compressive stiffness of the human lumbar intervertebral disc. J Biomech Eng 127(3):536–540

Kakutani K, Kanaji A, Asanuma K, Pichika R, An H, Yamada H, Masuda K (2008) Effect of IL-1 receptor antagonist and soluble TNF receptor on the anabolism of human intervertebral disc cells. In: 54th Annual Meeting of Orthopedic Research Society, San Francisco, p 442

Kang JD, Georgescu HI, McIntyre-Larkin L, Stefanovic-Racic M, Donaldson WF 3rd, Evans CH (1996) Herniated lumbar intervertebral discs spontaneously produce matrix metalloproteinases, nitric oxide, interleukin-6, and prostaglandin E2. Spine 21(3):271–277

Kang JD, Stefanovic-Racic M, McIntyre LA, Georgescu HI, Evans CH (1997) Toward a biochemical understanding of human intervertebral disc degeneration and herniation. Contributions of nitric oxide, interleukins, prostaglandin E2, and matrix metalloproteinases. Spine 22(10):1065–1073

Karppinen J, Korhonen T, Malmivaara A, Paimela L, Kyllonen E, Lindgren KA, Rantanen P, Tervonen O, Niinimaki J, Seitsalo S, Hurri H (2003) Tumor necrosis factor-alpha monoclonal antibody, infliximab, used to manage severe sciatica. Spine 28(8):750–753; discussion 753–754

Kato F, Mimatsu K, Kawakami N, Iwata H, Miura T (1992) Serial changes observed by magnetic resonance imaging in the intervertebral disc after chemonucleolysis. A consideration of the mechanism of chemonucleolysis. Spine 17(8):934–939

Kawaguchi Y, Osada R, Kanamori M, Ishihara H, Ohmori K, Matsui H, Kimura T (1999) Association between an aggrecan gene polymorphism and lumbar disc degeneration. Spine 24(23):2456–2460

Kawakami M, Matsumoto T, Hashizume H, Kuribayashi K, Chubinskaya S, Yoshida M (2005) Osteogenic protein-1 (osteogenic protein-1/bone morphogenetic protein-7) inhibits degeneration and pain-related behavior induced by chronically compressed nucleus pulposus in the rat. Spine 30(17):1933–1939

Kim DJ, Moon SH, Kim H, Kwon UH, Park MS, Han KJ, Hahn SB, Lee HM (2003) Bone morphogenetic protein-2 facilitates expression of chondrogenic, not osteogenic, phenotype of human intervertebral disc cells. Spine 28(24):2679–2684

Kim JH, Deasy BM, Seo HY, Studer RK, Vo NV, Georgescu HI, Sowa GA, Kang JD (2009) Differentiation of intervertebral notochordal cells through live automated cell imaging system in vitro. Spine 34(23):2486–2493. doi:10.1097/BRS.0b013e3181b26ed1

Kim JS, Ellman MB, An HS, van Wijnen AJ, Borgia JA, Im HJ (2010) Insulin-like growth factor 1 synergizes with bone morphogenetic protein 7-mediated anabolism in bovine intervertebral disc cells. Arthritis Rheum 62(12):3706–3715. doi:10.1002/art.27733

Kim JS, Ellman MB, An HS, Yan D, van Wijnen AJ, Murphy G, Hoskin DW, Im HJ (2012) Lactoferricin mediates anabolic and anti-catabolic effects in the intervertebral disc. J Cell Physiol 227(4):1512–1520. doi:10.1002/jcp.22867

Larson JW 3rd, Levicoff EA, Gilbertson LG, Kang JD (2006) Biologic modification of animal models of intervertebral disc degeneration. J Bone Joint Surg Am 88(Suppl 2):83–87

Le Maitre CL, Freemont AJ, Hoyland JA (2004) Localization of degradative enzymes and their inhibitors in the degenerate human intervertebral disc. J Pathol 204(1):47–54

Le Maitre CL, Freemont AJ, Hoyland JA (2005) The role of interleukin-1 in the pathogenesis of human intervertebral disc degeneration. Arthritis Res Ther 7(4):R732–R745

Le Maitre CL, Hoyland JA, Freemont AJ (2007a) Catabolic cytokine expression in degenerate and herniated human intervertebral discs: IL-1beta and TNFalpha expression profile. Arthritis Res Ther 9(4):R77. doi:10.1186/ar2275, ar2275 [pii]

Le Maitre CL, Hoyland JA, Freemont AJ (2007b) Interleukin-1 receptor antagonist delivered directly and by gene therapy inhibits matrix degradation in the intact degenerate human intervertebral disc: an in situ zymographic and gene therapy study. Arthritis Res Ther 9(4):R83. doi:10.1186/ar2282, ar2282 [pii]

Le Maitre CL, Frain J, Fotheringham AP, Freemont AJ, Hoyland JA (2008) Human cells derived from degenerate intervertebral discs respond differently to those derived from non-degenerate intervertebral discs following application of dynamic hydrostatic pressure. Biorheology 45(5):563–575

Li S, Jia X, Duance VC, Blain EJ (2011) The effects of cyclic tensile strain on the organisation and expression of cytoskeletal elements in bovine intervertebral disc cells: an in vitro study. Eur Cell Mater 21:508–522

Maclean JJ, Lee CR, Alini M, Iatridis JC (2004) Anabolic and catabolic mRNA levels of the intervertebral disc vary with the magnitude and frequency of in vivo dynamic compression. J Orthop Res 22(6): 1193–1200

Masuda K, An HS (2006) Prevention of disc degeneration with growth factors. Eur Spine J 15(Suppl 15):422–432

Masuda K, Hejna M, Thonar EJ-MA (2000) Alginate-recovered-chondrocyte method (ARC method): a novel two-step method for the formation of cartilage tissue. Ortho Res Soc Trans 25:620

Masuda K, Takegami K, An H, Kumano F, Chiba K, Andersson GB, Schmid T, Thonar E (2003) Recombinant osteogenic protein-1 upregulates extracellular matrix metabolism by rabbit annulus fibrosus and nucleus pulposus cells cultured in alginate beads. J Orthop Res 21(5):922–930

Masuda K, Oegema TR Jr, An HS (2004) Growth factors and treatment of intervertebral disc degeneration. Spine 29(23):2757–2769

Masuda K, Imai Y, Okuma M, Muehleman C, Nakagawa K, Akeda K, Thonar E, Andersson G, An HS (2006) Osteogenic protein-1 injection into a degenerated disc induces the restoration of disc height and structural changes in the rabbit anular puncture model. Spine 31(7):742–754

Mazzocca AD, McCarthy MB, Chowaniec DM, Cote MP, Romeo AA, Bradley JP, Arciero RA, Beitzel K (2012) Platelet-rich plasma differs according to preparation method and human variability. J Bone Joint Surg Am 94(4):308–316. doi:10.2106/JBJS.K.00430

Miyamoto H, Saura R, Harada T, Doita M, Mizuno K (2000) The role of cyclooxygenase-2 and inflammatory cytokines in pain induction of herniated lumbar intervertebral disc. Kobe J Med Sci 46(1–2):13–28

Miyamoto K, Pichika R, An H, Thonar E-M, Akeda K, Lenz M, Masuda K (2005) Tumor Necrosis Factor-a exhibits potent effects on the metabolism of human intervertebral disc cells. Trans Orthop Res Soc:188

Miyamoto K, An HS, Urban JP, Chujo T, Akeda K, Masuda K (2006a) Low oxygen tension enhances anabolic effects of osteogenic protein-1 on the extracellular matrix metabolism of bovine intervertebral disc cells. Trans Orthop Res Soc 31:1205

Miyamoto K, Masuda K, Kim JG, Inoue N, Akeda K, Andersson GB, An HS (2006b) Intradiscal injections of osteogenic protein-1 restore the viscoelastic properties of degenerated intervertebral discs. Spine J 6(6):692–703

Mwale F, Masuda K, Pichika R, Epure LM, Yoshikawa T, Hemmad A, Roughley PJ, Antoniou J (2011) The efficacy of Link N as a mediator of repair in a rabbit model of intervertebral disc degeneration. Arthritis Res Ther 13(4):R120. doi:10.1186/ar3423

Nagae M, Ikeda T, Mikami Y, Hase H, Ozawa H, Matsuda K, Sakamoto H, Tabata Y, Kawata M, Kubo T (2007) Intervertebral disc regeneration using platelet-rich plasma and biodegradable gelatin hydrogel microspheres. Tissue Eng 13(1):147–158

Nakashima S, Matsuyama Y, Takahashi K, Satoh T, Koie H, Kanayama K, Tsuji T, Maruyama K, Imagama S, Sakai Y, Ishiguro N (2009) Regeneration of intervertebral disc by the intradiscal application of cross-linked hyaluronate hydrogel and cross-linked chondroitin sulfate hydrogel in a rabbit model of intervertebral disc injury. Biomed Mater Eng 19(6):421–429. doi:10.3233/BME-2009-0608

Nasto LA, Seo HY, Robinson AR, Tilstra JS, Clauson CL, Sowa GA, Ngo K, Dong Q, Pola E, Lee JY, Niedernhofer LJ, Kang JD, Robbins PD, Vo NV (2012) ISSLS prize winner: inhibition of Nf-kb activity ameliorates age-associated disc degeneration in a mouse model of accelerated aging. Spine (Phila Pa 1976). doi:10.1097/BRS.0b013e31824ee8f7

Nishimura K, Mochida J (1998) Percutaneous reinsertion of the nucleus pulposus. An experimental study. Spine 23(14):1531–1538

Noponen-Hietala N, Virtanen I, Karttunen R, Schwenke S, Jakkula E, Li H, Merikivi R, Barral S, Ott J, Karppinen J, Ala-Kokko L (2005) Genetic variations in IL6 associate with intervertebral disc disease characterized by sciatica. Pain 114(1–2):186–194

Norcross JP, Lester GE, Weinhold P, Dahners LE (2003) An in vivo model of degenerative disc disease. J Orthop Res 21(1):183–188

Obata S, Akeda K, Imanishi T, Masuda K, Bae W, Morimoto R, Asanuma Y, Kasai Y, Uchida A, Sudo A (2012) Effect of autologous platelet-rich plasma-releasate on intervertebral disc degeneration in the rabbit anular puncture model: a preclinical study. Arthritis Res Ther 14(6):R241. doi:10.1186/ar4084

Okoro T, Tafazal SI, Longworth S, Sell PJ (2010) Tumor necrosis alpha-blocking agent (etanercept): a triple blind randomized controlled trial of its use in treatment of sciatica. J Spinal Disord Tech 23(1):74–77. doi:10.1097/BSD.0b013e31819afdc4

Okuda K, Kawase T, Momose M, Murata M, Saito Y, Suzuki H, Wolff LF, Yoshie H (2003) Platelet-rich plasma contains high levels of platelet-derived growth factor and transforming growth factor-beta and modulates the proliferation of periodontally related cells in vitro. J Periodontol 74(6):849–857

Okuma M, Mochida J, Nishimura K, Sakabe K, Seiki K (2000) Reinsertion of stimulated nucleus pulposus cells retards intervertebral disc degeneration: an *in vitro* and *in vivo* experimental study. J Orthop Res 18(6):988–997

Olmarker K (2008) Puncture of a lumbar intervertebral disc induces changes in spontaneous pain behavior: an experimental study in rats. Spine 33(8):850–855. doi:10.1097/BRS.0b013e31816b46ca, 00007632-200804150-00005 [pii]

Olmarker K, Larsson K (1998) Tumor necrosis factor alpha and nucleus-pulposus-induced nerve root injury. Spine 23(23):2538–2544

Osada R, Ohshima H, Ishihara H, Yudoh K, Sakai K, Matsui H, Tsuji H (1996) Autocrine/paracrine mechanism of insulin-like growth factor-1 secretion, and the effect of insulin-like growth factor-1 on proteoglycan synthesis in bovine intervertebral discs. J Orthop Res 14(5):690–699

Patel KP, Sandy JD, Akeda K, Miyamoto K, Chujo T, An HS, Masuda K (2007) Aggrecanases and aggrecanase-generated fragments in the human intervertebral disc at early and advanced stages of disc degeneration. Spine 32(23):2596–2603. doi:10.1097/BRS.0b013e318158cb85, 00007632-200711010-00014 [pii]

Pichika R, Penta K, Yoshikawa T, Hemmad A, Lenz ME, Szymkowski DE, Binette F, Masuda K (2011) A new approach for anti-TNF therapy: dominant-negative TNF effectively antagonizes IL-1β-induced catabolic changes in human intervertebral disc cells. Trans Orthop Res Soc 36:709, abstract

Pichika R, Yamaguchi T, Taborek A, Bae WC, Sah RL, Masuda K (2012) Interactive effect of IL-1 and BMP-7 on cytokines, matrix components and gene expression of human intervertebral disc cells: implications of pH and oxygen tension on biological therapy. Trans Orthop Res Soc 37:64

Pierce A, Feng M, Masuda K (2006) Distribution, pharmacokinetics and excretion of 125-Iodine labeled BMP-7 [OP-1] following a single-dose administration in lumbar IVD or knee joint of NZW rabbits. In: Sixth International Conference on Bone Morphogenetic Proteins, Cavtat, Croatia, 11–15 Oct 2006

Pratsinis H, Kletsas D (2007) PDGF, bFGF and IGF-I stimulate the proliferation of intervertebral disc cells in vitro via the activation of the ERK and Akt signaling pathways. Eur Spine J 16(11):1858–1866. doi:10.1007/s00586-007-0408-9

Pratsinis H, Constantinou V, Pavlakis K, Sapkas G, Kletsas D (2012) Exogenous and autocrine growth factors stimulate human intervertebral disc cell proliferation via the ERK and Akt pathways. J Orthop Res 30(6):958–964. doi:10.1002/jor.22017

Rajasekaran S, Babu JN, Arun R, Armstrong BR, Shetty AP, Murugan S (2004) ISSLS prize winner: a study of diffusion in human lumbar discs: a serial magnetic resonance imaging study documenting the influence of the endplate on diffusion in normal and degenerate discs. Spine 29(23):2654–2667

Rajasekaran S, Venkatadass K, Naresh Babu J, Ganesh K, Shetty AP (2008) Pharmacological enhancement of disc diffusion and differentiation of healthy, ageing and degenerated discs: results from in-vivo serial post-contrast MRI studies in 365 human lumbar discs. Eur Spine J 17(5):626–643

Rannou F, Corvol MT, Hudry C, Anract P, Dumontier MF, Tsagris L, Revel M, Poiraudeau S (2000) Sensitivity of anulus fibrosus cells to interleukin 1 beta. Comparison with articular chondrocytes. Spine 25(1):17–23

Reddi AH (2000) Morphogenetic messages are in the extracellular matrix: biotechnology from bench to bedside. Biochem Soc Trans 28(4):345–349

Sakuma M, Fujii N, Takahashi T, Hoshino J, Miyauchi S, Iwata H (2002) Effect of chondroitinase ABC on matrix metalloproteinases and inflammatory mediators produced by intervertebral disc of rabbit in vitro. Spine 27(6):576–580

Sawamura K, Ikeda T, Nagae M, Okamoto S, Mikami Y, Hase H, Ikoma K, Yamada T, Sakamoto H, Matsuda K, Tabata Y, Kawata M, Kubo T (2009) Characterization of in vivo effects of platelet-rich plasma and biodegradable gelatin hydrogel microspheres on degenerated intervertebral discs. Tissue Eng Part A 15(12):3719–3727. doi:10.1089/ten.TEA.2008.0697

Schollmeier G, Lahr-Eigen R, Lewandrowski KU (2000) Observations on fiber-forming collagens in the anulus fibrosus. Spine 25(21):2736–2741

Scott JE, Haigh M (1986) Proteoglycan-collagen interactions in intervertebral disc. A chondroitin sulphate proteoglycan associates with collagen fibrils in rabbit annulus fibrosus at the d-e bands. Biosci Rep 6(10):879–888

Seki S, Kawaguchi Y, Chiba K, Mikami Y, Kizawa H, Oya T, Mio F, Mori M, Miyamoto Y, Masuda I, Tsunoda T, Kamata M, Kubo T, Toyama Y, Kimura T, Nakamura Y, Ikegawa S (2005) A functional SNP in CILP, encoding cartilage intermediate layer protein, is associated with susceptibility to lumbar disc disease. Nat Genet 37(6):607–612

Seki S, Asanuma-Abe Y, Masuda K, Kawaguchi Y, Asanuma K, Muehleman C, Iwai A, Kimura T (2009) Effect of small interference RNA (siRNA) for ADAMTS5 on intervertebral disc degeneration in the rabbit anular needle-puncture model. Arthritis Res Ther 11(6):R166. doi:10.1186/ar2851

Shamji MF, Betre H, Kraus VB, Chen J, Chilkoti A, Pichika R, Masuda K, Setton LA (2007) Development and characterization of a fusion protein between thermally responsive elastin-like polypeptide and interleukin-1 receptor antagonist: sustained release of a local antiinflammatory therapeutic. Arthritis Rheum 56(11):3650–3661. doi:10.1002/art.22952

Shamji MF, Allen KD, So S, Jing L, Adams SB Jr, Schuh R, Huebner J, Kraus VB, Friedman AH, Setton LA, Richardson WJ (2009) Gait abnormalities and inflammatory cytokines in an autologous nucleus pulposus model of radiculopathy. Spine 34(7):648–654. doi:10.1097/BRS.0b013e318197f013, 00007632-200904010-00004 [pii]

Sinclair SM, Shamji MF, Chen J, Jing L, Richardson WJ, Brown CR, Fitch RD, Setton LA (2011) Attenuation of inflammatory eventsin human intervertebral disc cells with a tumor necrosis factor antagonist. Spine 36(15):1190–1196. doi:10.1097/BRS.0b013e3181ebdb43

Sobajima S, Shimer AL, Chadderdon RC, Kompel JF, Kim JS, Gilbertson LG, Kang JD (2005) Quantitative analysis of gene expression in a rabbit model of intervertebral disc degeneration by real-time polymerase chain reaction. Spine J 5(1):14–23

Solovieva S, Kouhia S, Leino-Arjas P, Ala-Kokko L, Luoma K, Raininko R, Saarela J, Riihimaki H (2004) Interleukin 1 polymorphisms and intervertebral disc degeneration. Epidemiology 15(5):626–633

Solovieva S, Lohiniva J, Leino-Arjas P, Raininko R, Luoma K, Ala-Kokko L, Riihimaki H (2006) Intervertebral disc degeneration in relation to the COL9A3 and the IL-1ss gene polymorphisms. Eur Spine J 15(5):613–619

Song YQ, Cheung KM, Ho DW, Poon SC, Chiba K, Kawaguchi Y, Hirose Y, Alini M, Grad S, Yee AF, Leong JC, Luk KD, Yip SP, Karppinen J, Cheah KS, Sham P, Ikegawa S, Chan D (2008) Association of the asporin D14 allele with lumbar-disc degeneration in Asians. Am J Hum Genet 82(3):744–747. doi:10.1016/j.ajhg.2007.12.017

Stoyanov JV, Gantenbein-Ritter B, Bertolo A, Aebli N, Baur M, Alini M, Grad S (2011) Role of hypoxia and growth and differentiation factor-5 on differentiation of human mesenchymal stem cells towards intervertebral nucleus pulposus-like cells. Eur Cell Mater 21:533–547

Studer RK, Gilbertson LG, Georgescu H, Sowa G, Vo N, Kang JD (2008) p38 MAPK inhibition modulates rabbit nucleus pulposus cell response to IL-1. J Orthop Res. doi:10.1002/jor.20604

Sugimura T, Kato F, Mimatsu K, Takenaka O, Iwata H (1996) Experimental chemonucleolysis with chondroitinase ABC in monkeys. Spine 21(2):161–165

Suzuki M, Inoue G, Gemba T, Watanabe T, Ito T, Koshi T, Yamauchi K, Yamashita M, Orita S, Eguchi Y, Ochiai N, Kishida S, Takaso M, Aoki Y, Takahashi K, Ohtori S (2009) Nuclear factor-kappa B decoy suppresses nerve injury and improves mechanical allodynia and thermal hyperalgesia in a rat lumbar disc herniation model. Eur Spine J. doi:10.1007/s00586-009-0940-x

Takahashi H, Suguro T, Okazima Y, Motegi M, Okada Y, Kakiuchi T (1996a) Inflammatory cytokines in the herniated disc of the lumbar spine. Spine 21(2):218–224

Takahashi T, Kurihara H, Nakajima S, Kato T, Matsuzaka S, Sekiguchi T, Onaya M, Miyauchi S, Mizuno S, Horie K, Fujita Y, Hirose T (1996b) Chemonucleolytic effects of chondroitinase ABC on normal rabbit intervertebral discs. Course of action up to 10 days postinjection and minimum effective dose. Spine 21(21): 2405–2411

Takahashi M, Haro H, Wakabayashi Y, Kawa-uchi T, Komori H, Shinomiya K (2001) The association of degeneration of the intervertebral disc with 5a/6a polymorphism in the promoter of the human matrix metalloproteinase-3 gene. J Bone Joint Surg Br 83(4):491–495

Takegami K, Thonar EJ, An HS, Kamada H, Masuda K (2002) Osteogenic protein-1 enhances matrix replenishment by intervertebral disc cells previously exposed to interleukin-1. Spine 27(12): 1318–1325

Takegami K, An HS, Kumano F, Chiba K, Thonar EJ, Singh K, Masuda K (2005) Osteogenic protein-1 is most effective in stimulating nucleus pulposus and annulus fibrosus cells to repair their matrix after chondroitinase ABC-induced in vitro chemonucleolysis. Spine J 5(3):231–238

Thompson JP, Oegema TJ, Bradford DS (1991) Stimulation of mature canine intervertebral disc by growth factors. Spine 16(3): 253–260

Tilkeridis C, Bei T, Garantziotis S, Stratakis CA (2005) Association of a COL1A1 polymorphism with lumbar disc disease in young military recruits. J Med Genet 42(7):e44

Tobinick EL, Britschgi-Davoodifar S (2003) Perispinal TNF-alpha inhibition for discogenic pain. Swiss Med Wkly 133(11–12):170–177, doi:2003/11/smw-10163

Tonomura H, Miyamoto K, Sah R, Urban J, Kubo T, Asanuma K, Lenz M, Masuda K (2007) Low oxygen tension and BMP-7 synergistically stimulate synthesis and deposition of proteoglycan by bovine articular chondrocytes in alginate beads. Ortho Res Soc Trans 32:257

Tozum TF, Demiralp B (2003) Platelet-rich plasma: a promising innovation in dentistry. J Can Dent Assoc 69(10):664

Trout J, Buckwalter J, Moore K, Landa S (1982) Ultrastructure of human intervertebral disc. I. Changes in notochordal cells with age. Tissue Cells 14:359–369

Urban JP (2002) The role of the physicochemical environment in determining disc cell behaviour. Biochem Soc Trans 30(Pt 6):858–864

Urban JP, Smith S, Fairbank JC (2004) Nutrition of the intervertebral disc. Spine 29(23):2700–2709

Videman T, Leppavuori J, Kaprio J, Battie MC, Gibbons LE, Peltonen L, Koskenvuo M (1998) Intragenic polymorphisms of the vitamin D receptor gene associated with intervertebral disc degeneration. Spine 23(23):2477–2485

Virtanen IM, Song YQ, Cheung KM, Ala-Kokko L, Karppinen J, Ho DW, Luk KD, Yip SP, Leong JC, Cheah KS, Sham P, Chan D (2007) Phenotypic and population differences in the association between CILP and lumbar disc disease. J Med Genet 44(4): 285–288. doi:10.1136/jmg.2006.047076, jmg.2006.047076 [pii]

Wallach CJ, Sobajima S, Watanabe Y, Kim JS, Georgescu HI, Robbins P, Gilbertson LG, Kang JD (2003) Gene transfer of the catabolic inhibitor TIMP-1 increases measured proteoglycans in cells from degenerated human intervertebral discs. Spine 28(20): 2331–2337

Walsh AJ, Bradford DS, Lotz JC (2004) In vivo growth factor treatment of degenerated intervertebral discs. Spine 29(2):156–163

Wei A, Williams LA, Bhargav D, Shen B, Kishen T, Duffy N, Diwan AD (2009) BMP13 prevents the effects of annular injury in an ovine model. Int J Biol Sci 5(5):388–396

Weibrich G, Kleis WK, Hafner G, Hitzler WE (2002) Growth factor levels in platelet-rich plasma and correlations with donor age, sex, and platelet count. J Craniomaxillofac Surg 30(2):97–102

Weiler C, Nerlich AG, Bachmeier BE, Boos N (2005) Expression and distribution of tumor necrosis factor alpha in human lumbar intervertebral discs: a study in surgical specimen and autopsy controls. Spine 30(1):44–53; discussion 54

Yamada K, Tanabe S, Ueno H, Oinuma A, Takahashi T, Miyauchi S, Shigeno S, Hirose T, Miyahara K, Sato M (2001) Investigation of

the short-term effect of chemonucleolysis with chondroitinase ABC. J Vet Med Sci 63(5):521–525
Yoon TS, Su Kim K, Li J, Soo Park J, Akamaru T, Elmer WA, Hutton WC (2003) The effect of bone morphogenetic protein-2 on rat intervertebral disc cells in vitro. Spine 28(16):1773–1780
Yurube T, Nishida K, Suzuki T, Kaneyama S, Zhang Z, Kakutani K, Maeno K, Takada T, Fujii M, Kurosaka M, Doita M (2010) Matrix metalloproteinase (MMP)-3 gene up-regulation in a rat tail compression loading-induced disc degeneration model. J Orthop Res 28(8):1026–1032. doi:10.1002/jor.21116

Tissue Engineering of the Intervertebral Disc

26

Rita Kandel, Paul Santerre, Eric Massicotte, and Mark Hurtig

Contents

R. Kandel, MD (✉)
Department of Pathology and Laboratory Medicine, Mount Sinai Hospital, University of Toronto, Toronto, ON, Canada

P. Santerre, PhD
Institute of Biomaterials and Biomedical Engineering, University of Toronto, Toronto, ON, Canada

E. Massicotte, MD
Department of Neurosurgery, Toronto Western Hospital, Toronto, ON, Canada

Department of Surgery, University of Toronto, Toronto, ON, Canada

M. Hurtig, DVM
Department of Clinical Studies, Ontario Veterinary College, University of Guelph, Guelph, ON, Canada

I.M. Shapiro, M.V. Risbud (eds.), *The Intervertebral Disc*, DOI 10.1007/978-3-7091-1535-0_26, © Springer-Verlag Wien 2014

26.1 Introduction

In an autopsy study, 97 % of individuals 50 years or older had histological evidence of intervertebral disc degeneration, a disease process that involves the annulus fibrosus, nucleus pulposus, and cartilaginous endplate (Miller et al. 1988). The back pain that can develop as a result of this disease has a lifetime prevalence of up to 80 % (Manchikanti et al. 2009; Takatalo et al. 2011, 2012). Approximately 1 in 50 Canadians becomes disabled by back pain which is responsible for 40 % of all workplace absences (Iron et al. 2004; Lee 1994; Rapoport et al. 2004). Although rarely life threatening, the annual total costs in 2002 in the USA as a result of back pain were over $100 billion (Asche et al. 2007; Dagenais et al. 2008; Iron et al. 2004; Lee 1994) (for a detailed discussion, see Chap. 9). It has been estimated that in the USA alone, there are up to four million adults with chronic back pain who have failed conservative therapy (Masuda and Lotz 2010) and although there are a number of surgical options for these individuals, they all have limitations (Chou et al. 2009; Kishen and Diwan 2010; Raj 2008). Discectomy which relieves pain (325,000 operations performed in 2004 in the USA) (2008) does not restore disc height or its original load-bearing capacity (Putzier et al. 2005). Spinal fusion (375,000 surgeries in 2004 in the USA) (2008) is another commonly performed treatment; as has been discussed earlier, this is not always successful, often leading to pseudoarthrosis and limited flexibility (Kishen and Diwan 2010; Mirza and Deyo 2007). Although controversial, some studies suggest that this type of treatment may induce degenerative changes in adjacent vertebrae (Huang et al. 2006; Javedan and Dickman 1999; Kim and Branch 2006; Lee et al. 2012a, b; Schulte et al. 2007). Disc replacement with a motion-preserving prosthesis, such as partial or total disc replacement, is another option (Fekete and Porchet 2010; Kishen and Diwan 2010; Shim et al. 2007; So et al. 2007; Vernengo et al. 2008).

However, there are numerous clinical contraindications to this treatment (Fekete and Porchet 2010; Shim et al. 2007), and these replacements do not fully restore kinematics (Fekete and Porchet 2010). This topic is discussed in considerable detail in Chap. 14. As well, disc prostheses can generate wear debris (van Ooij et al. 2007) and the reaction that this incites has the potential to be catastrophic given its location near major vessels and nerves. The long-term exposure to ions, such as cobalt and chromium, which can be detected in the serum after disc replacement is unknown (Zeh et al. 2009). Given all these issues, there has been great interest in developing new therapeutic options such as biological approaches for the treatment of chronic symptomatic disc disease (Bron et al. 2009; Kandel et al. 2008; Masuda and Lotz 2010; O'Halloran and Pandit 2007; Richardson et al. 2007). Cell-based therapies that regenerate the disc avoid the functional impact on the disc and/or adjacent tissues as well as the consequences of metal fatigue and the reaction to wear debris (Guyer et al. 2011; Tumialan and Gluf 2011). Importantly the regenerated tissue can remodel and respond to load in a way synthetic prostheses or fused discs cannot.

Box 26.1 What Is Regenerative Medicine?
Tissue engineering (regenerative medicine) is an interdisciplinary field that applies the principles of engineering (materials and biomedical engineering) and life sciences (genetics, cell and molecular biology) to the development of biological substitutes that can restore, maintain, or enhance tissue function that has been damaged by congenital abnormalities, disease, age, or trauma. It involves any combination of cells, materials, biomolecules, and/or mechanics (Langer and Vacanti 1993). First recognized as a field in the late 1980s, it has grown to incorporate the advances in basic science to enhance biological repair. Tissue-engineered products being used clinically now include skin and bladder and cartilage repair products are in clinical trials. Bioengineered tissues have other uses. For example, they can be used to investigate the mechanisms regulating tissue formation or for preclinical drug testing.

26.2 What Is the Goal for Cell-Based Therapies and Tissue Engineering?

The intervertebral disc is a specialized structure consisting of interdependent tissues: the annulus fibrosus which surrounds the centrally placed nucleus pulposus and is integrated into the cartilage endplate (Hukins 1994; Simon 1994). The outer annulus fibrosus is responsible for withstanding circumferential tensile forces while the nucleus pulposus and inner annulus fibrosus resist compressive forces (Hukins 1994; Simon 1994). Together these tissues can handle more load than each tissue alone, stressing the importance of properly integrated structures (Bogduk 1997). The intact cartilage endplate is also necessary. This tissue contributes to the maintenance of nucleus pulposus cell viability, absorbs the water that extrudes from the nucleus pulposus during loading, and prevents protrusion of the nucleus into the adjacent vertebral body (Benneker et al. 2005; Grunhagen et al. 2006; Horner and Urban 2001; Moore 2006; Roberts et al. 1996; Shirazi-Adl et al. 2010). The importance of a properly functioning cartilaginous endplate (Miller et al. 1988) is demonstrated by the fact that animal models of disc degeneration are created by damaging the endplate (Cinotti et al. 2005; Holm et al. 2004) or by endplate calcification (Gruber et al. 2007; Peng et al. 2001; Sahlman et al. 2001). A recent population study showed that the presence of Schmorl's nodes correlated with disc degeneration and low back pain (Takatalo et al. 2011, 2012). The organization of the intervertebral disc allows the disc to rotate, flex, and resist tensile and shear forces and is critical for proper disc function, especially, as the disc under certain conditions has to withstand up to ten times body weight. Thus, it would appear that for long-term success the goal should be repair and/or replacement of all the damaged tissues of the disc.

26.3 Intervertebral Disc Composition and Architecture: What Will Bioengineered Tissues Have to Recapitulate?

26.3.1 Annulus Fibrosus

While considerable information is provided elsewhere in the book concerning the detailed structure of the annulus, it is worthwhile reminding the reader that the annulus is a very well-engineered tissue and exquisitely adapted to its physiological role. It surrounds the nucleus pulposus and has a *cross-ply* laminate structure consisting of between 10 and 25 lamellae, each composed of collagen fibers oriented parallel to each other and about 65° from the vertical (Bron et al. 2009; Marchand and Ahmed 1990). The direction of the inclination alternates with each layer such that the fibers in one lamella are 65° to the right, while in the next lamella they are 65° to the left, so every second lamella has the same orientation. Lamella, which can be discontinuous, varies in thickness depending on the location in the disc and ranges from 100 to 600 μm (Marchand and Ahmed 1990). They have a unique insertion into the vertebral body and this differs somewhat between the outer and inner annulus (Nosikova et al. 2012). The collagen concentration is highest in the outer annulus and gradually decreases with progression towards the nucleus (Eyre 1979). The outer annulus fibrosus is composed predominately of collagen I with increasing amounts of collagen II present within the inner annulus. It also contains elastin both within the lamellae and between lamellae (Yu et al. 2002, 2005, 2007), a small amount of proteoglycans of which the most abundant is aggrecan (Inerot and Axelsson 1991) but others such as decorin, biglycan, versican, and fibromodulin are also present (Gotz et al. 1997). The proteoglycans have a differential distribution which is opposite to that of collagen so that the inner annulus fibrosus lamellae are separated by more proteoglycan-rich matrix than those in the outer annulus (Bron et al. 2009). The inner annulus fibrosus merges almost imperceptibly with the nucleus pulposus. The difference in composition between the inner and outer aspects of the annulus fibrosus may reflect the different functions of these regions (Bron et al. 2009; Hsieh and Twomey 2010). Translamellar bridges are seen in the outer annulus and recent work by Elliot et al. suggested that these represent areas of blood vessel regression (Melrose et al. 2008; Schollum et al. 2010; Schollum et al. 2009; Smith and Elliott 2011). It is not known whether they play a role in the biomechanical functioning of the disc. The interface of the annulus fibrosus with the vertebral body is complex, as a portion of the collagen fibers pass through the cartilage endplate into the calcified zone and the remainder sweep laterally to merge with the periosteum (Nosikova et al. 2012).

26.3.2 Nucleus Pulposus

Probably the most important tissue to be engineered in the disc is the nucleus pulposus. It consists of proteoglycans within a loose network of collagen that does not demonstrate the same level of organization as the annulus fibrosus (Bibby et al. 2001; Chan et al. 2011). Proteoglycans comprise up to 65 % of the dry weight of the nucleus. Aggrecan is the major proteoglycan and responsible for binding water thereby enabling the nucleus to resist compressive loads (Chan et al. 2011). Other proteoglycans such as versican, decorin, and fibromodulin are also present (Melrose et al. 2001; Singh et al. 2009; Smith et al. 2009). The nucleus contains predominately collagen II and lesser amounts of collagens III, VI, IX, and XI (Chan et al. 2011). The nucleus contains notochordal cells but the latter cell type either disappears or its morphology changes with age (for a detailed discussion of this topic, see Chaps. 3 and 21) (Choi et al. 2008; McCann et al. 2012; Risbud and Shapiro 2011; Weiler et al. 2010). The notochordal cells likely contribute to disc function and/or maintenance, but how this is achieved is not entirely known at this time (Abbott et al. 2012; Cappello et al. 2006; Risbud et al. 2010).

26.3.3 Cartilage Endplate

The cartilage endplate is a thin (about 1 mm) layer of hyaline cartilage, rich in collagen II. It is integrated with the vertebral body, nucleus pulposus, and annulus fibrosus (Moore 2006). Like articular cartilage, the plate consists predominately of water, proteoglycans, and collagen, but differs from that tissue in organization and amounts of these molecules (Gruber et al. 2007; Moore 2006). Vascular channels penetrate the cartilaginous endplate (Miller et al. 1988), but after growth has ceased, these are obliterated and nutrients and oxygen must diffuse from blood vessels in the vertebral body through the tissue (Benneker et al. 2005; Rajasekaran et al. 2004). In vitro studies suggest that the chondrocytes produce a factor that inhibits TNFα production by nucleus pulposus cells, and thus it may play a role in preventing many of the changes that are characteristic of aging (and degeneration) (Arana et al. 2010). The multiple functions of the cartilage layer in terms of nutrition and oxygen diffusion as well as protection of the nucleus stresses the necessity for an intact cartilage endplate when engineering a substitute tissue.

26.4 The Role of Tissue Architecture in Disc Function

Aside from addressing the needs of the molecular architecture briefly described above, the engineered disc will also need to replace many if not all of the functional requirements of the spine. As a major component of this functional unit, the annulus fibrosus can be viewed as an anisotropic, nonlinear, viscoelastic tissue (Hsieh and Twomey 2010). As discussed in detail in Chaps. 2 and 7, compressive loading causes disc narrowing and outward bulging, placing axial compressive forces as well as tensile (biaxial) strains along the circumference of the annulus fibrosus (Nerurkar et al. 2010a, b). Part of the compressive force is transmitted by the nucleus from one vertebral body to the next, decreasing the load borne by the annulus. Sudden increases in compressive stress are propagated through the vertebral column; because of interpositions of the intervertebral disc, changes in compressive stress are converted into tensile stain towards the outer annulus (Markolf and Morris 1974). This region experiences tensile strain with some compression in the inner aspect; the inner annulus fibrosus is compressed as it resists the circumferential expansion of the nucleus pulposus. With compression, collagen crimp angles change from outer to inner annulus fibrosus, resulting in both depth-dependent and linear region stiffness (Holzapfel et al. 2005). It has also been suggested that inter-collagen fiber shear is important in strain redistribution (Desrochers and Duncan 2010) which may affect nutrient diffusion (Ambard and Cherblanc 2009). These biomechanical events are relevant to the healthy disc; however, with degeneration of the nucleus pulposus, reorientation of the annulus fibrosus is compromised and tensile forces are transferred to the annulus fibrosus (Adams et al. 1996, 2009; Guerin and Elliott 2006). Finite element modeling suggests that strains in the inner annulus increase with degeneration and that with progressive disease this strain is transferred to the vertebral endplate (Schmidt et al. 2009). Thus, intact and properly oriented and interfaced annulus fibrosus lamellae are necessary for proper responses to loading (Adams et al. 2009; Guerin and Elliott 2006). Furthermore, it appears that annulus fibrosus fiber tension not only limits axial rotation (Krismer et al. 1996) but also limits susceptibility to degeneration (Lotz et al. 2008). These biomechanical principles are critical architectural features to be borne in mind in engineering a new intervertebral disc.

26.5 Tissue-Engineering Components

Diseases that afflict articulating joints in the appendicular skeleton involve cartilage and in some settings bone. In the disc, three tissues, the nucleus pulposus, the annulus fibrosus, and the cartilaginous endplate, are all impacted by the disease process (Miller et al. 1988). From this perspective, in order to achieve proper function, all of these tissues may require repair/replacement. Having to recapitulate three tissues, each with very different molecular architecture and function adds a level of complexity to successful biological disc repair.

The strategies for tissue engineering of disc tissues are similar to that of other tissues, namely, to use a combination of cells, scaffolds, growth factors, and/or mechanical signals. The choice is dictated by the tissue(s) under repair. Given that the disc is always loaded, the repair/replacement tissue will likely experience mechanical forces and signals immediately upon implantation.

26.5.1 Cells

One of the major issues limiting the clinical application of biological disc repair/replacement therapies is the identification of a suitable source of cells. Cells could be obtained from a number of tissues, such as the disc itself, cartilage, or bone marrow. It is not yet clear whether the cells used for nucleus pulposus repair must include notochordal cells. In vitro studies have shown that notochord cells produce factors, such as CTGF, which enhances matrix production by nucleus pulposus cells (Erwin 2008; Purmessur et al. 2011). Some investigations indicate that notochordal cells are critical for the maintenance of nucleus tissue (Risbud et al. 2010; Risbud and Shapiro 2011; Shapiro and Risbud 2010). If these cells are required, obtaining sufficient numbers from any of the sources listed above may be problematic, although recent studies in our laboratory suggest that under the appropriate culture conditions, notochord cell numbers in nucleus pulposus tissue can be increased in vitro (Kandel 2011, unpublished data).

Although nucleus pulposus cells would be ideal to use for tissue engineering, they are limited in number and would have to be expanded in culture to get sufficient numbers (Gruber et al. 1997; Maroudas et al. 1975). In the healthy nucleus, the cell density has been reported to be 4,000/mm^2; however, it may even been even lower since, with age, a proportion of the cells become senescent (Roberts et al. 2006). Not only do these cells have a slower proliferative rate, they also have an altered phenotype (Le Maitre et al. 2007). A sufficient number of cells may be obtained from herniated disc tissue; this approach may not be straightforward since these cells may be dedifferentiated with limited ability to regenerate tissue in vitro compared to cells obtained from the nucleus pulposus compartment (Hegewald et al. 2011a).

For the reasons stated above, it may be necessary to utilize allogeneic or xenogeneic sources; these cells carry the risk for immune reaction and disease transmission. If cells from the nucleus pulposus are to be used for tissue-engineering purposes, then genetic problems must be accommodated. As discussed in Chap. 10, polymorphism (Trp2 allele) in the COL9A2 gene encoding the alpha2 chain of collagen IX can predispose an individual to disc degeneration (Richardson and Hoyland 2008; Jim et al. 2005). Non-degenerated discs from these individuals were found to be mechanically inferior to non-degenerated normal discs (Aladin et al. 2007). This finding suggests that the use of genetically altered primary cells isolated from an otherwise healthy intervertebral disc may not be appropriate for regeneration of normal tissue. Use of nucleus pulposus cells also may be limited as they have been shown to lose their regenerative capacity with age (Kandel et al. 2007). A recent study demonstrated that matrix retention by nucleus pulposus cells obtained from adolescent cows is impaired and that compared to those obtained from younger animals (calves), matrix gene expression is decreased (Kandel et al. 2007). If similar alterations occur in human cells, it may not be appropriate to use nucleus pulposus cells from older patients unless conditions are identified that "prime" the cells and encourage reversion to a more juvenile geno/phenotype.

Box 26.2 Requirements of Cells for Regenerative Medicine

One of the factors preventing clinical application of regenerative medicine is a suitable source of cells to generate the tissue. Clearly primary cells are not an option. Stem cells will likely be critical to overcome this limitation. However, the mechanisms regulating differentiation to the appropriate cell types have yet to be fully elucidated. Delineation of the conditions to accomplish this in vitro is necessary, and factors such as the culture conditions, choice of culture media, presence of biomolecules, appropriate biomaterial, proper oxygenation status, and mechanical stimulation are all currently under investigation.

Many of the issues limiting the use of differentiated cells may be overcome using autologous stem cells. Developmentally, the annulus cells are derived from mesoderm, whereas nucleus pulposus cells are derived from the notochord (Chan et al. 2011; Choi et al. 2008; McCann et al. 2012). Thus, these cells could be obtained from a number of different tissue types, the most common being bone marrow (marrow stromal cells, MSCs) or adipose tissue (adipose-derived stem cells) (Ahmed et al. 2007; Bieback et al. 2008; Zuk et al. 2002). MSCs have the capability to commit to several different lineages including cartilage, bone, or adipose tissue in vitro, and it is speculated that they can also give rise to disc cells although the evidence for this is limited. Generating nucleus pulposus or annulus fibrosus cells from MSCs has been stymied by our lack of knowledge of tissue phenotype such as the characteristic molecular profile of these cells, a topic considered in detail in Chap. 11.

Despite an ever-increasing number of studies of stem cells and cells of the nucleus pulposus, difficulties still exist in confirming that a stem or stromal cell has differentiated along the disc lineage. For example, Steck et al. suggested that MSCs can adopt a gene expression profile resembling native disc cells but the molecules they examined are also present in the cartilage (Steck et al. 2005). It has been suggested that co-culturing MSC with disc or notochordal cells may be another way to effect conversion to a chondrogenic/discogenic phenotype (Korecki et al. 2010; Le Visage et al. 2006; Purmessur et al. 2011; Richardson et al. 2006; Strassburg et al. 2010; Vadala et al. 2008), possibly via paracrine effects or cell-cell interactions (Vadala et al. 2008). Given that MSC can differentiate to chondrocytes, ensuring that the MSC commit entirely to the nucleus pulposus phenotype has not yet been possible. An alternative approach is to use MSC to secrete factors that activate and stimulate nucleus pulposus cell matrix production and/or accumulation and thus potentiate tissue repair (Doorn et al. 2012; Miyamoto et al. 2010; Strassburg et al. 2010). However, there are further issues associated with the use of MSCs: with age they can lose their regenerative capability (Choumerianou et al. 2010; Erickson et al. 2011). Extensive culture and population doublings may promote senescence, and cell karyotype and gene expression can become altered (Wang et al. 2005; Wilson et al. 2010). For example, a subpopulation of cells in MSC culture was noted to appear morphologically distinct from typical human MSCs (Wang et al. 2005). These cells showed a high level of telomerase activity compared with typical MSCs and formed tumors when transplanted into NOD/SCID mice.

Embryonic stem cells (hESC), another potential source of cells, are derived from the inner cell mass of the embryo (Munoz et al. 2008). ESC can be readily maintained as undifferentiated cells under defined conditions, providing an unlimited supply of pluripotent stem cells. They are capable of differentiating into all three germ layers of the embryo and hence all cell types of the human body. While developing new approaches to use hESC as a source of chondrocytes is an area of intense investigation, little work has been done in this regard with disc cells. To date, deriving chondrocytes from embryonic stem cells that can form articular cartilage tissue has not been fully accomplished, suggesting that identifying conditions that induce differentiation of hESC to disc cells in cell culture is a long way off. Interestingly, in one study mouse ESC were differentiated in vitro to chondrocyte-type cells; these cells transdifferentiated to notochord cells following implantation into rabbit discs (Sheikh et al. 2009). These results suggest that ESC may be a source of notochordal cells, but this topic requires further study. Another issue associated with the use of ESC cells is that they can give rise to teratomas – an unacceptable complication for a treatment of a benign disease (Schriebl et al. 2012). To circumvent this problem, it will be necessary to ensure that there are no residual hESCs after induction of differentiation (Schriebl et al. 2012). Consideration will also have to be given to the ethical concerns related to the collection of these cells which could limit their application clinically.

Inducible progenitor cells (iPSC) hold much promise for disc repair and obviate the ethical issues related to the use of embryonic stem cells. iPSC can be generated by the transfection of the four transcription factors Oct3/4, Sox2, c-Myc, and Klf4 (Yamanaka factors) into somatic cells such as human fibroblasts (Maherali et al. 2008; Takahashi et al. 2007; Takahashi and Yamanaka 2006). The transduced cells return to an undifferentiated, pluripotent state and resemble ES cells (Takahashi et al. 2007). A new technology using virus-independent, transposon-mediated reprogramming of somatic cells into iPS cells has recently been developed (Woltjen et al. 2009), eliminating one of the potential contraindications to the clinical use of these cells. Successful differentiation into cell types such as chondrocytes and melanocytes suggests that iPSC have the potential to be an appropriate cell source for tissue engineering of the disc (Wei et al. 2012; Yang et al. 2011). However, recent studies have identified genetic and methylation changes in iPSCs and issues related to immunogenicity, all of which raise questions as to their suitability for tissue engineering (Barrilleaux and Knoepfler 2011; Lister et al. 2011; Zhao et al. 2011). Clearly, there is much work to be done before these cells can be used in clinical trials (Nakagawa et al. 2008; Yamanaka 2007).

Chondrocytes are another source of cells to use for nucleus pulposus repair. A study by Acosta et al. (2011) showed that juvenile chondrocytes formed cartilage tissue when implanted into porcine discs whereas MSC did not. However, the efficacy of these cells in the long term is not known. As there is increasing evidence that nucleus pulposus cells are different than chondrocytes, even though they produce many of the same molecules, perhaps they should not be used for nucleus repair (Mwale et al. 2004).

There has been little investigation into which cells are suitable to use for annulus fibrosus repair. MSC would seem to be an appropriate source of cells as the annulus fibrosus developmentally arises from the mesoderm. Annulus cells themselves could be used as when grown in monolayer culture, annulus cells maintain their phenotype for up to two passages (Chou et al. 2006). These cells would either have to be obtained from allogeneic or xenogeneic tissues similar to nucleus pulposus cells unless the entire disc is being replaced.

Another potential problem with growing the cells in vitro prior to implantation is their contact with animal products such as fetal calf serum (Tekkatte et al. 2011). Bovine proteins incorporated into the cell membrane could induce an immune response. There is also the risk of infection following implantation (Harrison et al. 2000). Interest in developing alternatives to animal serum to avoid these problems, such as growing cells in autologous serum (Harrison et al. 2000; Lange et al. 2007; Shahdadfar et al. 2005; Tekkatte et al. 2011) or human platelet plasma, is being investigated (Bieback et al. 2009; Schallmoser et al. 2007).

26.5.2 Scaffolds

For disc tissue engineering, roles for scaffolds include retention of cells in a desired location, provision of mechanical properties (sufficient for weight bearing while tissue is growing and maturing), and/or delivery of biochemical cues to the tissue as it is developing or to guide tissue ingrowth (Ikada 2006). Scaffold requirements are such that the material must be biocompatible and biodegradable at a rate that mirrors tissue regeneration. For the nucleus pulposus, a liquid-based scaffold would likely be preferable, whereas for the annulus fibrosus, a fiber-type scaffold would be better. The choice of scaffold is critical as it can affect the tissue that develops. Scaffold fiber diameter and stiffness have been shown to influence cell phenotype, function, proliferation, and orientation (Hadjipanayi et al. 2009; Hsia et al. 2011; Saino et al. 2011). These responses could be utilized in the design of disc scaffolds that enhance cell differentiation.

Adhesion molecules used to coat the scaffolds can also affect cell function (Attia et al. 2010). For example, as shown by Attia et al. (2010), polyurethane scaffolds coated with fibronectin result in an annulus fibrosus-like structure, cells that are aligned and elongated similar to native tissue, and importantly the newly synthesized collagen is also properly oriented parallel to the cell. In contrast if the scaffold is coated with collagen I, the cells assume a polygonal shape and collagen production is delayed and poorly oriented. In addition, the scaffold can influence the recipient tissue reaction after implantation. For example, breakdown products could induce fibrosis or lower the local pH; this is seen when polylactic/glycolic acid scaffolds degrade and release acid which negatively affects cell matrix synthesis (Razaq et al. 2003). One way to overcome some of the problems linked to cell source is to functionalize acellular scaffolds with biomolecules or genes. For example, in a study of intervertebral disc degeneration in rabbits, injection of platelet-rich plasma (containing growth factors) encapsulated in gelatin microspheres into the nucleus pulposus slowed down the disease process compared to untreated animals (Nagae et al. 2007).

26.5.3 Growth Factors

The role of growth factors in maintaining the disc phenotype during cell expansion in vitro and for tissue formation has not been studied extensively. Several studies have shown that growth factors, for example, OP-1 (BMP-7) (Masuda and Lotz 2010), enhance matrix production by nucleus pulposus and annulus fibrosus cells. Treatment of MSCs with growth factors may influence differentiation: one example is TGFβ3 treatment of MSCs maintained on a photo-cross-linked carboxymethyl cellulose hydrogel scaffold (Gupta et al. 2011). Whether the treated cells commit to a nucleus pulposus cell lineage or chondrocyte phenotype has yet to be determined. It has been shown that treatment with a growth factor, such as GDF5, or transduction with growth factor genes can enhance disc repair in vivo. These results lend strong support to the notion that growth factors have a major role to play in biological repair (Masuda 2008; Zhang et al. 2008). Further discussion of this topic is presented in Chaps. 23, 24, and 25.

26.6 Tissue-Engineering Approaches

26.6.1 Nucleus Pulposus Tissue Engineering

Repair of the nucleus pulposus by tissue engineering has received more attention than the annulus fibrosus for two reasons: the nucleus is a relatively less complex tissue and early disc degeneration can occur in the nucleus before being evident in the annulus. A number of different approaches have been taken to engineer the nucleus pulposus such as injections of cells (nucleus pulposus cells, chondrocytes, or mesenchymal stromal cells or stem cells) alone or in a scaffold or implantation of nucleus pulposus tissue formed in vitro prior to implantation.

26.6.1.1 Cell Therapy

A strategy for early disease repair is to inject cells into the disc at a time when only the nucleus pulposus is damaged and the annulus fibrosus and cartilaginous endplate (Miller et al. 1988) are intact. The implanted cells are postulated to work by one of two ways: either by synthesizing matrix or stimulating the endogenous remaining nucleus pulposus cells to synthesize matrix. There is increasing evidence that cell therapy for nucleus pulposus repair may be an appropriate approach. Injection of autologous nucleus pulposus cells or stem cells into the disc has been shown to delay degeneration in both small and large (dog and monkey) animal models (Allon et al. 2010; Crevensten et al. 2004; Ganey et al. 2003; Gruber et al. 2002; Hiyama et al. 2008; Meisel et al. 2007; Okuma et al. 2000; Sakai et al. 2005; Sheikh et al. 2009; Sobajima et al. 2008). In a rat study, the injection of a pellet of both nucleus pulposus cells and MSC was shown to preserve disc height, suggesting that the use of both cell types maybe advantageous (Allon et al. 2010). The duration of these individual studies was variable; the longest was a dog study in which the implant was assessed at 1 year (Ganey et al. 2003). Although the cells used in these trials were for the most part autologous, there were at least two studies that used allogeneic or xenogeneic cells. One was a rat study in which allogeneic MSC were used to repair the disc. There was no evidence of an immune reaction at 1 month, raising the possibility that the disc does provide an "immunoprivileged" environment and that it may be possible to use allogeneic or xenogeneic cells in this setting (Crevensten et al. 2004). In keeping with this premise, mouse ESC which were partially differentiated in vitro to chondrocytes were injected into rabbit degenerated discs: at 8 weeks no immune reaction was observed (Sheikh et al. 2009). Cell labeling studies confirmed that the injected cells remained in the disc. Since both of these studies were short term, longer-term studies are required.

Human cell therapy studies are ongoing. In one clinical trial cervical discs were injected with nucleus pulposus cells harvested from herniated disc tissue. While the 2-year results were promising (Hohaus et al. 2008), the longer-term outcome has yet to be reported. More recently, a pilot study was performed in which ten patients received intra-discal injections of MSCs; there was significant pain relief by 3 months and at 12 months there was increased water content in the disc even though disc height was not fully restored (Orozco et al. 2011).

Another approach to cellular repair is to inject MSC, not into the disc, but intravascularly (Alini M, personal communication 2012). It is expected that the cells would then home to the disc obviating the need for a delivery system or annulus fibrosus needle puncture, which has been shown in animals to alter disc mechanics and in humans to possibly promote disc degeneration (Carragee et al. 2009; Iatridis et al. 2009; Michalek et al. 2010; Zhang et al. 2009). Validation of this approach is lacking at this time, but an in vitro study showing that MSC can migrate into the disc is promising (Illien-Junger et al. 2012).

26.6.1.2 Cell-Seeded Scaffolds

A large number of scaffolds have been developed for nucleus pulposus repair and an overview of these have been published (see reviews) (O'Halloran and Pandit 2007; Yang and Li 2009). In summary, most have been shown to support cell growth and, in some cases, tissue formation. Agarose and alginate have been utilized, but the inability of agarose to degrade and the impurities in alginate may limit clinical application (Bron et al. 2011; Chou and Nicoll 2009). Other examples of scaffolds that have been developed for this purpose include collagen I, atelocollagen type II, collagen II enriched with hyaluronan and cross-linked with polyethylene glycol (4S-StarPEG), polylactic acid, combined thiol-modified hyaluronan and elastin-like polypeptide, chitosan-glycerophosphate, and collagen II/hyaluronan/chondroitin-6-sulfate copolymer sponge which have been seeded with either nucleus pulposus or MSC cells (Bowles et al. 2010; Collin et al. 2011; Halloran et al. 2008; Hegewald et al. 2011b; Huang et al. 2011; Lee et al. 2012a; Nettles et al. 2010; Richardson et al. 2008; Sakai et al. 2005). Some of these constructs have been evaluated in animal models. For example, nucleus pulposus cells seeded into collagen type II/hyaluronan/chondroitin-6-sulfate copolymer sponge were grown in culture for 1 week and then implanted into rabbit lumbar discs immediately after nucleotomy. At 6 months, the disc height was greater in rabbits that received the cell-seeded scaffold compared to scaffold alone; comparison to the normal unoperated disc was not provided. The implanted cells were present and there was evidence of tissue formation (Huang et al. 2011). However, as rabbit nucleus pulposus cells are predominately notochordal, the relevance of this study to humans is not clear. In another study, MSC were seeded into type I atelocollagen and implanted into rabbit discs 2 weeks after nucleus pulposus tissue aspiration. There was evidence of disc repair as the proteoglycan content returned to 83 % of normal. Cells were shown to be necessary as the scaffold alone resulted in only 13 % of the proteoglycan content of the native disc (Sakai et al. 2005). Studies in larger animals have not been performed. There has been increasing interest in hydrogels as they are injectable, able to swell and retain water, and thus withstand loading (Pereira et al. 2013). The plethora of scaffolds that have been generated would suggest that the ideal scaffold has yet to be identified.

26.6.1.3 Tissue Formation In Vitro

Nucleus pulposus tissue can be formed in the presence or absence of a scaffold in vitro prior to implantation. Supporting this approach, a study in rabbits showed that implantation of nucleus pulposus tissue was more effective in delaying disc degeneration than isolated cells (Nomura et al. 2001). There are several advantages to developing tissue prior to implantation. As the disc is always loaded in vivo, a formed tissue that is able to withstand some degree of loading after implantation is an obvious advantage. In addition, the tissue does not have to form in a harsh environment, e.g., presence of proinflammatory cytokines. Furthermore, this approach facilitates formation of more than one tissue type. For example, the authors have developed an in vitro system to form a portion of the intervertebral disc consisting of nucleus pulposus tissue adherent to a subjacent layer of cartilaginous tissue (representing the endplate), thus recreating the inner disc tissue (Hamilton et al. 2006).

26.6.2 Annulus Fibrosus Tissue Engineering

The annulus fibrosus experiences complex loading patterns, for example, under compression on the side of applied bending, there is both tensile radial and compressive axial strain, whereas the opposite side undergoes tensile axial strains (O'Connell et al. 2011). As the annulus fibrosus experiences residual strain even when unloaded (Michalek et al. 2012), it is not surprising that by midlife, about 50 % of individuals have annular tears (Videman and Nurminen 2004). However, the healing potential is limited and it is usually replaced by a fibrous tissue which is biomechanically inferior and herniation of the implant is not uncommon. Thus, once damaged, in order to restore its complex architecture, the annulus fibrosus requires repair and more likely replacement (Bron et al. 2009). Moreover, given the complex loading patterns of the annulus fibrosus, it is critical that the replacement tissue is engineered to closely match the original. Relevant to this issue, the inability of the annulus fibrosus to regenerate also influences the type of nucleus replacements that can be used.

26.6.2.1 Cell Therapy

Given the complexities of the engineered architecture of the annulus fibrosus and the continual strains it experiences, cell therapies are not suitable to use to repair this tissue.

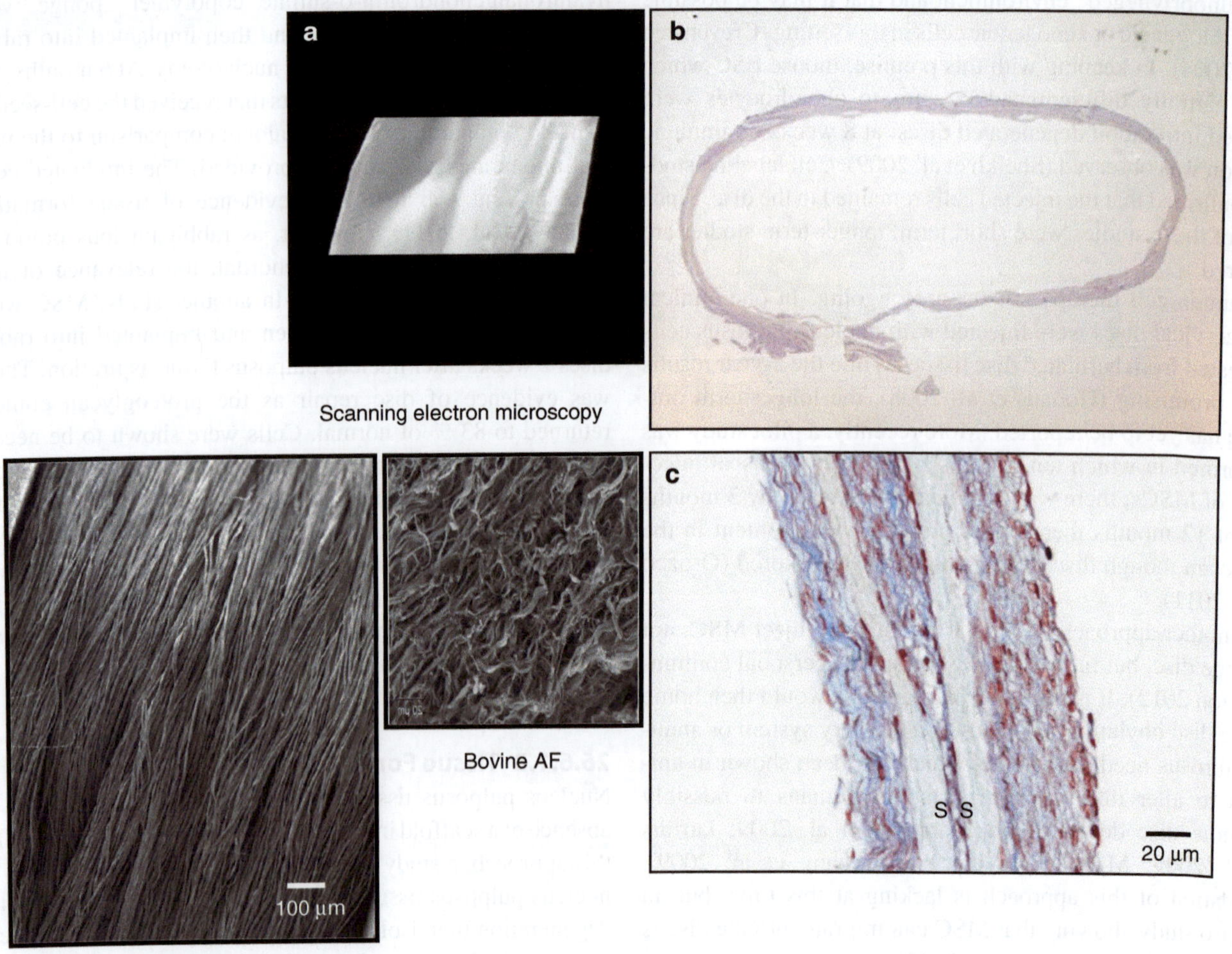

Fig. 26.1 Annulus fibrosus tissue engineering. (**a**) Appearance of electrospun nanofibrous scaffold grossly and by scanning electron microscopy. Bovine annulus fibrosus (*AF*) visualized by scanning electron microscopy shown as control. (**b, c**) Histological appearance of AF cell-seeded multilayer scaffold with AF tissue rich in collagen (*C* trichrome stain, *S* scaffold)

26.6.2.2 Cell-Seeded Scaffolds

A number of biological and synthetic scaffolds have been shown to support annulus fibrosus cell attachment and subsequent synthesis of extracellular matrix (Chang et al. 2007; Chou et al. 2008; Gruber et al. 2004; Helen and Gough 2008; Saad and Spector 2004; Shao and Hunter 2007; Yang et al. 2009). Contraction of a rat tail collagen solution around a polyethylene disc resulted in aligned collagen that supported growth of oriented annulus cells (Bowles et al. 2010). However, given the need to form multi-ply tissues with alternating angle of orientation (angle-ply multi-lamellated tissues), electrospinning has been gaining interest as a way to generate scaffolds suitable for the formation of annulus fibrosus tissue. Electrospun nanofibrous scaffolds can be generated on continually rotating circular mandrels, so they are aligned and resemble the scale of native fibrillar collagen, the major component of the annulus fibrosus matrix (see Fig. 26.1). Several studies have shown that annulus fibrosus cells will align on these scaffolds and produce a properly oriented matrix (Koepsell et al. 2011; Nerurkar et al. 2009; Vadala et al. 2012). A variety of biomaterials can be electrospun including polyurethane, polycaprolactone, poly(L-lactide), and poly-ε-caprolactone. As shown by Nerurkar et al., these cell-seeded scaffolds can form multi-lamellated structures and will be discussed further below (Nerurkar et al. 2009, 2010a). How to develop annulus fibrosus tissue with inner and outer zones has yet to be determined.

Box 26.3 Tissue Engineering of Articular Cartilage

Articular cartilage is very different than the intervertebral disc, as it is a simpler organ in that it is composed of only one tissue containing a small number of chondrocytes surrounded by a large amount of extracellular matrix rich in proteoglycans, collagen, and water. Although similar in some ways to the nucleus pulposus, the cells of these two tissues are very different and they can respond differently to stimuli. Tissue engineering of articular cartilage is further advanced than the disc, and the principles can be translated to engineering a functional endplate cartilage. However, both cartilage and disc tissue engineering have the same issue which is the recreation of the soft tissue to hard tissue (bone) interface. It is not yet clear whether this integration should be developed prior to implantation or whether it can be induced to develop in vivo, but it is a necessary goal if tissue-engineering approaches are to be successful.

26.7 Engineering the Cartilage Endplate

The cartilage endplate is critical to disc function and yet it has not been intensively studied. A recent study by Broom et al. demonstrated some of the features of collagen organization in this tissue (Wade et al. 2012). The authors have developed an in vitro system to form a layer of cartilaginous tissue (representing the cartilaginous endplate) which is integrated into the top surface of a biodegradable porous bone substitute material (calcium polyphosphate) (Waldman et al. 2002). The intent of the bone substitute is to allow for fixation of the construct into the vertebral body, an approach that has been used successfully in cartilage implant studies (Kandel et al. 2006). Generating nucleus pulposus tissue on this layer of cartilage, a composite structure is generated that exhibits enhanced interfacial shear strength to the bone substitute compared to nucleus pulposus tissue only (Hamilton et al. 2006).

26.8 Engineering the Intervertebral Disc

Although cell therapy studies have provided promising evidence in support of this approach in restoring disc function, the cellular and architectural aspects of the repair tissue formed have not been clarified. Moreover, it is likely that transplantation of tissue rather than cells may be a better approach. A study in rabbits demonstrated that insertion of nucleus pulposus tissue was more effective than nucleus pulposus cells in delaying disease (Nomura et al. 2001). However, implantation of cells alone, or even nucleus pulposus tissue, cannot reverse changes such as cartilaginous endplate calcification, which may be the cause of the disease process, nor will it be able to restore structural functionality when all three tissues are degenerated. In these settings the optimal approach would be to replace the entire disc.

Intervertebral disc and vertebral body graft transplants have been used successfully in animal models (Frick et al. 1994; Luk et al. 1997; Olson et al. 1991) and more recently in humans (Ruan et al. 2007) and serve as proof of concept for biological disc replacement. Autografts are not an option in humans, and the use of allografts is limited by tissue availability – they also generate their own problems, such as their ability to transmit disease. Hence, research groups have been developing methods to create a functional spinal unit using tissue-engineering principles. Mizuno et al. generated the first model of an intervertebral disc using nude mice as the bioreactor. They formed a disclike structure by generating a mesh of polyglycolic/polylactic acid polymers seeded with annulus fibrosus cells which was placed around an alginate hydrogel seeded with nucleus pulposus cells (Mizuno et al. 2006). This composite formed tissue only when grown subcutaneously in athymic mice. After 16 weeks, the biochemical properties approximated the mouse disc but the mechanical properties (Young's modulae) were inferior (Mizuno et al. 2006).

Since the inability to form tissues in vitro limited further study, Bowles et al. developed another model which uses collagen gels, rather than a synthetic polymer, to mimic the circumferential alignment of the annulus fibrosus

(Bowles et al. 2011). In this construct, annulus-seeded collagen surrounded a nucleus pulposus-seeded alginate plug. The cells used in this study were xenogeneic as they were obtained from sheep. Although this construct did not mimic the cross-ply alignment of the native annulus fibrosus, when implanted into rat caudal spines, there was integration with adjacent vertebral bodies, and disc height was restored. There was evidence of tissue formation while the modulus indicated that load-bearing properties were maintained. Interestingly, there was less energy dissipation which may be important for prevention of adjacent disc disease (Bowles et al. 2011). Although it could be argued that the implant was small and would not be subjected to the loads or nutritional demands of human discs, the study demonstrates that a biological disc replacement can integrate. To evaluate biological functionality and potential for use in a clinical setting, assessment in a large animal will be necessary.

A number of other groups have also generated biological discs in vitro, although these are yet to be evaluated in vivo. Mauck and Elliot have generated a composite disclike structure of cross-ply poly-ε-caprolactone aligned scaffolds cultured with mesenchymal stromal cells wrapped around an agarose plug containing MSCs (Nerurkar et al. 2010a). There was tissue formation after 6 weeks of culture which showed some resemblance to the native intervertebral disc. A construct measuring 8 mm, inner diameter of 3.5 mm, and a height of 3 mm using annulus fibrosus cell-seeded fibrous silk scaffolds surrounding a chondrocyte-seeded porous fibrin-hyaluronan hydrogel was engineered by Park et al. (2012). Likewise, Lazebnik et al. (2011) generated a disclike composite by electrospinning circumferentially orientated polycaprolactone fibers (an annulus fibrosus analog), seeding it with porcine chondrocytes which had been passaged three times and then gelling a chondrocyte (first passage cells)-agarose solution in the center (nucleus pulposus analog). Cells were present and remained viable in this construct, but no further characterization was performed. An electrospun poly(L-lactic acid) (PLLA) nanofibrous scaffold seeded with MSC was injected into the center of a MSC-containing slurry of hyaluronan to generate a composite structure. Nesti et al. (2008) showed that at 28 days, cells were embedded in a matrix rich in proteoglycans. The authors' group has taken a somewhat different approach to generating a disc. An annulus fibrosus cell-seeded aligned multi-lamellated polyurethane nanofibrous scaffold was wrapped around scaffold-free nucleus pulposus tissue which is integrated to the top surface of a porous bone substitute (see Fig. 26.2). The bone substitute will allow for fixation of the construct into the vertebral body by bone ingrowth into the pores. In aggregate, although these studies suggest that it will be possible to engineer biological disc replacements, further investigations are still required to generate an intervertebral disc that mimics the native tissue and is shown to be functional in a large animal model.

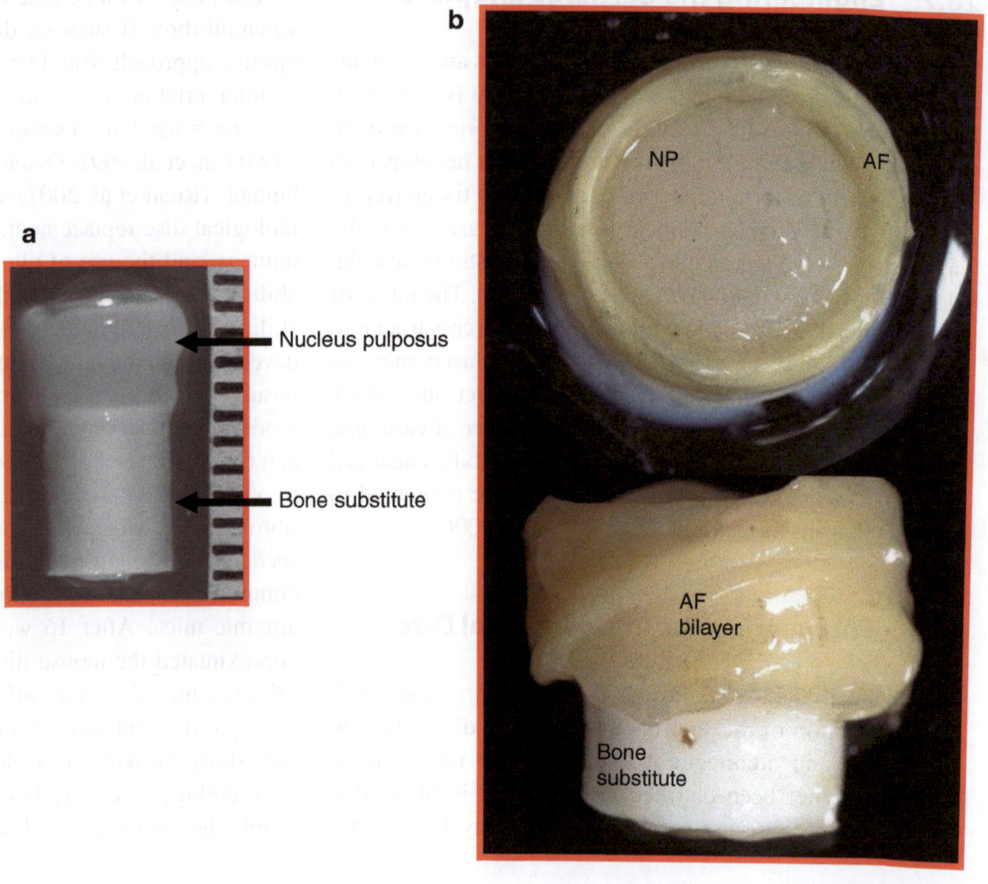

Fig. 26.2 Tissue-engineered intervertebral disc tissue. (**a**) Appearance of nucleus pulposus tissue on bone substitute. (**b**) Appearance of intervertebral disc model composed of nucleus pulposus surrounded by annulus fibrosus

26.9 Additional Challenges for Tissue Engineering a Functional Intervertebral Disc

A number of questions related to tissue engineering an intervertebral disc still need to be answered. Firstly, since the annulus fibrosus is composed of an inner and outer zone, will it be necessary to recapitulate both zones or will they form spontaneously in vivo? Attempts to address this are ongoing. For example, Wan et al. (2008) has developed a biphasic construct. The outer phase of the construct was a ring-shaped demineralized bone matrix gelatin scaffold extracted from cortical bone (rich in collagen I to mimic the outer annulus fibrosus) and an inner phase composed of poly(polycaprolactone triol malate) orientated in concentric sheets and seeded with chondrocytes to recapitulate the inner aspect of the annulus fibrosus (contains collagen II and proteoglycans). This in vitro study demonstrated that the cells on these scaffolds remain viable; no further characterization was performed.

Secondly, it is not known if the tissue-engineered disc tissue will exhibit the minimal mechanical properties necessary for survival following implantation. We have some rudimentary appreciation of the requirements for mature tissue, but little about the implanted tissue. Yao et al. (2006) predicted, using finite element modeling, that the nucleus pulposus should have a Young's modulus of between 5 and 10 MPa and be able to withstand compressive stress in excess of 1.67 MPa. It has been suggested that the annulus fibrosus should be able to withstand strains of up to 15 % (Bass et al. 2004). Cortes and Elliott (2012) demonstrated that the interlamellar tissue has an aggregate modulus of 10.2 ± 3.3 kPa; although nonlinearity was detected for compression less than 0.8. The contribution of the interlamellar tissue (defined as extrafibrillary matrix) to the total aggregate modulus of the annulus fibrosus decreased from 70 to 30 % for an applied compression of 50 % of the initial thickness. These data provide baseline information about what is desired from mature disc tissue.

Thirdly, it is not known at what rate the regenerating tissues will acquire the desired native mechanical properties. In a previous study, we demonstrated that in vitro-formed cartilage implanted into a focal articular joint defect in sheep with a compressive equilibrium modulus 1 % of native tissue survive showed a 30-fold improvement in mechanical properties by 9 months (Kandel et al. 2006). This raises the possibility that in vitro-formed disc tissue will remodel similarly in response to the mechanical environment into which it is placed as is seen in the maturation and growth of native disc tissue that occurs with aging (Fig. 26.3).

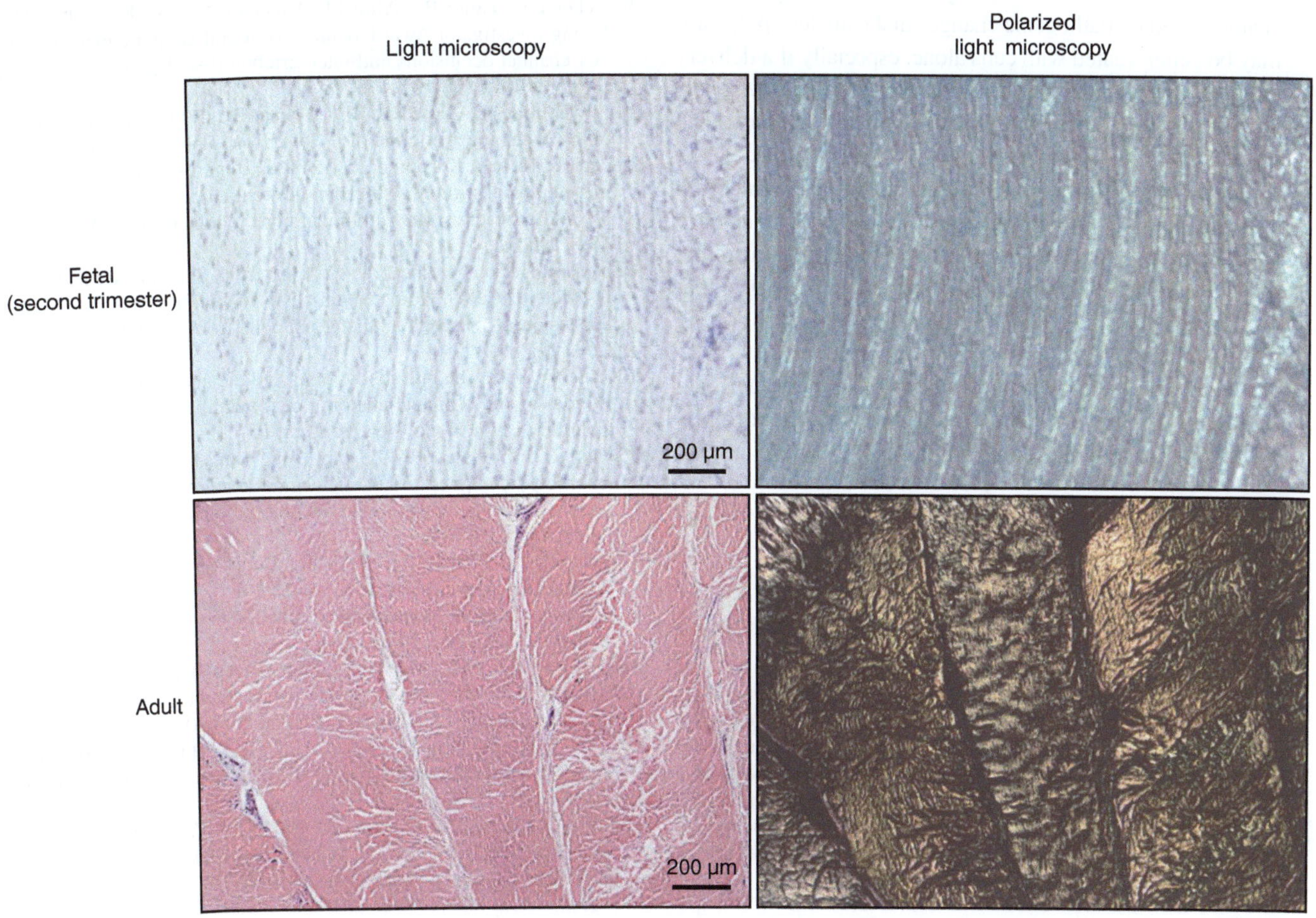

Fig. 26.3 Histological appearance of annulus fibrosus tissue in fetus and adult showing tissue growth with age (H&E stain)

Fourthly, the required strengths of the interlamellar interfaces and the nucleus pulposus-annulus fibrosus interface need to be determined; information that is critical for defining design parameters for tissues that will function in vivo.

Fifthly, the effect of the environment into which the disc will be placed has yet to be considered (Smith et al. 2011). It is likely that this will be unfavorable particularly if the disease process is long standing and the sclerotic osseous endplate is not replaced. Time to vascularization of the implant and nutrient diffusion are also unknown factors. Finally, clinical issues such as which individuals should receive an implant and how should these discs be implanted and the subsequent rehabilitation protocol need to be determined.

26.10 Summary of Critical Concepts Discussed in the Chapter

- No consensus exists as to which approach is optimal to treat symptomatic disc degeneration: implantation of cells, tissues, or an entire disc.
- The biological repair treatment paradigm will likely be personalized to the individual and influenced by extent of disease. For example, early symptomatic degeneration, characterized by pathogenic changes in the nucleus pulposus, may be better treated with cells alone, especially if a delivery method other than injection (needle puncture) is developed. However, when the disease affects the nucleus pulposus and annulus fibrosus, the entire disc may have to be replaced.
- Concomitant with the development of tissue-engineering approaches to biological repair, it will also be necessary to delineate the mechanism(s) leading to back pain so that the right patients are selected for treatment to ensure that biological treatment will be effective in ameliorating symptomatology.
- It will be necessary to determine how to best facilitate biological repair/replacement and what is the optimal posttreatment rehabilitation protocol.

Acknowledgements Canadian Institutes of Health Research (CIHR) Grant MOP114991

References

Abbott RD, Purmessur D, Monsey RD, Iatridis JC (2012) Regenerative potential of TGFbeta3 + Dex and notochordal cell conditioned media on degenerated human intervertebral disc cells. J Orthop Res 30:482–488

Acosta FL Jr, Metz L, Adkisson HD, Liu J, Carruthers-Liebenberg E, Milliman C, Maloney M, Lotz JC (2011) Porcine intervertebral disc repair using allogeneic juvenile articular chondrocytes or mesenchymal stem cells. Tissue Eng Part A 17:3045–3055

Adams MA, McNally DS, Dolan P (1996) 'Stress' distributions inside intervertebral discs. The effects of age and degeneration. J Bone Joint Surg Br 78:965–972

Adams MA, Dolan P, McNally DS (2009) The internal mechanical functioning of intervertebral discs and articular cartilage, and its relevance to matrix biology. Matrix Biol 28:384–389

Ahmed N, Stanford WL, Kandel RA (2007) Mesenchymal stem and progenitor cells for cartilage repair. Skeletal Radiol 36:909–912

Aladin DM, Cheung KM, Chan D, Yee AF, Jim JJ, Luk KD, Lu WW (2007) Expression of the Trp2 allele of COL9A2 is associated with alterations in the mechanical properties of human intervertebral discs. Spine (Phila Pa 1976) 32:2820–2826

Allon AA, Aurouer N, Yoo BB, Liebenberg EC, Buser Z, Lotz JC (2010) Structured coculture of stem cells and disc cells prevent disc degeneration in a rat model. Spine J 10:1089–1097

Ambard D, Cherblanc F (2009) Mechanical behavior of annulus fibrosus: a microstructural model of fibers reorientation. Ann Biomed Eng 37:2256–2265

Arana CJ, Diamandis EP, Kandel RA (2010) Cartilage tissue enhances proteoglycan retention by nucleus pulposus cells in vitro. Arthritis Rheum 62:3395–3403

Asche CV, Kirkness CS, McAdam-Marx C, Fritz JM (2007) The societal costs of low back pain: data published between 2001 and 2007. J Pain Palliat Care Pharmacother 21:25–33

Attia M, Santerre JP, Kandel RA (2010) The response of annulus fibrosus cell to fibronectin-coated nanofibrous polyurethane-anionic dihydroxyoligomer scaffolds. Biomaterials 32:450–460

Barrilleaux B, Knoepfler PS (2011) Inducing iPSCs to escape the dish. Cell Stem Cell 9:103–111

Bass EC, Ashford FA, Segal MR, Lotz JC (2004) Biaxial testing of human annulus fibrosus and its implications for a constitutive formulation. Ann Biomed Eng 32:1231–1242

Benneker LM, Heini PF, Alini M, Anderson SE, Ito K (2005) 2004 Young Investigator Award Winner: vertebral endplate marrow contact channel occlusions and intervertebral disc degeneration. Spine (Phila Pa 1976) 30:167–173

Bibby SR, Jones DA, Lee RB, Yu J, Urban JPG (2001) The pathophysiology of the intervertebral disc. Joint Bone Spine 68:537–542

Bieback K, Kern S, Kocaomer A, Ferlik K, Bugert P (2008) Comparing mesenchymal stromal cells from different human tissues: bone marrow, adipose tissue and umbilical cord blood. Biomed Mater Eng 18:S71–S76

Bieback K, Hecker A, Kocaomer A, Lannert H, Schallmoser K, Strunk D, Kluter H (2009) Human alternatives to fetal bovine serum for the expansion of mesenchymal stromal cells from bone marrow. Stem Cells 27:2331–2341

Bogduk N (1997) The inter-body joints and the intervertebral discs. In: Bogduk N (ed) Clinical anatomy of the lumbar spine and sacrum. Churchill Livingstone, New York, pp 13–31

Bowles RD, Williams RM, Zipfel WR, Bonassar LJ (2010) Self-assembly of aligned tissue-engineered annulus fibrosus and intervertebral disc composite via collagen gel contraction. Tissue Eng Part A 16:1339–1348

Bowles RD, Gebhard HH, Hartl R, Bonassar LJ (2011) Tissue-engineered intervertebral discs produce new matrix, maintain disc height, and restore biomechanical function to the rodent spine. Proc Natl Acad Sci U S A 108:13106–13111

Bron JL, Helder MN, Meisel HJ, Van Royen BJ, Smit TH (2009) Repair, regenerative and supportive therapies of the annulus fibrosus: achievements and challenges. Eur Spine J 18:301–313

Bron JL, Vonk LA, Smit TH, Koenderink GH (2011) Engineering alginate for intervertebral disc repair. J Mech Behav Biomed Mater 4: 1196–1205

Cappello R, Bird JL, Pfeiffer D, Bayliss MT, Dudhia J (2006) Notochordal cell produce and assemble extracellular matrix in a distinct manner, which may be responsible for the maintenance of healthy nucleus pulposus. Spine (Phila Pa 1976) 31:873–882; discussion 883

Carragee EJ, Don AS, Hurwitz EL, Cuellar JM, Carrino JA, Herzog R (2009) 2009 ISSLS Prize Winner: does discography cause accelerated progression of degeneration changes in the lumbar disc: a ten-year matched cohort study. Spine (Phila Pa 1976) 34: 2338–2345

Chan WC, Sze KL, Samartzis D, Leung VY, Chan D (2011) Structure and biology of the intervertebral disk in health and disease. Orthop Clin North Am 42:447–464, vii

Chang G, Kim HJ, Kaplan D, Vunjak-Novakovic G, Kandel RA (2007) Porous silk scaffolds can be used for tissue engineering annulus fibrosus. Eur Spine J 16:1848–1857

Choi KS, Cohn MJ, Harfe BD (2008) Identification of nucleus pulposus precursor cells and notochordal remnants in the mouse: implications for disk degeneration and chordoma formation. Dev Dyn 237:3953–3958

Chou AI, Nicoll SB (2009) Characterization of photocrosslinked alginate hydrogels for nucleus pulposus cell encapsulation. J Biomed Mater Res A 91:187–194

Chou AI, Bansal A, Miller GJ, Nicoll SB (2006) The effect of serial monolayer passaging on the collagen expression profile of outer and inner anulus fibrosus cells. Spine (Phila Pa 1976) 31:1875–1881

Chou AI, Reza AT, Nicoll SB (2008) Distinct intervertebral disc cell populations adopt similar phenotypes in three-dimensional culture. Tissue Eng Part A 14:2079–2087

Chou R, Baisden J, Carragee EJ, Resnick DK, Shaffer WO, Loeser JD (2009) Surgery for low back pain: a review of the evidence for an American Pain Society Clinical Practice Guideline. Spine (Phila Pa 1976) 34:1094–1109

Choumerianou DM, Martimianaki G, Stiakaki E, Kalmanti L, Kalmanti M, Dimitriou H (2010) Comparative study of stemness characteristics of mesenchymal cells from bone marrow of children and adults. Cytotherapy 12:881–887

Cinotti G, Della Rocca C, Romeo S, Vittur F, Toffanin R, Trasimeni G (2005) Degenerative changes of porcine intervertebral disc induced by vertebral endplate injuries. Spine (Phila Pa 1976) 30:174–180

Collin EC, Grad S, Zeugolis DI, Vinatier CS, Clouet JR, Guicheux JJ, Weiss P, Alini M, Pandit AS (2011) An injectable vehicle for nucleus pulposus cell-based therapy. Biomaterials 32:2862–2870

Cortes DH, Elliott DM (2012) Extra-fibrillar matrix mechanics of annulus fibrosus in tension and compression. Biomech Model Mechanobiol 11:781–790

Crevensten G, Walsh AJ, Ananthakrishnan D, Page P, Wahba GM, Lotz JC, Berven S (2004) Intervertebral disc cell therapy for regeneration: mesenchymal stem cell implantation in rat intervertebral discs. Ann Biomed Eng 32:430–434

Dagenais S, Caro J, Haldeman S (2008) A systematic review of low back pain cost of illness studies in the United States and internationally. Spine J 8:8–20

Desrochers J, Duncan NA (2010) Strain transfer in the annulus fibrosus under applied flexion. J Biomech 43:2141–2148

Doorn J, Moll G, Le Blanc K, van Blitterswijk C, de Boer J (2012) Therapeutic applications of mesenchymal stromal cells: paracrine effects and potential improvements. Tissue Eng Part B Rev 18:101–115

Erickson IE, van Veen SC, Sengupta S, Kestle SR, Mauck RL (2011) Cartilage matrix formation by bovine mesenchymal stem cells in three-dimensional culture is age-dependent. Clin Orthop Relat Res 469:2744–2753

Erwin WM (2008) The Notochord, Notochordal cell and CTGF/CCN-2: ongoing activity from development through maturation. J Cell Commun Signal 2:59–65

Eyre DR (1979) Biochemistry of the intervertebral disc. Int Rev Connect Tissue Res 8:227–291

Fekete TF, Porchet F (2010) Overview of disc arthroplasty-past, present and future. Acta Neurochir (Wien) 152:393–404

Frick SL, Hanley EN Jr, Meyer RA Jr, Ramp WK, Chapman TM (1994) Lumbar intervertebral disc transfer. A canine study. Spine (Phila Pa 1976) 19:1826–1834; discussion 1834–1835

Ganey T, Libera J, Moos V, Alasevic O, Fritsch KG, Meisel HJ, Hutton WC (2003) Disc chondrocyte transplantation in a canine model: a treatment for degenerated or damaged intervertebral disc. Spine (Phila Pa 1976) 28:2609–2620

Gotz W, Barnert S, Bertagnoli R, Miosge N, Kresse H, Herken R (1997) Immunohistochemical localization of the small proteoglycans decorin and biglycan in human intervertebral discs. Cell Tissue Res 289:185–190

Gruber HE, Stasky AA, Hanley EN Jr (1997) Characterization and phenotypic stability of human disc cells in vitro. Matrix Biol 16: 285–288

Gruber HE, Johnson TL, Leslie K, Ingram JA, Martin D, Hoelscher G, Banks D, Phieffer L, Coldham G, Hanley EN Jr (2002) Autologous intervertebral disc cell implantation: a model using Psammomys obesus, the sand rat. Spine (Phila Pa 1976) 27:1626–1633

Gruber HE, Leslie K, Ingram J, Norton HJ, Hanley EN (2004) Cell-based tissue engineering for the intervertebral disc: in vitro studies of human disc cell gene expression and matrix production within selected cell carriers. Spine J 4:44–55

Gruber HE, Gordon B, Williams C, Norton HJ, Hanley EN Jr (2007) Vertebral endplate and disc changes in the aging sand rat lumbar spine: cross-sectional analyses of a large male and female population. Spine (Phila Pa 1976) 32:2529–2536

Grunhagen T, Wilde G, Soukane DM, Shirazi-Adl SA, Urban JP (2006) Nutrient supply and intervertebral disc metabolism. J Bone Joint Surg Am 88(Suppl 2):30–35

Guerin HA, Elliott DM (2006) Degeneration affects the fiber reorientation of human annulus fibrosus under tensile load. J Biomech 39:1410–1418

Gupta MS, Cooper ES, Nicoll SB (2011) Transforming growth factor-beta 3 stimulates cartilage matrix elaboration by human marrow-derived stromal cells encapsulated in photocrosslinked carboxymethylcellulose hydrogels: potential for nucleus pulposus replacement. Tissue Eng Part A 17:2903–2910

Guyer RD, Shellock J, Maclennan B, Hanscom D, Knight RQ, McCombe P, Jacobs JJ, Urban RM, Bradford D, Ohnmeiss DD (2011) Early failure of metal-on-metal artificial disc prostheses associated with lymphocytic reaction: diagnosis and treatment experience in 4 cases. Spine (Phila Pa 1976) 36:E492–E497

Hadjipanayi E, Mudera V, Brown RA (2009) Close dependence of fibroblast proliferation on collagen scaffold matrix stiffness. J Tissue Eng Regen Med 3:77–84

Halloran DO, Grad S, Stoddart M, Dockery P, Alini M, Pandit AS (2008) An injectable cross-linked scaffold for nucleus pulposus regeneration. Biomaterials 29:438–447

Hamilton DJ, Seguin CA, Wang J, Pilliar RM, Kandel RA (2006) Formation of a nucleus pulposus-cartilage endplate construct in vitro. Biomaterials 27:397–405

Harrison PE, Ashton IK, Johnson WE, Turner SL, Richardson JB, Ashton BA (2000) The in vitro growth of human chondrocytes. Cell Tissue Bank 1:255–260

Hegewald AA, Endres M, Abbushi A, Cabraja M, Woiciechowsky C, Schmieder K, Kaps C, Thome C (2011a) Adequacy of herniated disc tissue as a cell source for nucleus pulposus regeneration. J Neurosurg Spine 14:273–280

Hegewald AA, Enz A, Endres M, Sittinger M, Woiciechowsky C, Thome C, Kaps C (2011b) Engineering of polymer-based grafts with cells derived from human nucleus pulposus tissue of the lumbar spine. J Tissue Eng Regen Med 5:275–282

Helen W, Gough JE (2008) Cell viability, proliferation and extracellular matrix production of human annulus fibrosus cells cultured within PDLLA/Bioglass composite foam scaffolds in vitro. Acta Biomater 4:230–243

Hiyama A, Mochida J, Iwashina T, Omi H, Watanabe T, Serigano K, Tamura F, Sakai D (2008) Transplantation of mesenchymal stem cells in a canine disc degeneration model. J Orthop Res 26: 589–600

Hohaus C, Ganey TM, Minkus Y, Meisel HJ (2008) Cell transplantation in lumbar spine disc degeneration disease. Eur Spine J 17(Suppl 4):492–503

Holm S, Holm AK, Ekstrom L, Karladani A, Hansson T (2004) Experimental disc degeneration due to endplate injury. J Spinal Disord Tech 17:64–71

Holzapfel GA, Schulze-Bauer CA, Feigl G, Regitnig P (2005) Single lamellar mechanics of the human lumbar anulus fibrosus. Biomech Model Mechanobiol 3:125–140

Horner HA, Urban JP (2001) 2001 Volvo Award Winner in Basic Science Studies: effect of nutrient supply on the viability of cells from the nucleus pulposus of the intervertebral disc. Spine 26:2543–2549

Hsia HC, Nair MR, Mintz RC, Corbett SA (2011) The fiber diameter of synthetic bioresorbable extracellular matrix influences human fibroblast morphology and fibronectin matrix assembly. Plast Reconstr Surg 127:2312–2320

Hsieh AH, Twomey JD (2010) Cellular mechanobiology of the intervertebral disc: new directions and approaches. J Biomech 43:137–145

Huang RC, Tropiano P, Marnay T, Girardi FP, Lim MR, Cammisa FP Jr (2006) Range of motion and adjacent level degeneration after lumbar total disc replacement. Spine J 6:242–247

Huang B, Zhuang Y, Li CQ, Liu LT, Zhou Y (2011) Regeneration of the intervertebral disc with nucleus pulposus cell-seeded collagen II/hyaluronan/chondroitin-6-sulfate tri-copolymer constructs in a rabbit disc degeneration model. Spine (Phila Pa 1976) 36:2252–2259

Hukins DW (1994) In: Ghosh P (ed) Biology of intervertebral disc. Disc Structure and Function. CRC Press, Boca Raton, p 2–37

Iatridis JC, Michalek AJ, Purmessur D, Korecki CL (2009) Localized intervertebral disc injury leads to organ level changes in structure, cellularity, and biosynthesis. Cell Mol Bioeng 2:437–447

Ikada Y (2006) Challenges in tissue engineering. J R Soc Interface 3:589–601

Illien-Junger S, Pattappa G, Peroglio M, Benneker LM, Stoddart MJ, Sakai D, Mochida J, Grad S, Alini M (2012) Homing of mesenchymal stem cells in induced degenerative intervertebral discs in a whole organ culture system. Spine (Phila Pa 1976) 37:1865–1873

Inerot S, Axelsson I (1991) Structure and composition of proteoglycans from human annulus fibrosus. Connect Tissue Res 26:47–63

Iron KS, Manuel DG, Williams J (2004) Using a linked data set to determine the factors associated with utilization and costs of family physician services in Ontario: effects of self-reported chronic conditions. Chronic Dis Can 24:124–132

Javedan SP, Dickman CA (1999) Cause of adjacent-segment disease after spinal fusion. Lancet 354:530–531

Jim JJ, Noponen-Hietala N, Cheung KM, Ott J, Karppinen J, Sahraravand A, Luk KD, Yip SP, Sham PC, Song YQ, Leong JC, Cheah KS, Ala-Kokko L, Chan D (2005) The TRP2 allele of COL9A2 is an age-dependent risk factor for the development and severity of intervertebral disc degeneration. Spine (Phila Pa 1976) 30:2735–2742

Kandel RA, Grynpas M, Pilliar R, Lee J, Wang J, Waldman S, Zalzal P, Hurtig M (2006) Repair of osteochondral defects with biphasic cartilage-calcium polyphosphate constructs in a sheep model. Biomaterials 27:4120–4131

Kandel RA, Hamilton D, Seguin C, Li SQ, Arana C, Pilliar R (2007) An in vitro tissue model to study the effect of age on nucleus pulposus cells. Eur Spine J 16:2166–2173

Kandel R, Roberts S, Urban JP (2008) Tissue engineering and the intervertebral disc: the challenges. Eur Spine J 17(Suppl 4):480–491

Kim PK, Branch CL Jr (2006) The lumbar degenerative disc: confusion, mechanics, management. Clin Neurosurg 53:18–25

Kishen TJ, Diwan AD (2010) Fusion versus disk replacement for degenerative conditions of the lumbar and cervical spine: quid est testimonium? Orthop Clin North Am 41:167–181

Koepsell L, Remund T, Bao J, Neufeld D, Fong H, Deng Y (2011) Tissue engineering of annulus fibrosus using electrospun fibrous scaffolds with aligned polycaprolactone fibers. J Biomed Mater Res A 99:564–575

Korecki CL, Taboas JM, Tuan RS, Iatridis JC (2010) Notochordal cell conditioned medium stimulates mesenchymal stem cell differentiation toward a young nucleus pulposus phenotype. Stem Cell Res Ther 1:18

Krismer M, Haid C, Rabl W (1996) The contribution of anulus fibers to torque resistance. Spine (Phila Pa 1976) 21:2551–2557

Lange C, Cakiroglu F, Spiess AN, Cappallo-Obermann H, Dierlamm J, Zander AR (2007) Accelerated and safe expansion of human mesenchymal stromal cells in animal serum-free medium for transplantation and regenerative medicine. J Cell Physiol 213:18–26

Langer R, Vacanti JP (1993) Tissue engineering. Science 260:920–926

Lazebnik M, Singh M, Glatt P, Friis LA, Berkland CJ, Detamore MS (2011) Biomimetic method for combining the nucleus pulposus and annulus fibrosus for intervertebral disc tissue engineering. J Tissue Eng Regen Med 5:e179–e187

Le Maitre CL, Freemont AJ, Hoyland JA (2007) Accelerated cellular senescence in degenerate intervertebral discs: a possible role in the pathogenesis of intervertebral disc degeneration. Arthritis Res Ther 9:R45

Le Visage C, Kim SW, Tateno K, Sieber AN, Kostuik JP, Leong KW (2006) Interaction of human mesenchymal stem cells with disc cells: changes in extracellular matrix biosynthesis. Spine (Phila Pa 1976) 31:2036–2042

Lee P (1994) The economic impact of musculoskeletal disorders. Qual Life Res 3(Suppl 1):S85–S91

Lee KI, Moon SH, Kim H, Kwon UH, Kim HJ, Park SN, Suh H, Lee HM, Kim HS, Chun HJ, Kwon IK, Jang JW (2012a) Tissue engineering of the intervertebral disc with cultured nucleus pulposus cells using atelocollagen scaffold and growth factors. Spine (Phila Pa 1976) 37:452–458

Lee MJ, Dettori JR, Standaert CJ, Brodt ED, Chapman JR (2012b) The natural history of degeneration of the lumbar and cervical spines: a systematic review. Spine (Phila Pa 1976) 37:S18–S30

Lister R, Pelizzola M, Kida YS, Hawkins RD, Nery JR, Hon G, Antosiewicz-Bourget J, O'Malley R, Castanon R, Klugman S, Downes M, Yu R, Stewart R, Ren B, Thomson JA, Evans RM, Ecker JR (2011) Hotspots of aberrant epigenomic reprogramming in human induced pluripotent stem cells. Nature 471:68–73

Lotz JC, Hadi T, Bratton C, Reiser KM, Hsieh AH (2008) Anulus fibrosus tension inhibits degenerative structural changes in lamellar collagen. Eur Spine J 17:1149–1159

Luk KD, Ruan DK, Chow DH, Leong JC (1997) Intervertebral disc autografting in a bipedal animal model. Clin Orthop Relat Res 337:13–26

Maherali N, Ahfeldt T, Rigamonti A, Utikal J, Cowan C, Hochedlinger K (2008) A high-efficiency system for the generation and study of human induced pluripotent stem cells. Cell Stem Cell 3:340–345

Manchikanti L, Singh V, Datta S, Cohen SP, Hirsch JA (2009) Comprehensive review of epidemiology, scope, and impact of spinal pain. Pain Physician 12:E35–E70

Marchand F, Ahmed AM (1990) Investigation of the laminate structure of lumbar disc anulus fibrosus. Spine (Phila Pa 1976) 15: 402–410

Markolf KL, Morris JM (1974) The structural components of the intervertebral disc. A study of their contributions to the ability of the disc to withstand compressive forces. J Bone Joint Surg Am 56:675–687

Maroudas A, Stockwell RA, Nachemson A, Urban J (1975) Factors involved in the nutrition of the human lumbar intervertebral disc: cellularity and diffusion of glucose in vitro. J Anat 120:113–130

Masuda K (2008) Biological repair of the degenerated intervertebral disc by the injection of growth factors. Eur Spine J 17(Suppl 4):441–451

Masuda K, Lotz JC (2010) New challenges for intervertebral disc treatment using regenerative medicine. Tissue Eng Part B Rev 16:147–158

McCann MR, Tamplin OJ, Rossant J, Seguin CA (2012) Tracing notochord-derived cells using a Noto-cre mouse: implications for intervertebral disc development. Dis Model Mech 5:73–82

Meisel HJ, Siodla V, Ganey T, Minkus Y, Hutton WC, Alasevic OJ (2007) Clinical experience in cell-based therapeutics: disc chondrocyte transplantation A treatment for degenerated or damaged intervertebral disc. Biomol Eng 24:5–21

Melrose J, Ghosh P, Taylor TK (2001) A comparative analysis of the differential spatial and temporal distributions of the large (aggrecan, versican) and small (decorin, biglycan, fibromodulin) proteoglycans of the intervertebral disc. J Anat 198:3–15

Melrose J, Smith SM, Appleyard RC, Little CB (2008) Aggrecan, versican and type VI collagen are components of annular translamellar crossbridges in the intervertebral disc. Eur Spine J 17:314–324

Michalek AJ, Funabashi KL, Iatridis JC (2010) Needle puncture injury of the rat intervertebral disc affects torsional and compressive biomechanics differently. Eur Spine J 19:2110–2116

Michalek AJ, Gardner-Morse MG, Iatridis JC (2012) Large residual strains are present in the intervertebral disc annulus fibrosus in the unloaded state. J Biomech 45:1227–1231

Miller JA, Schmatz C, Schultz AB (1988) Lumbar disc degeneration: correlation with age, sex, and spine level in 600 autopsy specimens. Spine 13:173–178

Mirza SK, Deyo RA (2007) Systematic review of randomized trials comparing lumbar fusion surgery to nonoperative care for treatment of chronic back pain. Spine (Phila Pa 1976) 32:816–823

Miyamoto T, Muneta T, Tabuchi T, Matsumoto K, Saito H, Tsuji K, Sekiya I (2010) Intradiscal transplantation of synovial mesenchymal stem cells prevents intervertebral disc degeneration through suppression of matrix metalloproteinase-related genes in nucleus pulposus cells in rabbits. Arthritis Res Ther 12:R206

Mizuno H, Roy AK, Zaporojan V, Vacanti CA, Ueda M, Bonassar LJ (2006) Biomechanical and biochemical characterization of composite tissue-engineered intervertebral discs. Biomaterials 27:362–370

Moore RJ (2006) The vertebral endplate: disc degeneration, disc regeneration. Eur Spine J 15(Suppl 3):S333–S337

Munoz M, Rodriguez A, De Frutos C, Caamano JN, Diez C, Facal N, Gomez E (2008) Conventional pluripotency markers are unspecific for bovine embryonic-derived cell-lines. Theriogenology 69: 1159–1164

Mwale F, Roughley P, Antoniou J (2004) Distinction between the extracellular matrix of the nucleus pulposus and hyaline cartilage: a requisite for tissue engineering of intervertebral disc. Eur Cell Mater 8:58–63, discussion 63–64

Nagae M, Ikeda T, Mikami Y, Hase H, Ozawa H, Matsuda K, Sakamoto H, Tabata Y, Kawata M, Kubo T (2007) Intervertebral disc regeneration using platelet-rich plasma and biodegradable gelatin hydrogel microspheres. Tissue Eng 13:147–158

Nakagawa M, Koyanagi M, Tanabe K, Takahashi K, Ichisaka T, Aoi T, Okita K, Mochiduki Y, Takizawa N, Yamanaka S (2008) Generation of induced pluripotent stem cells without Myc from mouse and human fibroblasts. Nat Biotechnol 26:101–106

Nerurkar NL, Baker BM, Sen S, Wible EE, Elliott DM, Mauck RL (2009) Nanofibrous biologic laminates replicate the form and function of the annulus fibrosus. Nat Mater 8:986–992

Nerurkar NL, Sen S, Huang AH, Elliott DM, Mauck RL (2010a) Engineered disc-like angle-ply structures for intervertebral disc replacement. Spine (Phila Pa 1976) 35:867–873

Nerurkar NL, Elliott DM, Mauck RL (2010b) Mechanical design criteria for intervertebral disc tissue engineering. J Biomech 43:1017–1030

Nesti LJ, Li WJ, Shanti RM, Jiang YJ, Jackson W, Freedman BA, Kuklo TR, Giuliani JR, Tuan RS (2008) Intervertebral disc tissue engineering using a novel hyaluronic acid-nanofibrous scaffold (HANFS) amalgam. Tissue Eng Part A 14:1527–1537

Nettles DL, Chilkoti A, Setton LA (2010) Applications of elastin-like polypeptides in tissue engineering. Adv Drug Deliv Rev 62:1479–1485

Nomura T, Mochida J, Okuma M, Nishimura K, Sakabe K (2001) Nucleus pulposus allograft retards intervertebral disc degeneration. Clin Orthop Relat Res (389):94–101

Nosikova YS, Santerre JP, Grynpas M, Gibson G, Kandel RA (2012) Characterization of the annulus fibrosus-vertebral body interface: identification of new structural features. J Anat 221:577–589

O'Connell GD, Vresilovic EJ, Elliott DM (2011) Human intervertebral disc internal strain in compression: the effect of disc region, loading position, and degeneration. J Orthop Res 29:547–555

O'Halloran DM, Pandit AS (2007) Tissue-engineering approach to regenerating the intervertebral disc. Tissue Eng 13:1927–1954

Okuma M, Mochida J, Nishimura K, Sakabe K, Seiki K (2000) Reinsertion of stimulated nucleus pulposus cells retards intervertebral disc degeneration: an in vitro and in vivo experimental study. J Orthop Res 18:988–997

Olson EJ, Hanley EN Jr, Rudert MJ, Baratz ME (1991) Vertebral column allografts for the treatment of segmental spine defects. An experimental investigation in dogs. Spine (Phila Pa 1976) 16:1081–1088

Orozco L, Soler R, Morera C, Alberca M, Sanchez A, Garcia-Sancho J (2011) Intervertebral disc repair by autologous mesenchymal bone marrow cells: a pilot study. Transplantation 92:822–828

Park SH, Gil ES, Cho H, Mandal BB, Tien LW, Min BH, Kaplan DL (2012) Intervertebral disk tissue engineering using biphasic silk composite scaffolds. Tissue Eng Part A 18:447–458

Peng B, Hou S, Shi Q, Jia L (2001) The relationship between cartilage end-plate calcification and disc degeneration: an experimental study. Chin Med J (Engl) 114:308–312

Pereira D, Silva-Correia J, Oliveira J, Reis R (2013) Hydrogels in acellular and cellular strategies for intervertebral disc regeneration. J Tissue Eng Regen Med 7:85–98

Purmessur D, Schek RM, Abbott RD, Ballif BA, Godburn KE, Iatridis JC (2011) Notochordal conditioned media from tissue increases proteoglycan accumulation and promotes a healthy nucleus pulposus phenotype in human mesenchymal stem cells. Arthritis Res Ther 13:R81

Putzier M, Schneider SV, Funk JF, Tohtz SW, Perka C (2005) The surgical treatment of the lumbar disc prolapse: nucleotomy with additional transpedicular dynamic stabilization versus nucleotomy alone. Spine (Phila Pa 1976) 30:E109–E114

Raj PP (2008) Intervertebral disc: anatomy-physiology-pathophysiology-treatment. Pain Pract 8:18–44

Rajasekaran S, Babu JN, Arun R, Armstrong BR, Shetty AP, Murugan S (2004) ISSLS prize winner: a study of diffusion in human lumbar discs: a serial magnetic resonance imaging study documenting the influence of the endplate on diffusion in normal and degenerate discs. Spine (Phila Pa 1976) 29:2654–2667

Rapoport J, Jacobs P, Bell NR, Klarenbach S (2004) Refining the measurement of the economic burden of chronic diseases in Canada. Chronic Dis Can 25:13–21

Razaq S, Wilkins RJ, Urban JP (2003) The effect of extracellular pH on matrix turnover by cells of the bovine nucleus pulposus. Eur Spine J 12:341–349

Richardson SM, Hoyland JA (2008) Stem cell regeneration of degenerated intervertebral discs: current status. Curr Pain Headache Rep 12:83–88

Richardson SM, Walker RV, Parker S, Rhodes NP, Hunt JA, Freemont AJ, Hoyland JA (2006) Intervertebral disc cell-mediated mesenchymal stem cell differentiation. Stem Cells 24:707–716

Richardson SM, Mobasheri A, Freemont AJ, Hoyland JA (2007) Intervertebral disc biology, degeneration and novel tissue

engineering and regenerative medicine therapies. Histol Histopathol 22:1033–1041
Richardson SM, Hughes N, Hunt JA, Freemont AJ, Hoyland JA (2008) Human mesenchymal stem cell differentiation to NP-like cells in chitosan-glycerophosphate hydrogels. Biomaterials 29:85–93
Risbud MV, Shapiro IM (2011) Notochordal cells in the adult intervertebral disc: new perspective on an old question. Crit Rev Eukaryot Gene Expr 21:29–41
Risbud MV, Schaer TP, Shapiro IM (2010) Toward an understanding of the role of notochordal cells in the adult intervertebral disc: from discord to accord. Dev Dyn 239:2141–2148
Roberts S, Urban JP, Evans H, Eisenstein SM (1996) Transport properties of the human cartilage endplate in relation to its composition and calcification. Spine (Phila Pa 1976) 21:415–420
Roberts S, Evans EH, Kletsas D, Jaffray DC, Eisenstein SM (2006) Senescence in human intervertebral discs. Eur Spine J 15(Suppl 3):S312–S316
Ruan D, He Q, Ding Y, Hou L, Li J, Luk KD (2007) Intervertebral disc transplantation in the treatment of degenerative spine disease: a preliminary study. Lancet 369:993–999
Saad L, Spector M (2004) Effects of collagen type on the behavior of adult canine annulus fibrosus cells in collagen-glycosaminoglycan scaffolds. J Biomed Mater Res A 71:233–241
Sahlman J, Inkinen R, Hirvonen T, Lammi MJ, Lammi PE, Nieminen J, Lapvetelainen T, Prockop DJ, Arita M, Li SW, Hyttinen MM, Helminen HJ, Puustjarvi K (2001) Premature vertebral endplate ossification and mild disc degeneration in mice after inactivation of one allele belonging to the Col2a1 gene for type II collagen. Spine (Phila Pa 1976) 26:2558–2565
Saino E, Focarete ML, Gualandi C, Emanuele E, Cornaglia AI, Imbriani M, Visai L (2011) Effect of electrospun fiber diameter and alignment on macrophage activation and secretion of proinflammatory cytokines and chemokines. Biomacromolecules 12:1900–1911
Sakai D, Mochida J, Iwashina T, Watanabe T, Nakai T, Ando K, Hotta T (2005) Differentiation of mesenchymal stem cells transplanted to a rabbit degenerative disc model: potential and limitations for stem cell therapy in disc regeneration. Spine (Phila Pa 1976) 30:2379–2387
Schallmoser K, Bartmann C, Rohde E, Reinisch A, Kashofer K, Stadelmeyer E, Drexler C, Lanzer G, Linkesch W, Strunk D (2007) Human platelet lysate can replace fetal bovine serum for clinical-scale expansion of functional mesenchymal stromal cells. Transfusion 47:1436–1446
Schmidt H, Heuer F, Wilke HJ (2009) Dependency of disc degeneration on shear and tensile strains between annular fiber layers for complex loads. Med Eng Phys 31:642–649
Schollum ML, Robertson PA, Broom ND (2009) A microstructural investigation of intervertebral disc lamellar connectivity: detailed analysis of the translamellar bridges. J Anat 214:805–816
Schollum ML, Appleyard RC, Little CB, Melrose J (2010) A detailed microscopic examination of alterations in normal anular structure induced by mechanical destabilization in an ovine model of disc degeneration. Spine (Phila Pa 1976) 35:1965–1973
Schriebl K, Satianegara G, Hwang A, Tan HL, Fong WJ, Yang HH, Jungbauer A, Choo A (2012) Selective removal of undifferentiated human embryonic stem cells using magnetic activated cell sorting followed by a cytotoxic antibody. Tissue Eng Part A 18:899–909
Schulte TL, Leistra F, Bullmann V, Osada N, Vieth V, Marquardt B, Lerner T, Liljenqvist U, Hackenberg L (2007) Disc height reduction in adjacent segments and clinical outcome 10 years after lumbar 360 degrees fusion. Eur Spine J 16:2152–2158
Shahdadfar A, Fronsdal K, Haug T, Reinholt FP, Brinchmann JE (2005) In vitro expansion of human mesenchymal stem cells: choice of serum is a determinant of cell proliferation, differentiation, gene expression, and transcriptome stability. Stem Cells 23:1357–1366
Shao X, Hunter CJ (2007) Developing an alginate/chitosan hybrid fiber scaffold for annulus fibrosus cells. J Biomed Mater Res A 82:701–710
Shapiro IM, Risbud MV (2010) Transcriptional profiling of the nucleus pulposus: say yes to notochord. Arthritis Res Ther 12:117
Sheikh H, Zakharian K, De La Torre RP, Facek C, Vasquez A, Chaudhry GR, Svinarich D, Perez-Cruet MJ (2009) In vivo intervertebral disc regeneration using stem cell-derived chondroprogenitors. J Neurosurg Spine 10:265–272
Shim CS, Lee SH, Shin HD, Kang HS, Choi WC, Jung B, Choi G, Ahn Y, Lee S, Lee HY (2007) CHARITE versus ProDisc: a comparative study of a minimum 3-year follow-up. Spine (Phila Pa 1976) 32:1012–1018
Shirazi-Adl A, Taheri M, Urban JP (2010) Analysis of cell viability in intervertebral disc: effect of endplate permeability on cell population. J Biomech 43:1330–1336
Simon SR (1994) In: Simon SR (ed) Orthopedic basic science. Kinesiology. Am Academy of Orthopedic Surgeons, Rosemont, pp 558–568
Singh K, Masuda K, Thonar EJ, An HS, Cs-Szabo G (2009) Age-related changes in the extracellular matrix of nucleus pulposus and anulus fibrosus of human intervertebral disc. Spine (Phila Pa 1976) 34:10–16
Smith LJ, Elliott DM (2011) Formation of lamellar cross bridges in the annulus fibrosus of the intervertebral disc is a consequence of vascular regression. Matrix Biol 30:267–274
Smith SM, Whitelock JM, Iozzo RV, Little CB, Melrose J (2009) Topographical variation in the distributions of versican, aggrecan and perlecan in the foetal human spine reflects their diverse functional roles in spinal development. Histochem Cell Biol 132: 491–503
Smith LJ, Chiaro JA, Nerurkar NL, Cortes DH, Horava SD, Hebela NM, Mauck RL, Dodge GR, Elliott DM (2011) Nucleus pulposus cells synthesize a functional extracellular matrix and respond to inflammatory cytokine challenge following long-term agarose culture. Eur Cell Mater 22:291–301
So K, Takemoto M, Fujibayashi S, Neo M, Kyomoto M, Hayami T, Hyon SH, Nakamura T (2007) Antidegenerative effects of partial disc replacement in an animal surgery model. Spine (Phila Pa 1976) 32:1586–1591
Sobajima S, Vadala G, Shimer A, Kim JS, Gilbertson LG, Kang JD (2008) Feasibility of a stem cell therapy for intervertebral disc degeneration. Spine J 8:888–896
Steck E, Bertram H, Abel R, Chen B, Winter A, Richter W (2005) Induction of intervertebral disc-like cells from adult mesenchymal stem cells. Stem Cells 23:403–411
Strassburg S, Richardson SM, Freemont AJ, Hoyland JA (2010) Co-culture induces mesenchymal stem cell differentiation and modulation of the degenerate human nucleus pulposus cell phenotype. Regen Med 5:701–711
Takahashi K, Yamanaka S (2006) Induction of pluripotent stem cells from mouse embryonic and adult fibroblast cultures by defined factors. Cell 126:663–676
Takahashi K, Tanabe K, Ohnuki M, Narita M, Ichisaka T, Tomoda K, Yamanaka S (2007) Induction of pluripotent stem cells from adult human fibroblasts by defined factors. Cell 131:861–872
Takatalo J, Karppinen J, Niinimaki J, Taimela S, Nayha S, Mutanen P, Sequeiros RB, Kyllonen E, Tervonen O (2011) Does lumbar disc degeneration on magnetic resonance imaging associate with low back symptom severity in young Finnish adults? Spine (Phila Pa 1976) 36:2180–2189
Takatalo J, Karppinen J, Niinimaki J, Taimela S, Mutanen P, Sequeiros RB, Nayha S, Jarvelin MR, Kyllonen E, Tervonen O (2012) Association of modic changes, Schmorl's nodes, spondylolytic defects, high intensity zone lesions, disc herniations, and radial tears with low back symptom severity among young Finnish adults. Spine (Phila Pa 1976) 37:1231–1239

Tekkatte C, Gunasingh GP, Cherian KM, Sankaranarayanan K (2011) "Humanized" stem cell culture techniques: the animal serum controversy. Stem Cells Int 2011:504723

Tumialan LM, Gluf WM (2011) Progressive vertebral body osteolysis after cervical arthroplasty. Spine (Phila Pa 1976) 36:E973–E978

Vadala G, Studer RK, Sowa G, Spiezia F, Iucu C, Denaro V, Gilbertson LG, Kang JD (2008) Coculture of bone marrow mesenchymal stem cells and nucleus pulposus cells modulate gene expression profile without cell fusion. Spine (Phila Pa 1976) 33:870 876

Vadala G, Mozetic P, Rainer A, Centola M, Loppini M, Trombetta M, Denaro V (2012) Bioactive electrospun scaffold for annulus fibrosus repair and regeneration. Eur Spine J 21(Suppl 1):S20–S26

van Ooij A, Kurtz SM, Stessels F, Noten H, van Rhijn L (2007) Polyethylene wear debris and long-term clinical failure of the Charite disc prosthesis: a study of 4 patients. Spine (Phila Pa 1976) 32:223–229

Vernengo J, Fussell GW, Smith NG, Lowman AM (2008) Evaluation of novel injectable hydrogels for nucleus pulposus replacement. J Biomed Mater Res B Appl Biomater 84:64–69

Videman T, Nurminen M (2004) The occurrence of anular tears and their relation to lifetime back pain history: a cadaveric study using barium sulfate discography. Spine (Phila Pa 1976) 29:2668–2676

Wade KR, Robertson PA, Broom ND (2012) On how nucleus-endplate integration is achieved at the fibrillar level in the ovine lumbar disc. J Anat 221:39–46

Waldman SD, Grynpas MD, Pilliar RM, Kandel RA (2002) Characterization of cartilagenous tissue formed on calcium polyphosphate substrates in vitro. J Biomed Mater Res 62:323–330

Wan Y, Feng G, Shen FH, Laurencin CT, Li X (2008) Biphasic scaffold for annulus fibrosus tissue regeneration. Biomaterials 29:643–652

Wang Y, Huso DL, Harrington J, Kellner J, Jeong DK, Turney J, McNiece IK (2005) Outgrowth of a transformed cell population derived from normal human BM mesenchymal stem cell culture. Cytotherapy 7:509–519

Wei Y, Zeng W, Wan R, Wang J, Zhou Q, Qiu S, Singh SR (2012) Chondrogenic differentiation of induced pluripotent stem cells from osteoarthritic chondrocytes in alginate matrix. Eur Cell Mater 23:1–12

Weiler C, Nerlich AG, Schaaf R, Bachmeier BE, Wuertz K, Boos N (2010) Immunohistochemical identification of notochordal markers in cells in the aging human lumbar intervertebral disc. Eur Spine J 19:1761–1770

Wilson A, Shehadeh LA, Yu H, Webster KA (2010) Age-related molecular genetic changes of murine bone marrow mesenchymal stem cells. BMC Genomics 11:229

Woltjen K, Michael IP, Mohseni P, Desai R, Mileikovsky M, Hamalainen R, Cowling R, Wang W, Liu P, Gertsenstein M, Kaji K, Sung HK, Nagy A (2009) PiggyBac transposition reprograms fibroblasts to induced pluripotent stem cells. Nature 458:766–770

Yamanaka S (2007) Strategies and new developments in the generation of patient-specific pluripotent stem cells. Cell Stem Cell 1:39–49

Yang X, Li X (2009) Nucleus pulposus tissue engineering: a brief review. Eur Spine J 18:1564–1572

Yang L, Kandel RA, Chang G, Santerre JP (2009) Polar surface chemistry of nanofibrous polyurethane scaffold affects annulus fibrosus cell attachment and early matrix accumulation. J Biomed Mater Res A 91:1089–1099

Yang R, Jiang M, Kumar SM, Xu T, Wang F, Xiang L, Xu X (2011) Generation of melanocytes from induced pluripotent stem cells. J Invest Dermatol 131:2458–2466

Yao J, Turteltaub SR, Ducheyne P (2006) A three-dimensional nonlinear finite element analysis of the mechanical behavior of tissue engineered intervertebral discs under complex loads. Biomaterials 27:377–387

Yu J, Winlove PC, Roberts S, Urban JP (2002) Elastic fibre organization in the intervertebral discs of the bovine tail. J Anat 201:465–475

Yu J, Fairbank JC, Roberts S, Urban JP (2005) The elastic fiber network of the anulus fibrosus of the normal and scoliotic human intervertebral disc. Spine (Phila Pa 1976) 30:1815–1820

Yu J, Tirlapur U, Fairbank J, Handford P, Roberts S, Winlove CP, Cui Z, Urban J (2007) Microfibrils, elastin fibres and collagen fibres in the human intervertebral disc and bovine tail disc. J Anat 210: 460–471

Zeh A, Becker C, Planert M, Lattke P, Wohlrab D (2009) Time-dependent release of cobalt and chromium ions into the serum following implantation of the metal-on-metal Maverick type artificial lumbar disc (Medtronic Sofamor Danek). Arch Orthop Trauma Surg 129:741–746

Zhang Y, Phillips FM, Thonar EJ, Oegema T, An HS, Roman-Blas JA, He TC, Anderson DG (2008) Cell therapy using articular chondrocytes overexpressing BMP-7 or BMP-10 in a rabbit disc organ culture model. Spine (Phila Pa 1976) 33:831–838

Zhang H, La Marca F, Hollister SJ, Goldstein SA, Lin CY (2009) Developing consistently reproducible intervertebral disc degeneration at rat caudal spine by using needle puncture. J Neurosurg Spine 10:522–530

Zhao T, Zhang ZN, Rong Z, Xu Y (2011) Immunogenicity of induced pluripotent stem cells. Nature 474:212–215

Zuk PA, Zhu M, Ashjian P, De Ugarte DA, Huang JI, Mizuno H, Alfonso ZC, Fraser JK, Benhaim P, Hedrick MH (2002) Human adipose tissue is a source of multipotent stem cells. Mol Biol Cell 13:4279–4295

About the Editors

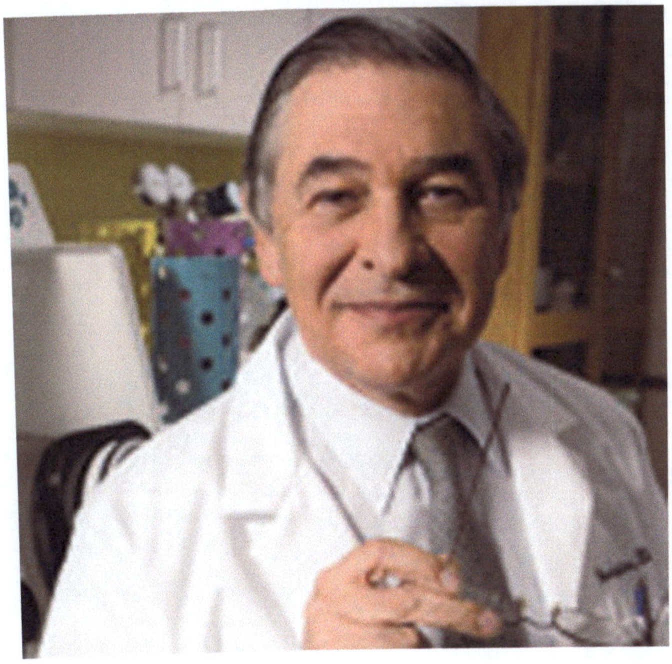

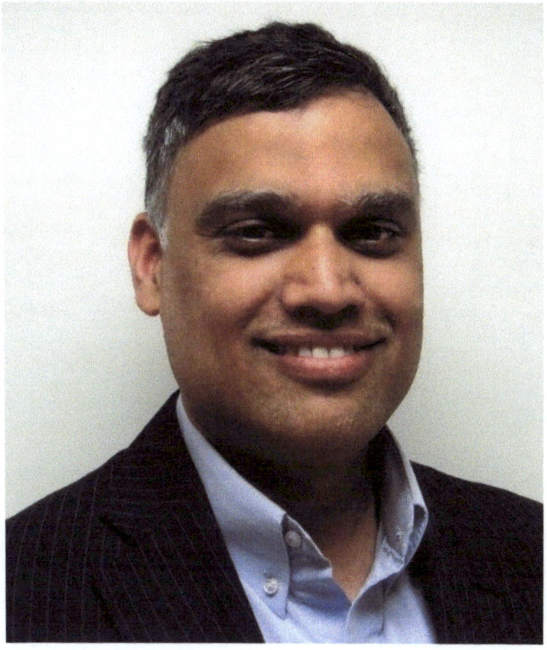

Irving M. Shapiro is the Director of the Division of Orthopaedic Research in the Department of Orthopaedic Surgery and the Anthony and Gertrude DePalma Professor of Orthopaedic Surgery, Jefferson Medical College, Philadelphia. Dr. Shapiro is a biochemist with a long term interest in skeletal tissues, especially the biology of bone, the growth plate and the intervertebral disc. His current work is focused on new approaches to restoring function to the degenerative disc.

Makarand V. Risbud is the leader of a team of investigators studying the pathogenesis of intervertebral disc disease. He is an international authority on the molecular biology of cells of the nucleus pulposus. Dr. Risbud did his post doctoral training at Harvard Medical School and is currently Professor of Orthopaedic Surgery at Jefferson Medical College in Philadelphia where he is also an active member of the program in Cell and Developmental Biology of the Graduate School of Biomedical Sciences.

I.M. Shapiro, M.V. Risbud (eds.), *The Intervertebral Disc*,
DOI 10.1007/978-3-7091-1535-0, © Springer-Verlag Wien 2014

Index

I.M. Shapiro, M.V. Risbud (eds.), *The Intervertebral Disc*,
DOI 10.1007/978-3-7091-1535-0, © Springer-Verlag Wien 2014

R

S

T

MIX
Papier aus verantwortungsvollen Quellen
Paper from responsible sources
FSC® C105338

If you have any concerns about our products,
you can contact us on
ProductSafety@springernature.com

In case Publisher is established outside the EU,
the EU authorized representative is:
Springer Nature Customer Service Center GmbH
Europaplatz 3, 69115 Heidelberg, Germany

Printed by Libri Plureos GmbH
in Hamburg, Germany